D0948951

The 5-Minute ICU Consult

The 5-Minute ICU Consult

Editor

Jose R. Yunen, MD
Emeritus Director, Cardiothoracic Intensive Care Unit
Assistant Professor of Medicine
Division of Critical Care Medicine
Department of Medicine
Albert Einstein College of Medicine
Montefiore Medical Center
Bronx, New York

Chief, Critical Care Medicine Department
Director, Critical Care Fellowship
Director, Infectious Diseases Division
CEDIMAT
Santo Domingo, Dominican Republic

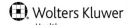 Wolters Kluwer | Lippincott Williams & Wilkins
Health
Philadelphia · Baltimore · New York · London
Buenos Aires · Hong Kong · Sydney · Tokyo

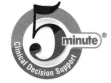

Acquisitions Editor: Brian Brown
Product Manager: Nicole Dernoski
Production Manager: Alicia Jackson
Senior Manufacturing Manager: Benjamin Rivera
Marketing Manager: Angela Panetta
Design Coordinator: Teresa Mallon
Production Service: Aptara, Inc.

Printed in China

Library of Congress Cataloging-in-Publication Data

978-1-60547-216-4
1-60547-216-6
CIP data available upon request

Care has been taken to confirm the accuracy of the information presented and to describe generally accepted practices. However, the authors, editors, and publisher are not responsible for errors or omissions or for any consequences from application of the information in this book and make no warranty, expressed or implied, with respect to the currency, completeness, or accuracy of the contents of the publication. Application of the information in a particular situation remains the professional responsibility of the practitioner.

The authors, editors, and publisher have exerted every effort to ensure that drug selection and dosage set forth in this text are in accordance with current recommendations and practice at the time of publication. However, in view of ongoing research, changes in government regulations, and the constant flow of information relating to drug therapy and drug reactions, the reader is urged to check the package insert for each drug for any change in indications and dosage and for added warnings and precautions. This is particularly important when the recommended agent is a new or infrequently employed drug.

Some drugs and medical devices presented in the publication have Food and Drug Administration (FDA) clearance for limited use in restricted research settings. It is the responsibility of the health care providers to ascertain the FDA status of each drug or device planned for use in their clinical practice.

To purchase additional copies of this book, call our customer service department at (800) 638-3030 or fax orders to (301) 223-2320. International customers should call (301) 223-2300.

Visit Lippincott Williams & Wilkins on the Internet: at LWW.com. Lippincott Williams & Wilkins customer service representatives are available from 8:30 am to 6 pm, EST.

10 9 8 7 6 5 4 3 2 1

CONTRIBUTORS

Aly Hemdan Abdalla, MD
Critical Care Director
Midstate Medical Center
Meriden, Connecticut

Avishai A. Alkalay, MD, MPH
Clinical Instructor
Department of Obstetrics & Gynecology
    and Women's Health
Albert Einstein College of Medicine
Maternal Fetal Medicine Fellow
Department of Obstetrics & Gynecology
    and Women's Health
Montefiore Medical Center/Weiler Division
Bronx, New York

Ram Sanjeev Alur, MD
Internist
Hahnemann University Hospital
Philadelphia, Pennsylvania

Devandra N. Amin, MD, FCCM, FCCP
Assistant Professor of Medicine
Department of Family Practice at Morton
    Plant Hospital Campus
University of South Florida
Medical Director of Critical Care
Department of Medicine
Morton Plant Hospital
Clearwater, Florida

Balaram Anandamurthy, MD
Critical Care Medicine Fellow
Department of Surgery
Mount Sinai School of Medicine
New York, New York
Associate Staff
Cardiothoracic Anesthesiology/
    CVICU
Cleveland Clinic
Cleveland, Ohio

Reza Askari, MD
Instructor in Surgery
Department of Surgery, Division of
    Trauma/Critical Care
Harvard Medical School
Associate Trauma Director
Department of Surgery
Brigham and Women's Hospital
Boston, Massachusetts

M. Kamran Athar, MD
Post Doctoral Fellow
Department of Medicine
Division of Critical Care Medicine
UMDNJ-Robert Wood Johnson Medical
    School
Cooper University Hospital/Medical
    Center
Camden, New Jersey

Muhammad N. Athar, MD
Pulmonologist
Nanticoke Memorial Hospital
Seaford, Delaware

Moses Bachan, MD
Critical Care Medical Fellow
Department of Surgery
Mount Sinai School of Medicine
New York, New York
Attending Physician
Department of Critical Care Medicine
Winchester Medical Center
Winchester, Virginia

Penelope Baez, MD
Infectious Disease Hospitalist
Department of Medicine
CEDIMAT
Santo Domingo, Dominican Republic

Erika Banks, MD
Associate Professor
Department of Obstetrics & Gynecology
    and Women's Health
Albert Einstein College of Medicine
Director of Gynecology
Department of Obstetrics & Gynecology
    and Women's Health
Montefiore Medical Center/Weiler
    Division
Bronx, New York

Paul Basciano, MD
Fellow in Hematology/Oncology
Department of Medicine
Weill Cornell Medical College
New York Presbyterian-Cornell Medical
    Center
New York, New York

Adel Bassily-Marcus, MD
Assistant Professor
Department of Surgery
Critical Care Division
Director
Surgical Critical Care Consultation
    Service
Director
Surgical Step Down Unit
Attending
Surgical Intensive Care Unit
Mount Sinai Medical Center
New York, New York

Francisco Eduardo Bautista, MD

Nrupen Baxi, MD
Student in Organized Health Care
    Education
Albert Einstein College of Medicine of
    Yeshiva University
Montefiore Medical Center
Bronx, New York

Ernest Benjamin, MD
Professor of Surgery and Anesthesiology
Department of Surgery
Mount Sinai School of Medicine
Director, Surgical ICU
Department of Surgery
Mount Sinai Hospital
New York, New York

Peter S. Bernstein, MD, MPH
Professor
Department of Obstetrics & Gynecology
    and Women's Health
Albert Einstein College of Medicine
Maternal Fetal Medicine Attending
Department of Obstetrics & Gynecology
    and Women's Health
Montefiore Medical Center/Weiler
    Division
Bronx, New York

Jose Diego Caceres, MD
General Physician
Department of Critical Care Medicine
CEDIMAT
Santa Domingo, Dominican Republic

Rodrigo Cavallazzi, MD
Pulmonary and Critical Care Fellow
Department of Medicine
Thomas Jefferson University
Philadelphia, Pennsylvania

David A. Chad, MD
Internist and Neurologist
Department of Neurology
Massachusetts General Hospital
Boston, Massachusetts

Sweta Chandela, MD
Internist
Coatesville Cardiology Clinic
Thorndale, Pennsylvania

Steven Chao, MD, FCCP
Critical Care Medicine Fellow
Department of Surgery
Mount Sinai School of Medicine
New York, New York

Sanjay Chawla, MD, FCCP
Assistant Professor of Medicine in Clinical
    Anesthesiology
Department of Anesthesia & Critical Care
    Medicine
Weill Cornell Medical College
Assistant Attending
Department of Anesthesiology & Critical
    Care Medicine
Memorial Sloane-Kettering Cancer
    Center
New York, New York

Cynthia Chazotte, MD
Professor & Vice Chair
Department of Obstetrics & Gynecology
    and Women's Health
Albert Einstein College of Medicine
Director of Obstetrics & Perinatology
Department of Obstetrics & Gynecology
    and Women's Health
Montefiore Medical Center/Weiler
    Division
Bronx, New York

Sreedhar Chintala, MD
Assistant Professor
The Saul R. Korey Department of
    Neurology
Albert Einstein College of Medicine of
    Yeshiva University
New York, New York
Department of Critical Care Medicine
Montefiore Medical Center
Bronx, New York

Brian Corbett, DO
Clinical Cardiologist
Department of Cardiology
Cooper University Hospital
Camden, New Jersey

Anahita Dabo-Trubelja, MD
Assistant Professor of Medicine in Clinical
    Anesthesiology
Department of Anesthesiology & Critical
    Care Medicine
Weill Cornell Medical College
Assistant Attending
Department of Anesthesiology & Critical
    Care Medicine
Memorial Sloane-Kettering Cancer Center
New York, New York

Rhonda D'Agostino, NP
Nurse Practitioner
Department of Anesthesiology & Critical
    Care Medicine
Memorial Sloan-Kettering Cancer Center
New York, New York

Maher Dahdel, MD
Pulmonary & Critical Care Division
UMDNJ-Cooper University Hospital
Camden, New Jersey

John C. D'Ambrosio, DO
Department of Emergency Medicine
Team Health East
Woodbury, New Jersey

Ashlesha K. Dayal, MD
Assistant Professor
Department of Obstetrics & Gynecology
    and Women's Health
Albert Einstein College of Medicine
Maternal Fetal Medicine Attending
Department of Obstetrics & Gynecology
    and Women's Health
Montefiore Medical Center/Weiler
    Division
Bronx, New York

Andrew Deroo, MD
Surgery Resident, 4th year
George Washington University School of
    Medicine
Washington, D.C.

Maria T. DeSancho, MD, MSc
Associate Professor of Medicine
Department of Medicine
Weill Cornell Medical College
Attending
Department of Medicine
New York Presbyterian-Cornell Medical
    Center
New York, New York

Sanjay Dhar, MD, FACP
Assistant Professor of Medicine
Department of Medicine
Pulmonary, Critical Care, Allergy and
    Immunologic Diseases Section
Wake Forest School of Medicine
Wake Forest Baptist Health
Winston-Salem, North Carolina

Fred DiBlasio, Jr., MD
Critical Care Practitioner, Internist
North Shore/Long Island Jewish Hospital
    System-Huntington Hospital
Huntington, New York

Karim Djekidel, MD
Assistant Professor of Medicine
Division of Pulmonary and Critical Care
    Medicine
Drexel University College of Medicine
Philadelphia, Pennsylvania

Ronen Dudaie, MD
Instructor in Medicine (Critical Care)
Albert Einstein College of Medicine
Montefiore Medical Center
Bronx, New York

Alina Dulu, MD
Assistant Professor
Attending Physician
Critical Care Medicine
Albert Einstein College of Medicine
Montefiore Medical Center
Bronx, New York

Qasim Durrani, MD
Assistant Professor
Department of Internal Medicine
University of North Dakota
Grand Forks, North Dakota

Lewis A. Eisen, MD
Assistant Professor of Clinical
    Medicine
Department of Medicine
Division of Critical Care Medicine
Albert Einstein School of Medicine
Director of the Medical Intensive
    Care Unit
Department of Medicine
Division of Critical Care Medicine
Montefiore Medical Center
Bronx, New York

Nelli Fisher, MD
Clinical Instructor
Department of Obstetrics & Gynecology
    and Women's Health
Albert Einstein College of Medicine
Maternal Fetal Medicine Fellow
Department of Obstetrics & Gynecology
    and Women's Health
Montefiore Medical Center/Weiler Division
Bronx, New York

James A. Gasperino, MD, PhD
Chief, Section of Critical Care
Director, Critical Care Medicine
Drexel University College of Medicine
Chairman, Performance Improvement
    Committee
Hahnemann University Hospital
Associate Professor, Department of
    Environmental and Occupational Health
    at the School of Public Health
Drexel University College of Medicine
Philadelphia, Pennsylvania

Juliana Gebb, MD
Clinical Instructor
Department of Obstetrics & Gynecology
    and Women's Health
Albert Einstein College of Medicine
Maternal Fetal Medicine Fellow
Department of Obstetrics & Gynecology
    and Women's Health
Montefiore Medical Center/Weiler
    Division
Bronx, New York

Shenaz Georgilis, RN, MSN, FNP
Nurse Practitioner
Department of Anesthesiology & Critical
    Care Medicine
Memorial Sloan-Kettering Cancer Center
New York, New York

Umesh Gidwani, MD
Assistant Professor of Medicine
Department of Medicine
Pulmonary, Critical Care, Cardiology
Mount Sinai School of Medicine
Chief
Cardiac Critical Care
Department of Cardiology
The Mount Sinai Hospital
New York, New York

Christopher R. Gilbert, DO
Fellow
Department of Pulmonary and Critical
    Care Medicine
Thomas Jefferson University
Thomas Jefferson University Hospital
Philadelphia, Pennsylvania

Hari Gnanasekeram, MD
Internist
Cardiologist
Cooper University Hospital
Camden, New Jersey

Ronaldo Collo Go, MD
Critical Care Medicine Fellow
Department of Surgery
Mount Sinai School of Medicine
New York, New York

Dena Goffman, MD
Assistant Professor
Department of Obstetrics & Gynecology
    and Women's Health
Albert Einstein College of Medicine
Maternal Fetal Medicine Attending
Department of Obstetrics & Gynecology
    and Women's Health
Montefiore Medical Center/Weiler
    Division
Bronx, New York

Sindhura Gogineni, MD

Oren N. Gottfried, MD
Assistant Professor of Surgery
Department of Surgery
Duke University of Medicine
Durham, North Carolina

Isaac Halickman, MD
Assistant Professor Coterminous
Clinical Cardiologist
Department of Cardiology
Cooper University Hospital
Camden, New Jersey

Stephen B. Heitner, MD
Internist
Cooper University Hospital
Camden, New Jersey

Timothy J. Henrich, MD
Instructor
Department of Medicine
Harvard Medical School
Associate Physician
Division of Infectious Diseases
Brigham and Women's Hospital
Boston, Massachusetts

Hye J. Heo, MD
Clinical Instructor
Department of Obstetrics & Gynecology
    and Women's Health
Albert Einstein College of Medicine
Maternal Fetal Medicine Fellow
Department of Obstetrics & Gynecology
    and Women's Health
Montefiore Medical Center/Weiler Division
Bronx, New York

Amya Hirani, MD
Pulmonary and Critical Care Fellow
Department of Medicine
Thomas Jefferson University
Philadelphia, Pennsylvania

Jennifer M. Howes, MD
Chief Fellow
Critical Care Medicine Fellowship
    Program
Albert Einstein College of Medicine
Montefiore Medical Center
Bronx, New York

Sherin M. Ibrahim, DO
Critical Care Medicine Fellow
Department of Surgery
Mount Sinai School of Medicine
New York, New York
Physician/Owner
Department of Internal Medicine/Sleep
    Medicine
The Pearl Clinic, LLC
Millsboro, Delaware

Javed Iqbal, Md, MPH, FCCP
Department of Medicine
Montefiore Medical Center
Bronx, New York

Sudhanshu Jain, MD
Internist
Department of Critical Care
Lakewood Hospital
Lakewood, Ohio

Ann Jakubowski, MD, PhD
Associate Professor of Medicine
Department of Medicine
Weill Cornell Medical College
Attending
Department of Medicine
Memorial Sloan-Kettering Cancer
    Center
New York, New York

Aditya Kasarabada, MD
Department of Pulmonary Critical
    Care
Hahnemann University Hospital
Philadelphia, Pennsylvania

Parul Kaushik, MD, MPH
Fellow
Division of Infectious Diseases and HIV
    Medicine
Drexel University College of Medicine
Hahnemann University Hospital
Philadelphia, Pennsylvania

Zinobia Khan, MD
Critical Care Medical Fellow
Department of Surgery
Mount Sinai School of Medicine
New York, New York
Staff Physician
Department of Medicine/Surgery
James J. Peters V.A. Medical Center
Bronx, New York

Claude Killu, MD, FCCP
Assistant Clinical Professor
Department of Medicine
University of California Los Angeles
Director
Department of Medical ICU
Cedars-Sinai Medical Center
Los Angeles, California

Keith Killu, MD
Assistant Clinical Professor
Wayne State University
Senior Staff/Critical Care
Department of Surgery
Henry Ford Hospital
Detroit, Michigan

Peter Y. Kim, MD
Assistant Professor
Department of Cardiology
M.D. Anderson Cancer Center
Houston, Texas

Merritt D. Kinon, MD
Preliminary Surgery
Neurological Surgery
Albert Einstein College of Medicine
Bronx, New York

Ari Klapholz, MD, FCCP
Clinical Assistant Professor
Active Attending
Department of Medicine
New York University Langone Medical
  Center
New York, New York

Roopa Kohli-Seth, MD, FCCP, FACP
Associate Professor of Surgery
Director
Central Venous Access Service
Division of Surgical Critical Care
  Medicine
Mount Sinai School of Medicine
New York, New York

Amanda Kolb, MD
University of Virginia School of Medicine
Charlottesville, Virginia

Sophia Koo, MD
Instructor in Medicine
Department of Medicine
Brigham and Women's Hospital
Harvard Medical School
Associate Physician
Department of Medicine
Division of Infectious Diseases
Brigham and Women's Hospital
Boston, Massachusetts

Neena Kumar, MD
Critical Care Fellow
Department of Surgery
Mount Sinai School of Medicine
New York, New York
Intensivist
Department of Medicine
Kingston Hospital
Benedictine Hospital
Kingston, New York

Negia Elisa Lalane, MD
Department of Internal Medicine PGY-3
Jacobi Medical Center
Bronx, New York

Ellen J. Landsberger, MD, MS
Assistant Professor
Department of Obstetrics & Gynecology
  and Women's Health
Albert Einstein College of Medicine
Maternal Fetal Medicine Attending
Department of Obstetrics & Gynecology
  and Women's Health
Montefiore Medical Center/Weiler
  Division
Bronx, New York

Damian Lee, RPA-C
Physician Assistant
North Central Bronx Hospital
Bronx, New York

Luciano Lemos-Filho, MD, MS
Assistant Professor of Medicine and
  Surgery
Surgical Critical Care
New York University School of Medicine
New York, New York

Ian A. Lentnek, MD, MA
Internist
Cooper University Hospital
Camden, New Jersey

Sharon S. Leung, MD
Assistant Professor in Medicine
  (Critical Care)
Albert Einstein College of Medicine
Montefiore Medical Center
Bronx, New York

Daniela Levi, MD, FCCP
Assistant Professor, Clinical Medicine and
  Neurology
Division of Critical Care Medicine
Albert Einstein College of Medicine
Director of Quality, Safety, and
  Development
Jay B. Langner Critical Care System
Montefiore Medical Center
Bronx, New York

Hady Lichaa, MD
Interventional Cardiology Fellow
Department of Cardiology
Cooper University Hospital
Camden, New Jersey

Terence P. Lonergan, MD
Emergency Physician
Camden, New Jersey

David J. Lundy, MD
Surgical Physician
Department of Surgery
Cooper University Hospital
Camden, New Jersey

Andria Lyn, NP
Nurse Practitioner
Department of Anesthesiology & Critical
  Care Medicine
Memorial Sloan-Kettering Cancer Center
New York, New York

Anthony Manasia, MD
Associate Professor of Surgery
Department of Surgery
Mount Sinai School of Medicine
Attending, Surgical ICU
Director
Critical Care Research
Surgery-Surgical ICU
Mount Sinai Hospital
New York, New York

Seth Manoach, MD
Chief Fellow
Crritical Care Medicine Fellowship
  Program
Albert Einstein College of Medicine
Montefiore Medical Center
Bronx, New York

Oveys Mansuri, MD
Clinical Fellow in Surgery
Department of Surgery
Harvard Medical School
Clinical Fellow in Surgery
Trauma, Burns, and Surgical Critical Care
Brigham and Women's Hospital
Boston, Massachusetts

Jeffrey Marcus, MD
Assistant Professor of Plastic Surgery
Department of Plastic, Maxillofacial and
  Oral Surgery
Duke University
Chief
Pediatric Plastic Surgery and Craniofacial
  Surgery
Duke Children's Hospital and Health
  Center
Durham, North Carolina

**Paul E. Marik, MBBCh, FRCP, FCCM,
  FCCP**
Professor of Medicine
Department of Medicine
Chief
Division of Pulmonary and Critical Care
Thomas Jefferson University
Philadelphia, Pennsylvania

Victor J. Matos, MD
Director
Department of Critical Care Medicine
Centro Medico Moderno
Santo Domingo, Domincan Republic

Paul H. Mayo, MD
Director
Medical Intensive Care Unit
Beth Israel Medical Center
New York, New York

Shilpi S. Mehta, MD
Clinical Instructor
Department of Obstetrics & Gynecology
  and Women's Health
Albert Einstein College of Medicine
Maternal Fetal Medicine Fellow
Department of Obstetrics & Gynecology
  and Women's Health
Montefiore Medical Center/Weiler
  Division
Bronx, New York

Eliany Mejia Lopez, MD
2nd year Internal Medicine Resident
Department of Medicine
Albert Einstein College of Medicine
Montefiore Medical Center
Bronx, New York

Vinia Mendoza, MD
Fellow
Department of Internal Medicine-
  Pulmonary and Critical Care
Thomas Jefferson University Hospital
Philadelphia, Pennsylvania

Nirav Mistry, MD
Hospitalist
Emergency Medical Associates
Nyack, New York

B. Sharmila Mohanraj, MD
Fellow
Department of Infectious Diseases
Drexel University College of Medicine
Philadelphia, Pennsylvania

Vicente San Martin Montenegro, MD
House Medical Staff
Department of Medicine
CEDIMAT
Santo Domingo, Dominican Republic

Saraswathi Devi. V. Muppana, MD
Fellow in Critical Care Medicine
Department of Anesthesiology & Critical
  Care Medicine
Weill Cornell Medical College
Memorial Sloan-Kettering Cancer Center
New York, New York

Sasikanth Nallagatla, MD
Critical Care Medicine Fellow
Department of Surgery
Mount Sinai School of Medicine
New York, New York
Pulmonary and Critical Care Doctor
Department of Internal Medicine
Christus Santa Rosa – Westover Hills
San Antonio, Texas

Tzvi Y. Neuman, MD
Assistant Professor in Medicine
  (Critical Care)
Albert Einstein College of Medicine
Montefiore Medical Center
Bronx, New York

Joseph Ng, MD
Intensivist
Department of Internal Medicine
Mather Hospital
Port Jefferson, New York

Themistoklis Nissirios, MD
Attending Cardiologist
Department of Cardiology
Orange Regional Medical Center
Middletown, New York

John M. Oropello, MD, FCCM
Co-Director, Neurosurgical ICU
Mount Sinai School of Medicine
New York, New York

Deborah Orsi, MD
Internal Medicine Physician
Saint Barnabas Hospital
Bronx, New York

David Oxman, MD
Assistant Professor
Department of Medicine
Drexel Medical College
Attending Intensivist
Division of Critical Care
Mercy Medical Center
Philadelphia, Pennsylvania

Monvasi Pachinburavan, MD
Fellow
Division of Pulmonary and Critical Care
Thomas Jefferson University Hospital
Philadelphia, Pennsylvania

Stephen M. Pastores, MD, FACP, FCCM
Professor of Medicine and
  Anesthesiology
Department of Anesthesiology & Critical
  Care Medicine
Weill Cornell Medical College
Director
CCM Fellowship Program
Department of Anesthesiology & Critical
  Care Medicine
Memorial Sloan-Kettering Cancer Center
New York, New York

Samir Peshimam, MD
Critical Care Medicine
Memorial Regional Hospital
Hollywood, Florida

Irina Petrenko, MD
Critical Care Medicine Fellow
Department of Surgery
Mount Sinai School of Medicine
New York, New York
Critical Care Medicine Attending
Department of Pulmonary and Critical
  Care Medicine
Staten Island University Hospital
Staten Island, New York

Nitin Puri
Attending Physician
Department of Critical Care
Inova Hospital
Falls Church, Virginia

Omar Rahman, MD
Director
Adult Intensive Care Shock Trauma Unit
Department of Critical Care Medicine
Geisinger Medical Center
Danville, Pennsylvania

Bindu Raju, MD
Assistant Professor
Department of Medicine/Pulmonary and
   Critical Care
Mount Sinai School of Medicine
New York, New York
Staff Physician
Department of Medicine/
   Surgery-Pulmonary and Critical
   Care Medicine
James J. Peters VA Medical Center
Bronx, New York

Madhusudanan Ramaswamy, MBBS,
   MS
Fellow in Critical Care Medicine
Department of Anesthesiology & Critical
   Care Medicine
Weill Cornell Medical College
Fellow in Critical Care Medicine
Department of Anesthesiology & Critical
   Care Medicine
Memorial Sloan-Kettering Cancer Center
New York, New York

Nina Raoof, MD, FCCP
Assistant Professor of Medicine
Department of Anesthesiology & Critical
   Care Medicine
Weill Cornell Medical College
Assistant Attending
Department of Anesthesiology & Critical
   Care Medicine
Memorial Sloan-Kettering Cancer Center
New York, New York

Ashraf O. Rashid, MD
Fellow in Critical Care Medicine
Department of Anesthesiology & Critical
   Care Medicine
Weill Cornell Medical College
Memorial Sloan-Kettering Cancer Center
New York, New York

Rajesh Rethnam, MD
Fellow in Critical Care Medicine
Department of Anesthesiology & Critical
   Care Medicine
Weill Cornell Medical College
Memorial Sloan-Kettering Cancer Center
New York, New York

Amy Rezak, MD
Assistant Professor
Department of Surgery
University of North Carolina School of
   Medicine
Trauma
Critical Care Surgeon
Department of Surgery
UNC Health Care
Chapel Hill, North Carolina

Miguel Angel Russo, MD
Infectious Disease Hospitalist
Department of Medicine
CEDIMAT
Santo Domingo, Dominican Republic

Sajjad A. Sabir, MD
Clinical Cardiologist
Department of Cardiology
Cooper University Hospital
Camden, New Jersey

Hayder Said, MD

Raghad H. Said, MD
Assistant Professor of Surgery and
   Medicine
NYU School of Medicine
New York, New York

Zaid Said, MD
Resident House Staff Physician
Department of Internal Medicine
Geisinger Medical Center
Danville, Pennsylvania

Lhissa Santana, MD
Hospitalist
Department of Medicine
Marlboro Park Hospital
Bennettsville, South Carolina

H. Christian Schumacher, MD
Doris & Stanley Tananbaum Stroke
   Center
Neurological Institute
Department of Interventional
   Neuroradiology
New York Presbyterian Hospital Columbia
   University
New York, New York

Raghu R. Seethala, MD
Clinical Fellow
Department of Anesthesia
Harvard Medical School
Critical Care Fellow
Department of Anesthesia, Brigham and
   Women's Hospital
Boston, Massachusetts

Arif M. Shaik, MD
HealthEast Critical Care
St. Joseph's Hospital
St. Paul, Minnesota

Brian Sherman, MD
Department of Ophthalmology
Division of Pediatric Ophthalmology
   Tallahassee
Memorial Hospital
Tallahassee, Florida

Ariel Shiloh, MD
Assistant Professor in Medicine
   (Critical Care)
Director, Critical Care Medicine Consult
   Services
Albert Einstein College of Medicine
Montefiore Medical Center
Bronx, New York

Hiren Shingala, MD
Pulmonary Critical Care Physician
Pulmonary Critical Care Medical
   Associates
Harrisburg, Pennsylvania

Robert E. Siegel, MD
Associate Professor of Medicine
Department of Pulmonary/Critical Care
Mount Sinai School of Medicine
New York, New York
Director
Pulmonary/Critical Care Section
Department of Pulmonary/CCM
James J. Peters VA Medical Center
Bronx, New York

Sivashankar Sivarman, MD
Department of Pulmonary Medicine
RML Specialty Hospital Chicago
Chicago, Illinois

Yoshita Shroff, MD
Fellow in Critical Care Medicine
Department of Anesthesiology & Critical
   Care Medicine
Weill Cornell Medical College
Memorial Sloan-Kettering Cancer Center
New York, New York

Rakesh Sinha, MD
Physician
Department of Medicine
Pomona Valley Hospital Medical
   Center
Pomona, California

Jina Sohn, MD
Assistant Professor
Department of Medicine-Cardiology
Georgetown University
Attending Physician
Department of Medicine-Cardiology
Georgetown University Hospital
Washington, DC

Mladen Sokiolovic, MD
Fellow in Critical Care Medicine
Department of Anesthesiology & Critical
   Care Medicine
Weill Cornell Medical College
Memorial Sloan-Kettering Cancer Center
New York, New York

Edgardo Soto, MD
Intensivist
Department of Pulmonary Critical Care
 Medicine
Division of Pulmonary Disease
Memorial Physicians Clinics
Gulf Coast Pulmonary Consultants
Gulfport, Mississippi

Graciela J. Soto, MD
Assistant Professor in Medicine
 (Critical Care)
Emeritus Director of CSICU
Weiler Division
Albert Einstein College of Medicine
Montefiore Medical Center
Bronx, New York

Jacqueline B. Sutter, DO
Department of Pulmonary Disease
Jefferson University Hospital
Philadelphia, Pennsylvania

Raghukumar Thirumala, MD
Fellow in Critical Care Medicine
Department of Anesthesiology & Critical
 Care Medicine
Weill Cornell Medical College
Memorial Sloan-Kettering Cancer Center
New York, New York

Pamela Tropper, MD
Associate Professor
Department of Obstetrics & Gynecology
 and Women's Health
Albert Einstein College of Medicine
Maternal Fetal Medicine Attending
Department of Obstetrics & College and
 Women's Health
Montefiore Medical Center/Weiler
 Division
Bronx, New York

Aditya Uppalapati, MD
Department of Internal Medicine
UPMC McKeesport Hospital
McKeesport, Pennsylvania

Urvashi Vaid, MD
Fellow
Pulmonary and Critical Care Medicine
Thomas Jefferson University
Philadelphia, Pennsylvania

Tajender S. Vasu, MD
Fellow
Pulmonary and Critical Care Medicine
Thomas Jefferson University Hospital
Philadelphia, Pennsylvania

Louis P. Voigt, MD, FCCP
Assistant Professor of Medicine in Clinical
 Anesthesiology
Department of Anesthesiology & Critical
 Care Medicine
Weill Cornell Medical College
Assistant Attending
Department of Anesthesiology & Critical
 Care Medicine
Memorial Sloan-Kettering Cancer Center
New York, New York

Patrick F. Walsh, DO, FCCP
Department of Critical Care Medicine
Geisinger Medical Center
Geisinger Wyoming Valley Medical Center
Select Specialty Hospital
Danville, Pennsylvania

Martin E. Weinand, MD
Professor
Division of Neurosurgery
Department of Surgery
University of Arizona College of Medicine
Program Director, Neurosurgery
 Residency
Division of Neurosurgery
Department of Surgery
University of Arizona Health Network
Tucson, Arizona

Stephanie Whitener, MD
Anesthesiology Resident
Department of Anesthesiology
Harvard, Brigham and Women's
 Hospital
Boston, Massachusetts

Jose R. Yunen, MD, FCCP
Emeritus Director, Cardiothoracic
 Intensive Care Unit
Assistant Professor of Medicine
Division of Critical Care Medicine
Department of Medicine
Albert Einstein College of
 Medicine
Montefiore Medical Center
Bronx, New York
Chief, Critical Care Medicine
 Department
Director, Critical Care Fellowship
Director, Infectious Diseases
 Division
CEDIMAT
Santo Domingo, Dominican
 Republic

Rafael Alba Yunen, MD
Resident
Department of Medicine
Lincoln Medical Center
Bronx, New York

Francisco Polanco Zacarias, MD
Hospitalist
Department of Medicine
Chesterfield General Hospital
Cheraw, South Carolina

FOREWORD

It is an honor and a pleasure to introduce *The 5-Minute ICU Consult* not only to the community of intensivists but also to all other medical professionals facing daily the challenges of managing acute illness in the emergency wards, recovery rooms, progressive care units, hospitalists wards, and all other areas. Critical care medicine is a well-recognized subspecialty with an independent board exam. It constitutes a significant part of economy of all hospitals, not only in the designated intensive care units, but over the past decade has diffused throughout most hospitals as the ICU Without Walls service responding to emergencies on the wards, in the radiology and procedural areas, as well as in the emergency wards and in the recovery rooms. The rapid response capability allows for early stabilization of patients using evidence-based ICU practice anywhere and to institute the proper care ranging from aggressive trial of ICU therapy to comfort care. The panel of experts contributing to this volume includes many old friends and acquaintances, some of the world authorities in their areas of expertise, to many young budding leaders of this specialty. The volume presents a rapid intellectual response to majority of critical care syndromes and conditions and is the most up-to-date effort to augment the clinical willingness of the dedicated critical care providers to provide excellent care anywhere that is needed.

VLADIMIR KVETAN, MD
Director, Jay B. Langner Critical Care System
Montefiore Medical Center
Director, Division of Critical Care Medicine
Department of Medicine
Professor of Anesthesiology and Clinical Medicine
Associate Professor of Surgery
Albert Einstein College of Medicine of
Yeshiva University
Bronx, New York

PREFACE

Critical Care has become a multidisciplinary specialty and *The 5-Minute ICU Consult* precisely reflects this approach. It is well established in the medical world that rapid access to critical care saves lives. However, concise formatted books and methods that will allow a clinician to respond timely to challenges are relatively recent. This book is intended to serve as a bedside tool to support the care of the acutely ill patient. This new addition to the 5-Minute Consult Series contains more than 200 entries covering all aspects of adult critical care. Each entry is presented on a two-page spread in a consistent format, with bulleted and listed information on definition of the disorder, pathophysiology, diagnosis, treatment, surgical interventions, and complications. Algorithms for common and complex diagnoses, procedures, and treatment options are presented in a special section.

Despite the plentitude of new books, this approach is still rarely offered as a text. This book is designed for critical care physicians, fellows, residents, interns, hospitalists, students, physician assistants, therapists, nurses, and the entire multidisciplinary critical care team. Our experienced authors prepared each topic to fit a precise and relevant summary of critical care diagnoses, procedures, and algorithms. Our aim is to continue to present accurate topics that will translate into evidence-based patient care.

JOSE R. YUNEN

ACKNOWLEDGMENTS

A book about Critical Care Medicine cannot be written by one person. There are so many aspects of the critically ill that one can't possibly learn all there is to know about the proper care without the help of a team. For this reason, the insights and research of many talented critical care physicians have gone into the making of this book.

I especially thank Dr. John Oropello, who provided valuable information in the guidance of this project. Dr. Ernest Benjamin, who inspired me to deliver the best care possible in the United States and in the Dominican Republic. Dr. Vladimir Kvetan, who taught me that critical care is a system and introduced me to a multidisciplinary approach. Honorable mention goes to all the nurses, technicians, students, and patients who inspired this bedside tool.

I am glad that my parents can now finally read about what I have been doing all these years. I thank them both for laying the fundaments for this work. I thank my stunning wife Laura for all the unconditional support. She has been my inspiration and motivation for continuing to improve my knowledge and move my career forward. Had I written this last sentence again, I couldn't have put it any better.

JOSE R. YUNEN

CONTENTS

The 5-Minute ICU Consult

ABDOMEN, ACUTE

Reza Askari
Amy Rezak

 ## BASICS

DESCRIPTION
- Abdominal pain is a common condition that calls for prompt diagnosis and treatment
- The term "acute abdomen" designates symptoms and signs of intra-abdominal disease that is usually best treated by surgical operation.

RISK FACTORS
Past surgical history (repeated abdominal surgeries) can help the differential diagnosis and give clues to the diagnosis of the present illness

PATHOPHYSIOLOGY
- Mesothelial cells cover the visceral and parietal peritoneal surfaces
- While irritation of the visceral peritoneum causes poorly localized pain, the irritation of the parietal peritoneum cause localized pain.

ETIOLOGY
- Stretching or distention of the peritoneum, bacterial or chemical peritoneal inflammation, and ischemia will lead to pain
- Abdominal pain can be visceral, parietal or referred

COMMONLY ASSOCIATED CONDITIONS
Multiple prior abdominal surgeries are common

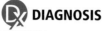 ## DIAGNOSIS

HISTORY
- Abdominal pain is the most common symptom.
- Characterize and document the pain.
- Location and duration of pain is important.
- Presence of nausea and vomiting
- Pain often precedes vomiting in a surgical abdomen.
- Bowel function, including history of constipation, diarrhea or recent changes can be important. Documentation should include the last bowel movement
- Anorexia may precede pain (it is essential to document timing of last meal).
- Menstrual history is important in women.
- Drug history is important: Corticosteroids can predispose to GI ulcers and possible perforation. They can also mask a surgical abdomen

PHYSICAL EXAM
- Fever, tachycardia, hypotension all can be signs of an acute abdomen
- Inspect (scars, hernias, masses, abdominal wall defects)
- Palpation is crucial, location of pain is very important
- Check for presence of guarding and rebound tenderness
- Tenderness upon percussion typically indicates inflammation (an intra-abdominal inflammatory process)

Pregnancy Considerations
Pain may be localized in an atypical location depending on gestational age, particularly with appendicitis

DIAGNOSTIC TESTS & INTERPRETATION
Lab
- Elevated wbc on CBC with left-shifted differential are common, chemistry panel, LFTs, Amylase and Lipase should be checked
- Check UA, and sediment
- Test β-HCG for women of childbearing age

Imaging
Initial approach
- CXR — to rule out free air
- Abdominal x-ray — Ileus, SBO, renal stones
- Ultrasound — provides safe, low cost evaluation of the liver and gallbladder, bile ducts, spleen, pancreas, kidneys, ovaries, adnexa and uterus
- CT scan — improves diagnostic accuracy, and reveals anatomic and pathologic details

Follow-Up & Special Considerations
Upper GI study, Barium enema

Diagnostic Procedures/Other
Laparoscopy can be both diagnostic and therapeutic

DIFFERENTIAL DIAGNOSIS
- Gastroenteritis
- Urinary tract infections
- Dysmenorrhea
- Ovarian torsion
- Irritable bowel syndrome
- MI
- Pneumonia, empyema, or pulmonary embolism can present with upper abdominal pain

 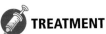

TREATMENT
MEDICATION
First Line
- Early broad spectrum antibiotic coverage
- Minimize pain medications until an abdominal exam is performed and status is documented

ADDITIONAL TREATMENT
General Measures
- IV fluid resuscitation
- Immediate surgical intervention, consider laparoscopy versus open abdominal exploration

Issues for Referral
Urgent surgical consult is needed

Additional Therapies
Foley, NG tube

SURGERY/OTHER PROCEDURES
Endoscopy, Laparoscopy, Exploratory Laparotomy

IN-PATIENT CONSIDERATIONS
Initial Stabilization
NPO, IV fluids, broad spectrum empiric antibiotics

Admission Criteria
Patients may require postop ICU care depending on comorbidities and severity of sepsis (if present)

IV Fluids
Crystalloids

Nursing
- Pain control, NPO, measure I/O
- Early ambulation, DVT prophylaxis
- Wound/Dressing care

Discharge Criteria
Afebrile, return of bowel function, tolerating diet

ONGOING CARE
FOLLOW-UP RECOMMENDATIONS
Follow-up with surgeon, call with signs and symptoms of infection

Patient Monitoring
Telemetry if cardiac disease is present

DIET
NPO initially and advance with return of bowel function

PATIENT EDUCATION
Signs and symptoms of infection

PROGNOSIS
Good with adequate source control

COMPLICATIONS
UTI, Surgical Site infections, ileus, intra-abdominal abscess, fistulas, DVT, MI, PE, Pneumonia

REFERENCES
1. Jones RS. Acute abdomen. In Sabiston Textbook of Surgery: The Biological Basis of Modern Surgical Practice, 17th ed.
2. Doherty GM. The acute abdomen. In Doherty GM, ed. CURRENT Diagnosis & Treatment: Surgery, 13th ed. Available at: http://www.accesssurgery.com/content.aspx?aID=5215706

CODES
ICD9
- 789.00 Abdominal pain, unspecified site
- 789.01 Abdominal pain, right upper quadrant
- 789.02 Abdominal pain, left upper quadrant

CLINICAL PEARLS
- Detailed history and abdominal exam is essential for early diagnosis
- Early diagnosis
- Early therapeutic intervention:
  - Surgical intervention for source control
  - Broad-spectrum antibiotics
  - IV fluid resuscitation

ABDOMINAL COMPARTMENT SYNDROME

JD Cohen

 BASICS

DESCRIPTION
Elevated intra-abdominal pressures (IAPs) leading to major organ dysfunction:
- Intra-abdominal hypertension is defined as IAPs >12 mm Hg
- Abdominal compartment syndrome (ACS) occurs when sustained abdominal pressures exceed 20 mm Hg:
  - Primary ACS is associated with injury or disease in the abdominopelvic region.
  - Secondary ACS is associated with conditions that do not originate from the abdominopelvic region.
  - Recurrent ACS is ACS that redevelops after initial improvement following medical or surgical treatment.

EPIDEMIOLOGY
Incidence
Varies significantly, 1–36% for at-risk populations
Prevalence
Varies between 4% and 8% in at-risk populations

RISK FACTORS
- Large volume resuscitation (>3.5 L/24 hrs)
- Hypothermia
- Acidosis
- Coagulopathy/massive transfusion
- Abdominal surgery/primary fascial closure

GENERAL PREVENTION
- Measuring IAPs for patients at significant risk for abdominal compartment syndrome:
  - Measure pressures upon admission and follow throughout hospital course
  - Important to take quick action if abdominal pressures are rising

PATHOPHYSIOLOGY
Abdominal compartment pressure rises above abdominal perfusion pressure, thereby decreasing blood flow to abdominal organs and IVC:
- Neurologic: High abdominal pressures transmitted to the thorax can decrease venous drainage from the jugulars and worsen intracranial pressure.
- Cardiac: High pressures can lead to collapse of the IVC and decreased venous return to the heart, therefore decreasing CO.

- Respiratory: Transfer of IAP can decrease FRC and thoracic wall compliance. Patients can have high measured peak inspiratory pressures.
- GI: Impaired flow through the mesenteric vessels leading to intestinal ischemia.
- Kidney: High pressures can markedly decrease renal function by compressing renal veins and renal cortical layer, leading to oliguria or eventual anuria. Additionally, high pressures have been shown to stimulate ADH secretion.

ETIOLOGY
- Decreased abdominal wall compliance:
  - Acute respiratory process causing increased intrathoracic pressures
  - Major abdominal trauma
  - Burns
  - Surgery with primary abdominal closure
- Increased abdominal content:
  - Tumors/masses or abscess
  - Obstruction with intestinal edema/distension
  - Ascites secondary to liver dysfunction, pancreatitis, or infection
- Increase permeability of abdominal vasculature or massive fluid resuscitation:
  - Sepsis, acidosis, hypothermia
  - Burns
  - Coagulopathies requiring massive transfusion

COMMONLY ASSOCIATED CONDITIONS
- Intra-abdominal surgery with primary closure
- High-volume fluid resuscitation
- Coagulopathy and massive transfusion
- Pulmonary, renal, or hepatic dysfunction
- Ileus

 DIAGNOSIS

HISTORY
Entertain a high clinical suspicion based on patient's underlying pathology and risk factors for intra-abdominal hypertension.

PHYSICAL EXAM
Often unreliable:
- Abdominal distension/tense abdomen
- Oliguria/anuria
- Increasing peak inspiratory pressures, difficulty ventilating
- High measured IAP

DIAGNOSTIC TESTS & INTERPRETATION
Diagnostic Procedures/Other
IAP measurements:
- Intravesicular pressure measurements:
  - Measured using transducer setup with Foley catheter. IAP measured in mm Hg should be measured at end expiration with the patient in the supine position.

Pathological Findings
- Sustained IAPs >20 mm Hg
- Ischemia of intra-abdominal organs

DIFFERENTIAL DIAGNOSIS
- Respiratory distress
- Acute renal failure
- Mesenteric/intestinal ischemia

 TREATMENT

ADDITIONAL TREATMENT
General Measures
Primary abdominal compartment syndrome generally requires surgical decompression with temporary abdominal closure to manage IAPs.

Issues for Referral
Once the compartment syndrome has resolved, the abdomen can be closed primarily, but it may require plastic surgery consultation:
- Nephrology consult to consider renal replacement therapy may be needed if renal failure is developing.

Additional Therapies
- Improve abdominal compliance (1)[C]:
  - Sedation/analgesia
  - Body position
  - Neuromuscular blockade
- Evacuate intraluminal or intra-abdominal contents:
  - NGT/OGT decompression
  - Rectal decompression
  - Prokinetic agents (Reglan, erythromycin, or neostigmine)
  - Paracentesis or percutaneous decompression
- Correct positive fluid balance:
  - Fluid restriction or diuretics
  - Colloids (3)[A]
  - Hemodialysis or ultrafiltration in renally compromised patients

SURGERY/OTHER PROCEDURES

- Surgical decompression is generally indicated as first-line treatment. Decompression is accomplished with laparotomy and temporary closure (1)[C].
- Abdominal decompression and temporary abdominal closures, such as towel clips, vacuum-assisted closures, or "Bogota bag":
  – It is important to keep in mind that abdominal compartment syndrome can still develop even with these temporary closure techniques.
- Definitive closure should be considered once the abdominal compartment syndrome has resolved.

IN-PATIENT CONSIDERATIONS

Initial Stabilization

- The patient should be stabilized hemodynamically with the goal of keeping the abdominal perfusion pressures high enough to perfuse abdominal organs (keep perfusion pressure >50 mm Hg), and IAPs should be measured.
- Baseline IAPs should be measured.

Admission Criteria

Patients at risk for abdominal compartment syndrome should be admitted to ICU for close monitoring.

IV Fluids

Massive fluid resuscitation is an independent risk factor for the development of abdominal compartment syndrome:

- Colloid resuscitation could be considered in the patient with elevated IAPs.

Nursing

- Periodic monitoring of IAPs
- Ensuring adequate sedation
- Monitoring for end-organ failure secondary to hypoperfusion of abdominal organs

Discharge Criteria

Resolution of ACS, elimination of the risk of associated organ failure

 ONGOING CARE

FOLLOW-UP RECOMMENDATIONS

Patient Monitoring

IAP measurement:

- In supine position at end-expiration with the transducer zeroed at the midaxillary line
- Use instillation volume no greater than 25 mL.
- Allow 30–60 sec after instillation of priming fluid for bladder detrusor muscle to relax.
- Should be performed in the absence of abdominal muscle contraction

DIET

Most patients with ACS are NPO due to primary abdominal cause of ACS or due to intolerance to enteral feeding.

PROGNOSIS

The mortality for patients with ACS may be as high as 40%.

COMPLICATIONS

- Renal failure requiring renal replacement therapy
- Bowel ischemia requiring bowel resection
- Respiratory failure
- Increased ICP
- Liver failure secondary to hypoperfusion

REFERENCES

1. Cheatham ML, et al. Results from the International Conference of Experts on Intra-abdominal Hypertension and Abdominal Compartment Syndrome. *Int Care Med*. 2007;33:951–962.
2. Vidal MG, et al. Incidence and clinical effects of intra-abdominal hypertension in critically ill patients. *Crit Care Med*. 2008;36:1823–1831.
3. O'Mara MS, et al. A prospective randomized evaluation of intra-abdominal pressures with crystalloid and colloid resuscitation in burn patients. *J Trauma*. 2005;58:1011–1018.

ADDITIONAL READING

- World Society of the Abdominal Compartment syndrome www.wsacs.org

 CODES

ICD9

729.73 Nontraumatic compartment syndrome of abdomen

CLINICAL PEARLS

- ACS is defined as sustained IAPs of >20 mm Hg, hence IAPs should be closely followed in high-risk patient populations.
- IAPs can be measured through the bladder and should be measured at end expiration and in the supine position.
- Primary ACS is treated with emergent surgical intervention/abdominal decompression.
- Secondary and recurrent ACS can be managed medically.

ACIDOSIS, LACTIC

Balaram Anandamurthy
Roopa Kohli-Seth

BASICS

DESCRIPTION
Lactic acidosis is elevated blood lactate levels
(>5 mmol/L) with metabolic acidosis. It is one of the
most common causes of metabolic acidosis.

EPIDEMIOLOGY
Incidence
Increased lactate is common among critically ill
patients, but the actual incidence is unknown. The
overall incidence varies between 0.5–3.8% in
published studies.

Prevalence
~1% of all hospitalized patients and ~44–49% in
ICUs.

RISK FACTORS
Genetics
- MELAS: Mitochondrial encephalopathy, lactic
  acidosis, and stroke-like syndromes have
  mitochondrial inheritance.
- The transmission is maternal, as the genes that code
  for mitochondrial proteins are inherited via the
  oocyte.
- Point mutations in mitochondrial t-RNA are present.

PATHOPHYSIOLOGY
- Lactate is produced by the reduction of pyruvate in
  anaerobic conditions.
- Lactate producers are skeletal muscle, the brain, the
  gut, the erythrocytes, and the injured lung.
- Lactate metabolizers are the liver (50%), the
  kidneys (20%), and the heart (20%).

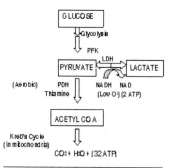

PFK-phospho fructo kinase; LDH- Lactate
Dehydrogenase; NAD (H): Nicotinamide
Adenine Dinucleotide (reduced); PDH- Pyruvate
Dehydrogenase.

- The ability of the liver to consume lactate is
  concentration dependent and progressively
  decreases as the blood lactate increases.
- When the normal physiology is disrupted either due
  to overproduction or under metabolism, lactic
  acidosis results.
- Normal pyruvate to lactate ratio is 10–20:1

ETIOLOGY
- Type A is associated with tissue hypoxia or hypo
  perfusion:
  – Cardiogenic, septic, or hemorrhagic shock.
  – Carbon monoxide or cyanide poisoning
- Type B is more common, with occult tissue ischemia
  without global hypoxemia or hypo perfusion. There
  are 3 types:
  – Type B1:
    ○ Associated with metabolic causes like DM,
      severe Iron deficiency anemia, liver disease,
      pancreatitis, malignancy, infection, renal failure,
      seizures, heat stroke, and parenteral nutrition
      without thiamine.
    ○ Patients with short bowel syndrome develop D-
      lactic acidosis (due to formation of D-lactate by
      the overgrowth of gut bacteria)
  – Type B2:
    ○ Medications: The important ones are
      acetaminophen, ethanol and glycols, nucleoside
      reverse transcriptase inhibitors used in the
      treatment of HIV, β agonists, cocaine, cyanide,
      5-flurouracil, biguanides, propofol, salicylates,
      linezolid, and epinephrine
  – Type B3:
    ○ Inborn errors of metabolism like Glucose 6
      phosphate deficiency, pyruvate kinase
      deficiency, and abnormalities in oxidative
      phosphorylation

COMMONLY ASSOCIATED CONDITIONS
- Shock (septic, cardiogenic, or traumatic)
- Hypoxemia
- Bowel ischemia
- Acute lung injury
- Liver disease
- Short bowel syndrome
- HIV infection and its treatment
- Seizures
- Medications

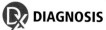

DIAGNOSIS

HISTORY
- The presenting symptom depends on the underlying
  etiology.
- A meticulous history including medications, chronic
  diseases like DM, seizure disorder, and HIV should
  be taken.

PHYSICAL EXAM
- Fever (>38.5°C) or hypothermia (<35°C)
- Hyperventilation
- Tachycardia
- Hypotension
- Altered sensorium.

DIAGNOSTIC TESTS & INTERPRETATION
Lab
- ABG:
  – pH <7.35
  – HCO_3 <15
  – Anion gap >15 mEq
- Absent serum ketones
- S. Lactate >5 mmol/L.

Imaging
Initial approach
- Depending on the initial clinical presentation:
  – Chest x-ray, CT scan of the chest in case of
    pneumonia or ARDS.
  – Echo in congestive heart failure.
- US of abdomen/CT scan (with contrast) if an
  abdominal process like cholecystitis, mesenteric
  ischemia, or pancreatitis is suspected

Follow-Up & Special Considerations
Depends on continuous clinical evaluation and status
of individual patient

Diagnostic Procedures/Other
- EEG for seizures.
- CT- or US-guided drainage of any abnormal
  collections, such as an abscess or effusion

DIFFERENTIAL DIAGNOSIS
- Diabetic ketoacidosis
- Alcoholic ketoacidosis
- Renal failure
- Hyperosmolar hyperglycemic nonketotic coma
- Poisoning
- Drug toxicity

TREATMENT

MEDICATION

First Line
Sodium bicarbonate: Use is controversial, may be considered if pH <7.2 (1)[C]:

- Initially, bicarbonate is given as a slow IV infusion, the dosage being $1/3$–$1/2$ of calculated base deficit.
- Base Deficit $= 0.4 \times$ Weight in Kg $\times$ (24 –Patient's HCO_3)
- Sodium bicarbonate can precipitate respiratory failure by increasing the CO_2 production.

Second Line
- Dichloroacetate: In a large RCT, reduced the arterial lactate concentration and increased pH but demonstrated no benefits on hemodynamics or mortality (2)[B]
- Tris-[hydroxymethyl] aminomethane, Carbicarb, carnitine, and riboflavin show no definitive demonstration of efficacy.
- Antimicrobials for D-lactic acidosis associated with short bowel syndrome (3)[C]
- Antibiotic treatment may result in overgrowth of lactobacillus and worsen the acidosis.

ADDITIONAL TREATMENT

Additional Therapies
Renal replacement therapy

SURGERY/OTHER PROCEDURES
Aimed at source control

IN-PATIENT CONSIDERATIONS

Initial Stabilization
- Establish airway and oxygenation.
- Treat primary cause with restitution of tissue oxygen delivery.

Admission Criteria
All patients with serum lactate above upper limit of normal reference value for the lab

IV Fluids
NS or Plasmalyte to correct the volume deficit

ONGOING CARE

FOLLOW-UP RECOMMENDATIONS
Frequent (q6h) measurement of blood lactate levels

Patient Monitoring
EKG, blood pressure, temperature, oxygen saturation, mixed venous oxygen saturation, cardiac output, and stroke volume variation

DIET
- Depending on the underlying condition, diet may be tailored.
- Low-carbohydrate diet for diabetic patients
- Renal diet for patients in renal failure
- Oxepa™ has been shown to be of benefit in patients with ARDS in a few smaller studies.

PROGNOSIS
- The clinical prognosis is directly proportional to the serum lactate levels; serum lactate >10 mmol/L is associated with 90% mortality.
- Patients who are critically ill and do not clear lactate by 48 hours have high mortality rate but the exact rate is unknown.

COMPLICATIONS
- Extreme acidemia may lead to:
  – Neurological: Altered mental status and seizures.
  – Cardiovascular: Arrhythmias (ventricular tachycardia/fibrillations) and decreased sensitivity to pressors.
  – Respiratory failure
  – Renal failure
- Multiorgan failure resulting in death

REFERENCES

1. Forsythe SM, et al. Sodium bicarbonate for the treatment of lactic acidosis. *Chest*. 2000;117(1): 260–7.
2. Stacpoole PW, et al. A controlled clinical trial of dichloroacetate for treatment of lactic acidosis in adults. *N Engl J Med*. 1992;327:1564–9.
3. Peterson C. D lactic acidosis. *Nutrit Clin Pract*. 2005;20(6):634–45.

ADDITIONAL READING

- Broder G, et al. Excess lactate: An index of reversibility of shock in human patients. *Science*. 1964;143(27):1457–9.
- Luft FC. Lactic acidosis update for critical care clinicians *J Am Soc Nephrol*. 2001;12:S15–S19.
- Otero RM, et al. Early goals directed therapy in severe sepsis and septic shock revisited; Concepts, controversies and contemporary findings. *Chest*. 2006;130;1579–95.

CODES

ICD9
276.2 Acidosis

CLINICAL PEARLS

- Lactic acid measurement involves sampling blood on iced fluoride tubes (gray top) to decrease in vitro red blood cells lactate production.
- Hypoalbuminemia should be factored in while measuring the anion gap.
- The risk of lactic acidosis with the use of metformin is increased in patients with renal failure, sepsis, and exposure to radiocontrast medium.
- The lactate level should be used in conjunction with other clinical markers of circulatory failure rather than as an ultimate indicator of disease severity.
- Increased lactate clearance during the initial stages of sepsis is associated with improved survival.

ACIDOSIS, METABOLIC

Ronaldo Collo Go
Sasikanth Nallagatla
Roopa Kohli-Seth

 BASICS

DESCRIPTION
Caused either by the loss of HCO_3^- or by the gain of acid

Geriatric Considerations
Older people are more prone to metabolic acidosis because of decreased renal function.

Pediatric Considerations
Newborns and infants are more vulnerable than older children and adults to developing acidosis because of low renal threshold for bicarbonate absorption.

EPIDEMIOLOGY
Incidence
The statistics are unknown. Overall, the incidence is more common in critically ill patients.

Prevalence
Prevalence is higher in patients with chronic kidney disease.

RISK FACTORS
- Septic shock
- Renal failure
- Uncontrolled diabetes
- Infusions like Ativan (1)[C] and propofol
- Ingestions/drugs: Salicylates, methanol, ethylene glycol, isoniazid, iron, toluene, metformin, linezolid
- Starvation, >3 days

Genetics
Some inborn errors of metabolism, such as pyruvate dehydrogenase dysfunction, are prone to lactic acidosis.

GENERAL PREVENTION
Metabolic acidosis is prevented by controlling the underlying causes and risk factors.

PATHOPHYSIOLOGY
- $H^+ + HCO_3^- <-> H_2CO_3 <-> CO_2 + H_2O$
- Aberrancy of the buffering symptom above.
- Due to increased acid production:
  - Lactate secondary to reduced cell oxygenation, cytopathic hypoxia, thiamine deficiency, hepatic insufficiency, or cyanide toxicity
  - Ketosis (acetones and β-hydroxybutyrate); metabolites of free fatty acids
  - Glycolic acid
  - Formic acid
- Decreased acid secretion, such as renal failure
- Decreased bicarbonate production
- Compensation: Respiratory compensation for metabolic acidosis is hyperventilation.
- Expected $PaCO_{2+} = 1.5 \times (HCO_3^-) + 8 +/- 2$ (Winter's formula)

- Nonanion and anion gap (AG) metabolic acidosis:
  - AG: Difference between measured anions and cations
  - $AG = Na^+ - (Cl^- + HCO_3^-)$; normal 12 ± 4
  - Unmeasured cations include calcium, magnesium, γ-globulins, and potassium.
  - Unmeasured anions include albumin, phosphate, lactate, and organic anions.
  - AG is decreased in hypoalbuminemia, lithium toxicity, bromide intoxication, multiple myeloma.
  - Adjusted AG = observed gap + 2.5 × (normal–measured albumin)
  - Elevated AG occurs when an unmeasured anion is produced or exogenously gained.
  - Normal AG occurs when increased plasma chloride replaces plasma bicarbonate, secondary to renal or extrarenal (GI) losses.
- Urinary AG is used to differentiate the causes of non-AG acidosis:
  - Increased renal $NH4^+Cl^-$ excretion to enhance H^+ removal is a normal physiologic response to metabolic acidosis.
  - Urinary AG reflects the ability of the kidney to excrete NH_4Cl.
  - Urinary AG = $(Na^+ + K^+) - Cl^-$
  - Urine AG >0 occurs in types 1 and 4 RTA
- Osmolar gap = (Measured Plasma Osmolarity − Calculated Plasma Osmolarity)
  - Calculated $P_{osm} = (2 \times Na) + (glucose/18) + (BUN/2.8)$
  - Normal osmolar gap = 10 mOsm/kg
  - AG metabolic acidosis with high osmolar gap is associated with ethylene glycol, methanol, ESRD, DKA, ETOH ketoacidosis, lactic acidosis, formaldehyde, paraldehyde.

ETIOLOGY
- AG metabolic acidosis (metabolic anion, endogenous):
  - Diabetic ketoacidosis
  - Alcoholic ketoacidosis
  - Lactic acidosis
  - Renal insufficiency
  - Starvation
  - Massive rhabdomyolysis.
- Drugs/chemical anion (exogenous)
  - Salicylate intoxication
  - Methanol (formic acid)
  - Ethylene glycol (oxalic acid)
  - Sodium carbenicillin therapy
- Non-AG metabolic acidosis (hyperchloremic acidosis):
  - Extrarenal causes (GI disorders):
    ○ Diarrhea
    ○ Pancreatic biliary fistula
    ○ Laxatives
    ○ Ureterointestinal diversions
  - Renal causes:
    ○ Type 2 RTA (proximal)
    ○ Type 1 RTA (distal)
    ○ Hypoaldosteronism (type 4 RTA)
    ○ Hyperkalemia
    ○ Acetazolamide

- Exogenous acids:
  - Ammonium chloride
  - Hydrochloric acid
  - Amino acids (L-arginine and L-lysine)

COMMONLY ASSOCIATED CONDITIONS
- Septic shock
- Renal failure
- Uncontrolled type 1 diabetes

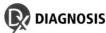 **DIAGNOSIS**

HISTORY
Symptoms of metabolic acidosis are mainly those of underlying disorder. Important points in the history include the following:
- Infection leads to sepsis leads to lactic acidosis.
- Diarrhea leads to GI loss of HCO_3^-.
- Polyuria, increased thirst, epigastric pain, vomiting leads to diabetic ketoacidosis.
- Ingestion of drugs or toxins from salicylates, methanol, ethylene glycol
- Renal stones lead to RTA or chronic diarrhea.

PHYSICAL EXAM
- Kussmaul's respiration: Deep, regular, sighing respiration is seen in severe cases
- Xerosis, pallor, drowsiness, fetor, asterixis, pericardial rub: Renal failure
- Papilledema and retinal hemorrhage: Methanol

DIAGNOSTIC TESTS & INTERPRETATION
Lab
- ABG analysis: Low pH, low PCO_2, low HCO_3^-
- Complete metabolic panel: Measure AG and elevated glucose seen in DKA.
- Urine analysis: pH >5.5 with acidemia is consistent with type 1 RTA and calcium oxalate crystals seen with ethylene glycol toxicity.
- Urine Na, K, Cl to calculate urine AG
- Plasma osmolarity to calculate osmolar gap
- Lactate (pathologic if >2)
- Drug levels if poisoning is suspected
- Cultures if sepsis is suspected

Imaging
- Renal sonogram to find cause for renal failure
- CT scans to find infectious source or ischemic bowel causing lactic acidosis

Diagnostic Procedures/Other
Surgery may be indicated if ischemia is the cause of lactic acidosis and to remove the septic foci in shock patients.

Pathological Findings
Calcium phosphorous stones are common in distal renal tubular acidosis.

DIFFERENTIAL DIAGNOSIS
- Acute renal failure
- Chronic renal failure
- Dialysis complications

 ## TREATMENT

MEDICATION
First Line
- The key to treatment is reversing the pathogenesis of endogenous production and eliminating excess acid:
  - Bicarbonate therapy remains controversial in the setting of AG acidosis (especially lactic acidosis). (2)[C]
  - Adverse effects:
    - Hypernatremia
    - Hyperosmolality
    - Worsening intracellular acidosis
  - Might be considered in severe metabolic acidosis with a pH <7.10 and in salicylate intoxication
- Calculation of HCO_3^- deficit = $0.5 \times$ body weight $\times (24 - HCO_3^-)$
- Treatment for non-AG acidosis:
  - Acute therapy: IV HCO_3^- therapy
  - Chronic therapy: PO HCO_3^-/citrate
  - Fludrocortisone: In hypoaldosteronism

Second Line
Treat the underlying causes and risk factors that cause the metabolic acidosis.

ADDITIONAL TREATMENT
Issues for Referral
Referral to hemodialysis is indicated in severe refractory acidosis and in drug/toxin ingestions.

SURGERY/OTHER PROCEDURES
- Surgery may be needed to remove the source of sepsis.
- Shock wave lithotripsy is the choice for removal of stones formed in distal renal tubular acidosis.

IN-PATIENT CONSIDERATIONS
Initial Stabilization
Maintain ABCs and correct electrolytes aggressively.

Admission Criteria
All patients with metabolic acidosis may need admission for further workup.

IV Fluids
Plasmalyte is preferred for fluid resuscitation because of its neutral pH (3)[B].

Nursing
Frequent monitoring of vitals, EKG, blood glucose

Discharge Criteria
Cause for acidosis is resolved

 ## ONGOING CARE

FOLLOW-UP RECOMMENDATIONS
Frequent follow-up in clinic is recommended for patients with renal failure, diabetes, and heart failure.

Patient Monitoring
Monitor complete metabolic panel, urine analysis, and ABG as necessary.

DIET
- Low-calorie ADA diet is recommended in diabetic patients.
- Low-protein diet in renal failure patients

PROGNOSIS
- Prognosis is directly related to the underlying etiology and the ability to treat or correct that particular disorder.
- Very poor in severe acidosis with pH <7.0

COMPLICATIONS
Severe acidosis can predispose to:
- Fatal ventricular arrhythmias
- Reduced cardiac contractility
- Decreased inotrope response to catecholamines
- Decreased mentation leading to coma
- Chronic acidemia may cause osteomalacia or osteopenia in adults.

REFERENCES

1. Arbour R. Propylene glycol toxicity occurs during low dose infusions of lorazepam. *Crit Care Med*. 2003;31:664–5.
2. Forsythe SM, et al. Sodium bicarbonate for the treatment of lactic acidosis. *Chest*. 2000;117:260–7.
3. Gauthier PM, et al. Metabolic acidosis in the intensive care unit. *Crit Care Clin*. 2002;18:289–308.

ADDITIONAL READING

- Gunnerson KJ, et al. Acid-base and electrolyte analysis in critically ill patients. *Curr Opin Crit Care*. 2003;9:468–73.
- Rose BD, et al. *Clinical Physiology of Acid-Base and Electrolyte Disorders*. New York: McGraw-Hill, 2000.

 ## CODES

ICD9
- 276.2 Acidosis
- 775.7 Late metabolic acidosis of newborn

CLINICAL PEARLS
- Decreased HCO_3^- with acidemia
- Divided into high AG acidosis and normal AG acidosis.
- The highest AG acidoses are seen in lactic acidosis, ketoacidosis, or in the presence of toxins.
- Normal AG acidosis is mainly caused by GI HCO_3^- loss or renal tubular acidosis. Urinary AG may help distinguish between these causes.

ACIDOSIS, RENAL TUBULAR

Sindhura Gogineni
Aditya Uppalapati
Roopa Kohli-Seth

BASICS

DESCRIPTION
- Development of nonanion gap hyperchloremic metabolic acidosis due to impairment in the renal tubular function. Typically, renal function (GFR) is unimpaired.
- 4 major subgroups
  - Type I or distal
  - Type 2 or proximal
  - Type 3 or mixed
  - Type 4 or hypoaldosteronism

EPIDEMIOLOGY
Incidence and prevalence of RTA in ICU population is unknown.

RISK FACTORS
- Severe Illness in ICU patients may lead to hypoaldosteronism.
- Deep venous thrombosis prophylaxis with heparin or low-molecular-weight heparin (LMWH)
- Renal transplantation

Genetics
- Type 1:
  - Autosomal dominant:
    - Mutations in the SLC4A1 gene, Cl^-/HCO_3^- exchanger, AE1 (anion exchanger) gene
  - Autosomal recessive
  - Mutations in the proton pump ($H+{-}$ATPase) in α-intercalated cells.
  - The genes involved ATP6V1B1 (with deafness) ATP6V0A4 (preserved hearing)
- Type 2:
  - Associated with Fanconi syndrome (autosomal recessive), Dent syndrome, cystinosis, tyrosinemia, galactosemia, Wilson disease
  - Autosomal recessive:
    - Mutations in the gene CA2 (carbonic anhydrase)
  - Autosomal dominant:
    - Seen in multiple family members (case reports) but no gene association found
- Type 3 RTA:
  - Recessive mutation in the CA2 gene on chromosome 8q22
- Type 4 RTA:
  - PHA1 (pseudohypoaldosteronism): Autosomal dominant or autosomal recessive
  - PHA2: Autosomal dominant pseudohypoaldosteronism
  - Gordon syndrome: Results in a renal aldosterone resistance (1)

GENERAL PREVENTION
- Patients with known or history of RTA in family should be monitored with serum chemistry.
- The latter can be screened for RTA.
- Type 1 and 2 patients should be given oral bicarbonate and potassium as needed and monitored with serum chemistry.
- Patients with type 4 should be on low-potassium diet and monitored with serum chemistry.

PATHOPHYSIOLOGY
- RTA 1: Impaired ability to acidify the urine in the distal tubule
- RTA 2: Impaired proximal reabsorption of bicarbonate
- RTA 3: Mixed
- RTA 4: Aldosterone deficiency or resistance causes hyperkalemia and in turn leads to suppression of ammonium ion excretion and mild metabolic acidosis.

ETIOLOGY
- Type 1:
  - Autoimmune diseases: Rheumatoid arthritis, Sjögren syndrome
  - Drugs: Analgesic abuse, amphotericin B, trimethoprim, lithium
  - Calcium disorders causing nephrocalcinosis: Primary hyperparathyroidism, vitamin D intoxication
  - Others: Obstructive uropathy, chronic UTIs, sickle cell disease, primary biliary cirrhosis, hypergammaglobulinemia, cryoglobulinemia, renal transplant rejection
- Type 2:
  - Multiple myeloma, renal transplantation, carbonic anhydrase inhibitors, ifosfamide hyperparathyroidism, familial disorders (e.g., glycogen storage disorders)
- Type 4:
  - Aldosterone deficiency:
    - Primary: Primary adrenal insufficiency, congenital adrenal hyperplasia, heparin and LMWH
    - Hyporeninemic hypoaldosteronism: Diabetic nephropathy, ACE inhibitors, NSAIDs, obstructive uropathy, renal transplant rejection, cyclosporine, HIV infection
  - Aldosterone resistance:
    - Drugs: Amiloride, triamterene, spironolactone, trimethoprim, pentamidine
    - Tubulointerstitial disease
    - Pseudohypoaldosteronism

COMMONLY ASSOCIATED CONDITIONS
See Genetics and Etiology

DIAGNOSIS

- Detailed history and physical exam to be obtained regarding the etiology
- History of fever, chills, burning micturition (UTI symptoms)
- History of renal stones, hematuria, analgesic abuse, diabetes, renal transplantation
- Physical exam:
  - Costovertebral angle tenderness
  - Bone tenderness, muscle strength

DIAGNOSTIC TESTS & INTERPRETATION
Lab
Initial lab tests
- Serum chemistry:
  - Normal or minimally affected glomerular filtration rate
  - Hypokalemia: Type 1 & 2
  - Hyperkalemia: Type 4
- Anion gap normal
- CBC (anemia, myeloma)
- Liver function tests:
  - Elevated enzymes, decreased albumin:
    - Hypergammaglobulinemia, cirrhosis
- ABG
- Urine analysis, urine pH
- Urine electrolytes:
  - NA^+, K^+, Cl^-
- Urine anion gap (Ur AG)
- Urine (Na + K^- Chloride):
  - Positive Ur AG: Indicative of low NH_{4+} (ammonia) excretion:
    - Only need to rule out type of RTA
  - Negative Ur AG: Indicative of High NH_{4+} excretion:
    - Need to rule out causes other than RTA (e.g., GI bicarbonate loss)

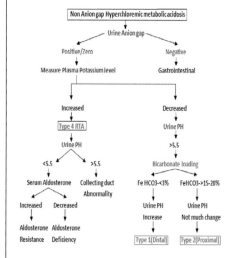

Follow-Up & Special Considerations
- Types 1 and 2 RTA:
  - Bicarbonate loading (0.5–1.0 mEq/Kg/hr) to raise serum HCO_3 to normal (18–20 mEq/L) and calculate fractional excretion of bicarbonate ($FeHCO_3$):
    - (Ur HCO_3 × Pl Cr)/(Pl HCO_3 × Ur Cr) × 100
    - Where Ur is Urine, Pl is plasma
  - Type 2: Urine pH will increase from baseline to as high as >7.5, $FeHCO_3$ – >15–20%
  - Type 1: Urine pH not much changed from baseline, $FeHCO_3$ – <3%
- Type 4 RTA:
  - Transtubular potassium gradient (TTKG)
    - TTKG = [Urine K ÷ (Urine osmolality/Plasma osmolality)] ÷ Plasma K
    - TTKG <7 suggest hypoaldosteronism
  - Serum aldosterone
  - Serum random cortisol if relative adrenal insufficiency is suspected
  - After the type of RTA is diagnosed, further lab tests should be directed to its possible etiology.

Imaging
Initial approach
- X-ray of skeletal system in suspected multiple myeloma, rheumatoid arthritis, skeletal abnormalities
- X-ray of abdomen to evaluate for nephrocalcinosis
- US: If cirrhosis, obstructive uropathy is suspected
- Renal sonogram can be used to evaluate renal size or presence of stones.
- CT abdomen: If adrenal hyperplasia is suspected

Diagnostic Procedures/Other
IV pyelogram: Stone, medullary sponge kidney, nephrocalcinosis, obstructive uropathy

DIFFERENTIAL DIAGNOSIS
- Other causes of nonanion gap acidosis
- Acid infusion: Amino acid, hydrochloric acid, ammonium chloride, excessive resuscitation with NS, use of hypertonic saline
- Bicarbonate losses:
  - Transplanted pancreas (with bladder anastomosis)
  - GI causes: Diarrhea or intestinal losses; fistula
  - Urethral diversion: Ileal loop
- Toluene ingestion
- Carbonic anhydrase inhibitor

TREATMENT
MEDICATION
First Line
- Type 1 RTA: Sodium bicarbonate (650–1300 mg 2 to 4 times daily) or potassium citrate (15 mL b.i.d. or t.i.d.) (2,3)[C]
- Type 2 RTA: 10–15 mEq of alkali/Kg/d. Potassium citrate or sodium bicarbonate can be used (2,3)[C].
- Thiazide diuretics to promote proximal tubule HCO_3 absorption
- Type 4 RTA: Alkali therapy for acidosis; loop diuretics and dietary restriction of potassium (4)[B]; fludrocortisone (100–300 μg/d) may be used to correct hyperkalemia and acidosis.

Second Line
- Type 2: If associated with Fanconi syndrome, replace vitamin D, calcium, phosphate
- Type 4: Primary adrenal insufficiency; mineralocorticoid administration
- If hypokalemia, potassium citrate

ADDITIONAL TREATMENT
General Measures
Avoid the offending medications.

Issues for Referral
Nephrology for dialysis in case of symptomatic or severe hyperkalemia (>7.5 mEq/L) in RTA type 4

Additional Therapies
CVVH or dialysis for severe hyperkalemia (RTA type 4)

SURGERY/OTHER PROCEDURES
- If severe hyperkalemia: Large-bore catheter for CVVH/dialysis if needed
- If severe Hypokalemia: Central venous catheter might be needed to replete with IV potassium chloride
- Lithotripsy if symptomatic renal stones
- Percutaneous decompression (nephrostomy) for hydronephrosis secondary to renal stones, obstruction

IN-PATIENT CONSIDERATIONS
Initial Stabilization
Correction of electrolyte abnormalities

Admission Criteria
- Shock
- Altered mental status
- Respiratory distress from hypokalemia
- Muscular paralysis, weakness, neural paralysis from hypokalemia
- Cardiac arrhythmias from hypo- or hyperkalemia

IV Fluids
- Sodium bicarbonate
- Plasmalyte (Isolyte) if hypokalemia and acidosis

Nursing
- Cardiac monitoring, telemetry
- Frequent neural exam in case of weakness

Discharge Criteria
Stable electrolytes

ONGOING CARE
FOLLOW-UP RECOMMENDATIONS
Long-term follow-up is required to monitor for kidney and bone complications.

Patient Monitoring
In severe hyperkalemic and hypokalemic patients, serial potassium measurement q3–4h until potassium level stabilize to 3.5–4.0

DIET
- If hyperkalemia (type 4): Low-potassium diet
- If hypokalemia (type 1 or 2): Potassium-rich diet

PATIENT EDUCATION
- Dietary consultation
- Education about RTA

PROGNOSIS
If RTA occurs in the ICU and is recognized, it can be corrected and treated.

COMPLICATIONS
- Type 1: Hypercalciuria, hypocitraturia, nephrolithiasis (calcium phosphate), nephrocalcinosis, skeletal abnormalities.
- Type 2: Nephrolithiasis uncommon. However, calcium stones are common with acetazolamide therapy, skeletal abnormalities
- Myopathy (due to electrolyte abnormalities)

REFERENCES
1. Pereira PC, et al. Molecular pathophysiology of renal tubular acidosis. *Curr Genomics*. 2009;10:51–59.
2. Brown AS. Renal tubular acidosis. *Dimens Crit Care Nurs*. 2010;29(3):112–119.
3. Rodriguez Soriano J. Renal tubular acidosis: The clinical entity. *J Am Soc Nephrol*. 2002;13:2160.
4. Weisberg LS. Management of hyperkalemia. *Crit Care Med*. 2008;36:3246–51.

ADDITIONAL READING
- Troels Ring, et al. Clinical review: Renal tubular acidosis: Physicochemical approach. *Crit Care*. 2005;9:573–80.

CODES
ICD9
- 255.5 Other adrenal hypofunction
- 588.89 Other specified disorders resulting from impaired renal function

CLINICAL PEARLS
- RTA is an important cause of nonanion gap, hyperchloremic metabolic acidosis.
- Treat the underlying cause of RTA.
- Aggressively treat the electrolyte imbalances associated with RTA.

ACIDOSIS, RESPIRATORY

Sanjay Dhar
Roopa Kohli-Seth

 BASICS

DESCRIPTION

- Acid–base disorder with primary increase in the arterial partial pressure of carbon dioxide (PCO_2) and a compensatory increase in bicarbonate concentration (HCO_3)
- Acute respiratory acidosis: $PaCO_2$ is elevated above the upper limit of reference range (>45 mm Hg), with accompanying acidemia (pH <7.35)
- Chronic respiratory acidosis: $PaCO_2$ is elevated above the upper limit of reference range with near normal blood pH (7.35–7.45) secondary to renal compensation with an elevated bicarbonate (HCO_3 >30 mm Hg).

EPIDEMIOLOGY

Incidence
Increased in associated conditions

Prevalence
- Increased in associated conditions
- In a 1-year period, prevalence study of respiratory acidosis in acute exacerbations of COPD were 75/100,000 per year for men (45–79) and 57/100,000 per year (46–69) for women (1)[B].

RISK FACTORS
- Hypercapnia attributed to increased production of CO_2:
  - ICU patients
  - Increased metabolic rate
- Hypercapnia attributed to decreased elimination of CO_2:
  - COPD
  - Restrictive lung disease
  - Deformity of chest wall
  - Neuromuscular disease
  - Trauma
  - Anesthesia

Genetics
- Severe α1-antitrypsin (AAT) deficiency (e.g., protease inhibitor [PI] Z) proven genetic risk factor for COPD.
- Mutations in the ALS2, SETX, SOD1, and VAPB genes linked to amyotrophic lateral sclerosis (ALS)
- Mutations in dystrophin linked to Duchenne muscular dystrophy

GENERAL PREVENTION
- Smoking cessation, especially in COPD patients
- Weight loss is helpful in obesity hypoventilation syndrome and obstructive sleep apnea.

PATHOPHYSIOLOGY
- Metabolism rapidly generates large quantities of volatile acid (CO_2), which combines with water to form carbonic acid (H_2CO_3). Lungs normally excrete this through ventilation, and acid accumulation does not occur. Significant alterations in alveolar ventilation that limits elimination of CO_2 results in respiratory acidosis.
- Ventilation is influenced and regulated by chemoreceptors for $PaCO_2$, PaO_2, and pH located in the brainstem, as well as by neural impulses from lung-stretch receptors and impulses from the cerebral cortex. Failure of ventilation quickly increases the $PaCO_2$.

- In acute respiratory acidosis, the body's compensation occurs in 2 steps:
  - The initial response is cellular buffering that occurs over minutes to hours. Cellular buffering elevates plasma bicarbonate values, but only slightly (~1 mEq/L foreach 10 mm Hg increase in $PaCO_2$).
  - The 2nd step is renal compensation that occurs over 3–5 days. With renalcompensation, renal excretion of carbonic acid is increased and bicarbonate reabsorption is increased.

ETIOLOGY
- Acute respiratory acidosis:
  - Airway obstruction: Laryngospasm
  - Respiratory center depression: General anesthesia, head injury, sedatives
  - Circulatory collapse: Cardiac arrest, pulmonary edema
  - Neurogenic causes: Cervical spine injury, Guillain-Barré syndrome, myasthenia gravis, organophosphates
  - Restrictive defects: Flail chest, hemothorax, pneumothorax, ARDS
- Chronic respiratory acidosis:
  - Airway obstruction: COPD
  - Respiratory center depression: Pickwickian syndrome, chronic sedative overdose, brain tumor
  - Neurogenic causes: Muscular dystrophy, ALS, myxedema, phrenic nerve palsy
  - Restrictive defects: Hydrothorax, fibrothorax, ascites

COMMONLY ASSOCIATED CONDITIONS
- Cardiopulmonary arrest
- COPD
- Guillain Barré syndrome
- Myasthenic crisis
- Obesity hypoventilation syndrome
- Sedative overdose
- Muscular dystrophies

DIAGNOSIS

HISTORY
- Specific to underlying cause (e.g., CNS disease, sedatives, COPD, obesity hypoventilation syndrome, neuromuscular disease, or related to airway obstruction)
- Depends on severity of underlying disorder and rate of development of hypercapnia

PHYSICAL EXAM
Related to underlying cause:
- With airway obstruction: Dyspnea labored breathing, wheezing, hyperresonance on percussion, prolonged expiration
- With Hypoxemia: Cyanosis
- With respiratory center depression: Shallow or apneustic breathing, asterixis, myoclonus or seizures
- Mild respiratory acidosis: Nonspecific symptoms; like headache, tremors, weakness
- Marked respiratory acidosis: Fatigue, confusion
- Severe respiratory acidosis: Papilledema, stupor, coma

Geriatric Considerations
Assess underlying cause. Hypercapnia is well tolerated in those with chronic respiratory acidosis.

Pediatric Considerations
Early assessment of acuity of event and degree of hypoxemia is critical to outcome.

Pregnancy Considerations
Maternal hypercapnia results in fetal respiratory acidosis. Institute careful fetomaternal monitoring.

DIAGNOSTIC TESTS & INTERPRETATION
Lab
Initial lab tests
- ABGs and serum chemistries: Acidemic pH (<7.35) and elevated $PaCO_2$ (>45 mm Hg) in the presence of appropriate HCO_3. Hypoxemia in pulmonary disease causing respiratory acidosis.
- CBC: Chronic hypoxemia leading to polycythemia
- Thyroid function tests: Obesity
- Drug screens: Opiates, barbiturates benzodiazepines

Follow-Up & Special Considerations
- Expected change in serum bicarbonate concentration
- Acute respiratory acidosis: Bicarbonate increases by 1 mEq/L for each 10 mm Hg rise in $PaCO_2$.

$$HCO_3 = 0.1 \times PCO_2$$

- Chronic respiratory acidosis: Bicarbonate increases by 3.5 mEq/L for each 10 mm Hg rise in $PaCO_2$.

$$HCO_3 = 0.35 \times PCO_2$$

- Expected change in pH:
  - Acute respiratory acidosis:Change in pH = 0.008 $\times$ (40 − $PaCO_2$)
  - Chronic respiratory acidosis:Change in pH = 0.003 $\times$ (40 − $PaCO_2$)
- Electrolytes:
  - Increased ionized calcium
  - Extracellular shift of potassium
  - Renal ammonia production increased
  - Increased hydrogen ion secretion
  - Fall in urine pH

Imaging
Initial approach
- Based on cause
- Chest x-ray: Airway obstruction, flail chest, hemothorax, pneumothorax, ARDS
- CAT scan: C spine, head injury, stroke (pons + medulla)
- MRI brain: If CAT scan is inconclusive, to detect stroke in pons and medulla
- Fluoroscopy: Sniff test: Paradoxical elevation of paralyzed diaphragm with inspiration in unilateral diaphragmatic palsy

Follow-Up & Special Considerations
To assess resolution of primary cause resulting in respiratory acidosis

Diagnostic Procedures/Other
Related to primary cause
- Pulmonary function testing:
  - Obstructive lung disease: Ratio of FEV_1/FVC reduced, TLC increased; DLCO severely reduced in emphysema.
  - Restrictive lung disease: Ratio of FEV_1/FVC normal or increased, TLC decreased; hallmark of restrictive lung disease
  - Neuromuscular disease: Decreased vital capacity, NIF
- Electromyography and nerve conduction velocity:
  - Useful in diagnosing myasthenia gravis, ALS, and Guillain Barré syndrome
- Transdiaphragmatic pressure measurements:
  - Decreased in diaphragmatic dysfunction and paralysis

Pathological Findings
Related to primary cause

DIFFERENTIAL DIAGNOSIS
- Asthma
- Botulism
- COPD
- Diaphragmatic paralysis
- Obesity
- Opioid use
- May mimic pseudotumor cerebri (increased CSF pressure and papilledema)
- Sedative use
- Myasthenia gravis
- ALS

 TREATMENT

MEDICATION
First Line
- Supplemental oxygen to correct hypoxemia to maintain saturation >90–92%
- Bronchodilators to relieve airway obstruction
- Steroids to reduce airway inflammation
- Hypercapnia is instrumental in improving outcomes of patients with acute lung injury and ARDS (2,3)[A].

Second Line
Administration of antagonists to opiates or benzodiazepines is helpful if respiratory depression from these agents is suspected.

ADDITIONAL TREATMENT
General Measures
- Establish effective airway: Suctioning to remove secretions, stimulation of cough, chest percussion, postural drainage.
- Establish definitive airway: Endotracheal intubation and mechanical ventilation, tracheostomy.

Issues for Referral
- Depends on cause of hypercapnic respiratory failure
- Respiratory failure requiring mechanical ventilation: ICU referral
- Neuromuscular dysfunction: Early referral to neurology should be obtained.

Additional Therapies
- Noninvasive positive-pressure ventilation
- Aerobic exercises
- Breathing retraining technique: Pursed lip breathing techniques in COPD

COMPLEMENTARY & ALTERNATIVE THERAPIES
Stress relaxation techniques may help to alleviate dyspnea.

SURGERY/OTHER PROCEDURES
- Tracheostomy
- Bullectomy
- Lung volume reduction surgery
- Lung transplant
- Video assisted thoracoscopic biopsy
- Plasmapheresis

IN-PATIENT CONSIDERATIONS
Initial Stabilization
- ABCs
- Monitor oxygenation, ECG.

Admission Criteria
- ICU admission criteria: Respiratory muscle fatigue, confusion, lethargy, low pH, monitoring on NIPPV, hemodynamic instability
- Invasive diagnostic and therapeutic procedures

IV Fluids
Maintain euvolemia.

Nursing
- Standard bundle approach to prevent hospital acquired infections.
- Aggressive suctioning
- Incentive spirometry
- Pulmonary rehab

Discharge Criteria
- Correction of underlying primary admitting cause.
- Hemodynamic stability
- Resolution of severe acidosis

 ONGOING CARE

FOLLOW-UP RECOMMENDATIONS
- Oxygen therapy:
  - Criteria for long-term oxygen therapy: PaO_2 of <55 mm Hg or PaO_2 of <59 mm Hg with evidence of polycythemia or cor pulmonale
- Noninvasive ventilation:
  - Nasal bilevel positive-pressure ventilation can be used long-term to treat patients with neuromuscular disorders, COPD with hypercapnia, primary alveolar hypoventilation, and obesity hypoventilation syndrome.

Patient Monitoring
- ABG determinations
- Pulmonary function tests
- Pulmonary rehab

DIET
- Aspiration precautions
- Speech swallow evaluation should be done in those with neuromuscular disorders.

PATIENT EDUCATION
- Multidisciplinary approach:
  - Smoking cessation, aerobic exercise, breathing retraining, stress relaxation, bronchial hygiene, physical therapy, immunization, vocational and psychosocial support

PROGNOSIS
- Varies, depending on severity of underlying condition
- Early recognition of signs and symptoms and underlying etiology is critical in prognostication.

COMPLICATIONS
- Chronic hypoxemia leading to polycythemia
- Chronic hypoxia leading to pulmonary vasoconstriction, pulmonary hypertension, and right-heart failure
- Apnea hypopnea leading to increased risk for ventricular fibrillation
- Acute respiratory acidemia leading to increased cerebral blood flow. High levels of $PaCO_2$ (>70 mm Hg) can lead to confusion, loss of consciousness, and seizures (4)[A].
- Acute hypercapnia can lead to depression of diaphragmatic contractility.

REFERENCES
1. Plant PK, et al. One year period prevalence study of respiratory acidosis in acute exacerbations of COPD: Implications for the provision of non-invasive ventilation and oxygen administration. *Thorax.* 2000;55:550–4.
2. Kallet RH, et al. Management of acidosis during lung-protective ventilation in acte respiratory distress syndrome. *Respir Care Clin North Am.* 2003;9:437–56.
3. Thorensj-B, et al. Effects of rapid permissive hypercapnia on hemodynamics, gas exchange, and oxygen transport and consumption during mechanical ventilation for the acute respiratory distress syndrome. *Intensive Care Med.* 1996;22:182–91.
4. Kregenow DA, et al. Hypercapnic acidosis and mortality in acute lung injury. *Crit Care Med.* 2006;34;1–7.

ADDITIONAL READING
- Feihl F, et al. Permissive hypercapnia: How permissive should we be? *Am J Respir Care Med.* 1994;150:1722–37.
- Laffey JG, et al. Buffering hypercapnic acidosis worsens acute lung injury. *Am J Respir Crit Care Med.* 2000;161:141–6.

 CODES

ICD9
276.2 Acidosis

CLINICAL PEARLS
- Search for underlying cause of acid–base disorder.
- Normal pH, serum bicarbonate, and PCO_2 do not necessarily exclude acid–base disorders.
- Acidemia represents changes in pH, whereas acidosis denotes underlying pathological process.
- In patients with COPD, rather than target a $PaCO_2$ of 40 mm Hg, manipulate the ventilator to target the patient's baseline serum bicarbonate or a pH of 7.35–7.38 to prevent ventilator-associated alveolar overdistention and lung injury.

ADVANCED CARDIAC LIFE SUPPORT

Victor Matos
Vicente San Martín

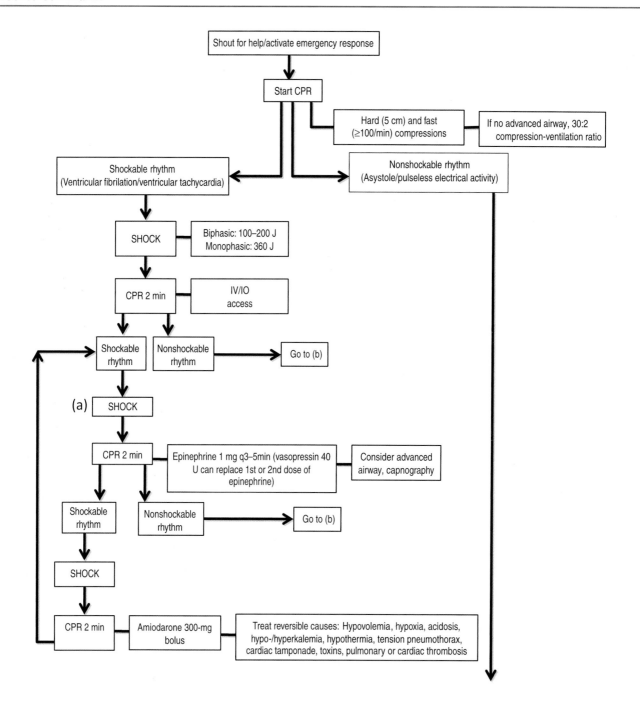

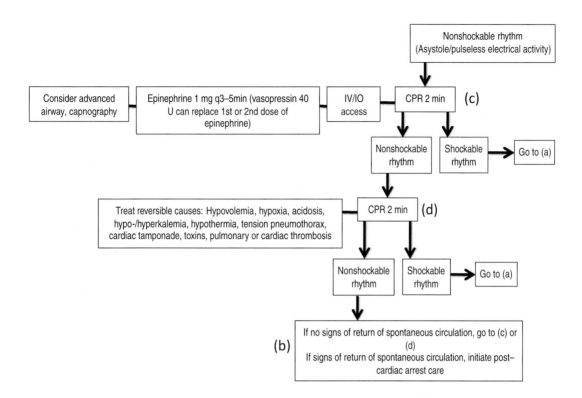

ADDITIONAL READING

- Neumar RW, et al. Part 8: Adult advanced cardiovascular life support: 2010 American Heart Association Guidelines for Cardiopulmonary Resuscitation and Emergency Cardiovascular Care. *Circulation*. 2010;122;S729-S767.

ACINETOBACTER

Jose Diego Caceres
Jose R. Yunen

 BASICS

DESCRIPTION
- Infection caused by the organism *Acinetobacter calcoaceticus-baumannii* complex, mostly nosocomial
- Remains an opportunistic pathogen in the critically ill patient:
  - Ventilator-associated pneumonia
  - Bacteremias
  - Wound infections
  - Urinary tract infections in patient with indwelling urinary catheter
  - Meningitis in neurosurgical patients

PATHOPHYSIOLOGY
- Isolated from hospital equipment, bedding, furniture, and medical staff:
  - Contamination of hospital devices with *A. baumannii* isolates has been documented for ventilator tubing, suction catheters, humidifiers, multidose vials of medication, potable water, bedding, and arterial lines.
  - Can colonize skin, wounds, and the respiratory and GI tracts
- "Multidrug resistant" strains are defined as those found resistant to ≥3 classes of drug that would otherwise serve as treatment. Critically ill patients have increased risk.
- "Panresistant *Acinetobacter*" are strains found resistant to all standard antimicrobial agents tested (except colistin).

ETIOLOGY
- *Acinetobacter* is a genus of coccobacillus strictly aerobic, nonmotile, gram-negative, nonfermentative, oxidase-negative, catalase-positive organism. There are currently 32 Acinetobacter named and unnamed species:
  - *A. baumannii* is responsible for the majority of the infections.
  - Minority are caused by *A. calcoaceticus*, *A. junii*.
  - Also referred to as *A. calcoaceticus- A. baumannii* complex, encompasses these 2 species, plus 2 other unnamed species, 3 and 13TU, due to the close relatedness of these strains; this complex is primarily responsible for clinical pathogenesis.

COMMONLY ASSOCIATED CONDITIONS
- Alcoholism
- Diabetes mellitus
- Chronic obstructive pulmonary disease (COPD)
- Immunocompromised host
- Invasive procedures
- Mechanical ventilation
- Central venous or urinary catheters
- Prolonged ICU stay
- Use of broad-spectrum antibiotics

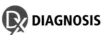 **DIAGNOSIS**

HISTORY
- Patient under prolonged mechanical ventilation
- Long ICU stay, particularly during outbreaks
- Wide-spectrum antibiotic therapy or antibiotics with little antimicrobial activity against *Acinetobacter* in colonized patient

PHYSICAL EXAM
- Fever or hypothermia
- Tachycardia
- Tachypnea
- Hypotension
- Hypoxia
- Decreased breath sounds
- Pleural friction rub
- Rales
- Rhonchi
- Altered mental status
- Neck rigidity
- Signs of wound infection: Tumor, rubor, calor, and pain
- Signs related to underlying chronic medical conditions

DIAGNOSTIC TESTS & INTERPRETATION
Lab
Initial lab tests
- CBC count usually presents with leukocytosis with left shift.
- ABG analysis
- Serum lactate
- Serum electrolytes
- BUN and creatinine
- Blood cultures
- Sputum culture and gram stain.
- Cultures body fluids or secretions.

Follow-Up & Special Considerations
- Repeat CBC count, BUN, creatinine and electrolyte q24h.
- Repeat ABG if in distress or mechanically ventilated patient
- Endotracheal secretions and urine isolation in patient with Foley catheter does not indicate active infection.
- Isolate monitoring devices, medical staff, and multiple patients during outbreaks.

Imaging
Initial approach
- Chest x-ray is first line imaging study to identify the extent of the infiltrations.
- Chest CT scan is not useful.
- Head CT scan or MRI is useful if meningeal involvement is suspected.

Follow-Up & Special Considerations
- Chest x-ray q24h in patient with ventilator-associated pneumonia to evaluate response to treatment
- Chest CT scan in 48 hours after initiating treatment if the patient is not improving
- Head CT after 48 hours of initial treatment or in 24 hours if the patient is not found to improve
- Consider EEG in patient with low level of conscious.

Diagnostic Procedures/Other
Reserve only for treatment and follow-up related to specific organ involvement.

Pathological Findings
Gram-negative short coccobacilli with diplococcal features. Strictly aerobic and nonfermenting.

DIFFERENTIAL DIAGNOSIS
- Community-acquired pneumonia
- Pulmonary edema
- ARDS
- Meningoencephalitis
- Aseptic meningitis
- Other cause of SIRS or septicemia

 TREATMENT

MEDICATION
First Line
Imipenem 500 mg IV q6h or Meropenem 0.5–1 g IV q8h or a fluoroquinolone + Amikacin 15 mg/kg/d IV/IM divided b.i.d./t.i.d.; not to exceed 1.5 g/d regardless of higher BW or ceftazidime 1–2 gm IV q8–12h

Second Line
- Ampicillin-sulbactam 1.5–3 g IV q8h
- Colistin 2.5–5 mg/kg/day divided in 2 to 4 doses (max 800 mg/day)
- Tigecycline 100 mg IV loading dose, then 50 mg IV q12h

ADDITIONAL TREATMENT
Additional Therapies
- Acetaminophen 1 g PO q6h
- Nebulizations ipratropium bromide and normal saline q6h
- Supportive care for fever, dehydration, and respiratory distress

SURGERY/OTHER PROCEDURES
- Central and peripheral lines should be changed or removed if evidence of infection or positive line cultures are found.
- Intraventricular ICP monitoring devices should be removed if no signs of elevated ICP.
- Consider tracheostomy in patients with prolonged (7–10 days) need for mechanical ventilation.

IN-PATIENT CONSIDERATIONS
Initial Stabilization
- Patient isolation
- Suctioning of upper airway, nasogastric or orogastric tube placement
- Oxygen supplementation
- Cardiac monitoring and pulse oximetry
- Consider endotracheal intubation in patients with acute respiratory distress, shock, or unable to protect airway.
- Central line placement
- Further hemodynamic monitoring in patients with shock or ARDS using transthoracic or transesophageal echo, pulse contour analysis or pulmonary artery catheter

IV Fluids
- Normosol or NS solutions, maintaining input and output balance
- Electrolyte replacement

 ONGOING CARE

DIET
Enteral nutrition is preferred.

PROGNOSIS
Variable data among different studies in critical patients:
- Overall mortality ranges between 19% and 54%.

ADDITIONAL READING
- Bassetti M, et al. Drug treatment for multidrug-resistant Acinetobacter baumannii infections. *Future Microbiology*. 2008;3(6):649–60.
- Gootz TD, et al. Acinetobacter baumannii: An emerging multidrug-resistant threat. *Expert Rev Anti Infect Ther*. 2008;6(3):309–25.
- Hartzell JD, et al. Acinetobacter pneumonia: A review. *Medscape Gen Med*. 2007;9(3):4.
- Munoz-Price LS, et al. Acinetobacter infection. *N Engl J Med*. 2008;358:1271–81.
- Van de Beek D, et al. Nosocomial Bacterial Meningitis. *N Engl J Med*. 2010;362:146–54.

 CODES

ICD9
- 041.85 Other specified bacterial infections in conditions classified elsewhere and of unspecified site, other gram-negative organisms
- 136.9 Unspecified infectious and parasitic diseases
- 486 Pneumonia, organism unspecified

CLINICAL PEARLS
- *A. baumannii* is a nosocomial infection more prevalent in mechanically ventilated patients.
- Multidrug resistant strains are becoming more frequent in the hospital setting.
- Isolate monitoring devices, medical staff, and multiple patients during outbreaks.

ACUTE RESPIRATORY DISTRESS SYNDROME

Arif M. Shaik
Anthony Manasia

 BASICS

DESCRIPTION
- Acute respiratory distress syndrome (ARDS) is characterized by noncardiogenic pulmonary edema, lung inflammation, hypoxemia, and decreased lung compliance.
- American-European consensus conference criteria includes a PaO_2 to FiO_2 ratio of <200 mm Hg, bilateral pulmonary infiltrates, and no clinical evidence of left atrial hypertension. Acute lung injury is defined by a PaO_2 to FiO_2 ratio of <300.

EPIDEMIOLOGY
Incidence
The reported incidence of ARDS ranges from 75 per 100,000 populationto as low as 1.5 per 100,000.

Prevalence
10–15% of patients admitted to the ICU and 20% of all mechanically ventilated patients meet the criteria for ARDS.

RISK FACTORS
- Sepsis, major trauma, pancreatitis, aspiration of gastric contents, and multiple transfusions (>15 units per 24 hours in one study) are associated with the highest risk of developing ARDS.
- The risk of developing ARDS may be especially high among septic patients with a history of alcoholism.

Genetics
A small association between a polymorphism in the gene for surfactant protein B and angiotensin-converting enzyme may have an effect on the incidence and outcome of ARDS patients.

GENERAL PREVENTION
- Avoid unnecessary transfusions
- Aspiration precautions
- Early diagnosis and treatment of sepsis

PATHOPHYSIOLOGY
- ARDS is a disorder of increased alveolar-capillary permeability leading to protein-rich edema fluid that fills the alveoli.
- Proinflammatory cytokines such as TNF, interleukin (IL)-1, IL-6, and IL-8 are released in response to a variety of precipitants.
- Alveolar filling leads to decreased respiratory system compliance, as well as right-to-left shunting and profound hypoxemia.
- Injury to type II alveolar epithelial cells results in loss of surfactant production, leading to a decrease in lung compliance.
- ARDS has classically been described using three overlapping and sequential stages:
  - Exudative phase: Hyaline membranes and protein-rich fluid in the alveolar spaces, as well as epithelial disruption, infiltration of the interstitium, and air spaces with neutrophils resulting in diffuse alveolar damage. This phase lasts for 5–7 days.
  - Proliferative phase: Obliteration of pulmonary capillaries and deposition of interstitial and alveolar collagen may be observed along with a decrease in the number of neutrophils and the amount of pulmonary edema. This phase lasts 1–2 weeks.
  - Fibrotic phase: Some patients develop diffuse interstitial fibrosis.

ETIOLOGY
- Sepsis is the most common cause of ARDS. It should be considered first in any patient who develops otherwise unexplained ARDS.
- Aspiration of gastric contents: ~1/3 of hospitalized patients who experience a clinically recognized episode of gastric aspiration subsequently develop the syndrome.
- Infectious pneumonia: Pneumonia is probably the most common cause of ARDS in outpatients.
- Acute pancreatitis: Common cause of noninfectious ARDS.
- Major abdominal surgery
- Severe trauma and surface burns
- Massive blood transfusion: Transfusion of >15 units of blood is an important risk factor for the development of ARDS.
- Transfusion-related acute lung injury (TRALI) can occur following even 1 unit of blood product.
- Lung and bone marrow transplantation; common in first 2–3 weeks
- Drugs and alcohol: ARDS can be caused by overdose of several common drugs including aspirin, cocaine, opioids, phenothiazines, and tricyclic antidepressants.
- Others: Cardiopulmonary bypass, pneumonectomy, and near drowning.

COMMONLY ASSOCIATED CONDITIONS
Sepsis, blood product transfusions, and pancreatitis

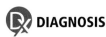 **DIAGNOSIS**

HISTORY
Recent history of aspiration, pneumonia, trauma, abdominal surgery, blood transfusion, or drug overdose

PHYSICAL EXAM
- Fever or hypothermia
- Look for sources of infection or signs of trauma.
- Tachypnea, use of accessory muscles
- Coarse breath sounds/rales bilaterally
- Epigastric tenderness if pancreatitis suspected

DIAGNOSTIC TESTS & INTERPRETATION
Lab
Initial lab tests
- ABGs: Elevated alveolar-arterial oxygen gradient, severe hypoxemia and respiratory alkalosis
- CBC: Leukocytosis with left shift if infectious etiology
- Panculture if sepsis is suspected
- Serum lipase if pancreatitis is suspected
- Brain natriuretic peptide (BNP): A BNP level <100 pg/mL identifies ARDS/ALI with a sensitivity, specificity, positive predictive value, and negative predictive value of 27, 95, 90, and 44%, respectively. BNP is less specific in critically ill patients with sepsis and systemic inflammation.
- Transthoracic or transesophageal echocardiography: To assess cardiac contractility and volume status, and to rule out cor pulmonale.
- Pulmonary artery catheter is no longer indicated. A multicenter trial found no improvement in survival or organ function, but reported more complications (1)[A].

Follow-Up & Special Considerations
Diagnostic bronchoscopy: If the cause of ARDS cannot be determined, consider bronchoscopy for inspection of the airways and for bronchoalveolar lavage.

Imaging
Initial approach
Chest x-ray shows diffuse bilateral alveolar infiltrates.
Follow-Up & Special Considerations
- CT scan of chest generally demonstrates patchy abnormalities with increased density in dependent lung zones.
- CT of abdomen and pelvis if infectious source is suspected

Diagnostic Procedures/Other
Lung biopsy is done only when other diagnostic tests are inconclusive.

Pathological Findings
Heavy, boggy lungs with microscopic alveolar damage and edema, neutrophilic infiltration, and formation of hyaline membrane in exudative phase

DIFFERENTIAL DIAGNOSIS
- Diffuse alveolar hemorrhage
- Acute interstitial pneumonia (Hamman-Rich syndrome)
- Idiopathic acute eosinophilic pneumonia (IAEP)

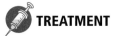 **TREATMENT**

MEDICATION
First Line
- Treat underlying cause.
- Early broad-spectrum antibiotics in sepsis and septic shock
- Intubation and sedation
- Paralysis may be required to improve oxygenation and decrease airway pressures, but should be minimized to prevent prolonged neuromuscular weakness.
- Mechanical ventilation with low tidal volume (VT) and PEEP
- Pressure-regulated volume control (PRVC) combines a pressure limit while assuring volume by manipulating inspiratory time and flow, thus reducing risk of barotrauma.
- Airway pressure release ventilation (APRV) is described as CPAP (continuous positive airway pressure) with an intermittent release phase. It may be beneficial in severely hypoxemic patients by maintaining an adequate lung volume while recruiting collapsed alveoli.
- Conservative fluid management: Maintain euvolemia or negative fluid balance, which may improve oxygenation (2)[A].
- FiO_2: Initially 1.0 and quickly reduce as tolerated to ≤0.6 to achieve adequate oxygenation and prevent oxygen toxicity and pulmonary fibrosis.
- Tidal volume: Set initial tidal volume at 6 mL/kg of predicted body weight (PBW = 50.0 + 0.91 [height in cm, 152.4] for men, PBW = 45.5 + 0.91 [height in cm, 152.4] for women). Lung size strongly correlates with height and gender. PBW normalizes the tidal volume to lung size. Aim to maintain plateau pressure (Pplat) at <30 mm Hg to prevent alveolar overdistention and barotrauma.
- PEEP (positive end expiratory pressure) to recruit alveoli and prevent further alveolar collapse. PEEP should be applied in small increments of 3–5 cm H_2O to achieve acceptable arterial saturation (>0.9) with nontoxic FiO_2 values (<0.6) to prevent pulmonary fibrosis, and acceptable airway Pplat

($>30-<30$ cm H_2O) to prevent barotrauma. Comparison of low to high PEEP demonstrated no significant differences in mortality, ventilator-free days, or ICU stay in patients with ARDS (ARDS Network).

- Ventilator rate: High ventilatory rates of 18–24 breaths/min are often necessary in patients with ARDS due to increased physiologic dead space and smaller lung volumes.
- Low VT or APRV may lead to elevated PCO_2 levels (permissive hypercapnia). This is contraindicated in patients with intracranial hypertension.

Second Line

- Corticosteroids given early have shown to increase ventilator-free days and possibly infer a survival benefit. Recent meta-analysis did not demonstrate any definitive benefit (3)[B].
- Starting steroids >2 weeks after onset may increase risk of death.
- Inhaled vasodilators can selectively dilate vessels that perfuse well-ventilated lung zones, resulting in improved V/Q matching and better oxygenation. However, no improvement was seen in the duration of mechanical ventilation or 28-day mortality in a meta-analysis (4)[A].
- Different modes of mechanical ventilation can be used if conventional methods fail, such as APRV and high-frequency ventilation (HFV).
- Prone positioning improves oxygenation rapidly and allows a reduction in FiO_2, but trials have not demonstrated any survival benefit.

ADDITIONAL TREATMENT
General Measures
- Start nutrition early; enteral is preferred over parenteral nutrition.
- Daily sedation breaks and neurological assessment
- GI and DVT prophylaxis

Issues for Referral
Ventilator management and critical illness require a critical care or pulmonary/critical care consult. Infectious disease consult may be beneficial.

Additional Therapies
Muscular paralysis will decrease the work of breathing and oxygen consumption in severe cases, resulting in an improvement in oxygenation.

COMPLEMENTARY & ALTERNATIVE THERAPIES
- Extracorporeal membrane oxygenation (ECMO) and extracorporeal CO_2 removal (ECCO2R) are only available in a few centers and have not demonstrated a survival benefit.
- Nitric oxide causes pulmonary vasodilatation, which may improve V/Q matching and decrease pulmonary HTN, but has not improved outcome.
- Prostacyclin has a similar profile as nitric oxide.
- PGE1, ketoconazole, ibuprofen have not improved survival in ARDS patients.
- Antioxidants: N-acetylcysteine (NAC) did not prove beneficial.
- Surfactant replacement: Numerous clinical trials have demonstrated no improvement in survival in adults.
- Liquid ventilation. Experimental.
- β-agonists: IV or inhaled β-agonists decrease alveolar edema but do not improve survival.
- Activated protein C: Study stopped due to futility

SURGERY/OTHER PROCEDURES
Exploratory laparotomy or drainage of abscess is necessary if source of infection is in abdomen or pelvis.

IN-PATIENT CONSIDERATIONS
Initial Stabilization
- Endotracheal intubation
- Use of vasopressors for hemodynamic instability
- Central venous catheter
- Arterial line for BP and ABG monitoring

Admission Criteria
- Severe hypoxemia
- Hemodynamic instability
- Need for intubation and mechanical ventilation

IV Fluids
- Crystalloids are fluid of choice for initial resuscitation.
- Following adequate volume resuscitation, limit the amount of IVF administered to prevent further pulmonary edema and to improve pulmonary function.

Nursing
- General nursing care and pulmonary toilet
- Frequent turning of the patient to avoid decubitus ulcers
- Keep head end of bed >30 degrees.
- Wrist and ankle splints

Discharge Criteria
- Hemodynamically stable condition
- Extubated or posttracheostomy on trach collar
- Respiratory care unit for patients with prolonged mechanical ventilation and weaning

 ## ONGOING CARE

FOLLOW-UP RECOMMENDATIONS
- Once acute phase of ARDS resolves, rehabilitation and physical therapy may be required due to prolonged ventilatory support, and to regain muscle strength.
- If patient continues to have dyspnea, yearly PFT recommended.

Patient Monitoring
- Arterial catheters for exact measurement of blood pressure
- Pulmonary artery catheter is not indicated for hemodynamic monitoring of patients with ARDS.
- TTE or TEE is beneficial in determining cardiac contractility and ventricular volume status.
- Noninvasive continuous pulse contour monitoring using pressure variability (SBP or PP) with respiration and calibrated cardiac output (transpulmonary thermodilution or lithium dilution) may be beneficial in monitoring the response to therapy.

DIET
- ARDS patients develop a proinflammatory state and protein catabolism.
- Overfeeding may lead to hypercapnia. Indirect calorimetry (IC) may be beneficial in determining daily caloric requirement. IC is inaccurate when FiO_2 >60%.
- A low-carbohydrate high-fat enteral formula containing components that are anti-inflammatory and vasodilating (eicosapentaenoic acid and linoleic acid) with antioxidants has been demonstrated to improve outcome in ARDS patients.
- Enteral nutrition is the preferred route.

PATIENT EDUCATION
ARDS Support Center (www.ards.org)

PROGNOSIS
- The mortality rate varies with the underlying cause, with most patients dying of multisystem organ failure rather than isolated respiratory failure and hypoxemia.

- Overall mortality of ARDS ranges from 25–58% and has been trending downward due to earlier recognition and intervention.

COMPLICATIONS
- Ventilator-associated pneumonia (VAP) represents a complication of prolonged mechanical ventilation in ARDS patients and is an important cause of morbidity and mortality.
- Barotrauma: Excessive tidal volumes and/or high PEEP predisposes to pneumothorax, subcutaneous emphysema, and pneumomediastinum.
- Ventilator-induced lung injury secondary to repetitive alveolar expansion and collapse
- Critical illness polyneuromyopathy develops mostly in patients with prolonged mechanical ventilation, prolonged sedation, and use of paralytics and corticosteroids.

REFERENCES

1. Wheeler AP, et al. Pulmonary artery versus central venous catheter to guide treatment of acute lung injury. N Engl J Med. 2006;354:2213.
2. Wiedemann HP, et al. Comparison of two fluid-management strategies in acute lung injury. N Engl J Med. 2006;354(24):2564–75.
3. Peter JV, et al. Corticosteroids in the prevention and treatment of acute respiratory distress syndrome (ARDS) in adults: Meta-analysis. Brit Med J. 2008;336(7651):1006–9.
4. Adhikari NK, et al. Effect of nitric oxide on oxygenation and mortality in acute lung injury: Systematic review and meta-analysis. Brit Med J. 2007;334(7597):779.
5. Ardsnet.org.

ADDITIONAL READING

- Johnson ER, et al. Acute lung injury: Epidemiology, pathogenesis and treatment. J Aeorsol Med Pulm Drug Deliv. 2010;23(4):243–2.
- ARDS Network (www.ardsnet.org):
  – Fluid Algorithm
  – Lower Tidal Volume/Higher PEEP
  – Ventilator Protocol

 ## CODES

ICD9
- 518.5 Pulmonary insufficiency following trauma and surgery
- 518.82 Other pulmonary insufficiency, not elsewhere classified

CLINICAL PEARLS

- Hypoxemia and bilateral infiltrates on chest x-ray 24–36 hours following primary predisposing insult (including major surgery) equals ARDS until proven otherwise.
- IV fluid resuscitation should be limited to prevent further alveolar edema and decreased lung compliance.
- The use of corticosteroids to treat ARDS remains controversial and may increase infection rate and impair neuromuscular function.

ADRENAL INSUFFICIENCY AND CIRCI

Paul E. Marik

 BASICS

DESCRIPTION
- The stress system receives and integrates a diversity of cognitive, emotional, neurosensory, and peripheral somatic signals.
- The stress response is normally adaptive and time limited.
- The stress response is mediated largely by activation of the hypothalamic-pituitary-adrenal (HPA) axis with the release of cortisol.

- There is a graded cortisol response to the degree of stress (i.e., type of surgery).
- Cortisol has several important physiologic actions on metabolism, cardiovascular function, and the immune system.
- Cortisol increases the synthesis of catecholamines and catecholamine receptors which is partially responsible for its positive inotropic effects.
- Cortisol has potent anti-inflammatory actions including the reduction in number and function of various immune cells, such as T and B lymphocytes, monocytes, neutrophils, and eosinophils at sites of inflammation.

PATHOPHYSIOLOGY
- The HPA axis and the release of cortisol are possibly impaired in many critically ill patients.
- The overall incidence of adrenal insufficiency in critically ill medical patients approximates 10–20%, with an incidence as high as 60% in patients with septic shock.

- The major impact of adrenal insufficiency is on the systemic inflammatory response (excessive inflammation) and cardiovascular function (hypotension).
- A complex syndrome referred to as *critical illness related corticosteroid insufficiency* (CIRCI) (2,3) is characterized by exaggerated pro-inflammatory response with systemic inflammation.

- CIRCI is defined as inadequate corticosteroid activity for the severity of the patients' illness.
- CIRCI manifests with insufficient corticosteroid mediated downregulation of inflammatory transcription factors.
- Similar to type II diabetes (relative insulin deficiency), CIRCI arises due to corticosteroid tissue resistance, together with inadequate circulating levels of free cortisol.

ETIOLOGY
- CIRCI is most common in patients with severe sepsis (septic shock) and patients with ARDS.
- Patients with liver disease have a high incidence of AI (hepatoadrenal syndrome).
- CIRCI should also be considered in patients with pancreatitis.

- A subset of patients may suffer structural damage to the adrenal gland from either hemorrhage or infarction and this may result in long-term adrenal dysfunction.
- A number of drugs are associated with adrenal failure.

 CODES

ICD9
255.41 Glucocorticoid deficiency

AIRWAY MANAGEMENT

Ulf Hemprich
Andrew Leibowitz

The Basics

Indications for intubation: Hypoxemia, hypercarbia, need to "protect" airway (e.g., coma), shock

Assess urgency of situation, potential for noninvasive ventilator support (e.g., BiPAP)

Quick Assessment

Does patient appear difficult to manually ventilate?: Elderly, edentulous, obese, history of sleep apnea, beard, oral–pharyngeal pathology, cervical spine pathology

Does patient appear difficult to intubate: Mallampati Score*, small mouth opening, receding chin, short thyromental distance, large neck circumference, oral–pharyngeal pathology, cervical spine pathology

Do I need help? Know your limitations!

Is there a full stomach (e.g., recent oral intake, bowel obstruction, known GERD)?

Preparation I

Apply 100% oxygen to patient before proceeding.

Equipment

Intubating device: Mac vs. Miller Blades, Video Laryngoscope (e.g., Glidescope), Intubating Laryngeal Mask Airway, etc.

Endotracheal tube: In adults, use size 7.0–8.0; use 8.0 if bronchoscopy or aggressive suctioning will be required

Suction preferable with Yankauer tip

Manually inflating resuscitation bag (e.g., AMBU)

Oral airways: Various sizes and note that an oral airway with a center channel (e.g., Guedel) is more effective

End-tidal CO_2 detector

Pulse oximeter preferably applied before procedure

Stethoscope

Securing device (e.g., tape, tie)

Mallampati Score: Class 1–4; 4 = most difficult. Maneuver: Open mouth fully and protrude tongue. Class 1: Full visualization of tonsils, uvula, and soft palate; Class 2: Visible hard and soft palate, only tip of uvula not seen; Class 3: Only base of the uvula visible, soft and hard palate are visible; Class 4: Soft palate and uvula not seen; only hard palate visible.

Preparation II

Drugs:

Short-acting hypnotics:

Etomidate (0.2–0.3 mg/kg) most hemodynamically stable, associated with myoclonus, pain on injection and adrenal suppression

Propofol (2–3 mg/kg) most associated with hypotension. Suggest using a reduced dose (e.g., 1–1.5 mg/kg) in ICU patients.

Ketamine (1–5 mg/kg) usually hemodynamically stable unless catecholamine depleted, associated with tachycardia and increased secretions.

All doses should be reduced in the presence of hypotension, hypovolemia, nonsinus rhythm, and advanced age (e.g., > 70 years old).

Adjuncts to short-acting hypnotics:

Midazolam (1–2 mg)

Fentanyl (50–250 mcg)

Lidocaine (1–1.5 mg/kg)

Paralytics (if experienced):

Depolarizing agent:

Succinylcholine (1.5 mg/kg) most rapid acting, usually < 60 seconds, avoid in de-innervating injuries, massive burns

Nondepolarizing agents:

Rocuronium (0.6-1.2 mg/kg) most rapid onset, usually <90 seconds

Vecuronium (0.1 mg/kg) onset at least 90–120 seconds

Cisatracurium (0.2 mg/kg) onset at least 90–120 seconds

Preparation for postintubation hemodynamic instability:

Consider fluid bolus (e.g., simultaneous NS or LR 500 mL).

Have a vasopressor available (e.g., ephedrine bolus dose 5–10 mg, phenyephrine bous dose of 50–200 mcg or infusion of 50–200 mcg/min, norepinephrine bolus dose of 1–5 mcg or infusion of 1–5 mcg/min).

Consider pre intubation anticholinergic (e.g., glycopyyrolate 0.2–0.4 mg or atropine 0.4 mg) if bradycardic or with copious secretions.

Working IV running wide open.

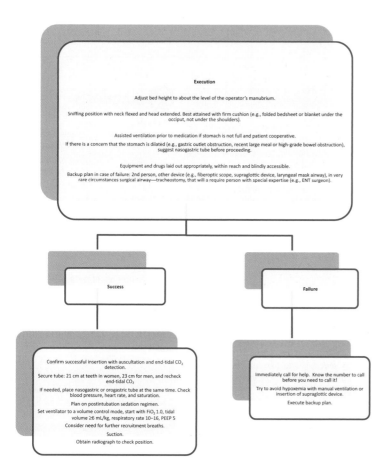

Execution

Adjust bed height to about the level of the operator's manubrium.

Sniffing position with neck flexed and head extended. Best attained with firm cushion (e.g., folded bedsheet or blanket under the occiput, not under the shoulders).

Assisted ventilation prior to medication if stomach is not full and patient cooperative.

If there is a concern that the stomach is dilated (e.g., gastric outlet obstruction, recent large meal or high-grade bowel obstruction), suggest nasogastric tube before proceeding.

Equipment and drugs laid out appropriately, within reach and blindly accessible.

Backup plan in case of failure: 2nd person, other device (e.g., fiberoptic scope, supraglottic device, laryngeal mask airway), in very rare circumstances surgical airway—tracheostomy, that will a require person with special expertise (e.g., ENT surgeon).

Success

Failure

Confirm successful insertion with auscultation and end-tidal CO_2 detection.

Secure tube: 21 cm at teeth in women, 23 cm for men, and recheck end-tidal CO_2

If needed, place nasogastric or orogastric tube at the same time. Check blood pressure, heart rate, and saturation.

Plan on postintubation sedation regimen.

Set ventilator to a volume control mode, start with FiO_2 1.0, tidal volume ≥6 mL/kg, respiratory rate 10–16, PEEP 5

Consider need for further recruitment breaths.

Suction.

Obtain radiograph to check position.

Immediately call for help. Know the number to call before you need to call it!

Try to avoid hypoxemia with manual ventilation or insertion of supraglottic device.

Execute backup plan.

REFERENCES

1. Langeron O, et al. Clinical review: management of difficult airways. *Crit Care* 2006;10(6):243.
2. Jaber S, et al. An intervention to decrease complications related to endotracheal intubation in the intensive care unit: a prospective, multiple-center study. *Intensive Care Med* 2010;36(2): 248–55.
3. Jaber S, et al. Clinical practice and risk factors for immediate complications of endotracheal intubation in the intensive care unit: a prospective, multiple-center study. *Crit Care Med* 2006;34(9): 2355–61.

ADDITIONAL READING

• Leibowitz AB. Tracheal intubation in the intensive care unit: extremely hazardous even in the best of hands. *Crit Care Med* 2006;34(9):2497–8.

 CODES

CPT
31500 – Endotracheal Intubation

ICD9
518.81 – Respiratory Failure / Acute

CLINICAL PEARLS

• Any fool with a plan will outperform a genius without one.
• 4 hands are always better than 2.
• In elective situations, 1/100 patients may be difficult to intubate and 1/1000 impossible to intubate. In critically ill patients, these incidences are about 10 times more likely.
• In elective situations, intubation is associated with severe hemodynamic compromise in <1/1000 patients and death in <1/500,000 patients. In critically ill patients, these incidences are >100 times and 5000 times more likely, respectively.
• Hope for the best; prepare for the worst.
• It may be better to be lucky than good, but good people are naturally luckier.

ALKALOSIS, METABOLIC

Ronaldo Collo Go
Sasikanth Nallagatla
Roopa Kohli-Seth

 BASICS

DESCRIPTION
- Metabolic alkalosis results from an elevation in the plasma bicarbonate concentration and is associated with increase in plasma pH.
- It can be caused by either a gain of HCO_3^- or a loss of fixed acid from the extracellular fluid.

EPIDEMIOLOGY
Incidence
Metabolic alkalosis is the most common acid–base disorder in hospitalized patients.
Prevalence
Accounts up to 50% of all acid–base disorders in hospitalized patients.

RISK FACTORS
- Drug use: Diuretics, antacids, calcium carbonate, glucocorticoids, licorice
- Recurrent vomiting, nasogastric or orogastric suctioning
- RL, blood transfusions, TPN
- Electrolyte abnormalities: Hypokalemia
Genetics
Occurs in familial disorders like Bartter syndrome and congenital adrenal hyperplasia

GENERAL PREVENTION
- Early identification of endocrine and genetic disorders causing metabolic alkalosis
- Careful monitoring of fluid and electrolyte status of each patient
- Stop gastric fluid losses.
- Encourage enteral feeds as early as possible.
- Limit the use of diuretics.
- H_2 receptor antagonists

PATHOPHYSIOLOGY
- To maintain the alkalosis, renal bicarbonate excretion must be impaired. This occurs in the setting of depleted chloride or effective circulatory volume, excessive mineralocorticoid activity, or severe renal insufficiency
- Hypokalemia: Intracellular potassium leaves the cell to replete extracellular stores while hydrogen ions move intracellularly to maintain electroneutrality.
- Gastric losses, via vomiting or nasogastric tube: Production of HCl by gastric parietal cells leads to increased HCO₃ in serum. This is countered by bicarbonate secretion of the pancreas upon gastric acid stimulation of duodenum; loss of this mechanism leads to sustained HCO₃, and chloride loss stimulates renal HCO₃ reabsorption in proximal tubules.

- Diuretics: Remove fluid through natriuresis, which is accompanied by chlorosis; HCO₃ is reabsorbed.
- Volume depletion: Avidity for Na and subsequent HCO₃ renal reabsorption increase as a consequence of secondary hyperaldosteronism.
- Anions of organic acids (lactate, citrate, acetate): Bicarbonate ion is formed as anion metabolized to CO_2 and H_2O.
- Posthypercapnic state: To maintain normal pH, increased renal HCl excretion and bicarbonate reabsorption occurs.
- Respiratory compensation for metabolic alkalosis involves respiratory suppression and increase in PCO_2.
- For every 1 mEq increase in HCO_3^-, PCO_2 changes by 0.7 mm Hg.

ETIOLOGY
- Chloride-sensitive (urine chloride <20 mEq/L):
  - GI causes: NG suction, vomiting, chloride diarrhea
  - Renal: Postdiuretic therapy, penicillins, citrate therapy
  - Exogenous alkali: Baking soda (sodium bicarbonate), sodium citrate, transfusions, antacids, bicarbonate infusions, parenteral nutrition (acetate, glutamate)
  - Post-hypercapnic metabolic alkalosis: Caused by abrupt treatment of chronic respiratory acidosis
- Chloride-resistant (urine chloride >20 mEq/L):
  - Hypertensive:
    ○ Renovascular hypertension
    ○ Primary hyperaldosteronism
    ○ Cushing syndrome
    ○ Liddle syndrome
    ○ Glycyrrhizic acid
    ○ Licorice
  - Normotensive:
    ○ Diuretics (thiazides and loop diuretics)
    ○ Bartter, Gitelman syndromes
    ○ Severe potassium depletion (K <2 mEq/L)
    ○ Hypercalcemia
    ○ Hypomagnesemia
    ○ Hypoparathyroidism
    ○ Refeeding alkalosis

COMMONLY ASSOCIATED CONDITIONS
- Endocrine disorders like hyperaldosteronism, Cushing syndrome, hypoparathyroidism.
- Genetic disorders like Liddle syndrome, Bartter syndrome, Gitelman syndrome, and congenital adrenal hyperplasia.

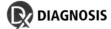 DIAGNOSIS

HISTORY
- Symptoms related to volume depletion: Weakness, muscle cramps, postural dizziness
- Hypokalemia: Polyuria, polydipsia, muscle weakness
- Neurologic symptoms: Headaches, stupor, tetany
- Cardiac symptoms: Arrhythmias
- Obtain detailed history of medication use.

PHYSICAL EXAM
- Observe for signs of hypocalcemia (e.g., tetany, Chvostek sign, Trousseau sign)
- Evaluate for hypertension, tachycardias, and fluid status assessment.
- Look for erosions of teeth enamel and dental caries in patients with bulimia.
- Obesity, moon face, hirsutism, acne, and violaceous skin striae seen in Cushing syndrome.

DIAGNOSTIC TESTS & INTERPRETATION
Lab
- Serum electrolytes with focus on CO_2, Cl, K
- ABG analysis
- Urine chloride ion concentration might be more helpful in setting of normal renal function, and results might be misleading with recent diuretic use. If nondiagnostic, a trial of saline infusion to see if metabolic alkalosis resolves might help with diagnosis (3)[B].
- Plasma renin and aldosterone levels to evaluate for hyperaldosteronism
- Plasma cortisol levels and dexamethasone suppression test to exclude Cushing syndrome
- Urine diuretic screen to exclude surreptitious diuretic use in patients with unexplained hypokalemic metabolic alkalosis

Imaging
- Renal Doppler US, MRI to evaluate for renovascular hypertension
- MRI/CT of adrenal glands to evaluate for primary hyperaldosteronism

Diagnostic Procedures/Other
- Renal angiography to evaluate for renovascular hypertension
- Gene analysis is helpful in diagnosing inherited causes of hypokalemic alkalosis.

DIFFERENTIAL DIAGNOSIS
- Acute respiratory acidosis
- Chronic respiratory acidosis
- Respiratory alkalosis

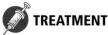

TREATMENT

MEDICATION

First Line
- Mild alkalosis is well tolerated.
- Severe or symptomatic alkalosis pH >7.60 requires urgent treatment.
- Saline responsive:
  - Aim at correction of extracellular volume deficit with 0.9% NS.
  - Correction of Cl depletion with 0.9% NS will promote alkaline diuresis (1)[A]. Chloride deficit: 0.2 × body weight (kg) × desired increase in plasma Cl (mmol/L)
  - Acetazolamide 250 mg once or twice a day; inhibits bicarbonate reabsorption in proximal tubules.
    - ○ Caution in patients with hypokalemia since it will induce diuresis as well.
    - ○ Efficacy of therapy can be estimated by monitoring urine pH (3)[A].
  - Correct hypokalemia with potassium chloride.
  - HCL infusion 150 mEq/L over 8–24 hours through a central vein catheter in severe metabolic alkalosis (pH >7.55), refractory to conventional measures and fluid overload.
    - ○ Formula used is: 0.5 × body weight (kg) × desired reduction in plasma bicarbonate (mmol/L). Initial goal is half normal bicarbonate level (2)[B].
  - Ammonium chloride: Hepatic conversion
  - Arginine monohydrochloride: Combines with ammonia and forms urea and HCl: May induce severe hyperkalemia and hyperglycemia
- Saline unresponsive:
  - Surgical removal of mineralocorticoid-producing tumor.
  - ACE inhibitors and spironolactone to block the effects of aldosterone.
  - Amiloride and triamterene are useful in managing the rare patient with Liddle syndrome.

Second Line
Discontinue diuretics and administer H_2 blockers, proton pump inhibitors in alkalosis secondary to gastric aspiration (2)[B].

ADDITIONAL TREATMENT

General Measures
Discontinuation of diuretic use and licorice is indicated if that is the cause for alkalosis.

Issues for Referral
Referral to hemodialysis is considered in patients with severe metabolic alkalosis.

SURGERY/OTHER PROCEDURES
Surgical removal of mineralocorticoid-producing tumor

IN-PATIENT CONSIDERATIONS

Initial Stabilization
Prompt resuscitation with NS is required in metabolic alkalosis secondary to volume depletion.

Admission Criteria
- All patients with metabolic alkalosis pH >7.5 need hospital admission.
- Patients with pH >7.55 need ICU admission as mortality is high.

IV Fluids
0.9% NS is the fluid of choice for resuscitation in patients with metabolic alkalosis.

Nursing
Frequent monitoring of vitals, EKG, urine output

Discharge Criteria
- Cause for alkalosis has been identified
- Adequate treatment of the underlying cause of metabolic alkalosis

ONGOING CARE

FOLLOW-UP RECOMMENDATIONS
Upon discharge from ICU, follow-up is necessary to monitor electrolytes.

Patient Monitoring
Frequent electrolyte and ABG monitoring throughout the day

DIET
No dietary recommendations.

PROGNOSIS
Alkalemia in critically ill patients is associated with increased mortality, up to 40% with pH >7.55 and up to 80% with pH >7.65.

COMPLICATIONS
- Metabolic alkalosis suppresses ventilation, leading to CO_2 retention and relative hypoxemia.
- Acutely increases hemoglobin oxygen affinity; shifts oxyhemoglobin desaturation curve to left and decreases tissue oxygen delivery.
- Decreased ionized calcium: Paresthesias, tetany, and seizures
- Confusion/obtundation secondary to decreased oxygen delivery to brain
- Hypokalemia and hypomagnesemia lead to arrhythmias.
- Patients with hepatic disease and hypokalemia can be predisposed to high ammonia levels.

REFERENCES

1. Friedman BS, et al. Prevention and management of metabolic alkalosis. *J Intensive Care Med*. 1990;5:S22–S27.
2. Rimmer JM, et al. Metabolic alkalosis. *J Intensive Care Med*. 1997;2:137–50.
3. Shah N, et al. Metabolic alkalosis in the intensive care unit. *Netherlands J Crit Care*.2008;12:113–9.

ADDITIONAL READING

- DuBose TD. Acid-base disorders. In Brenner BM, ed., *Brenner & Rector's The Kidney*, 7th ed. Philadelphia: Saunders, 2004.
- www.acidbase.com

 CODES

ICD9
276.3 Alkalosis

CLINICAL PEARLS
- High HCO_3^- occurs with alkalemia.
- Check potassium and chloride levels.
- Metabolic alkalosis is divided into saline-responsive and saline-unresponsive types.
- Urinary chloride concentration might not be helpful in renal failure or recent diuretic use.

ALKALOSIS, RESPIRATORY

Sanjay Dhar
Roopa Kohli-Seth

BASICS

DESCRIPTION
- Primary decrease in arterial partial pressure of carbon dioxide (hypocapnia) indicates respiratory alkalosis
- Clinical disturbance secondary to alveolar hyperventilation
- Alveolar hyperventilation resulting in decreased arterial partial pressure of carbon dioxide (PCO_2) represent the primary disturbance, and compensation occurs by changes in plasma bicarbonate (HCO_3) (1)[A].

EPIDEMIOLOGY
Incidence
Most common acid–base abnormality observed in the critically ill

Prevalence
Varies according to the etiology

RISK FACTORS
- Hypoxemia
- CNS disorders
- Excessive mechanical ventilation
- Hyperventilation secondary to anxiety/pregnancy/salicylate toxicity
- Sepsis

Genetics
Gitelman's variant of Bartter's syndrome, inherited hypokalemic alkalosis, is caused by mutations in the thiazide-sensitive Na—Cl cotransporter (2)[A].

GENERAL PREVENTION
Iatrogenic hyperventilation secondary to excessive mechanical ventilation must be corrected by decreased tidal volumes/decreased rate or sedatives or paralysis, depending on clinical situation (3)[A].

PATHOPHYSIOLOGY
Hyperventilation refers to an increase in the rate of alveolar ventilation that is disproportionate to the rate of carbon dioxide production. PCO_2 is normally maintained in the range of 37–43 mm Hg. Chemoreceptors in the brain (central chemoreceptors) and in the carotid bodies (peripheral chemoreceptors) sense hydrogen concentrations and influence ventilation to adjust the PCO_2, PO_2, and pH. When these receptors sense an increase in hydrogen ions, breathing is increased to "blow off" carbon dioxide and subsequently reduce the amount of hydrogen ions. Hyperventilation, if persistent, leads to hypocapnia.

ETIOLOGY
Underlying basic mechanism:
- Direct CNS stimulation of respiration
- Hypoxia
- Metabolic acidosis

COMMONLY ASSOCIATED CONDITIONS
- CNS:
  - Pain
  - Anxiety
  - Fever
  - Cerebrovascular accident
  - Meningitis/encephalitis
  - Tumor
  - Trauma
  - High altitude
  - Right-to-left shunts
- Pulmonary:
  - Pneumothorax/hemothorax
  - Pneumonia
  - Pulmonary edema
  - Pulmonary embolism
  - Asthma
  - Emphysema
  - Interstitial lung disease
- Endocrine:
  - Hyperthyroidism
  - Pregnancy
  - Diabetic ketoacidosis
- Drug intake:
  - Salicylates
  - Nicotine
  - Progesterone
  - Catecholamines
  - Methylxanthines
  - Propanidid
  - Analeptics
- Miscellaneous:
  - Congestive heart failure
  - Hepatic failure
  - Sepsis
  - Mechanical ventilation
  - Heat exhaustion
  - Anemia

DIAGNOSIS

HISTORY
- Clinical manifestations depend on underlying disease process, duration, and severity.
- Hypocapnia leading to cerebral vasoconstriction may result in dizziness, confusion, numbness, paresthesias, syncope, and seizures
- Hypoxia leading to hypocapnia may result in chest pain, anxiety, and dyspnea.
- Electrolyte disturbances may lead to tetany.

PHYSICAL EXAM
Related to underlying pathological process
- CNS: Fever, irritability, decreased cerebral perfusion, focal neurological signs, depressed level of consciousness, vertigo, and syncope
- Pulmonary: Tachypnea, crackles, rhonchi, and cyanosis if hypoxic
- Cardiovascular: Tachycardia, hypotension

Geriatric Considerations
Central causes via direct action on the respiratory center: For example, head injury, stroke, psychogenic or anxiety hyperventilation syndrome or drug intake to be ruled out.

Pediatric Considerations
Early/neonatal respiratory distress syndrome (RDS) and ventilator mismanagement of tidal volumes and respiratory rate are common causes in children.

Pregnancy Considerations
Mild, fairly well-compensated respiratory alkalosis is the usual finding in pregnancy.

DIAGNOSTIC TESTS & INTERPRETATION
Lab
Initial lab tests
- ABGs: pH >7.44 and PCO_2 <35 in the presence of normal or decreased HCO_3
- CBC and serum chemistries
- Thyroid function and liver function tests
- Urine toxicology

Follow-Up & Special Considerations
- The expected change in serum bicarbonate concentration can be estimated as follows:
  - Acute respiratory alkalosis: Bicarbonate (HCO_3^-) falls 2 mEq/L for each decrease of 10 mm Hg in the PCO_2.
  - Chronic respiratory alkalosis: Bicarbonate (HCO_3^-) falls 5 mEq/L for each decrease of 10 mm Hg in the PCO_2.

- Plasma bicarbonate level rarely drops below 12 mm Hg secondary to compensation for respiratory alkalosis: If it does so, a secondary cause for acidosis (metabolic) exists.
- Intracellular shift of sodium potassium phosphate and decrease in free calcium due to increased protein bound fraction

Imaging
Initial approach
- Based on history and etiology
- Chest x-ray
- CT scan chest
- CT scan brain
- ECG: ST-segment or T wave flattening or inversion
- EEG: Normal or increase in number of slow high-voltage waves

Follow-Up & Special Considerations
- CTA chest
- V/Q scan
- Brain MRI

Diagnostic Procedures/Other
- Lumbar puncture
- End-tidal CO_2 measurements
- Cerebral blood flow

Pathological Findings
Related to underlying etiology

DIFFERENTIAL DIAGNOSIS
Carefully search for the associated conditions:
- Metabolic acidosis with respiratory compensation
- Salicylate overdose, which can cause primary metabolic acidosis and primary respiratory alkalosis simultaneously

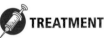 TREATMENT

MEDICATION
Directed toward underlying causative disorder

First Line
- Increase inspired oxygen concentration if patient is hypoxemic
- Sedatives
- Antidepressants
- β-Blockers

Second Line
- Blood transfusion, if anemia is present
- Treatment for sepsis, if present
- Treatment of liver failure
- Treatment of underlying CNS disorder

ADDITIONAL TREATMENT
General Measures
- Respiratory alkalosis encountered during mechanical ventilation is corrected by reducing the tidal volume or rate, or using sedation or paralysis in the case of patient-triggered ventilator breaths.
- Reassurance, rebreathing into paper bag during acute episode, and treatment of underlying psychological state

Issues for Referral
- Based on underlying etiology
- Neurology: For CNS disorders (stroke/SAH/meningitis)
- Pulmonary: Pulmonary embolism/pneumonia/ARDS
- Cardiology: For cardiovascular disorders (arrhythmia/hypotension)

Additional Therapies
Behavioral therapy

COMPLEMENTARY & ALTERNATIVE THERAPIES
- Stress relaxation techniques to reduce anxiety
- Behavioral therapy to reduce anxiety

SURGERY/OTHER PROCEDURES
Related to treatment of causative disorder

IN-PATIENT CONSIDERATIONS
Initial Stabilization
- ABCs
- Monitor oxygenation, ECG.

Admission Criteria
- Based on underlying etiology
- ICU admission: SAH, stroke, severe meningitis, need for mechanical ventilation, arrhythmias, hypotension

IV Fluids
- Maintain euvolemia.
- Treat underlying cause.

Nursing
Standard bundle approach to prevent hospital acquired infections

Discharge Criteria
- Correction of underlying primary admitting cause
- Hemodynamic stability
- Resolution of severe alkalosis pH >7.5

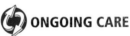 ONGOING CARE

FOLLOW-UP RECOMMENDATIONS
Once underlying cause is corrected, the acid–base disorder resolves.

Patient Monitoring
Psychosocial support groups

DIET
- As tolerated
- Aspiration precautions

PATIENT EDUCATION
In hyperventilation syndrome, reassurance/relaxation/breathing techniques

PROGNOSIS
Related to underlying disorder

COMPLICATIONS
- Related to underlying disorder
- Potential for tetany and seizures

REFERENCES

1. Laffey JG, et al. Hypocapnia. N Engl J Med. 2002; 347:43–53.
2. Simon DB, et al. Gitelman's variant of Barter's syndrome: Inherited hypokalaemic alkalosis, is caused by mutations in the thiazide-sensitive Na-Cl cotransporter. Nature Genetics. 1996;12:24–30.
3. Myrianthefs PM, et al. Hypocapnic but not metabolic alkalosis impairs alveolar fluid reabsorption. Am j Respir Crit Care Med. 2005;171: 1267–71.

ADDITIONAL READING

- Laffey JG, et al. Carbon dioxide and the critically ill: Too little of a good thing? Lancet. 1999;354: 1283–6.
- Wise RA, et al. Respiratory physiologic changes in pregnancy. Immunol Allergy Clin North Am 2006;26:1–12.

CODES

ICD9
276.3 Alkalosis

CLINICAL PEARLS
- In both respiratory alkalosis and metabolic acidosis. PCO_2 is reduced and HCO_3 is low.
- In respiratory alkalosis, low $PaCO_2$ is the primary disturbance and pH is above normal; whereas in metabolic acidosis, low HCO_3 is the primary disturbance and pH is in the acidic range.
- Iatrogenic hyperventilation owing to excessive mechanical ventilation needs to be appropriately treated.

ALVEOLAR HEMORRHAGE, DIFFUSE

Edgardo Soto
John Oropello

 BASICS

DESCRIPTION
- Diffuse alveolar hemorrhage (DAH) is a rare yet serious and frequently life-threatening complication of a variety of conditions characterized by bleeding into the alveolar spaces.
- Early recognition is crucial because the prompt institution of supportive measures and immunosuppressive therapy is required for survival.

PATHOPHYSIOLOGY
Bleeding into the alveolar spaces due to disruption of the alveolar-capillary basement membrane caused by injury or inflammation of the arterioles, venules, or alveolar septal capillaries.

ETIOLOGY
- There are 3 general patterns:
- With capillaritis:
  - Systemic vasculitis:
    - Wegener granulomatosis (WG)
    - Microscopic polyangiitis (MPA)
    - Isolated pauci-immune pulmonary capillaritis
    - Henoch-Schönlein purpura
    - Immunoglobin A nephropathy
    - Pauci-immune glomerulonephritis
    - Immune complex-associated glomerulonephritis
    - Urticaria-vasculitis syndrome
  - Connective tissue diseases:
    - Polymyositis
    - Primary antiphospholipid antibody syndrome
    - Systemic lupus erythematosus
    - Systemic sclerosis
    - Goodpasture's syndrome
    - Mixed connective tissue disease
    - Rheumatoid arthritis
  - Drugs (associated with capillaritis):
    - Diphenylhydantoin
    - Propylthiouracil
    - Retinoic acid syndrome
  - Other conditions with capillaritis:
    - Autologous hematopoietic cell transplantation
    - Idiopathic pulmonary hemosiderosis
    - Infective endocarditis
    - Isolated pulmonary capillaritis
    - Leptospirosis
    - Lung transplant rejection

- Bland hemorrhage (without capillaritis or vasculitis):
  - Anticoagulants, antiplatelets or thrombolytics
  - Disseminated intravascular coagulation
  - Mitral stenosis and mitral regurgitation
  - Pulmonary veno-occlusive disease
  - Infections: HIV, infective endocarditis
  - Toxins: Trimellitic anhydride, isocyanates, crack cocaine, pesticides, detergents.
  - Drugs: Diphenylhydantoin, amiodarone mitomycin D-penicillamine, sirolimus, methotrexate, haloperidol, nitrofurantoin, gold, all-trans-retinoic acid, bleomycin (especially with high oxygen concentrations), montelukast, zafirlukast, infliximab
  - Idiopathic pulmonary hemosiderosis
- Alveolar bleeding associated with another process or condition:
  - Diffuse alveolar damage
  - Pulmonary embolism
  - Sarcoidosis
  - HAPE (high-altitude pulmonary edema)
  - Infections: Invasive aspergillosis, cytomegalovirus, legionellosis, herpes simplex virus, mycoplasmosis, hantavirus, leptospirosis, other bacterial pneumonia
  - Malignant conditions
  - Lymphangioleiomatosis
  - Tuberous sclerosis
  - Pulmonary capillary hemangiomatosis
  - Lymphangiography

COMMONLY ASSOCIATED CONDITIONS
Most common diseases that cause DAH:
- WG: 17–50% DAH
- MPA: 10–50% DAH
- Goodpasture's: 80–94% DAH
- SLE: 4–20% DAH
- Idiopathic pulmonary hemosiderosis: 100% DAH
- Allogeneic bone marrow transplant: 3–7% DAH.
- Catastrophic antiphospholipid antibody syndrome

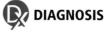 **DIAGNOSIS**

HISTORY
- Hemoptysis is the most common clinical manifestation—30% will have DAH without evidence of hemoptysis
- Shortness of breath
- Cough
- Fever
- Acute respiratory failure—50% require mechanical ventilation.

PHYSICAL EXAM
Nonspecific unless there are physical signs of an underlying systemic vasculitis or connective tissue vascular disorder:
- Oropharynx, nose, and sinuses should be carefully evaluated for signs suggestive of WG.
- Other symptoms of vasculitis: Rash, purpura, eye lesions, hepatosplenomegaly and clubbing

DIAGNOSTIC TESTS & INTERPRETATION
Lab
Initial lab tests
- Serial CBCs: To assess rate of progression
- PTT, PT/INR
- Assess for signs of glomerulonephritis:
  - Serum chemistry
  - Urine Analysis
  - Urine microscopy
- Blood cultures
- ESR, CRP
- Drug screening—suspected cocaine use

Follow-Up & Special Considerations
- PR3 (proteinase 3)-ANCA: 80–90% in active WG
- p-ANCA: 50–80% with MPA
- Anti-GMB antibodies
- ANA, anti-dsANA, complement levels: SLE
- RA
- IgG and IgM anticardiolipin antibodies
- Rheumatoid factor
- ASO titers: Poststreptococcal glomerulonephritis

Initial approach
- Chest x-ray:
  - Diffuse alveolar infiltrates
  - Rarely ground glass opacities
  - Infiltrates are mainly perihilar or predominate in the middle and lower pulmonary fields.
- Chest CT:
  - Ground glass or airspace-filling opacities that are usually diffuse and bilateral
  - Occasionally they present as unilateral

Follow-Up & Special Considerations
- Complete resolution of chest x-ray may take 3–4 days.
- 2D echo: Cardiomegaly from myocarditis or pericardial effusion may be seen in DAH with some systemic vasculitides and connective tissue diseases:
  - Evaluation of mitral valve stenosis or regurgitation

Diagnostic Procedures/Other
- Bronchoscopy with BAL:
  - Performed to rule out infection and evaluate the presence of DAH
  - Diagnostic yield is higher if performed in the first 48 hours of symptoms.
  - Persistent and increasing blood in 3 or more sequential aliquots from a single affected area of the lung.
- Lung biopsy:
  - Should only be considered if potential diagnostic tissue cannot be obtained from other sites
  - No role for transbronchial biopsy.
  - Tissue can be obtained by VATS if the respiratory status permits collapse of one lung.
- Renal biopsy including immunofluorescence if laboratory abnormalities suggestive of renal insufficiency or glomerulonephritis.

Pathological Findings
- Pulmonary capillaritis (most common histologic pattern in DAH)
- Neutrophilic infiltration of the alveolar interstitium with subsequent fibrinoid necrosis. Loss of integrity of the epithelial–endothelial basement membranes and leakage of red blood cells.
- Bland pulmonary hemorrhage: Hemorrhage into the alveolar spaces without inflammation or destruction of the alveolar structures
- Diffuse alveolar damage: Main underlying lesion of the acute respiratory distress syndrome characterized by formation of intra-alveolar hyaline membranes that line the alveolar spaces.

DIFFERENTIAL DIAGNOSIS
- Broad range of diagnosis:
  - Neoplasms
  - Tuberculosis
  - Necrotizing pneumonia
  - Vasculitis
  - Fungal infections (Aspergillus and mucor)
- Bronchiectasis

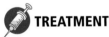 TREATMENT

MEDICATION
- Immunosuppressive agents are mainstay of treatment:
  - IV methylprednisolone up to 500 mg q6h for 4–5 days.
  - Cyclophosphamide: Preferred adjunctive immunosuppressive drug (2 mg/kg/day, adjusted to renal function), may be continued for several weeks or until adverse effects occur.
  - Other agents: CellCept, Etanercept, Imuran
- Plasmapheresis:
  - Most useful in the ANCA-associated vasculitides.

ADDITIONAL TREATMENT
Additional Therapies
Intrapulmonary administration of recombinant activated factor VIIa has been used in patients not responding to conventional haemostatic therapy

SURGERY/OTHER PROCEDURES
Selective arterial embolization and surgery are not options for DAH.

IN-PATIENT CONSIDERATIONS
Initial Stabilization
- Airway management:
  - WG involves the upper respiratory: 16% of cases results in subglottic stenosis:
    - Potentially difficult intubation requiring a smaller diameter endotracheal tube
    - Tracheostomy may be required in ~50% of cases (80% will need some form of surgical intervention)
  - Patients may develop acute respiratory distress syndrome requiring mechanical ventilation:
    - Use protective ventilation strategy (tidal volumes of 6 mL/kg and inspiratory plateau pressures below 30 cm H_2O
  - Intubation with bronchial tamponade
  - NIV (noninvasive ventilation) may be used in patients with respiratory failure due to a rapidly treatable cause.
- Reversal of coagulopathy
- Cardiovascular:
  - Hypotension due to large amounts of bleeding combined with dehydration from vasculitis.
  - May require inotropic/vasopressor support.

IV Fluids
- Blood transfusion may be necessary.
- Use of crystalloids for resuscitation from hypovolemia or sepsis

 ONGOING CARE

DIET
Not restricted

PROGNOSIS
- Very poor prognosis if left untreated
- Depends on the underlying cause:
  - Churg-Strauss Syndrome (CSS) 50% death within a year.
  - With treatment, 5-year survival is around 70–80%.
  - Around 25–50% survival for ICU patients.
  - Mortality of hematopoietic stem cell transplant recipients with DAH approximates 80%.

COMPLICATIONS
- Up to 50% of women given cyclophosphamide for WG become infertile or amenorrheic.
- Prolonged oral cyclophosphamide carries a life-long increased risk for bladder cancer, cutaneous squamous cell cancer, myelodysplasia, and lymphoma.

- Irreversible organ damage before treatment is effective
- End-stage renal disease occurs in up to 20–25% of patients with WG or MPA
- Recurrent episodes may lead to various degrees of interstitial fibrosis.

REFERENCES
1. Ioachimescu OC, et al. Diffuse alveolar hemorrhage: diagnosing it and finding the cause. *Cleve Clin J Med*. 2008;75(4):258, 260, 264–5 passim. Review.
2. Jin SM, et al. Aetiologies and outcomes of diffuse alveolar haemorrhage presenting as acute respiratory failure of uncertain cause. *Respirology*. 2009;14(2):290–4.
3. Papiris SA, et al. Bench-to-bedside review: pulmonary-renal syndromes—an update for the intensivist. *Crit Care*. 2007;11(3):213.
4. Specks U. Diffuse alveolar hemorrhage syndromes. *Curr Opin Rheumatol*. 2001;13(1):12–7. Review.
5. Semple D, et al. Clinical review: Vasculitis on the intensive care unit – part 2: treatment and prognosis. *Crit Care*. 2005;9(2):193–7.
6. Yildirim H, et al. Recombinant factor VIIa treatment for life-threatening hemoptysis. *Respirology*. 2006;11(5):652–4.

 CODES

ICD9
- 446.0 Polyarteritis nodosa
- 446.4 Wegener's granulomatosis
- 786.30 Hemoptysis, unspecified s

CLINICAL PEARLS
Up to 30% of patients with DAH will present without hemoptysis

AMINOGLYCOSIDES

B. Sharmila Mohanraj

 BASICS

DESCRIPTION

- Aminoglycosides have been utilized to treat susceptible infections for >50 years.
- Aminoglycosides are derived from substances produced by soil Actinobacteria. Amikacin, gentamicin, tobramycin, and streptomycin are the most clinically relevant aminoglycosides in use in the US.
- Aminoglycosides bind to the 30S subunit of prokaryotic ribosomes, interfering with mRNA translation and protein synthesis. It is hypothesized that further mechanisms correlating to bactericidal activity have yet to be identified.
- In vitro antimicrobial characteristics:
  - Concentration-dependent killing: The rate of bactericidal activity increases as the initial concentration of antibiotic increases, regardless of the size of inoculum. This observation led to the rational for high-dose, extended interval dosing.
  - Postantibiotic effect: Bacterial growth is suppressed for several hours after drug levels drop below the MIC. The higher the initial concentration is, the longer the effect will be (again, supporting the use of once-daily dosing). The mechanism for this effect is thought to relate to inhibition of protein synthesis.
  - Antimicrobial synergy: Using a cell wall-active antibiotic in combination with an aminoglycoside leads to a more than additive antimicrobial effect. The mechanism appears to relate to enhancement of intracellular aminoglycoside uptake.

 TREATMENT

- Aminoglycosides are active against aerobic gram-negative bacilli. When used in combination with other antibiotics (β-lactams, vancomycin), they are also effective for treating *Enterococcus spp.*, *Viridans streptococci*, and in some circumstances MSSA. Notably, they have no practical utility against pneumococci, anaerobics microbes, or MRSA. Occasionally, they are used in combination treatment of mycobacteria.
- Based on demonstration of increased potency, gentamicin is the drug of choice for *Serratia spp,* infections, whereas tobramycin is preferred for *P. aeruginosa*. Because parenteral aminoglycosides achieve poor concentrations in bronchial secretions, inhaled formulations may be substituted. Inhaled tobramycin is a staple of management of patients with cystic fibrosis.
- Resistance to aminoglycosides may be intrinsic or acquired. Mechanisms include inhibition of drug uptake, efflux pump activity, and enzymatic drug modification.
- Resistance patterns are dependent upon multiple factors including the specific drug, the particular pathogen, and variations in the patient population and patterns of antibiotic use.

- Clinical indications:
  - Despite their toxicities, aminoglycosides are important tools in the arsenal of antimicrobials. Their potent bactericidal activity makes them useful agents for empiric therapy for severe infections, usually in combination with other antibiotics.
  - Examples of empiric indications include bacteremia, infective endocarditis, intra-abdominal infection, malignant otitis externa, meningitis, neutropenic fever, ocular infection, osteomyelitis, septic arthritis, pneumonia, pyelonephritis, and sepsis.
  - In severe infections, empiric double gram-negative therapy is recommended to increase the likelihood of covering the pathogenic organism with an active drug. Currently, guidelines do recommend narrowing antibiotics once susceptibility data is known (1). Thus, aminoglycosides are often employed for short empiric courses of 3–4 days, which limits their toxic potential.

- Interestingly, a recent study suggests that early combination therapy reduces mortality compared to monotherapy for patients with septic shock, even when the pathogen is susceptible to all drugs used (2). However, this approach is not currently endorsed by guidelines.
- Increasingly, aminoglycosides are being called upon for treatment of nosocomial multidrug-resistant microbes such as *Klebsiella pneumoniae* carbapenamase-producing organisms, in which aminoglycosides and colistin may be the only options.
- Dosing:
  - High-dose, extended interval dosing is preferable when possible. Currently, it is not recommended in morbid obesity and pregnancy. Its use in meningitis and osteomyelitis is not well studied.
  - For gentamicin or tobramycin, initial dosing with normal renal function is 5 mg/kg (IBW) q24h. Whereas for amikacin and streptomycin, initial dosing is 15 mg/kg q24h. As GFR declines, the dosing interval is extended.
  - There is no standardized method for drug monitoring; a common approach is to draw serum levels 6–14 hours postdosing and assess the result with a nomogram designed to help determine the optimal dosage interval. Drug dosing and monitoring may be complicated, especially in the setting of renal dysfunction, and pharmacy consultation is advised.
  - Traditional multiple daily dosing regimens may start with a loading dose for severe infections.
  - For maintenance in normal renal function, 1.7 mg/kg q8h is recommended for gentamicin and tobramycin, whereas 7.5 mg/kg q8h is given for amikacin. Similar to once-daily dosing, the dosing interval is extended as GFR declines. For critically ill patients or patients receiving >3 days therapy, peak and trough levels should be monitored.
  - When using aminoglycosides for synergy, initially dosing with normal renal function of 1 mg/kg q8h is advised for gentamicin, whereas 7.5 mg/kg q8h is recommended for amikacin. Peak and trough levels should be followed if receiving treatment for several days.

ADDITIONAL TREATMENT
Issues for Referral
- Infectious diseases consultation is recommended for management of severe infections, especially when considering prolonged aminoglycoside use.
- Consider pharmacy assistance when dosing for patients with renal dysfunction or morbid obesity. Also nephrology input is prudent in patients on CRRT.

ONGOING CARE
COMPLICATIONS
Adverse Effects
- Nephrotoxicity: 99% of a dose of aminoglycoside is excreted through the kidneys. Toxicity occurs through damage to proximal tubular cells. Reported incidences vary, but typically range from 5–10% for significant declines in GFR. Oliguric renal failure requiring dialysis is rare. The risk increases with longer duration of antibiotic use, older age, preexisting renal dysfunction, and use of concomitant nephrotoxins. Notably, tubular injury is usually reversible once the drug is held.
- Ototoxicity: Both cochlear and vestibular toxicity are possible. Ototoxicity is particularly concerning as it is irreversible and may develop even after discontinuation of the medication. Risk increases with the cumulative dose and duration of treatment. When anticipating using aminoglycosides for an extended course, baseline and serial audiometry exams are advisable when feasible.
- Neuromuscular blockade: Though a rare adverse effect, flaccid paralysis and respiratory muscle weakness are possible. For this reasons, aminoglycosides are typically contraindicated with neuromuscular blocking agents or anesthetics.

ADDITIONAL READING
- Craig WA . Optimizing aminoglycoside use. *Crit Care Clin*. 2011;27:107–21.
- Dellinger RP, et al. Surviving Sepsis Campaign: International guidelines for management of severe sepsis and septic shock: 2008. *Crit Care Med*. 2008;36:296–337.
- Kumar A, et al. Early combination antibiotic therapy yields improved survival compared with monotherapy in septic shock: A propensity-matched analysis. *Crit Care Med*. 2010;38(9):1775–83.
- Mandell GL, et al. *Principles and Practice of Infectious Diseases. Aminoglycosides*. New York: Churchill Livingstone Elsevier; 2010:359–84.

CODES

ICD9
- 421.0 Acute and subacute bacterial endocarditis
- 567.9 Unspecified peritonitis
- 790.7 Bacteremia

AMNIOTIC FLUID EMBOLUS (AFE)

Avishai A. Alkalay
Peter S. Bernstein

 BASICS

DESCRIPTION
- A foreign substance is introduced into maternal circulation that leads to an acute onset of cardiovascular and pulmonary collapse with a coagulopathy.
- Usually occurs during labor, delivery, or within 30 minutes after delivery
- Classic story is cardiopulmonary arrest in a previously healthy pregnant, laboring, or immediately postpartum patient.
- Also known as anaphylactoid syndrome of pregnancy.
- System(s) affected: Cardiovascular; Pulmonary; Hematologic; Renal

EPIDEMIOLOGY
Incidence
1 in 8000–30,000 pregnancies

Prevalence
- 70% of cases occur during labor
- 11% occur postpartum
- Accounts for 5–10% of maternal deaths in the U.S.

RISK FACTORS
- Increased maternal age
- Multiple gestation (uterine overdistension)
- Cesarean section
- Uterine rupture
- High cervical laceration
- Placental abruption
- Intrauterine fetal demise
- Intense uterine contractions (oxytocin use)
- Meconium-stained fluid
- Abdominal trauma

GENERAL PREVENTION
Unpredictable

PATHOPHYSIOLOGY
- Breach in the barrier between the maternal circulation and amniotic fluid:
  – Possibly in the endocervical veins, placental site, or site of uterine trauma
- Amniotic fluid enters systemic and pulmonary circulation.
- Pulmonary vasculature exposure to soluble (leukotrienes, surfactant, thromboxane A2, endothelin, etc.) and insoluble components (hair, vernix, squames, mucin, etc.) leads to capillary leak, negative inotropism, and bronchospasm:
  – Manifests as hypoxia, cyanosis, and respiratory distress.
- Decrease in cardiac contractility becomes prevalent, leading to an increase in pulmonary venous pressure (congestion) and a drop in cardiac output:
  – Manifests as pulmonary edema, hypotension, and shock.

- Exposure of intravascular compartment to amniotic fluid thromboplastin and other mediators induces a consumptive coagulopathy:
  – Manifests as disseminated intravascular coagulation and severe uterine bleeding.
- Resultant systemic hypotension decreases uterine perfusion:
  – Manifests as fetal heart rate abnormalities and fetal distress/death.
- Respiratory and hemodynamic compromise leads to neurological response:
  – Manifests as seizures, confusion, or coma.
- Prolonged hypoxia or arrest can result in permanent neurological disability and/or maternal and fetal death.

ETIOLOGY
Uncertain/unpredictable

COMMONLY ASSOCIATED CONDITIONS
- Pregnancy: Usually 2nd stage of labor, or immediately postpartum
- Following amniocentesis (rare)
- 1st or 2nd trimester abortions (rare)

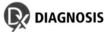 DIAGNOSIS

- Clinical diagnosis
- Spectrum of disease from mild form to sudden cardiopulmonary arrest

HISTORY
- Hypoxia: 93% of Cases (1)[C]:
  – Related to respiratory failure initially followed by cardiogenic pulmonary edema
- Hypotension with shock: 100% of Cases (1)[C]:
  – Most commonly cardiogenic shock from left ventricular failure
- Coagulopathy/DIC: 83% of Cases (1)[C]:
  – Occurs within 4 hours of initial presentation, and presents with profound bleeding
- Altered mental status: >70% of cases (1)[C]:
  – Encephalopathy likely secondary to hypotension and hypoxia
  – Seizure activity in >50% of cases, which may exacerbate brain injury
  – Confusion
  – Agitation
- Constitutional symptoms (fever, chills, headache, nausea, vomiting) (1)[C]

DIAGNOSTIC TESTS & INTERPRETATION
Lab
- ABG:
  – Determines adequacy of ventilation
- Chemistry including calcium, magnesium
- Complete blood count
- Coagulation studies:
  – INR, PTT, fibrinogen

Imaging
- Portable anterior/posterior chest radiograph:
  – Evaluate for pulmonary edema, cardiomegaly
- 12-lead ECG:
  – Evaluate for ischemia, arrhythmia
- Transthoracic echocardiogram may identify left heart failure, or less commonly obstructive shock with right ventricular dysfunction.

Pathological Findings
Postmortem: Fetal squamous cells and other elements of fetal debris in the pulmonary vessels

DIFFERENTIAL DIAGNOSIS
- Respiratory distress:
  – Pulmonary embolism (thrombus, fluid, air, fat)
  – Pulmonary edema
  – Anesthesia complication
  – Aspiration
- Hypotension and shock symptoms:
  – Septic shock
  – Hemorrhagic shock
  – Anaphylactic shock
  – Myocardial infarction
  – Cardiac arrhythmias
- Hemorrhage and bleeding disorders:
  – DIC
  – Placental abruption
  – Uterine rupture
  – Uterine atony
- Neurological and seizure-related conditions:
  – Eclampsia
  – Epilepsy
  – Cerebrovascular accident
  – Hypoglycemia

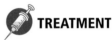 TREATMENT

ALERT
May be called for maternal cardiopulmonary arrest in the setting of AFE. The treatment is prompt initiation of BLS/ACLS with attention to modifications for pregnancy (2)[C]:
- Airway:
  – Continuous cricoid pressure during positive pressure ventilation
  – Secure airway early.
  – Use a smaller endotracheal tube than in nonpregnant (airway edema).
- Breathing:
  – Hypoxemia develops rapidly; be prepared to support oxygenation/ventilation.
  – Ventilation volumes may need to be reduced due to elevated diaphragm.
- Circulation:
  – Chest compressions higher on the sternum to adjust for elevation of the diaphragm and abdominal contents by gravid uterus.
  – Uterine displacement (wedge under hip) is required for effective resuscitation.
  – Remove fetal/uterine monitors before defibrillation.
- Perimortem cesarean section should be initiated within several minutes of asystole, if maternal condition is refractory to ACLS.

MEDICATION
- Hypoxia (1,3)[C]:
  - Treat with 100% oxygen.
- Hypotension (1,3)[C]:
  - Treat with fluid resuscitation (isotonic fluid).
  - Vasopressors for refractory hypotension
  - Norepinephrine: Ideal secondary to α-adrenergic and β-adrenergic effects; IV 2–4 μg/min
- Left ventricular diminished contractility (1)[C]:
  - Treat with isotonic fluids.
  - Inotropic therapy (dobutamine)
  - Dobutamine: IV 2–40 μg/kg
- DIC (1)[C]:
  - Treat with fresh frozen plasma.
  - Cryoprecipitate
  - Fibrinogen
  - Factor replacement
- Hemorrhage (1)[C]:
  - Treat with fluid resuscitation (isotonic fluid).
  - Packed RBCs transfusion
  - Platelets
- Uterine atony (1)[C]:
  - Treat with oxytocin 20–40 U in 1000 mL of isotonic fluid.
  - Methergine 0.2 mg IM q2–4h
  - Hemabate 250 μg IM q15min (up to 8 doses)
  - Cytotec 1000 μg rectally
  - Blood products
- Fetal distress (1)[C]:
  - Correct hypoxia.
  - Displace uterus to left.
  - Deliver once mother is stabilized.

ADDITIONAL TREATMENT
- In 65% of cases of AFE, delivery has not yet occurred.
- Prompt delivery should be achieved to prevent fetal hypoxemia once maternal condition is stabilized (1)[C].

ALERT
Maternal stabilization and resuscitation should be 1st priority before proceeding to delivery.

General Measures
- Continuous cardiac telemetry
- Respiratory monitoring with pulse oximetry
- BP monitoring:
  - Serial BPs or intra-arterial catheter
- Continuous fetal monitoring (if undelivered)

- IV access
  - Central venous catheter or pulmonary artery catheter as clinically indicated
- Supportive care:
  - Usually in the ICU (1)[C]

Issues for Referral
- Maternal fetal medicine specialist should be involved in the management.
- Renal failure rarely requires hemodialysis.

 ## ONGOING CARE

FOLLOW-UP RECOMMENDATIONS
Patient Monitoring
- Monitor for hypoxia.
- Monitor for hypotension.
- Monitor for hemorrhage, evidence of DIC.
- Provide neurological evaluation.
- Monitor for oliguria/renal failure.

PATIENT EDUCATION
No additional risk in subsequent pregnancies

PROGNOSIS
- Catastrophic and unpredictable
- Prognosis is improved with early detection and resuscitation efforts.
- Maternal mortality ranges from 26–86%.
- Neurologic deficits occur in up to 85% of survivors.
- Fetal mortality is 21%.
- Fetal neurologic complications, 50%.

COMPLICATIONS
- Cardiogenic: Cardiac failure with left ventricular impairment, myocardial ischemia, myocardial infarction, cardiogenic pulmonary edema.
- Respiratory: Respiratory failure, refractory bronchospasm, noncardiogenic pulmonary edema
- Hematologic: DIC, hemorrhage, thrombosis
- Neurologic: Seizure, altered mental status, coma, neurological deficits
- Renal: Oliguric renal failure
- Fetus: Hypoxemia, nonreassuring fetal status, neurological handicap

REFERENCES
1. Moore J, et al. Amniotic fluid embolus. *Crit Care Med.* 2005;33(10 Suppl):279–85.
2. American Heart Association. Cardiac arrest associated with pregnancy. *Circulation.* 2005;112: IV150–3.
3. Gei G, et al. Amniotic fluid embolism: An update. *Contemp Ob/Gyn.* 2000;45:53–66.
4. Tuffnell DJ. Amniotic fluid embolism. *Curr Opin Obstet Gynecol.* 2003;15;119–22.
5. Clark SL, et al. Amniotic fluid embolism: Analysis of the national registry. *Am J Obstet Gynecol.* 1995; 172:1158–67.

 ## CODES

ICD9
- 673.10 Amniotic fluid embolism, unspecified as to episode of care
- 673.12 Amniotic fluid embolism, with delivery, with mention of postpartum complication

CLINICAL PEARLS
- Unpredictable and catastrophic
- Suspect AFE if called for maternal cardiopulmonary arrest in a previously healthy pregnant or recently postpartum patient.
- Immediate recognition and diagnosis of AFE is essential to improve maternal and fetal outcomes.
- Aggressive supportive care in an ICU is often necessary.

ANEMIA, SICKLE CELL

Yoshita Shroff
Sanjay Chawla

 BASICS

DESCRIPTION
- A chronic hemolytic anemia associated with acute and chronic vaso-occlusion
- Most common intensive care management problems include acute chest syndrome, severe anemia, sepsis, stroke, and priapism.
- System(s) affected: Hematologic, Pulmonary, Cardiac, Renal, Nervous, and Bone

Pregnancy Considerations
- Worsening anemia, vaso-occlusive crises, and acute chest syndrome may occur during pregnancy.
- Fetuses are at increased risk of prematurity, low birth weight, or even death.
- Prophylactic transfusion to maintain a hemoglobin concentration >9 g/dL is recommended.

Pediatric Considerations
- Sequestration crises and hand-foot syndrome are seen only in infants/young children.
- Functional asplenia in later childhood
- Prophylactic penicillin and appropriate pneumococcal vaccination schedule must be followed.
- Consider periodic transcranial Doppler US in all children ages 2–16.

EPIDEMIOLOGY
Incidence
- 1/500 African American infants.
- Common in individuals of African, Caribbean, Mediterranean, Arab, and other Middle Eastern descent

Prevalence
>60,000 people in the U.S. (1)[A]

RISK FACTORS
- Hypoxemia
- Acidosis
- Infection
- Dehydration

Genetics
- Autosomal recessive disorder of hemoglobin
- Homozygous disease (Hb SS): Most common
- Heterozygous carrier state (sickle trait): Usually asymptomatic.

GENERAL PREVENTION
- Avoid exposure to cold, fever, dehydration, and stress.
- Genetic counseling
- Yearly influenza vaccination

PATHOPHYSIOLOGY
- Substitution of a valine residue for glutamic acid at position 6 in the β-subunit of hemoglobin forming hemoglobin sickle (Hb S).
- Deoxygenated Hb S tends to polymerize noncovalently into long strands that deform the erythrocyte, giving the characteristic "sickle cell" morphology.

- Vaso-occlusive crisis or acute pain crisis is caused by tissue ischemia and infarction.
- Bones are affected due to ischemia and infarction of bone marrow and inflammation of periosteum.
- Acute chest syndrome is due to infection (*Chlamydia*, *Mycoplasma*, respiratory syncytial virus, *Staphylococcus aureus*, and *Streptococcus pneumoniae*), vascular infarction, and fat emboli (1).
- Stroke: Mostly thrombotic (mainly in children), but may be hemorrhagic in adults.
- Sepsis: Higher predisposition due to splenic dysfunction; mainly susceptible to encapsulated organisms (e.g., *Pneumococcus*)
- Pulmonary hypertension: Due to increased nitric oxide (NO) consumption and decreased NO synthesis (2)[B].
- Priapism: Exact mechanism unknown. Penile venous outflow is obstructed by sickled cells.
- Hemolytic anemia: Mostly extravascular and due to increased red cell fragility

ETIOLOGY
Autosomal recessive genetic disorder in which polymerized deoxygenated Hb S causes red cells to become distorted into a sickled shape and leads to increased viscosity, stasis, obstruction of small arterioles and capillaries, and tissue ischemia.

COMMONLY ASSOCIATED CONDITIONS
- Fluid overload.
- Renal dysfunction

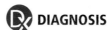 DIAGNOSIS

HISTORY
- Vasoocclusive pain crisis: Severe deep pain in the extremities, involving long bones and back. Abdominal pain may mimic acute abdomen.
- Pain may be accompanied by fever, malaise, and leukocytosis.
- Acute chest syndrome: Chest pain, fever, tachypnea, wheezing, or cough.
- Stroke: Childhood and adolescence; varying degrees of deficit
- Sepsis: Fever with high-grade leucocytosis
- Priapism: Painful prolonged erection
- Chronic hemolytic anemia

PHYSICAL EXAM
- Nonspecific; may include scleral icterus, pale mucous membranes
- Systolic murmur may be heard over the entire precordium.
- In childhood, splenomegaly is present, but not in adults due to autosplenectomy.

DIAGNOSTIC TESTS & INTERPRETATION
Lab
- Hemoglobin electrophoresis establishes the diagnosis of sickle cell disease.
- CBC: Microcytic anemia with hemoglobin of 7–9 g/dL
- Leucocytosis, thrombocytosis
- Reticulocytosis of 3–15%.
- Peripheral blood smear shows the presence of sickled erythrocytes, polychromasia indicative of reticulocytosis, and Howell-Jolly bodies reflecting hyposplenia.
- Unconjugated hyperbilirubinemia, elevated serum LDH, and low serum haptoglobin

Imaging
- Painful crisis: Radiograph may demonstrate areas of infarction for painful bones.
- MRI demonstrates areas of avascular necrosis for the femoral and humeral heads and may distinguish between osteomyelitis and bony infarction for painful bones.
- Acute chest syndrome: Chest x-ray shows new pulmonary infiltrate involving at least 1 complete lung segment. Infiltrates are often in the upper lobes in children and lower lobes in adults. Multilobar disease suggests a worse prognosis.
- Stroke: Transcranial Doppler US; patients at risk are those with time-averaged mean blood flow velocity >200 cm/sec in the internal or middle carotid arteries.
- Pulmonary hypertension: Doppler echocardiography to estimate pulmonary artery pressure and right-heart function.
- Abdominal sonogram is useful to document spleen size and the presence of biliary stones.

Pathological Findings
- In moderate to severe cases, hyposplenism due to autosplenectomy is common.
- Hypoxia/infarction in multiple organs

DIFFERENTIAL DIAGNOSIS
- Anemia: Other hemoglobinopathies (e.g., Hb SC disease, Hb C disease, sickle cell-β thalassemia)
- Hemolytic anemia
- Painful crises: Other causes of acute pain in bones, joints, and abdomen

TREATMENT

MEDICATION

First Line
- Pain control: Morphine is the drug of choice. Narcotic dosing needs to be individualized:
  - Administer parenteral morphine (0.1–0.15 mg/kg IV q2–4h), hydromorphone (1–4 mg IV q3–6h), or fentanyl as a continuous IV infusion. Give additional smaller doses for breakthrough pain. PCA pump may be useful. Reassess pain frequently.
- Acute chest syndrome: Judicious hydration, oxygen, pain management (2):
  - Incentive spirometry to prevent atelectasis.
  - Antibiotic coverage for *Streptococcus pneumoniae*
  - Include macrolide or quinolone for coverage of atypical pathogens *Chlamydia pneumoniae* and *Mycoplasma pneumoniae*.
  - Transfuse RBCs but do not exceed hemoglobin >10 g/dL
  - Exchange transfusion should be considered for severe cases.
- Stroke: Ischemic stroke mandates immediate exchange transfusion to limit further infarction.
- Priapism: IV hydration, analgesia, α-adrenergic agonists (etilefrine or phenylephrine), exchange transfusion

Second Line
- Painful crisis: Ketorolac 30 mg IV q6h, methylprednisolone (15 mg/kg/d IV in 2 doses) (3)
- Acute chest syndrome: Dexamethasone pulse therapy (0.3 mg/kg IV q12h in 4 doses in children) or inhaled nitric oxide
- Pulmonary hypertension: No proven treatment. Regular blood transfusions or long-term anticoagulation may be necessary:
  - Prostacyclin analogues, endothelin-1 receptor antagonists, phosphodiesterase inhibitors (including sildenafil), and calcium channel blockers are being evaluated.

ADDITIONAL TREATMENT

General Measures
- Oxygen therapy
- Careful fluid management
- Adequate pain control

Issues for Referral
- Hematology consult should be sought early.
- Infectious disease for sepsis
- Pain management
- Psychiatry

Additional Therapies
Prevention of acute episodes:

- Hydroxyurea elevates fetal hemoglobin and decreases frequency of painful crises and acute chest syndrome (3)[B].
- Bone marrow transplantation: Only curative therapy but not widely available and associated with significant morbidity and mortality.

SURGERY/OTHER PROCEDURES
- Skin grafts can help heal chronic leg ulcers.
- Hip replacement or other orthopedic procedures can be used to treat avascular necrosis.
- Resistant priapism may require surgical draining of the penile corpora.

IN-PATIENT CONSIDERATIONS

Initial Stabilization
Adequate oxygenation, hydration, and pain control

Admission Criteria
- Severe pain requiring IV medications
- Infection
- Acute chest syndrome
- Severe anemia

IV Fluids
- IV fluids should be of sufficient quantity to correct dehydration and to replace continuing losses, both insensible and due to fever.
- Frequent assessment for signs of fluid overload is necessary.

Nursing
- Provision of adequate pain medications
- Adequate hydration and strict monitoring of input and output
- Correction of hypoxemia
- Monitoring for infection

Discharge Criteria
- Painful crisis resolved
- Stable hemoglobin (patient's baseline Hb)
- No signs of infection

ONGOING CARE

FOLLOW-UP RECOMMENDATIONS
- Outpatient clinic follow-up is required for all SCD patients.
- Immunization for *S. pneumoniae, Haemophilus influenzae* type B, *Meningococcus*, and influenza virus

Patient Monitoring
Annual follow-up investigations: Blood counts, hepatic and renal tests, transcranial Doppler US for children, heart and liver US.

DIET
- Daily folate supplementation.
- Avoid alcohol (leads to dehydration)

PATIENT EDUCATION
- Educate all patients to recognize signs of infection, worsening anemia, and organ failure.
- Genetic counseling and prenatal diagnosis may be offered to at-risk couples.

PROGNOSIS
- Anemia is lifelong. In 2nd decade of life, patient usually experiences fewer crises, but complications are more frequent.
- Median age of death is 42 for men and 48 for women.
- Common causes of death are infections, thrombosis, pulmonary emboli, pulmonary hypertension, and renal failure.

COMPLICATIONS
- Septicemia, meningitis
- Osteomyelitis
- Acute chest syndrome
- Stroke
- Repeated vaso-occlusive crises
- Acute aplastic anemia

REFERENCES

1. Steinberg MH. Sickle cell anemia, the first molecular disease: Overview of molecular etiology, pathophysiology, and therapeutic approaches. *Sci World J*. 2008; 8:1295–1324.
2. de Montalembert M. Management of sickle cell disease. *BMJ*. 2008;337:a1397.
3. Ballas SK. Pain management of sickle cell disease. *Hematol Oncol Clin N Am*. 2005;19:785–802.

ADDITIONAL READING

- Frenette PS, et al. Sickle cell disease: Old discoveries, new concepts, and future promise. *J Clin Invest*. 2007;117:850–8.
- National Heart Lung and Blood Institute. The management of sickle cell disease. 2004. Accessed at www.nhlbi.nih.gov/health/prof/blood/sickle

See Also (Topic, Algorithm, Electronic Media Element)

- http://www.cdc.gov/ncbddd/sicklecell/faq_sicklecell.htm
- http://www.scinfo.org/

 CODES

ICD9
- 282.5 Sickle-cell trait
- 282.61 Hb-ss disease without crisis
- 282.62 Hb-ss disease with crisis

CLINICAL PEARLS

- Sickle cell anemia is an autosomal recessive disorder of hemoglobin associated with chronic hemolytic anemia and vaso-occlusive crises.
- ICU admission and management is indicated for acute chest syndrome, sepsis, stroke, and severe vaso-occlusive pain crisis.
- Adequate pain control, IV hydration, oxygen therapy, RBC transfusion, and antibiotics are key management strategies for ACS.

ANEURYSM, CEREBRAL

Damian Lee

BASICS

DESCRIPTION
- Abnormal bulging or ballooning of a cerebral blood vessel, typically an artery
- Aneurysms appear in different shapes and sizes, such as saccular or berry.
- Giant berry aneurysms may expand to >2 cm in diameter (1).
- Can occur anywhere in the brain
- May be saccular or berry (rounded or pouch-like), lateral (bulge on one side of vessel), or fusiform (widened along all walls of vessel).

EPIDEMIOLOGY
Incidence
- Unknown
- ~30,000 cases of aneurysmal SAH occur annually in the U.S.

Prevalence
~2–5% of the population at any given time will possess some form of cerebral aneurysm (1,2).

RISK FACTORS
- Family history
- Arteriovenous malformations (AVM).
- Genetic predisposition in persons with PCKD, Ehlers-Danlos Type IV, and coarctation of aorta.
- Risk of rupture increases in:
  - As above
  - Trauma
  - Alcohol abuse
  - Sickle cell anemia
  - Uncontrolled hypertension
  - Cocaine use
  - Oral contraceptives (3)

GENERAL PREVENTION
- No known ways to prevent an aneurysm from forming
- To minimize chances of rupture:
  - Avoid smoking
  - Treat hypertension
  - Screening by CTA, MRI, or MRA is suggested for individuals with significant risk factors, such as family history and genetic predisposition.

PATHOPHYSIOLOGY
- Congenital abnormality or weakening of a portion of the cerebral artery wall that, over time, balloons and fills with blood
- Trauma, hypertension, infection (mycotic aneurysm), tumors, atherosclerosis, tobacco, and cocaine use all compromise the integrity of the layers of the arterial wall from overstretching or inflammation. This can lead to aneurysm formation (3).

ETIOLOGY
Unknown

COMMONLY ASSOCIATED CONDITIONS
- Polycystic kidney disease (PCKD)
- Coarctation of the aorta

DIAGNOSIS

HISTORY
- For nonruptured aneurysms:
  - Asymptomatic
  - Headache
  - Eye or neck pain
  - Facial numbness, weakness or paralysis
  - Visual changes
- Rupture aneurysm, e.g., SAH:
  - "Thunderclap" headache (worst headache of life)
  - Symptoms of nonrupture
- Changes in mentation
- Neurologic deficits
- Nausea/vomiting with or without neck stiffness
- Numbness, weakness, and/or paralysis (typically contralateral to the side of rupture/bleed)
- Changes in mood or temperament
- Seizures

ALERT
Most unruptured aneurysms are asymptomatic. Symptoms typically occur when the aneurysm compresses nerves or blood vessels.

PHYSICAL EXAM
Pupil exam may reveal sluggish, nonreactive, and/or blown (fixed and dilated) pupil. Anisocoria (unequal pupils) is typical.

DIAGNOSTIC TESTS & INTERPRETATION
Lab
Initial lab tests
Spinal tap revealing xanthochromia is diagnostic for ruptured aneurysm (SAH).
Follow-Up & Special Considerations
- Cerebral aneurysm <7 mm in size has an ~0.1% annual chance of rupture.
- Cerebral aneurysm >7 mm in size has an ~0.5–1% annual chance of rupture.
- Cerebral aneurysm >2 cm in size has an ~5% annual chance of rupture.

ALERT
A ruptured aneurysm is a medical/surgical emergency. Delay in diagnosis and treatment could result in death.

Imaging
Initial approach
- Often found incidentally on imaging for other purposes
- Noncontrast CT of brain is primary to evaluate for bleed. This would indicate rupture.
- Cerebral angiogram is gold standard, and remains the diagnostic test of choice. It can diagnose and treat via coiling if aneurysm found.

- CT angiogram (CTA) is a suitable alternative and has become more common over recent years. However, it can only diagnose; it offers no treatment modality.
- Magnetic resonance angiography (MRA) is also utilized in some centers. It offers slightly better sensitivity and specificity than CTA. However, exam requires more time to perform and more technical difficulty.
- EEG may be required to rule-out or rule-in seizure activity in ruptured aneurysms, especially if subclinical.

Follow-Up & Special Considerations
Post-treatment angiogram to evaluate for filling defects or residual aneurysm

Diagnostic Procedures/Other
ECG may exhibit abnormalities, especially in rupture.

Pathological Findings
Nonspecific.

DIFFERENTIAL DIAGNOSIS
- Migraine headache
- Intracranial infection

TREATMENT

MEDICATION
First Line
- Nimodipine is the only drug that has been studied and proved to help reduce the incidence of postbleed vasospasm in SAH.
- Antihypertensive infusions may be needed in the ruptured, pretreatment phase to control blood pressure, thus preventing further bleeding. Nicardipine has been found to be ideal and is common in many neuro ICUs. Other common agents are labetalol, hydralazine.

Second Line
- Tylenol to prevent fevers and for pain. Hyperthermia will put further demands on an already compromised brain.
- Stool softeners (Colace, senna) to prevent constipation and thus increase ICP during Valsalva or straining

ADDITIONAL TREATMENT
General Measures
- Aneurysm risk of rupture based on size and location. This determines need for treatment; see Follow-up & Special Consideration section
- Aneurysms in frontal cerebral vessels (MCA and ACA) <7 mm in diameter have a low risk of rupture (2).
- May require external ventricular drain (EVD) insertion to monitor for and treat intracranial hypertension or hydrocephalus.
- Aneurysm are usually coiled (interventional radiology/endovascular surgery) or clipped (intra-op via craniotomy) to prevent bleed or rebleed.

Issues for Referral
Referral is based on symptoms or complications and could involve a wide range of specialists.

Additional Therapies
Based on symptoms or complications

COMPLEMENTARY & ALTERNATIVE THERAPIES
Unknown

SURGERY/OTHER PROCEDURES
- Craniotomy with clipping of aneurysm (10–15% mortality)
- Coiling of aneurysm via intra-arterial catheter placed in interventional radiology suite or intraop

IN-PATIENT CONSIDERATIONS
Initial Stabilization
- Pay attention to ABCs.
- IV access and intra-arterial catheter is desirable for close blood pressure monitoring.

Admission Criteria
- All ruptured aneurysms require admission for emergent neurosurgical intervention.
- Symptomatic unruptured aneurysm may require admission for treatment. Urgency is based on severity of symptoms.

IV Fluids
- Pretreatment: Avoid excess IVF or fluid overload as this may result in increased blood pressure. This could potentially increase risk of rupture or increase bleeding if already ruptured.
- Posttreatment: During vasospasm period, increased doses of IVF are usually infused in an attempt to prevent vasospasm. There is no specific volume for this, and this is not necessarily proved to work.

Nursing
- Bed rest for ruptured aneurysm and activity as tolerated for noncomplicated elective aneurysm treatment.
- Close neurologic monitoring is required, especially for ruptured aneurysm, in an ICU setting for at least 10–14 days postbleed. It is during this period that the risk of postbleed vasospasm is highest (1).
- Persons with neurological deficits will need assistance with ADLs.

Discharge Criteria
- Based on level of disability. Some will require prolonged occupational, physical, and speech therapy to regain lost function, and it may be best to discharge to rehabilitation facility.
- Other may be discharged home with services or to a skilled nursing facility.

 ONGOING CARE

FOLLOW-UP RECOMMENDATIONS
Monitor for neurologic deficits that could indicate rerupture.

Patient Monitoring
- Gradual increase in activity posttreatment, based on clinical condition. Some patients may require physical or occupational therapy to regain function.
- Patients with moderate to severe residual neurologic deficits may require skilled nursing facility.

DIET
- Varies, based on clinical status
- Aspiration risk must be considered in all patients postbleed.

PATIENT EDUCATION
- Avoid triggers of aneurysm rupture such as smoking, uncontrolled hypertension, alcohol abuse, head trauma, oral contraceptives, or cocaine use.
- Seek emergency medical attention if symptoms recur.

PROGNOSIS
- Ruptured aneurysms are often fatal.
- ~25% of those with ruptured aneurysm die within 24 hours; 25% die within 3 months of presentation; 50% of survivors experience permanent disability (1).

COMPLICATIONS
- Complications tend to occur from ruptured aneurysm, iatrogenic injury during the treatment of a nonruptured aneurysm, or nonruptured aneurysm compressing or occluding nerves or blood vessels.
- Most feared complication is vasospasm resulting in ischemic stroke.
- Physical or mental disability
- Death

REFERENCES

1. Medline Plus Medical Encyclopedia. (09/2008). Aneurysm in the brain. Retrieved March 9, 2009 from http://www.nlm.nih.gov/medlineplus/ency/article/001414.htm
2. Mayo Foundation for Education and Research. Cerebral aneurysms. 2009. Retrieved March 9, 2009 from http://www.mayoclinic.org/cerebral-aneurysm/
3. National Institute of Neurologic Disorders and Stroke. Cerebral aneurysm fact sheet. August 2008. Retrieved March 9, 2009 from http://www.ninds.nih.gov/disorders/cerebral_aneurysm/detail_cerebral_aneurysm.htm

ADDITIONAL READING

- Brain Aneurysm Foundation: http://www.bafound.org
- American Association of Neurologic Surgeons: http://www.aans.org
- Cerebral Aneurysm-eMedicine Neurosurgery: http://emedicine.medscape.com/article/252142

 CODES

ICD9
- 430 Subarachnoid hemorrhage
- 437.3 Cerebral aneurysm, nonruptured

CLINICAL PEARLS

- Patient presenting with complaint of the worst headache of life or thunder-clap headache is indicative of a ruptured cerebral aneurysm (SAH) until proved otherwise.
- Postbleed vasospasm in SAH patients occurs commonly between days 4–14; highest around day 10.

ANTIBIOTIC THERAPY

David Oxman

 BASICS

DESCRIPTION

- Infections in ICU patients are common, and often necessitate the prompt initiation of appropriate antibiotics.
- However, low specificity of signs/symptoms and diagnostic tests (e.g., fever and chest x-ray for the diagnosis of ventilator-associated pneumonia) may lead to overdiagnosis of infectious syndromes.
- Always balance the need to treat potential infections early and aggressively with harm of unnecessary antibiotics.
- Overuse of antibiotics leads to individual complications (e.g., colonization with resistant organisms and *Clostridium difficile* colitis) and increased rates of antimicrobial resistance in the ICU.

 TREATMENT

- Empiric treatment:
  - Acuity of illness often requires early antibiotic treatment before it is clear if infection is present or what the infecting organism is.
  - Many studies have demonstrated worse outcomes for variety of infections (e.g., ventilator-associated pneumonia, severe sepsis, bloodstream infection) with even minor delays (hours) in appropriate antimicrobial treatment.
  - Antibiotic choice must be based on the site of infection, knowledge of the likely pathogens, and likelihood of antibiotic resistance.

- Common empiric antibiotic regimens in ICU:
  - Ventilator-associated pneumonia:
    - As the chance of antibiotic-resistant organisms is high and specific resistance patterns are unpredictable, empiric therapy must include multiple agents to maximize chances of giving appropriate therapy early.
    - 1 drug must be directed to gram-positive coverage including MRSA (e.g., vancomycin or linezolid); *AND*
    - Empiric coverage for gram negative bacteria requires two drugs from different classes. Recommended regimens include
      1) a broad-spectrum beta-lactam (e.g. cefepime or piperacilin-tazobactam) + an aminoglycoside (e.g. gentamicin)
      2) a carbapenem (e.g. imipenem) + a quinolone (e.g. ciprofloxacin)
  - Catheter-related bloodstream infection:
    - Gram-positive organisms, including MRSA, cause the majority of infections, and vancomycin is the first-line agent.
    - In the immunocompromised or septic patient, empiric treatment should be broadened to cover typical nosocomial gram-negative organisms. Burn patients also are at high risk from gram-negative infections.
    - Fungal CRBSI, although increasing in incidence, is still relatively uncommon, and empiric antifungal coverage should be reserved for high-risk patients. In ICU patients with possible fungal line sepsis, an echinocandin (e.g., caspofungin, micafungin) is first-line empiric agent.

ANTIBIOTIC RESISTANCE

- Factors leading to high rates of antimicrobial resistance in the ICU:
  - High rates of previous exposure to broad-spectrum antibiotics
  - High use of invasive catheters
  - High rates of comorbid conditions
- The most commonly encountered antibiotic-resistant infections in the ICU are:
  - Methicillin-resistant *Staphylococcus aureus* (MRSA): Most ICUs report >50% of *S. aureus* isolates to be MRSA.
  - Vancomycin-resistant enterococcus (VRE): Increasingly common pathogen in ICU patients
- Resistant gram-negative organisms include extended-spectrum β-lactamase (ESBLs) and carbepenamase-producing organisms; these are resistant to most, and sometimes all, available antibiotics.
- Resistance patterns vary from hospital to hospital, and intensivists must be familiar with their own hospital antibiogram and local antibiotic resistance profiles.

ANTIBIOTIC DE-ESCALATION
Description
- Antibiotic de-escalation is an approach that emphasizes the early treatment of infection with broad-spectrum agents followed by:
  – Stopping antibiotics entirely when it is clear no infection is actually present
  – Tailoring antibiotics when sensitivity of infecting organism is known
  – Minimizing duration of treatment
- With very few exceptions, monotherapy with a single antibiotic is sufficient once sensitivity patterns of the pathogen are known.
- Antibiotic duration should be appropriate for given infection (e.g., 8 days for ventilator-associated pneumonia; 4–7 days for uncomplicated intra-abdominal abscess).
- Biomarkers, such as procalcitonin, may be useful in assessing response to therapy and deciding if antibiotics should be continued or changed.

PHARMOCOKINETIC CONSIDERATIONS
- Careful attention should be paid to antibiotic dosing. Inadequate antibiotic dosing can lead to treatment failure and the promotion of resistance.
- Physiologic changes in critically ill patients, such as increased volume of distribution due to edema or increased clearance due to hyperdynamic states, can affect drug levels.
- Hypoalbuminemia can reduce drug levels of protein-bound antibiotics.
- Tissue penetration of antibiotics in septic patients may be impaired.
- Kill characteristics of antibiotics vary. For example, β-lactam antibiotics depend on time above MIC, whereas aminoglycosides kill bacteria in concentration-dependent manner.

ADDITIONAL READING
- Depuydt P, et al. Antibiotic therapy for ventilator-associated pneumonia: de-escalation in the real world. *Crit Care Med*. 2007;35(2):632–3.
- Kollef MH, et al. Antibiotic resistance in the intensive care unit. *Ann Intern Med*. 2001;134(4):298–314.

- Laupkand KB, et al. Occurrence and outcome of fever in critically ill adults. *Crit Care Med*. 2008; 36(5):1531–35.
- Roberts JA, et al. Pharmokinetic issues for antibiotics in the critically ill patient. *Crit Care Med*. 2009;37(3):840–51.

 CODES

ICD9
- 041.12 Methicillin resistant Staphylococcus aureus
- 136.9 Unspecified infectious and parasitic diseases
- 997.31 Ventilator associated pneumonia

AORTIC DISSECTION

Nitin Puri

 BASICS

DESCRIPTION
A potentially catastrophic condition due to a tear in the wall of the aorta that can cause the layers of the vessel to separate, potentially leading to rupture.

EPIDEMIOLOGY
- Predominant age: 6th–8th decade
- Male > Female 2:1
- Women diagnosed are older than men.

Incidence
2.6–3.5 per 100,000 people per year (1)

RISK FACTORS
- Hypertension
- Smoking
- Dyslipidemia
- Prior aortic aneurysm
- Cocaine use
- Vasculitic diseases
- Prior cardiac or aortic surgery
- Prior aortic surgery
- Cardiac catheterization
- Dissection in pregnancy (3rd trimester) has been described, but pregnant patients likely have a unrecognized genetic cause (2)

Genetics
- Marfan syndrome: Autosomal dominant
- Ehlers-Danlos syndrome type IV: Autosomal dominant
- Annuloaortic ectasia
- Familial aortic dissection
- Bicuspid aortic valve
- Coarctation of aorta
- Turner syndrome

PATHOPHYSIOLOGY
- Tear in the intima layer of the aorta in which blood can enter and create a false lumen between the intima and the media or adventitia (3)
- Tear can propagate either anterograde or retrograde.
- Both genetic and acquired comorbidities have the same common pathway.
- Both aortic intramural hematoma (blood in wall of aorta) and aortic ulcers are precursors to aortic dissection.
- When symptomatic, concern for rupture
- Classification:
  - Stanford classification:
    - Type A: All dissections involving the ascending aorta, irrespective of site of origin
    - Type B: All dissections not involving the ascending aorta
  - DeBakey classification:
    - Type I: Originates in ascending aorta and goes to at least aortic arch
    - Type II: Originates and confined to ascending aorta
    - Type III: Originates and confined to descending aorta

ETIOLOGY
- Trauma:
  - Decelerating injury such as car crash
- Aortitis:
  - Syphilitic, Takayasu or giant cell arteritis
- Iatrogenic:
  - Cardiac surgery
  - Aortic surgery
  - Aortic valve replacement
- Drug use (cocaine, amphetamines, other)

COMMONLY ASSOCIATED CONDITIONS
- Patient <40 years:
  - ~50% have Marfan syndrome
  - Bicuspid aortic valve
- Patient >40 years:
  - Hypertension
  - Dyslipidemia

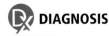 **DIAGNOSIS**

HISTORY
- Diverse clinical presentation
- Severe pain with abrupt onset
- Pain more often described as sharp rather than tearing or ripping
- Chest pain:
  - More likely in type A (79%) vs. type B (63%)
  - Anterior chest pain more commonly associated with type A
- Abdominal pain;
  - More likely in type B (43%) vs. (22%)
- Back pain:
  - More likely in type B (64%) vs. type A (47%)
- Syncope (9.4%)
- Congestive heart failure (6.6%)
- Cerebral vascular accident (4.7%)
- Painless (4.5%)

PHYSICAL EXAM
- Vital signs:
  - Hypertension more likely associated with type B dissection (70%) vs. type A (35%)
  - Hypotension type A (25%)
- Pulse deficit type A > type B
- Type A
  - Clinical signs of cardiac tamponade
  - Systolic blood pressure (BP) variation between arms of ≥20 mm Hg
  - Acute aortic regurgitation murmur will occur in a significant minority of patients with type A dissection.
  - Neurologic deficits due to dissection into carotid artery
  - Horner syndrome: Miosis, ptosis, anhydrosis due to compression of superior cervical ganglion

DIAGNOSTIC TESTS & INTERPRETATION
Lab
- EKG should be done, but often normal (31%). Nonspecific ST, T-wave changes in 42%, ischemic changes in 15%
- No diagnostic lab test currently exists:
  - Smooth muscle myosin, which is released from damaged aortic medial muscle, may have promise, but requires further clinical evaluation.
  - CK, troponin I, CBC, D-dimer, LDH, PT, PTT, INR, BUN, Cr, type and screen, lactic acid

Imaging
- Chest x-ray:
  - Widening of mediastinum is classic finding present in 63% of type A and in 56% of type B
  - No abnormalities (12.4%)
  - Left pleural effusion is of concern due to possible rupture of dissection
- Transthoracic echocardiogram (TTE):
  - Inability to visualize distal ascending, transverse, and descending aorta limits utility to diagnose dissection.
  - Useful for cardiac complications of dissection
  - Useful for tamponade and to rule out other causes of shock
- Transesophageal echocardiogram (TEE):
  - Good visualization of thoracic aorta due to proximity of aorta to esophagus without lung or chest interference
  - Sensitivity 99%, specificity 89%, increased specificity to 100% with M mode imaging
  - Can be done quickly, but requires experienced operator
  - Requires intubation of patient and may be difficult to perform in hemodynamically unstable patients
- CT scan:
  - Most frequently used modality to diagnose dissection
  - Standard CT scan: Sensitivity 83–98%, specificity 87–100%; limited ability to detect intimal injury
  - Spiral CT: Improved sensitivity and specificity; most accurate method of detecting aortic arch injury
  - CT requires the use of potentially nephrotoxic contrast
- MRI:
  - Highest sensitivity, specificity
  - Contrast has better safety profile than CT contrast
  - Disadvantages are associated claustrophobia, inability to perform on patients with pacemakers or metal devices
- Aortography:
  - Historically, the gold standard of diagnosis
  - Sensitivity approximately 90%, specificity >95%
  - Limitations include time required to do procedure and its invasive nature

Pathological Findings
- Cystic medial degeneration is a histopathologic degenerative change that occurs in the wall of the aorta, specifically the tunica media.
- It is a degeneration of collagen and elastin that can occur genetically or through acquired secondary conditions (atherosclerosis).
- This leads to weakening of the wall of the aorta and possible dissection.
- See Pathophysiology.

DIFFERENTIAL DIAGNOSIS
- Myocardial Infarction
- Pericarditis
- Pleuritis
- Pulmonary embolism
- Aortic aneurysm without dissection
- Valvular aortic regurgitation
- Musculoskeletal pain
- Pancreatitis

TREATMENT

MEDICATION

First Line
- IV β-blocker (3)[A]:
  - Systolic BP <120 mm Hg and pulse to <60
  - Decrease shearing force (dP/dT) to decrease dissection extension and to decrease rupture.
  - Titrate BP and pulse to lowest physiological level tolerated by patient while maintaining vital organ perfusion. Aim for SBP <120 mm Hg and pulse <60
  - Labetalol
  - Esmolol is useful due to its short half-life.
- Analgesia:
  - Aggressive control of pain is important using morphine sulfate or other opiates

Second Line
- Vasodilators (3)[A]:
  - IV nitroprusside should be used in conjunction with a β-blocker to avoid enhanced ventricular contraction (thus increased aortic shear stress).
  - Prolonged use can lead to cyanide toxicity, especially in patients with renal failure
  - Hydralazine should be avoided in acute setting due to unpredictable effect on BP and decreased reversibility.
- Calcium channel blockers: Diltiazem, verapamil, nicardipine can all effectively lower BP,

ADDITIONAL TREATMENT

General Measures
- Hemodynamically unstable patients should be intubated.
- Bedside TEE is imaging procedure of choice in unstable patients due to its portability.

Issues for Referral
- Type A dissection if a cardiothoracic surgeon is not available
- Type B dissection if a vascular surgeon is not available

SURGERY/OTHER PROCEDURES
- Type A is a surgical emergency.
- Endovascular stent grafts are being used in some centers in selected patients for type A dissections.
- Type B without end-organ dysfunction can be managed medically most of the time:
  - Most such patients have comorbidities that increase the risk of surgery.
  - Minimally invasive catheter-based therapies are useful for chronic type B dissections.
  - Minimally invasive therapies have shown promising results in type B dissections with malperfusion in selected patients with appropriate anatomy (4)[C]

IN-PATIENT CONSIDERATIONS

Initial Stabilization
- Admit to ICU.
- Ensure proper IV access.
- Most merit placement of arterial catheter.
- Place indwelling bladder catheter
- Draw initial labs.
- Consult specialists as needed.
- Determine if further radiographic tests are needed.

Admission Criteria
All patients with acute dissection should be admitted.

IV Fluids
IV fluids should be used as needed to optimize perfusion, watching carefully for pulmonary edema.

Nursing
- Pulse checks
- Neurological checks
- Pain control
- Monitor urine output
- Control BP
- 2 large-bore IVs or large-bore central catheter
- Arterial catheter may be required for BP monitoring.

Discharge Criteria
- Type B dissection
- Patient able to tolerate oral medications
- No pain
- No signs or lab studies indicating malperfusion

ONGOING CARE

FOLLOW-UP RECOMMENDATIONS
Continue to minimize aortic wall shear stress:
- Aggressive control of BP <120/80
- Follow-up imaging
- Assessment of aorta 1, 3, 6, 9,12 months after discharge and every 6–12 months afterward
- Reoperation as needed

PATIENT EDUCATION
Patients must understand that the whole aorta is at risk. Maintaining adequate BP control is crucial.

PROGNOSIS
- In both types of dissection, in-hospital mortality is 24%.
- 5-year survival is 32% vs. Olmstead County, MN 1966–1980 population study (5), which showed 5 year survival of 5%:
  - Type A:
    - Without intervention, mortality is 24% at 24 hours and 49% at day 14.
    - With surgical intervention, in-hospital mortality is 10% at 24 hours and 20% at day 14.
  - Type B:
    - Without end-organ dysfunction, 30-day mortality is 10%.
    - With end-organ dysfunction (renal failure, visceral ischemia, etc.) 20% mortality at day 2 and 25% mortality at day 30.
- Aortic intramural hematoma: In ascending aorta, prognosis is similar to type A dissection; in descending aorta, prognosis is similar to type B dissection.

COMPLICATIONS
- Acute coronary syndrome
- Aortic valve insufficiency
- Pericardial tamponade
- Hemothorax
- Extremity dysfunction
- Paraplegia
- Bowel ischemia
- Renal failure

REFERENCES

1. Hagan PG, et al. The International Registry of Acute Aortic Dissection (IRAD) new insights into an old disease. *JAMA*. 2000;283:897–903.
2. Nienabar CA, et al. Aortic dissection: New frontiers in diagnosis and management. Part I: From etiology to diagnostic strategies. *Circulation*. 2003;108: 628–35.
3. Tsai TT, et al. Acute aortic syndromes. *Circulation*. 2005;112:3802–13.
4. Lombardi JV, et al. Endovascular management of type B aortic dissection: Fenestration, stents and endografts. *Adv Vasc Surg*. 2006;12:109–30.
5. Clouse WD, et al. Acute aortic dissection: Population-based incidence compared with degenerative aortic aneurysm rupture. *Mayo Clinic Proc*. 2004;79:176.

ADDITIONAL READING

- Dake MD, et al. Endovascular stent-graft placement for the treatment of acute aortic dissection. *N Engl J Med*. 1999;340:1546–52.
- Meszaros I, et al. Epidemiology and clinicopathology of aortic dissection. *Chest*. 2000;117:1271–8.

CODES

ICD9
- 441.00 Dissection of aorta, unspecified site
- 441.01 Dissection of aorta, thoracic
- 441.02 Dissection of aorta, abdominal

CLINICAL PEARLS
- Type A dissection is a surgical emergency.
- Patient complaining of persistent chest or abdominal pain without satisfactory diagnosis deserves imaging to rule of aortic dissection.
- Imaging must be done promptly; chest x-ray to rule out dissection is unsatisfactory.
- β-Blockers are the initial treatment of choice for patients with acute presentation, provided the patient is not hemodynamically unstable.

AORTIC STENOSIS
Qasim Durrani

 BASICS

DESCRIPTION
- Aortic stenosis (AS) is characterized by abnormal narrowing of the valve.
- The severity of AS is described by aortic valve (AV) area. Normal AV area is 4–5 cm^2. AS can be classified into mild, moderate, and severe; this is explained under initial approach.

EPIDEMIOLOGY
Incidence
- Congenital AS: 4 in 1000
- About 1–2% of the population have bicuspid aortic valves (high risk for AS).
- Unicuspid aortic valve (high risk for AS) is a rare, but well-described pediatric congenital anomaly.

Prevalence
- 1/4 of all patients with chronic valvular heart disease
- In older adults, mild thickening, calcification, or both of a trileaflet aortic valve without restricted leaflet motion (i.e., aortic sclerosis) affects about 25% of the population older >65.
- Calcific aortic stenosis, however, affects ~2–3% of those >75 years.

RISK FACTORS
- Age
- Male sex
- Hypertension
- Smoking
- Serum LDL and lipoprotein(a) levels
- DM

Genetics
- Congenital AS occurs in 4 in 1000. A small number of candidate genes have been identified but need to be confirmed in larger samples:
  - VDR (Vitamin D receptor gene)
  - APOE (Apolipoprotein E)
  - APOB (Apolipoprotein B)
  - IL10 (interleukin 10)
  - ESR1 (estrogen receptor-α)
- Defects in the Notch1 signaling pathway causes aortic valve diseases in a restricted number of families.

GENERAL PREVENTION
- AS usually cannot be prevented.
- Prevention of rheumatic fever may prevent secondary AS.

PATHOPHYSIOLOGY
- AS causes pressure gradient between left ventricle and aorta.
- With disease progression, left ventricular hypertrophy (LVH) develops to overcome increased afterload.
- Though initially beneficial, this compensatory LVH later results in complications:
  - Diastolic dysfunction
  - CHF
  - Decrease coronary blood flow
  - Increased sensitivity to ischemia
  - Inappropriate LVH resulting in high perioperative morbidity and mortality

ETIOLOGY
- Congenital
- Bicuspid valve: Presents in 3rd–5th decade
- Rheumatic: Presents in 4th–5th decade
- Degenerative (calcific): Usually age >65
- Rare causes:
  - Homozygous type II hyperlipoproteinemia
  - Alkaptonuria
  - Fabry's disease

COMMONLY ASSOCIATED CONDITIONS
- CAD
- Mitral valve disease
- Infective endocarditis
- AV nodal block

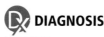 **DIAGNOSIS**

HISTORY
- Usually prolonged latent period.
- When symptomatic, may present with:
  - Angina (during exercise or at rest)
  - Syncope
  - Dyspnea (during exercise or at rest)
  - CHF
  - Atrial fibrillation

PHYSICAL EXAM
- Delayed and diminished carotid upstroke (pulsus parvus et tardus). Anacrotic notch (shudder on upstroke) may be felt. Systolic thrill may be present develops later with LV dilatation and failure.
- Sustained apical impulse. Classically, nondisplaced with isolated LVH, but may be lateral/inferior with marked hypertrophy.

- Auscultation:
  - Soft S2 as A2 is diminished; may be single or paradoxically split.
  - Normal S2 implies absence of severe AS; (narrow) or paradoxical splitting of 2nd heart sound in severe AS.
  - Ejection click at base after S1. Can be lost as increased severity renders valve immobile; S3 and/or S4
  - Ejection systolic murmur best heard at aortic area, which increases with augmentation of preload (squatting/leg raising); peaks later with increasing severity
  - Amplitude of murmur not especially useful as index of severity, as it decreases later with decreasing cardiac output.

DIAGNOSTIC TESTS & INTERPRETATION
Lab
- No specific biochemistry
- EKG: LVH with or without a strain pattern
- 13% have conduction defects.
- Left atrial enlargement

Imaging
Initial approach
- 2D echocardiogram is recommended for diagnosis and assessment of AS, LV wall thickness and function, and hemodynamic severity.
- Indicators of AS are valve area (calculated using the continuity equation), jet velocity, and mean gradient. Based on these indicators, the AS is classified as:
  - Mild: Valve area >1.5 cm^2 OR jet velocity <3 m/s OR mean gradient <25 mm Hg
  - Moderate: Valve area 1–1.5 cm^2 OR jet velocity 3–4 m/s OR mean gradient 25–40 mm Hg
  - Severe: Valve area <1 cm^2 OR jet velocity >4 m/s OR mean gradient >40 mm Hg

Follow-Up & Special Considerations
Regular clinical follow-up is mandatory in all patients with asymptomatic mild to moderate AS.

Diagnostic Procedures/Other
- In patients with low-flow/low-gradient AS and LV dysfunction, dobutamine stress echocardiography is reasonable to distinguish decreased valvular opening due to low stroke volume (pseudo-obstruction) from severe AS.
- Exercise stress test can be considered in asymptomatic but not in symptomatic patients.
- Cardiac catheterization:
  - To evaluate degree of concomitant CAD before aortic valve replacement (AVR)
  - Assessment of severity of AS when noninvasive tests are inconclusive

Pathological Findings
- Stenosis of AV leading to LVH: Concentric hypertrophy
- AS is an active disease process characterized by lipid accumulation, inflammation, and calcification, with many similarities to atherosclerosis.
- Rheumatic AS due to fusion of the commissures with scarring and eventual calcification of the cusps is less common and is invariably accompanied by MV disease.

DIFFERENTIAL DIAGNOSIS
- Hypertrophic obstructive cardiomyopathy
- MI
- Other valvular diseases causing ejection systolic murmurs:
  - Pulmonary stenosis

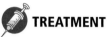 TREATMENT

MEDICATION
There is no effective medical treatment for AS; relief of obstruction is the only therapy.

ADDITIONAL TREATMENT
General Measures
- Maintain preload
- Manage anemia

Issues for Referral
Surgical evaluation for AVR

SURGERY/OTHER PROCEDURES
- AVR is only reliable treatment to relieve obstruction
- Indications:
  - Symptomatic patients with moderate to severe AS
  - Patients with severe (or moderate in some cases) AS undergoing CABG or other cardiac surgery
  - Severe AS with LV dysfunction
  - Aortic balloon valvotomy might be reasonable as a bridge to surgery in hemodynamically unstable adult patients with AS who are at high risk for AVR, or for palliation in adult patients with AS in whom AVR cannot be performed because of serious comorbid conditions. Results are generally modest, and benefits transient.
  - Aortic valves that can be placed percutaneously (or surgically through the LV apex) are under development, but are currently experimental.

Geriatric Considerations
Age by itself is not a contraindication to AVR. LV function and coronary artery anatomy are the most important predictors of outcome after AVR in this population.

IN-PATIENT CONSIDERATIONS
Initial Stabilization
- Preload maintenance
- Management of CHF:
  - Patients with evidence of pulmonary congestion can benefit from cautious treatment with digitalis (in patients with depressed LV function or AF), diuretics, and ACE inhibitors.
  - In patients with acute pulmonary edema due to AS, nitroprusside infusion may be used to reduce congestion and improve LV performance.
  - Such therapy should be performed in an ICU under the guidance of invasive hemodynamic monitoring, as excessive preload reduction can depress cardiac output and thus decrease blood pressure.

Admission Criteria
- Any new heart failure, chest pain, or syncope.
- Exacerbations of CHF
- Acute pulmonary edema

IV Fluids
- Judicious use, especially in preload-depleted patients
- Avoid in pulmonary edema

Nursing
General patient care.

Discharge Criteria
Resolution of CHF.

 ONGOING CARE

FOLLOW-UP RECOMMENDATIONS
- Depending upon severity, transthoracic echocardiography is recommended for reevaluation of asymptomatic patients:
  - Every year for severe AS
  - Every 1–2 years for moderate AS
  - Every 3–5 years for mild AS

Patient Monitoring
As in follow-up recommendation

PATIENT EDUCATION
- Recommendations for physical activity are based on the clinical exam, with special emphasis on the hemodynamic severity of the stenotic lesion.
- Physical activity is not restricted in asymptomatic patients with mild AS; these patients can participate in competitive sports.
- Patients with moderate to severe AS should avoid competitive sports that involve high dynamic and static muscular demands.

PROGNOSIS
- Exertional angina: Death within 3 years (if untreated)
- Effort syncope: Death within 2 years
- Exertional dyspnea: Death within 1 year
- Overt cardiac failure: Death within 6 months

COMPLICATIONS
- Acute heart failure
- CHF
- Infective endocarditis
- Tachy/brady arrhythmias
- Sudden death due to complete heart block or ventricular tachycardia/fibrillation

ADDITIONAL READING
- 2008 Focused update incorporated into the ACC/AHA 2006 Guidelines for the management of patients with valvular heart disease. *J Am Coll Cardiol.* 2008;52:1–142.
- Bossé Y, et al. Genomics: The next step to elucidate the etiology of calcific aortic valve stenosis. *J Am Coll Cardiol.* 2008;5:1327–36.
- Carabello BA, et al. Aortic stenosis. *Lancet.* 2009;373(9667):956–66. Epub 2009 Feb 21. Review.
- Dal-Bianco JP, et al. Management of asymptomatic severe aortic stenosis. *J Am Coll Cardiol.* 2008; 52(16):1279–92. Review.

 CODES

ICD9
- 395.0 Rheumatic aortic stenosis
- 424.1 Aortic valve disorders
- 746.3 Congenital stenosis of aortic valve

CLINICAL PEARLS
- Systolic hypertension does not exclude severe stenosis.
- Murmurs may become inaudible in patients with cardiac failure.
- After clinical evaluation, echocardiography is the 1st diagnostic test to assess severity of aortic stenosis.

ACTIVATED PROTEIN C

Oveys Mansuri

BASICS

DESCRIPTION
- Activated protein C (APC) promotes fibrinolysis and inhibits thrombosis.
- FDA approved for use in patients with sepsis and shock:
  - Brand name: Xigris (manufactured by Eli Lilly)
  - Generic name: Activated drotrecogin alfa

Genetics
- Gene symbol: PROC
- Located 2nd chromosome

Action
- Protein C (a serine protease) promotes anticoagulation by inhibiting Factor V and providing additional cytoprotection:
  - Bound to endothelial protein C receptor (EPCR), it produces a cytoprotective effect.
  - Not bound to EPCR, it produces anticoagulative effects.
- APC also inhibits tumor necrosis factor production, blocks leukocyte adhesion to selectins, and limits inflammatory responses.

DIAGNOSIS

HISTORY
History of new-onset septic shock refractory to medical/surgical management;
- Apace II score ≥25

PHYSICAL EXAM
- Fever
- Hypotension

DIAGNOSTIC TESTS & INTERPRETATION
Lab
- Pretreatment CBC to evaluate for increased WBC and Hgb/Hct/Plt levels
- Coagulation studies
- Chemistry panel

Imaging
As required for the diagnosis of sepsis/septic shock

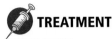 TREATMENT

MEDICATION
- Continuous infusions for 96 hours in 12-hour periods
- Maximum duration of each infusion is 12 hours.
- Dosing formula: mg of APC = (patient weight in kg) × (24 mcg/kg/hr) × (hours of infusion)/1,000

ADDITIONAL TREATMENT
General Measures
APC maybe coadministered with subcutaneous heparin.

Issues for Referral
- Pharmacy consultation
- ICU consultation

Additional Therapies
For the complex management of sepsis and septic shock, see Dellinger et al., 2004.

COMPLEMENTARY & ALTERNATIVE THERAPIES
See Dellinger et al., 2004.

> **ALERT**
> - Contraindications: Active internal bleeding, recent hemorrhagic stroke, recent head trauma, trauma patients with risk for bleeding, epidural catheter, brain mass/malignancy
> - Caution when using other drugs that may affect coagulation.
> - No strong evidence against concomitant use of prophylactic heparin unless other concern for bleeding is present.

Pediatric Considerations
Per manufacturer warning issued for contraindication of use in pediatric patient population

Pregnancy Considerations
Pregnancy Category C: Adverse effect on fetus in animal studies, no adequate studies in humans; potential benefits may warrant use in pregnant women regardless of potential risks.

IN-PATIENT CONSIDERATIONS
Initial Stabilization
Evaluate risk of bleeding and any contraindications before administering APC.

Admission Criteria
APC should be administered in ICU setting with close monitoring given risks for bleeding. Most patients eligible to receive APC have high acuity and severity and are in need of ICU care.

IV Fluids
- Adequate fluid resuscitation with use of crystalloid replacement (i.e., 0.9% NS or LR)
- Ensure appropriate central venous access; also monitor volume status (CVP), and central venous oxygenation for these patients.

Nursing
Close monitoring for signs of bleeding

Discharge Criteria
Resolution or significant improvement in sepsis and septic shock

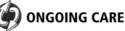 ONGOING CARE

FOLLOW-UP RECOMMENDATIONS
- Continue to monitor hematologic indicators if any concern for bleeding: CBC, coagulation studies
- At discharge from ICU, compile detailed sign-out to assure safe and seamless transfer of care to floor or for discharge to home and follow-up with primary care physician.

Patient Monitoring
Continue close monitoring while in ICU

PROGNOSIS
PROWESS trial: 28-day mortality: 24.7%, statistically insignificant increase in bleeding:
- 6.1% decrease in mortality in severe sepsis
- 13% decrease in mortality when Apache II $\geq$24

COMPLICATIONS
- Bleeding
- Death

ADDITIONAL READING

- Bernard GR, et al. Efficacy and safety of recombinant human activated protein C for severe sepsis. N Engl J Med. 2001;699–709.
- Dellinger RP , Carlet JM, Masur H, et al. Surviving Sepsis Campaign guidelines for management of severe sepsis and septic shock. Crit Care Med. 2004;32:858–73.
- Khan A, et al. Prevalence of serious bleeding events and intracranial hemorrhage in patients receiving activated protein C: A systematic review and meta-analysis. Respir Care. 2010;55(7):901–10.
- Rivers E, et al. Early goal-directed therapy in the treatment of severe sepsis and septic shock. N Engl J Med. 2001;345:1368–77.
- Steingrub JS, et al. A prospective, observational study of Xigris use in the United States (XEUS). J Crit Care. 2010;25:660.e9–660.e16.
- Wheeler A, et al. A retrospective observational study of drotrecogin alfa (activated) in adults with severe sepsis: Comparison with a controlled clinical trial. Crit Care Med. 2008;36:14–23.

 CODES

ICD9
- 038.9 Unspecified septicemia
- 785.50 Shock, unspecified
- 785.52 Septic shock

CLINICAL PEARLS

- APC is still undergoing research to determine its role in sepsis/shock.
- Indications vary; general guidelines suggest best for septic shock refractory to medical/surgical management and/or Apache II score $\geq$25
- Must weigh risk vs. benefit of bleeding complications
- Review contraindications carefully.
- ICU monitoring and care is key.

APPENDICITIS

Andrew Deroo

BASICS

DESCRIPTION
Acute appendicitis is an inflammation of the appendix leading to localized peritonitis and possible appendical rupture if left untreated.

EPIDEMIOLOGY
Incidence
250,000 reported cases a year in the US

PATHOPHYSIOLOGY
Obstruction of the appendical orifice leads to bacterial overgrowth, infection, and inflammation.

ETIOLOGY
• Fecalith
• Lymphoid hyperplasia
• Neoplasm
• Parasites

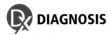

DIAGNOSIS

HISTORY
• Timing and duration of abdominal pain is an important part of the history.
• Migration of pain from periumbical to right lower quadrant is common.
• Many patients will have accompanying symptoms including nausea, vomiting, diarrhea, and anorexia.
• It is important to elicit other symptoms that may point to another diagnosis, especially gynecologic symptoms in women.
• Presentation and location of pain can be atypical in pregnant women.

PHYSICAL EXAM
• Focused abdominal exam
• Localized pain and peritonitis over McBurney's point
• Guarding, rebound, psoas sign, and Rovsing's sign have low sensitivity and specificity.

DIAGNOSTIC TESTS & INTERPRETATION
Lab
• CBC often elevated
• UA
• Pregnancy test in women
• 10% of patients will have normal WBC

Imaging
Initial approach
• Considered a clinical diagnosis
• US with overall accuracy of 90–94%, but appendix is unable to be visualized in most patients
• US most useful in young children
• CT scan with overall accuracy of 90–94%

Follow-Up & Special Considerations
If appendix is not visualized on CT and clinical concern is low, can monitor patient with serial abdominal exams

Diagnostic Procedures/Other
• Diagnostic laparoscopy with appendectomy if work-up equivocal and clinical suspicion is high
• Perforated appendicitis with periappendicular abscess requires surgical or IR drainage and interval appendectomy.

Pathological Findings
Inflamed, injected appendix with periappendiceal fat changes

DIFFERENTIAL DIAGNOSIS
• Meckel's diverticulitis
• Mesenteric adenitis
• Intussusception
• Appendical/colonic diverticulitis
• Crohn disease
• Ureteral colic/kidney stones
• Pyelonephritis
• Gastroenteritis/GERD/PUD
• PID
• Ectopic pregnancy
• Ovarian torsion/cyst
• UTI

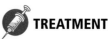

TREATMENT

MEDICATION
Antibiotics to cover enteric gram-negative bacteria and anaerobes

ADDITIONAL TREATMENT
General Measures
Like all forms of sepsis, prompt and appropriate antibiotic coverage and surgical source control of the infection is key.

Issues for Referral
If appendical abscess is treated with IR drainage, patient will need IR follow-up for drain removal and surgical referral for interval appendectomy.

SURGERY/OTHER PROCEDURES

- Laparoscopic or open appendectomy
- Diagnostic laparoscopy for diagnostic dilemmas
- IR drainage of ruptured appendicitis with periappendicular abscess
- Laparoscopic and open procedures are associated with similar hospital LOS, morbidity, and mortality, but a higher wound infection rate is found with open appendectomies.

IN-PATIENT CONSIDERATIONS

Initial Stabilization

- Fluid resuscitation
- Antibiotics

IV Fluids

Resuscitative fluids with either LR or NS

Nursing

Routine nursing care

Discharge Criteria

- Patients with nonperforated appendicitis usually can be discharged within 24 hours when tolerating PO.
- Patients with perforated appendicitis may require prolonged hospital stay for IV antibiotic and IV fluids until resolution of possible ileus, resolution of leukocytosis, and pain.

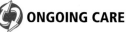 ONGOING CARE

FOLLOW-UP RECOMMENDATIONS

Routine postop follow-up in 1–2 weeks

DIET

Regular diet as soon as tolerating POs

PATIENT EDUCATION

- Routine postop care
- Avoid heavy lifting or strenuous exercise
- Warn of signs of abscess and wound infection

PROGNOSIS

- Good; low-mortality in nonperforated cases
- Higher morbidity and mortality in elderly patients

COMPLICATIONS

- Wound infection is most likely in open appendectomy for perforated appendicitis; <5% in laparoscopic cases for nonperforated appendicitis.
- Intra-abdominal abscess

ADDITIONAL READING

- Appendicitis. In: Townsend CM, et al., eds. *Sabiston Textbook of Surgery*, 18th ed. Philadelphia: WB Saunders, 2007.
- Humes DJ, et al. Acute appendicitis. *BMJ*. 2006;333: 530–4.
- Paulson EK, et al. Suspected appendicitis. *NEJM*. 2003;348(3):236–42.

 CODES

ICD9

- 540.0 Acute appendicitis with generalized peritonitis
- 540.9 Acute appendicitis without mention of peritonitis
- 541 Appendicitis, unqualified

CLINICAL PEARLS

- In equivocal cases based on history, laboratory values, and imaging, observation is acceptable.
- In patients >50 years of age, assume neoplasm as cause until proven otherwise. Patients should have colonoscopy after discharge for colon cancer screening.

ARRHYTHMIAS, VENTRICULAR AND DIRECT CURRENT DEFIBRILLATION

Stephen B. Heitner
Isaac Halickman

 BASICS

DESCRIPTION
- Defective myocardial conduction resulting from the origin of cardiac impulses anywhere distal to the His bundle, and resulting in sequences of rapidly conducted ventricular beats
- Subtypes:
  - Premature ventricular beats (PVCs): Wide-complex QRS beats in isolation or couplets.
  - Ventricular tachycardia (VT): Wide-complex tachycardia ranging from 100–250 bpm:
    o Nonsustained (NSVT): 3 beats to 30 seconds.
    o Sustained (VT): >30 second duration or requiring immediate therapy due to hemodynamic collapse
    o Monomorphic
    o Polymorphic
    o Torsades de pointes (discussed elsewhere)
  - Ventricular fibrillation (VF) is an uncoordinated contraction of the cardiac muscle of the ventricles in the heart, making them tremble rather than contract properly, resulting in hemodynamic collapse.
- System(s) affected: Cardiovascular

EPIDEMIOLOGY
Incidence
- The overall incidence is 0.1–0.2%/year (1).
- Up to 3% of healthy men have PVC/NSVT (2).
- Up to 80% of post-MI patients will have PVCs, 6.8% of patients have NSVT, and 0.1% will have VT in first 24 hours post-MI (3).
- 48% of patients with an implantable cardiac defibrillator (ICD) for cardiomyopathy and left ventricular ejection fraction (LVEF) <30% will have VT/VF within the 1st year post-implantation (4).

RISK FACTORS
- Structural heart disease:
  - Recent MI (polymorphic VT/VF) or remote MI (monomorphic VT/VF)
  - Both ischemic and nonischemic cardiomyopathy with depressed LVEF (highest incidence with LVEF <30%) (5,6)
  - Prior surgery for congenital heart disease (tetralogy of Fallot)
  - LV hypertrophy/hypertrophic obstructive cardiomyopathy (HOCM)
  - Valvular heart disease
  - Arrhythmogenic right ventricular (RV) dysplasia
- Prior history of cardiac arrest
- Family history of sudden cardiac death
- Coexisting congenital or genetic syndrome (e.g., trisomy 21)

Genetics
- Brugada syndrome:
  - Mutations in a gene responsible for the sodium channel (SCN5A) have been identified in ~20% of families with Brugada syndrome.
- Catecholaminergic polymorphic ventricular tachycardia (CPVT):
  - Autosomal recessive mutation of cardiac ryanodine receptor type 2 (RyR2) or calsequestrin 2 (CASQ2) gene mutations

- HOCM:
  - Autosomal dominant mutation in genes that encode protein constituents of the sarcomere
  - >450 different mutations have been identified within 13 myofilament-related genes.
- Channelopathies: Discussed under long-QT syndromes

PATHOPHYSIOLOGY
- Reentrant arrhythmia:
  - Responsible for most VT/VF in patients with ischemic and structural heart disease
  - Surviving myocardial tissue separated by connective tissue provides serpentine routes of activation traversing infarcted areas that can establish reentry pathways
- Triggered activity:
  - Catecholamine-dependent
  - Terminated by the Valsalva maneuver, adenosine, and verapamil
  - Generally located in the RV outflow tract
- Increased automaticity:
  - Unusual cause of VT/VF, but should be considered for electrophysiologic evaluation if the arrhythmia is not associated with structural heart disease and is not suppressed with adenosine

ETIOLOGY
- Myocardial scar tissue reentry:
  - Most frequently in post-infarction and surgical patients, particularly at the infarct border zone
  - Typically monomorphic VT
- Sarcoplasmic reticulum calcium channel disorders (RyR2 and CASQ2):
  - Exercise-induced monomorphic VT that progresses to polymorphic VT/VF
  - Seen in catecholaminergic polymorphic ventricular tachycardia
- Early after-depolarizations (EADs):
  - Catecholamine-dependent
  - Seen in idiopathic RV and LV outflow tract (RVOT and LVOT) VT
- QT prolongation: Discussed elsewhere

COMMONLY ASSOCIATED CONDITIONS
- Hypokalemia
- Hypomagnesemia
- Ephedrine containing medications
- Psychotropic medications are frequently associated with QT prolongation.
- Chronic obstructive pulmonary disease
- Thyrotoxicosis
- Pericarditis
- CHF
- Muscular or myotonic dystrophies
- Sarcoidosis
- Cardiac sarcoidosis
- Myocarditis
- Muscular dystrophies
- Any systemic illness with underlying myocardial substrate for VT will predispose to arrhythmogenesis

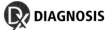 DIAGNOSIS

HISTORY
- Palpitations, syncope, presyncope, chest pain or a history of MI
- Shortness of breath or symptoms suggestive of CHF
- Onset during emotional or physical stress may suggest a catecholamine-dependent mechanism.
- Family history of premature or death

PHYSICAL EXAM
- Signs of shock necessitating urgent treatment need to be sought immediately; the presence of a pulse and measurable blood pressure effectively exclude VF.
- Heart rate is typically >100 bpm (occasionally may have "slow VT"). VT rates generally do not exceed 250 bpm.
- Blood pressure and pulse intensity may show variation, and jugular venous pressure may show cannon A-waves indicative of atrioventricular (AV) dissociation.
- Valsalva maneuver or carotid sinus massage can cause a transient increase in vagal tone and disrupt 1:1 AV relationships, helping to demonstrate AV dissociation.
- Pulmonary rales, peripheral edema, and cyanosis indicating CHF.

DIAGNOSTIC TESTS & INTERPRETATION
Resting 12-lead ECG is essential for the diagnosis (1)[A]:
- Wide-complex tachycardia with QRS duration >120 ms (the wider the complex, the more likely VT)
- Monomorphic VT can frequently be classified as either LBBB or RBBB pattern.
- AV dissociation: P-wave activity independent of QRS complexes. The use of vagal maneuvers may help demonstrate this.
- VT beats may be identical to those of PVCs during sinus rhythm on a prior ECG.
- If there is a preexisting bundle branch block, a contralateral bundle branch block pattern suggests VT.
- It is important to differentiate supraventricular tachycardias (SVT) with aberrant conduction from stable VT. Patients with a history of ischemic heart disease most likely have VT.

Lab
Cardiac enzymes (cardiac-specific troponins with or without CK and CK-MB), serum electrolytes, thyroid function tests, brain natriuretic peptide

Imaging
Initial approach
Echocardiography is essential for the evaluation of all patients with a history of VT/VF, for assessment of LV function and the presence of structural heart disease (I) (7)[B].

Follow-Up & Special Considerations
- Exercise or pharmacologic stress testing with and without an imaging modality (echo or nuclear) is recommended when ischemia is suspected (I)(7)[B].
- Coronary angiography is recommended in life-threatening events, or when there is a high probability of underlying ischemic disease (7)(IIa)[C]
- Cardiac MRI and CT can be useful when echocardiography is not helpful (7)(IIa)[B].

Diagnostic Procedures/Other
- Ambulatory ECG (I)[A], event monitors (I)[B], and implantable recorders (I)(7)[B]
- Signal averaged ECG and T-wave alternans are specialized techniques (IIa) (7)[A].
- Electrophysiological testing is recommended in patients with a history of MI and symptoms suggestive of VT/VF (I)[B], VT ablation (I)[B], and undiagnosed wide complex rhythms (I)(7)[C].

DIFFERENTIAL DIAGNOSIS
- SVT with aberrant conduction
- Tachyarrhythmia with underlying preexcitation (Wolf-Parkinson-White syndrome)

TREATMENT

MEDICATION
- Antiarrhythmic drugs are largely relegated to supportive role in patients with ICD:
  - IV β-blockers are recommended in hemodynamically stable ischemic, sustained polymorphic VT (I) (7)[B].
  - Consider amiodarone for sustained monomorphic (IIa) [C] sustained polymorphic VT (I)[C], and incessant VT (7) (IIa)[B].
  - Consider procainamide for sustained monomorphic (IIa)[B] and incessant VT (IIa) (7)[B].
  - Consider lidocaine for monomorphic VT suspected to be ischemic (IIb)[C], or in sustained polymorphic VT (IIb) (7)[C].

ADDITIONAL TREATMENT
- Defibrillation: Monophasic dose of 360 J or biphasic dose of 150–200 J:
  - Direct-current cardioversion with appropriate sedation as necessary for sustained monomorphic (I)[B] and polymorphic VT (I)[B].
  - Automatic external defibrillator should be used in out-of-hospital VT/VF (I)[C].
- Implantable cardiac defibrillators
  - Secondary prevention for sudden cardiac death in patients with dilated cardiomyopathy (I)[A], HOCM (I)[B], Arrhythmogenic RV cardiomyopathy (I)[B], VT/VF survivors with an EF <40% (I)[A], Brugada syndrome (I)[C], and idiopathic VT (IIb)[C].
  - Primary prevention with ICD is indicated for depressed LV systolic function in both ischemic and nonischemic cardiomyopathies, and the primary VTs.
- Consider catheter ablation in patients at low risk for arrhythmia-associated death and sustained monomorphic VT (I)[C], bundle branch reentrant arrhythmia (I)[C], and incessant VT (I)[C].
- Surgical therapy in arrhythmias resistant to ablation and medical modalities

General Measures
- Standard supportive measures as indicated by the hemodynamic scenario
- Telemetry monitoring
- ICU-level care if hemodynamically compromised
- Correct electrolyte imbalances (IIb)[B].
- Revascularization (percutaneous or surgical) if ischemic VT/VF or incessant VT (I)[C]

Issues for Referral
- All patients with malignant arrhythmias should be seen by a cardiologist.
- Electrophysiology referral for primary, secondary prevention with ICD placement, as well as for possible VT ablation in certain instances

IN-PATIENT CONSIDERATIONS
Initial Stabilization
- Hospitalization in most cases
- Close telemetry and hemodynamic monitoring
- Remove causal agent (e.g., ischemia, vasopressors, electrolyte imbalance, digoxin toxicity).
- Sustained VT: IV amiodarone, lidocaine, or procainamide, followed by an infusion.
- For VT that is refractory, hemodynamically significant, or associated with angina, immediate DC cardioversion is indicated.

ONGOING CARE

FOLLOW-UP RECOMMENDATIONS
Outpatient cardiologist follow-up is almost always indicated.

Patient Monitoring
- Ambulatory ECG to monitor response to therapy or disease burden. Regular ICD interrogation (in office q3–6mon or monthly via telephone)
- LFTs, thyroid functions, renal function, electrolytes, and serial ECGs in patients requiring antiarrhythmic medications

PATIENT EDUCATION
ICD-specific education regarding shock therapy, and limitations with regards to having implantable hardware (MRI, metal detectors, etc.)

PROGNOSIS
Prognosis varies according to the type of VT.

COMPLICATIONS
- Syncope, anoxic brain injury, MI, end-organ hypoperfusion, and sudden death in the acute setting
- Tachycardia-induced cardiomyopathy in primary untreated VT

REFERENCES
1. Libby P, et al., eds. *Braunwald's Heart Disease: A Textbook of Cardiovascular Medicine*, 8th ed. Philadelphia: Saunders, 2007.
2. Jouven X, et al. Long-term outcome in asymptomatic men with exercise-induced premature ventricular depolarizations. *N Engl J Med*. 2000;343:826–33.
3. Maggioni AP, et al., on behalf of GISSI-2 Investigators. Prevalence and prognostic significance of ventricular arrhythmias after acute myocardial infarction in the fibrinolytic era: GISSI results. *Circulation*. 1993;87:312–22.
4. Freedberg NA, et al. Recurrence of symptomatic ventricular arrhythmias in patients with implantable cardioverter defibrillator after the first device therapy: Implications for antiarrhythmic therapy and driving restrictions. CARE Group. *J Am Coll Cardiol*. 2001;37:1910–15.
5. Moss AJ, et al., the Multicenter Automatic Defibrillator Implantation Trial II Investigators. Prophylactic implantation of a defibrillator in patients with myocardial infarction and reduced ejection fraction. *N Engl J Med*. 2002;346:877–83.
6. Bardy GH, et al., Sudden Cardiac Death in Heart Failure Trial (SCD-HeFT) Investigators. Amiodarone or an implantable cardioverter-defibrillator for congestive heart failure. *N Engl J Med*. 2005;352:225–37.
7. Zipes D, et al. ACC/AHA/ESC 2006 Guidelines for Management of Patients With Ventricular Arrhythmias and the Prevention of Sudden Cardiac Death—Executive Summary. *Circulation*. 2006;114;1088–132.

ADDITIONAL READING
- 2005 American Heart Association Guidelines for Cardiopulmonary Resuscitation and Emergency Cardiovascular Care. *Circulation*. 2005;112(Suppl I):IV-1–IV-5.

 CODES

ICD9
- 427.1 Paroxysmal ventricular tachycardia
- 427.69 Other premature beats
- 427.9 Cardiac dysrhythmia, unspecified

CLINICAL PEARLS
- Ventricular dysrhythmias are usually life-threatening, and in most instances are secondary to an underlying cardiomyopathy. Initial investigation for ischemic and nonischemic cardiomyopathy is mandatory.
- Initial therapy is electrical cardioversion in the hemodynamically unstable patient, but stable patients may require antiarrhythmic medication (e.g., amiodarone, lidocaine, procainamide) for suppression in the acute setting.
- Therapy is usually multimodal, and may include medications, devices (ICD), ablation, and/or surgery, but the underlying etiology always needs careful elucidation.

ARTERIAL BLOOD GAS ANALYSIS (ABG)

Aditya Uppalapati
Roopa Kohli-Seth

Values needed: pH, PCO_2, Bicarbonate (HCO_3), Sodium (Na^+), Chloride (Cl^-), Albumin

Normal values: pH = 7.40, PCO_2 = 40 mm Hg, HCO_3 = 24 mEq/L, Na^+ = 135–145 mEq/L, Cl^- = 96–106 mEq/L, Albumin = 4 g/dL

1) Assess the clinical scenario in the interpretation of ABGs

2) Validate PH

$(H^+) = 24 \times PCO_2/HCO_3$

40 nm = pH 7.40

If represented pH as 7.xx, 80 − xx = nm

pH	NmH^+
7.50	32
7.40	40
7.30	50
7.20	63

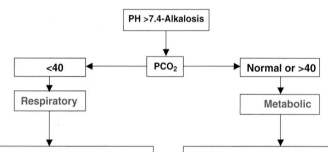

PH >7.4-Alkalosis

PCO_2

<40 → → **Respiratory**

Normal or >40 → **Metabolic**

---

1) Calculate expected change in pH for changes in PCO_2

Acute: pH = (40 − measured PCO_2) × 0.008

Chronic: pH = (40 − measured PCO_2) × 0.003

2) Calculate compensatory metabolic change

Acute: Every 10 decr. PCO_2, HCO_3 decr. 2

Chronic: Every 10 decr. PCO_2, HCO_3 decr. 5

Act > Cal: Concomitant metabolic alkalosis
Act = Cal: Appropriate compensation
Act < Cal: Concomitant metabolic acidosis

(Act, actual; Cal, Calculated, decr., decrease.)

---

1) Check urine Chloride (Cl^-)

Urine Cl <20: Chloride responsive

Urine Cl >20: Chloride resistant

2) Calculate compensatory PCO_2

Expected PCO_2 = 0.7 × (Measured HCO_3 − 24)

Act = Cal: Appropriate
Act < Cal: Concomitant respiratory alkalosis
Act > Cal: Concomitant respiratory acidosis

(Act, actual; Cal, Calculated)

CODES

ICD9
V72.69 Other laboratory examination

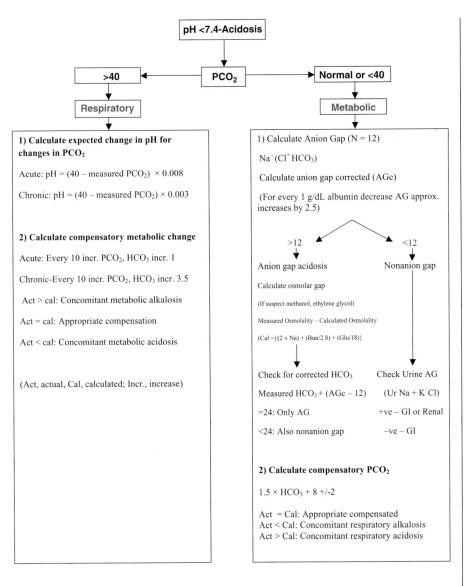

pH <7.4-Acidosis

PCO₂

>40 → **Respiratory**

Normal or <40 → **Metabolic**

Respiratory side:

1) Calculate expected change in pH for changes in PCO₂

Acute: pH = (40 – measured PCO₂) × 0.008

Chronic: pH = (40 – measured PCO₂) × 0.003

2) Calculate compensatory metabolic change

Acute: Every 10 incr. PCO₂, HCO₃ incr. 1

Chronic-Every 10 incr. PCO₂, HCO₃ incr. 3.5

Act > cal: Concomitant metabolic alkalosis

Act = cal: Appropriate compensation

Act < cal: Concomitant metabolic acidosis

(Act, actual, Cal, calculated; Incr., increase)

Metabolic side:

1) Calculate Anion Gap (N = 12)

Na⁻ (Cl⁺ HCO₃)

Calculate anion gap corrected (AGc)

(For every 1 g/dL albumin decrease AG approx. increases by 2.5)

>12 → Anion gap acidosis

<12 → Nonanion gap

Anion gap acidosis:

Calculate osmolar gap

(If suspect methanol, ethylene glycol)

Measured Osmolality – Calculated Osmolality

(Cal ={(2 × Na) + (Bun/2.8) + (Glu/18)}

Check for corrected HCO₃

Measured HCO₃ + (AGc – 12)

=24: Only AG

<24: Also nonanion gap

Nonanion gap:

Check Urine AG

(Ur Na + K⁻Cl)

+ve – GI or Renal

–ve – GI

2) Calculate compensatory PCO₂

1.5 × HCO₃ + 8 +/-2

Act = Cal: Appropriate compensated
Act < Cal: Concomitant respiratory alkalosis
Act > Cal: Concomitant respiratory acidosis

ARTERIAL LINE CANNULATION

Jose R. Yunen
Vicente San Martín

PROCEDURE

INDICATIONS

- Need for continuous blood pressure monitoring
- Need for access to the arterial circulation for measurement of arterial oxygenation, arterial carbon dioxide, and/or frequent blood sampling
- Hemodynamic instability requiring the use and titration of vasopressors or inotropes

CONTRAINDICATIONS

- Systemic anticoagulation (relative)
- Infection in the skin or subcutaneous tissues around cannulation site
- Compromised flow distal to cannulation site
- Injury distal to cannulation site

TECHNIQUE

See algorithm.

```
┌──────────────────────────────────────────────┐
│ Obtain patient or next of kin written consent │
└──────────────────────────────────────────────┘
                      ↓
┌──────────────────────────────────────────────┐
│            Perform universal protocol          │
└──────────────────────────────────────────────┘
                      ↓
┌──────────────────────────────────────────────┐
│             Identify cannulation site          │
└──────────────────────────────────────────────┘
```

Perform Allen test to confirm collateral circulation

Based on patient's anatomy, clinical situation, and/or the use of real-time ultrasound

```
┌──────────────────────────────────────────────┐
│                  Preparation                    │
└──────────────────────────────────────────────┘
```

Recommended: 2% aqueous chlorhexidine-gluconate solution

If not available, use alcohol swabs or povidone-iodine antiseptics (do not use if an allergy to iodine is known); both of them should dry

```
┌──────────────────────────────────────────────┐
│                 Drape (full body)               │
└──────────────────────────────────────────────┘
                      ↓
┌──────────────────────────────────────────────────────────────────┐
│ Infiltrate skin and tissue around the vessel with a local anesthetic │
└──────────────────────────────────────────────────────────────────┘
```

1% or 2% lidocaine solution

Use alternative local anesthetics if an allergy to lidocaine is known

```
┌──────────────────────────────────────────────┐
│          Identify artery with gentle pressure.  │
└──────────────────────────────────────────────┘
                      ↓
┌──────────────────────────────────────────────────────────────┐
│ Small-gauge finder needle angled 45 degrees toward the artery   │
└──────────────────────────────────────────────────────────────┘
```

Enter skin just distal to palpated artery site

```
┌──────────────────────────────────────────────┐
│      Thread the guide wire into the gauge needle │
└──────────────────────────────────────────────┘
                      ↓
```

Seldinger technique

52

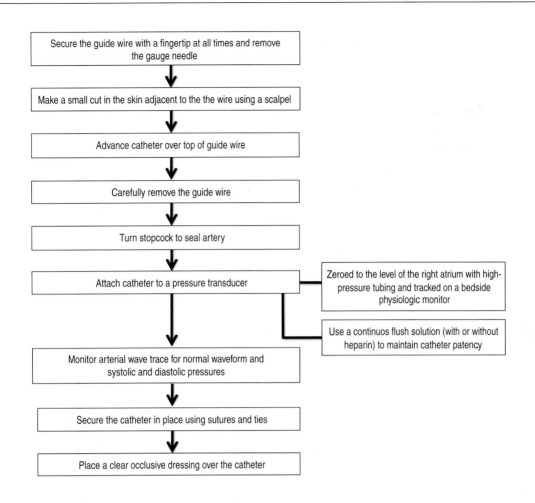

Secure the guide wire with a fingertip at all times and remove the gauge needle

↓

Make a small cut in the skin adjacent to the the wire using a scalpel

↓

Advance catheter over top of guide wire

↓

Carefully remove the guide wire

↓

Turn stopcock to seal artery

↓

Attach catheter to a pressure transducer → Zeroed to the level of the right atrium with high-pressure tubing and tracked on a bedside physiologic monitor

Use a continuos flush solution (with or without heparin) to maintain catheter patency

↓

Monitor arterial wave trace for normal waveform and systolic and diastolic pressures

↓

Secure the catheter in place using sutures and ties

↓

Place a clear occlusive dressing over the catheter

COMPLICATIONS
- Arterial vasospasm
- Infection
- Dissection
- Transection
- Thrombosis
- Embolization (clot or air during catheter flushing)
- Hematoma
- Aneurysm formation

ADDITIONAL READING
- Tegtmeyer K, et al. Placement of an arterial line. *N Engl J Med*. 2006; 354:e13

ASCITES

Kagan Ilya

 BASICS

DESCRIPTION
- Ascites is an abnormal accumulation of fluid within the peritoneal cavity.
- High serum-ascites albumin gradient (SAAG >1.1 g/dL) ascites: Portal hypertension, portal vein occlusion, congestive heart failure
- Low SAAG <1.1 g/dL: Diseased peritoneum (malignant conditions, infections), hypoalbuminemia, miscellaneous conditions.
- Grading:
  – Grade 1: Mild ascites detectable only by US examination
  – Grade 2: Moderate ascites manifested by moderate symmetrical distension of abdomen
  – Grade 3: Large ascites with marked abdominal distention
- Refractory ascites: Lack response to high dose of diuretics
- System(s) affected: Liver/Cardiovascular

EPIDEMIOLOGY
- Most common cause of ascites is cirrhosis or other forms of severe liver disease; 85% of cases
- Within 10 years after diagnosis of compensated cirrhosis, 58% of patients will have developed ascites.

PATHOPHYSIOLOGY
- Portal hypertension:
  – Increased hepatic resistance to portal flow due to cirrhosis causes development of portal hypertension and collateral vein formation. As portal hypertension develops, splanchnic vasodilatation occurs due to the enhance production of nitric oxide and other vasodilators.
  – The combination of portal hypertension and splanchnic arterial vasodilatation alters intestinal capillary pressure and permeability, which facilitates the accumulation of the retained fluid in the abdominal cavity
- Hypoalbuminemia:
  – Extravasation of fluid from plasma to the abdominal cavity is caused by reduced plasma oncotic pressure.
- Malignant conditions:
  – Blockage of the draining lymphatic channels (ovarian or urinary bladder cancer)
  – Obstruction or compression of portal veins or liver failure due to metastases (colonic, lung, pancreatic cancer)

ETIOLOGY
- Portal hypertension (SAAG >1.1 g/dL):
  – Liver disease:
    ◦ Liver cirrhosis
    ◦ Alcoholic hepatitis
    ◦ Portal vein thrombosis
    ◦ Liver metastases
  – Hepatic congestion:
    ◦ Congestive heart failure
    ◦ Constrictive pericarditis
    ◦ Tricuspid insufficiency
    ◦ Budd-Chiari syndrome

- Hypoalbuminemia (SAAG <1.1 g/dL):
  – Nephrotic syndrome
  – Protein-losing enteropathy
  – Severe malnutrition with anasarca
- Infections (SAAG <1.1 g/dL):
  – Bacterial peritonitis
  – Tuberculous peritonitis
  – Fungal peritonitis
  – HIV-associated peritonitis
- Malignancy (SAAG <1.1 g/dL):
  – Peritoneal carcinomatosis
  – Primary mesothelioma
  – Pseudomyxoma peritonei
  – Hepatocellular carcinoma
- Other conditions (SAAG <1.1 g/dL):
  – Chylous ascites
  – Bile ascites
  – Urine ascites
  – Pancreatic ascites
  – Ovarian disease
  – Familial Mediterranean fever
  – Vasculitis
  – Granulomatous peritonitis
  – Eosinophilic peritonitis
  – Myxedema

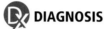 **DIAGNOSIS**

HISTORY
- Increasing abdominal girth
- Abdominal and flank pain
- Anorexia
- Nausea
- Early satiety
- Dyspnea
- Weigh gain
- Risk factors of liver disease
  – Ethanol consumption
  – History of viral hepatitis
  – Transfusions
  – Tattoos
  – Jaundice
  – Birth in an area endemic for hepatitis
- History of cancer: Malignant ascites
- Fever: Primary or secondary peritonitis
- Immigrants/immunocompromised patients/severe malnourished alcoholics/history of tuberculosis; tuberculous peritonitis.
- Risk factors of CHF
- Family history of liver disease
- Risk factors for nonalcoholic steatohepatitis (obesity, diabetes and hypolipidemia)

PHYSICAL EXAM
- Abdominal distension
- Bulging flanks
- Tightly stretched skin
- Everted umbilicus/umbilical hernia
- Abdominal fluid wave
- Shifting dullness
- Puddle sign

- Signs of liver disease and cirrhosis:
  – Vascular spiders
  – Palmar erythema
  – Jaundice
  – Muscle wasting
  – Gynecomastia
  – Dupuytren's contracture
- Signs of CHF:
  – Anasarca
  – Pleural effusion
  – Elevated jugular venous pressure

DIAGNOSTIC TESTS & INTERPRETATION
Lab
- Abdominal paracentesis should be performed in all adult patient presenting with new-onset ascites (1,2)[C].
- Routine studies of ascites fluid:
  – Cell count:
    ◦ >250/mm³ neutrophils are highly suggestive bacterial peritonitis
  – Albumin in ascites fluid and serum:
    ◦ High SAAG (>1.1 g/dL) ascites (portal hypertension, portal vein occlusion, congestive heart failure)
  – Low SAAG <1.1 g/dL: Diseased peritoneum (malignant conditions, infections), hypoalbuminemia, miscellaneous conditions
- Of use in specific circumstances:
  – Total protein:
    ◦ Value >1 g/dL suggests secondary peritonitis.
  – Bacterial cultures in blood culture bottles (10 mL of fluid)
  – Glucose:
    ◦ Values <50 mg/dL suggest secondary peritonitis instead of SBP.
  – Lactate dehydrogenase:
    ◦ Values greater than the upper limit of normal for serum suggest secondary peritonitis instead of SBP.
  – Amylase:
    ◦ Values markedly elevated (often >2000 U/liter or 5× serum levels) in patients with pancreatic ascites or hollow viscus perforation
  – Triglyceride:
    ◦ Values >200 mg/dL suggest chylous ascites
  – Carcinoembryonic antigen:
    ◦ Values >5 ng/mL suggest hollow viscus perforation
  – Cytology
  – Mycobacterial culture
- Blood tests:
  – Liver function test
  – Coagulation test
  – Serum creatinine
  – Electrolytes
- Urinary tests:
  – Sodium (preferably from a 24-hour urine collection)
  – Protein (preferably from a 24-hour urine collection)

Imaging
Abdominal US or CT scan

Diagnostic Procedures/Other
- Endoscopy of upper GI tract
- Doppler US
- Liver biopsy for selected patients (liver disease of unclear type or cause)
- Diagnostic laparoscopy

Pathological Findings
Peritoneal biopsy may demonstrate tuberculosis or malignancy.

DIFFERENTIAL DIAGNOSIS
- Obesity
- Intestinal obstruction
- Pregnancy
- Ovaries cyst or carcinoma
- Ascites fluid type:
  - High SAAG (>1.1 g/dL)
  - Low SAAG (<1.1 g/d)

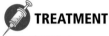 # TREATMENT

MEDICATION
- Diuretics:
  - Spironolactone 50–100 mg/d (or amiloride 5–10 mg/d) to reach goal of weigh loss: 300–500 g/d (C). If needed, doses to be increased every 7 days up to 400 mg/d (1,2)[C].
  - Furosemide 20–40 mg/d (up to 160 mg/d if need)
- Precautions and adverse reactions:
  - Renal failure of prerenal origin
  - Hyperkalemia due to spironolactone
  - Hypokalemia due to furosemide
  - Muscle cramps due to diuretic therapy
  - Gynecomastia due to spironolactone
- Possible interactions:
  - ACE inhibitors and spironolactone
  - Spironolactone and potassium supplements.
- Ascites caused by peritoneal carcinomatosis does not respond to diuretics.

ADDITIONAL TREATMENT
General Measures
- Low-sodium diet of ∼2000 mg/d (90 mmol)
- Fluid restriction (1000 mL/d) only in patient with dilutional hyponatremia (<125 mmol/L)
- For large-volume ascites: Total paracentesis plus IV albumin (8 g per L of ascites removed) followed be sodium restriction and diuretics (1–3)[C]
- For refractory ascites: Total paracentesis plus IV albumin (8 g per L of ascites removed):
  - Increased risk of type-1 hepatorenal syndrome and hemodynamic instability
- Treat causes of ascites (for example tumor-target therapy)

Issues for Referral
- Recommended weigh loss to prevent prerenal renal failure is 300–500 g/d (1,2)[C]
- Monitor of renal function, electrolytes in serum.
- Routine measurement of urine sodium is not necessary.
- Spontaneous bacterial peritonitis in patients with ascetic-fluid protein concentration <15 g/L: PO norfloxacin (400 mg/d); oral ciprofloxacin (750 mg/wk), or trimethoprim-sulfamethoxazole (169 mg and 800 mg, respectively, 5 days per week) (C).

SURGERY/OTHER PROCEDURES
- Transjugular intrahepatic portosystemic shunt (TIPS) significantly improves transplant-free survival of cirrhotic patients with refractory ascites (4)[A].

- Surgical portacaval shunt
- Liver transplantation for decompensated liver disease

 # ONGOING CARE

FOLLOW-UP RECOMMENDATIONS
Patient Monitoring
- Recommended weigh loss to prevent prerenal renal failure is 300–500 g/d.
- Monitor renal function, electrolytes in serum.
- Routine measurement of urine sodium is not necessary.
- Monitor mental status to assess for encephalopathy.

DIET
- Low-sodium diet of ∼2000 mg/d (90 mmol)
- Fluid restriction (1000 mL/d) only in patient with dilutional hyponatremia (<125 mmol/L)

PROGNOSIS
Varies depending on underlying cause

COMPLICATIONS
- Medical treatment complications:
  - Hypo- and hyperkalemia
  - Prerenal renal failure
  - Worsening encephalopathy
  - Volume depletion
- Paracentesis complications:
  - Circulatory dysfunction (large-volume paracentesis)
  - Hepatorenal syndrome
  - Death
  - Persistent leakage of ascetic fluid
  - Localized infection
  - Abdominal wall hematoma
- Spontaneous bacterial peritonitis
- Dilutional hyponatremia

REFERENCES

1. Gines P, et al. Management of cirrhosis and ascites. *N Engl J Med*. 2004;350:1646–54.
2. Gines P, et al. The management of ascites and hyponatremia in cirrhosis. *Semin Liver Dis*. 2008;28:43–58.
3. Thomsen TW, et al. Paracentesis. *N Engl J Med*. 2006;355:e21
4. Salerno F, et al. Transjugular intrahepatic portosystemic shunt for refractory ascites: A meta-analysis of individual patient data. *Gastroenterology*. 2007;133:825–34.

 # CODES

ICD9
- 452 Portal vein thrombosis
- 572.3 Portal hypertension
- 789.59 Other ascites

CLINICAL PEARLS

- The SAAG is the best diagnostic measure for the classification of ascites.
- Ascites is characterized by 3 grades of severity, and treatment is based on grade.
- Diagnostic paracentesis must be performed in all patients with new ascites.

ASPIRATION

Roopa Kohli-Seth
Adel Bassily-Marcus

 BASICS

DESCRIPTION
Aspiration is defined as entry of a foreign body or inhalation of oropharyngeal, gastric contents, or fumes and vapors into the lower respiratory tract:

- Aspiration pneumonitis, often witnessed, is caused by acute chemical damage to the tracheobronchial tree by inhaled sterile contents.
- Aspiration pneumonia, often unwitnessed, is an infectious process caused by chronic inhalation of small amounts oropharyngeal contents.
- Most studies use the above 2 terms interchangeably although their treatment is different.

EPIDEMIOLOGY
Incidence
- Varies from 5.7–53% in different studies
- 5–15% of cases of community-acquired pneumonia result from aspiration.
- 10% of patients who are hospitalized after drug overdoses have an aspiration pneumonitis

Prevalence
The overall prevalence of aspiration pneumonia is 0.8%:
- Varies among hospitals, by surgical procedure, and by patient characteristics.

PATHOPHYSIOLOGY
- Aspiration pneumonitis, also known as Mendelson syndrome, is a chemical parenchymal burn caused by inhalation of large volume, acidic, sterile gastric contents:
  - The acute inflammatory response causes massive recruitment of neutrophils and release of powerful cytokines, especially tumor necrosis factor-α and Interleukin-8, cyclooxygenase and lipoxygenase products, and reactive oxygen species.
- Aspiration pneumonia is an infectious process that develops after the inhalation of colonized oropharyngeal material:
  - Anaerobic and/or aerobic and/or microaerophilic organisms play an important role.
  - Colonization of organisms in the oropharynx, sedation, endotracheal intubation, host factors (as in alcoholism) that suppress mucociliary clearance and phagocytic efficiency, and periodontal disease determine pathogenesis.

ETIOLOGY
- Almost all patients who develop aspiration have ≥ 1 of the risk factors listed below. While all the risk factors predispose the patient to aspiration pneumonitis, altered consciousness and periodontal disease specifically predispose the patient to aspiration pneumonia:
  - Male > Female
  - Extremes of age
  - Critically ill patients due to spine position, gastroparesis, and nasogastric intubation (causes gastroesophageal reflux.
  - Dental problems
  - Altered mental status due to:
    ○ Sedatives
    ○ Anesthesia
    ○ CVA
    ○ Alcohol abuse
    ○ Drug overdose
    ○ Intracranial mass lesion
    ○ Head trauma
    ○ seizures
  - Neuromuscular disorders, such as Guillain-Barré syndrome
  - Anatomic abnormalities, such as laryngeal tumor, achalasia, esophageal dilatation or stricture, esophageal web
  - Nursing home patients
- Patients chronically fed by a feeding tube

COMMONLY ASSOCIATED CONDITIONS
- Alcoholism and drug overdose
- Head trauma, CVA, seizures
- Esophageal strictures, neoplasm, web, gastroesophageal reflux disease, tracheoesophageal fistula
- Multiple sclerosis, pseudobulbar palsy, Parkinson disease, dementia, myasthenia gravis, Guillain-Barré syndrome

℞ DIAGNOSIS

HISTORY
- Clinical presentation varies from minimal symptoms to acute respiratory failure, acute respiratory distress syndrome (ARDS), and septic shock.
- Symptoms may include:
  - Fever
  - Cough
  - Pleuritic chest pain
  - Shortness of breath
  - Symptoms related to underlying predisposing risk factors.

PHYSICAL EXAM
- Fever or hypothermia
- Tachycardia
- Tachypnea
- Hypotension
- Hypoxia
- Decreased breath sounds
- Pleural friction rub
- Rales
- Rhonchi
- Egophony
- Decreased breath sounds
- Altered mental status
- Signs related to underlying chronic medical conditions.

DIAGNOSTIC TESTS & INTERPRETATION
Lab
Initial lab tests
- CBC with differential
- ABGs
- Serum lactate
- Serum electrolytes
- BUN and creatinine
- Blood cultures
- Sputum culture and Gram stain may not be helpful and only identify colonized organisms

Follow-Up & Special Considerations
- Repeat ABGs and serum lactate within 6 hours to assess response to oxygen supplementation and fluids
- Repeat serum electrolytes, BUN, creatinine within 24 hours
- Repeat blood cultures in 48 hours if the patient continues to be febrile, deteriorating, and there is no identifiable organism in the 1st blood culture.

Imaging
Initial approach
- Chest x-ray is the first-line imaging study to identify the extent and location of infiltrate:
  - RML and RLL most often involved
  - Posterior segments of upper lobe and apical segments of lower lobe are involved in recumbent aspiration.
  - RUL is implicated in patients who aspirate in prone position.
  - Bilateral lower lung lobes more commonly involved in patients who aspirate standing or sitting up.
  - Left-sided infiltrates more likely in patients who aspirate in left lateral decubitus position.
- CT chest is not emergent but the best test to localize and characterize infiltrate, for identifying loculated pleural effusion, empyema, abscess, or foreign body in the tracheobronchial tree
- MRI is more sensitive than x-ray but no better than CT scan.

Follow-Up & Special Considerations
- Repeat CXR within 24 hours to determine the complete extent of the aspiration:
  - Initial study may be limited by patient's hydration status, ability to mount inflammatory response, nature, and amount of aspiration.
    - CT chest may be repeated if patient's condition is not improving or continues to deteriorate.

Diagnostic Procedures/Other
- Bronchoscopy with protected brush or bronchoalveolar lavage is helpful in guiding and discontinuing antibiotic therapy in aspiration pneumonia (1)[A].
- Thoracentesis to drain pleural fluid or diagnose empyema
- Chest tube placement to drain empyema

DIFFERENTIAL DIAGNOSIS
- Community acquired pneumonia
- Pulmonary edema
- ARDS due to nonaspiration pneumonia
- Asthma, bronchitis, COPD, emphysema
- Pulmonary hemorrhage
- Squamous cell carcinoma
- Bronchoalveolar carcinoma

 TREATMENT

MEDICATION
First Line
- Antibiotics are not indicated for aspiration pneumonitis unless there is superinfection (2)[A].
- Various antibiotic regimens are indicated for aspiration pneumonia according to the severity of the disease and location of the patient:
  - For nontoxic patient from the community:
    - Azithromycin + ceftriaxone
    - Levofloxacin
    - Moxifloxacin
  - Add vancomycin or linezolid for suspected MRSA
  - For non-penicillin allergic toxic appearing patient ≥48 hours of hospital stay:
    - Cefepime + Flagyl
    - Piperacillin/tazobactam
    - Imipenem/cilastatin
  - For true penicillin-allergic toxic-appearing patient ≥48 hours of hospital stay:
    - Levaquin

ADDITIONAL TREATMENT
General Measures
- Elevate head of the bed between 30 and 45 degrees.
- Monitor endotracheal and tracheal cuff inflation pressures; maintain between 25 and 34 cm of H_2O.
- In ARDS, mechanical ventilation using low tidal volume strategy(6 mL/kg) to keep plateau pressure <30 cm of water (3)[A].
- Continuous veno-venous hemofiltration(CVVH) in hemodynamically unstable patients who develop acute renal failure

SURGERY/OTHER PROCEDURES
- Video-assisted thoracoscopic surgery (VATS) in patients with loculated empyema
- Consider tracheostomy in patients with prolonged (7–10 days) need for mechanical ventilation.

IN-PATIENT CONSIDERATIONS
Initial Stabilization
- Suctioning of upper airway, nasogastric or orogastric tube placement
- Oxygen supplementation
- Cardiac monitoring and pulse oximetry
- Consider endotracheal intubation in patients with acute respiratory distress, shock, or unable to protect airway.
- Arterial and central line placement
- Further hemodynamic monitoring in patients with shock or ARDS using transthoracic or transesophageal echo, pulse contour analysis, or pulmonary artery catheter

IV Fluids
- Aggressive fluid resuscitation with crystalloids such as plasmalyte or RL
- Colloids if patient continues to be hypotensive despite adequate crystalloid infusion
- Electrolyte replacement

 ONGOING CARE

DIET
Early enteral nutrition is preferred over parenteral nutrition.

PROGNOSIS
- Mortality associated with aspiration pneumonia is 25%.
- Uncomplicated aspiration pneumonitis has a mortality of 5%.
- In severe aspiration pneumonitis, mortality is reported as high as 70%.

COMPLICATIONS
- Acute respiratory failure
- Empyema
- Necrotizing pneumonia
- Abscess
- Acute respiratory distress syndrome
- Septic shock
- Acute renal failure
- Multisystem organ dysfunction

REFERENCES
1. Kollef MH, et al. Antibiotic utilization and outcomes for patients with clinically suspected ventilator-associated pneumonia and negative quantitative BAL culture results. *Chest*. 2005;128:2706–13.
2. Marik PE. Aspiration pneumonitis and aspiration pneumonia. *N Engl J Med*. 2001;344:665–71.
3. The Acute Respiratory Distress Syndrome Network. Ventilation with lower tidal volumes as compared with traditional tidal volumes for acute lung injury and the acute respiratory distress syndrome. *N Engl J Med*. 2000;342:1301–8.

ADDITIONAL READING
- Irwin RS. Aspiration. In: Irwin RS et al., eds. *Irwin and Rippe's intensive care medicine*, 4th ed. Vol. 1. Philadelphia: Lippincott–Raven, 1999:685.
- Torres A, et al. Severe community-acquired pneumonia: Epidemiology and prognostic factors. *Am Rev Respir Dis*. 1991;144:312–8.
- Drakulovic MB, et al. Supine body position as a risk factor for nosocomial pneumonia in mechanically ventilated patients: A randomised trial. *Lancet*. 1999;354:1851–8.

 CODES

ICD9
- 507.0 Pneumonitis due to inhalation of food or vomitus
- 934.9 Foreign body in respiratory tree, unspecified
- 997.39 Other respiratory complications

CLINICAL PEARLS
- Aspiration pneumonia is one of the most common causes of ARDS.
- Prophylactic antibiotics are not recommended for aspiration pneumonitis unless there is superinfection.
- Antibiotics can be safely discontinued after 72 hours with culture-negative BAL.

ASTHMA/STATUS ASTHMATICUS

Sherin M. Ibrahim
Bindu Raju

 BASICS

DESCRIPTION
- Airflow obstruction caused by a chronic inflammatory disorder of the tracheobronchial tree
- Acute symptoms result from narrowing of airways, hyperreactivity of bronchial muscles, and inflammation of the mucosa and production of mucus.
- Medical emergency if symptoms are refractory to initial bronchodilator therapy
- System(s) affected: Pulmonary

Pregnancy Considerations
- 50% have no change in symptoms, 25% improve, 25% worsen
- Preventing stress can decrease symptoms.
- Safe to use β agonists and inhaled corticosteroids
- Must weigh risk vs. benefits of oral steroids

EPIDEMIOLOGY
Prevalence
Increased prevalence in inner-city populations:
- 9.3% among U.S. adults in 2000

GENERAL PREVENTION
Prophylactic management:
- Anti-inflammatory agents
- Inhaled steroids
- Cromolyn
- Leukotriene modifiers

PATHOPHYSIOLOGY
- Influx of eosinophils during early-phase reaction and a mixed cellular infiltrate composed of eosinophils, mast cells, lymphocytes and neutrophils during the late-phase reaction
- Leads to inflammatory cascade
- Airway hyperreactivity
- Mucus secretion
- Structural changes

ETIOLOGY
- Allergic:
  – Pollen
  – Mold
  – Dust mites
  – Dander
  – Feather pillows
- Others:
  – Smoke
  – Air pollution
  – Infections (viral)
  – Aspirin
  – Cold Air
  – Sinusitis
  – GERD

COMMONLY ASSOCIATED CONDITIONS
- Reflux esophagitis
- Sinusitis
- Nasal polyps
- ASA allergy
- Atopy

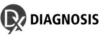 **DIAGNOSIS**

HISTORY
- Prior history of intubation, frequent ER visits and use of systemic corticosteroids
- Present with audible wheezing
- With status asthmaticus, severe dyspnea develops over hours to days.
- Triggers
- Excessive use of inhalers

PHYSICAL EXAM
- Tachypnea in early stages with significant wheezing:
  – Initially only on expiration, later in both inspiration and expiration
- Hyperexpanded chest, accessory muscle use:
  – As constriction worsens, wheezing may disappear.
- Pulsus paradoxus does not exceed 15 mm Hg:
  – In severe asthma >25 mm Hg

DIAGNOSTIC TESTS & INTERPRETATION
Lab
- Normal CBC
- Peripheral eosinophilia
- Nasal eosinophils
- ABG

Imaging
Initial approach
- CXR
- CT chest

Diagnostic Procedures/Other
- Spirometry: Decreased FEV_1
- Pulmonary function tests
- Allergy testing
- PPD
- Laryngoscopy to diagnose vocal cord dysfunction

Pathological Findings
- Smooth muscle hyperplasia
- Thickened basement membrane
- Inflammatory response
- Hyperinflated lungs
- Mucus plugging

DIFFERENTIAL DIAGNOSIS
- Foreign body aspiration
- COPD
- Recurrent pulmonary emboli
- Congestive heart failure
- Vocal cord dysfunction
- Viral respiratory infection (croup, bronchiolitis)
- Tuberculosis
- Epiglottis
- Bronchopulmonary aspergillosis
- Hypersensitivity pneumonitis
- Tracheobronchomalacia
- Cystic fibrosis

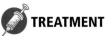

TREATMENT

MEDICATION

- Frequent nebulized β-agonists:
  - Ipratropium nebulizer if not responding
- Steroids:
  - Methylprednisolone 2 mg/kg IV once then 1 mg/kg IV q6h
- Mast cell stabilizers
- Methylxanthines
- Anticholinergics
- Leukotriene modifiers

COMPLEMENTARY & ALTERNATIVE THERAPIES

- Ketamine
- Halothane or enflurane in combination with propofol or ketamine
- Nitric oxide
- H1-Antagonists
- Troleandomycin (TAO)
- Methotrexate
- IVIG
- Lasix

IN-PATIENT CONSIDERATIONS

Initial Stabilization

- Oxygen therapy to maintain Hb-O_2 sat >92%:
  - Respiratory failure: A pCO_2 of 40 is not normal
  - Intubation and mechanical ventilation
  - Monitor ABG to adjust ventilator settings
  - Permissive hypercapnia to avoid auto PEEP leading to high airway pressures and barotrauma
  - Sedation to achieve patient–ventilator synchrony and adequate expiratory time; may add paralytic agent if needed, but deep sedation is preferred
- Short acting β-adrenergic agonists: Onset of action in 5 minutes, peak effect in 30–60 minutes, duration of action 4–6 hours:
  - Albuterol MDI-HFA 90 mcg/puff or liquid for nebulization 0.63, 1.25, or 2.5 mg/vial
  - Levalbuterol (Xopenex) MDI-HFA 45 microgram/puff or liquid for nebulization 0.31, 0.63, or 1.25 mg/vial
  - Pirbuterol (Maxair) MDI-CFC 200 mcg/puff
- Inhaled corticosteroids:
  - Beclomethasone (Qvar) MDI-HFA 40 or 80 mcg
  - Budesonide (Pulmicort) DPI 90 or 80 mcg, nebulizer 250 or 500 mcg
  - Fluticasone (Flovent) MDI-HFA 44, 110, or 220 mcg, DPI 50 or 100 mcg

- Inhaled corticosteroids in combination with long-acting β-agonists:
  - Budesonide and formoterol (Symbicort) MDI-HFA 80 or 160 mcg with 4.5 mcg of formoterol
  - Fluticasone with salmeterol (Advair) MDIHFA 45, 115, or 230 (with 21 mcg), DPI 100, 250, or 500 (with 50 mcg)
  - Long-acting β-agonist bronchodilators: Sustained activity >12 hours.
  - Formoterol (Foradil) single dose DPI 12 mcg per capsule; onset of action is 5 minutes
  - Salmeterol (Serevent) DPI 50 mcg/inhalation; onset of action is 15–20 minutes
- Leukotriene modifiers: Bronchodilate within hours, maximal effect within first few days:
  - Montelukast (Singulair) 4, 5, or 10 mg/d
  - Zafirlukast (Accolate) 10 or 20 mg b.i.d.
  - Zileuton (Zyflo) 600 mg ii tabs b.i.d.
- Omalizumab (Xolair) subcutaneous injection every 2–4 weeks depending on dose.
  - Positive RAST test
  - IgE 30–700 IU/mL

IV Fluids
As needed to ensure euvolemia

ONGOING CARE

DIET
Avoid food allergies

PROGNOSIS

- Excellent, with attention to general health, avoidance of environmental triggers and compliance with medications
- <50% of children outgrow asthma.
- Mortality increases with:
  - >3 ER visits per year
  - Nocturnal symptoms
  - History of ICU admission
  - Mechanical ventilation
  - >2 hospitalizations per year
  - Systemic steroid dependence
  - History of syncope with asthma
  - History of noncompliance

COMPLICATIONS

- Respiratory failure requiring intubation and mechanical ventilation
- Air leak syndromes (pneumothorax)
- Atelectasis in 25% of hospitalized patients
- Steroid myopathy
- Flaccid paralysis (severe exacerbation treated with paralytic agents + steroids)
- SIADH

ADDITIONAL READING

- Fanta CP. Asthma. *NEJM*. 2009;360:1002–14.
- Han P, et al. Evolving differences in the presentation of severe asthma requiring intensive care unit admission. *Respiration*. 2004;71(5):458–62.
- National Asthma Education and Prevention Program. Expert Panel Report 3: Guidelines for the Diagnosis and Management of Asthma. National Institutes of Health; 2007.
- Rodrigo GJ, et al. Elevated plasma lactate level associated with high dose inhaled albuterol therapy in acute severe asthma. *Emerg Med J*. 2005;22(6): 404–8.

 See Also (Topic, Algorithm, Electronic Media Element)

- American Lung Association (www.lungusa.org)
- Asthma and Allergy Foundation (www.aafa.org)
- Allergy and Asthma Network (www.aanma.org)

 CODES

ICD9

- 493.90 Asthma, unspecified, unspecified
- 493.91 Asthma, unspecified type, with status asthmaticus

CLINICAL PEARLS

- Not all asthma wheezes, and not all that wheezes is asthma.
- Secure airway as a first priority; intubate if refractory to medical therapy. BiPAP has not been shown to be beneficial in asthmatics.
- Rule out foreign body aspiration as a culprit, especially in children.

ATRIAL ARRHYTHMIAS/FIBRILLATION/FLUTTER

Brian Corbett

BASICS

DESCRIPTION
- Atrial fibrillation (AF) is defined as an irregularly irregular supraventricular tachycardia characterized by disorganized atrial activation.
- Atrial flutter (AFL):
  - Defined as a supraventricular tachycardia with a regular rate between 250 and 350 bpm
  - "Typical": Negative, sawtooth-like P wave deflections in leads II, III and AVF with positive P wave deflections in lead V_1 and negative deflections in lead V_6
  - "Atypical": Positive, notched P wave deflections in the inferior leads with negative P wave deflections in V_1 and positive deflections in V_6
- System(s) affected: Cardiovascular/Neurologic

EPIDEMIOLOGY
Incidence
- AF is the most common sustained arrhythmia; the estimated prevalence is 0.4–1% in the general population (1).
- Highest in people >85 (11–12%) and lower in people <55 (0.1–0.2%) (1).
- Likely underestimated due to the incidence of asymptomatic paroxysmal AF/AFL.

Prevalence
- Male > Female
- Whites > African Americans

RISK FACTORS
- Age
- Prior myocardial infarction
- Coronary artery disease
- Congestive heart failure
- Valvular heart disease
- Cardiomyopathy
- Hypertension
- Male gender
- Diabetes
- Binge alcohol abuse
- Postoperative cardiac surgical period
- Hyperthyroidism
- Obesity
- Pulmonary embolism
- Medications
- Atrial septal defects

Genetics
Chromosomal abnormalities have been associated with AF/AFL (2,3).

GENERAL PREVENTION
Modification of risk factors

PATHOPHYSIOLOGY
- AF is triggered by rapidly firing foci usually from the pulmonary vein (less often from the right atrium, the superior vena cava, or coronary sinus).
- AFL is activation of an atrial reentrant circuit.

ETIOLOGY
- Atrial enlargement
- Age
- CAD/Previous MI
- Hypertension
- Hyperthyroid
- CHF
- Valvular heart disease
- Pulmonary embolism
- Alcohol
- Medications
- Atrial septal defects

COMMONLY ASSOCIATED CONDITIONS
- Hyperthyroidism
- Pulmonary embolism
- Myocardial ischemia
- Rheumatic/nonrheumatic valve disease
- Hypertension
- Atrial septal defects
- WPW

DIAGNOSIS

HISTORY
- Length of symptoms (first episode, paroxysmal, persistent or permanent)
- Palpitations
- Fatigue/effort intolerance
- Chest pain
- Dyspnea
- Dizziness
- Syncope
- Stroke
- Medications
- Family history of heart disease
- Alcohol intake

PHYSICAL EXAM
- Heart rate
- Irregular jugular venous pulsations
- Blood pressure; for possible cardioversion
- Irregular pulse
- Variation in the intensity of the first heart sound
- Absence of a 4th heart sound heard on previous exams
- Neurological assessment: Hx stroke/TIA

DIAGNOSTIC TESTS & INTERPRETATION
Lab
- Thyroid-stimulating hormone
- Markers of ischemia
- Serum electrolytes
- Renal
- Hepatic function

Imaging
- Chest radiography: Assess for cardiac hypertrophy, signs of heart failure or lung disease.
- Echocardiography: Left atrial size, left ventricular hypertrophy (LVH), ejection fraction, valvular disease, pulmonary artery pressure estimate (pulmonary disease), and pericardial disease

Diagnostic Procedures/Other
- Electrocardiogram: Necessary to confirm the diagnosis and *must be performed on every patient being evaluated for AF/AFL*:
  - AF is diagnosed by the absence of P waves and irregularly irregular usually narrow QRS complexes. The atrial rate is 400–700 bpm. The ventricular rate depends on conduction through the AV node and usually is 120–180 bpm.
  - Regular, narrow complex tachycardia at 150 bpm should raise suspicion for the presence of AFL with 2:1 conduction.
- Holter monitoring for evaluation of possible PAF
- Exercise testing: Test adequacy of rate control.
- Transesophageal echocardiogram: Identify LA thrombus and guide cardioversion.

Pathological Findings
- Atrial dilation (4)
- Atrial patchy fibrosis juxtaposed with normal atrial fibers and loss of atrial muscle mass (4)

DIFFERENTIAL DIAGNOSIS
- Premature atrial contractions (PAC)
- Supraventricular tachycardia (SVT)
- Sick sinus syndrome (SSS)
- Sinus tachycardia/bradycardia
- Multifocal atrial tachycardia (MAT)

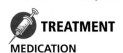

TREATMENT

MEDICATION

- IV β-blockers or calcium channel antagonists to control the ventricular response (<100 bpm) (5)[B]:
  - β-Blockers include: Esmolol (500 mcg/kg bolus, then 50 mcg/kg infusion, titrated to 200 mcg/kg in 50 mcg/kg increments as needed), metoprolol (2.5–5 mg bolus over 2 minutes up to 3 boluses), labetalol (40–80 mg q10min), atenolol (50–100 mg/d PO), propranolol (0.15 mg/kg IV), and carvedilol (3.25–25 mg PO b.i.d.).
  - Nondihydropyridine calcium channel blockers include: Diltiazem (0.25 mg/kg over 2 minutes) and verapamil (0.075–0.15 mg/kg IV over 2 minutes)
- Digoxin: Especially with LV dysfunction:
  - Rarely useful as a single agent in rate-controlled AF (5) [Level B when used in conjunction with other agents].

ALERT
- Calcium channel antagonists and β-blockers are contraindicated in patients with concomitant Wolff-Parkinson-White syndrome as this can lead to ventricular fibrillation.
- Use with caution in patients with relative hypotension or heart failure.

Second Line

- Anticoagulation (5)[A]:
  - Aspirin (81–325 mg) for patients at low risk for thromboembolism (CHADS score 0–1, see General Measure section)
  - Warfarin (INR 2.0–3.0) for patients at high risk of thromboembolism (CHADS score >2)
  - Dabigatran (150 mg BID) is an alternative to warfarin that does not require INR monitoring
  - Moderate-risk patients (CHADS score 1 or 2) should be weighed on an individual basis regarding bleeding risk, stroke risk, and inconvenience of anticoagulation.

Third Line

- Antiarrhythmics (rhythm control strategies)
- Trials indicate similar outcome in patients managed with either rate or rhythm control (6,7). Treatment should be individualized at the physician's discretion.
- Vaughn Williams classification:
  - Type 1A (5)[B]: Quinidine, procainamide, disopyramide
  - Type 1B (5)[B]: Lidocaine, mexiletine
  - Type 1C (5)[B]: Flecainide, propafenone
  - Type II (5)[C]: β-Blockers
  - Type III (5)[B]: Amiodarone, dofetilide, ibutilide, sotalol
- Type IV (5)[C]: Nondihydropyridine calcium channel antagonists

ADDITIONAL TREATMENT
General Measures

- Synchronized cardioversion for AF/AFL not responsive to pharmacologic agents in patients with ongoing ischemia, symptomatic hypotension, angina or HF (5)[A]:
  - Also for WPW with hemodynamic instability or very rapid tachycardia (5)[A]
  - Long-term management in appropriate patients with AF/AFL (5)[B]
- CHADS score: Stroke risk stratification of AF/AFL patients (8):
  - 1 point each: CHF, HTN, age >75, DM
  - 2 points each: Prior ischemic stroke, TIA
  - Low risk = CHADS 0
  - Moderate risk = CHADS 1 or 2
  - High risk = CHADS >2

Issues for Referral
Cardiology

Additional Therapies
- AV nodal ablation with permanent pacemaker
- Circumferential pulmonary vein ablation: 60–85% success in paroxysmal AF; 40–70% in chronic AF (4)[B]

COMPLEMENTARY & ALTERNATIVE THERAPIES
ACE inhibitors and HMG CoA-reductase inhibitors may decrease the incidence of AF (10,11).

SURGERY/OTHER PROCEDURES
Surgical ablation (the MAZE procedure): In conjunction with cardiac surgery; success is 70–90%

IN-PATIENT CONSIDERATIONS
Initial Stabilization

Evaluate hemodynamic stability. All patients with evidence of symptomatic hypotension or angina as a result of AF/AFL should undergo immediate synchronized electrical cardioversion (200 J in monophasic mode) (5)[A].

Admission Criteria
- Rapid ventricular response (>150 bpm)
- Signs and/or symptoms of heart failure
- Neurological symptoms
- Angina
- Syncope
- Hypotension

IV Fluids
Individualized to meet the patient's needs

Discharge Criteria
- Controlled ventricular response
- Hemodynamically stable
- Evaluation for stroke risk/anticoagulation

 ## ONGOING CARE

FOLLOW-UP RECOMMENDATIONS
Continued care is provided on an outpatient basis.

Patient Monitoring
- Routine follow-up is required
- Exercise testing if myocardial ischemia is suspected and prior to initiating type IC antiarrhythmic drug therapy
- Evaluate adequacy of rate control at maximal activity.

DIET
Cardiac diet

PATIENT EDUCATION
Modification of risk factors

PROGNOSIS
Associated with an increased risk of stroke, CHF, and doubled all-cause mortality (12)

COMPLICATIONS
- Embolic stroke
- Tachycardia-induced cardiomyopathy
- Bleeding (secondary to anticoagulation)

REFERENCES

1. Laksminarayn K, et al. Clinical epidemiology of atrial fibrillation and related cerebrovascular events in the United States. *Neurologist.* 2008;3(14):143–50.
2. Gudbjartsson DF, et al. Variants conferring risk of atrial fibrillation on chromosome 4q25. *Nature.* 2007;448:353–7.
3. Fox CS, et al. Parental atrial fibrillation as a risk factor for atrial fibrillation in offspring. *JAMA.* 2004;291:2851–5.
4. Allessie M, et al. Electrical, contractile and structural remodeling during atrial fibrillation. *Cardiovasc Res.* 2002:54:230–46.
5. ACC/AHA/ESC 2006 guidelines for the management of patients with atrial fibrillation JACC. 2006;48(4):149–246.
6. Corley SD, et al. Relationships between sinus rhythm, treatment, and survival in the Atrial Fibrillation Follow-Up Investigation or Rhythm Management (AFFIRM) Study. *Circulation.* 2004;109:1509–13.
7. Van Gelder IC, et al. A comparison of rate control and rhythm control in patients with recurrent persistent atrial fibrillation. *N Engl J Med.* 2002;347:1834–40.
8. Gage BF, et al. Validation of clinical classification schemes for predicting stroke: Results from the national registry of atrial fibrillation. *JAMA.* 2001;285:2864–70.
9. Chen SA, et al. Initiation of atrial fibrillation by ectopic beats originating from the pulmonary veins: Electrophysiological characteristics, pharmacological responses and effects of radiofrequency ablation. *Circulation.* 1999;100: 1879.
10. Vermes E, et al. Enalapril decreases the incidence of atrial fibrillation in patients with left ventricular dysfunction: Insights from the Studies of Left Ventricular Dysfunction trials. *Circulation.* 2003;107:2926–31.
11. Siu CW, et al. Prevention of atrial fibrillation recurrence by statin therapy in patients with lone atrial fibrillation after successful cardioversion. *Am J Cardiol.* 2003;92:1343–5.
12. Kannel WB, et al. Coronary heart disease and atrial fibrillation: The Framingham Study Stroke. *Am Heart J.* 1983;106:389–96.

 ## CODES

ICD9
- 427.9 Cardiac dysrhythmia, unspecified
- 427.31 Atrial fibrillation
- 427.32 Atrial flutter

CLINICAL PEARLS

- AF is the most common sustained arrhythmia.
- Evaluation of the patient should assess hemodynamic stability, determine the duration of AF (to determine need for anticoagulation), and evaluate for preexisting cardiac disease and risk factors for systemic emboli.
- The initial treatment should focus on control of the ventricular response, treatment of reversible causes, anticoagulation, and consideration for cardioversion with or without antiarrhythmic therapy.

BASICS

DESCRIPTION
- Air trapping or stacking
- Incomplete alveolar emptying during expiration
- AutoPEEP is the difference between the end expiratory alveolar pressure (intrinsic) and the end expiratory airway pressure (applied) (PEEP)

EPIDEMIOLOGY
Incidence
Up to 35% of critically ill patients on mechanical ventilation (1)

Prevalence
Not known; common in patients with obstructive airway disease

RISK FACTORS
- Disease factor:
  - Obstructive airway disease (asthma, COPD)
  - Excessive secretions
- Ventilator factors:
  - High tidal volume
  - Rapid respiratory rate
  - Inverse I:E ratio
  - Small endotracheal tube diameter

GENERAL PREVENTION
- Avoid large tidal volumes.
- Avoid rapid respiratory rates.
- The effect of external PEEP in COPD and asthmatic patients should be monitored carefully.

PATHOPHYSIOLOGY
- End expiratory pressure in the alveoli relative to the proximal airway is positive
- Dynamic hyperinflation with intrinsic expiratory flow limitation (1):
  - Obstructive airway disease
  - Excessive thick secretions
- Dynamic hyperinflation without intrinsic expiratory flow limitation:
  - Fast respiratory rate
  - High tidal volume
  - Small endotracheal tube diameter
- Without dynamic hyperinflation:
  - Recruitment of expiratory muscles

ETIOLOGY
Inability to exhale all of the inspired air before the next breath is delivered:
- Airway constriction or obstruction
- Rapid respiratory rate:
  - Decrease in exhalation time
- High tidal volume, 10–12 mL/kg
- Inverse I:E ratio:
  - Decrease in exhalation time

COMMONLY ASSOCIATED CONDITIONS
- Obstructive airway disease (common)
- High minute ventilation (e.g., fever, sepsis); common

DIAGNOSIS

HISTORY
- History of obstructive airway disease
- Delayed weaning from the ventilator in previous admissions

PHYSICAL EXAM
- Wheezing
- Diminished air entry
- Exhalation that continues until the next breath starts (1)
- A delay between the start of the inspiratory effort and the drop in airway pressure
- Failure of peak airway pressure to change when external PEEP is applied
- In a heavily sedated patient, a decrease in plateau pressure after a prolonged exhalation
- Patient–ventilator asynchrony

DIAGNOSTIC TESTS & INTERPRETATION
Lab
ABGs:
- Possible hypoxemia if autoPEEP is severe.
- Hypercarbia if airway obstruction

Imaging
Chest x-ray: Hyperinflated lung fields

Diagnostic Procedures/Other
- Monitor the flow–time curve, which fails to return to baseline (zero) (2,3) (Fig. 1)

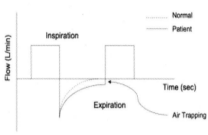

Fig. 1 The expiratory flow rate does not return to zero at the time of the next inspiration indicating that expiration is not complete, i.e., air trapping is present.

- End expiratory pause can identify the presence of autoPEEP (2,3,5) (Fig. 2):
  - Observe the pressure–time curve.
  - The pressure at end expiration is measured by end expiratory pause.
  - AutoPEEP is the total pressure obtained minus the set PEEP.

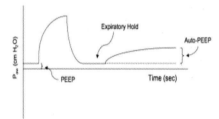

Fig. 2 At the end of expiration, placing an 'expiratory hold' prevents any further expiration, i.e., air outflow ceases. If air trapping is present, the airway pressure will increase.

DIFFERENTIAL DIAGNOSIS
Dynamic hyperinflation

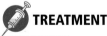
TREATMENT

MEDICATION
- B_2 agonists for bronchoconstriction (2,4)
- Ipratropium

ADDITIONAL TREATMENT
General Measures
- Control minute ventilation by treating the underlying cause.
- Decrease tidal volume.
- Decrease respiratory rate; may control the rate with sedation if tolerated.
- Increase flow rate.
- Correct I:E ratio if reversed.
- Suction for secretion clearance.
- Switch to a larger-bore endotracheal tube if needed.

- Increase external PEEP by 85% of the autoPEEP value:
  - This should be done only in patients with airflow obstruction and dynamic airway compression.
  - If increasing external PEEP does not increase the peak airway pressure, then it might be helpful to allow triggering of the ventilator with less patient effort.

Additional Therapies
In certain conditions, disconnecting the patient from the ventilator can eliminate autoPEEP, but this will lead to loss of recruitment and should not be considered as a routine practice. Although it may be used diagnostically, particularly in an emergency, autoPEEP will eventually return with ventilator reconnection unless the treatment measures noted above are successfully instituted.

 ONGOING CARE

FOLLOW-UP RECOMMENDATIONS
Patient Monitoring
- Flow–time curve
- Synchrony with the ventilator
- Plateau and peak airway pressure
- Patient ability to trigger the ventilator comfortably
- Hemodynamics

COMPLICATIONS
- Increase work of breathing:
  - Increase the pressure needed to trigger the ventilator
- Barotrauma

- Hemodynamic compromise:
  - Decrease cardiac output
  - Decrease venous return
  - Decrease ventricular compliance
  - Increase right ventricular outflow impedance
  - External ventricular constraint
- Misinterpretation of CVP, PCWP, and erroneous calculation of respiratory compliance

REFERENCES

1. Mugghal MM, et al. Auto-positive end-expiratory pressure: Mechanisms and treatment. *Cleve Clin J Med*. 2005;72(9):801–9.
2. Koh Y. Ventilatory management in patients with chronic airflow obstruction. *Crit Care Clin*. 2007;23:169–81.
3. Bekos V, et al. Monitoring the mechanically ventilated patient. *Crit Care Clin*. 2007;23: 575–611.
4. Blanch L, et al. Measurement of air trapping, intrinsic positive expiratory pressure, and dynamic hyperinflation in mechanically ventilated patients. *Resp Care*. 2005;50:110–23.
5. Stather DR, et al. Clinical review: Mechanical ventilation in severe asthma. *Crit Care*. 2005;9:581–7.

ADDITIONAL READING

- Pepe PE, et al. Occult positive end-expiratory pressure in mechanically ventilated patients with airflow obstruction: The auto-PEEP effect. *Am Rev Respir Dis*. 1982:126;166–70.
- Santanilla JI, et al. Mechanical ventilation. *Emerg Med Clin N Am*. 2008;26:849–62.
- Tobin MJ. Advances in mechanical ventilation. *N Engl J Med*. 2001;344;26:1986–96.

 CODES

ICD9
- 493.90 Asthma, unspecified, unspecified
- 516.9 Unspecified alveolar and parietoalveolar pneumonopathy
- 786.9 Other symptoms involving respiratory system and chest

CLINICAL PEARLS

- Monitoring the flow–time curve in mechanically ventilated patients can help in detecting autoPEEP.
- Measures should be taken to prolong expiratory phase and eliminate airway obstruction.
- AutoPEEP can lead to hemodynamic compromise and delay the weaning process.

BACTEREMIA, CENTRAL LINE ASSOCIATED
Rafael Alba Yunen

 BASICS

DESCRIPTION
A central line is a tube placed into a patient's large vein, usually in the neck, chest, arm, or groin. It may be left in place for several weeks. A bloodstream infection can occur when bacteria or other germs travel down a central line and enter the blood. The patient with a catheter-associated bloodstream infection becomes ill with fevers and chills or the skin around the catheter may become sore and red.

EPIDEMIOLOGY
Incidence
- Intravascular catheter-related infections remain one of the top 3 causes of nosocomial sepsis.
- ~48% of patients in ICUs have a central line, accounting for 15 million central line-days per year (2,3):
  - 75% of all catheter-related infections are due to the use of a central line.
  - >250,000 CVC-related infections per year in the U.S. (1)

RISK FACTORS
- Central lines disrupt the integrity of the skin, making patients vulnerable to bacterial and fungal infections, including central line-associated bloodstream infections (CLABSI). The CDC defines CLABSI as an infection in a patient who had a central line in place within the 48-hour period before the onset of infection (4).
- Any patient with a central line is at risk of developing a CLABSI. General risk depends on a number of patient-level factors, including:
  - Patient's illness (e.g., those receiving chemotherapy or with burn wounds)
  - ICU care setting
  - Patient's general care setting (patients in academic [teaching] hospitals with medical trainees may be at greater risk than patients in private nonteaching hospitals).
  - Particular risk in diabetics, immunosuppressive therapy, immunodeficiency diseases, skin diseases at the insertion site, and the presence of sepsis from a distinct source

- Catheter-specific risk factors related to the vein that is catheterized, the type of catheter used, and how the catheter is used:
  - The specific vein that has been cannulated; e.g., neck veins are associated with a lower risk than groin veins, likely because of urine and stool exposure. Nonrandomized studies suggest that use of the subclavian vein for insertion of vascular catheters is associated with a lower risk for infection compared with internal jugular vein catheterization.
  - Whether the catheter is tunneled (tunneling is associated with reduced risk)
  - Duration of catheter use (the longer the duration, the greater the risk for infection)
  - Specific uses of the catheter (e.g., multiple entries for drawing blood increases risk)
  - Physical properties of the catheter (i.e., length, number of lumens, presence of subcutaneous cuffs, anti-infective coatings)
- Physician and environmental factors increasing risk of catheter infections:
  - Catheter placement under emergency or nonsterile conditions
  - Insertion of large or multilumen catheters
  - Catheterization of a central vein
  - Prolonged catheterization at a single site
  - Placement by surgical cutdown
  - Inexperienced operator

Genetics
The extent to which genetic factors (e.g., polymorphisms in basic host defense mechanisms) or endovascular co-pathogens (e.g., endothelial cytomegalovirus infection) contribute to an increased risk for vascular access device infections is not known.

GENERAL PREVENTION
See Guidelines for the Prevention of Intravascular Catheter-related Infections from the CDC's Healthcare Infection Control Practices Advisory Committee (HICPAC) (5):
- Education of personnel
- Hand hygiene
- Maximal sterile barriers precautions during catheter insertion
- Chlorhexidine to prepare catheter insertion site
- Daily assessment of the need for central lines
- Weekly dressing changes
- Use of antiseptic or antimicrobial-impregnated vascular catheters

PATHOPHYSIOLOGY
Central lines disrupt the integrity of the skin, making patients vulnerable to bacterial and fungal infections, including CLABSI.

ETIOLOGY
Assuming catheter is not contaminated on insertion, infection can be multifactorial; potential causes ranging from more common:
- Bacteria colonizing the skin site
- Catheter hub(s)
- Hematogenous seeding
- Infusated (IV fluid) contamination

COMMONLY ASSOCIATED CONDITIONS
- Septic shock
- Bacterial endocarditis
- Suppurative thrombophlebitis
- Common microorganisms:
  - Most common are the skin contaminant, *Staphylococcus aureus*, *S. epidermitis*, *Candida* spp. (especially in the diabetic). If *Enterococcus* spp., *E. coli*, *Pseudomonas* spp., or *Klebsiella* spp., this suggests contaminated IV solution.

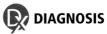 **DIAGNOSIS**

HISTORY
48-hour period after initial insertion is an important part of history

PHYSICAL EXAM
Unexplained fever, chills, mental status changes, hypotension, tachycardia, shock, pus, and erythema at the central line site

DIAGNOSTIC TESTS & INTERPRETATION
Lab
- Sepsis workup is warranted.
- CBC
- BMP: Unexplained hyperglycemia
- Blood cultures, including several sets over hours to days from a site separate from the catheter insertion site. Obtaining the same organism from a blood culture at a distant site is a strong evidence of catheter-related infection.
- Tip of the catheter is sent for culture and Gram stain.
- If >15 colonies of a single organism are isolated, infection is more likely than colonization.

B

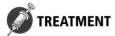 TREATMENT

MEDICATION

- First line of treatment is line removal.
- Antibiotics for 7–14 days.
- Considering the high incidence of MRSA in many ICUs, empiric antibiotic therapy with vancomycin is warranted. Additional coverage for gram-negative, antipseudomonal as well; if *Candida* is present, then parenteral amphotericin B, fluconazole, or caspofungin. Vancomycin-resistant organisms may respond to linezolid.

ADDITIONAL TREATMENT
General Measures
Line removal

COMPLEMENTARY & ALTERNATIVE THERAPIES

- New catheter technologies with antibiotic and antiseptic coated.
- A central line can be changed over a wire when there is fever without obvious external signs (pus or erythema at central line site) of infection. Send tip of catheter to the lab for culture.
- A central line changed over a wire can be left in place if culture of previous line returns <15 CFU.
- A central line changed over a wire should be pulled and a central line placed at a different site if the previous line culture returns >15 CFU.
- Multiple studies have shown that guidewire exchanges neither decrease nor increase infections risk.

IN-PATIENT CONSIDERATIONS
When patients are transferred out of ICUs to medical wards, each catheter should be assessed to determine its need to remain in place. All catheters determined to be absolutely unnecessary should be removed.

 ONGOING CARE

FOLLOW-UP RECOMMENDATIONS
Patient Monitoring
Approach to the febrile patient with a central line:

- Catheter no longer needed; remove and culture tip
- Severe sepsis or septic shock with catheter in for >72 hours: Remove catheter and culture tip
- Severe sepsis or septic shock with catheter in for <72 hours: Antibiotics, remove catheter if no improvement in 12–24 hours and no other source identified
- Stable patient, catheter in for >72 hours: Guidewire exchange with tip culture; if culture >15 CFU, remove catheter

PROGNOSIS
- Mortality ranges from 10–30%
- Morbidity and mortality are impacted by many variables like the type of ICU, type of catheter and composition, duration of catheterization, and site.

COMPLICATIONS
- Septic shock
- Bacterial endocarditis
- Suppurative thrombophlebitis

REFERENCES

1. Mermel LA. Prevention of intravascular catheter-related infections. *Ann Intern Med.* 2000;132:391–402.
2. Soufir L, et al. Attributable morbidity and mortality of catheter-related septicemia in critically ill patients: A matched, risk-adjusted, cohort study. *Infect Control Hosp Epidemiol.* 1999;20:396–401.
3. CDC. Guidelines for the prevention of intravascular catheter-related infections. *MMWR.* 2002;51 (No. RR–10):1–26.
4. CDC. Central line-associated bloodstream infection (CLABSI) event. Available at: http://www.cdc.gov/nhsn/PDFs/pscManual/4PSC_CLABScurrent.pdf. Date accessed: June 22, 2009.
5. O'Grady NP, et al. Centers for Disease Control and Prevention. Guidelines for the prevention of intravascular catheter-related infections. *MMWR.* 2002;51:1–26.

CODES

ICD9
- 790.7 Bacteremia
- 996.62 Infection and inflammatory reaction due to other vascular device, implant, and graft

CLINICAL PEARLS

- CLABSI are a common problem, not only in ICUs, but also in other specialty care areas (e.g., hematology/oncology wards, bone marrow transplant units, solid organ transplant units, inpatient dialysis units, long-term acute care areas), neonatal ICUs, and any other patient care location in an institution (e.g., medical or surgical wards).
- The biology of these infections and pathogenesis-driven prevention measures have been extensively studied. Many interventions are extremely effective, so much so that most if not all CLABSI should be preventable. The use of chlorhexidine for skin preparation, patient cleansing, catheter coating, and impregnated catheter-skin sponges has been shown to be important for prevention of CLABSI.
- In conclusion, hand hygiene and hub care represent a "back to basics" approach to preventing central line-associated bacteremia, and any evidence of phlebitis or cellulitis or any suspicion of septic complications caused by IV cannulas should lead to prompt removal of the cannulas.

BLAST CRISIS

Alina Dulu
Stephen M. Pastores

BASICS

DESCRIPTION

- Advanced phase of chronic myelogenous leukemia (CML) characterized by >20% of peripheral blood or bone marrow blasts, or presence of extramedullary blastic infiltrates, and associated with rapid progression and short survival (1)[A]

- System affected: Hematologic

EPIDEMIOLOGY

Incidence
- Almost all untreated CML and 7% of treated CML progress to blast crisis at 5 years.
- 10–15% CML patients initially present in blast crisis.

Prevalence
- More common in untreated CML and CML resistant to tyrosine kinase inhibitors
- Median age at presentation is 67 years, but can present in all age groups.

Pediatric Considerations
Course of disease in children is similar to that in adults; however, response to hematopoietic cell transplantation (HCT) is better.

RISK FACTORS
Accelerated phase of CML

Genetics
- Philadelphia (Ph) chromosome, a reciprocal balanced translocation between the long arms of chromosome 9 and 22, t(9;22) (q34;q11.2) with new BCR-ABL gene formation
- BCR-ABL gene encodes a protein with deregulated tyrosine kinase activity (2).
- Cytogenetic evolution with acquisition of new chromosomal changes:
  - Additional chromosomal abnormalities, such as a double Ph(+Ph), trisomy (+8), (+19), or isochromosome 17
  - Additional chromosome translocations t(3;21)(q26;q22), which generates AML1–EVI1, translocation t(8;21)(q22;q22) with AML1–ETO gene, t(7;11)(p15;p15) and NUP98–HOXA9 gene, inv(16)(p13;q22) with CBFβ–SMMHC gene
  - New point mutations in the p53 tumor suppression gene, RB, and CDKN2A; deletions in the p16 tumor suppressor gene; overexpression of genes such as EVI1 and Myc

PATHOPHYSIOLOGY
Genetic abnormality results in a unique gene, BCR-ABL, producing a constitutively active tyrosine kinase that increases proliferation, affects differentiation, and blocks apoptosis of the clonal cells.

ETIOLOGY
- Increased susceptibility of the BCR–ABL-expressing clone to additional genetic and molecular changes
- Uncontrolled production of neutrophils with gradual progression to impaired and then failure of differentiation.

COMMONLY ASSOCIATED CONDITIONS
CML

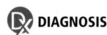

DIAGNOSIS

HISTORY
- Fever, fatigue, weight loss, bone pain
- Abdominal discomfort, easy satiety, left upper quadrant fullness or pain
- Frequent mucosal bleeding and infections
- Leukostatic symptoms if WBC >100,000: Dyspnea, drowsiness, confusion, priapism
- Gouty arthritis and uric nephropathy (elevated uric acid levels)
- Upper GI ulceration and bleeding (from elevated histamine levels due to basophilia)

PHYSICAL EXAM
Pallor, petechiae, hepatosplenomegaly, lymphadenopathy

DIAGNOSTIC TESTS & INTERPRETATION

Lab
Initial lab tests
- CBC:
  - Leukocytosis: Granulocytes at all stages of differentiation
  - >20–30% blasts:
    - In 60% of cases, blasts have a myeloid or undifferentiated-like phenotype (MBC) whereas in 30% the blasts appear lymphoid-like (LBC)
  - Absolute eosinophil and basophil count >20%
  - Mild anemia
  - Thrombocytosis or thrombocytopenia
- Chemistry profile: K, phosphorus, Ca, renal function
- Serum levels of vitamin B_{12}, lactate dehydrogenase, uric acid, and lysozyme are often increased.
- Bone marrow aspiration: Hypercellular with marked myeloid hyperplasia; myeloid-to-erythroid ratio is 20:1; >20% blasts

Follow-Up & Special Considerations
- Cytogenetics: Measures number and structure of chromosomes in bone marrow
- Fluorescence in situ hybridization (FISH) of fusion genes in blood samples
- Reverse-transcription polymerase chain reaction (RT-PCR) for BCR-ABL mRNA
- Flow cytometry
- Cytochemistry: Peroxidase, TdT
- HLA typing for possible allogeneic hematopoietic cell transplantation (HCT)

Imaging
Initial approach
- Abdominal US or CT for evaluation of hepatosplenomegaly
- Head CT for patients with neurologic symptoms and leukostasis to evaluate for ischemic strokes

Diagnostic Procedures/Other
- Bone marrow aspiration and biopsy
- Possible bone marrow donor evaluation

Pathological Findings
- Bone marrow biopsy: Large clusters of blasts, increased reticulin and fibrosis
- Extramedullary blastic infiltrates (myeloid sarcoma, also known as granulocytic sarcoma or chloroma) (2)
- Spleen: Infiltration of the cords of the red pulp with granulocytes at different stages of maturation
- Liver: Infiltration with granulocytic cells in the portal areas and hepatic sinusoids

DIFFERENTIAL DIAGNOSIS
- Leukemoid reactions
- Ph positive acute myeloid leukemia (AML), acute lymphoblastic leukemia (ALL)

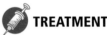

TREATMENT

MEDICATION

First Line
- Attempt to return to a chronic phase and proceed with allogeneic HCT after an initial response.
- Tyrosine kinase inhibitors(TKI): Potent and specific inhibitor of BCR-ABL tyrosine kinase (3):
  - Imatinib 600 mg/d PO
  - Dasatinib 70 mg PO b.i.d. or nilotinib 400 mg PO b.i.d. for patients resistant or intolerant to imatinib
- TKI toxicity: Nausea, vomiting, diarrhea, fluid retention, rash, hepatotoxicity, neutropenia, thrombocytopenia, anemia
- Combination modalities:
  - TKIs plus AML regimens (idarubicin + cytarabine + imatinib) in myeloblastic blast crisis
  - TKIs plus ALL regimens (hyper-CVAD + imatinib or dasatinib) in lymphoblastic blast crisis + CNS prophylaxis: 30% of patients may develop CNS disease

- Allogeneic HCT if feasible, after maximum response to combination therapy:
  - Eligibility criteria for allogeneic HCT vary by institution; age, comorbidities, uncontrollable infections, psychosocial problems, donor availability

Pregnancy Considerations
Risk of miscarriage and birth defects while taking imatinib are uncertain; men and women are strongly advised to use a birth control method during treatment.

Second Line
If patient has resistance or intolerance to TKIs and is not an HCT candidate:
- Interferon α-based regimens and/or
- Cytarabine-based regimens

ADDITIONAL TREATMENT
General Measures
- Monitor for tumor lysis syndrome (TLS).
- Prevent TLS:
  - Aggressive IV hydration
  - Allopurinol 300 mg/d PO
  - Rasburicase if serum uric acid level >9 mg/dL and/or elevated serum creatinine

Issues for Referral
- Consultation with a hematologist is imperative once a diagnosis has been established.
- Consult with bone marrow transplant specialist.
- Consult with renal specialist if TLS is complicated, requiring hemodialysis.

Additional Therapies
- Platelet transfusion to keep platelet count >10,000/mm^3 or > 50,000/mm^3 with clinically evident bleeding
- Myeloid growth factors for fever and absolute neutrophil count <500/mm^3
- Hemodialysis for complicated TLS
- Symptomatic leukocytosis:
  - TKIs, hydroxyurea
  - Emergency leukapheresis in patients who cannot start chemotherapy immediately

COMPLEMENTARY & ALTERNATIVE THERAPIES
- Clinical trials:
  - Autologous HCT for patients ineligible for allogeneic HCT
  - Donor lymphocyte infusion after relapsed allogeneic HCT

SURGERY/OTHER PROCEDURES
Lumbar puncture for CNS disease evaluation

IN-PATIENT CONSIDERATIONS
Initial Stabilization
- Initial diagnosis and management require hospitalization.
- Monitor for spontaneous or chemotherapy- induced TLS.

Admission Criteria
- ICU admission for patient at risk for TLS before starting chemotherapy
- ICU admission for patients with symptomatic leukocytosis:
  - Medical emergency: Efforts should be made to lower the WBC count rapidly

IV Fluids
Iso- or hypotonic IV saline to maintain urine output >2.5 L/d

ONGOING CARE

FOLLOW-UP RECOMMENDATIONS
Disease monitoring to assess response to therapy: CBC, cytogenetic evaluation by FISH and molecular evaluation by RT-PCR

Patient Monitoring
- Hematologic response:
  - Complete: Normalization of WBC, no immature cells, normal platelets count, no splenomegaly
  - Partial: Normal WBC, persistent immature cells, thrombocytosis, splenomegaly
- Cytogenic response:
  - Complete: No Ph + metaphases
  - Partial: <34% Ph + metaphases
  - Minor: >34% Ph +metaphases
- Molecular response:
  - Complete: BCR-ABL mRNA undetectable
  - Major: >3 log reduction BCR-ABL mRNA
- Mutational analysis: ABL kinase domain mutations for patients not responding to TKIs

DIET
Neutropenic diet: Avoid raw or rare-cooked meat, fish, and eggs; avoid fresh and uncooked fruit and vegetables; drink only pasteurized milk, yogurt, cheese; eat fruit that you can peel thick skin off.

PATIENT EDUCATION
- Activity: Avoid mild trauma, bleeding precautions.
- Given the difficult and complex nature of treatment of blast crisis, consultation with a specialist is critical.

PROGNOSIS
- Poor: Median survival is 12–15 months
- Better survival after allogeneic HCT (5–15%):
  - HCT: Only curative treatment for patients who achieve 2nd chronic phase before transplantation
  - While the patient remains in blast crisis, HCT has poor results, with <10% long-term survival.

COMPLICATIONS
- Leukostasis syndrome
- Tumor lysis syndrome:
  - Hyperkalemia, hyperphosphatemia, secondary hypocalcemia, hyperuricemia
  - Acute renal failure
  - Arrhythmia, seizure, sudden death
- Pancytopenia:
  - Neutropenic sepsis
  - Thrombocytopenia with bleeding

REFERENCES
1. Vardiman JW, et al. The World Health Organization (WHO) classification of the myeloid neoplasms. *Blood*. 2002;100(7):2292–302.
2. Druker BJ, et al. Activity of a specific inhibitor of the BCR-ABL tyrosine kinase in the blast crisis of chronic myeloid leukemia and acute lymphoblastic leukemia with the Philadelphia chromosome. *N Engl J Med*. 2001;344(14):1038–42.
3. Jabbour E, et al. Current and emerging treatment options in chronic myeloid leukemia. *Cancer*. 2007;109:2171–81.

ADDITIONAL READING
- Kantarjian H, Cortes J. Chronic myeloid leukemia. In: Abeloff MD, et al., eds. Clinical Oncology. 4th ed. Philadelphia, PA: Elsevier; 2008:2279–2289.
- Bhatia R, Radich JP. Chronic myeloid leukemia. In: Hoffman R, et al., eds., Hematology Basic Principles and Practice, 5th ed. (Chapter 69). New York: Churchill Livingstone Elsevier, 2008.
- National Comprehensive Cancer Network Guidelines 2009.

CODES

ICD9
205.10 Myeloid leukemia, chronic, without mention of having achieved remission

CLINICAL PEARLS
- Blast crisis of CML is characterized by the presence of >20% of peripheral blood or bone marrow blasts, large foci of blasts on bone marrow biopsy, and/or presence of extramedullary blastic infiltrates.
- Progression to blast crisis requires additional chromosomal or cytogenetic abnormalities other than the Ph chromosome translocation.
- First-line treatment includes imatinib followed by allogeneic HCT for eligible patients.
- Prognosis is poor in patients with CML in blast crisis who are not candidates for HCT.

BOTULISM
Alina Dulu

 BASICS

DESCRIPTION
A rare but potentially life-threatening paralyzing disease caused by the potent neurotoxin of the bacterium *Clostridium botulinum*.

Pediatric Considerations
- Infantile botulism (IB) is the most common form presently.
- Occurs in the first 6 months of life
- Consumption of spores that germinate in the immature GI tract forming organisms that produce small quantities of toxin over a prolonged period
- Attributed in the past to contaminated honey ingestion; presently more frequent from ingestion of environmental dust
- Constipation and lethargy
- Feeding and respiratory difficulties
- Weakness of the neck and limbs
- Poorly reactive pupils
- Hypoactive tendon reflexes
- Dry mouth, tachycardia, hypotension, neurogenic bladder
- Most patients require ventilatory support.
- A human-derived antitoxin immunoglobin is available for infants aged <1 year (BIG-IV).
- BIG shortens the duration and reduces the complications of adverse symptoms.

EPIDEMIOLOGY
Incidence
- 24 cases per year of food-borne botulism (FB), 3 cases per year of wound botulism (WB), and 71 cases per year of infant botulism (IB)
- More than 12,000 cases of FB have been reported worldwide since 1951.

RISK FACTORS
- The ingestion of contaminated home-canned fruits, vegetables, and fish
- Restaurant-associated outbreaks are small (2%).
- Subcutaneous or intramuscularinjection drug abusers may harbor *C. botulinum* at sites of small abscesses.
- Cocaine snorting and sinusitis can be the source of *C. botulinum*.
- The use of botulinum toxin for the treatment of dystonia, hemifacial spasm, and spasticity

GENERAL PREVENTION
Do not eat food from bulging cans.

PATHOPHYSIOLOGY
- The spores of *C. botulinum* produce a very potent toxin.
- The toxin, a polypeptide, is absorbed into the circulation from a mucosal surface or wound:
  - FB is caused by ingestion of preformed toxin
  - WB is both an infection and an intoxication; toxin is elaborated by organisms that contaminate a wound.
  - In IB, toxin is produced by organisms in the GI tract.
- The toxin binds to a specific receptor (synaptotagmin II) on the presynaptic sides of peripheral cholinergic synapses at ganglia and neuromuscular junctions.
- Toxin blocks the release of acetylcholine from the presynaptic motor nerve terminal, resulting in autonomic dysfunction and skeletal muscle paralysis.
- Recovery from the toxin involves sprouting of nerve terminals, which form new synapses and take months.
- The toxin does not permeate the blood–brain barrier; therefore the central nervous system is not affected.

ETIOLOGY
- *C. botulinum* is an anaerobic, gram-positive bacillus found in soil, on fruits and vegetables.
- It proliferates under anaerobic conditions and produces a powerful toxin.
- It generates spores that survive extreme temperature and are relatively heat-resistant.
- It produces 8 immunologically distinct neurotoxins (usually A, B, or E) that are heat labile.

Pregnancy Considerations
The fetus is not at risk of neonatal botulism when the mother is afflicted (1).

COMMONLY ASSOCIATED CONDITIONS
Disorder of GI tract (Crohn disease) is associated with hidden botulism (HB).

 DIAGNOSIS

HISTORY
- Neuromuscular symptoms begin 12–36 hours after ingestion of contaminated food.
- Severity of illness is related to the quantity of toxin ingested:
  - Nausea, vomiting, abdominal pain, diarrhea
  - Blurred vision, diplopia,
  - Dysphagia
  - Dysarthria
- Weakness progresses for several days and then reaches a plateau.

PHYSICAL EXAM
- Cranial nerve palsies:
  - Ptosis, extraocular paresis
  - Impaired pupillary reflex (fixed dilated pupils)
  - Tongue weakness
  - Impaired speech
  - Decreased gag reflex
- Symmetrical descending flaccid paralysis:
  - Reduction of tendon reflex responses
- Autonomic dysfunction:
  - Dry mouth, constipation, urinary retention
  - Postural hypotension,
- Fatal respiratory paralysis may occur rapidly.
- No sensory abnormalities with intact mental status

DIAGNOSTIC TESTS & INTERPRETATION
Lab
Initial lab tests
- Cultures of suspected food, wound, stool for *C. botulinum*
- Toxin assay in suspected food, serum, and stool
- Normal CSF analysis

Follow-Up & Special Considerations
The toxin type can be identified using mouse bioassay studies with antitoxin neutralization.

Diagnostic Procedures/Other
- Electrophysiologic testing:
  - Normal sensory nerve amplitudes, velocities, and latencies
  - Normal motor conduction velocities and latencies
- Abnormal stimulation single-fiber EMG:
  - Reduced compound muscle action potentials (CMAP) amplitude in at least 2 muscles
  - At least 20% facilitation of CMAP amplitude during tetanic stimulation
  - Persistence of facilitation for at least 2 minutes after activation
  - No postactivation exhaustion
  - Repetitive nerve stimulation shows increment with rapid repetitive stimulation.
- Needle EMG shows increased number of brief polyphasic motor unit action potentials and fibrillation potentials.
- ECG: Sinus arrhythmia, R-R interval variation

Pathological Findings
Nonspecific

DIFFERENTIAL DIAGNOSIS
- Myasthenia gravis
- Hypermagnesemia
- Guillain-Barré syndrome (Miller-Fisher variant)
- Basilar artery CVA
- Lambert-Eaton myasthenic syndrome
- Diphtheritic neuropathy
- Tick paralysis

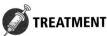 TREATMENT

MEDICATION
First Line
- Trivalent equine serum botulinum antitoxin must be given early (A, B, E):
  – Antitoxin administration is controversial (2).
  – It may decreased fatality rates.
  – One vial by IM injection and one vial IV
  – Derived from horse serum
  – Significant incidence of serum sickness
  – Skin testing (conjunctival instillation and observation for 15 minutes) and possible desensitization, before treatment

Second Line
Anticholinesterase drugs and plasmapheresis are not proved in clinical trials.

ADDITIONAL TREATMENT
General Measures
- Antibiotic use is unproved by clinical trialbut recommended in WB.
- WB: Penicillin 2 million U IV q4h or metronidazole 500 mg IV q8h
- WB: Tetanus boosters as well, if it has been >5 years since last immunization

Issues for Referral
- Physical and occupational therapy for rehabilitation, including supportive devices
- ENT/surgery for early tracheotomy and feeding gastrectomy for patients who require prolonged ventilatory support

Additional Therapies
Pentavalent vaccine available

SURGERY/OTHER PROCEDURES
Surgically debride wound and remove devascularized tissue that might facilitate anaerobic conditions.

IN-PATIENT CONSIDERATIONS
Admission Criteria
- Patients with suspicion for botulism should be hospitalized.
- Patients with rapidly evolving weakness should be monitored in ICU for signs of respiratory failure until the maximum extent of progression has been established.
- Respiratory monitoring: Bedside measurements of forced vital capacity (FVC) and negative inspiratory force (NIF)
- Close monitoring in ICU if:
  – Rapid disease progression
  – FVC <20 mL/kg
  – NIF <30% normal
- Mechanical ventilation may be needed:
  – FVC is <12–15 mL/kg,
  – FVC decline by 30% from baseline
  – FVC is rapidly decreasing
  – NIF <−20 cm H_2O
  – PaO_2 is <70
  – Early signs of respiratory fatigue
  – Difficulty clearing respiratory secretions

IV Fluids
Normal saline

Nursing
- Frequently reposition patient to minimize formation of pressure sores.
- Prevent exposure keratitis in cases of facial plegia by using artificial tears and by taping the eyelids closed at night.
- Laxative, enema to avoid fecal impactions
- Foley for urine retention
- When severe ileus is present, parenteral hyperalimentation may be required.

Discharge Criteria
Neurologically stable

 ONGOING CARE

PATIENT EDUCATION
- Boil the food at 250°F for 30 minutes when preparing canned food to destroy the spores.
- Avoid honey in the 1st year of life.

PROGNOSIS
- Death occurs in 70% of untreated cases and 9% in modern ICU times.
- Recovery begins within a few weeks; it is prolonged and usually complete.
- Recovery of autonomic function takes longer.

COMPLICATIONS
- Long-term ventilatory support
- Aspiration pneumonia

REFERENCES
1. Moser E, et al. Botulinum toxin A (Botox) therapy during pregnancy. *Neurology*. 1997;48(suppl): A399.
2. Hibbs RG, et al. Experience with the use of an investigational F(ab')2 heptavalent botulism immune globulin of equine origin during an outbreak of type E botulism in Egypt. *Clin Infect Dis*. 1996;23:337–40.

ADDITIONAL READING
- Bradley WG, et al., eds. *Neurology in Clinical Practice*, 5th ed. New York: Elsevier, 2008.
- Goetz G. *Textbook of Clinical Neurology*, 3rd ed. New York: Elsevier, 2007.

 CODES

ICD9
- 005.1 Botulism food poisoning
- 040.41 Infant botulism
- 040.42 Wound botulism

CLINICAL PEARLS
- Not all people who ingest the contaminated food become symptomatic.
- Aminoglycosides are contraindicated, since they induce neuromuscular blockade, potentiating the effects of the toxin.
- Inhalational botulism is the form that would occur if aerosolized toxin was released in an act of bioterrorism.

BRADYARRHYTHMIAS/PACING INDICATIONS

Ian A. Lentnek

 BASICS

DESCRIPTION
- Bradycardia is defined as heart rate <60 bpm.
- Bradyarrhythmias include: Sinus bradycardia, sinus arrhythmia/arrest, junctional bradycardia, 1st-degree heart block (PR >200 ms), 2nd-degree heart block (Mobitz Type 1, aka Wenckebach, with successive prolongation of PR interval leading to a nonconducted P wave; Mobitz Type 2, with stable PR interval and sudden nonconducted P wave), and 3rd-degree (aka complete) heart block with no conducted P waves and atrial and ventricular contraction dependent on different pacemakers (atrioventricular dissociation)
- Causes include:
  - Physiologic: Resting heart rate of well-trained athletes, normal heart during sleep, carotid massage/hypersensitivity, any cause of elevated intracranial pressure, vasovagal syncope, vomiting
  - Medications: AV nodal blocking agents (β-blockers, calcium channel blockers), antiarrhythmic toxicity
  - Primary cardiac disease: Sinus node dysfunction (e.g., sick sinus syndrome), AV node dysfunction, conduction system disturbance, myocardial infarction (especially inferior), congestive heart failure, pericardial disease
  - Metabolic/other: Electrolyte abnormality (e.g., hyperkalemia), hypoxia, myxedema, connective tissue disease, idiopathic

EPIDEMIOLOGY
Incidence
Incidence of temporary or permanent pacing varies widely depending on underlying disease.

Prevalence
Prevalence of permanent pacing varies widely depending on underlying disease.

RISK FACTORS
- Structural heart disease
- Causative medications
- Systemic disease

Genetics
- Genetics of underlying disease or conduction abnormality; examples include:
  - Kearns-Sayre syndrome: An inherited disorder due to deletions in a gene of mitochondrial DNA that results in ophthalmologic abnormalities in young people and can cause heart block
  - Muscular dystrophies:
    - Duchenne muscular dystrophy: X-linked recessive disorder of the DMD gene that encodes the protein dystrophin
    - Becker's muscular dystrophy: A less rapidly progressive form of Duchenne

  - Systemic lupus erythematosus:
    - In utero transmission of anti-Ro and anti-La antibodies causes infant myocardial inflammation and conduction system fibrosis resulting in an increased incidence of congenital complete AV block.
    - In afflicted patients, vasculitis and fibrosis of nodal or conductive tissue may result in varying degrees of heart block or bundle branch block; however, complete AV block is rare.

GENERAL PREVENTION
- Prevent structural heart disease.
- Avoid antiarrhythmic toxicity.
- Prevent sequelae of underlying disease.

PATHOPHYSIOLOGY
- Bradycardia may be due to dysfunction of or abnormal effects on the sinus node, AV node, or atrial or ventricular conduction tissue.
- Elevated parasympathetic tone or depressed sympathetic tone may also cause bradycardia.

ETIOLOGY
- Idiopathic
- Exogenous source (e.g., medication)
- Interruption of intrinsic pacemakers or conductive tissue:
  - Lenègre disease: Fibrosis of His-Purkinje system
  - Lev disease: Extrinsic fibrosis that damages the His-Purkinje system
- Abnormal chemical milieu inhibiting normal cellular function

COMMONLY ASSOCIATED CONDITIONS
- Athletic training
- Structural heart disease
- Ingestion of causative medications
- Associated systemic disease
- Acute myocardial infarction, especially inferior

 DIAGNOSIS

HISTORY
- Asymptomatic
- Lightheadedness/dizziness (presyncope)
- Palpitations
- Fatigue
- Syncope
- Findings of congestive heart failure
- Always obtain history of:
  - Symptom onset, termination, and frequency
  - Past medical history
  - Medications
  - Family history

PHYSICAL EXAM
- Normal exam
- Pulse <60 beats/min (>60 beats/min if intrinsic pacemaker overtakes slow sinus beats)
- Regularity of heart rhythm
- Orthostatic hypotension
- Chronotropic incompetence
- Findings of congestive heart failure
- "Cannon" A waves with AV dissociation
- Carotid massage

DIAGNOSTIC TESTS & INTERPRETATION
Lab
Initial lab tests
- 12-lead ECG (no additional studies with benign arrhythmia)
- Electrolyte panel
- Consider drug level

Follow-Up & Special Considerations
- Assess hemodynamic stability.
- Pacing pads if high risk for hemodynamic compromise due to bradyarrhythmia

Imaging
Initial approach
- Benign arrhythmias do not require imaging.
- Echocardiogram: Rule-out structural heart disease
- Chest x-ray: Evaluate for congestive heart failure

Follow-Up & Special Considerations
Coronary angiography if acute infarction

Diagnostic Procedures/Other
- Benign bradyarrhythmias do not require additional testing.
- Exercise testing (chronotropic competence)
- ECG monitoring (e.g., Holter, event recording, implanted loop recorders, device interrogation)
- Upright tilt-table testing
- Intracardiac electrograms

Pathological Findings
- High-degree AV block
- Sinus node dysfunction/arrest:
  - Prolonged AV conduction or His-V interval
  - Prolonged sinoatrial conduction time (SACT)
- Carotid hypersensitivity

DIFFERENTIAL DIAGNOSIS
Potential causes and rhythms listed under "Basics"

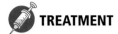

TREATMENT

MEDICATION

First Line
- Benign arrhythmias do not require treatment.
- Treat reversible causes (1)[A]
- Atropine 1 mg IV (repeat up to total dose of 3 mg) (1)[A]

Second Line
- Epinephrine 1 mg IV (repeat) (1)[A]
- Dopamine 2–10 mcg/kg/min IV (1)[A]

ADDITIONAL TREATMENT

General Measures
- Hemodynamic instability secondary to bradyarrhythmia will require temporary pacing (1)[A]:
  – Can be done via external pads or temporary venous pacing
- For permanent pacing indications, see "Surgery/Other Procedures"

Issues for Referral
- Cardiologists or electrophysiologists can identify complex arrhythmias, recommend appropriate testing, and review appropriateness, indication, and device selection for permanent pacing.
- Device implantation by cardiologists, electrophysiologists, or surgeons

SURGERY/OTHER PROCEDURES
- Permanent pacing indications, summarized below, are published by the American College of Cardiology/American Heart Association (2)[A]:
  – Symptomatic bradycardia or chronotropic incompetence
  – Type 2 2nd- and 3rd-degree heart block
  – After catheter ablation of AV node
  – Postoperative AV block not expected to recover
  – In patients with muscular dystrophies and high-degree block (e.g., Becker, Emery-Dreifuss, myotonic dystrophy)
  – Asystole >3.0 seconds
  – Minimally symptomatic patients with chronic heart rate <30 bpm while awake
  – Primary sinus node dysfunction or due to essential drug therapy resulting in symptomatic bradycardia with heart rate <40 bpm

IN-PATIENT CONSIDERATIONS

Initial Stabilization
- ACLS protocol for hemodynamically unstable patients
- Treat underlying disease state.

Admission Criteria
- Symptomatic bradycardia usually due to conduction abnormality, drug toxicity, or ventricular arrhythmia secondary to bradycardia require admission
- Underlying disease or reversible cause of arrhythmia may necessitate admission.

IV Fluids
No specific indications (electrolyte repletion and blood pressure support)

Nursing
Hemodynamic and continuous cardiac monitoring

Discharge Criteria
Following appropriate therapy for arrhythmia, drug toxicity treatment, or stabilization of underlying disease with resolution of bradycardia

ONGOING CARE

FOLLOW-UP RECOMMENDATIONS
- Benign arrhythmias do not require follow-up.
- Patients requiring temporary pacing during acute illness with resolution of their arrhythmia do not usually require specific follow-up.
- Patients with sinus node dysfunction or conduction disease not requiring permanent pacing require regular follow-up to evaluate for disease progression.
- Patients treated with devices require scheduled follow-up and device interrogation to monitor battery-life and arrhythmia events and optimize device settings (telephonic monitoring acceptable with at least an annual office visit).
- Follow-up as required for underlying disease

Patient Monitoring
- Hemodynamically unstable or high-risk patients require a critical care setting.
- Stable patients with high degree of block may be monitored on a telemetry ward.
- Electrolyte normalization protocol should be initiated.

DIET
No specific diet; recommendations as indicated for underlying disease state

PATIENT EDUCATION
- Patients should be taught adverse effects of medications.
- Patients can be taught to monitor their heart rate during episodes suggestive of bradyarrhythmia and to avoid injurious falls.
- Patients requiring device implantation should be taught appropriate instructions regarding follow-up, surgical site care, and avoidance of potentially damaging environmental exposures.

PROGNOSIS
- Benign bradyarrhythmias generally do not progress.
- Arrhythmia secondary to structural heart disease may progress.
- Patients requiring temporary pacing in the setting of myocardial infarction have a worse prognosis not clearly improved with permanent pacing.

COMPLICATIONS
Short- and long-term adverse effects of pacemakers are well described; some chronic complications may be alleviated by biventricular pacing.

REFERENCES

1. ECC Committee, Subcommittees, Task Forces of the American Heart Association: 2005 American Heart Association Guidelines for Cardiopulmonary Resuscitation and Emergency Cardiovascular Care. *Circulation.* 2005;112 [Suppl]: IV1.
2. Gregoratos G, et al. ACC/AHA guidelines for implantation of cardiac pacemakers and antiarrhythmia devices: A report of the American College of Cardiology/American Heart Association Task Force on Practice Guidelines (Committee on Pacemaker Implantation). *J Am Coll Cardiol.* 1998;31:1175–1206.

ADDITIONAL READING
- Libby P, ed. *Braunwald's Heart Disease: A Textbook of Cardiovascular Medicine*, 8th ed. Philadelphia: Saunders Elsevier, 2008.
- Nixon JV, ed. *The AHA Clinical Cardiac Consult*, 2nd ed. Philadelphia: Lippincott Williams and Wilkins, 2007.

CODES

ICD9
- 426.6 Other heart block
- 427.81 Sinoatrial node dysfunction
- 427.89 Other specified cardiac dysrhythmias

CLINICAL PEARLS
- Correct identification of the rhythm is essential to determine further evaluation, treatment, and prognosis.
- Some bradyarrhythmias reflect a normal, healthy, athletically trained heart.
- Structural heart disease is closely linked to abnormal cardiac rhythms.

BRAIN DEATH

Daniela Levi

 BASICS

DESCRIPTION
- A consequence of complete brain failure
- Synonyms: Death by neurologic criteria, whole brain death
- Requires absence of brainstem reflexes, motor responses, and respiratory drive in a comatose patient with a known irreversible brain lesion.
- The equivalence of brain death with death is largely, although not universally, accepted.

RISK FACTORS
- Traumatic brain injury
- Subarachnoid hemorrhage
- Hypoxemic-ischemic brain insult
- Hepatic encephalopathy
- Intracranial tumors

Pediatric Considerations
Child abuse is the most common cause of brain death in children, followed by motor vehicle accident and asphyxia, meningitis, encephalitis.

PATHOPHYSIOLOGY
- The brain has a function–supply-dependent blood flow.
- The decrease in blood flow to the brain is impeded by mass-occupying lesions and brain herniations.
- With severe brain injury, the brain tissue function decreases first, followed by decreased blood flow.

ETIOLOGY
- Hypoxic-hypotensive injury
- Infectious causes,
- Mass occupying lesions
- Bleeding
- Cerebral edema

COMMONLY ASSOCIATED CONDITIONS
- Brain aneurysm, brain masses, encephalitis or meningitis, drug overdose, poisoning
- Cardiovascular instability (hypotension-hypertension, arrhythmias)
- Diabetes Insipidus
- Hypernatremia
- Hypo or hyperthermia
- Acid–base disturbances

DIAGNOSIS

HISTORY
Need to know the cause of coma. This is a permissive diagnostic:
- A reason sufficient to explain death
- Hypothermia and drug intoxication must be excluded or corrected.
- Must have intact neuromuscular transmission (no paralytic agents)
- Ascertainment of irreversibility

PHYSICAL EXAM
- Comatose patient
- Absence of motor responses
- Absence of brainstem reflexes:
  - Pupillary (absence of pupillary responses to light and pupils in midposition with respect to dilation 4–6 mm)
  - Corneal
  - Cervico-ocular
  - Vestibulo-ocular
  - Gag reflex
  - Cough (absence of coughing in response to suctioning)
  - Response to noxious stimuli applied to face

ALERT
Spontaneous and reflex movement in brain death may be present in the form of spinal reflexes and reflexes that originate from medulla oblongata.

DIAGNOSTIC TESTS & INTERPRETATION
Diagnostic tests are performed for determining or confirming the cause of coma.

Lab
- ABG, serum chemistry and electrolytes, liver function tests, urine or serum drug screen if overdose is suspected, cultures, spinal tap if infection/meningitis or encephalitis is suspected
- Apnea testing is another brainstem reflex test.
- An arterial blood gas on 100% FiO_2 should be sent prior to starting the apnea testing:
  - The patient has to be adequately preoxygenated with 6–10 L/min oxygen flow by way of a tracheal catheter
  - A repeat ABG needs to be sent after 8 minutes of apnea.
- The patient should not breath when pCO_2 increases from 40 to 60 mm Hg:
  - This value has been arbitrarily set in U.S. as pCO_2 of 60 mm Hg or >20 mm Hg rise from baseline pCO_2
- If the patient fails the apnea test or this test cannot be performed due to contraindications, then the physician should proceed to ordering other confirmatory tests.
- The patient has to be monitored for breathing, hypoxia, hypotension, arrhythmia:
  - Presence of any respiratory movement, desaturation or hemodynamic instability during the apnea testing mandates failure, and the test should be stopped immediately.

Imaging
Initial approach
Imaging techniques are used to diagnose the cause or ascertain irreversibility of coma:
- CT of the brain can reveal a mass lesion, herniation, or edema.
- CT of the head can be normal early postcardiopulmonary arrest or in meningitis/encephalitis.

Follow-Up & Special Considerations
- Ascertainment of irreversibility
- Repeat neurological exam
- For adults, there is no specific time interval:
  – Repeat testing is hospital- or state-dependent in the U.S.
  – The number of observers and the speciality of physicians is also hospital- or state-dependent.

Pediatric Considerations
- Children do not have fully developed cranial nerves.
- Need to observe for a minimum of 48 hours after initial exam confirming brain death

Diagnostic Procedures/Other
Confirmatory tests (not mandatory in adults with sufficient clinical criteria):
- EEG is rarely performed because of multiple artifacts due to interference
- Cerebral blood flow studies:
  – Angiogram
  – TCD
  – Scintigraphy, nuclear scan

DIFFERENTIAL DIAGNOSIS
- Locked-in syndrome
- Minimally conscious disease
- Persistent vegetative state
- Guillain-Barré syndrome
- Hypothermia
- Drug intoxications:
  – Sedatives, neuromuscular blocking agents, anesthetics

ALERT
- Tricyclic antidepressants agents, cyanide, lithium, fentanyl may not be detected in routine drug screens.
- Observe the patient for >4 times the half-time of the drug or >48 hours, and then use confirmatory testing.

 TREATMENT

ADDITIONAL TREATMENT
Issues for Referral
- After clinical criteria of brain death have been met, the physician should inform the next of kin.
- The physician should not approach the family for organ donation.
- In U.S., organ-procurement agencies must be notified to request the donation of organs.
- If the legal next of kin declines to donate organs, it is good medical judgment to discontinue mechanical ventilation.
- When mechanical ventilation and support are continued because of ethical or legal objections, cardiac arrest occurs commonly.
- The period between the occurrence of brain death and procurement of donated organs is punctuated by profound hemodynamic instability.

ADDITIONAL READING
- Bernat JL. The concept and practice of brain death. *Prog Brain Res*. 2005;150:369–79.
- Truog RD. *J Law Med Ethics*. 2007;summer:35:273.
- Wijdicks EFM. *Neurology*. 2008;70:1234.
- Wijdicks EFM. The diagnosis of brain death. *N Engl J Med*. 344:1215–21.
- Wood K, Laureys S. Care of the potential organ donor. Nature Rev/Neurosci. 2005;6:899

 CODES

ICD9
- 348.1 Anoxic brain damage
- 348.89 Other conditions of brain
- 854.00 Intracranial injury of other and unspecified nature, without mention of open intracranial wound, with state of consciousness unspecified

CLINICAL PEARLS
- A comatose patient with absent brainstem reflexes may be dead by neurologic criteria.
- Presence of spinal reflexes does not rule out brain death.
- Failure or inability to perform an apnea test should lead to confirmatory testing.
- Confirmatory tests are not mandatory in adults.
- Referral to organ donor network is mandatory.

BRAIN INJURY, ANOXIC

Raghad Said
Hayder Said

 BASICS

DESCRIPTION
- Anoxic injury occurs when oxygen supply to the brain cells is disrupted
- Anoxic brain injury is suspected after cardiac arrest when patient is in a coma after ROSC.
- Coma is defined as a state of pathologic unconsciousness; patients are unaware of their environment and are unarousable.

EPIDEMIOLOGY
Incidence
80% patients remain comatose for a variable period after cardiac arrest (1):
- Of those comatose patients, 80% remain unconscious due to hypoxic ischemic cerebral dysfunction and progress to brain death or persistent vegetative state.
- Only 20% of these will survive and regain consciousness.

RISK FACTORS
- Premorbid conditions(1):
  - Age >70
  - Poor functional status prior to arrest
  - APACHE II score of ≥25
  - H/o Renal failure, CVA, CHF, CA, pneumonia
- Periarrest conditions:
  - Long duration of arrest (>10 minutes)
  - PEA arrests and asystole vs. pulseless VT/VF arrest
  - Unwitnessed arrest
  - Absence of a CPR-trained individual
  - In-hospital arrest
  - Arrests in unmonitored wards
  - ICU or a general ward location vs. ER or CCU
  - Arrest at night or weekends
- Postarrest conditions:
  - Hypotension and high pressor and/or inotrope dose needed
  - Hypoxia initial PO_2 <50 mm Hg after ROSC
  - Hyperglycemia within first 24 hours
  - Fever within the first 48 hours

GENERAL PREVENTION
Community training in BLS with emphasis on correct and uninterrupted chest compressions

PATHOPHYSIOLOGY
- Ischemia, rather than hypoxia, is primary cause of neuronal damage after cardiac arrest.
- There is no clear distinction between ischemic and hypoxic injury, and the term *anoxic brain injury* is often used to describe both.
- Anoxia causes brain injury by:
  - Reducing energy stores
  - Ion pump failure
  - Activation of excitatory neurotransmitters(glutamate)
  - Increase in intracellular calcium
  - Oxygen free-radical generation after reperfusion injures cell membranes(2)

ETIOLOGY
- Cardiopulmonary arrest of any cause
- Head trauma
- CO poisoning
- Drug overdose
- Childbirth complications
- Anesthesia complications
- Strangulation and or suffocation
- Drowning

COMMONLY ASSOCIATED CONDITIONS
- Acute MI
- Respiratory failure
- Shock
- Intracranial hypertension (in 30% after severe anoxic injury)
- Central DI reported in pediatrics

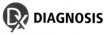 **DIAGNOSIS**

HISTORY
- Prearrest details: History of drugs and medication use, prodromal symptoms
- Circumstances surrounding CPR: The time and place of onset, anoxia time; duration of CPR; cause of the cardiac arrest (cardiac vs. noncardiac); type of cardiac arrhythmia

PHYSICAL EXAM
- Serial neurological exam is the most useful means of predicting individual outcome following ROSC.
- The Glasgow Coma Scale (GCS) score of ≤8 or an absent or extensor motor response at 72 hours is suggestive of poor outcome but does not provide an absolute prognostic prediction.
- Loss of brainstem reflexes: The prognosis is poor in comatose patients with absent pupillary or corneal reflexes 72 hours after cardiac arrest (3)[A].
- Myoclonic status epilepticus present within the 1st day after a circulatory arrest confers a poor prognosis.
- Only features consistent with brain death at any time provide an absolute prediction for brain death.

DIAGNOSTIC TESTS & INTERPRETATION
Lab
Initial lab tests
- ABG: No correlation between initial pH and survival
- S. lactate: Levels >16 mmol/L correlate with poor neurologic outcome
- Chem 7
- CBC
- Urine and/or blood drug toxicology

Follow-Up & Special Considerations

Serum neurone-specific enolase: Levels >33 μg/L at days 1–3 post-CPR accurately predict poor outcome (1)[B].

Imaging
- CT:
  - Rule out other causes of come (e.g., CVA)
  - Loss of distinction between gray and white matter on CT predicts poor outcome especially at the cerebral cortex and basal ganglia level (1)[C].
- MRI:
  - Strong correlation between MRI findings and long-term outcome for infants suffering hypoxic ischemic encephalopathy.
- Role of MRI and PET scan for prognostic assessment of adults with anoxic-ischemic brain is still investigational.

Diagnostic Procedures/Other
- EEG:
  - Rule out status epilepticus
  - Complete or near complete suppression, burst-suppression, generalized periodic complexes, and the α-θ pattern are associated with poor prognosis (3)[B].
  - Variability and reactivity are favorable signs.
  - There is disagreement on classification systems and recording intervals for EEG.
  - EEG is affected by subjective interpretation, electrical interference, sedative medications, and septic or metabolic encephalopathies.
- Somatosensory evoked potentials (SSEPs):
  - Noninvasive bedside test
  - High reproducibility
  - Less susceptible to electrical interference
  - Less affected by sedation or septic or metabolic encephalopathy than EEGs
  - Absence of bilaterally cortical SSEPs (N20 response) within 1–3 days indicates poor prognosis (3)[B].
  - Hypothermia may slow conduction velocities and alter the predictive ability of SSEP.
  - The availability of SSEP is limited.

Pathological Findings
- Ischemic changes in the boundary zones between major cerebral arteries in the cerebral cortex (mostly in the parieto-occipital region), mainly in layers 3–6, basal ganglia, cerebellum, and spinal cord
- Petechial hemorrhages are also seen because of reperfusion injury.
- Severe hypoxia causes preferential damage to the medial temporal lobe.

DIFFERENTIAL DIAGNOSIS
- Locked-in syndrome
- Akinetic mutism
- Dementia

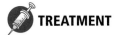 TREATMENT

ADDITIONAL TREATMENT

General Measures

- Head of the bed elevation
- DVT prophylaxis with SQ heparin and/or compression boots
- Valproate or clonazepam to treat myoclonic status epilepticus, although treatment does not improve outcome
- Prevention and treatment of nosocomial infections

Issues for Referral

- Some states mandate transfer of patients after cardiac arrest to centers with induced hypothermia capability.
- The complexity of evaluation and various options of decision making require neurologic professional expertise.

Additional Therapies

- Induced hypothermia: The early induction of mild to moderate hypothermia to a target temperature 32–34°C for up to 24 hours improves the neurologic outcome of patients successfully resuscitated after cardiac arrest, when the patient remains comatose following resuscitation (grade IIa for V fib arrests and IIb for non Vfib or in-hospital arrests) (4)[A]:
  – Sedation and sometimes paralysis are needed to counteract shivering.

IN-PATIENT CONSIDERATIONS

Initial Stabilization

- Intubation for airway protections
- Maintaining MAP of 60 mm Hg with fluids and vasopressors as needed

Admission Criteria

All patients after cardiac arrest require ICU admission initially.

IV Fluids

Avoid hypotonics if signs of high ICP.

Nursing

Avoid moving and bathing hypothermic patients to avoid ventricular arrhythmias.

Discharge Criteria

If severe anoxic brain injury diagnosis is established, physicians are obligated to discuss goals of care with the family or proxy; options are:

- Rethink resuscitation orders or even adjust the level of care to comfort measures only.
- Discharge to a chronic nursing home facility after tracheotomy and feeding tube placement.
- These decisions should be made after multiple meetings with well-informed family members or proxy and with the best interpretation of advance directives or the previously voiced wishes of the patient.

 ONGOING CARE

FOLLOW-UP RECOMMENDATIONS

Patient Monitoring

- ICP monitoring if young patients with favorable neurological exam; benefit is unclear
- Jugular bulb venous (SjO$_2$) oxygen saturation: In nonsurvivors SjO$_2$ steadily increases due to reduced cerebral oxygen consumption secondary to loss of functional tissue.

DIET

- No enteral feeds if hypothermia is used, due to high incidence of ileus.
- GI ulcer prophylaxis in all intubated patients

PATIENT EDUCATION

Explain to family or proxy that the prognosis is largely based on clinical exam with some help from laboratory tests. Also, articulate that the chance of error is very small.

PROGNOSIS

- 57–68% die after cardiac arrest, in general due to primary neurologic failure secondary to anoxic injury, only 9% died because of multiorgan failure.
- 50% of patients discharged after out-of-hospital arrest had some neurologic deficit, compared to 80% after in-hospital cardiac arrest.
- Old age did not negate good cerebral outcome after cardiorespiratory arrest.
- Comorbidity and premorbid performance status are good individual predictors of poor outcome following cardiorespiratory arrest, but they do not predict awakening in survivors.
- Prolonged resuscitation (>10 minutes) is associated with poor outcome. However, it is impossible to absolutely predict poor outcome from arrest duration alone once ROSC is achieved.

COMPLICATIONS

- Persistent vegetative state
- Disability
- Brain death

REFERENCES

1. Kaye P. Early prediction of individual outcome following cardiopulmonary resuscitation: Systematic review. *Emerg Med J*. 2005;22:700–5.
2. Traystman RJ. Oxygen radical mechanisms of brain injury following ischemia and reperfusion. *J Appl Physiol*. 1991;71(4):1185–95.
3. Zandbergen EG, et al. Systematic review of early prediction of poor outcome in anoxic-ischemic coma. *Lancet*. 1998;352:1808.
4. 2005 American Heart Association Guidelines for Cardiopulmonary Resuscitation and Emergency Cardiovascular Care. *Circulation*. 2005; 112(24 Suppl):IV1–IV203.

ADDITIONAL READING

- Holzer M, et al. on behalf of the Collaborative Group on Induced Hypothermia for Neuroprotection After Cardiac Arrest. Hypothermia for neuroprotection after cardiac arrest: Systematic review and individual patient data meta-analysis. *Crit Care Med*. 2005; 33(2):414–8.

 CODES

ICD9

- 348.1 Anoxic brain damage
- 780.01 Coma

CLINICAL PEARLS

- Absent pupillary or corneal reflexes, or absent or only extensor motor responses at 3 days after cardiac arrest are invariably associated with a poor outcome.
- A serum enolase level >33 mcg/L or bilaterally absent somatosensory evoked responses bilaterally at 24–72 hours may be useful to identify those with a poor prognosis.
- Induced hypothermia with a target temperature of 32–34°C for 24 hours for patients who are unconscious after successful resuscitation from a ventricular fibrillation arrest is recommended (1)[A].

BRAIN INJURY, TRAUMATIC

Omar Rahman

 BASICS

DESCRIPTION
- Injury to brain tissue due to trauma
- Primary TBI occurs at the time of initial impact and can be classified as:
- TBI according to mechanism of injury:
  - Direct blunt impact
  - Acceleration-deceleration injury
  - Penetration by low- or high-velocity projectile (pTBI)
  - Blast wave injury (bTBI)
- TBI according to type of parenchymal effect:
  - Concussion injury
  - Brain contusion
  - Intracranial hemorrhage: Epidural hematoma (EDH), subdural hematoma (SDH), subarachnoid hemorrhage (SAH)
  - Diffuse axonal injury (DAI)
- TBI according to severity of injury:
  - Mild: Glasgow Coma Scale (GCS) 14–15
  - Moderate: GCS 9–13
  - Severe: GCS <9
- Secondary brain injury: Damage to neuronal tissue occurring after initial event:
  - Can be early or delayed
  - Determinant of neurological and overall outcome
  - Influenced by local (intracranial) and systemic factors
  - Treatment strategies are mainly directed toward preventing or treating secondary brain injury.

EPIDEMIOLOGY
Incidence
- ~1.5 million cases/year are reported in the U.S. Incidence is 180–250/100,000 people.
- Incidence rising in low- to middle-income countries.

Prevalence
- High-risk age groups: Children 5–9 and adults >80 years
- Peak incidence: 15–24 years of age
- Major cause of mortality and disability in the population aged 1–44.
- Leading cause of morbidity and mortality amongst military/war-related injuries
- Males have 2-fold higher incidence and 4-fold higher risk of fatal injury. Women >50 years have higher rates of cerebral edema and worse outcomes.

RISK FACTORS
- Falls
- Substance and alcohol abuse
- Motor vehicle accidents, particularly bicycle- and motorcycle-related
- Sports and outdoor recreational activities
- Firearm violence and explosion blasts
- Child abuse and domestic violence

GENERAL PREVENTION
- Fall screening for high-risk populations
- Utilization of safety equipment and procedures in high-risk sports and physical activities
- Adherence to traffic safety laws regulations
- Use of protective gear for military or other personnel at risk of exposure to blast injuries
- Child and domestic abuse screening

PATHOPHYSIOLOGY
- Brief physiology:
  - The brain weighs 1400 g (3 lb) and is 80% of cranial vault volume, the rest is blood volume and cerebrospinal fluid (CSF)
  - Cerebral blood flow (CBF) is 15% of cardiac output
  - Brain CSF content is 130–150 mL
  - CBF is constant over a range of systemic blood pressures due to autoregulation.
  - Monroe-Kellie doctrine: Due to skull incompressibility, volume equilibrium exists between blood, CSF, and brain tissue. Increase in volume of one of these must be compensated by a decrease in volume of another, resulting in increased intracranial pressure (ICP).
  - Loss of autoregulation causes cerebral perfusion pressure (CPP) dependence on mean arterial pressure (MAP) and ICP
    - $CPP = MAP - ICP$
- Primary TBI according to mechanism of external mechanical force:
  - Neuron cell body, axonal, and vascular damage occurs due to direct impact and shear injury in both direct and opposite plane of motion against the inner skull bone (coup-contrecoup pattern).
  - pTBI: Dural integrity is breached by foreign object, resulting in tearing injury. Tissue cavitation is seen with high-velocity objects
  - bTBI: Concussion-percussion wave, high- energy, and toxic fumes from explosive blasts cause injury.
- Primary TBI according to parenchymal effect:
  - Concussion: Transient white matter fiber stretch and alteration in neurotransmitters without persistent pathologic changes
  - Contusions: Heterogeneous distribution of hemorrhage. Local mass effect, edema, and blood–brain barrier disruption is seen.
  - EDH: Laceration of meningeal vessels following low-velocity impact leads to accumulation of mostly arterial blood in the epidural space and subsequent mass effect.
  - SDH: Cortical vessel damage causing diffuse accumulation of mostly venous blood in the subdural space and subsequent mass effect
  - SAH: Cerebral vasospasm and hydrocephalus
  - DAI: Microscopic diffuse disruption of axon projections in the white matter
- Secondary brain injury:
  - Intracellular and extracellular pathologic processes starting after primary injury
  - Local factors: Inflammation, ischemia, reperfusion, excitatory neurotransmitters, compressive lesions, seizures, intracranial hypertension, cerebral edema
  - Systemic determinants: Hypoperfusion, hypoxia, anemia, temperature dysregulation, acid–base disorders, hyper/hypocapnia
- Cerebral edema:
  - TBI causes vasogenic and cytotoxic edema
- Herniation syndromes:
  - Transtentorial (central and lateral): Due to supratentorial mass effect or temporal lesion
  - Subfalcine: Due to frontal or parietal convexity mass lesion
  - Cerebellar: Cerebellum/posterior fossa lesion

ETIOLOGY
- Trauma
- Systemic causes of secondary brain injury:
  - Shock states: Hypovolemic, cardiogenic, hemorrhagic, obstructive, spinal/neurogenic
  - Severe hypoxemia and hypercapnia
  - Hyperpyrexia
  - Seizures

COMMONLY ASSOCIATED CONDITIONS
- Trauma-related:
  - Spine fractures and spinal cord injury
  - Pulmonary contusions and rib fractures
  - Hemopneumothorax (tension or simple)
  - Abdominal trauma
  - Depressed, open or simple skull fractures including basilar skull fractures
  - Long-bone fractures (open or closed)
  - Cardiac contusion and tamponade
  - Carotid and/or vertebral arterial injury
- Nontrauma conditions:
  - Acute MI
  - Cardiac arrhythmias
  - ARDS and pulmonary edema
  - Rhabdomyolysis
  - Acute kidney injury
  - Coagulopathy
  - Electrolyte imbalance: Hyponatremia, hypernatremia, hypokalemia
  - Hypoglycemia and hyperglycemia

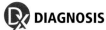 **DIAGNOSIS**

HISTORY
Trauma patient history protocol:
- **A**llergies, **M**edication, **P**ast medical history, **L**ast meal, **E**vent (mechanism of injury)

PHYSICAL EXAM
- Primary survey: Identify life-threatening injury
- Secondary survey with neurological exam
- GCS
- Scalp lacerations and open wounds
- Signs of basilar skull fracture:
  - Periorbital ecchymosis (raccoon eyes sign)
  - CSF otorrhea and rhinorrhea
  - Postauricular ecchymosis (Battle's sign)
- Signs of increased ICH and herniation syndromes (1)[B]:
  - Cushing's triad: Bradycardia, irregular respirations, and widened pulse pressure
  - Transtentorial:
    - Anisocoria and ipsilateral CN III palsy
    - Contralateral hemiparesis (75%)
    - Ipsilateral hemiparesis (25%, Kernohan's notch effect)
    - Coma, decorticate to decerebrate posturing
  - Subfalcine: Asymmetric motor posturing with preserved oculocephalic reflex
  - Cerebellar: Bilateral motor posturing, coma

ALERT
- EDH patients: "Talk & die" phenomena due to initial lucid interval followed by herniation (2)[B]
- Children and adolescents: "Secondary impact syndrome" after initial concussion may be fatal.

DIAGNOSTIC TESTS & INTERPRETATION
Lab
Initial lab tests
- CBC, metabolic panel, PT/INR, PTT
- ABG, urine, and serum toxicology screen
- CPK, serum osmolality

Follow-Up & Special Considerations
- CSF chemistry and culture
- Correct coagulopathy

Imaging
Initial approach
CT scan:
- High sensitivity and specificity
- EDH: Convex, lentiform appearance
- SDH: Concave diffuse appearance
- Midline shift can be detected
- Minor hemorrhages, contusions, and early ischemia may not be evident

Follow-Up & Special Considerations
- Cerebral angiography, MRI, and MRA
- Radionuclide blood flow scans

Diagnostic Procedures/Other
- ICP monitoring
- Brain tissue oxygen monitoring (PbrO$_2$)
- Jugular venous O$_2$ saturation (SjO$_2$)
- EEG
- Cerebral microdialysis
- Somatosensory evoked potentials

DIFFERENTIAL DIAGNOSIS
- Metabolic encephalopathy
- Nonconvulsive seizures
- Cerebrovascular accident
- Aneurysmal SAH

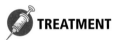 TREATMENT

MEDICATION
See elevated ICP management

ADDITIONAL TREATMENT
General Measures
- ABCs
- C-spine collar
- Pain control (fentanyl, remifentanil)
- DVT prophylaxis with sequential compression device and stockings:
  - SC low-molecular-weight heparin (LMWH) or heparin if no active bleeding; no guidelines for timing of initiation
  - IVC filter if not candidate for LMWH/heparin
- Stress gastric ulcer prevention
- Nosocomial infection prevention

Issues for Referral
Early transfer to neurosciences trauma center

IN-PATIENT CONSIDERATIONS
Initial Stabilization
- Airway control and rapid sequence intubation
- Large-bore IV access; central venous catheter
- Hemodynamic monitoring; arterial catheter
- Maintain euvolemia.
- Avoid hypotension (keep SBP >90 mm Hg).
- Avoid hypoxia (goal PaO$_2$ >60 mm Hg).
- Antibiotics for pTBI or basal skull fractures
- Avoid fever, maintain normothermia:
  - If hypothermic, may need active rewarming
- Treat active seizures: Benzodiazepines, phenytoin, levetiracetam
  - Prophylaxis prevents only early seizures; routine prophylaxis 1 week post TBI is not recommended.
- Surgical evacuation of compressive lesions
- ICP monitoring indications (3)[A]:
  - GCS $\leq$8
  - Abnormal CT scan
  - Age >40 years
  - SBP <90 mm Hg
- Elevated ICP management (3)[A]:
  - ICP goal is <20–25 mm Hg
  - Head of bed elevated 30–45 degrees
  - Mannitol 20% 1–1.5 g/kg IV bolus
  - Role of hypertonic saline is less clear
  - Sedation: Propofol, pentobarbital
  - Elevate CPP if <60 mm Hg (norepinephrine, phenylephrine, or dopamine)
  - Hyperventilation (PaCO$_2$ 28–32) only for impending herniation as a temporary measure; sustained use is deleterious
  - Hypothermia to 32–34°C for refractory ICP:
    ○ No impact on overall mortality
  - Cranial decompression: CSF drainage or hemicraniectomy may be definitive treatment.

Admission Criteria
Moderate to severe TBI, concomitant trauma, or hemodynamic/respiratory compromise, shock, ICP monitoring, other organ failure

IV Fluids
- NS (0.9%)
- Hypertonic saline (3%, 7.5%, 23.4%)

Nursing
Standard ICU nursing per local protocols

Discharge Criteria
Per ICU protocols to step-down units, rehabilitation, or skilled facilities

 ONGOING CARE

FOLLOW-UP RECOMMENDATIONS
Speech, physical, neuropsychiatric therapy
Patient Monitoring
- ICU care and monitoring as described
- ICP monitoring: Better outcomes (3)[B]

DIET
Early enteral feeding may improve outcome.

PATIENT EDUCATION
Fall prevention, relevant safety guidelines

PROGNOSIS
Factors impacting prognosis:
- Initial GCS (<9: 25–75% mortality)
- CT scan findings
- Age (>60 or <2 years)
- Hypotension, hypoxemia, acidosis, hyperglycemia

COMPLICATIONS
- Hydrocephalus
- Central DI, SIADH, cerebral salt wasting
- Nosocomial infections: VAP, BSI, and UTI
- Chronic respiratory failure, DVT/PE, CHF
- Late post-traumatic seizures
- Motor, sensory, and psychological disabilities

REFERENCES

1. Cushing H. Physiological and anatomical observations of the influence of brain compression on intracranial circulation and some other related. *Mitteilungen aus den Grenzgebieten der Medizin und Chirurgie.* 1902;9:773–808.
2. Lobato RD, et al. Head injured patients who talk and deteriorate into coma. Analysis of 211 cases by CT. *J Neurosurg.* 1992;75(2):256–61.
3. Bratton SL, et al. Guidelines for the management of severe traumatic brain injury. *J Neurotrauma.* 2007;24(Suppl 1):S1–S106.

ADDITIONAL READING

- Heegard W, et al. Traumatic brain injury. *Emerg Med Clin N Am.* 2007;25:655–78.

 CODES

ICD9
- 850.9 Concussion, unspecified
- 854.00 Intracranial injury of other and unspecified nature, without mention of open intracranial wound, with state of consciousness unspecified
- 854.10 Intracranial injury of other and unspecified nature, with open intracranial wound, with state of consciousness unspecified

CLINICAL PEARLS
- Early cranial decompression may be indicated.
- Antiepileptics do not prevent late seizures.
- No role for corticosteroids
- Prevent secondary brain injury.

BURNS

Ariel L. Shiloh

 BASICS

DESCRIPTION

- Burns are classified based on their depth and size.
- Burns are often associated with additional trauma and inhalation injury.
- Burn type:
  - Mild (outpatient):
    - <10% TBSA (<5% elderly)
    - <2% full-thickness burn
  - Moderate (inpatient):
    - 10–20% TBSA (5–10% elderly)
    - 2–5% full thickness burn
    - High-voltage injury
    - Suspect inhalation injury
    - Circumferential burn
    - Medical predisposition to infection
  - Major (burn center):
    - >20% TBSA (>10% elderly)
    - >5% full-thickness burn
    - High-voltage burn
    - Known inhalation injury
    - Involvement of face, eyes, ears, genitalia, joints
    - Associated injury/trauma

EPIDEMIOLOGY

Incidence

- 500,000 burn injuries receiving medical treatment per year
- 4,000 fire and burn deaths per year
- 75% of deaths occur at the scene or during transport
- 40,000 hospitalizations for burn injury per year of which 25,000 admissions to burn centers
- 70% male
- Burn Cause:
  - Flame: 46%
  - Scald/immersion: 32%
  - Hot object contact: 4%
  - Electrical: 4%
  - Chemical: 3%
  - Other: 6%

DIAGNOSIS

PHYSICAL EXAM

- Remove all clothing and debris to diminish further injury and evaluate the extent of burns and any associated trauma.
- Assess the extent of the burn.
- Size (total body surface area):
  - "Rules of nine"/Lund and Browder chart:
    - Each arm: 9%
    - Each leg: 18%
    - Anterior trunk: 18%
    - Posterior trunk: 18%
    - Head: 9%
    - Genitalia: 1%
- Depth:
  - Superficial (1st degree):
    - Painful
    - Dry, red, blanching
    - 3–6 days healing
  - Superficial partial thickness (2nd degree):
    - Intact pain sensation
    - Blisters, erythema, capillary refill
    - 7–20 days healing
  - Deep partial-thickness (3rd degree):
    - Absent pain sensation
    - Moist blisters, pale white/yellow, no capillary refill
    - >21 days healing
  - Full-thickness (4th degree):
    - Absent pain sensation
    - Waxy, inelastic, leathery, charred, dry, no capillary refill
    - Does not heal
- Changes in mental status may indicate smoke inhalation, carbon monoxide toxicity, and cyanide toxicity.

DIAGNOSTIC TESTS & INTERPRETATION

Assess ABCs and assess for smoke inhalation injury:

- Evaluate for signs and symptoms of respiratory distress and have a high suspicion for smoke inhalation injury when the following are present:
  - Cough, stridor, wheeze, hoarseness
  - Tachypnea and accessory muscle use
  - Face and circumferential neck burns
  - Oropharyngeal/nasopharyngeal injury
  - Hypoxia and hypercapnia
- Complete airway obstruction due to laryngeal edema is possible, and intubation should not be delayed.
- Evaluate the cardiovascular status, establish vascular access, and initiate resuscitation.

Diagnostic Procedures/Other

- CXR, EKG
- Fiberoptic laryngoscopy/bronchoscopy for airway evaluation
- ABGs with co-oximetry to assess carbon monoxide toxicity
- End-tidal CO_2, serum lactate, and cyanide level to assess cyanide toxicity and organ perfusion
- CPK

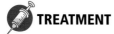

TREATMENT

ADDITIONAL TREATMENT

General Measures
- Supplemental oxygen:
  - Bronchodilators are administered for bronchospasm related to inhalation injury.
  - Avoid corticosteroids due to the high risk of secondary infection.
- Provide airway protection and mechanical ventilation as required.
- Initiate fluid resuscitation.
- Transfer to a burn center for major burns or if there is associated trauma and/or inhalation injury.

Additional Therapies
- Fluid resuscitation:
  - Patients with >15% TBSA nonsuperficial burns require formal fluid resuscitation.
  - Burn shock consists of decreased capillary tone and myocardial depression:
    - Two large-bore IVs or central access, preferably through nonburned skin
    - Arterial catheter for blood pressure management and frequent ABGs and serum lactate level
    - Bladder catheter to evaluate adequate fluid resuscitation and end organ perfusion via urine output
  - Parkland formula calculates the initial 24-hour fluid requirement (most widely used formula):
    - Fluid requirements = TBSA burned(%) × Wt (kg) × 4 mL
    - Administer 1/2 of total calculated requirements over 8 hours and the remainder over 16 hours.
  - Use LR solution.
  - Keep urine output at 0.5 mL/kg/hr.
  - Avoid excessive resuscitation, which may lead to pulmonary edema and compartment syndrome.

- Secondary management:
  - Clean cool burns with cold water and saline-soaked gauze but avoid excessive hypothermia:
    - Avoid the use of ice and ice water.
  - Administer pain control with IV opiates.
  - Assess tetanus immunization status and administer if necessary.
  - Apply topical antibiotics to nonsuperficial burns (i.e., silver sulfadiazine):
    - There is no evidence for the use of empiric parenteral antibiotics.
  - Avoid causing circulatory impairment with dressings:
    - Biologic dressings may be beneficial for wound healing and pain control.
  - Deep partial- and full-thickness burns require surgical excision and skin grafting.
  - Provide nutrition to match catabolic demands.
- Decompressive escharotomy:
  - Escharotomy is used to treat elevated compartment pressures that compromise perfusion in circumferential burns.
  - Constriction of the chest and neck preventing adequate ventilation require escharotomy.
  - Fasciotomy is required to treat compartment syndrome.
- Carbon monoxide toxicity:
  - Administer 100% oxygen to displace carbon monoxide from hemoglobin.
  - Hyperbaric oxygen is administered for most patients if carboxyhemoglobin is >40%.
  - Hyperbaric oxygen is administered regardless of level for:
    - Unconscious patients
    - Pregnant patients/fetal distress

- Cyanide toxicity:
  - In the setting of smoke inhalation, administer empiric treatment if there is unexplained lactic acidosis, low end-tidal CO_2, depressed mental status, or cardiac complications.
  - Antidote: Sodium thiosulfate and hydroxocobalamin:
    - In burn patients, avoid therapy with nitrates due to methemoglobinemia.

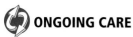

ONGOING CARE

PROGNOSIS
- If early organ failure is avoided, survival after near-total burns is not uncommon.
- ~95% overall survival rate

ADDITIONAL READING
- American Burn Association: burn incidence fact sheet www.ameriburn.org
- Monafo WW. Initial management of burns. N Engl J Med. 1996;335:1581–6.
- Singer AJ, et al. Current management of acute cutaneous wounds. N Engl J Med. 2008;359:1037–46.

CODES

ICD9
- 949.0 Burn of unspecified site, unspecified degree
- 949.1 Erythema due to burn (first degree), unspecified site
- 949.2 Blisters with epidermal loss due to burn (second degree), unspecified site

CANDIDURIA

Miguel Angel Russo

 BASICS

DESCRIPTION

Candida spp. are frequent colonizers of the lower urinary tract. *C. albicans* represents ~1/2 of the fungal isolates in urine. Non-albicans species of *Candida* including *C. glabrata*, *C. tropicalis*, and *C. krusei* may also cause funguria, especially in patients previously treated with antifungal agents. Of particular concern is the use of fluconazole in hospitalized patients.

EPIDEMIOLOGY

In an ICU surveillance study, candiduria developed in 22% of patients admitted for >7 days. In that same study, independent risk factors for candiduria included age >65, female sex, length of hospital stay before ICU admission, diabetes mellitus, total parenteral nutrition, mechanical ventilation, and previous antimicrobial use.

RISK FACTORS

Candiduria have been associated with:
- Antibiotics
- Diabetes mellitus
- Foley catheters

GENERAL PREVENTION

Prevention can be addressed in three stages: prevention of catheterization; once the catheter is in place, prevention of candiduria; and once candiduria occurs, prevention of complications.

PATHOPHYSIOLOGY

- *Candida* spp., particularly *C. albicans*, colonize the human GI, respiratory, and reproductive tracts and the skin. Invasive disease occurs when host defenses break down or are breached.
- A variety of adhesins facilitate attachment of the fungus to epithelial and endothelial surfaces.
- The ability of *Candida* spp. to form biofilm on surfaces such as catheters has contributed to the emergence of these fungi as major pathogens of patients with indwelling medical devices.
- Biofilm-associated infections are frequently refractory to antifungal therapy.

ETIOLOGY

- *C. albicans* is the cause in 90% of patients.
- *C. glabrata*, *C. krusei*, *C. tropicalis*, and *C. pseudotropicalis* produce infection in recurrent cases and in women with HIV infection.

COMMONLY ASSOCIATED CONDITIONS

Factors predisposing to candiduria include:
- Diabetes mellitus
- Urinary tract abnormalities
- Malignancy

 DIAGNOSIS

DIAGNOSTIC TESTS & INTERPRETATION
Diagnostic Procedures/Other

- The diagnosis of fungal UTI represents a challenge to the clinician.
- The presence of *Candida* spp. in urine does not necessarily signify true infection and may instead merely represent colonization or even contamination of the urinary sample.
- The lack of specific signs and symptoms complicates the process of diagnosing fungal UTI, and some patients with infection are asymptomatic.
- The presence of pyuria and colony counts of 10,000–15,000 *Candida* spp. per milliliter of urine may suggest infection; however, the predictive value of these findings when urinary catheters are in place is not known. Indeed, studies in experimental renal candidiasis demonstrate that CFUs are not a reliable predictor of renal candidiasis.

TREATMENT

- There are various options for management of candiduria. In the absence of an underlying chronic medical condition, the identification of *Candida* spp. in the urine may represent colonization or low-grade infection that often resolves without specific therapy or with removal of the urinary catheter. All indwelling urinary instrumentation should be removed if possible.
- Candiduria should be treated in symptomatic patients, low-birth-weight infants, patients with neutropenia, and persons expected to undergo urinary tract instrumentation.

MEDICATION
First Line
Oral fluconazole (200 mg), in non-krusei candidal cystitis

Second Line
In patients with intact renal function, flucytosine (25 mg/kg/d) may be an option, although resistance can develop rapidly when this agent is used as monotherapy.

COMPLEMENTARY & ALTERNATIVE THERAPIES
Amphotericin B bladder irrigation (50 mg/L over 24 hours or 50 mg/L for 7 days) has been used for candiduria. Short-term eradication rates with this type of therapy are comparable with fluconazole, but the technique is cumbersome, and patients may complain of bladder fullness.

 ONGOING CARE

COMPLICATIONS
Papillary necrosis, fungus ball formation, and perinephric abscess can result from ascending infection, particularly in the presence of urinary tract obstruction, renal stones, or diabetes mellitus.

ADDITIONAL READING

- Alvarez-Lerma F, et al. Candiduria in critically ill patients admitted to intensive care medical units. Intensive *Care Med*. 2003;29:1069–76.

 CODES

ICD9
112.2 Candidiasis of other urogenital sites

C

CARBON MONOXIDE

Ram Sanjeev Alur
James Gasperino

 BASICS

DESCRIPTION
- Systemic toxic inhalant
- Colorless, odorless, nonirritating

EPIDEMIOLOGY
Incidence
- During 1999–2004, carbon monoxide (CO) poisoning was listed as a contributing cause of death on 16,447 death certificates in the U.S.
- During 2004–2006, an estimated average of 20,636 ED visits for nonfatal, unintentional, non–fire-related CO exposures occurred each year.
- The annual average age-adjusted death rate in the US was 1.5 deaths per million persons.
- 3rd cause of unintentional poisoning deaths in US

Prevalence
- ~15,200 emergency department visits each year during 2001–2003
- An average of 439 persons died annually from unintentional, non–fire-related CO poisoning.

RISK FACTORS
- For exposure:
  - Poor ventilation
  - Use of raw material in metallurgy
  - Engine exhaust
  - Use of wood or coal
  - Use of propane heaters
- For toxicity:
  - Fetus of pregnant woman, cardiorespiratory comorbidity

GENERAL PREVENTION
- Have heating systems, water heaters, and any other gas-, oil-, or coal-burning appliances serviced by a qualified technician every year.
- Install battery-operated CO detectors in homes, and check or replace batteries when changing the time on clocks each spring and fall.

PATHOPHYSIOLOGY
- Tissue hypoxia due to decreased arterial oxygen content; CO binds to both Hb and Mb with high affinity.
- CO has an ~250 × higher affinity for Hb than does oxygen.
- Carboxyhemoglobin does not carry oxygen.
- Decreased oxygen delivery to tissues shifts oxy-Hb dissociation curve to the left.
- Inhibits cytochrome oxidase, causing impaired mitochondrial utilization of oxygen.
- ATP production is impaired.
- Free radical formation induces lipid peroxidation in CNS, leading to neurologic changes.

ETIOLOGY
- Tissue hypoxia from decreased arterial oxygen content, delivery, and impaired utilization of oxygen
- Exposure scenarios: Environmental, occupational, and intentional

COMMONLY ASSOCIATED CONDITIONS
- CNS: Altered mental status
- Cardiovascular: Tachyarrhythmia, hypotension, myocardial ischemia
- Pulmonary: ARDS
- Renal: Acute tubular necrosis
- Ocular: Blindness
- Musculoskeletal: Rhabdomyolysis

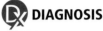 **DIAGNOSIS**

HISTORY
- Exposure
- Headaches, confusion, muscle aches, fatigue, dyspnea, chest pain, nausea, vomiting, palpitations, seizures
- Nonspecific: Underdiagnosed, could be misdiagnosed as viral syndrome
- Symptoms associated with levels:
  - COHb (%) 10–20: Flu-like symptoms
    - 30: Severe headache
    - 50: Loss of consciousness
    - 60–70: Seizure, hemodynamic collapse
    - 80: Rapidly fatal
    - Any level >50% can be lethal

PHYSICAL EXAM
- Nearly unremarkable to coma or death
- Tachypnea, diaphoresis, lethargy
- Ataxia
- Decreased MMSE
- Cherry red discoloration of skin, lips (rare)

DIAGNOSTIC TESTS & INTERPRETATION
Lab
Initial lab tests
- Co-oximetry of arterial blood-COHb level
- Pulse oximeters overestimate arterial blood oxygenation.
- ABG, CPK, serum electrolytes, CBC, ECG

Follow-Up & Special Considerations
- Pregnancy testing in all women of childbearing age
- Pulse oximetry misleading
- COHb does not correlate with clinical severity.

Imaging
Initial approach
- Chest radiograph, CT, and MRI of the brain
- CO can produce different patterns of brain injury in the acute and delayed stages. The globus pallidus is the most common site of involvement in CO poisoning.

Pregnancy Considerations
- Fetal COHb levels are higher than mother's.
- Fetal death and brain damage are real concerns.
- ABG and co-oximetry must be calibrated for fetal Hb.

Follow-Up & Special Considerations
Pregnant women are high risk; increased fetal morbidity and mortality

Pathological Findings
- Features of tissue ischemia
- Basal ganglia infarction
- Similar to anoxic brain injury

DIFFERENTIAL DIAGNOSIS
Viral syndrome, TIA, acute coronary syndrome, acute lung injury

 TREATMENT

Remove from exposure

MEDICATION
First Line
- Initial stabilization
- 100% supplemental oxygen by face mask as soon as diagnosis is suspected
- Hyperbaric oxygen if evidence shows end-organ damage independent of COHb level, COHb >25%, >15% if pregnant woman, child

- Improves neurologic outcomes
- Hyperbaric oxygen decreases half-life of COHb, increases arterial oxygen content, decreases lipid peroxidation.
- 3 hyperbaric oxygen treatments within a 24-hour period appeared to reduce the risk of cognitive sequelae 6 weeks and 12 months after acute CO poisoning.

Second Line
Seizures: Use of antiepileptic medications

ADDITIONAL TREATMENT
General Measures
- ABCs
- IV fluids

Issues for Referral
- Transfer to a facility with hyperbaric chamber should not be delayed.
- Organ transplant considerations

IN-PATIENT CONSIDERATIONS
Initial Stabilization
- ICU monitoring
- ABCs

Admission Criteria
- Symptoms
- Signs of end-organ damage
- Need for hyperbaric oxygen therapy

Discharge Criteria
- COHb <10%
- ECG normal for the patient
- Baseline mental status

 ONGOING CARE

FOLLOW-UP RECOMMENDATIONS
Neuropsychiatric testing for neuropsychological complications

Patient Monitoring
- Delayed neurologic sequelae
- Neuropsychiatric testing

PATIENT EDUCATION
- Awareness
- Home CO monitoring
- Improve ventilation

PROGNOSIS
Hypotension or syncope at presentation indicates likely neurological sequelae.

COMPLICATIONS
As above

ADDITIONAL READING

- Butler FK, et al. Hyperbaric oxygen therapy and the eye. *Undersea Hyperb Med*. 2008;35:333–87.
- Carbon monoxide-related deaths—United States, 1999–2004. *MMWR Morb Mortal Wkly Rep*. 2007;56:1309–12.
- Hampson N. Pulse oximetry in severe carbon monoxide poisoning. *Chest*. 1998;114:1036–41.
- Lo C, et al. Brain injury after acute carbon monoxide poisoning: early and late complications. *AJR Am J Roentgenol* 2007;189:W205–W211.
- Non-fatal unintentional, non-fire-related carbon monoxide exposures—United States, 2004–2006. *MMWR Morb Mortal Wkly Rep*. 2008;57:896–9.
- Unintentional non-fire-related carbon monoxide exposures in the United States, 2001–2003. *MMWR Morb Mortal Wkly Rep*. 2005;54:36–9.
- Weaver LK, et al. Hyperbaric oxygen for acute carbon monoxide poisoning. *N Engl J Med*. 2002;347:1057–67.

 CODES

ICD9
986 Toxic effect of carbon monoxide

CLINICAL PEARLS

- Entertain a low index of suspicion.
- Levels do not correlate with severity.

C

CARDIAC TAMPONADE

Hari Gnanasekeram

 BASICS

DESCRIPTION
- Cardiac tamponade is a clinical syndrome caused by the accumulation of fluid in the pericardial space, resulting in reduced ventricular filling and impaired cardiac diastolic filling, which can lead to hemodynamic compromise
- Fluid accumulation can be global or loculated within the pericardium:
  - Acute tamponade involves rapid filling of fluid within a stiff noncompliant pericardium.
  - Subacute tamponade allows an existing effusion to accumulate gradually, with pericardial stretching to allow accommodation of larger amounts of fluid.

EPIDEMIOLOGY
Incidence and Prevalence
- Most common cause of acute pericardial tamponade is penetrating trauma (seen in approximately 2% of cases); it is rarely seen in blunt chest trauma.
- Malignancy is the most common etiology of pericardial effusions in developed countries.
- Tuberculosis should be considered in endemic areas.

RISK FACTORS
High-risk patients:
- Large circumferential pericardial effusion (echocardiographic depth >2 cm) (1)
- Recent anticoagulant treatment
- Concurrent malignancy, particularly lung, breast, lymphoma and leukemia
- Internal or external chest trauma or catheter manipulation
- Fever >38°C
- Immunosuppressive states, HIV
- Atypical ECG evolution
- Significant leukocytosis and elevated cardiac biomarkers (1)

Genetics
Unknown

PATHOPHYSIOLOGY
- Accumulation of fluid within pericardial space, which consists of an outer fibrous layer and an inner serous layer
- Gradual collection fluid leads to impairment of diastolic cardiac filling and eventually circulatory collapse.
- Rapid accumulation leads to circulatory collapse more commonly than gradual accumulation, which allows for pericardial stretch and adaptive compliance (2).

- When sufficient fluid accumulates, and a critical point on the compliance curve is reached, intrapericardial pressure rises rapidly. When this happens, transmural pressures in the intracardiac chambers decrease, and venous return is impeded in diastole.
- Finally, when diastolic equalization of the left and right ventricles occurs, cardiac output falls (2).
- Low-pressure tamponade occurs when intravascular volume depletion causes significant hemodynamic changes as the intracardiac chambers equalize at lower pressures (3).
- Hypertensive cardiac tamponade has all of the features of classic tamponade, but can occur at very high systolic pressures (often >200 mm Hg), often associated with excessive sympathetic drive in a patient with pre-existing hypertension

ETIOLOGY
- Acute:
  - Penetrating or blunt chest trauma, usually causing hemopericardium
  - Myocardial rupture post-MI or ruptured myocardial aneurysm
  - Dissecting ascending aortic aneurysm
  - Recent thrombolytic therapy (4)
  - Complication of percutaneous coronary intervention or spontaneous coronary artery rupture (5)
  - Recent coronary artery bypass graft surgery.
  - Iatrogenic causes, including central line or pacer wire insertion (6)
- Subacute:
  - Iatrogenic secondary to instrumentation
  - Idiopathic pericarditis, usually of undiagnosed viral origin
  - Use of thrombolysis in acute myocardial infarction.
  - Infections:
    ○ Viral: Commonly Coxsackie group and HIV.
    ○ Bacterial: Commonly *Staphylococcus* species (4)
    ○ Fungal less common
  - Hypothyroidism
  - Connective tissue disease: SLE, rheumatoid arthritis, scleroderma, acute rheumatic fever (4)
  - End-stage renal disease and uremic states

COMMONLY ASSOCIATED CONDITIONS
- Cardiogenic shock with cardiovascular collapse
- Change in mental status or loss of consciousness secondary to cranial hypoperfusion

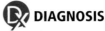 **DIAGNOSIS**

HISTORY
- Most common presenting symptom is dyspnea with respiratory distress
- Concomitant symptoms can include chest pain, nausea, and abdominal pain from hepatic congestion.
- For acute presentations, investigate for recent trauma, surgery, or recent instrumentation.
- Subacute presentations usually have underlying effusions of chronic etiologies.

PHYSICAL EXAM
- Beck's triad (hypotension, elevated systemic venous pressure, jugular venous distention) is commonly seen (6).
- Distant heart sounds with a friction rub may be heard.
- Common findings:
  - Tachycardia (2,6):
    ○ Tachypnea.
    ○ Pulsus paradoxus (2)
  - Elevation of jugular venous pressure during inspiration; Kussmaul sign
  - Cardiogenic shock with hemodynamic compromise or pulseless electrical activity (2)
- Lower extremity edema

DIAGNOSTIC TESTS & INTERPRETATION
ECG:
- Sinus tachycardia.
- Low-voltage QRS complex in precordial and limb leads (6)
- Electrical alternans: Beat-to-beat variation of QRS amplitude (7)
- Diffuse upward ST-segment elevation; may progress from initial ST elevation to diffuse T wave inversions and finally ST-T normalization

Lab
- Acute tamponade:
  - CBC, chemistry, and coagulopathic factors
- Subacute tamponade:
  - Elevated creatine kinase and troponin
  - Increased ESR and elevated C-reactive protein
  - Leukocytosis, tuberculosis and rheumatoid factor screen, ANA, and HIV serology
  - Viral serologies when appropriate

Imaging
- CXR:
  - Enlarged cardiac silhouette (with >200 mL of effusion) can suggest pericardial effusion on CXR (2,6).
- Echocardiogram:
  - Significant pericardial effusion causing tamponade
  - Swinging heart within the effusion (7)
  - Tissue Doppler:
    - Mitral inflow E velocity decrease of >25% with inspiration
    - Tricuspid inflow E velocity increase of >40% with inspiration
    - These findings are the echocardiographic equivalent of pulsus paradoxus and indicate that a pericardial effusion is hemodynamically significant.
  - Right ventricular diastolic collapse is the echocardiographic hallmark of tamponade. Right atrial collapse is more sensitive, but a much less specific sign (7).
  - IVC distension indicative of elevated right-sided pressures
- CT and MRI:
  - Both studies may be useful in characterizing the cause of tamponade by identifying the nature of effusion (2).
  - Can identify involvement of surrounding vascular structures
  - MRI use is limited in acute presentations.

Diagnostic Procedures/Other
- Right-heart catheterization:
  - Hemodynamic hallmark of tamponade is elevation and equalization of right-sided heart pressures in diastole.
  - Biphasic (plateau and trough) pattern of constriction or restriction is usually absent.
- Left-heart catheterization:
  - Aortogram can show a double barrel sign for aortic dissection.
  - Contrast in pericardial space can differentiate hemopericardium from aortic dissection.

DIFFERENTIAL DIAGNOSIS
- MI infarction with rupture of papillary muscle or myocardium
- Aortic dissection with pericardial involvement
- Pulmonary embolism
- Pneumothorax

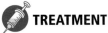

TREATMENT
MEDICATION
- Drugs are temporizing measures only; definitive therapy is removal of pericardial fluid.
- Initial temporizing measure is fluid infusion by boluses (3).
- Inotropes, such as dopamine, or vasopressors, such as norepinephrine, may be needed for hypotension refractory to fluids, but such hypotension is an indication for urgent fluid removal.
- Avoid diuretics, vasodilators, and β blockers as these can lead to hemodynamic collapse.

ADDITIONAL TREATMENT
Issues for Referral
- Patients should be referred for drainage.
- Acute drainage can be attempted blindly by pericardiocentesis using a subxiphoid approach with ECG or echocardiographic guidance.
- Fluoroscopy may allow pericardiocentesis to be performed more safely if it is readily available and time permits (2)[A].
- If a penetrating wound is the cause of tamponade, immediate thoracotomy is indicated for exploration and repair.
- Open thoracotomy is also indicated for failed percutaneous drainage (1)[B].

IN-PATIENT CONSIDERATIONS
- Frequently need ICU monitoring (2)
- Pericardial drainage is mainstay of treatment.
- Swan-Ganz catheter may be useful for close evaluation of hemodynamics when necessary.
- Endotracheal intubation should be undertaken with great trepidation, as positive pressure ventilation increases resistance to venous return and usually exacerbates hypotension, sometimes dramatically.

ONGOING CARE
FOLLOW-UP RECOMMENDATIONS
Follow-up echocardiography is indicated for recurrence of effusion (8)[A].
PROGNOSIS
- Acute tamponade patients at tertiary hospitals and level-1 trauma centers have a 75% survival rate (2).
- Fluoroscopy-guided drainage has 90% survival rate.
- Echocardiography-guided drainage has 60–90% survival rate, depending on size and etiology of effusions.
- Blind approach has 65% success rates.

COMPLICATIONS
- Myocardial puncture
- Pneumothorax
- Arrhythmias secondary to epicardial irritation

REFERENCES
1. Spodick D. Risk prediction in pericarditis: Who to keep in the hospital? *Heart.* 2008;94:398–9.
2. Spodick D. Acute cardiac tamponade. *N Engl J Med.* 2003;349(7):684–90.
3. Sagrista J, et al. Hemodynamic effects of volume expansion in patients with cardiac tamponade. *Circulation.* 2008;19(4):13–7.
4. Imazio M, et al. Aetiological diagnosis in acute and recurrent pericarditis: when and how. *J Cardiovasc Med.* 2009;10(3):217–30.
5. Moonen MI, et al. The blue man: an unusual happy end of a spontaneous rupture of a coronary artery. *Eur J Cardiothorac Surg.* 2008;34(6):1265–7.
6. Forauer AR. Pericardial tamponade in patients with central venous catheters. *J Infus Nurs.* 2007;30(3):161–7.
7. Olearczk BM, et al. The swinging heart: Cardiac alternans and right ventricular collapse in classic tamponade. *Can J Cardiol.* 2009;25(4):240.
8. Simmons JD, et al. Is there a role for secondary thoracic ultrasound in patients with penetrating injuries to the anterior mediastinum? *Am Surg.* 2008;74(1):11–4.

CODES
ICD9
- 423.3 Cardiac tamponade
- 423.9 Unspecified disease of pericardium

CARDIOMYOPATHY, HYPERTROPHIC

Qasim Durrani

BASICS

DESCRIPTION
- Ventricular hypertrophy of the left (and sometimes right) ventricle that is primary (i.e., without an obvious cause like HTN or aortic stenosis)
- Abnormal ventricular wall stiffness causes impaired diastolic filling.
- Hypertrophic cardiomyopathy (HCM) may not always be obstructive. When it is, the term hypertrophic obstructive cardiomyopathy (HOCM) is used.

EPIDEMIOLOGY
Prevalence
- 1 in 500 of general population
- Slightly more prevalent in males.

RISK FACTORS
Positive family history in 1/3 of cases
Genetics
- Generally inherited as autosomal dominant trait with variable penetrance.
- >400 mutations in 11 genes:
  - The mutations are in genes that encode constituents of the sarcomere.
  - Most common is cardiac β myosin heavy
  - chain gene on Chromosome 14.
  - The mutations have different manifestations, and they do not all go together. Prominent hypertrophy may or may not be associated with a high risk of arrhythmic death.

GENERAL PREVENTION
No prevention for development of HCM.

PATHOPHYSIOLOGY
- Diastolic dysfunction may be caused by:
  - Abnormal chamber geometry, myocyte hypertrophy, myocyte and myofibrillar disarray, abnormal intracellular calcium metabolism, and myocardial ischemia.
  - Collagen turnover is increased, with collagen type I synthesis prevailing over degradation; there is also evidence for abnormal inhibition of matrix metalloproteinases (MMP-1 and MMP-2).
  - Patients with HCM have prolonged isovolumic relaxation, delayed peak filling, reduced relative volume during the rapid filling period, increased atrial contribution to filling, and regional heterogeneity in the timing, rate, and degree of left ventricular (LV) relaxation and diastolic filling.

- LV outflow tract (LVOT) obstruction:
  - ~25% of patients with HCM have a resting pressure gradient in the outflow tract of LV caused by systolic anterior motion (SAM) of the mitral valve leaflets.
  - SAM may result as septal hypertrophy and consequent outflow tract narrowing produces a high-velocity stream anterior to the mitral valve that causes the tip of the anterior mitral valve leaflet to be sucked against the septum by the Venturi effect.
  - Clinically significant obstruction should only be considered when the outflow gradient is at least 30 mm Hg and probably >50 mm Hg.
- Myocardial ischemia can be explained by:
  - Small-vessel disease, reduced capillary density, epicardial coronary compression, and increased oxygen demand caused by myocardial hypertrophy and myocyte disarray. Atrial Fibrillation

ETIOLOGY
- Genetic: Familial or nonfamilial
- Idiopathic

DIAGNOSIS
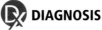

HISTORY
- Exertional dyspnea
- Angina
- Dizziness/lightheadedness
- Syncope
- Palpitations
- Sudden cardiac death:
  - Angina in the absence of epicardial coronary
  - artery disease usually occurs with exertion and may result from inability of the coronary microcirculation to supply the hypertrophied myocardium and, in HOCM, high myocardial oxygen demand associated with elevated LV systolic pressure.

PHYSICAL EXAM
- Brisk carotid upstroke:
  - Pulsus bisferiens
- Double or triple apical impulse
- Loud 4th heart sound
- Harsh diamond-shaped murmur of outflow obstruction (increases with Valsalva maneuver)
- Holosystolic murmur of mitral regurgitation

DIAGNOSTIC TESTS & INTERPRETATION
Lab
EKG: LVH, A-Fib, LA enlargement or p-mitrale, Prominent septal Q waves due to hypertrophy (may be confused with septal infarction), deep T waves, especially in case of apical hypertrophy

Imaging
Initial approach
- CXR: Normal lung fields, cardiomegaly
- Echo:
  - LV hypertrophy
  - Septal thickness >1.3 × posterior LV free wall achieves criteria for asymmetric septal hypertrophy ASH
  - Systolic anterior motion of mitral valve
  - Ground-glass appearance in areas of fibrosis
  - Spade-shaped LV cavity in apical hypertrophy
  - May have dynamic outflow tract gradient by Doppler; peaks late in systole:
    - Can worsen with Valsalva

Follow-Up & Special Considerations
Regular clinical follow-up is mandatory in all patients. This should include serial echocardiography for development or progression of LV obstruction.

Diagnostic Procedures/Other
- Cardiac MRI to accurately locate regions of hypertrophy and fibrosis
- Genetic test: Not routine, but helpful to identify family members who need to be followed by an echo.

Pathological Findings
- The principal histological hallmarks of HCM are myocyte disarray, hypertrophy, and interstitial fibrosis.
- The asymmetrical variant of HCM may be associated with a subaortic mitral impact lesion, but this is not pathognomonic of HCM.

DIFFERENTIAL DIAGNOSIS
- HTN and aortic stenosis
- Aortic stenosis:
  - Valvular
  - Subaortic
- Restrictive cardiomyopathies, such as amyloidosis or Fabry disease
- Inherited metabolic cardiomyopathies, such as glycogen storage cardiomyopathy or Friedreich's ataxia

TREATMENT

MEDICATION
First Line
- β-blockers (e.g., propranolol, metoprolol):
  - May decrease outflow obstruction and improve symptoms. Some evidence suggests they may increase ventricular compliance.
  - No clear evidence that they reduce incidence of sudden death.
  - If patient tolerates, may titrate up to 320 mg/d of propranolol to obtain clinical effect.

- Nondihydropyridine calcium-channel blockers (primarily verapamil):
  - Alternative to propranolol and may have better effect on exercise performance
  - Decreases LVOT gradient owing to negative inotropic and chronotropic actions.
  - Improves diastolic filling by improved diastolic relaxation

Second Line
In face of LVOT gradient or persistent symptoms, might add disopyramide, which has negative inotropic and antiarrhythmogenic properties.

ADDITIONAL TREATMENT
General Measures
- Avoid excessive exertion and volume depletion.
- Avoid alcohol.

Issues for Referral
- High risk for SCD/need ICD placement:
  - History of cardiac arrest
  - Recurrent syncope
  - VT/NSVT
  - Septal hypertrophy >30 mm
  - Failure to raise SBP >20 mm Hg with exercise
  - Certain mutations and family history
- Mechanical relief of obstruction

Additional Therapies
- Anticoagulation in case of atrial fibrillation (AF)
- Amiodarone for AF
- Infective endocarditis (IE) prophylaxis only if previous history of endocarditis

COMPLEMENTARY & ALTERNATIVE THERAPIES
None proved to be beneficial.

SURGERY/OTHER PROCEDURES
- Septal myectomy (2) is reserved for:
  - Patients having severe symptoms refractory to medical therapy
  - Patients with greater outflow gradient (>50 mm Hg).
- Alcohol ablation is a potential alternative to septal myectomy. Complications may include:
  - Heart block
  - Ventricular arrhythmias
  - MI
- DDD pacemaker therapy is another alternative to surgery, especially for those at risk for invasive therapy.
- ICD may prevent SCD in high-risk patients (3).

IN-PATIENT CONSIDERATIONS
Initial Stabilization
- Management of arrhythmias as needed
- Correction of electrolytes and fluids
- Avoid diuresis in CHF presentations

Admission Criteria
- CHF exacerbation
- Syncope
- Arrhythmias

IV Fluids
NS may be used as needed, depending on the clinical scenario.

Nursing
Appropriate bed rest as needed

Discharge Criteria
Resolution of acute problems and hemodynamic stability

 ## ONGOING CARE

FOLLOW-UP RECOMMENDATIONS
Regular follow-up and patient education

Patient Monitoring
- Monitor for signs/symptoms of arrhythmias:
  - Consider Holter monitoring to screen for nonsustained ventricular tachycardia.

DIET
Regular

PATIENT EDUCATION
- Avoid sudden exertion/strenuous exercise.
- Avoid dehydration or volume loss.
- Avoid medications like nitrates, diuretics, digoxin, and vasodilators.
- Make patient aware of possibility of SCD.

PROGNOSIS
- Many remain asymptomatic throughout life.
- Most common cause of mortality is SCD.
- 5–10% of HCM progress to dilated cardiomyopathy called "burnt out HCM." May result in CHF, which can be difficult to treat.
- Infective endocarditis occurs in <10% of patients.
- AF is common in later course of disease.

COMPLICATIONS
- SCD
- AF
- Infective endocarditis
- Recurrent chest pains, syncope +/– falls.

REFERENCES
1. Fifer MA, et al. Management of symptoms in hypertrophic cardiomyopathy. *Circulation*. 2008;117:429–39.
2. Monteiro PF. Effects of surgical septal myectomy on left ventricular wall thickness and diastolic filling. *Am J Cardiol*. 2007;100(12):1776–8.
3. Maron BJ, et al. Implantable cardioverter-defibrillators and prevention of sudden cardiac death in hypertrophic cardiomyopathy. *JAMA*. 2007;298:442–45.
4. Morgan JF. Psychiatric disorders in hypertrophic cardiomyopathy. *Gen Hosp Psychiatry*. 2008;30(1): 49–54.

ADDITIONAL READING
- Hughes SE, McKenna WJ. New insights into the pathology of inherited cardiomyopathy. *Heart*. 2005;91(2):257–64. Review.
- Kelly BS. HCM: Electrocardiographic manifestations and other important considerations for emergency physicians. *Am J Emerg Med*. 2007;25(1):72–9.
- Ricksten S. Refractory shock in the intensive care unit: Don't fail to spot obstruction of the left ventricular outflow tract! *Crit Care Med*. 2009; 37(2);793–4.

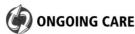 ### See Also (Topic, Algorithm, Electronic Media Element)

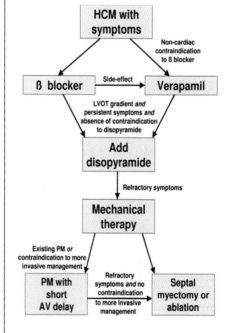

 ## CODES

ICD9
- 425.11 Hypertrophic obstructive cardiomyopathy
- 425.18 Other hypertrophic cardiomyopathy

CLINICAL PEARLS
- HOCM and mitral valve prolapse are 2 conditions in which the intensity of murmur increases with Valsalva maneuver or inhalation of amyl nitrate.
- It is important to evaluate family members of the patient with HOCM.
- Patients should avoid strenuous exercise, especially competitive sports.

CARDIOMYOPATHY, PERIPARTUM (PPCM)

Hye Jung Heo
Peter Bernstein

BASICS

DESCRIPTION
- Heart failure during last month of pregnancy or up to 5 months postpartum
- Absence of prior heart disease or identifiable cause for cardiac failure
- Left ventricular (LV) systolic dysfunction (LVEF <45% or a reduced shortening fraction <30%)
- System(s) Affected: Cardiac

EPIDEMIOLOGY
Incidence
Wide geographical variation:
- 1:3000–1:4000 live births in the U.S.
- 1:1000 in South Africa
- 1:300 in Haiti
- 1:100 in Zaire, Nigeria

Prevalence
Varies significantly

RISK FACTORS
- Multiparity
- African American
- Older maternal age (>30)
- Preeclampsia/gestational hypertension
- Multiple gestation
- Long-term oral tocolytic therapy (terbutaline)
- Maternal cocaine abuse

Genetics
Familial clustering has been observed:
- Could reflect genetic and/or environmental factors

GENERAL PREVENTION
Avoidance of pregnancy with prior history of peripartum cardiomyopathy

PATHOPHYSIOLOGY
Hemodynamic factors:
- Significant increase in blood volume and cardiac output, which results in transient LV remodeling

ETIOLOGY
- Exact etiology unknown
- Possible etiologies:
- Viral trigger: Enterovirus, coxsackie virus, parvovirus B19, adenovirus, and herpes virus
- Inflammatory cytokines:
  - Tumor necrosis factor (TNF)-α, interleukin-6, Fas/Apo-1, and C-reactive protein are associated with more severe disease.
- Myocarditis:
  - Endomyocardial biopsies with evidence of interstitial inflammation

- Abnormal immune response:
  - Maternal immunologic response to a fetal antigen (microchimerism)
  - High titers of autoantibodies against normal human cardiac tissue proteins (including myosin), adenine nucleotide translocator, and branched chain α-ketoacid dehydrogenase

COMMONLY ASSOCIATED CONDITIONS
- Preeclampsia/gestational hypertension
- Multiple gestation

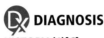

DIAGNOSIS

HISTORY (1)[C]
- Dyspnea
- Cough
- Orthopnea
- Paroxysmal nocturnal dyspnea
- Hemoptysis
- Persistent weight retention or weight gain
- Most patients present in NYHA Class III or IV functional status.

PHYSICAL EXAM (1)[C]
- Signs of congestion:
  - Peripheral edema
  - Jugular venous distention
  - Rales or pleural effusion
  - Hepatic enlargement
  - Ascites
- Signs of diminished perfusion:
  - Cool extremities
  - Hypotension
  - Decreased pulse pressure
  - Decreased urine output
  - Mental status changes

DIAGNOSTIC TESTS & INTERPRETATION
Lab
Initial lab tests (1)[C]
- CBC
- Urinalysis
- Serum electrolytes (including calcium and magnesium)
- BUN
- Serum creatinine
- Blood glucose
- ABG
- Liver function test
- Thyroid-stimulating hormone

Imaging
Initial approach
- Echocardiography (1)[C]:
  - Reduction in contractility and LV enlargement without hypertrophy
  - LVEF <45% and/or fractional shortening <30%
  - LV end-systolic dimension >2.7 cm/m^2
- Chest x-ray:
  - Enlargement of the cardiac silhouette, pulmonary venous congestion, and/or interstitial edema
  - Pulmonary edema
  - Not necessary to make a diagnosis

Follow-Up & Special Considerations
Systemic and pulmonary embolization seen more frequently than in other forms of cardiomyopathies

Diagnostic Procedures/Other
- Cardiac catheterization (right heart) (1)[C]:
  - Rarely needed (cardiac pressures measured with Doppler)
  - May be helpful in critically ill patients
- Pulmonary artery catheter is rarely needed but can be used for hemodynamic management during labor in difficult cases.
- Measurement of inotropic contractile reserve during dobutamine-stress echocardiography is shown to accurately correlate with subsequent recovery of LV function.

Pathological Findings
Endomyocardial biopsy (1)[C]:
- Myocarditis, myofiber hypertrophy and/or degeneration, fibrosis, and interstitial edema
- No pathognomonic findings

DIFFERENTIAL DIAGNOSIS
- Idiopathic dilated cardiomyopathy
- Acute or chronic heart failure due other causes of LV systolic dysfunction

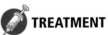

TREATMENT

MEDICATION
First Line
- Improving cardiac function by reducing afterload and preload and increasing contractility

- Diuretics decrease preload and relieve pulmonary congestion (1)[A].
- Digoxin may improve myocardial contractility and facilitate rate control when atrial fibrillation is present (1)[A].
- ACE inhibitors for afterload reduction postpartum (1)[A]:
  - Recommended for all patients (after delivery)
  - Improves symptoms, functional class, ejection fraction, exercise tolerance, quality of life
  - Prevent progressive ventricular remodeling and hospitalization and improves survival
  - Contraindicated in pregnancy

- Hydralazine: Afterload reduction before delivery
- β-Blockade in stable, euvolemic patients has demonstrated improvement in cardiac function and survival outside of pregnancy (1)[A].

Second Line
Myocarditis: Immunosuppressive treatment only with proven myocarditis

ADDITIONAL TREATMENT
General Measures
Pain control decreases cardiac work and reduces tachycardia:
- A carefully dosed epidural is appropriate.

Additional Therapies
- Anticoagulation with heparin (antepartum) or warfarin (postpartum) should be considered with EF <35% (1)[B].
- Mechanical circulatory support when refractory to conventional pharmacologic therapy while awaiting cardiac transplant

COMPLEMENTARY & ALTERNATIVE THERAPIES
Immune modulatory therapy not clear (2)[C]

SURGERY/OTHER PROCEDURES
- Intra-aortic balloon counterpulsation may be needed as a bridge to cardiac transplant.
- Surgical support with ventricular assist devices may be indicated (3)[C]:
  - Recovery of myocardial function can occur in ~15% on ventricular assist device support; these may not require transplant.
- Cardiac transplantation for those who remain refractory to conventional pharmacologic therapy (4)[C]
- Cesarean delivery is reserved for obstetric indications.
- Early fetal delivery may be necessary in women needing hospitalization for heart failure with hemodynamic instability; however, if stabilized, goal is delivery at term.

IN-PATIENT CONSIDERATIONS
Initial Stabilization
- Pharmacologic therapy
- Acute heart failure:
  - With congestion and adequate perfusion: IV diuretic/vasodilators (nitroglycerin, nitroprusside, or nesiritide)
  - With diminished perfusion: Inotropic drugs (IV dobutamine or milrinone)

Admission Criteria
- Exacerbation of congestive heart failure
- Acute respiratory failure
- Supraventricular or ventricular arrhythmias
- Syncope
- Pulmonary or systemic emboli

IV Fluids
Fluid restriction

Discharge Criteria
Pharmacologic stabilization of cardiac homodynamic status

ONGOING CARE
FOLLOW-UP RECOMMENDATIONS
Patient Monitoring
- Echocardiography repeated at 3 and 6 months after diagnosis
- Subsequent serial assessments of LV function at least annually
- Optimal treatment of coexisting conditions (i.e., anemia, thyroid disease, and diabetes)

DIET
- Sodium restriction (2 g sodium-restricted diet)
- Fluid restriction (<2 L in 24 hours)

PATIENT EDUCATION
- Lifestyle modifications
- Smoking cessation and avoidance of alcohol

PROGNOSIS
- Normalization of ventricular function in ~50% of patients is more likely if the ejection fraction is >30% at time of diagnosis.
- Most physicians counsel against a 2nd pregnancy.
- Recurrence rate: ~30% of cases
- Transplant rate: 4–7%

COMPLICATIONS
- Mortality 4–19% when LV dysfunction has not resolved:
  - 85% 5-year mortality rate in patients with persistent LV dysfunction (5)
  - Kaiser Permanente Southern California from 1996–2005: 60 with diagnosis, with mortality rate of 3.3% with mean follow-up of 4.7 years (6).
- Mortality up to 2% in patients with normal function
- Death is usually due to progressive congestive heart failure, arrhythmia, or thromboembolism.

REFERENCES

1. Hunt SA, et al. ACC/AHA 2005 guideline update for the diagnosis and management of chronic heart failure in the adult: A report of the American College of Cardiology/American Heart Association Task Force on the practice guidelines (Writing Committee to Update the 2001 Guidelines for the Evaluation and Management of Heart Failure: Developed in collaboration with the American College of Chest Physicians and the International Society for Heart and Lung Transplantation: Endorsed by the Heart Rhythm Society. Circulation. 2005;112(12):e154–235.
2. Murali S, Baldisseri M. Peripartum cardiomyopathy. Crit Care Med. 2005;3(10):S340–S346.
3. Oosterom L, et al. Left ventricular assist device as a bridge to recovery in a young woman admitted with peripartum cardiomyopathy. Neth Heart J. 2008;16(12):426–8.
4. Habli M, et al. Peripartum cardiomyopathy: Prognostic factors for long-term maternal outcome. Am J Obstet Gynecol. 2009;199(4):415.e1–5.
5. Sutton M, et al. Effects of subsequent pregnancy on left ventricular function in peripartum cardiomyopathy. Am Heart J. 1991;121:1776.
6. Brar S, et al. Incidence, mortality, and racial differences in peripartum cardiomyopathy. Am J Cardio. 2007;100(2):302–4.

ADDITIONAL READING

- Borna S, et al. Pregnancy outcomes in women with heart disease. Int J Gynecol Obstet. 2006;92:122–3.
- Elkayam U, et al. Pregnancy-associated cardiomyopathy: Clinical characteristics and a comparison between early and late presentation. Circulation. 2005;111:2050–55.
- Elkayam U, et al. Maternal and fetal outcomes of subsequent pregnancies in women with peripartum cardiomyopathy. N Engl J Med. 2001;344:1567–71.
- Mielniczuk LM, et al. Frequency of peripartum cardiomyopathy. Am J Cardiol. 2006;97:1765–68.
- Pearson GD, et al. Peripartum cardiomyopathy. National heart, Lung, and blood Institute and Office of Rare Diseases (National Institute of Health) Workshop recommendations and review. JAMA. 2000;283:1183–88.
- Sliwa K, et al. Peripartum cardiomyopathy. Lancet. 2006;368:682–93.

CODES
ICD9
- 674.50 Peripartum cardiomyopathy, unspecified as to episode of care or not applicable
- 674.51 Peripartum cardiomyopathy, delivered, with or without mention of antepartum condition
- 674.52 Peripartum cardiomyopathy, delivered, with mention of postpartum condition

CLINICAL PEARLS
- Nonspecific fatigue, chest discomfort, peripheral edema, or abdominal pain may be confused with normal symptoms of pregnancy.
- Most physicians counsel against a 2nd pregnancy.
- Peripartum cardiomyopathy will recur in ~30% of cases.
- Mortality rates depends on persistence of LV dysfunction.

CARDIOTOXICITY, ANTINEOPLASTIC DRUG-INDUCED

Ashraf O. Rashid
Andria Lyn
Stephen M. Pastores

 BASICS

DESCRIPTION
- Majority of chemotherapy-induced cardiotoxicities are related to preexisting heart disease.
- Commonest agents with cardiac toxicity:
  - Anthracyclines: Doxorubicin, daunorubicin, idarubicin, and epirubicin
  - Monoclonal antibodies: Trastuzumab, bevacizumab, and alemtuzumab
  - Antimetabolites: 5-fluorouracil (FU)/capecitabine and cytarabine
  - Antitumor antibiotics: Bleomycin and mitomycin C
  - Alkylating agents: Cyclophosphamide, ifosfamide, cisplatin
  - Microtubule-targeting drugs: Paclitaxel

EPIDEMIOLOGY
Incidence
Variable:
- Anthracyclines: 3–18%
- Monoclonal antibodies: Trastuzumab 2–7%, bevacizumab 2%
- Fluorouracil: 1–19%
- Bleomycin: <3%
- Cyclophosphamide: 1–28%
- Paclitaxel: <5%

RISK FACTORS
- General:
  - Older age
  - Chest irradiation
  - Underlying heart disease
  - Synergistic effect with other chemotherapy
- Cumulative dose:
  - Doxorubicin: >550 mg/m^2
  - Mitomycin C: >30 mg/m^2
- High-dose protocol:
  - Cyclophosphamide: >1.5 g/m^2
  - Ifosfamide: 6.25–10 g/m^2

GENERAL PREVENTION
- Screening before, during, and after treatment protocols (Echo/MUGA)
- Anthracyclines:
  - Limit cumulative dose:
    ○ Doxorubicin <550 mg/m^2
  - Use of dexrazoxane (cardioprotective)
  - Liposome encapsulation formulation
  - Use continuous infusion rather than bolus dosing.
- Trastuzumab should be avoided in patients with an abnormal baseline cardiac function.
- Fluorouracil: Prophylactic use of calcium channel blockers may be of benefit.
- Cyclophosphamide: Use infusion protocol or b.i.d. dosing.

PATHOPHYSIOLOGY (1)
- Anthracyclines: Reactive oxygen species and mitochondrial dysfunction
- Trastuzumab: May involve human epidermal growth factor receptor (HER2) blockade
- Fluorouracil: Coronary vasospasm
- Cyclophosphamide: Endothelial capillary damage

COMMONLY ASSOCIATED CONDITIONS (2)
- Anthracyclines: Cardiomyopathy, arrhythmias (supraventricular and ventricular) and CAD. Can be acute (during or immediately following the infusion), subacute (up to 3–8 months after therapy), and late (5–15 years).
- Monoclonal antibodies:
  - Trastuzumab: Asymptomatic decreased ejection fraction (EF), symptomatic CHF (less common)
  - Bevacizumab: MI and CHF
  - Alemtuzumab: CHF and arrhythmia
- Antimetabolites:
  - 5-FU: Chest pain/angina and MI. Many have silent EKG changes.
  - Cytarabine: Pericarditis and tamponade
- Antitumor antibiotics:
  - Bleomycin: Acute chest pain associated during infusion, CAD, and pericarditis
  - Mitomycin C: CHF
- Alkylating agents:
  - Cyclophosphamide: ↓ QRS amplitude, complete heart block, cardiomyopathy, hemorrhagic myopericarditis
  - Ifosfamide: Arrhythmia and CMP
- Paclitaxel: Bradycardia and A/V block

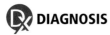 DIAGNOSIS

HISTORY
- Depends on clinical presentation
- Coronary artery disease: Chest pain, dyspnea
- Cardiomyopathy: Dyspnea, paroxysmal nocturnal dyspnea, lower extremity edema, fatigue
- Arrhythmia: Palpitation, syncope

PHYSICAL EXAM
- CVS: S$_3$ or S$_4$ gallop, leg edema
- Lungs: Bilateral rales

DIAGNOSTIC TESTS & INTERPRETATION
Lab
BNP, cardiac enzymes, and ESR

Imaging
CXR: Cardiomegaly, pulmonary edema

Diagnostic Procedures/Other
- EKG: ST/T wave changes, premature atrial and ventricular contractions, Mobitz type I and II and complete heart block
- Echo (class I): ↓ EF, dilated ventricles, pericardial effusion, wall motion abnormalities
- MUGA scan: ↓ EF
- Coronary angiography may be necessary to rule out atherosclerotic heart disease.

Pathological Findings
- Anthracyclines: Sarcotubular dilation, disruption of mitochondria, and myofibrillar loss of actin and myosin
- 5-FU: Inflammatory cells, diffuse interstitial edema, intracytoplasmic vacuolization of myocytes
- Mitomycin C: Similar to radiation-induced cardiac injury
- Cyclophosphamide: Endothelial capillary damage

DIFFERENTIAL DIAGNOSIS
- Valvular heart disease
- Pulmonary embolism
- Pulmonary toxicity of chemotherapy
- Radiation-induced heart diseases
- Anemia

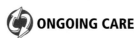 TREATMENT

MEDICATION

First Line

- Cardiomyopathy from anthracyclines: ACE inhibitors (1st choice) and diuretics
- Trastuzumab (3):
  – Asymptomatic: Hold if EF ↓ by >15–20% to a level <40% and repeat in 2 weeks
  – Symptomatic: Hold if EF ↓ by >10% and repeat in 2 weeks. Treat with β-blockers and ACE inhibitors
- Antimetabolites:
  – 5-FU: Discontinue
  – Cytarabine: Steroids
  – Cyclophosphamide: Hemorrhagic myopericarditis may respond to steroids.

Second Line

- β-blockers, spironolactone, and digitalis for cardiomyopathy.
- Nitrates and calcium channel blockers may reverse vasospasm from 5-FU.

ADDITIONAL TREATMENT

General Measures (4)

- Trastuzumab: Many patients improve after discontinuation of therapy.
- Fluorouracil: Many patients improve after discontinuation of therapy.
- Bleomycin: May be continued since the acute chest pain usually does not recur during future infusions.

Issues for Referral

Cardiology consultation for symptomatic CHF refractory to conventional therapy

SURGERY/OTHER PROCEDURES

Heart transplantation in refractory severe cases

IN-PATIENT CONSIDERATIONS

Initial Stabilization

- Oxygen supplementation
- Treatment of arrhythmia:
  – SVT: Adenosine
  – Ventricular tachycardia: Amiodarone
  – Unstable arrhythmia: Cardioversion

Admission Criteria

- Unstable angina/MI
- Symptomatic CHF
- Unstable arrhythmia

Nursing

- Monitor input and output closely with CHF
- Telemetry monitoring

Discharge Criteria

- Stable class I/II CHF
- Stable heart rhythm
- Resolution of chest pain/MI

 ONGOING CARE

FOLLOW-UP RECOMMENDATIONS

Cardiology out-patient follow-up

Patient Monitoring

- Anthracyclines (echo/MUGA):
  – Before starting therapy
  – After 100, 300, and 400 (high risk) or 450 mg/m^2 (low risk)
  – Troponin and B-type natriuretic peptide elevation may correlate with toxicity.
- Trastuzumab (echo/MUGA):
  – Before starting therapy
  – At 3, 6, and 12 months after starting therapy
- Mitomycin C: Risk ↑ after a cumulative doses >30 mg/m^2

DIET

Cardiomyopathy: Low Na, low cholesterol

PATIENT EDUCATION

Detailed discussion of cardiac side effects should be carried out before starting chemotherapy.

PROGNOSIS

- Anthracyclines:
  – Symptomatic patients carry a worse prognosis than asymptomatic ones; 80% of symptomatic patients may improve with medical therapy.
  – Can progress to death
- Trastuzumab: Cardiac toxicity is reversible in many patients; rechallenge could be safe in some.
- Fluorouracil: Angina symptoms usually resolve after stopping treatment. Rechallenge is controversial.
- Ifosfamide: Toxicities are generally reversible.
- Paclitaxel: Cardiac rhythm abnormalities are typically reversible.

COMPLICATIONS

Irreversible and progressive loss of cardiac function and death

REFERENCES

1. Howard B, et al. Chemotherapy and cardiotoxicities. *Rev Cardiovasc Med.* 2008;9(2):75–83.
2. Justin DF, et al. Cardiotoxicity of cancer therapy. *J Clin Oncol.* 2005;23:7685.
3. Steven ME, Michael SE. Cardiotoxicity profile of trastuzumab. *Drug Safety.* 2008;31(6):459–67.
4. Yeh ET, et al. Cardiovascular complications of cancer therapy: diagnosis, pathogenesis, and management. *Circulation.* 2004;109:3122.

CODES

ICD9

- 423.8 Other specified diseases of pericardium
- 425.4 Other primary cardiomyopathies
- 963.1 Poisoning by antineoplastic and immunosuppressive drugs

CLINICAL PEARLS

- The spectrum of cardiac events associated with different chemotherapy classes is variable and includes asymptomatic decrease in ejection fraction to severe irreversible loss of cardiac function leading to death.
- Cardiac toxicity is higher with coadministration of antineoplastic agents due to synergistic effect.
- Monitoring treatment protocols using different cardiac imaging techniques may help detect potential cardiac complications earlier.
- Most of the cardiac toxicities are managed by stopping the offending agents and supportive care.

C

CENTRAL VENOUS CATHETERIZATION

Jose R. Yunen
Vicente San Martin

PROCEDURE

INDICATIONS

- Central venous pressure monitoring
- Administration of drugs that cause phlebitis or pain in peripheral veins
- Alternative access when peripheral veins are unavailable
- Parenteral nutrition

CONTRAINDICATIONS

- Skin infection
- Coagulopathy
- Contralateral carotid disease (internal jugular cannulation contraindicated)
- Diseased or absent contralateral lung (subclavian cannulation contraindicated)
- Ipsilateral pneumothorax (subclavian cannulation contraindicated)

TECHNIQUE

See algorithm.

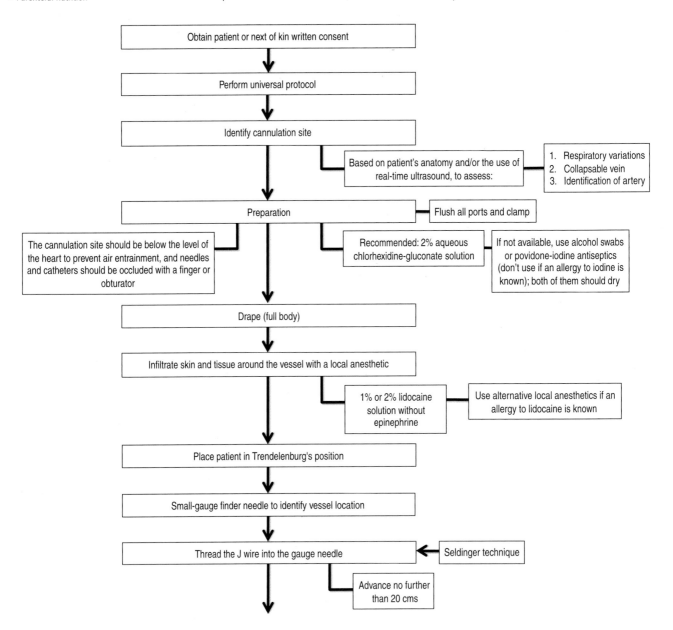

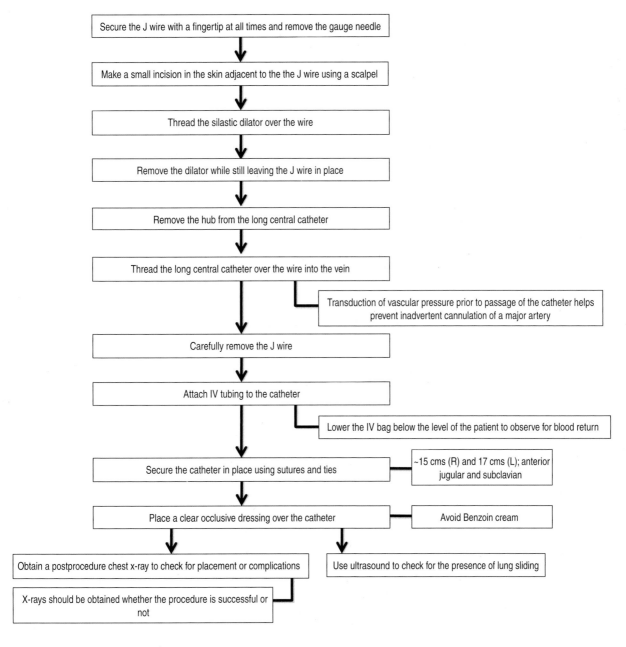

Secure the J wire with a fingertip at all times and remove the gauge needle

↓

Make a small incision in the skin adjacent to the the J wire using a scalpel

↓

Thread the silastic dilator over the wire

↓

Remove the dilator while still leaving the J wire in place

↓

Remove the hub from the long central catheter

↓

Thread the long central catheter over the wire into the vein → Transduction of vascular pressure prior to passage of the catheter helps prevent inadvertent cannulation of a major artery

↓

Carefully remove the J wire

↓

Attach IV tubing to the catheter → Lower the IV bag below the level of the patient to observe for blood return

↓

Secure the catheter in place using sutures and ties → ~15 cms (R) and 17 cms (L); anterior jugular and subclavian

↓

Place a clear occlusive dressing over the catheter → Avoid Benzoin cream

↓ ↓

Obtain a postprocedure chest x-ray to check for placement or complications | Use ultrasound to check for the presence of lung sliding

X-rays should be obtained whether the procedure is successful or not

COMPLICATIONS
- Air embolism
- Pneumothorax
- Arterial puncture (if arterial cannulation do not remove the catheter; vascular surgery advice)
- Infection and thrombosis (delayed complications)

ADDITIONAL READING
- Braner D, et al. Central venous catheterization—subclavian vein. *N Engl J Med*. 2007;357:e26.
- Graham A, et al. Central venous catheterization. *N Engl J Med*. 2007;356:e21.
- Ortega R, et al. Ultrasound-guided internal jugular vein cannulation. *N Engl J Med*. 2010;362:e57.

CEREBRAL SALT WASTING SYNDROME (CSWS)

Damian Lee

 BASICS

DESCRIPTION
- Cerebral salt wasting syndrome (CSWS) is one of the most common causes of hyponatremia in patients with intracranial pathology.
- Due to excessive renal loss of sodium with resultant dehydration and hyponatremia
- Must be differentiated form SIADH; may be difficult, but main point of differentiation is intravascular volume state

EPIDEMIOLOGY
Incidence
Unknown. However, ~60% of children with brain injury or tumor develop hyponatremia during hospitalization (1).

Prevalence
Can occur at any age; most commonly seen between infancy and mid 60s.

RISK FACTORS
Common in individuals with intracranial pathology such as trauma, tumor, infection

Genetics
No specific genetic link

GENERAL PREVENTION
- No specific prevention measures as it usually is a result of a primary pathology or injury. Mainstay would involve preventing primary pathology or injury, which is not always possible.
- Early recognition and intervention is best to prevent progression and complications.

PATHOPHYSIOLOGY
- Not fully understood
- Impaired sodium resorption of proximal nephron
- Possibly natriuresis with hyponatremia from decreased sympathetic input to the kidney with resultant increased level of circulating natriuretic peptides. Causes increased GFR/perfusion pressure and dopamine with decreased sodium reabsorption in the medullary collecting duct (2).

ETIOLOGY
- Brain surgery
- Intracranial or intracerebral trauma or hemorrhage (SAH).
- Brain tumor
- CVA
- Infections: Encephalitis and meningitis

COMMONLY ASSOCIATED CONDITIONS
SIADH; often difficult distinguishing the two disorders

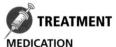 **DIAGNOSIS**

HISTORY
- No specific historical element.
- May include features of intravascular volume depletion such as thirst and inappropriately excessive urination when compared with intake.
- May include features of hyponatremia:
  – Mild: Nausea, headache, lethargy, malaise
  – Severe: Confusion, stupor, seizure, coma

PHYSICAL EXAM
- No specific physical finding
- May manifest features of intravascular volume depletion: Dry mucous membranes, tachycardia, orthostatic hypotension, tachypnea, sunken anterior fontanel and eyeballs in infants
- May manifest features of hyponatremia, such as altered mentation, seizures, and coma in extreme cases
- If patient has central venous pressure (CVP) monitoring, this is usually low.

DIAGNOSTIC TESTS & INTERPRETATION
Lab
Initial lab tests
- Serum sodium level revealing hyponatremia (<135). Must rule out pseudohyponatremia in hyperglycemia and hypertriglyceridemia. Also check TSH, cortisol, and BUN to rule out other causes. The BUN-to-creatinine ratio is normally increased.
- Serum and urine osmolarity: Serum osmolarity is usually normal or high (>275); urine osmolarity is usually low (<100).
- Urine lytes (Na): Inappropriate urine sodium loss (>20 mmol/L). This is not a gold standard as this may also be seen in SIADH.
- Uric acid: Normal or low in CSWS and low in SIADH. In CSWS, uric acid remains low after sodium correction, whereas in SIADH it tends to normalize (3).
- BNP may be elevated; must rule out cardiac origin (2).

Follow-Up & Special Considerations
- Frequent monitoring of serum sodium until normalized
- Hyponatremia that improves with volume repletion suggests a diagnosis of CSWS as opposed to SIADH.
- Some nephrologists suggest that one cannot distinguish CSWS and SIADH in intracranial pathology and that the correct treatment is the same for both: hypertonic saline solution (4).

Imaging
Initial approach
Noncontrast head CT to evaluate for intracranial pathology or injury.

Follow-Up & Special Considerations
If intracranial pathology is suspected but not clearly delineated on CT scan, MRI may be employed and/or contrast CT imaging.

Diagnostic Procedures/Other
Chest radiograph to rule-out CHF

Pathological Findings
Intracranial injury, mass, or infection

DIFFERENTIAL DIAGNOSIS
- SIADH
- Excessive loop or thiazide diuretic use
- Addison disease (hypoadrenalism)
- Thyroid disease (hypothyroidism)
- Liver/renal failure
- CHF

TREATMENT

MEDICATION
First Line
- Volume replacement with normal or hypertonic saline solution to maintain a positive salt balance (5)
- Mineralocorticoids such as fludrocortisone (Florinef), in complicated cases, promotes increased resorption of sodium and loss of potassium by renal distal tubules. Typical dose 0.05–0.2 mg/d PO (1).

ALERT
Too rapid correction of sodium can lead to central pontine myelinolysis. Maximum recommended correction is 15 mEq in 24-hour period.

Second Line
Sodium chloride tablets: Typically 1–4 g q6h

ADDITIONAL TREATMENT
General Measures
- Intravascular volume repletion and correction of hyponatremia
- Maintain positive salt balance.
- Stop any diuretic therapy.
- Typical treatment of CSWS (volume repletion) is the opposite that of SIADH (volume restriction).

ALERT
Incorrect therapy from failure to distinguish between CSWS from SIADH could worsen patient's clinical condition.

Issues for Referral
May be needed, but based on etiology

SURGERY/OTHER PROCEDURES
Only if necessary to treat underlying pathological process

IN-PATIENT CONSIDERATIONS
Initial Stabilization
- Monitor ABC: Endotracheal intubation for airway protection if indicated for airway protection.
- Correct hypovolemia as previously stated: Administer hypertonic saline in severe and/or symptomatic cases.
- Diagnose and treat underlying pathological process.

Admission Criteria
- Generally, all patients with moderate to severe symptoms should be admitted for workup of underlying cause.
- Admission is also required for severe dehydration for IV fluid repletion.
- Anyone presenting with seizure or confusion
- All symptomatic infants and elderly

IV Fluids
- NS
- Hypertonic saline in more severe cases

Nursing
- Nursing needs will vary with symptoms and patient.
- High-risk patients (very young or very old) or those who are symptomatic should be observed closely and frequently.

Discharge Criteria
- Euvolemia attained
- Symptom-free or minimal symptoms
- Able to tolerate sodium chloride tablets and/or mineralocorticoids enterally
- Able to comply with discharge instructions

 ## ONGOING CARE

FOLLOW-UP RECOMMENDATIONS
- Monitor serum sodium level as necessary to adjust or stop therapy.
- Evaluate underlying cause.

Patient Monitoring
High-risk patients (very young or very old) or those who are symptomatic should be in an ICU setting for signs of neurologic deterioration.

DIET
- Normal or modified based of preference or risk factors. Encourage fluid intake
- Do not restrict sodium.

PATIENT EDUCATION
- Recognition of early signs of hyponatremia
- Education about the type and need for therapy; this often increases compliance.

PROGNOSIS
- Occurs weeks 1–4 after brain insult. May last several months (1).
- Varies based on underlying causative factor

COMPLICATIONS
- Symptomatic hyponatremia: Altered mentation, seizure, stupor, and coma
- Prolonged, untreated CSWS may lead to severe dehydration and death from herniation.

REFERENCES

1. Springate J. Endocrinology. In *Cerebral Salt-Wasting Syndrome*. Retrieved March 10, 2009 from http://emedicine.medscape.com/article/919609.
2. Lenhard T, et al. Cerebral salt-wasting syndrome in a patient with neuroleptic malignant syndrome. *Arch Neurol*. 2007;64:122–5.
3. Momi J, et al. Hyponatremia in a patient with Cryptococcal meningitis: SIADH or Cerebral salt wasting? *Internet J Endocrinol*. 2009;5(1). Retrieved March 16, 2009, from Internet Scientific Publications database.
4. Sterns RH, et al. Cerebral salt wasting versus SIADH: What difference? *J Am Soc Nephrol*. 2008;19:194–6.
5. Cerda-Esteve M, et al. Cerebral salt wasting syndrome: Review. *Eur J Intern Med*. 2008; 19(4):249–54. Abstract retrieved March 10, 2009, from PubMed database. Abstract No. 18471672.

ADDITIONAL READING

- Okutan V, et al. Cerebral Salt Wasting Syndrome in a brain injury caused by acute dehydration. *Int Pediatr*. 2000;15(2):110–3.
- Brimioulle S, et al. Hyponatremia in neurological patients: Cerebral salt wasting versus inappropriate antidiuretic hormone secretion. *Int Care Med*. 2008;34:125–31.

 ## CODES

ICD9
- 276.1 Hyposmolality and/or hyponatremia
- 593.9 Unspecified disorder of kidney and ureter

CLINICAL PEARLS

- Not all cases of CSWS are hypovolemic.
- If hyponatremia improves with fluid resuscitation, this suggest a diagnosis of CSWS, not SIADH.
- Uric acid level remains low in CSWS even after sodium correction, whereas it tends to normalize in SIADH.
- CSWS patients are typically volume depleted.
- Serum osmolarity tends to be high or normal in CSWS but low in SIADH.
- Urine output tends to increase in CSWS but decrease in SIADH.

CEREBRAL VASOSPASM

Raghad Said
Zaid Said

 BASICS

DESCRIPTION
Neurological and/or cerebral angiographic changes that happen day 3–14 after subarachnoid hemorrhage(SAH); those changes cannot be attributed to other causes:

- Peak velocity on transcranial Doppler (TCD) >120 m/sec might predict and/or define vasospasm.
- Symptomatic vasospasm is defined as permanent or reversible focal neurological deficit associated with radiographic vasospasm.
- Severe angiographic vasospasm is defined as >50% reduction in arterial diameter
- Delayed cerebral ischemia (DCI) is symptomatic vasospasm or cerebral infarct due to vasospasm.

EPIDEMIOLOGY
Incidence
Radiographic vasospasm develops in 70% after SAH, but only 30% develop symptomatic vasospasm.

RISK FACTORS
- Presence of large volume of blood or thick clot on initial head CT (high Fisher grade)
- Presence of intraventricular or intraparenchymal blood in addition to SAH
- Duration of CT: Apparent SAH (slow clearing)
- Poor neurological grade on presentation
- Older age

Genetics
APOE4 allele may increase the risk of a negative outcome.

GENERAL PREVENTION
- Nimodipine 60 mg PO q4h; start within 96 hours and continue for 14–21days (1)[A]:
  - Voltage-gated calcium channel blocker with neuroprotective properties
  - Causes selective relaxation of cerebral arterial smooth muscle by increasing intracellular Ca
  - Decreases poor outcome after SAH, NNT = 20
  - Decreases death/disability due to DCI
  - No significant decrease in all-cause mortality
  - No decrease in angiographic vasospasm

- Statins: Anti-inflammatory effect (2)[B]
- IV magnesium to maintain a level of 2.4–4.8 mg/dL for 14 days reduced DCI and poor outcome (3).

PATHOPHYSIOLOGY
- Pathological contraction of vascular smooth muscles in response to inflammatory reaction to hemoglobin metabolites and other RBC components in the CSF
- Ischemia results from:
  - Global reduction in cerebral blood flow
  - Narrowing of the spastic vessels
  - Embolization of intraluminal microthrombi

ETIOLOGY
- Constriction of cerebral arterial smooth muscles caused by presence of blood in the subarachnoid space
- Typically involves large vessels of circle of Willis but may involve smaller branches too

COMMONLY ASSOCIATED CONDITIONS
Cerebral salt wasting

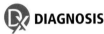 **DIAGNOSIS**

HISTORY
- Usually begins 3–4 days after SAH
- Hyperacute vasospasm <48 hours is seen in <10% of patients
- Reaches a peak at day 6–8
- Resolves by day 12–14

PHYSICAL EXAM
- Decline in mental status and delirium
- Focal neurological deficit:
  - Minor changes in neurological exam could indicate vasospasm in comatose or poor-grade SAH patients.
  - No monitoring modality replaces frequent neurological exams.

DIAGNOSTIC TESTS & INTERPRETATION
Lab
Initial lab tests
- Blood glucose, serum Na, and serum Mg
- Hct

Follow-Up & Special Considerations
- Serial neurological exam
- Noncontrast head CT to rule out rebleeding, edema, CVA, or hydrocephalus
- CXR prior to starting HHH therapy
- EEG to rule out seizure in comatose patients

Imaging
Initial approach

- Serial TCD (4)[A]:
  - Insonation of MCA, ACA, basilar artery
  - Flow velocity proportional to blood flow and inversely proportional to vessel diameter
  - Velocity >120 cm/s NPV of vasospasm: 94%
  - Velocity >200 cm/s highly suggestive of vasospasm with PPV: 87%
  - Increase in velocity >50% in 24 hours is worrisome.
  - Velocity is also altered by anemia, intracranial pressure, systemic BP, and volume.
  - Lindegaard ratio: Ratio of the velocity in the brain vessel to that of the ipsilateral extracranial ICA; ratio >3 is suggestive of vasospasm and >6, severe vasospasm
  - Lindegaard ratios did not improve predictive value of TCD.
  - It has not been demonstrated yet that SAH outcome is changed by utilizing TCD

Follow-Up & Special Considerations
Catheter angiography is gold standard for diagnosis (5)[A].

Diagnostic Procedures/Other
- CT and MR angiography
- Diffusion perfusion MRI
- Xenon-CT cerebral perfusion
- Continuous EEG monitoring
- Jugular venous bulb oximetry
- Cerebral microdialysis
- Brain tissue oximetry

Pathological Findings
- Intraluminal platelet aggregation and thrombosis
- Intimal proliferation and fibrosis begins within a week of SAH

DIFFERENTIAL DIAGNOSIS
- Aneurysmal rebleed
- Nonconvulsive seizure
- CVA related to coiling or clipping
- Infection: Meningitis, ventriculitis
- Cerebral edema
- Hydrocephalus

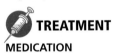 **TREATMENT**

MEDICATION
First Line
Triple H therapy: Hypertensive, Hypervolemic, Hemodilution (6)[A]:

- Increase MAP by 20–40% over baseline, typically with phenylephrine
- Hypervolemia CVP 10–12 and/or PCWP 15–18 is achieved with isotonic crystalloids or colloids.
- Hemodilution to Hct of 28–32 improves blood viscosity but lowers oxygen-carrying capacity.
- Complication rate is 24%.
- Hypertensive hypervolemic therapy (HH) and even hypertensive therapy (H) alone are used to treat vasospasm in many centers with comparable results.

Second Line
Augmentation of cardiac output with inotropic agents and/or IABP can reverse vasospasm independent of blood pressure (7).

ADDITIONAL TREATMENT
General Measures
Prevent secondary injury by avoiding:

- Hypovolemia (8)[A]
- Hypotension
- Hyponatremia
- Hypomagnesemia
- Hyperglycemia
- Seizures
- Intracranial hypertension
- Hypoxia
- Fever
- Sepsis

Issues for Referral

Early referral to a high-volume center that has both experienced endovascular specialist and neurosurgeons is reasonable (6)[B].

Additional Therapies

- Steroids are not effective and increase mortality.
- IV nicardipine did not improve outcome due to systemic hypotensive effect; intrathecal nicardipine is associated with many complications.
- Enoxaparin, ASA, and tirilazad (21-aminosteroid, inhibitor of lipid peroxidation) do not decrease vasospasm.
- Endothelin-1 antagonist showed dose-dependent reduction in angiographic spasm but no effect of clinical outcome at 3 months.

COMPLEMENTARY & ALTERNATIVE THERAPIES

- Prophylactic HHH therapy has not clearly been shown to prevent symptomatic vasospasm (9).
- Prophylactic angioplasty is associated with high incidence of vessel rupture.
- Removal of clot: Pharmacologically with intrathecal thrombolytics or during craniotomy, rendered conflicting results

SURGERY/OTHER PROCEDURES

- Balloon angioplasty (6)[B]:
  - Mechanical disruption of intima and media results in sustained increase in vessel diameter.
  - Effective for large proximal vessels, but not safe for distal perforating branches beyond 2nd-order segments.
  - Reversal of DCI in 30–70%
  - Decrease in hospital death by 16%
  - Most effective when deployed within 2 hours of onset of symptoms
  - Complications occur in 5%, including vessel rupture and aneurysm clip displacement
- Intra-arterial vasodilators (6)[B]:
  - High doses of papaverine, nicardipine, or verapamil injected into the artery involved
  - Treat 3rd- or 4th-order spastic cerebral vessels.
  - Temporary improvement in vessel diameter
  - Clinical response in 20–50%
  - Complications in 5%, including high ICP

IN-PATIENT CONSIDERATIONS

Initial Stabilization

- Maintain ABC
- Interventions to decrease ICP if signs and symptoms of intracranial hypertension are present

Admission Criteria

All patients are kept in a monitored setting for "vasospasm watch" for 10–14 days after SAH.

IV Fluids

5% albumin administration was associated with improved 3-month outcome (10)[B].

Discharge Criteria

Clinical stability and decreasing TCD velocities

 ONGOING CARE

FOLLOW-UP RECOMMENDATIONS

Patient Monitoring

- CAP and arterial line for patients on HHH or HH therapy
- PA catheter to monitor patients with preexisting cardiac disorders or myocardial stunning after SAH decreases frequency of pulmonary edema (11)[B].
- Echocardiography and noninvasive cardiac monitoring devices can be used to monitor CO.

PROGNOSIS

- Vasospasm is an independent risk factor for death and disability.
- Primary cause of death in 28% of patients and disability in 40% of SAH patients
- Increases SAH mortality from 17–31%
- Reduces the frequency of good outcome among survivors from 70–44%

COMPLICATIONS

- Ischemic stroke 5%
- Complications from HHH or HH therapy:
  - Pulmonary edema
  - Dilutional hyponatremia
  - Cerebral edema
  - Increase ICP
  - Rebleeding
  - Reversible leukoencephalopathy syndrome

REFERENCES

1. Dorhout Mees SM, et al. Calcium antagonists for aneurysmal subarachnoid haemorrhage. *Cochrane Database Syst Rev.* 2007;(3):CD000277.
2. Lynch JR, et al. Simvastatin reduces vasospasm after aneurysmal subarachnoid hemorrhage. *Stroke.* 2005;36:2024–6.
3. Van den Bergh WM, et al. Magnesium sulfate in aneurysmal subarachnoid hemorrhage: A randomized controlled trial. *Stroke.* 2005;36: 1011–15.
4. Sloan MA, et al. Assessment: transcranial Doppler ultrasonography: report of the Therapeutics and Technology Assessment Subcommittee of the American Academy of Neurology. *Neurology.* 2004;62:1468–81.
5. Lysakowski C, et al. Transcranial Doppler versus angiography in patients with vasospasm due to a ruptured cerebral aneurysm: A systemic review. *Stroke.* 2001;32:2292–8.
6. Bederson JB, et al. Guidelines for the management of aneurysmal subarachnoid hemorrhage: A statement for healthcare professionals from a special writing group of the Stroke Council, American Heart Association. *Stroke.* 2009;40(3):994–1025.
7. Joseph M, et al. Increase in cardiac output can reverse flow deficit form vasospasm independent of blood pressure. *Neurosurgery.* 2004;55(4): 1008–10.
8. Wijdicks EF, et al. Volume depletion and natriuresis in patients with ruptured intracranial aneurysm. *Ann Neurol.*1985;18:211–6.
9. Egge A. Prophylactic hyperdynamic postoperative fluid therapy after subarachnoid hemorrhage. *Neurosurgery.* 2001;49(3):593–605.
10. Suarez JL, et al. Effect of human albumin administration on clinical outcome and hospital cost in patients with subarachnoid hemorrhage. *J Neurosurg.* 2004;100:585–90.
11. Kim DH, et al. Reduction of pulmonary edema after SAH with a pulmonary artery catheter-guided hemodynamic management protocol. *Neurocrit Care.* 2005;3(1):11–15.

ADDITIONAL READING

- Naval NS, et al. Controversies in the management of aneurysmal subarachnoid hemorrhage. *Crit Care Med.* 2006;34:511–24.

 See Also (Topic, Algorithm, Electronic Media Element)

Subarachnoid Hemorrhage

 CODES

ICD9

- 430 Subarachnoid hemorrhage
- 435.9 Unspecified transient cerebral ischemia

CLINICAL PEARLS

Treatment of cerebral vasospasm starts with early clipping or coiling of the ruptured aneurysms and maintaining normovolemia.

CHEST SYNDROME, ACUTE

Madhusudanan S. Ramaswamy
Louis P. Voigt

 BASICS

DESCRIPTION
- Acute chest syndrome (ACS) is an acute pulmonary complication of sickle cell disease (SCD) characterized by the presence of chest pain, fever, cough and wheezing in children, and by shortness of breath and pain at the extremities in adults (1).
- System(s) affected: Respiratory

Pediatric Considerations
Common complication in children with SCD, with peak incidence between 2 and 4 years (25.3/100 patient-years)

EPIDEMIOLOGY
Incidence
- ACS is the leading cause of death among patients with SCD.
  – 12.8 hospitalizations per 100 patient years (2)
- 8.8/100 patient-years in adults (2)
- Incidence is inversely proportional to concentration of fetal hemoglobin and degree of anemia, and directly proportional to the WBC count.

Prevalence
- Higher prevalence during winter months
- Second most common cause of hospitalization for patients with SCD

RISK FACTORS
- Young age
- Type of sickle cell variant
- Winter season

Genetics
- Patients with SS type at much higher risk compared to SC type
- Less frequently, may affect S-beta thalassemia patients

PATHOPHYSIOLOGY
- Complex; results from deoxygenation of hemoglobin S, leading to Hgb S polymerization and sickling of red blood cells
- Contributory factors include inflammation due to infection or fat embolus; hypoventilation from atelectasis, pulmonary edema, bronchospasm, pain from vasoocclusive crisis, or administration of excessive opiods; and endothelial dysfunction of the pulmonary microvasculature.

ETIOLOGY
- Infections (viruses, Mycoplasma, Chlamydia, and other bacteria)
- Pulmonary fat embolism
- Pulmonary infarction

COMMONLY ASSOCIATED CONDITIONS
- Sickle cell crisis
- Postoperative state (especially after abdominal surgery)
- Asthma
- Chronic hypoxemia

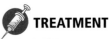 **DIAGNOSIS**

HISTORY
- Chest pain
- Extremity pain
- Shortness of breath
- Wheezing
- Cough
- Fever
- Hemoptysis
- Chills

DIAGNOSTIC TESTS & INTERPRETATION
Lab
- CBC: Search for anemia, thrombocytopenia, and leukocytosis
- Reticulocyte count
- ABG: Hypoxemia
- Blood cultures
- Sputum cultures
- Urine legionella antigen
- Mycoplasma antibody titers
- Parvovirus B-19 antibody titers
- Intracellular lipid from alveolar macrophages on samples of bronchoalveolar lavage (BAL) fluid.

Imaging
- Chest x-ray: new infiltrate (may need serial films, if initial film is negative)
- Perfusion lung scan: consider in patients with high clinical suspicion but negative chest x-ray.

Diagnostic Procedures/Other
Bronchoscopy with bronchial washings and BAL fluid obtained for cultures and for detection of intracellular lipids in alveolar macrophages

Pathological Findings
Intracellular lipid from alveolar macrophages

DIFFERENTIAL DIAGNOSIS
- Sickle cell crisis
- Bronchial asthma
- Pneumonia
- Pulmonary embolism
- Deep venous thrombosis

TREATMENT

MEDICATION
- Oxygen
- Bronchodilators
- Broad-spectrum antibiotics including macrolide
- IV corticosteroids in mild to moderate cases

- Hydroxyurea for recurrent ACS (2)[B]
- Inhaled nitric oxide: Promising but randomized studies needed (3)[B]

ADDITIONAL TREATMENT
General Measures
- Adequate hydration with IV fluids (isotonic or hypotonic saline preferred)
- Pain control: Ketorolac, morphine; PCA pump may be useful
- Incentive spirometry
- Blood transfusion
- Exchange transfusion to decrease Hgb S level to <30% of total hemoglobin concentration
- Noninvasive and invasive mechanical ventilation for respiratory failure
- Vaccines against influenza, Streptococcus pneumoniae, and respiratory syncytial virus

Issues for Referral
- Critical care medicine consultation is recommended whenever ACS is considered.
- Hematology consultation is also warranted.

IN-PATIENT CONSIDERATIONS
Initial Stabilization
- ACS diagnosis requires in-hospital management.
- Attention to hypoxemia
- Early transfusion and antibiotics in high-risk patients

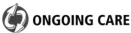

ONGOING CARE

FOLLOW-UP RECOMMENDATIONS
- Referral to hematology service and possibly hematopoietic stem cell transplantation service
- Immunization against prevalent organisms associated with ACS

Patient Monitoring
- Monitoring for increased respiratory rate and hypoxia
- Monitoring for other organ failure
- Monitoring for worsening anemia and thrombocytopenia
- Serial chest x-rays, if initial imaging is negative
- Treat infections early.
- Monitor patients receiving chronic transfusions for hepatitis and hemosiderosis.

DIET
- Normal if stable
- NPO if respiratory insufficiency worsens, as patient may require intubation
- Folic acid supplementation
- Maintain hydration.

PATIENT EDUCATION
- Early activity once pain is adequately controlled
- Incentive spirometry
- Deep breathing
- Physical therapy
- Pulmonary toilet
- Reassurance

PROGNOSIS
- Early recognition and aggressive care is associated with good prognosis.
- Prognosis is worse in patients with worsening anemia, thrombocytopenia, and acute respiratory distress syndrome.

COMPLICATIONS
- 25% mortality rate
- Older patients are more likely to have complications and to die.
- Respiratory complications are the leading cause of death:
  – Pulmonary embolism
  – Bronchopneumonia
  – Pulmonary hypertension
- Neurologic events:
  – Altered mental status
  – Seizures
  – Posterior leukoencephalopathy syndrome
  – Necrotizing encephalitis
  – Neuromuscular abnormalities
- Cardiac events:
  – Congestive heart failure
  – Arrhythmias
  – Hypotension
- Renal insufficiency/failure

REFERENCES
1. Vichinsky EP, et al. Causes and outcomes of the acute chest syndrome in sickle cell disease. National Acute Chest Syndrome Study Group. *N Engl J Med.* 2000;342(25):1855–65.
2. Steinberg MH, et al. Effect of hydroxyurea on mortality and morbidity in adult sickle cell anemia: Risks and benefits up to 9 years of treatment. *JAMA.* 2003;289(13):1645–51.
3. Bonds DR. Three decades of innovation in the management of sickle cell disease: The road to understanding the sickle cell disease clinical phenotype. *Blood Rev.* 2005;19:99–110.

ADDITIONAL READING
- Stuart MJ, et al. Sickle-cell disease. *Lancet.* 2004;364:1343–60.

See Also (Topic, Algorithm, Electronic Media Element)
- http://www.scinfo.org/chest.htm
- http://jama.ama-assn.org/cgi/reprint/300/22/2690.pdf

CODES

ICD9
- 282.60 Sickle-cell disease, unspecified
- 282.62 Hb-ss disease with crisis
- 517.3 Acute chest syndrome

CLINICAL PEARLS
- ACS is the leading cause of death and hospitalization among patients with SCD.
- Pathogenesis and pathophysiology involves deoxygenation of hemoglobin S by an inciting process, leading to polymerization of Hgb S and sickling of RBCs within the pulmonary vasculature, resulting in vaso-occlusion, ischemia, and endothelial injury.
- Adequate hydration, analgesia, and respiratory support with supplemental oxygen; bronchodilators; transfusion support; and use of broad-spectrum antibiotics are recommended.
- Hydroxyurea may decrease the frequency of ACS; hematopoietic stem cell transplantation may become necessary for patients who develop multiple ACS events and who have an HLA-matched sibling donor.

CHEST TUBE THORACOSTOMY

Jose R. Yunen
Vicente San Martín

PROCEDURE

INDICATIONS
- Aspiration of air from a pneumothorax or with bronchopleural fistula
- Therapeutic drainage of serous, malignant, or infected fluid from chest
- Postoperative drainage of the chest following thoracic or cardiac surgery
- Trauma

CONTRAINDICATIONS
- Coagulopathy
- Pleural adhesions

TECHNIQUE
See algorithm.

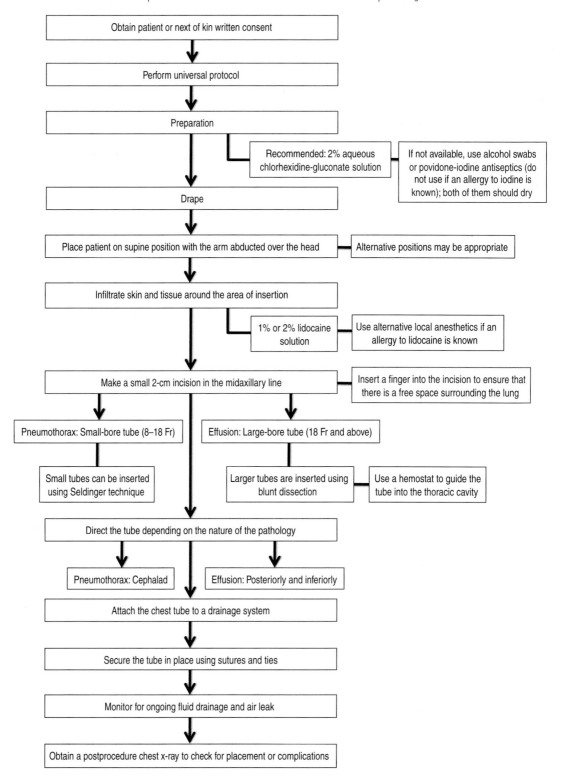

Obtain patient or next of kin written consent

↓

Perform universal protocol

↓

Preparation → Recommended: 2% aqueous chlorhexidine-gluconate solution → If not available, use alcohol swabs or povidone-iodine antiseptics (do not use if an allergy to iodine is known); both of them should dry

↓

Drape

↓

Place patient on supine position with the arm abducted over the head → Alternative positions may be appropriate

↓

Infiltrate skin and tissue around the area of insertion → 1% or 2% lidocaine solution → Use alternative local anesthetics if an allergy to lidocaine is known

↓

Make a small 2-cm incision in the midaxillary line → Insert a finger into the incision to ensure that there is a free space surrounding the lung

↓

Pneumothorax: Small-bore tube (8–18 Fr) → Small tubes can be inserted using Seldinger technique

Effusion: Large-bore tube (18 Fr and above) → Larger tubes are inserted using blunt dissection → Use a hemostat to guide the tube into the thoracic cavity

↓

Direct the tube depending on the nature of the pathology

↓

Pneumothorax: Cephalad

Effusion: Posteriorly and inferiorly

↓

Attach the chest tube to a drainage system

↓

Secure the tube in place using sutures and ties

↓

Monitor for ongoing fluid drainage and air leak

↓

Obtain a postprocedure chest x-ray to check for placement or complications

COMPLICATIONS
• Lung laceration

• Misplacement relative to the pathology

ADDITIONAL READING

• Dev S, et al. Chest-tube insertion. *N Engl J Med*. 2007;357:e15.

C

CHOLECYSTITIS, ACALCULOUS
Andrew Deroo

 BASICS

DESCRIPTION
Acalculous cholecystitis (ACC) is defined as an inflammation of the gallbladder without the presence of gallstones.

EPIDEMIOLOGY
Incidence
Incidence varies based on underlying illness or injury but is reported to range from 2–15%.

RISK FACTORS
ACC has been associated with critical illness, trauma, burns, MOF, positive-pressure ventilation, and opioid and TPN administration.

PATHOPHYSIOLOGY
- Exact pathophysiology is unknown but thought to be secondary to biliary stasis, gallbladder distention, and hypoperfusion of the gallbladder resulting in ischemia.
- Inflammation of the gallbladder occurs in the absence of gallstones in ACC.

COMMONLY ASSOCIATED CONDITIONS
- Critical illness
- Burns
- Trauma
- TPN administration
- Hyperalimentation
- Positive-pressure ventilation

 DIAGNOSIS

HISTORY
- Difficult to illicit in many cases but clinical symptoms are similar to acute cholecystitis with abdominal pain, nausea, vomiting, anorexia, and fever.
- In sedated patients in which a history is unable to be elucidated, fever, elevated WBC, elevated alkaline phosphatase, and elevated bilirubin should prompt further evaluation for ACC.

PHYSICAL EXAM
- Physical exam findings are unreliable in most cases.
- Depending on responsiveness of patient, it might be possible to elicit RUQ or upper abdominal pain with localized or generalized peritonitis.

DIAGNOSTIC TESTS & INTERPRETATION
Lab
- WBC elevated
- LFT elevated
- Amylase, lipase
- Leukocytosis or elevated LFTs with unknown cause should lead to suspicion of ACC but are not specific in critically ill patients.

Imaging
- US is most accurate initial diagnostic test; look for GB wall thickening/edema, sludge, and pericholecystic fluid.
- HIDA scan can be used for stable patients but is less specific in critically ill patients.
- CT scan of abdomen can diagnose ACC while evaluating for other intra-abdominal sources as cause of symptoms or laboratory abnormalities.

Pathological Findings
Inflamed GB wall with areas of patchy necrosis

DIFFERENTIAL DIAGNOSIS
- Acute cholecystitis
- Ascending cholangitis
- Hepatitis
- Intrahepatic cholestasis
- Drug toxicity
- Fatty liver from TPN

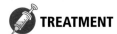 **TREATMENT**

MEDICATION
- Empiric antibiotics to cover enteric gram-negatives and anaerobes
- Antibiotics should cover *E. coli*, *Klebsiella*, *Enterococcus*, and other nosocomial bacteria such as *Pseudomonas*, *MRSA*, and *VRE*.

ADDITIONAL TREATMENT
General Measures
As for all causes of sepsis, adequate source control and empiric antibiotic treatment is imperative.

Issues for Referral
- Surgical referral for cholecystectomy or removal of cholecystostomy tube if ACC treated surgically
- IR referral for placement of percutaneous cholecystostomy tube

COMPLEMENTARY & ALTERNATIVE THERAPIES
Some small series describe a bedside laparoscopy procedure under local anesthesia and IV sedation as means of diagnosis (for critically ill patients).

SURGERY/OTHER PROCEDURES
- Percutaneous drainage via IR is usual first-line treatment if ACC is suspected.
- IR drainage is successful in 90% of cases, but if there is no improvement, surgical intervention for possible GB perforation/necrosis/gangrene is warranted.
- Surgical options include open/laparoscopic cholecystostomy tube placement or cholecystectomy.

IN-PATIENT CONSIDERATIONS
Initial Stabilization
Aggressive fluid resuscitation, prompt antibiotic coverage, and source control

Admission Criteria
Although some evidence of ACC is seen in outpatients, most patients are already admitted to the ICU.

IV Fluids
Resuscitative fluids with LR or NS

 ONGOING CARE

FOLLOW-UP RECOMMENDATIONS
- Percutaneous cholecystostomy tubes can be removed once sepsis resolves and cystic duct is demonstrated to be patent.
- Those treated with percutaneous cholecystostomy tube do not need interval cholecystectomy.

PROGNOSIS
- 30% associated mortality
- 85–90% of ACC cases are treated with percutaneous cholecystostomy tube placement.

COMPLICATIONS
- GB necrosis/gangrene/perforation
- Emphysematous cholecystitis
- Hepatic abscess
- Bile peritonitis

REFERENCES
1. Babb RR. Acute acalculous cholecystitis. *J Clin Gastroenterol*. 1992;15(3):238–241.
2. Barie PS, Fischer E, Eachempati S. Acute acalculous cholecystitis. *Curr Opin Crit Care*. 1999;5(2).
3. Barie PS, et al. Surgical infections. In: Gabrielli A, Layon AJ, Yu M, eds. *Civetta, Taylor, & Kirby's Critical Care, 4th ed*. Baltimore: Lippincott, 2009.
4. Oddsdottir M, et al. Gallbladder and extrahepatic biliary system. In: Brunicardi FC, Andersen DK, et al, eds. *Schwartz's Manual of Surgery*, 8th ed. New York: McGraw-Hill, 2006.
5. Posther KE, et al. Acute cholecystitis. In: Cameron JL, ed. *Current Surgical Therapy*, 8th ed. Philadelphia: Elsevier Mosby, 2004.
6. Raunest J, et al. Acute cholecystitis: A complication in severely injured intensive care patients. *J Trauma*. 1992;32(4):433–440.
7. Ryu JK, et al. Clinical features of acute acalculous cholecystitis. *J Clin Gastroenterol*. 2003;36(2):166–169.

 CODES

ICD9
- 575.0 Acute cholecystitis
- 575.10 Cholecystitis, unspecified
- 576.1 Cholangitis

CLINICAL PEARLS
- ACC should be high on the differential for undiagnosed sepsis in critically ill patients.
- Elevated WBC and abnormal LFTs might lead to discussion of ACC, but are not sensitive or specific enough in the critically ill patient.
- History and physical exam are usually of limited use in ACC; the diagnosis should be based on high clinical suspicion with laboratory and radiologic evidence suggestive of ACC.

CHOLECYSTITIS, ACUTE

Andrew Deroo

 BASICS

DESCRIPTION
Acute cholecystitis is an inflammation of the gallbladder caused by cystic duct obstruction.

EPIDEMIOLOGY
Incidence
10% of people in the Western word have gallstones.

Prevalence
- 80% of people with gallstones are asymptomatic.
- 1–3% of people with gallstones develop acute cholecystitis.

RISK FACTORS
- 3 times more common in women
- Increased gallstone formation in:
  - Obesity
  - Pregnancy
  - Dietary factors
  - Crohn disease
  - Terminal ileal resection

Genetics
Increased risk of developing gallstones in sickle cell disease, thalassemia, and hereditary spherocytosis

PATHOPHYSIOLOGY
- Obstruction results in increased intraluminal pressure, gallbladder distention/edema, and an inflammatory response.
- Secondary bacterial superinfection occurs in 20–50% of cases.

ETIOLOGY
- 90% result from obstruction of the cystic duct by biliary sludge or gallstones.
- Extrinsic compression from tumor is a less common cause of obstruction.

COMMONLY ASSOCIATED CONDITIONS
- Gallstones
- Gallbladder wall diverticulum

DIAGNOSIS

HISTORY
- Persistent upper abdominal pain often localized to RUQ
- Nausea, vomiting, and anorexia are common.
- Often have history of biliary colic or history of gallstones
- Referred pain to scapula or shoulder
- Systemic symptoms including fever, mild tachycardia, chills, and rigors

PHYSICAL EXAM
- Murphy's sign: Pain and inspiratory arrest with deep palpation of RUQ
- Can have localized peritonitis with associated guarding in RUQ

DIAGNOSTIC TESTS & INTERPRETATION
Lab
Initial lab tests
- WBCelevated
- LFTelevated (particularly the alkaline phosphatase)
- Amylase, lipase:
  - May have mild leukocytosis and bilirubin with uncomplicated cholecystitis; higher elevation should cause concern for choledocholithiasis and ascending cholangitis

Follow-Up & Special Considerations
If LFTs are elevated on admission, they should be trended to ensure no CBD obstruction is present.

Imaging
- US
- HIDA
- CT scan
- US is first choice for imaging; has 95% sensitivity and 97% specificity.
- Signs of acute cholecystitis on US include pericholecystic fluid, GB wall thickening (>3.5 mm), biliary sludge, GB distension, sonographic Murphy's sign, and gallstones.
- HIDA has a 100% sensitivity and 95% specificity.
- HIDA is positive if radionucleotide goes through CBD but not into GB, suggesting cystic duct obstruction.
- HIDA has high false-positive rate if patient has been fasting for >5 days.
- CT scan can show perforation, abscess, phlegmon, or cholecyst-enteric fistula.

Diagnostic Procedures/Other
MRCP or ERCP may be needed if concern exists for CBD stone.

Pathological Findings
Inflammatory changes with subserosal hemorrhage and patchy necrosis

DIFFERENTIAL DIAGNOSIS
- Biliary colic
- Choledocholithiasis
- Gallstone pancreatitis
- Regional enteritis
- Bowel obstruction
- Hepatitis
- Pyelonephritis
- Right heart failure with hepatic congestion
- PUD
- GERD

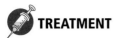 TREATMENT

MEDICATION
Antibiotics to cover gram-negatives and anaerobes including *E. coli*, *Klebsiella*, *Streptococcus*, *Clostridium*, *Proteus*, and *Enterobacter*

ADDITIONAL TREATMENT
Issues for Referral
If treated medically with IV antibiotics and fluids, the patient will need referral to surgeon in 4–6 weeks for cholecystectomy

Additional Therapies
IR percutaneous cholecystostomy tube or open cholecystostomy tube in those deemed inappropriate for surgery secondary to comorbidities or clinical picture

SURGERY/OTHER PROCEDURES
* Laparoscopic vs. open cholecystectomy associated with similar mortality, cost, hospital LOS, and complications
* Patients can have cholecystectomy if they present early in the course of inflammation; however, there is a high conversion rate to open procedure if done in acute inflammatory stage.
* Interval cholecystectomy in 6–8 weeks is recommended if patient presents late in course of illness (after 3–4 days).

IN-PATIENT CONSIDERATIONS
Initial Stabilization
* IVF resuscitation
* Appropriate antibiotic coverage

Admission Criteria
Acute pain with localized peritonitis and clinical, laboratory, and radiologic evidence suggestive of acute cholecystitis as opposed to biliary colic

IV Fluids
Resuscitative IV fluids/crystalloids

Discharge Criteria
* Normalized laboratory values if abnormal on admission
* Resolution of pain
* Tolerating oral diet

 ONGOING CARE

FOLLOW-UP RECOMMENDATIONS
* Surgical follow-up to discuss cholecystectomy if treated medically
* Routine postsurgical follow-up if cholecystectomy is performed while hospitalized

DIET
No restrictions, although some may recommend a low-fat diet

PROGNOSIS
Low morbidity/mortality

COMPLICATIONS
* Ascending cholangitis
* Gallstone pancreatitis
* Cholecystenteric fistula
* Gallstone ileus
* Gallbladder necrosis/gangrene
* Gallbladder rupture with bile peritonitis

ADDITIONAL READING
* Barie PS, et al. Surgical infections. In: Gabrielli A, et al., eds. *Civetta, Taylor, & Kirby's Critical Care*, 4th ed. Baltimore: Lippincott Williams & Wilkins; 2009.
* Indar A, et al. Acute cholecystitis. *BMJ*. 2002;325: 639–643.
* Oddsdottir M, et al. Gallbladder and extrahepatic biliary system. In: Brunicardi FC, et al., eds. *Schwartz's Manual of Surgery*, 8th ed. New York: McGraw-Hill, 2006.
* Posther KE, et al. Acute cholecystitis. In: Cameron JL, ed. *Current Surgical Therapy*, 8th ed. Philadelphia: Elsevier Mosby, 2004.
* Trowbridge R, et al. Does this patient have acute cholecystitis? *JAMA*. 2003;289(1):80–86.

 CODES

ICD9
* 574.00 Calculus of gallbladder with acute cholecystitis, without mention of obstruction
* 574.21 Calculus of gallbladder without mention of cholecystitis, with obstruction
* 575.0 Acute cholecystitis

CLINICAL PEARLS
* Acute cholecystitis should be differentiated from biliary colic, and patients with active cholecystitis should be admitted for IV antibiotics and possible surgical intervention.
* Patients admitted for acute cholecystitis that fails to improve with conservative medical management should have surgical (or IR) referral for cholecystostomy tube placement or cholecystectomy.

CHRONIC OBSTRUCTIVE PULMONARY DISEASE (COPD)

Rakesh Sinha
John Oropello

 ## BASICS

DESCRIPTION
- COPD is a preventable and treatable disease state characterized by airflow limitation that is not fully reversible. The airflow limitation is usually progressive and is associated with an abnormal inflammatory response of the lungs to noxious particles or gases, primarily caused by cigarette smoking (1):
  - Chronic bronchitis and emphysema are part of COPD disease state
- System(s) affected: Primarily lung, but COPD produces significant systemic consequences.
- COPD exacerbation is an event in the natural course of the disease and is defined as acute change in a patient's baseline dyspnea, cough, and/or sputum beyond day-to-day variability sufficient to warrant a change in therapy.
- Exacerbations are a common cause of morbidity and mortality in COPD patients.

PATHOPHYSIOLOGY
Inflammation, imbalance of proteinases and antiproteinases and oxidative stress in lung causes:
- Mucous hypersecretion and ciliary dysfunction
- Airflow limitation and hyperinflation
- Gas exchange abnormalities
- Pulmonary hypertension and cor pulmonale

ETIOLOGY
- Exposures: Cumulative over life:
  - Tobacco smoke: Cigarette smoking is most important. Pipe, cigar, and environmental tobacco smoke also predispose
  - Occupational dusts and chemicals
  - Environmental pollution
- Perinatal events, childhood illnesses, recurrent bronchopulmonary infections, socioeconomic status, diet, airway hyperreactivity, and atopy influence individual's risk
- α-1 antitrypsin (AAT) deficiency causes early COPD.
- COPD exacerbations are frequently associated with infections.

COMMONLY ASSOCIATED CONDITIONS
- Coronary artery disease (CAD)
- Lung cancer
- Asthma

DIAGNOSIS

HISTORY
- Current or ex-smoker with:
  - Cough with or without sputum production
  - Dyspnea: Progressive, usually worse with exercise, and persistent (present every day)
  - Hemoptysis (rare, seen in chronic bronchitis)

PHYSICAL EXAM
- Early disease: Normal except prolonged expiration or wheeze on forced expiration
- Advanced disease:
  - Signs of wasting or cachexia
  - Tachypnea with use of accessory muscles
  - Pursed lip breathing
  - Facial plethora related to polycythemia
  - Cyanosis
  - Barrel chest
  - Wheezing and crackles
  - Markedly diminished breath sounds
  - Asterixis due to hypercapnia
  - Confusion, lethargy and coma

DIAGNOSTIC TESTS & INTERPRETATION
Lab
Initial lab tests
ABG: Respiratory failure if PaO_2 <60 mm Hg or $PaCO_2$ >50 mm Hg on room air
Follow-Up & Special Considerations
AAT deficiency screening in patients <45 or with strong family history of COPD

Imaging
- Chest x-ray: Seldom diagnostic but valuable to exclude alternative or coexisting diagnoses such as pneumonia, tuberculosis, and cancer.
- In advanced disease it may show flattening of diaphragm, increased retrosternal space, small tubular cardiac silhouette, pruning of pulmonary arteries, and presence of bullae.

Diagnostic Procedures/Other
Spirometry with bronchodilator reversibility is required for diagnosis of COPD (1,2) but is not performed during exacerbation or ICU stay:
- A postbronchodilator forced expiratory volume in 1 second (FEV_1) to forced vital capacity (FVC) ratio ≤ 0.7 confirms the presence of airflow limitation.
- Stages of COPD is based on spirometry:
  - Stage I: Mild COPD; FEV_1 $\geq$80% predicted, subjects may be unaware of lung function being abnormal
  - Stage II: Moderate COPD; FEV_1 50–80% predicted, shortness of breath present, typically on exertion
  - Stage III: Severe COPD; FEV_1 30–50% predicted, reduced exercise capacity, exacerbations impact quality of life
  - Stage IV: Very severe COPD; FEV_1 <30% predicted OR FEV_1 <50% predicted plus chronic respiratory failure, poor quality of life, exacerbations are life-threatening

Pathological Findings
Central airways, peripheral airways, lung parenchyma, and pulmonary vasculature are affected.

DIFFERENTIAL DIAGNOSIS
- Asthma
- Congestive heart failure
- Bronchiectasis
- Tuberculosis
- Obliterative bronchiolitis
- Diffuse panbronchiolitis

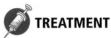 ## TREATMENT

MEDICATION
First Line
- Treatment of severe exacerbation:
  - Nebulizer, cautious use of oxygen in patients with hypercapnia:
    - Albuterol: Start 2.5–5 mg q20min then 2.5–10 mg q1–4h OR 10–15 mg/h continuous
    - Ipratropium: Start 500 μg q1h then 500 μg q4–6h
  - MDI with spacer:
    - Albuterol 90 μg: Start 4–8 puffs q20min, then 4–8 puffs q1–4h
    - Ipratropium 17 μg: 4–8 puffs q4–6h
- Systemic corticosteroids for exacerbations:
  - IV methylprednisolone 125 mg, 1 dose followed by 60 mg q6h, switch to oral
  - PO prednisone 30–40 mg q24h for 10–14 days
- Treatment of stable COPD:
  - Short-acting β_2-agonists (3)[A]:
    - Albuterol MDI 90 μg: 2 puffs q4–6h p.r.n.
  - Long-acting β_2-agonists (3)[A]:
    - Salmeterol DPI 50 μg: 1 dose q12h
    - Formoterol DPI 12 μg: 1 dose q12h
  - Short-acting anticholinergics (3)[A]:
    - Ipratropium MDI 17 μg: 2 puffs q6h
  - Long-acting anticholinergics (3)[A]:
    - Tiotropium DPI 18 μg: 1 dose q24h
  - Inhaled corticosteroids in combination with long-acting inhaled β-agonists (3)[A]:
    - Fluticasone/Salmeterol DPI 100/50, 250/50, 500/50 μg: 1 dose q12h OR MDI 45/21,115/21, 230/21 μg: 2 puffs q12h
- Budesonide/Formoterol MDI 80/4.5, 160/4.5 μg: 2 puffs q12h

Second Line
- Antibiotics for exacerbations: Recommended when dyspnea is present with increased sputum volume and purulence or when on ventilator.
- Based on local bacteria resistance pattern:
  - Levofloxacin 750 mg/d for 5 days
- Theophylline IV
  - Healthy nonsmoker: 0.4 mg/kg/h; load 5 mg/kg if no theophylline within 24 hours
  - Smoker: 0.7 mg/kg/h; load 5 mg/kg if no theophylline within 24 hours

Geriatric Considerations
Theophylline IV 0.3 mg/kg/h; load 5 mg/kg if no theophylline within 24 hours

ADDITIONAL TREATMENT
Additional Therapies
- Chest physiotherapy
- DVT prophylaxis
- Vaccination: Influenza vaccine reduces serious illness and death in COPD patients by 50% (2)[A].
- Pneumococcal vaccine is recommended.
- Smoking cessation is single most effective (and cost effective) intervention to reduce risk of developing COPD and slow its progression 2[A]:
  - Even brief 3-minute counseling is effective.
  - Pharmacotherapy (avoid if patient smokes <10 cigarettes/day or pregnant): Varenicline, bupropion (avoid in seizures), nicotine replacement patch, gum or nasal spray (avoid in unstable CAD, recent myocardial infarction, or stroke; untreated peptic ulcer)
- Pulmonary rehabilitation
- Long-term oxygen improves survival, exercise, and cognitive performance in Stage IV (2)[A]:
  - Indications: PaO_2 <55 mm Hg or PaO_2 55–60 mm Hg with cor pulmonale or polycythemia with optimized medications
  - Goal: Keep SpO_2 >90% during rest, sleep, and exertion by titrating flow rate

SURGERY/OTHER PROCEDURES
- Surgery in COPD:
  - Smoking cessation recommended for at least 4–8 weeks prior for elective procedures
  - Lung resection should be performed only after evaluation for predicted postoperative lung function
- Surgery for COPD:
  - Bullectomy is useful in patients with rapidly progressive dyspnea with large bulla.
  - Lung volume reduction surgery improves survival in patients with upper lobe emphysema and low exercise capacity.
- Lung transplantation improves quality of life in select patients with very advanced disease.

IN-PATIENT CONSIDERATIONS
Initial Stabilization
- Controlled oxygen: Titrate to keep SpO_2 >90%; check ABG in 30–60 minutes to assess satisfactory oxygenation without CO_2 retention and acidosis.
- Determine if exacerbation is life-threatening and admit to ICU accordingly.
- Bronchodilators: Albuterol/Ipratropium; use nebulizer or MDI with spacer (2)[A]
- Systemic steroids (2)[A]
- Antibiotics (2)[B]
- Methylxanthines intravenously (2)[B]
- Noninvasive positive pressure ventilation (NIPPV) is a first-line intervention for the respiratory failure due to COPD exacerbation:
  - NIPPV can be administered on the ward or high-dependency respiratory care unit but requires the same level of monitoring as invasive mechanical ventilation during the first few hours.
  - Selection criteria for NIPPV:
    - Moderate to severe dyspnea with use of accessory muscles and paradoxical abdominal motion

- Moderate to severe acidosis (pH $\leq$7.35) and/or hypercapnia ($PaCO_2$ >45 mm Hg)
- Respiratory frequency >25 breaths/minute
- Exclusion criteria for NIPPV:
  - Respiratory arrest
  - Hypoxemic respiratory failure
  - Cardiovascular instability (hypotension, arrhythmias, myocardial infarction)
  - Changes in mental status; uncooperative
  - High aspiration risk or copious secretions
  - Burns or craniofacial trauma
  - Fixed nasopharyngeal abnormalities
  - Extreme obesity
- NIPPV settings:
  - PSV 8–12 cm H_2O (IPAP 12–20 cm H_2O)
  - CPAP 4–8 cm H_2O (EPAP 4–8 cm H_2O)
  - Monitor ABG
- Invasive mechanical ventilation:
  - Indications:
    - Unable to tolerate NIPPV or NIPPV failure
    - Needs ventilation but meets exclusion criteria for NIPPV
    - Severe dyspnea with use of accessory muscles and paradoxical abdominal motion
    - Respiratory frequency >35 breaths/minute
    - Life-threatening hypoxemia
    - Severe acidosis (pH <7.25) and/or hypercapnia ($PaCO_2$ >60 mm Hg)
    - Coexisting complications (sepsis, pulmonary embolism, pneumonia, etc.)

Admission Criteria
Indications of ICU admission for exacerbation:
- Severe dyspnea that responds inadequately to initial emergency therapy
- Changes in mental status (confusion, lethargy, coma)
- Persistent or worsening hypoxemia (PaO_2 <40 mm Hg), and/or severe/worsening hypercapnia ($PaCO_2$ >60 mm Hg), and/or severe/worsening acidosis (pH <7.25) despite supplemental oxygen and optimal medical therapy
- Need for invasive mechanical ventilation
- Hemodynamic instability; need for vasopressors

IV Fluids
Crystalloids

 ## ONGOING CARE

DIET
- Nutritional screening is recommended.
- Underweight patients have increased mortality risk.

PROGNOSIS
- Risk of dying from an acute exacerbation is related to development of respiratory acidosis, need for ventilatory support, and presence of significant comorbidities but no clinical features can identify patients who will experience more burden than benefit from life-supportive care.
- BODE index correlates with risk of death:
  - B: **B**ody Mass Index (BMI), inverse relationship
  - O: Airflow **O**bstruction (measured by FEV_1 % predicted), inverse relationship
  - D: Modified Medical Research Council **D**yspnea scale; higher dyspnea score entails worse prognosis
  - E: **E**xercise capacity (measured by 6-minute walk distance), inverse relationship

COMPLICATIONS
- Frequent exacerbations with need for mechanical ventilation
- Mechanical ventilator dependence
- Pulmonary hypertension
- Cor pulmonale and heart failure
- Sleep disturbance and memory deficits
- Anxiety and depression
- Weight loss and muscular atrophy
- Osteoporosis

REFERENCES
1. Celli BR , MacNee W, and committee members. Standards for the diagnosis and treatment of patients with COPD: A summary of the ATS/ERS position paper. *Eur Respir J*. 2004;23:932–46.
2. Rabe KF, et al. Global strategy for the diagnosis, management and prevention of chronic obstructive pulmonary disease: GOLD executive summary. *Am J Respir Crit Care Med*. 2007;176:532–55.
3. Celli BR. Update on the management of COPD. *Chest*. 2008;133:1451–62.

ADDITIONAL READING
- http://www.copd-ats-ers.org/
- http://goldcopd.com/

 See Also (Topic, Algorithm, Electronic Media Element)

Mechanical Ventilation

 CODES

ICD9
- 491.9 Unspecified chronic bronchitis
- 492.8 Other emphysema
- 496 Chronic airway obstruction, not elsewhere classified

CLINICAL PEARLS
- COPD is a preventable and treatable disease with significant systemic complications and can have frequent exacerbations needing hospitalization.
- Smoking cessation is the most effective intervention to reduce risk of developing COPD and to slow its progression.
- Pharmacologic treatment can prevent and control symptoms, reduce the frequency and severity of exacerbations, improve health status, and improve exercise tolerance.
- Noninvasive positive pressure ventilation should be considered as the first-line intervention, in addition to optimal medical therapy, for the management of respiratory failure due to exacerbation of COPD. It requires the same level of monitoring as conventional mechanical ventilation during the first few hours.
- Risk of dying from an acute exacerbation is related to development of respiratory acidosis, need for ventilatory support, and presence of significant comorbidities, but no clinical features can identify patients who will experience more burden than benefit from life-supportive care.

CHRONIC RESPIRATORY FAILURE AND WEANING

Ronaldo Go
John M. Oropello

 BASICS

DESCRIPTION
- There is no universally accepted definition for chronic respiratory failure (CRF).
- In 2005, a consensus conference defined CRF as the need for prolonged mechanical ventilation (PMV) for $\geq$6 hrs/d for at least 21 days.
- CRF may also be defined by ABGs as a PaO_2 <60 on room air (or requires supplemental oxygen to maintain PaO_2 $\geq$60) or $PaCO_2$ >50 that develops over time (weeks) and is persistent.
- Relevant to ICU practice, the two main categories of chronic respiratory failure are:
  - Acute respiratory failure transitioning to chronic respiratory failure (i.e., the need for PMV); most of these patients also have a syndrome termed *chronic critical illness* (CCI).
  - Patients with pre-existing permanent chronic respiratory failure due to severe progressive or irreversible disorders (e.g., end-stage COPD, neuromuscular diseases, etc.):
    ○ Patients in the 2nd category usually have a pre-existing tracheotomy or an early tracheotomy within days of ICU admission and are never expected to wean off the ventilator. Intensive care consists of treating the acute processes, (e.g., sepsis, GI bleed, etc.) and returning the patient to a long-term care facility.
- This chapter is focused on patients in category 1 with PMV, usually as the hallmark of CCI.
- PMV occurs in about 5–10% of mechanically ventilated patients and may be higher depending on the ICU population.

PATHOPHYSIOLOGY
- Load and capacity imbalance: Decreased respiratory muscle capacity in relation to breathing load (demand); this is clinically determined by high respiratory rate or increased respiratory frequency to tidal volume ratios, and reduced maximal inspiratory pressure. It is a consequence of a combination of factors that increase the work of breathing and decease overall strength:
  - Neuromuscular weakness
  - Hypoxemia secondary to ventilation/perfusion mismatch or shunts
  - Obstructive airways disease; dynamic hyperinflation
  - Asynchronous breathing or dysfunctional respiratory drive
  - Anasarca
  - Morbid obesity
  - Psychological factors (e.g., anxiety)
- Renal compensation for hypercapnia occurs over 2–3 days; diuretics and steroids may further induce metabolic alkalosis.

ETIOLOGY
- Usually multifactorial
- Systemic effects of infection:
  - Sepsis, severe sepsis, septic shock
  - Multiple organ failure
  - Inflammatory polymyoneuropathy
  - Atrophy and remodeling; loss of mean body mass
  - Impaired anabolism; enhanced catabolism
  - Acute lung injury/ARDS
  - Hepatic dysfunction
  - Acute kidney injury

- Encephalopathy
- Obstructive lung disease
- Interstitial lung disease
- Cardiovascular disease (e.g., ischemia including silent, heart failure-cardiogenic pulmonary edema, pulmonary hypertension)
- Liver cirrhosis
- Chronic renal failure
- Malnutrition due to chronic critical illness
- General debilitation due to chronic disease and cancer
- Dementia
- CVA
- Anxiety
- Medications (steroids, neuromuscular blockers, aminoglycosides)
- Continued aspiration despite tracheotomy
- Iatrogenic: Inappropriate assessment of ventilator liberation capabilities, unnecessary sedation strategies, sleep deprivation

COMMONLY ASSOCIATED CONDITIONS
- Poor prior functional status
- Severe deconditioning
- Skin breakdown and decubitus ulcers
- Infection with multidrug resistant organisms
- Unrecognized (occult) sources of sepsis

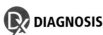 **DIAGNOSIS**

HISTORY
- Symptoms: Anxiety, depression, pain, thirst, dyspnea
- Pre-ICU functional status
- Social history
- Oxygen dependency
- Chronic diseases

PHYSICAL EXAM
- General survey: Elements of deconditioning, such as muscle wasting and cachexia; morbid obesity; anasarca; note admission weight vs. current weight; catheter site inspection
- Skin: Breakdown associated with malnutrition, edema, coagulopathy, incontinence; frank decubitus ulcers
- HEENT: Nasogastric, orogastric tubes, endotracheal tube, tracheotomy
- Chest: Deformities (e.g., kyphoscoliosis), hyperinflation, paradoxical breathing, breath sounds, wheezing, crackles and/or rhonchi
- Cardiovascular: Hyperdynamic vs. hypodynamic circulation, murmurs, systolic blood pressure variability with respiration, JVD distention, hepatojugular reflex
- Abdomen: Wounds, distension, ileus, ascites, tenderness, PEG site
- Genitourinary: Foley, scrotal edema, skin breakdown
- Extremities: Edema (upper and lower), vascular insufficiency, unequal size right vs. left
- Neurological: Encephalopathy, dementia, muscle weakness
- Psychological: Anxiety, depression

DIAGNOSTIC TESTS & INTERPRETATION
Lab
ABG, serum electrolytes, BUN, Cr, LFTs, CBC, lactate if hemodynamically unstable or metabolic acidosis

Imaging
CXR

Diagnostic Procedures/Other
- ECG
- Blood cultures
- Duplex US to rule out DVT (e.g., in extremities of unequal size)
- CT scan head, chest, abdomen, pelvis: Rules out CVA, occult source of sepsis
- Echocardiogram: Systolic or diastolic dysfunction, regional wall motion abnormalities; ischemia, valvular disorders, pulmonary hypertension
- Nerve conduction study or electromyogram (EMG) (assess for critical illness polymyoneuropathy)
- Lung biopsy via bronchoscopy or video assisted thoracotomy in selected cases with uncertain but possibly treatable interstitial lung diseases \ infection

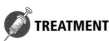 **TREATMENT**

MEDICATION
First Line
- Bronchodilators
- β_2 agonists:
  - Albuterol: Nebulizer MDI-HFA 90 mcg/puff or liquid for nebulization 0.63, 1.25, or 2.5 mg/vial
  - Levalbuterol: Less sinus and supraventricular tachycardia than albuterol is controversial
  - MDI-HFA 45 mcg/puff or liquid for nebulization 0.31, 0.63, or 1.25 mg/vial
- Anticholinergics:
  - Ipratropium: 500 mcg/2.5 mL NEB q6–8h; MDI 2–5 puffs q6h
- Steroid trial in select patients with COPD/asthma: Solu-Medrol 30–40 mg PO/IV daily with taper, monitoring response
- N-acetylcysteine: Mucolytic; may aggravate bronchospasm so monitor lung through auscultation/airway pressures before and after:
  - 3–5 mL 20% nebulizer q6h
  - 6–10 mL 10% nebulizer q6h
  - 1–2 mL 10–20% via tracheotomy q1–4h
- Diuretics: In patients with pulmonary edema or volume overload:
  - Furosemide 40 mg = torsemide 20 mg = bumetanide 1 mg
  - GI prophylaxis (H_2 blocker; e.g., famotidine 40 mg/d, decrease in renal failure: 20 mg/d)
  - DVT prophylaxis (sequential compression decompression devices, SQ heparin 5000 q8h)

Second Line
- Antibiotics (suspected or documented infection)
- Multidrug resistance is common; antibiotic use should be limited to hemodynamically unstable sepsis and specific documented clinical infections.

ADDITIONAL TREATMENT
- Tracheostomy:
  - Consider when the patient remains ventilator dependent for 7–10 days and is not expected to be liberated within the next week (1)[B].
  - The timing is still debated; however, recent trends are toward earlier tracheotomy (e.g., 14–21 days vs. >21 days).
  - Benefits include less translaryngeal and vocal cord injury, more comfort and less risk of tube

dislodgement, leading to less sedation, better oral hygiene, and earlier ability to phonate.
- Although studies are ongoing, it appears that there is an easier weaning process and reduced length of stay in ICU with earlier tracheotomy.
- May be performed open (surgically) at the bedside or in the operating room, or at the bedside via percutaneous dilation. The most important factor determining the type of tracheotomy is patient anatomy and the expertise of the staff performing the procedure.
- Chest physiotherapy:
  - Indirect removal of mucous by percussion or clapping the back, anterior chest, and under arms of patients
- Weaning in prolonged mechanical ventilation:
  - The earliest possible pathway to liberation from the ventilator depends on an organized approach using weaning protocols that consist of:
  - Daily reduction of the depth of continuous sedation, limitation of excessive bolus sedation, and avoidance of long-acting sedatives
  - Spontaneous breathing trials (SBT) conducted using the pressure support (PS) mode beginning at half the pressure delivered during full support. (e.g., 10–15 cm H_2O) for 30–120 minutes, followed by reductions in PS or trach collar trials for progressively longer periods each day as tolerated (1)[B].
  - Successful trials are determined by objective markers such as patient comfort and lack of dyspnea with stable gas exchange and hemodynamics (e.g., SaO_2 >90, PaO_2 >60 on FiO_2 40–50% and increase in $PaCO_2$ <10 mm Hg. Other parameters may include a decrease in pH <0.10, respiratory rate <35 per minute, heart rate <140 or <20% increase from baseline, SBP <160 or >80 mm Hg.)
  - There is no consensus on what period of time constitutes successful weaning after PMW; 48 hours, 7 days, or until discharge from ICU have been used (2)[B].
- Anemia:
  - Weaning increases oxygen consumption due to increased work of breathing.
  - Patients with anemia and CRF due to COPD have a higher mortality; however, there is no data supporting improved outcome with transfusion.
  - Unnecessary transfusions may impair weaning due to complications such as acute lung injury and volume overload (3)[B].
- Renal failure:
  - Successful weaning is less likely in patients with renal dysfunction.
  - Renal replacement therapy can be used to treat uremia, acidemia, electrolyte disturbances, and manage fluid overload.
  - Administer erythropoietin in patients with anemia of chronic renal insufficiency and Hb <10
- When and where to transfer:
  - Patients who resolve the acute illnesses but remain chronically critically ill and cannot be weaned are candidates for ICU alternatives that focus more on rehabilitation and comfort than life support. There is no longer a need for pressors or inotropes, and tracheotomy has already been performed (1)[C].
  - Transfer facilities (e.g., long-term acute care; LTAC) have requirements for transfer, including failed weaning attempts and ability to benefit from rehabilitation.

- Possible venues for transfer include:
  - LTAC
  - Skilled nursing facility
  - Rehabilitation hospital
  - Subacute hospital
  - Inpatient rehabilitation facilities
- The optimal time to consider and plan for the possibility of eventual transfer to LTAC is at the time of tracheotomy, since the process can take several weeks.
- Palliative services:
  - For relief of pain, anxiety, and family counseling since most patients have multiple comorbidities
  - To determine goals of care and the patient's preferences for treatment
- Early mobilization:
  - Includes range of motion, sitting up, OOB in chair, exercises, progressive weight-bearing
  - May mitigate development, severity, and/or duration of ICU weakness
  - Physical therapy may be limited by profound weakness or encephalopathy
- Decubitus ulcer:
  - Tissue pressure in excess of capillary filling pressure of 32 mm for prolonged periods of time, usually on dependent bony protuberances while lying in bed or sitting in chair
  - Patient repositioning every 2 hours to alternately decompress susceptible areas
  - Specialized support surfaces should be used in patients at highest risk (e.g., elderly, immobile, poor nutritional status, debilitated)
- Psychological support:
  - Frequent conversations among patient, family, and medical staff
  - Television, books, music
  - Improve sleep environment (reduce noise, light, and minimize interruptions)

SURGERY/OTHER PROCEDURES
- Percutaneous gastrostomy or jejunostomy:
  - Indicated for patients who will require nasogastric enteral nutrition for >30 days.
- Plastic surgery: For poorly healing wound management, decubitus ulcer debridement, and skin grafting

IN-PATIENT CONSIDERATIONS
Initial Stabilization
- Goal oxyhemoglobin saturation >88–90%
- Adjust mechanical ventilation to maintain PaO_2 and PCO_2 at baseline, avoid posthypercapnic metabolic alkalemia in patients with chronic CO_2 retention.
- Fluid challenges, pressors as appropriate if hemodynamically unstable

IV Fluids
- Adjusted to basal needs; depends on the degree of hemodynamic stability and assessment of current intravascular volume status
- In general, these patients are edematous with acute lung injury of varying severity and may benefit from avoidance of continued positive fluid balance and institution of negative balance via volume restriction and diuretics.

 ONGOING CARE

DIET
- Patients are usually in malnourished Kwashiorkor-like state.
- Goals: Metabolic supplementation to minimize loss of lean body mass while avoiding overfeeding,

which can lead to or worsen hyperglycemia and may increase CO_2 load.
- Enteral feeding is preferred.
- TPN is warranted if GI dysfunction prevents use of the enteral route.

PROGNOSIS
- Some degree of functional disability, with only 10% of patients returning to functional independence in 1 year
- Mortality depends on comorbidities, age, and prior functional status and varies from 39–75%.

COMPLICATIONS
- Persistent CCI with unavoidable nosocomial complications (e.g., recurrent infections, progressive neuromuscular deterioration, delirium, organ failure)
- Permanent ventilator dependence

REFERENCES

1. MacIntyre NR, et al. Evidence-based guidelines for weaning and discontinuing ventilatory support: A collective task force facilitated by the American College of Chest Physicians; the American Association for Respiratory Care; and the American College of Critical Care Medicine. *Chest.* 2001;120: 375S–95S.
2. MacIntyre NR, et al. Management of patients requiring prolonged mechanical ventilation: Report of NAMDRC Consensus Conference. *Chest.* 2005; 128:3937–54.
3. Herbert PC, et al. Do blood transfusions improve outcomes related to mechanical ventilation? *Chest.* 2001;119:1850–7.
4. Nelson JE, et al. Chronic critical illness. *Am J Respir Care Med.* 2010;182:446–54.
5. Garnacho-Montero J, et al. Effect of critical illness polyneuropathy on the withdrawal from mechanical ventilation and the length of stay in septic patients. *Crit Care Med.* 2005;33:349–54.
6. Lima DF, et al. Potentially modifiable predictors of mortality in patients treated with long-term oxygen therapy. *Respir Med.* 2011;105:470–6.

CODES

ICD9
- 496 Chronic airway obstruction, not elsewhere classified
- 518.81 Acute respiratory failure
- 518.83 Chronic respiratory failure

CLINICAL PEARLS
- PMV is a hallmark of CCI.
- Infections are common and include lower respiratory tract, urinary tract, *Clostridium difficile*, and central line infection.
- Length of stay and time to wean are significantly longer in patients with apparent infection.
- The SBT is superior to any combination of weaning parameters in determining the earliest time to ventilator liberation.
- Between 30% and 53% of CCI patients are liberated from mechanical ventilation (defined as discharged alive and breathing without assistance) in the acute care hospital.
- Begin planning for PMV-focused care when tracheotomy is first considered.

CIRRHOSIS

Ben Ari Ziv

BASICS

DESCRIPTION
- Cirrhosis is the histological development of regenerative nodules surrounded by fibrous bands in response to chronic liver injury.
- Characterized by an asymptomatic phase ("compensated" cirrhosis) and a rapidly progressive phase ("decompensated cirrhosis"): Complications of portal hypertension and/or liver dysfunction
- Upon decompensation, median survival time is ~2 years
- Liver transplantation remains the only curative option for a selected group of patients
- Staging:
  - Stage 1: Absence of esophageal varices and of ascites.
  - Stage 2: The presence of esophageal varices without ascites and without bleeding
  - Stage 3: Ascites with or without esophageal varices in a patient who has never bled
  - Stage 4: GI bleeding with or without ascites
- System(s) affected: Liver/Cardiovascular/Kidney/Brain/Adrenal

EPIDEMIOLOGY
- Cirrhosis prevalence is estimated at 0.15% or 400,000 in the U.S.
- Cirrhosis is the 9th leading cause of death in the U.S.
- ~40% of patients with cirrhosis are asymptomatic.

PATHOPHYSIOLOGY
- Cirrhosis is an advanced stage of liver fibrosis accompanied by distortion of the hepatic vasculature.
- Impaired hepatocyte (liver) function, an increased intrahepatic resistance (portal hypertension), and the development of hepatocellular carcinoma (HCC) are characteristic.
- The general circulatory abnormalities in cirrhosis are linked to the hepatic vascular alterations and the resulting portal hypertension.
- Enhanced bacterial translocation from the intestine is a major infective source in cirrhotics.

ETIOLOGY
- Viral infections:
  - Chronic hepatitis C infection
  - Chronic hepatitis B infection
- Alcoholic liver disease
- Nonalcoholic fatty liver disease:
  - Nonalcoholic steatohepatitis
- Autoimmune hepatitis
- Cholestatic liver disease:
  - Primary sclerosing cholangitis
  - Primary biliary cirrhosis
- Metabolic disorders:
  - Wilson disease
  - Hemochromatosis
  - α-1-antitrypsin deficiency
- Vascular liver disease:
  - Budd-Chiari syndrome
  - Veno-occlusive disease
  - Chronic hepatic congestion due to right-sided heart failure
- Drugs toxicity:
  - Amiodarone (Cordarone)
  - Isoniazid (INH)
  - Methotrexate
- Miscellaneous:
  - Granulomatous liver disease (e.g., sarcoidosis)
- 10–15% of cases remain "cryptogenic"; no etiology can be Identified.

DIAGNOSIS

HISTORY
- Fatigue and weakness
- Anorexia, weight loss
- Abdominal pain
- Swelling of legs and/or abdomen
- Risk factors of liver disease:
  - Ethanol consumption
  - History of viral hepatitis
  - Transfusions
  - Illicit drugs use
- Jaundice
- Fever
- Family history of liver disease
- Risk factors for nonalcoholic steatohepatitis (obesity, diabetes type 2, and hyperlipidemia)
- Loss of libido
- Hemorrhage: Nose, alimentary tract

PHYSICAL EXAM
- Abdominal wall vascular collaterals (caput medusa)
- Ascites
- Asterixis
- Clubbing and hypertrophic osteoarthropathy
- Dupuytren's contracture
- Fetor hepaticus: A sweet, pungent breath odor
- Gynecomastia
- Hepatomegaly
- Jaundice
- Palmar erythema
- Vascular spiders (spider angiomata)
- Purpura
- White nails
- Splenomegaly
- Testicular atrophy
- Loss of male hair pattern
- Muscle wasting
- Anasarca
- Right-sided pleural effusion
- Neurological changes: Mental function

DIAGNOSTIC TESTS & INTERPRETATION
Lab
- CBC: Hemoglobin, leucocyte, and platelet count
- Coagulation tests: INR
- Serum biochemistry: Bilirubin, transaminase, alkaline phosphatase, γ-glutamyl-transpeptidase, albumin and globulin, immunoglobulins
- Serology: Hepatitis B antigen, anti-HCV, smooth muscle, mitochondrial and nuclear antibodies, anti-liver kidney membrane; anti soluble liver antigen, anti-pANCA
- Ceruloplasmin, urinary Cu (24-hour), slit-lamp: Corneal Cu deposits, ATP7B gene mutation
- Transferrin saturation, ferritin, HFE mutation
- Tumor markers: α-Fetoprotein
- Serum creatinine
- Uric acid, fasting glucose/insulin/triglycerides
- Electrolytes
- Urinary tests

Imaging
Abdominal US, CT, or MRI and MRCP

Diagnostic Procedures/Other
- Endoscopy of upper GI tract
- Doppler US
- Contrast-enhanced US
- Noninvasive tests: Fibroscan and Fibrotest
- Liver biopsy for selected patients (liver disease of unknown cause)

Pathological Findings
Regenerative nodules surrounded by fibrous bands. In selected cases, etiology can be detected (fatty changes, ground-glass hepatocytes, pas-positive globules, onion skin).

DIFFERENTIAL DIAGNOSIS
- Malignancy
- Cardiomyopathy
- Myxedema
- Lymphoma
- Protein losing enteropathy
- Glomerulopathy: Nephrotic syndrome

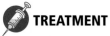 TREATMENT

MEDICATION
- Primary approaches focus on treatment of the underlying disease:
  - HCV-cirrhosis: PEGinterferon-based antiviral treatment or,
  - HBV: Long-term treatment with oral nucleoside/nucleotide analogues
  - Autoimmune hepatitis: Long-term treatment with corticosteroids-PBC:URSO
- Secondary approach: Pharmacotherapy focused on the mechanism of fibrogenesis; antifibrotic drugs
- Precautions and adverse reactions:
  - Decompensation due to interferon treatment
  - Viral resistance due to nucleotide/side analogues treatment
  - Steroid side effects

ADDITIONAL TREATMENT
General Measures
- Abstinence from alcohol
- Nonimmunized cirrhotic patients should receive vaccinations for hepatitis A and B, influenza, and pneumococcus.
- Cirrhotic patients with cholestatic conditions should be screened for osteoporosis.

SURGERY/OTHER PROCEDURES
- Transjugular intrahepatic portosystemic shunt (TIPS) for cirrhotic patients with refractory ascites or uncontrolled bleeding esophageal varices
- Liver transplantation for decompensated liver disease

 ONGOING CARE

FOLLOW-UP RECOMMENDATIONS
Patient Monitoring
Screening every 6 months for the development of hepatocellular carcinoma with α-fetoprotein level and an imaging study (ultrasound, MRI, or CT scan).

DIET
- No protein restriction.
- In patients with ascites sodium restriction who are obese and have NAFLD, modest and sustained weight reduction should be practiced.

PROGNOSIS
- Depends on both the etiology and treatment of the underlying cause.
- Once decompensation has occurred, mortality without transplant is as high as 85% over 5 years.
- Prediction of prognosis in patients with cirrhosis:
- The Child-Pugh-Turcotte (CPT) classification
- The Model for End Stage Liver Disease (MELD)

COMPLICATIONS
- Variceal bleeding
- Ascites
- Spontaneous bacterial peritonitis
- Hepatic encephalopathy
- Hepatorenal syndrome type 1 and 2
- Bacterial infections
- Hepatopulmonary syndrome
- Portopulmonary hypertension
- Cirrhotic cardiomyopathy
- Hepatocellular carcinoma
- Death

ADDITIONAL READING

- Groszmann RJ, et al. Portal hypertension. From bedside to bench. *J Clin Gastroenterol.* 2005; 39(suppl 2):S125–30.
- Schiff ER, et al., eds. *Schiff's Diseases of the Liver*, 9th ed. Philadelphia, PA: Lippincott, Williams & Wilkins, 2003.
- Schuppan D, et al. Liver cirrhosis. *Lancet.* 2008;371: 838–51.
- Sherlock S, et al, eds. *Diseases of the Liver and Biliary System*, 11th ed. Oxford, UK, and Malden, MA: Blackwell Science, 2002.

CODES

ICD9
- 571.2 Alcoholic cirrhosis of liver
- 571.5 Cirrhosis of liver without mention of alcohol
- 571.8 Other chronic nonalcoholic liver disease

CLINICAL PEARLS
- Cirrhosis regression or even reversal is possible in selected cases.
- Liver transplantation remains the only curative option for a selected group of patients, once decompensation has occurred.
- Cirrhosis is a major risk factor for hepatocellular carcinoma.

CLOSTRIDIUM DIFFICILE

Negia E. Lalane

 BASICS

DESCRIPTION
- Described initially in the 1950s, pseudomembranous colitis was conferred to *Staphylococcus aureus* or *Candida alabamans*. It was not until 1974 when *Clostridium difficile* (C Diff) was attributed to be the causative agent of antibiotic-associated diarrhea.
- *C. difficile* causes antibiotic-associated diarrhea, pseudomembranous colitis, toxic membranous colitis, sepsis, and even death.
- It is one of the most common nosocomial infections and a significant cause of morbidity and mortality in the elderly population.
- It is also seen in peripartum women, children.
- Prevalence and virulence have increased in the past years due to mutations that confer antibiotic resistance, being responsible for several outbreaks in health care centers throughout the world.

EPIDEMIOLOGY
Incidence
- C Diff incidence has experienced dramatic increase in the last year, with outbreaks in countries all over the world, such as Canada, UK, and the U.S., mostly due to a hypervirulent strain (BI/NAP1/027).
- From 1987–1998 the reported cases of C Diff was 12.2 cases per 10,000 patient/days. Data from the CDC reported that, compared with 1996, in 2003 CDI increased almost 2-fold from 31/100,000 to 61/100,000 population.
- The minimum annual incidence of community-associated CDI was estimated to be 7.6 cases/100,000 population.

Prevalence
- *C. difficile* has been implicated as the causative organism in 10–25% of patients with antibiotic-associated diarrhea, 50–75% of those with antibiotic-associated colitis, and 90–100% of those with antibiotic-associated pseudomembranous colitis.
- Mortality of *C. difficile*-associated disease (CDAD) ranges from 6–30% when pseudomembranous colitis is shown to be present.
- Recent studies have suggested that mortality has been highest in persons >65 years.

RISK FACTORS
- Antibiotic use is one of the main risk factors.
- Frequently associated are clindamycin, fluoroquinolones, penicillins (broad-spectrum), cephalosporins (broad-spectrum)
- Occasionally associated: Macrolides, TMTSMX.
- Rarely associated: Aminoglycosides, tetracycline, chloramphenicol, metronidazole, vancomycin
- Other risk factors are gastric acid suppression, enteral feeding, GI surgery, cancer chemotherapy, and hematopoietic stem cell transplantation.

GENERAL PREVENTION
Judicious use of antibiotics, isolation of the patient, use of contact precautions such as gloves, gowns, soap and water (alcohol-based lotions are not that effective against spore-forming bacteria), and the use hypochlorite-based disinfectant for cleaning purposes.

PATHOPHYSIOLOGY
- 2 events take place in the development of C Diff: Colonization of the intestinal tract, which occurs via the fecal-oral route, and the disruption of normal intestinal flora due to antimicrobial therapy.
- *C. difficile* produces two potent exotoxins, toxin A (enterotoxin) and toxin B (cytotoxin). Toxin A causes intestinal inflammation and fluid secretion; the role of toxin B not quite understood, since there is controversy regarding the pathogenicity of it.

ETIOLOGY
C. difficile is an anaerobic spore-forming gram-positive bacillus; it is a commensal of the human intestines.

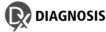 **DIAGNOSIS**

HISTORY
Diarrhea, recent antibiotic use, recent hospitalizations. Nevertheless, high suspicion for community acquired C Diff infection should be held on low-risk populations such as peripartum women, children, and people with no recent antibiotic exposure.

PHYSICAL EXAM
- Profuse watery, foul-smelling diarrhea, abdominal pain, fever (low grade), leukocytosis
- In cases of fulminant colitis, the abdominal pain becomes more severe, diffuse, with abdominal distention, hypovolemia, lactic acidosis, and marked leukocytosis (up to 40,000 WBC).
- Rare cases of appendicitis, cellulites, and small bowel involvement have been described in the literature.

DIAGNOSTIC TESTS & INTERPRETATION
Lab
Initial lab tests
- The tissue culture cytotoxic assay is the gold standard diagnostic test but is limited by slow turnaround time (at least 48 hours), work intensity, and cost (sensitivity 94–100%).
- The enzyme immunoassay for detection of toxins A and B is the most commonly used test because of its ease of use and rapidity. This test is highly specific, it has a lower sensitivity (70–87%) than the cytotoxic assay. Testing 3 stool specimens can increase the yield by 10% or more.
- In 2009, the FDA approved the Xpert *C. difficile* test (Cepheid),

Diagnostic Procedures/Other
- CT scan. Patients with pseudomembranous colitis show thickening of the colonic wall.
- Colonoscopy can show ulceration in the colonic mucosa, pseudomembranes, which are yellow plaques, bowel wall edema, erythema

DIFFERENTIAL DIAGNOSIS
- Infectious diarrhea: *E. coli, Salmonella, Shigella, S. aureus*
- Noninfectious diarrhea: Lactose intolerance, IBS

TREATMENT

- First, stop the offending agent.
- Do not use antimotility agents, as there is evidence that it may cause toxic megacolon.
- Do not treat carriers without any symptoms.

MEDICATION
First Line
Metronidazole 500 mg q6–8h hours for 7–10 days. If patient cannot tolerate PO, use IV metronidazole. Do not use if patient is pregnant or allergic.

Second Line
PO vancomycin 125 mg q6h.

ADDITIONAL TREATMENT
General Measures
- In between 8–50% of patients CDAD recurs.
- The recommended treatment for a 1st recurrence is a 2nd course of the initial therapy with either metronidazole or vancomycin.
- Probiotics (most commonly *Lactobacillus* spp. or *Saccharomyces boulardii*) as adjuvant treatment
- Stool transplants from a healthy donor through colonoscopy have been reported as effective in refractory cases.
- Human IV immunoglobulin containing the toxoid for toxin A and B. (There is lack of data to fully support this.)

SURGERY/OTHER PROCEDURES
Surgery is indicated in cases of toxic megacolon, or when patients have perforation, massive hemorrhage, worsening signs of toxicity.

 ONGOING CARE

COMPLICATIONS
- Pseudomembranous colitis
- Toxic megacolon
- Perforations of the colon
- Sepsis
- Death (rarely)

ADDITIONAL READING

- Bulusu M, et al. Leukocytosis as a harbinger and surrogate marker of Clostridium difficile infection in hospitalized patients with diarrhea. *Am J Gastroenterol*. 2000;95:3137.
- Carignan A, et al. Risk of Clostridium difficile infection after perioperative antibacterial prophylaxis before and during an outbreak of infection due to a hypervirulent strain. *Clin Infect Dis*. 2008;46:1838.
- Gould CV, McDonald LC. Bench-to-bedside review: Clostridium difficile colitis. Prevention and Response Branch, Division of Healthcare Quality Promotion, Centers for Disease Control and Prevention, Clifton Road NE, Atlanta, GA 30333, USA. *Critical Care*. 2008;12:203 (doi:10.1186/cc6207).
- CDC. Guidelines for environmental infection control in health-care facilities. *MMWR. Morb Mortal Wkly Rep*. 2003;52(RR10):1–42. Also available at: http://www.cdc.gov/ncidod/hip/enviro/guide.htm
- CDC. Severe Clostridium difficile-associated disease in populations previously at low risk: Four states, 2005. *MMWR Morb Mortal Wkly Rep*. 2005;54: 1201–5.

- Huang H, et al. Comparison of a commercial multiplex real-time PCR to the cell cytotoxicity neutralization assay for diagnosis of clostridium difficile infections. *J Clin Microbiol*. 2009;47:3729.
- McDonald LC, et al. Clostridium difficile infection in patients discharged from US short-stay hospitals, 1996–2003. *Emerg Infect Dis*. 2006;12:409–15.
- Rubin MS, et al. Severe Clostridium difficile colitis. *Dis Colon Rectum*. 1995;38:350.
- Saima A, et al. Treatment of Clostridium difficile-associated disease: Old therapies and new strategies. *Lancet Infect Dis*. 2005;5:549–57.
- Thomas C, et al. Antibiotics and hospital-acquired Clostridium difficile-associated diarrhoea: a systematic review. *J Antimicrob Chemother*. 2003; 51:1339.
- Wanahita A, et al. Clostridium difficile infection in patients with unexplained leukocytosis. *Am J Med*. 2003;115:543.
- Wistrom J, et al. Frequency of antibiotic-associated diarrhoea in 2462 antibiotic-treated hospitalized patients: a prospective study. *J Antimicrob Chemother*. 2001;47:43.
- Zar FA, et al. A comparison of vancomycin and metronidazole for the treatment of Clostridium difficile-associated diarrhea, stratified by disease severity. *Clin Infect Dis*. 2007;45:302–7.

 CODES

ICD9
- 008.45 Intestinal infection due to clostridium difficile
- 009.0 Infectious colitis, enteritis, and gastroenteritis
- 787.91 Diarrhea

COAGULOPATHY

Paul Basciano
Maria T. DeSancho

 BASICS

DESCRIPTION
- Inability of the blood to coagulate normally as a result of depletion, dilution, or inactivation of circulating clotting factors.
- System(s) affected: Hematologic

EPIDEMIOLOGY
Incidence
- Up to 2/3 of critically ill patients show laboratory indicators of coagulopathy (1).
- ~15% of general ICU patients have clinical evidence of coagulopathy (1).

Prevalence
- 45% of trauma patients die from exsanguination.
- 20% in neurosurgical ICU
- 30% in severe thermal injuries
- 20–50% in cardiothoracic surgical patients

RISK FACTORS
- Medications, especially antiplatelet agents, mainly clopidogrel and IIb/IIIa antagonists
- Antithrombotics: Vitamin K antagonists (VKAs), unfractionated heparin, low-molecular-weight heparin, pentasaccharides, and direct thrombin inhibitors
- Thrombolytic therapy
- Renal and liver dysfunction
- Peptic ulcer
- Malignancy
- Sepsis
- Recent complex or emergent surgery

Genetics
- Factor V Leiden mutation (Arg506Gln) may decrease mortality in ARDS.
- TLR2, OMIM 603028: Reduction of bleeding after cardiac surgery
- Tumor necrosis factor beta (TNF-β) development of posttraumatic sepsis
- Plasminogen activator inhibitor 1 (PAI-1) 4G/4G associated with poor survival rate after severe trauma

PATHOPHYSIOLOGY
- Primary hemostasis:
  - Quantitative or qualitative disorders of platelets and/or von Willebrand factor (vWF) can cause failure of platelet adhesion, aggregation, activation, cross-linking, and/or activation of secondary hemostasis.
- Secondary hemostasis:
  - Abnormalities of coagulation factors caused by quantitative, qualitative deficiencies, acquired inhibitors that cause delayed or abnormal fibrin clot formation
- Tertiary hemostasis:
  - Disorders of Factor XIII (hereditary and most commonly acquired) that impair cross-links in fibrin to stabilize clots
- Fibrinolytic system:
  - Abnormalities may cause accelerated degradation of fibrin clots.

ETIOLOGY
- Genetic
- Acquired:
  - Platelets: Medications, consumption, underproduction, metabolic (uremia)
  - Coagulation factors: Deficiencies, increased consumption, abnormal synthesis, metabolic causes, toxins/venoms

COMMONLY ASSOCIATED CONDITIONS
- Infection/sepsis
- Massive thrombosis (consumption)
- Malignancy
- Trauma
- Postsurgical (complex or emergent)
- Cirrhosis, liver dysfunction
- Uremia
- Hypocalcemia
- Hypothermia
- Acidemia
- Malabsorptive disorders
- Complications of pregnancy (abruptio, severe preeclampsia)
- Autoimmune disorders (systemic lupus erythematosus, thrombotic thrombocytopenic purpura)
- Vascular diversions/prostheses:
  - Cardiopulmonary bypass
  - ECMO
  - LVAD
  - Dilutional coagulopathy
  - Hemodilution
  - Use of fractionated blood products
  - DIC

DIAGNOSIS

HISTORY
- Personal or family history of excessive bleeding diathesis:
  - Postprocedural, including minor procedures
  - Menorrhagia
  - Intra- or postpartum
  - Spontaneous epistaxis, other mucosal bleeding, hematomas
- Medication use:
  - ASA, other NSAIDs
  - Clopidogrel, ticlopidine, dipyridamole, prasugrel, cangrelor, ticagrelor
  - IIB/IIIA inhibitors, thrombolytics
  - Vitamin K antagonists: Warfarin
  - Antibiotics
  - Chemotherapy
  - Angiogenesis inhibitors
  - Oral direct thrombin inhibitor (dabigatran)
  - Oral direct Xa inhibitor (rivaroxaban)
- Recent/ongoing infection, complications of pregnancy, malignancy, surgery
- Dietary habits, intestinal/malabsorptive disorders
- Recent animal or insect bites
- Concerning symptoms:
  - Headache
  - Back or abdominal pain (retroperitoneal
  - bleed)
  - Throat pain (retropharyngeal bleed in hemophiliacs)
  - Focal muscular pain

PHYSICAL EXAM
- Gross evidence of bleeding
- Petechiae, purpura, ecchymoses
- Hemorrhagic bullae
- Acral cyanosis
- Lymph node and spleen examination

DIAGNOSTIC TESTS & INTERPRETATION
Lab
- CBC, peripheral blood smear, reticulocyte count:
  - Quantification and qualitative appearance of platelets
  - Evidence of intravascular hemolysis (RBC fragments)
- PT and aPTT:
  - Abnormalities in PT or APTT do not necessarily mean an increased risk of bleeding.
- PT and aPTT mixing studies:
  - Perform only when initial PT or aPTT is abnormal.
  - Abnormalities due to factor deficiency correct when patient plasma is mixed with normal plasma.
  - Abnormalities due to factor inhibitors do not correct upon mixing studies.
- Measurement of coagulation factor levels:
  - Specific combinations of factor deficiencies can suggest underlying etiology:
    - Warfarin use or vitamin K deficiency: FII, FVII, FIX, FX
    - Hepatic dysfunction: FII, FVII, FIX, FX, FV
    - DIC/consumption: FII, FVII, FIX, FX, FV, FVIII (FVIII may be normal in early DIC)
- Quantitative fibrinogen levels
- Thrombin time and reptilase time (RT):
  - Evaluate for heparin effect (abnormal TT, normal RT)
  - Detection of dysfibrinogenemias (TT and RT both abnormal)
- D-dimer and fibrin split products (elevated in renal and liver insufficiency)
- Platelet function assays (PFA100) to screen for thrombocytopathies
- Platelet aggregation studies (gold standard for diagnosis of thrombocytopathies):
  - Bleeding times are no longer recommended due to poor reproducibility.
- vWF Antigen (quantitative), vWF activity: Ristocetin cofactor (qualitative), vWF multimers
- Euglobulin clot lysis time:
  - Measure of fibrinolytic system activity
- Urea clot solubility
  - Assesses integrity of FXIII activity

Imaging
Based on clinical assessment of bleeding to monitor size/extent of hematomas, as well as angiography to evaluate for culprit vessels for intervention

Diagnostic Procedures/Other
Interventions to control bleeding: Open surgical, endoscopies, or embolizations may be employed for large-vessel bleeding.

Pathological Findings
Depends on the etiology of bleeding

DIFFERENTIAL DIAGNOSIS
Diverse and includes infection, metabolic or autoimmune disorders, massive transfusion, malignancy, postsurgical and trauma-associated bleeding

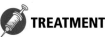 TREATMENT

MEDICATION
Blood components:
- Packed red blood cells (RBC):
  - Transfusion to a Hct of 10 g/dL is recommended in severe bleeding to enhance rheostatic support of platelets (1)[C].
- Platelets:
  - If platelet count is <10,000 or when platelet is <50,000 and bleeding
- Fresh frozen plasma:
  - For replacement of multiple factor efficiencies with bleeding; e.g., DIC (2)[C]
  - For coagulopathy and bleeding associated with liver disease (2)[C]
  - For reversal of VKA with significant bleeding and only in conjunction with IV vitamin K (2)[C]
  - Dose: 10–20 mL/kg
- Cryoprecipitate: Contains concentrated fibrinogen, FVIII, FXIII, vWF and fibronectin:
  - For replacement of fibrinogen in hypo- or dysfibrinogenemias; contains 200 mg/bag
  - For replacement of FXIII; 1 bag/10 kg once
  - For vWD if bleeding and no other source available; 1 bag/10 kg q6–12h
- Factor concentrates:
  - Used to replace isolated deficiencies of FVIII, FIX, FXIII, and vWF
  - Multiple sources and types available
- Prothrombin complexes:
  - Mainly for hemophiliacs with known inhibitors
  - For reversal of warfarin
  - Can induce DIC
- Recombinant factor VIIa (NovoSeven):
  - Approved for use in hemophiliacs with known inhibitors and significant bleeding (5)[A]
  - Unlabeled uses: Warfarin toxicity, intracerebral bleeding, bleeding in cardiothoracic surgery, and other major and/or uncontrolled bleeds
  - Increased risk of arterial thrombosis (3)

First Line
- Vitamin K (phytodione):
  - Used for reversal of warfarin and for suspected vitamin K deficiency
  - Each route of administration has potential pitfalls:
    ○ Oral: Erratic absorption, especially in malabsorptive state
    ○ Subcutaneous (least reliable) not recommended
    ○ IV may cause severe anaphylactic-type reactions; slow IV infusions of up to 5 mg are used

- DDAVP (desmopressin):
  - Used in type 1 vWD to induce release of vWF stores, uremic patients with bleeding and mild hemophilia A
  - Tachyphylaxis develops with repeated use
  - May induce hyponatremia; fluid intake should be controlled and electrolytes monitored carefully.
  - Dose: 0.3 mcg/kg IV infusion (20–30 minutes)
- Aminocaproic acid:
  - Inhibit fibrinolysis to control mucocutaneous bleeding
  - Contraindicated in upper genitourinary bleeding due to risk of urinary obstruction
  - 4–5 g IV or PO over 1 hour, followed by 1 g qh. up to 30 g

Second Line
Conjugated estrogens

ADDITIONAL TREATMENT
General Measures
- Avoid medications that can worsen bleeding.
- Avoid unnecessary invasive procedures.

Issues for Referral
- Inpatient consultation with a hematologist should be obtained for complex or refractory bleeding cases.
- Outpatient follow-up with hematologist recommended for:
  - Congenital disorders of platelets
  - Hemophilia
  - Acquired inhibitors
- Referral for genetic counseling for hemophiliacs and other inherited coagulopathies

IN-PATIENT CONSIDERATIONS
Initial Stabilization
Early control of bleeding; transfusion support with FFP, cryoprecipitate, platelets and RBC as needed

 ONGOING CARE

FOLLOW-UP RECOMMENDATIONS
Patient Monitoring
Depends on underlying etiology of coagulopathy

DIET
Encourage well-balanced diet unless restrictions are needed for warfarin therapy.

PATIENT EDUCATION
- Avoidance of NSAIDs and antithrombotics if continued coagulopathy
- Nutritional education for those on warfarin or with vitamin K deficiency
- Self-monitoring for overt bleeding and microvascular bleeding (purpura)
- Avoidance of high-impact activities if coagulopathy continues; fall prevention

PROGNOSIS
Varies widely depending on type, severity, and reversibility of underlying disorder

COMPLICATIONS
- Multisystem involvement may be seen in DIC, and may be catastrophic.
- Hematomas may lead to organ compromise through direct mass-effect or via compromise of blood supply.

REFERENCES
1. Chakraverty R, et al. The incidence and cause of coagulopathies in an intensive care population. *Br J Haem*. 1996;93:460–3.
2. Lauzier F, et al. Fresh frozen plasma transfusion in critically patients. *Crit Care Med*. 2007;35: 1655–59.
3. Levi M, et al. Safety of recombinant activated factor VII in randomized clinical trials. *N Engl J Med* 2010;363:1791–1800.

ADDITIONAL READING
- Drews RE. Critical issues in hematology: anemia, thrombocytopenia, coagulopathy, and blood product transfusions in critically ill patients. *Clin Chest Med*. 2003;24:607–22.

CODES

ICD9
- 286.9 Other and unspecified coagulation defects
- 289.81 Primary hypercoagulable state

CLINICAL PEARLS
- Coagulopathic disorders are common in ICU patients and are associated with significant morbidity.
- Treatment of the underlying cause and supportive transfusions of plasma, cryoprecipitate, platelets, and RBC are often required.

C

COAGULOPATHY, DISSEMINATED INTRAVASCULAR (DIC)

Anahita Dabo-Trubelja
Stephen M. Pastores

 BASICS

DESCRIPTION
- Syndrome resulting in both thrombosis and hemorrhage
- Propensity for activation of blood coagulation, fibrin deposition, and vasoocclusion, which may lead to ischemia and multisystem organ failure
- System affected: Hematologic

EPIDEMIOLOGY
Incidence
- Most complex coagulation disorder in intensive care
- Overall incidence 10–15%

Prevalence
- May be as high as 22% in obstetric disorders
- 50% in gram-negative sepsis
- 70% in severe trauma
- 15% in malignancy
- 1% with large aortic aneurysm

RISK FACTORS
- Sepsis
- Trauma
- Malignancy
- Obstetrical emergencies
- Vascular disorders: Giant hemangiomas, large aortic aneurysms

GENERAL PREVENTION
Prompt treatment of conditions known to lead to DIC

PATHOPHYSIOLOGY
- Generalized activation of the coagulation cascade is initiated by the increased presence of tissue factor resulting from enhanced expression by inflammatory cells, vascular epithelial injury, and release of thromboplastins into the systemic circulation.
- Tissue factor-mediated generation of thrombin, along with impairment of normal anticoagulant pathways (decreased antithrombin II, protein C, and tissue factor pathway inhibitor) results in formation of fibrin and thrombosis of small and midsize vessels.
- Impaired fibrinolysis results from increased production of plasminogen-activator inhibitor (PAI-1) and leads to inadequate removal of fibrin.

ETIOLOGY
Acquired disorder resulting from an underlying condition that leads to increased production of thrombin and widespread activation of the coagulation cascade, as well as platelet and coagulation factor consumption that can result in hemorrhagic complications (1).

COMMONLY ASSOCIATED CONDITIONS
- Sepsis
- Malignancy
- Brain injury
- Trauma
- Burn and crush injuries
- Obstetric complications
- Vascular disorders: Giant hemangiomas, large aortic aneurysms
- Snake bites

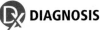 **DIAGNOSIS**

HISTORY
- Varies depending on underlying predisposing clinical disorder
- Bleeding occurs in about 60% of patients.
- May be acute or chronic

PHYSICAL EXAM
- Signs of venous and arterial thromboses: Venous limb gangrene, deep venous thrombosis, pulmonary embolism, transient ischemic attack
- Signs of bleeding: Petechiae, ecchymoses, diffuse oozing of blood from line sites, surgical wounds, mucosal surfaces lung, and GI tract
- Mental status changes, coma or focal neurologic deficits in case of CNS bleeding
- Jaundice

DIAGNOSTIC TESTS & INTERPRETATION
Lab
Initial lab tests (2)
- Thrombocytopenia: $<100,000/mm^3$ or rapid drop in platelet count
- Prolongation of PT and aPTT
- Elevated levels of fibrin degradation products and D-dimer
- Decreased levels of fibrinogen, antithrombin III, protein C, and protein S
- Decreased levels of factors V, VII, and VIII

Follow-Up & Special Considerations
- Hemolysis with evidence of schistocytes on peripheral blood smear
- Renal failure is common due to ischemia of the renal parenchyma.

Imaging
Appropriate venous and arterial imaging studies to search for thrombus (US, echocardiography, CT, MRI)

Pathological Findings
Related to venous and arterial thromboses

DIFFERENTIAL DIAGNOSIS
- Sepsis
- Bone marrow disease
- Primary fibrinolysis
- HELLP syndrome (hemolysis with microangiopathic anemia, elevated liver enzymes, and low platelets in pregnancy)
- HIT (heparin-induced thrombocytopenia)
- Liver disease
- TTP (thrombotic thrombocytopenic purpura)
- Chemotherapy-induced hypoplasia
- Massive transfusions
- Heparin therapy

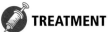

TREATMENT

MEDICATION
First Line
Specific and aggressive treatment of the underlying disorder

Second Line
- Unfractionated heparin: 300–500 units/kg/hr for patients with catastrophic thromboembolism or purpura fulminans (3)
- Antithrombin III and protein C concentrates have been used with variable success.
- Recombinant activated factor VII for patients who are bleeding and not responsive to other treatments.

ADDITIONAL TREATMENT
General Measures
Supportive therapy with platelets, fresh frozen plasma and cryoprecipitate for active bleeding or prior to invasive procedures.

Issues for Referral
- Complex cases of DIC should be referred to a hematology consultant.
- Limb-threatening thrombosis should prompt vascular surgery consultation.

IN-PATIENT CONSIDERATIONS
Initial Stabilization
- Initial diagnosis and management require intensive care admission.
- Prompt administration of IV antibiotics and source control in patients with sepsis
- Secure ABC and hemorrhage control in trauma patients

 ONGOING CARE

FOLLOW-UP RECOMMENDATIONS
- Chronic DIC: May require long-term anticoagulation
- Outpatient clinic follow-up while on anticoagulation

Patient Monitoring
- Monitor platelet count, fibrinogen level and coagulation tests (PT, INR, aPTT) during treatment.
- Monitor coagulation tests at periodic intervals while on anticoagulation.
- Dose adjustments made depending on clinical signs and coagulation test results.

PROGNOSIS
- Severity of underlying condition and intensity of coagulation disorder contributes to morbidity and mortality.
- Generally poor with multisystem organ failure.

COMPLICATIONS
- Patients with mild DIC may experience bleeding following surgery or chemotherapy.
- Cerebrovascular accident (stroke or bleeding)
- Acute renal failure
- Pulmonary hemorrhage
- GI bleeding

REFERENCES

1. Bick RL. Disseminated intravascular coagulation, current concepts of etiology, pathophysiology, diagnosis, and treatment. *Hematol Oncol Clin N Am*. 2003;17:149–76.
2. DeLoughery TG. Critical care clotting catastrophes. *Crit Care Clin*. 2005;21(3): 531–62.
3. Levi M. Disseminated intravascular coagulation. *Crit Care Med*. 2007;35(9):2191–5.

ADDITIONAL READING
- Franchini M, Manzato F. Update on the treatment of disseminated intravascular coagulation. *Hematology*. 2004;9:81–85.

 CODES

ICD9
286.6 Defibrination syndrome

CLINICAL PEARLS
- DIC is an acquired syndrome secondary to an underlying disorder that can cause both thrombosis and bleeding.
- Pathophysiology involves widespread activation of coagulation cascade, impaired fibrinolysis, and consumption of coagulation factors and platelets.
- Laboratory criteria include thrombocytopenia, prolonged PT and aPTT, decreased fibrinogen, and elevated D-dimer and fibrin degradation products.
- Primary treatment is directed to the underlying condition causing the DIC, transfusion of blood products when active bleeding occurs, and use of heparin for catastrophic thromboembolism or purpura fulminans.

COLONIC PSEUDO-OBSTRUCTION (OGILVIE SYNDROME)
Shaul Lev

 BASICS

DESCRIPTION
Functional dilatation of the colon in the absence of true mechanical bowel obstruction or colonic disease.

RISK FACTORS
- Anticholinergic or opiates use
- Old age
- Critically ill patients

PATHOPHYSIOLOGY
Unknown disturbance to the autonomic innervation of the colon

COMMONLY ASSOCIATED CONDITIONS
- Trauma
- Infection
- Myocardial infarction
- Heart failure
- Parkinson disease
- Spinal cord injury
- Multiple sclerosis
- Alzheimer disease
- Orthopedic surgery, neurosurgery
- Potassium depletion

 DIAGNOSIS

- Distended abdomen
- Dilatation of cecum or hemicolon
- Constipation or diarrhea
- Association with severe illness
- Association with electrolytes imbalance
- Association with medications

DIAGNOSTIC TESTS & INTERPRETATION
Lab
Hypokalemia, hypocalcemia, and hypomagnesemia should be looked for and corrected.

Imaging
Initial approach
Radiographs reveal a dilated colon from the cecum to the splenic flexure, and occasionally to the rectum with well-defined septa and haustral markings and very little fluid, making air–fluid levels uncommon.

Follow-Up & Special Considerations
Supportive care and removal of possible precipitants (electrolytes, opiates, and anticholinergics)

DIFFERENTIAL DIAGNOSIS
- Toxic megacolon
- Mechanical obstruction

 TREATMENT

ADDITIONAL TREATMENT
General Measures
- Treat underlying disease.
- Oral intake should be avoided.
- Correct electrolyte imbalances.
- Insert a nasogastric tube allow drainage.
- Insert a rectal tube and attach to gravity drainage.
- Discontinue opiates, sedatives, anticholinergic drugs, calcium channel blockers.
- Avoid oral laxatives.
- 1–2 mg IV neostigmine as a single dose in patients at risk for perforation:
  - No improvement in 24 hours
  - Cecal dilation >12 cm

ALERT
Done with careful cardiac monitoring (bradycardia), colonoscopic decompression in patients who fail or who have contraindications to neostigmine

SURGERY/OTHER PROCEDURES
Tube cecostomy should be done in patients who fail conservative treatment.

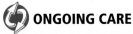 **ONGOING CARE**

FOLLOW-UP RECOMMENDATIONS
- Patients should get serial physical exams and plain abdominal radiographs (assess cecal size).
- Watch for abdominal tenderness.

PROGNOSIS
Most cases are caused by medications or underling condition, and patient symptoms improve with decompression. Prognosis related to underling condition.

COMPLICATIONS
- Peritonitis due to colonic perforation.
- Colonic ischemia

ADDITIONAL READING
- Eisen GM, et al. Acute colonic pseudo-obstruction. *Gastrointest Endosc.* 2002;56:789.
- Saunders MD, et al. Acute colonic pseudo-obstruction. *Best Pract Res Clin Gastroenterol.* 2007;671–87.

 CODES

ICD9
- 560.89 Other specified intestinal obstruction
- 560.9 Unspecified intestinal obstruction
- 564.7 Megacolon, other than hirschsprung's

CLINICAL PEARLS
- For acute colonic distension think:
  – Toxic megacolon infection
  – Mechanical obstruction
  – Acute colonic pseudo-obstruction
- Use neostigmine when indicated! It is effective even in lower doses than reported (0.75 mg).
- Monitor closely patients on neostigmine treatment; prepare atropine.

C

COMA

Lewis A. Eisen

 BASICS

DESCRIPTION
- Unresponsiveness, unarousable to any stimulus, at least some brainstem reflexes intact
- System affected: Neurologic

EPIDEMIOLOGY

Incidence
In cardiac arrest survivors, 80–90% become comatose at least temporarily (1).

Prevalence
- 15–20% of ventilated patients are comatose (2,3).
- 16% of septic patients are comatose (4).

RISK FACTORS
- Toxic or metabolic disturbance
- Structural CNS lesions
- Head trauma

Genetics
No genetic predilection for ICU coma

GENERAL PREVENTION
Avoid toxins, maintain normal metabolic profile.

PATHOPHYSIOLOGY
- Structural lesions, toxins, or metabolic insults may affect the reticular activating system in upper brainstem.
- Bilateral cortical insults may also produce coma.
- Insults impair oxygen delivery or impair neuronal excitation in brain.

ETIOLOGY
- Drugs
- Trauma
- Primary CNS disease
- Toxins
- Metabolic
- Infectious
- Diffuse ischemia
- Hypothyroidism

COMMONLY ASSOCIATED CONDITIONS
- Hepatic failure
- Renal failure
- Sepsis
- Drug or toxin ingestion
- Primary cerebral disorders
- Period of hypoxia

DIAGNOSIS

HISTORY
- Information from family or friends may provide clues to etiology.
- Time course of loss of consciousness (abrupt or gradual)
- History of trauma?
- Were focal signs or seizures present?
- Drug or toxin ingestion?
- Signs of recent infection?

PHYSICAL EXAM
- Vital signs, including temperature and pulse oximetry
- Inspection (signs of trauma, evidence of vasculitis, evidence of drug use)
- Level of consciousness
- Brainstem reflexes
- Pupillary size, position, and responsiveness
- Motor responses (posturing, asymmetry on exam implies structural cause)
- Breathing pattern (Cheyne-Stokes, apneustic)
- Funduscopic exam (papilledema, subhyaloid hemorrhage seen in subarachnoid hemorrhage)
- Glasgow Coma Scale 3–15 (add eyes, verbal, motor scores):
  - Eyes:
    - 1: Does not open eyes
    - 2: Opens eyes to painful stimulus
    - 3: Opens eyes to voice
    - 4: Opens eyes spontaneously
  - Verbal:
    - 1: No sounds
    - 2: Incomprehensible sounds
    - 3: Inappropriate words
    - 4: Confused, disoriented
    - 5: Oriented, converses normally
  - Motor:
    - 1: No movement
    - 2: Extension to painful stimulus
    - 3: Flexion to painful stimulus
    - 4: Withdraws to painful stimulus
    - 5: Localizes to painful stimulus
    - 6: Obeys commands

DIAGNOSTIC TESTS & INTERPRETATION

Lab

Initial lab tests
- Serum electrolytes (especially Na+), glucose, urea, creatinine
- ABG
- Drug screens
- Adrenal and thyroid function

Follow-Up & Special Considerations
- Ammonia level if liver disease, hereditary or secondary hyperammonemia is suspected
- Infectious workup, including blood cultures if infection is suspected
- Carboxyhemoglobin if possible exposure

Imaging

Initial approach
Noncontrast CT scan

Follow-Up & Special Considerations
MRI may be needed if brainstem lesion is suspected.

Diagnostic Procedures/Other
- EEG to rule out nonconvulsive status epilepticus (8% of comatose patients with no clinical seizures have nonconvulsive status epilepticus on EEG) (5)[B]
- Lumbar puncture after imaging if cause of coma is unclear or meningitis/encephalitis suspected

Pathological Findings
Depends on underlying cause

DIFFERENTIAL DIAGNOSIS
- Brain death (absence of cortical and brainstem response)
- Minimally conscious state (occasional purposeful responses)
- Pontine lesion (locked-in syndrome): Voluntary blinking will remain intact
- Akinetic mutism (injury to premotor cortex, inability to initiate movements): Patient will track with the eyes
- Vegetative state: Patient lacks consciousness; has no awareness of self or environment
- Psychogenic coma: Sometimes resists passive movements, may demonstrate pseudoseizures as well

C

TREATMENT

MEDICATION

First Line
- 25 g 50% dextrose IV if cause of coma is unknown (2.5 mg/kg of 10% dextrose in children)
- Thiamine if alcohol ingestion is possible.

Second Line
- Naloxone 0.4–2 mg IV if opiate ingestion is suspected (0.1 mg/kg for child <5 years or <20 kg)
- Flumazenil 0.2 mg IV if acute benzodiazepine ingestion suspected (0.01 mg/kg in child)
- Phenytoin or fosphenytoin 15–20 mg/kg IV if seizures suspected
- Vancomycin 2 mg/kg/day IV, ceftriaxone 2 g IV q12h, acyclovir 10 mg/kg IV q8h if meningitis or encephalitis suspected
- For children, vancomycin IV 60 mg/kg/day in 4 divided doses, ceftriaxone IV 100 mg/kg/d), acyclovir 20 mg/kg/dose q8h IV)
- Mannitol 1 g/kg IV if signs of herniation present

ADDITIONAL TREATMENT

General Measures
- Intubation if airway protection compromised
- Definitive treatment depends on diagnosis.
- Control fluid and electrolyte balance.
- Control blood pressure.
- Avoid any sedating medicines if possible.
- Treat hyperthermia as it can exacerbate brain damage.

Issues for Referral
- Consider ID consult for undiagnosed meningitis or encephalitis.
- Neurosurgical consult for brain lesion, hemorrhage, or increased intracranial pressure
- Neurology consult for intractable seizures, complex or inconsistent neurologic exam, focal infarct or hemorrhage, prognosis after prolonged coma:
  – Poison control consult if toxicologic cause
  – Palliative care consult if consistent with goals of care after discussion of prognosis with surrogate

Additional Therapies
- Passive range of motion or splinting may be required to prevent contractures.
- Thromboembolic prophylaxis

COMPLEMENTARY & ALTERNATIVE THERAPIES
None proved

SURGERY/OTHER PROCEDURES
CSF drainage or hemicraniectomy may be required for increased intracranial pressure

IN-PATIENT CONSIDERATIONS

Initial Stabilization
- Focus on ABCs
- Stabilize cervical spine if history unclear or trauma suspected

Admission Criteria
Patients with new coma will generally require ICU monitoring.

IV Fluids
- Keep patient euvolemic.
- Avoid hypotonic fluids if patient is at risk for brain edema.

Nursing
- Eye care to prevent corneal damage
- Decubitus ulcer prevention

Discharge Criteria
Once medically stable, with stable long-term airway and feeding plans, patient should be discharged to rehab facility.

ONGOING CARE

FOLLOW-UP RECOMMENDATIONS
Frequent neurological exams

Patient Monitoring
- Tracheotomy care
- Thromboembolic prophylaxis
- Stasis ulcer prevention
- Eye care to prevent corneal ulceration

DIET
Feeding through gastric tube

PATIENT EDUCATION
Family should be informed about prognosis and potential complications.

PROGNOSIS
Depends on etiology of coma; hypoxic encephalopathy has worse prognosis than uncomplicated drug ingestion.

COMPLICATIONS
- Progression to brain death
- Pneumonia
- Thromboembolism
- Stasis ulcer

REFERENCES

1. Vos PE, et al. Glial and neuronal proteins in serum predict outcome after severe traumatic brain injury. *Neurology*. 2004;62:1303–10.
2. Ely EW, et al. Delirium as a predictor of mortality in mechanically ventilated patients in the intensive care unit. *JAMA*. 2004;201:1753–62.
3. Esteban A, et al. How is mechanical ventilation employed in the intensive care unit? An international utilization review. *Am J Respir Crit Care Med*. 2000;161:1450–8.
4. Nelson JE, et al. Brain dysfunction: Another burden for the chronically critically ill. *Arch Intern Med*. 2006;166:1993–9.
5. Towne AR, et al. Prevalence of non-convulsive status epilepticus in comatose patients. *Neurology*. 2000;54:340–5.

ADDITIONAL READING

- Stevens RD, Nyquist PA. Coma, delirium, and cognitive dysfunction in critical illness. *Crit Care Clin*. 2007;22:787–804.

See Also (Topic, Algorithm, Electronic Media Element)

Delirium

CODES

ICD9
780.01 Coma

CLINICAL PEARLS

- Causes of coma include structural, systemic disease, metabolic disorders, and toxins.
- Asymmetry on neurologic exam implies structural cause.
- Always consider nonconvulsive status epilepticus in the comatose patient in the ICU.
- Consider prolonged effect of sedation in critically ill patients with organ dysfunction.
- Evaluate etiologies promptly, as several causes are treatable emergencies.

COMPARTMENT SYNDROME

Deborah Orsi

 BASICS

DESCRIPTION
- Compartment syndrome is a surgical emergency that occurs when tissue pressure in a confined space (compartment) rises to a point of compromising perfusion.
- It can occur acutely (trauma) or chronically, with insidious onset (athletes).

EPIDEMIOLOGY
- Traumatic injury:
  - More common in young men (due to relative larger muscle mass within fascia)
  - Long bone fracture: 75% (tibia > forearm)
  - Sport
  - Crush injury
  - Burns
- Nontraumatic:
  - Ischemia-reperfusion injury: From revascularization procedure and treatment (bypass surgery, embolectomy); can occur in few hours as well in days.
  - Recreational drug, bleeding, thrombosis

PATHOPHYSIOLOGY
- Occurs in anatomic compartments bound by fascia (extremities, abdomen, thorax)
- Extrinsic pressure that compresses the compartment (cast, crush injury) or increased volume inside the compartment (edema or bleeding) impede perfusion, with subsequent cellular anoxia.
- Nerve tissue is more sensitive than muscle to ischemic insult.
- Normal pressure of a tissue compartment is around 0–8 mm Hg. Capillary blood flow becomes affected at 20 mm Hg; pain occurs at pressures between 20 and 30 mm Hg, and ischemic injuries become evident >30 mm Hg.

DIAGNOSIS

- Clinical, with serial physical exams in patient at risk
- Confirmed by direct measurement of compartment pressure

PHYSICAL EXAM
- Severe pain out of proportion to apparent injury
- Paresthesia (ischemic manifestation of nerve compromise about 30 minutes to 2 hours of onset of symptoms)
- Pain with passive motion
- Muscle weakness (2–4 hours)
- Tense compartment

DIAGNOSTIC TESTS & INTERPRETATION
Measurement of compartment pressure:
- Manometry, serial measurements:
- Diagnosed by:
  - Tissue pressure >45 mm Hg
  - A difference of 30 mm Hg between diastolic and compartment pressures
- When chronic compartment syndrome is suspected, measurement must be performed immediately after the activity that causes pain.

Lab
- CPK to evaluate for rhabdomyolysis (CPK >10,000 IU)
- Basic metabolic panel
- Creatinine

TREATMENT

- Remove cast, splint, eschar if extrinsic compartment pressure
- Fasciotomy to fully decompress the compartment is the definite treatment.

ONGOING CARE

COMPLICATIONS
- Permanent nerve injury and loss of muscle
- Unconscious and heavily sedated patient are at increased risk.
- In more severe cases, amputation may be necessary.
- If left untreated, mortality can reach 15%.

ADDITIONAL READING

- Garner AJ, Handa A. Screening tools in the diagnosis of acute compartment syndrome. *Angiology*. 2010;61(5):475–81.
- Rizvi S, et al. Responding promptly to acute compartment syndrome. *Emerg Med*. 2008;40:12.

CODES

ICD9
- 958.8 Other early complications of trauma
- 958.91 Traumatic compartment syndrome of upper extremity
- 958.92 Traumatic compartment syndrome of lower extremity

CLINICAL PEARLS

- Diagnosis requires high index of suspicion.
- Serial physical exams and compartment pressure measurements are of utmost importance.

C

COMPARTMENT SYNDROME, ABDOMINAL

Sivashankar Sivaraman

 BASICS

DESCRIPTION
- Intra-abdominal pressure (IAP) is the steady-state pressure contained within the abdominal cavity.
- Normal IAP is ~5–7 mm Hg in critically ill adults.
- Abdominal perfusion pressure (APP) = mean arterial pressure (MAP) - IAP
- Intra-abdominal hypertension (IAH) is defined by a sustained or repeated pathologic elevation of IAP ≥12 mm Hg.
- Abdominal compartment syndrome (ACS) is defined as a sustained IAP >20 mm Hg (with or without an APP <60 mm Hg) that is associated with new organ dysfunction or failure.

EPIDEMIOLOGY
Incidence
- Incidence of IAH and ACS in critically ill patients on ICU admission is 32.1% and 4.2%, respectively.
- Male = Female

Prevalence
Prevalence of IAH and ACS in critically ill patients is 58.8% and 8.2%, respectively.

ETIOLOGY
- Patients should be screened for IAH/ACS risk factors upon ICU admission and in the presence of new or progressive organ failure.
- Etiology/Risk factors include:
  – Diminished abdominal wall compliance including abdominal Surgery, ARDS, trauma, central obesity
  – Increased intraluminal contents
  – Increased abdominal contents, including hemoperitoneum, ascites
  – Capillary leak/massive fluid resuscitation

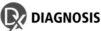 DIAGNOSIS

HISTORY
- Abdominal distension
- Dyspnea/hypoxemia
- Oliguria or anuria
- Dizziness/syncope
- Nausea and vomiting
- Trauma
- Pancreatitis
- Post abdominal surgery

PHYSICAL EXAM
- Increase in abdominal girth
- Hypotension
- Rales, increased respiratory rate, low oxygen saturation
- Increased peak/plateau pressures on ventilator

DIAGNOSTIC TESTS & INTERPRETATION
- Bladder pressure is the gold-standard for measuring IAP.
- If IAH is present, serial IAP measurements should be performed throughout the patient's critical illness.

Lab
- Comprehensive metabolic panel
- CBC
- Liver function test along with amylase and lipase
- Coagulation profile
- Cardiac markers
- Urine analysis and electrolytes
- ABG
- Serum lactate level

Imaging
- Chest radiography to determine pulmonary edema, pneumonia
- Abdominal CT or abdominal US to identify any intraluminal or extraluminal lesions

Diagnostic Procedures/Other
- Measure IAP at least every 4–6 hours or continuously.
- Titrate therapy to maintain IAP <15 mm Hg and APP >60 mm Hg

DIFFERENTIAL DIAGNOSIS
- The differential is:
  – Abdominal Trauma
  – Appendicitis
  – Cholangitis
  – Congestive Heart Failure and Pulmonary - Generalized Edema
  – Aortic pathology
  – Intestinal Disease
  – Foreign Bodies
  – Urinary Obstruction

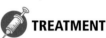 TREATMENT

The management of patients with IAH is based on the following 4 principles:
- Specific procedures to reduce IAP and the consequences of ACS
- General supportive care
- Surgical decompression
- Optimization after surgical decompression

MEDICATION

- If patient has IAP >12 mm Hg, begin medical management to reduce IAP.
- Evacuate intraluminal contents:
  – Insert nasogastric tube.
  – Trial prokinetic drugs.
  – Minimize enteral nutrition.
  – Enemas
  – Colonic decompression
- Evacuate intra-abdominal contents:
  – Abdominal US/CT scan to identify lesions
  – Percutaneous catheter drainage/paracentesis
  – Surgical evacuation
- Improve abdominal wall compliance:
  – Maintain adequate sedation and analgesia.
  – Neuromuscular blockade if needed
  – Avoid abdominally constrictive dressings.
  – Avoid head of bed >20 degrees.
- Optimize fluid administration:
  – Avoid excessive fluid resuscitation.
  – Resuscitate with hypertonic fluids or colloids.
  – Remove fluid by diuresis or hemodialysis once stable.
- Optimize systemic/regional perfusion:
  – Goal-directed fluid therapy with close hemodynamic monitoring
  – Maintain APP >60 mm Hg; if needed use vasopressors.

ADDITIONAL TREATMENT

Issues for Referral

Surgical consult for surgical decompression of abdomen

SURGERY/OTHER PROCEDURES

- The timing of this procedure still remains controversial.
- Consider strongly surgical abdominal decompression if:
  – If IAP >25 mm Hg (and/or APP <50 mm Hg) and new organ dysfunction is present
  – Patient's IAH/ACS is refractory to medical management

IN-PATIENT CONSIDERATIONS

Admission Criteria

- Suspicion for IAH
- Elevated bladder pressure
- Organ failure

Discharge Criteria

- IAH resolved
- Stable hemodynamically

 ## ONGOING CARE

FOLLOW-UP RECOMMENDATIONS

IAP measurement can be discontinued when the:

- Risk factors for IAH are resolved.
- The patient has no signs of acute organ dysfunction.
- IAP <12 mm Hg for 24–48 hours.
- Consider diuresis if volume overloaded.

ADDITIONAL READING

- Cheatham ML, et al. Is the evolving management of intra-abdominal hypertension and abdominal compartment syndrome improving survival? *Crit Care Med.* 2010;38(2):402–7.
- Malbrain ML, et al. Prevalence of intra-abdominal hypertension in critically ill patients: A multicentre epidemiological study. *Int Care Med.* 2004; 30:822–9.
- Malbrain ML, et al. Incidence and prognosis of intraabdominal hypertension in a mixed population of critically ill patients: A multiple-center epidemiological study. *Crit Care Med.* 2005;33(2): 315–22.
- Sugrue M, et al. Clinical examination is an inaccurate predictor of intraabdominal pressure. *World J Surg.* 2002;26(12):1428–31.

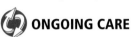 ### See Also (Topic, Algorithm, Electronic Media Element)

- The World Society on Abdominal Compartment Syndrome (www.wsacs.org)
- www.abdominal-compartment-syndrome.org

 ## CODES

ICD9

- 729.73 Nontraumatic compartment syndrome of abdomen
- 958.93 Traumatic compartment syndrome of abdomen

CONGESTIVE HEART FAILURE

Terence P. Lonergan

 BASICS

DESCRIPTION
- CHF is a clinical syndrome of various causes.
- Abnormal left ventricular function resulting in:
  - Decreased cardiac output
  - Pulmonary edema
  - Salt and water retention
- 2 major functional subtypes:
  - Systolic: Decreased ejection fraction (EF)
  - Diastolic: Preserved systolic function
- Classification: Four stages of chronic CHF:
  - Stage A: Patient with risk factors but no structural heart disease
  - Stage B: Structural heart disease present, no symptoms
  - Stage C: Structural disease with previous or current symptoms
  - Stage D: Refractory symptoms despite maximal medical therapy

EPIDEMIOLOGY
Incidence
- >65, incidence 10/1000 persons/yr
- Diastolic heart failure more common in elderly; up to 50% of cases >70

Prevalence
- ~5 million in the U.S.
- 1 million U.S. hospital admissions annually

RISK FACTORS
- Hypertension
- Coronary artery disease/myocardial infarction
- Diabetes
- Smoking
- Dyslipidemia/metabolic syndrome
- Peripheral vascular disease
- Valvular heart disease
- Rheumatic fever
- Myopathy
- History of mediastinal radiation
- Exposure to cardiotoxic drugs:
  - Alcohol
  - Bleomycin, other chemotherapeutics
- Collagen vascular disease
- Thyroid disease

Genetics
Several inherited cardiomyopathies have been identified.

GENERAL PREVENTION
- Control of modifiable risk factors (lifestyle)
- Treat hypertension/diabetes.
- Treat ischemic heart disease.
- Appropriate treatment of valvular disease

PATHOPHYSIOLOGY
- Multiple mechanisms of chronic CHF; most salient:

  - Activation of rennin/angiotensin/aldosterone
  - Sympathetic up-regulation/catecholamines
  - Circulating cytokines
  - Ongoing myocardial ischemia
  - Vasopressin
  - Bradykinin, prostaglandins, nitric oxide
  - Brain natriuretic peptide (BNP)

- These have both systemic and local effects:
  - Endocrine/paracrine effects on myocardium
    - Apoptosis, increased interstitial fibrosis
    - Ventricular remodeling (dilatation or hypertrophy)
    - Loss of normal LV shape/dimensions
    - Tachycardia
  - Systemic effects:
    - Increased vascular tone/afterload
    - Renal salt/water retention
    - Decreased systemic perfusion with further up-regulation of these mechanisms
  - LV dilatation may lead to:
    - Abnormal mitral geometry/regurgitation
    - Atrial enlargement +/– atrial fibrillation (a-fib)
  - Diastolic failure; impaired ventricular relaxation with increased filling pressure
- Acute myocardial ischemia:
  - Myocardial death/stunning
  - Ischemic papillary muscle; acute mitral regurgitation
- Myocarditis with reduced systolic function
- Other valve failure:
  - Ruptured mitral chordae tendineae
  - Infectious endocarditis (mitral or aortic)
  - Aortic dissection
  - Aortic stenosis
  - Mitral stenosis

ETIOLOGY
- Hypertension
- Myocardial Ischemia
- Valvular heart disease
- Cardiotoxic drugs/radiation
- Cardiac myopathies/myocarditis

COMMONLY ASSOCIATED CONDITIONS
- Hypertension
- Coronary artery/peripheral vascular disease
- Diabetes/metabolic syndrome/dyslipidemia
- Smoking
- Thyroid disease
- Atrial fibrillation (a-fib)
- Renal dysfunction

Pregnancy Considerations
- Caution: ACE inhibitors (see Treatment below) teratogenic
- Peripartum dilated cardiomyopathy occurs in 1/13,000–4000 births

 DIAGNOSIS

HISTORY
- Chronic/acute-on-chronic:
  - Progressive dyspnea
  - Fatigue
  - Orthopnea/paroxysmal nocturnal dyspnea
  - Dependent edema
  - Medication noncompliance
  - Assess for chest pain/angina
- Sudden/acute onset:
  - Severe dyspnea
  - Chest pain (MI)
  - Diaphoresis, nausea, vomiting (MI)
  - Pain radiating to the back/shoulders (aortic dissection)

PHYSICAL EXAM
- All or none may be present
- Cardiovascular findings:
  - S3 gallop
  - Evidence of volume overload
    - Jugular venous distension
    - Hepato-jugular reflux
    - Dependent edema
  - Valve involvement: Aortic or mitral murmur
  - Cardiogenic shock: Decreased perfusion:
    - Cool, clammy skin
    - Altered mental status
- Pulmonary findings:
  - Rales
  - Wheezing ("cardiac asthma")

DIAGNOSTIC TESTS & INTERPRETATION
Lab
Initial lab tests
- Electrolytes
- BUN/creatinine
- CBC
- Cardiac biomarkers
- BNP/pro-BNP
- Liver function testing
- TSH, free T4

Follow-Up & Special Considerations
- Closely monitor renal function, potassium if diuresing.
- Consider trending BNP/pro-BNP as index of response to therapy.

Imaging
Initial approach
- Chest x-ray:
  - Pulmonary vascular congestion/edema
  - Kerley B lines
  - Pleural effusions
- Echocardiography:
  - Urgent in acute presentations/cardiogenic shock
  - Evaluate overall systolic function
  - Evidence of valvular dysfunction
  - Evidence of muscular hypertrophy/impaired relaxation
  - Pericardial fluid/tamponade
  - Evidence of right ventricular failure (see chapter)

Follow-Up & Special Considerations
Other imaging guided by clinical scenario

Diagnostic Procedures/Other
Electrocardiogram (all patients):
- Left ventricular hypertrophy
- Myocardial ischemia
- Rhythm disturbances

Pathological Findings
Myocardial biopsy in select cases may show:
- Myocarditis
- Vasculitis
- Myocardial infiltration

DIFFERENTIAL DIAGNOSIS
- Decreased cardiac output/shock:
  - Hypovolemia
  - Distributive (sepsis, anaphylaxis)
  - Obstructive (tamponade)

C

- Dyspnea/hypoxemia:
  - COPD/asthma/restrictive lung disease
  - Pneumonia
  - Pulmonary embolism
- Volume overload:
  - Cirrhosis/hypoproteinemia
  - Nephrosis

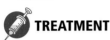
TREATMENT
MEDICATION
First Line
- ACE inhibitors (ACE-I) improve survival, reduce hospitalizations and symptoms, and reverse remodeling (1,2)[A]:
  - Start low dose and titrate to maximum tolerated based on BP, renal function
- β-Blockers in stabilized patients not recently requiring inotropic therapy improve survival, symptoms, ejection fraction, and reduce sudden death (1,2) [A]:
  - May initiate once stable off pressors/inotropes
  - Should already be on ACE-I/ARB
  - Start low dose and titrate every 2–4 weeks to maximum tolerated dose
  - Watch for worsening CHF, hypotension, bradycardia
- Loop diuretics (e.g., furosemide) if clinical evidence of volume overload:
  - Furosemide: Start 20–40 mg IV and titrate dose to response.
  - Consider continuous infusion if inadequate response to intermittent dosing.
  - Assess renal function, potassium frequently.

Second Line
- Angiotensin II receptor blockers (ARB) if unable to tolerate ACE inhibitor
- Spironolactone: In patients with NY Heart Association class III or IV disease (severe symptoms or symptoms at rest)
- Digoxin: Reduces morbidity/hospitalizations, no effect on mortality; use with caution in renal impairment, avoid in diastolic dysfunction
- Nesiritide: Promotes natriuresis and lowers pulmonary artery pressures; concern over lack of outcome data and effects on renal function (2)[B]
- Hydralazine/nitrate combination: RCTs support; use if unable to tolerate ACE-I/ARB

ADDITIONAL TREATMENT
General Measures
Control of precipitating/coexisting factors

Issues for Referral
Multidisciplinary teams have been shown to reduce hospital admissions.

Additional Therapies
- Left ventricular assist devices in select patients as a bridge to heart transplantation
- Consider ultrafiltration for acute volume overload refractory to medical management (1).

SURGERY/OTHER PROCEDURES
- Coronary revascularization in patients with ischemic cardiomyopathy
- Heart transplantation evaluation for select patients
- Biventricular pacing/implantable defibrillators in select patients

IN-PATIENT CONSIDERATIONS
Initial Stabilization
- IV access, supplemental oxygen, monitor
- Continuous pulse oximetry
- Positive pressure ventilation (PPV):
  - Noninvasive PPV is often an option; do not delay endotracheal intubation in patients with depressed mental status, inability to tolerate mask, aspiration risk, or frank shock.
  - PPV decreases preload, afterload, and work of breathing.
- Priority is to categorize/treat the acute CHF patient in 1 of 5 groups (3)[C]:
  - Group 1: Systolic pressure (SBP) >140:
    - Usually component of diastolic dysfunction with prominent pulmonary edema
    - Symptoms often developed abruptly
    - PPV
    - Nitrates; sublingually until IV available
    - IV nitroglycerine at 10–20 mcg/min and titrated up at 5 mcg/min increments every 5 minutes until desired effect
  - Group 2: SBP 100–140:
    - Typical of gradually developing exacerbation of chronic systolic dysfunction
    - PPV, nitrates, diuretics if systemic volume overload on exam
  - Group 3: SBP <100:
    - Hypoperfusion is the main concern; pulmonary edema may be minimal.
    - Consider initial volume loading with isotonic fluid; if oxygenation worsens, adjust ventilation settings (FiO$_2$, PEEP).
    - Inotropes if perfusion is not improved (dobutamine, milrinone).
    - Vasopressors (norepinephrine, dopamine, Neo-Synephrine) if blood pressure remains low
    - Invasive hemodynamic monitoring with pulmonary artery catheter and arterial line
  - Group 4: CHF and evidence of ACS:
    - Treat CHF as above according to blood pressure.
    - Treat ACS according to current guidelines.
    - Cardiogenic shock warrants consideration of intra-aortic balloon pump (IABP)
  - Group 5: Right heart failure (see Right Heart Failure chapter)

Admission Criteria
- Significant respiratory distress/hypoxia
- Anasarca or significant edema
- Syncope
- Concomitant medical illness
- Poor social support
- Evidence of active myocardial ischemia
- Failure of outpatient management
- CHF of new onset/unknown cause

IV Fluids
Restrict in volume overloaded patients

Nursing
- Daily weights as a measure of fluid status
- Deep vein thrombosis prophylaxis
- Mobilize patients as able

Discharge Criteria
Based on patient stability and resolution of admission criteria.

ONGOING CARE
FOLLOW-UP RECOMMENDATIONS
Close follow-up for all CHF patients within several weeks of discharge, according to stability

Patient Monitoring
- At each visit, assess volume status, BP, severity of symptoms.
- Closely monitor electrolytes, renal function.
- May be useful to trend BNP/pro-BNP.

DIET
Low-sodium cardiac diet is recommended.

PATIENT EDUCATION
- Adherence to medication schedules
- Self assessment for weight changes
- Prompt medical care for worsening symptoms.

PROGNOSIS
Depends on stage; 5-year mortality for symptomatic heart failure remains ~50%

COMPLICATIONS
- Arrhythmias; a-fib, ventricular tachycardia
- Intracardiac thrombus formation
- Cardio-renal syndrome: Compromised renal function resulting from poor renal perfusion

REFERENCES

1. Jessup M, et al. 2009 Focused Update: ACCF/AHA Guidelines for the diagnosis and management of heart failure in adults. *Circulation*. 2009;119: 1977–2016.
2. Dickstein K, et al. ESC Guidelines for the diagnosis and treatment of acute and chronic heart failure. *Eur Heart J*. 2008;29:2388–2442.
3. Mebazaa A, et al. Practical recommendations for prehospital and early in-hospital management of patients presenting with acute heart failure syndromes. *Crit Care Med*. 2008;36(1):S129–39.

ADDITIONAL READING
- Topalian S, et al. Cardiogenic shock. *Crit Care Med*. 2008;36(1):S66–74.

See Also (Topic, Algorithm, Electronic Media Element)

- Acute Coronary Syndromes
- Valvular Heart Diseases

CODES

ICD9
- 428.0 Congestive heart failure, unspecified
- 428.20 Systolic heart failure, unspecified
- 428.30 Diastolic heart failure, unspecified

CLINICAL PEARLS
- CHF may occur with normal systolic function.
- Obtain an echocardiogram early.
- Identify and treat factors contributing to acute decompensated CHF (e.g., myocardial ischemia).
- Diuretics are reserved for systemic volume overload.
- PPV and nitrates (if BP allows) are first-line therapies in acute, decompensated CHF.

CONTINUOUS VENOVENOUS HEMOFILTRATION (CVVH)

Aditya Uppalapati
Sindhura Gogineni
Roopa Kohli–Seth

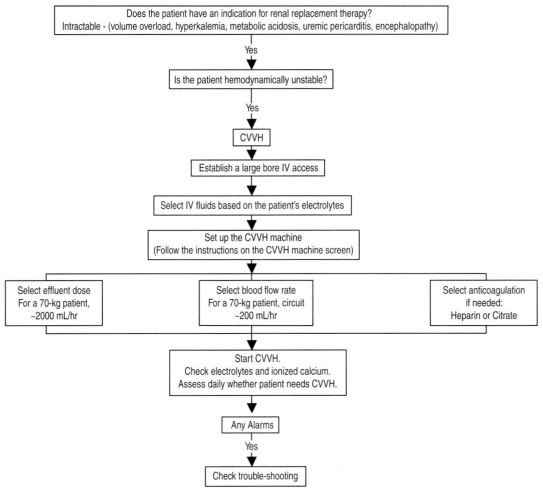

Does the patient have an indication for renal replacement therapy?
Intractable - (volume overload, hyperkalemia, metabolic acidosis, uremic pericarditis, encephalopathy)

↓ Yes

Is the patient hemodynamically unstable?

↓ Yes

CVVH

↓

Establish a large bore IV access

↓

Select IV fluids based on the patient's electrolytes

↓

Set up the CVVH machine
(Follow the instructions on the CVVH machine screen)

↓

Select effluent dose
For a 70-kg patient,
~2000 mL/hr

Select blood flow rate
For a 70-kg patient, circuit
~200 mL/hr

Select anticoagulation
if needed:
Heparin or Citrate

↓

Start CVVH.
Check electrolytes and ionized calcium.
Assess daily whether patient needs CVVH.

↓

Any Alarms

↓ Yes

Check trouble-shooting

CVVH is a technique of continuous renal replacement therapy. Blood is driven through a highly permeable membrane by a peristaltic pump and via an extracorporeal circuit. The extracorporeal circuit originates through a large-bore catheter in a vein and terminates through the same large-bore catheter into the vein.

PRINCIPLE

- Pressure generated by the pumped blood induces the passage of plasma water (the solvent) across the membrane. This process is called *ultrafiltration*.
- Ultrafiltrate produced during the transit of blood through the membrane contains all molecules to which the membrane is permeable. As the solvent moves across the membrane, it drags solutes along with it (solvent drag) in response to a positive transmembrane pressure. This process is called *convection*.
- The fluid loss is in part replaced by replacement solution.
  – The replacement fluid can be given prefilter (predilution) or postfilter (postdilution).
- Fluid balance is maintained by the difference between fluid input (replacement fluid) and output (effluent/ultrafiltrate).
  – A net negative, zero, or positive balance can be maintained.

INDICATIONS FOR CVVH

- Symptomatic AKI especially in hemodyamically unstable patient. No significant data on exactly when. As AKI-RIFLE failure associated with greater mortality, may consider initiating when patient reached AKI-RIFLE failure.
- Renal Indications:
  – Intractable volume overload
  – Hyperkalemia
  – Metabolic acidosis
  – Uremic pericarditis
  – Encephalopathy.
- Other indications:
  – Drug and toxin removal
    ○ Methanol
    ○ Isopropanol
    ○ Ethylene glycol
    ○ Lithium
    ○ Salicylate
    ○ Theophylline
    ○ Valproic acid
    ○ Tricyclic antidepressants
  – contrast agents
  – cytokines removal
  – sepsis
  – liver transplantation

VASCULAR ACCESS AND FILTER

- Large-bore catheter (11.5–14.0 Fr gauge) with 2 lumens.
  – One lumen for outflow of blood and the other for inflow of blood.
  – The length of the catheters varies from 13–20 cm.
  – Typically these catheters are inserted in the internal jugular or femoral veins.
  – Blood flow of 150–300 mL/min can be achieved with these catheters.
- Filter: Tubular-shaped device that is made of plastic casing and the capillary fibers of the semipermeable membrane within.

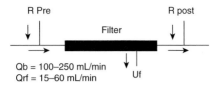

Qb = 100–250 mL/min
Qrf = 15–60 mL/min

CVVH
R pre-replacement solution pre filter
R post-replacement solution post
Qb-Blood flow
Qrf-replacement solution
Uf-Ultrafilteration

INTENSITY AND EFFICACY OF RRT

Intensity of RRT:

- Product of clearance (K) × time.
  – No difference between low intensity (20–25 mL/kg/hr) vs. high intensity (35–40 mL/kg/hr) in terms of mortality, recovery of kidney function.
  – Profound hypophosphatemia with high intensity.
  – Not recommended to exceed 25 mL/kg/hr intensity (2)[A],(3)[A].

Efficacy of RRT:

- Kt/V where V is volume of distribution of the marker molecule in the body.
  – It is a dimensionless number.
  – It is an established measure of dialysis dose.
  – 25 mL/kg/hr roughly correspond to Kt/V of 1.0 (e.g., 70-kg patient, 25 mL × 70 kg × 24 hr = 42 L/day, V = 70 kg × 0.6 = 42 L; Kt/V = 1).
  – 35 mL/kg/hr corresponds to a Kt/V of 1.4.
    ○ For intermittent hemodialysis, a Kt/V of minimum 1.2 is required.
    ○ However, for CVVH, it is suggested to deliver no less than 20 mL/kg/hr × 24 hr.

The most common practice involves prefilter dilution with replacement fluid, median effluent dose of 2 L/hr and median blood flow of 200 mL/min (1)(A).

Pre- vs. Postfilter dilution:

- Prefilter dilution: Decreases the membrane polarization and results in an improved mass transfer.
  – Also increases the mass transfer by increasing the flow secondary to mixing with replacement fluid.
  – However, the low efficiency (clearance) leading to high replacement fluid requirements.
- Postfilter dilution:
  – Increased clearance but
  – increased risk of filter clotting.

WHEN TO STOP CVVH
No clear cut guidelines. Clinical decision.

Creatinine Clearance	Management of RRT
<12 mL/min	Continue RRT
12–20 mL/min	Clinical Judgment
>20 mL/min	Discontinue RRT

FLUIDS FOR CVVH

- Sodium is kept in the normal range of 135–145 mEq/L.
- Chloride, bicarbonate, and potassium are adjusted based on the patient's electrolytes.
- Generally about 9 bags (1 L each) of fluid are used.
- Plasmalyte, half-normal saline with sodium bicarbonate 60–70 mEq and commercially available renal replacement solutions are generally used.
- Normal saline is rarely used. (It can cause hyperchloremic metabolic acidosis)

Fluid	Plasmalyte/ Isolyte	Normal Saline	1/2 Normal Saline + 70 mEq Sodium Bicarbonate
Na mEq/L	140	154	147
Cl mEq/L	98	154	77
K mEq/L	5	0	0
Ca mEq/L	—	0	0
Mg mEq/L	3	0	0
Buffers	Acetate (27)		Bicarbonate (70)

TROUBLE-SHOOTING

- CVVH monitor, low arterial or high venous pressure alarm:
  – Suspect malfunctioning catheter, kinking, obstruction;
    ○ Check the flow from the catheter, unkink if catheter kinked, flush the catheter; if good flow, then reconnect,
    ○ If still a problem, swap the tubing connections on the 2 ports of the catheter.
    ○ If no improvement, then the catheter needs to be changed.
- Monitor air alarm: Follow the instructions on the monitor.
- Circuit clogging:
  – May need more heparin in the circuit,
  – Blood flow rate should be adjusted,
  – Prefilter dilution instead of post filter,
  – Suspect DIC in appropriate clinical setting.

REFERENCES

1. Bellomo R, et al. Renal study investigators. Renal replacement therapy for acute kidney injury in Australian and New Zealand intensive care units: a practice survey. *Crit Care Resusc*. 2008;10(3):225–30.
2. Bellomo R, et al. The renal replacement therapy study investigators. Intensity of Continuous Renal-Replacement Therapy in Critically Ill Patients. *N Engl J Med*. 2009;361:1627–38.
3. Palevsky PM. The VA/NIH Acute Renal Failure Trial Network. Intensity of renal support in critically ill patients with acute kidney injury. *N Engl J Med*. 2008;359:7–20.

 CODES

ICD9
- 276.2 Acidosis
- 276.7 Hyperpotassemia
- 866.00 Unspecified injury to kidney without mention of open wound into cavity

CRITICAL CARE OF THE GENERAL SURGERY PATIENT

Seth Manoach

 BASICS

DESCRIPTION

- Neuroendocrine response to surgery, operative complexity, and patient characteristics combine to define perioperative risk and subsequent need for critical care.
- Treatment of hemodynamic and other derangements:
  - Diagnostic evaluation for bleeding
  - Myocardial ischemia/failure
  - Sepsis
  - Pulmonary embolus
  - Intra-abdominal hypertension
  - Anastomotic leaks
  - Fistula formation
  - Abscess formation

EPIDEMIOLOGY

- 264 adults/100,000 population/year admitted to ICU in Calgary, Canada.
- 59% general and cardiac surgery patients.

ETIOLOGY

- Fluid shifts:
  - Major open body cavity surgery results in insensible loss of ~1 L/cavity/hr.
  - Postoperative edema ("third spacing")
  - 1–4 days postop: "Third spaced" fluid → back into vascular compartment.
  - Bleeding, fluid loss from drains, fistulas, and other sources, increase volume requirement.
  - Positive fluid balance:
    - Congestive heart failure
    - Renal insufficiency
    - Hypoalbuminemia
- Catabolic state and ileus:
  - Loss of integrity of gut–blood barrier → enteric bacterial translocation, sepsis
  - Negative nitrogen balance, protein loss:
    - Immunosuppression
    - Poor wound healing
    - Dehiscence
    - Fistula formation
    - Abscess formation

DIAGNOSIS

Signs and symptoms are specific to the many common problems of surgical patients:

- Particularly important signs: Unexplained tachycardia and hemodynamic instability, altered mental status, abdominal distension, abdominal pain, respiratory distress
- Increased minute ventilation may result from bleeding, sepsis, ischemia, anastomotic leak, other nonrespiratory metabolic crises.

HISTORY

- History is problem-specific.
- The hand-off from anesthesia-surgical team to the intensivist is crucial:
  - Most patients requiring postoperative critical care are unable to provide detailed history.
- Initial presentation + evaluation and operative records must be reviewed.
  - Intensivist should verify written data with OR team as information may be missing or inaccurate (e.g., "estimated blood loss").
  - Critical information: OR time, fluid and blood totals, ventilatory parameters, detailed account of complications.

PHYSICAL EXAM

- Physical exam is problem-specific.
- Monitoring equipment, intubation/sedation, restraints, ancillary tests, contact infection precautions often limit ICU physical exam:
  - Co-management, covered wounds compound problem in surgical patient:
    - Failure to perform adequate physical exam leads to missed systemic infection source, wound complications, limb ischemia, other grave outcomes.

DIAGNOSTIC TESTS & INTERPRETATION

- Essential workup is problem-specific.
- Targeted evaluation of hemodynamically or otherwise unstable perioperative patient is of paramount importance:
  - Hemorrhage requiring reoperation or intervention is 1st target of evaluation.
- Failure to resolve postoperative hyperdynamic state after 3–4 days should prompt search for anastomotic leak, abscess/fistula formation, intra-abdominal compartment syndrome, other complications mentioned above.

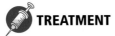 **TREATMENT**

- Hemodynamic instability should be treated with volume and/or blood products unless there is clear evidence of volume overload, cardiogenic, or neurogenic shock:
  - Vasopressor agents are to be used only when the intensivist has ruled out bleeding and adequately resuscitated the patient.
- Broad-spectrum antibiotics must be started as soon as sepsis is suspected:
  - Most general surgical patients require coverage for gram-positive, gram-negative, and anaerobic bacteria.
  - Enterocutaneous fistulae leads to suspect fungal infection.
  - Empiric antibiotic therapy can later be narrowed based on culture results.

IN-PATIENT CONSIDERATIONS
Discharge Criteria
Discharge from ICU to appropriate medical or surgical service after achieving:
- Hemodynamic stability
- Liberation from mechanical ventilation and/or tracheostomy
- Control of life-threatening postoperative conditions

 ONGOING CARE
DIET
In general, enteral feeding should be started as soon as possible:
- Postoperative ileus may be prolonged by abstention from enteral feeding.

ADDITIONAL READING

- Cheatham ML, et al. Is the evolving management of intra-abdominal hypertension and abdominal compartment syndrome improving survival? *Crit Care Med*. 2010;38:402–7.
- Laupland KB. Population-based epidemiology of intensive care: Critical importance of ascertainment of residency status. *Crit Care*. 2004;8:R431–6.
- Lee TH, et al. Derivation and prospective validation of a simple index for predication of cardiac risk for major noncardiac surgery. *Circulation*. 1999;100: 1043–9.

- Moore FA, et al. Early enteral feeding, compared with parenteral, reduces post-operative septic complications: The results of a meta-analysis. *Ann Surg*. 1992;216:172–83.
- Noordzji PG, et al. Postoperative mortality in the Netherlands: A population-based analysis of surgery-specific risk in adults. *Anesthesiology*. 2010;112:1110–15.

 CODES

ICD9
- 038.9 Unspecified septicemia
- 414.8 Other specified forms of chronic ischemic heart disease
- 998.89 Other specified complications of procedures not elsewhere classified

CLINICAL PEARLS

- Early postoperative hemodynamic compromise is assumed to be bleeding until proved otherwise.
- Downstream measures of inadequate end-organ perfusion, such as $\uparrow$ lactate or $\downarrow$ $SvcO_2$ are often earliest indicators of bleeding, sepsis, other crises.
- Thoroughly review preoperative and operative course of any surgical ICU patient by data review and direct communication with OR team.
- Intensivist must maintain a collaborative relationship with the surgical team at all times.

C

CRITICAL CARE OF THE VASCULAR SURGERY PATIENT

Jennifer M. Howes

 BASICS

DESCRIPTION
- Vascular disease affects all circulatory beds.
- Vascular patients often have many comorbidities:
  - Ischemic heart disease
  - Hypertension
  - Diabetes mellitus
  - Chronic obstructive pulmonary disease
  - Renal insufficiency
- Critical care management of the postoperative vascular surgery patient requires management of potential postoperative complications and sequelae of preexisting conditions.

EPIDEMIOLOGY
- Risk for vascular disease increases with age
- Male > Female
- Risk factors include:
  - Metabolic syndrome
  - Hypertension
  - Diabetes mellitus
  - Tobacco

 ONGOING CARE

COMPLICATIONS
- General potential postoperative complications:
  - Hemorrhage
  - Acute myocardial ischemia
  - Acute renal failure
  - Prolonged mechanical ventilation
- Specific vascular diseases and potential postoperative complications:
- Aortic aneurysmal disease
  - Most commonly, infrarenal aorta
  - Natural history is continual expansion and eventual rupture.

- Surgical repair when diameter ≥5.5 cm:
  - Endovascular:
    - Postoperative complications include hematoma at device insertion site; distal embolization of dislodged plaque
  - Open:
    - Postoperative complications include prolonged ileus; bowel ischemia occurs in 0.6% of patients; presents with bloody stools, fever, abdominal pain, leukocytosis, lactic acidosis; requires surgical resection of infarcted bowel
    - Lower extremity ischemia occurs in 2–5% of patients due to intraoperative aortic occlusion; requires immediate surgical exploration.

- Aortic dissection:
  - Stanford type A:
    - Ascending aorta
    - Management with immediate surgical repair
  - Stanford type B:
    - Descending aorta
    - Medical management with aggressive blood pressure control
    - Surgical management if distal vessel perfusion defects, uncontrolled hypertension, unrelenting pain, aneurysm development
- Postoperative complications:
  - Prolonged ileus
  - Bowel ischemia
  - Lower extremity ischemia

- Carotid occlusive disease/stenosis:
  - Carotid endarterectomy when symptomatic or high-grade stenosis (>60–70%)
  - Postoperative complications:
    - Cerebrovascular accidents:
      - Ischemic: Inadequate intraoperative perfusion
      - Watershed: Increased perfusion to areas with altered baroreceptor response
      - Thromboembolic: Graft-related
    - Altered baroreceptor responses (hypotension, hypertension, bradycardia)
- Peripheral occlusive disease/stenosis:
  - Revascularization with bypass when severe disability or failure of nonsurgical treatment
  - Postoperative complications:
    - Graft occlusion:
      - Prevention with anticoagulation in high risk grafts (small caliber distal target arteries, conduit of multiple vein segments sewn together)
      - Treatment with anticoagulation and surgical re-exploration
    - Compartment syndrome (see Compartment Syndrome)

ADDITIONAL READING

- Freezor RJ, et al. *Vascular surgery in the intensive care unit.* In: Gabrielli A et al., eds., 4th ed. Philadelphia: Lippincott, Williams, & Wilkins, 2009:1237–45.
- Gopalan PD, et al. Critical care of the vascular surgery patient. *Crit Care Clin.* 2003;109–25.

 CODES

ICD9
- 401.9 Unspecified essential hypertension
- 414.9 Chronic ischemic heart disease, unspecified
- 997.2 Peripheral vascular complications

C

CYTOMEGALOVIRUS

Jose Diego Caceres Maceo
Jose R. Yunen

 BASICS

DESCRIPTION
- Cytomegalovirus (CMV) infection is a late-appearing entity in the critically ill patient, commonly between the 4th and 12th day in ICU.
- Common cause of allograft rejection
- Usually acquired during childhood or teenage years, remaining as latent disease; clinical manifestations are due to reactivation of latent disease and in some newly acquired disease:
  - Commonly associated with long ICU stay, mechanical-associated pneumonia.

EPIDEMIOLOGY
- Among U.S. population, 60% have been exposed. Prevalence of 90% among high-risk groups.
- In critically ill patients, infection is reported to occur in up to 36% of immunocompetent patients with a 5-fold increase with severe sepsis.
- CMV disease occurs in 11–17% up to 3 months in posttransplanted patients.

PATHOPHYSIOLOGY
- Infection usually is asymptomatic, but remains latent. Latent infection is diagnosed when viral protein or nucleic acid is isolated from any body fluid.
- Transmitted from person to person via close contact. Can also occur via blood transfusion, organ transplantation, through the placenta and breast milk. Medical personal can also transmit the disease.
- Can affect almost any organ; produces well-defined clinical syndromes:
  - Pneumonia and ARDS
  - Pericarditis and myocarditis
  - Neurological disease or meningoencephalitis
  - Gastroenteritis
  - Hematological disorders, mostly cytopenias and hemolytic anemia
  - Hepatitis (transaminitis)
  - Retinitis

ETIOLOGY
Double-stranded DNA virus family of the Herpesviridae. Grows only in human cells, and replicates best in fibroblasts.

COMMONLY ASSOCIATED CONDITIONS
- Severe sepsis
- Long ICU stay
- Transfusion in the last 24 hour of admission
- AIDS patient
- Solid organ transplanted patients
- Bone marrow transplanted patients
- Severe burn injuries
- Immunosuppression therapy in patients with rheumatoid arthritis, systemic lupus, Crohn disease.

DIAGNOSIS

HISTORY
- A patient with associated conditions that predispose to CMV reactivation or new infection presents with flu-like symptoms and malaise.
- Commonly presents in patients with severe sepsis, prolonged mechanical ventilation, multiple transfusion, solid organ receptor, or immunocompromised with worsening target organ dysfunction.
- Shortness of breath, dyspnea with or without cough
- Painful dysphagia, abdominal pain
- Confusion, irritability, severe headache
- Palpitations, chest pain
- Decreased visual acuity, floaters, unilateral vision loss

PHYSICAL EXAM
- Pharyngitis
- Cervical lymphadenopathy
- Prolonged fever
- Fine lung crackles to absent breath sound, rales, and wheezing
- Splenomegaly
- Hepatomegaly, right upper quadrant tenderness
- Oral ulcerations, abdominal tenderness, nausea, vomiting, diarrhea, melena, hematemesis
- Ophthalmological exam shows yellow areas with perivascular exudates.

DIAGNOSTIC TESTS & INTERPRETATION
Lab
Initial lab tests
- CMV IgM and IgG
- PCR from bronchoalveolar lavage or sputum
- CBC, ABG
- BUN, creatinine
- Liver function tests: AST, ALT, GGT, total bilirubin, indirect bilirubin
- Haptoglobin
- Total creatine phospho kinase and mb fraction, troponin
- Viral panel: Anti HIV 1 & 2, HBsAg, HBeAg, anti HBV, anti HCV

Follow-Up & Special Considerations
- False-positive of CMV IgM in patients with high rheumatic factor, EBV, or HHV-6 infection
- Serum antibodies are usually not present early in the course.
- Qualitative and quantitative PCR is positive before serum antibodies.
- Test for HHV-6, because it occurs in up to 57% of patients with multiple organ failure.
- Follow CBC and ABG with CMV pneumonia.
- Follow BUN and creatinine if renal dysfunction is present.

Imaging
Initial approach
- Chest x-ray must always be obtained if CMV is suspected because asymptomatic pneumonia may occur. Bilateral pulmonary infiltrates are commonly seen.
- Chest CT scan is more sensitive in identifying pulmonary infiltrates and can be performed if no clear involvement is seen on CXR.
- Abdominal x-ray can identify presence of pneumoperitoneum associated with colonic rupture.
- Abdominal US can help assess integrity and sizes of spleen and liver; also can rule out structural damage to kidneys.
- Head CT scan and/or MRI scan if meningoencephalitis is suspected or neurological findings are present.
- Electrocardiography should be performed if the patient presents with irregular pulses and/or heart sounds. Echocardiography can identify possible pericarditis.

Follow-Up & Special Considerations
- If ventilator-associated pneumonia or ARDS, chest x-ray must be obtained every 24 hours.
- In patient with threat of renal graft rejection, obtain serial renal graft Doppler and US.
- After initial treatment of meningoencephalitis, CT or MRI scan may be obtained after 1 week or whenever neurological status worsens.

Diagnostic Procedures/Other
- Tissue biopsy may be obtained if no clear diagnosis is obtained.
- Bronchoalveolar lavage can be obtained in patients with pulmonary findings.

Pathological Findings
Classic hallmark is the presence of cells with intranuclear inclusion with a clear halo, commonly referred as "owl's eyes."

DIFFERENTIAL DIAGNOSIS
- Fever of unknown origin
- Bacterial pneumonia
- Bacterial meningitis
- Peptic ulcer disease
- Active SLE
- Viral and autoimmune hepatitis
- HIV disease

C

 TREATMENT

MEDICATION

First Line
- Ganciclovir and immunoglobulin (CytoGam):
  - Ganciclovir: Induction: 5 mg/kg IV b.i.d. plus immunoglobulin 500 mg/kg 3 times/wk for the first 2 weeks. Maintenance: 5 mg/kg IV for 1 month plus immunoglobulin 500 mg/kg every week for 1 month.
  - CytoGam: 400 mg/kg CMV-IG in combination with ganciclovir on days 1, 2, 7, followed by 200 mg/kg CMV-GIVE on days 14 and 21
- Valganciclovir: Induction: 900 mg PO q12h. Maintenance dose: 900 mg PO q.d.

Second Line
- Foscarnet
- Cidofovir

ADDITIONAL TREATMENT
General Measures
Prophylaxis in patient with positive CMV serology undergoing organ transplantation:
- Ganciclovir: 5 mg/kg IV q12h for 7–14 days, followed by 5 mg/kg daily 7 days/wk or 6 mg/kg daily 5 days/wk for 100 days.
- Valganciclovir: Used in heart, kidney, kidney-pancreas transplant recipients; start 900 mg PO daily beginning within 10 days of transplant and continue for 100 days posttransplant.

SURGERY/OTHER PROCEDURES
- Colonic or small bowel resection may be needed in patients with bowel perforation or uncontrolled GI bleeding.
- Spinal tap should be obtained if meningoencephalitis is suspected and CMV IgM and PCR is measured on obtained CSF.

IN-PATIENT CONSIDERATIONS
Initial Stabilization
- Patient isolation
- Suctioning of upper airway, nasogastric or orogastric tube placement
- Oxygen supplementation
- Cardiac monitoring and pulse oximetry
- Central line placement
- Consider endotracheal intubation in patients with acute respiratory distress, shock, or unable to protect airway

- Consider hemodialysis catheter placement in patient with impending renal failure
- Further hemodynamic monitoring in patients with shock or ARDS using transthoracic or transesophageal echo, pulse contour analysis, or pulmonary artery catheter

IV Fluids
- Normosol R or NS solutions to maintain proper input and output balance; increase solutions if fever is recurrent.
- Electrolyte replacement

 ONGOING CARE

DIET
- Enteral nutrition is preferred if no GI involvement is present.
- Consider low-protein regimen if hepatic failure is present.
- Parenteral nutrition must be used if there is evidence of bowel perforation or profuse GI bleeding.

PROGNOSIS
Varies widely; data are very heterogenous. Recent data suggest an overall mortality between 5% and 71%.

ADDITIONAL READING

- Bowden RA, et al. A comparison of filtered leukocyte-reduced and cytomegalovirus (CMV) seronegative blood products for the prevention of transfusion-associated CMV infection after marrow transplant. *Blood*. 1995;86(9):3598–603.
- Collier AC, et al. Cytomegalovirus infection in homosexual men. Relationship to sexual practices, antibody to human immunodeficiency virus, and cell-mediated immunity. *Am J Med*. 1987; 82(3 Spec No):593–601.
- Cunha BA. Cytomegalovirus pneumonia: community-acquired pneumonia in immunocompetent hosts. *Infect Dis Clin North Am*. 2010;24(1):147–58.
- Deayton JR, et al. Importance of cytomegalovirus viraemia in risk of disease progression and death in HIV-infected patients receiving highly active antiretroviral therapy. *Lancet*. 2004;363(9427): 2116–21.
- Guinan ME, et al. Heterosexual and homosexual patients with the acquired immunodeficiency syndrome. A comparison of surveillance, interview, and laboratory data. *Ann Intern Med*. 1984;100(2): 213–8.
- Hayden FG, et al. Herpesvirus infections in burn patients. *Chest*. 1994;106(1 Suppl):15S–21S.

- Heininger, et al. Human cytomegalovirus infections in nonimmunosuppressed critically ill patients. *Crit Care Med*. 2001;29(3):541–7.
- Kutza AS, et al. High incidence of active cytomegalovirus infection among septic patients. *Clin Infect Dis*. 1998;26(5):1076–82.
- Nichols WG, et al. Transfusion-transmitted cytomegalovirus infection after receipt of leukoreduced blood products. *Blood*. 2003; 101(10):4195–200.
- Osawa R, et al. Cytomegalovirus infection in critically ill patients: A systematic review. *Crit Care*. 2009;13(3):R68.
- Paudice N, et al. Preemptive therapy for the prevention of cytomegalovirus disease in renal transplant recipients: Our preliminary experience. *Transplant Proc*. 2009;41(4):1204–6.
- Razonable RR, et al. Selective reactivation of human herpesvirus 6 variant A occurs in critically ill immunocompetent hosts. *J Infect Dis*. 2002; 185(1):110–3.
- Rennekampff H-O, et al. Cytomegalovirus infection in burns: A review. *J Med Microbiol*. 2006; 55(Pt 5):483–7.
- Ziegler TR. Parenteral nutrition in critically ill patient. *N Engl J Med*. 2009;361:1088–97.

CODES

ICD9
- 078.5 Cytomegaloviral disease
- 480.8 Pneumonia due to other virus not elsewhere classified
- 518.5 Pulmonary insufficiency following trauma and surgery

CLINICAL PEARLS

- CMV infection should be suspected in patients with long ICU stay and mechanical ventilation pneumonia with no identifiable bacterial cause.
- CMV infection commonly is diagnosed by serologic studies after ≥2 weeks. PCR testing is usually positive earlier in the course.
- Multiple organ failure is commonly associated with CMV infection.

DELIRIUM, ICU

Fred DiBlasio Jr.
Roopa Kohli-Seth

BASICS

DESCRIPTION
- Delirium is defined by the DSM IV as a disturbance of consciousness with inattention accompanied by a change in cognition or perceptual disturbance that develops over a short period (hours to days) and fluctuates over time.
- Delirium is frequent complication encountered in the ICU.
- Independent risk factor for prolonged length of stay and >6-month mortality rates.
- Many ICU survivors have persistent cognitive deficits months to years later.

EPIDEMIOLOGY
Incidence
- 20–50% of lower severity ICU patients or those not receiving mechanical ventilation
- 60–80% of ICU patients receiving mechanical ventilation.
- 78–87% among older ICU patients; complicates hospital stay of more than 2–3 million elderly patients per year in the U.S.
- Involves over 17.5 million in-patient days
- Accounts for >$4 billion in Medicare expenditures.
- Rates between 5% and 52% in postoperative patients, with highest rates among hip fracture and aortic surgery patients
- In perioperative setting, untreated pain and inadequate analgesia are also strong risk factors for delirium.

Prevalence
- Predominant age: Older persons
- Male = Female

RISK FACTORS
- ICU patients, especially older persons, are among the most vulnerable hospitalized patients for the development of delirium.
- Baseline risk factors include:
  - Advanced age
  - Dementia
  - Smoking and alcoholism
  - Prior cognitive impairment
  - Functional impairment
  - High BUN:Cr ratio
  - Dehydration
  - Malnutrition
  - Hearing or vision impairment
  - Frailty
- Precipitating risk factors:
  - Severe illness in any organ system(s)
  - Need for urinary catheter
  - >3 medications
  - Pain
  - Any adverse iatrogenic event
  - Long acting sedative hypnotics
  - Narcotics (esp. meperidine)
  - Anticholinergics (e.g., diphenhydramine)
  - Corticosteroids
  - Sleep deprivation and loss of circadian rhythm
  - ICU patients average 2 hours sleep q24h
  - MODS
  - ARDS
  - Immobilization (restraints, catheters)
  - Anemia (phlebotomy)

GENERAL PREVENTION
Follow treatment approach.

PATHOPHYSIOLOGY
- Neuropathology is not clearly defined.
- Multicomponent approach addressing contributing factors can reduce incidence and complications.

ETIOLOGY
- Multifactorial
- Interaction between predisposing and precipitating factors

COMMONLY ASSOCIATED CONDITIONS
- New medicine or medicine changes
- Infections (lung, urine, meningitis)
- Toxic-metabolic (hyponatremia, hypercalcemia, renal failure, hepatic failure)
- Heart attack
- Stroke
- Alcohol or drug withdrawal

DIAGNOSIS

- Gold standard criteria used to diagnose delirium is the clinical history and exam as guided by DSM-IV:
  - Exam is lengthy and time consuming.
  - Not appropriate for many ICU patients
- CAM-ICU is well validated and requires less time for full assessment.
- Confusion assessment method (CAM) developed so that nonpsychiatrists could assess key delirium features and identify patients with delirium quickly and accurately.
- Four features:
  - An acute onset of mental status changes and a fluctuating course.
  - Inattention
  - Disorganized thinking
  - A level of consciousness other than alert
- Patients are determined to be delirious (i.e., CAM positive) if they have both features 1 and 2 and either feature 3 or 4.
- This is the most widely implemented and user-friendly method of objectively measuring delirium, with sensitivity of 94–100%, specificity between 90–95%, excellent interobserver reliability (κ of 0.81–1.0).
- Best combination of ease, speed of use, data acquisition, reliability, and validity
- Any medical condition can precipitate delirium in a susceptible host; multiple underlying conditions are often found. The conditions noted most include:
  - Infections (urinary tract, respiratory tract, skin and soft-tissue)
  - Fluid and electrolyte disturbances (dehydration, hyponatremia/hypernatremia)
  - Drug toxicity
  - Metabolic disorders (hypoglycemia, hypercalcemia, uremia, liver failure)
  - Low perfusion states (shock, heart failure)
  - Withdrawal from alcohol and sedatives.

HISTORY
- Time course of mental status changes
- Recent medication changes
- Symptoms of infection
- New neurologic signs

ALERT
- Key diagnostic features of CAM-ICU
- Acute change in mental status that fluctuates
- Abnormal attention and either disorganized thinking or altered level of consciousness
- Any of the following nondiagnostic symptoms may be present:
- Short- and long-term memory problems
- Sleep–wake cycle disturbances'
- Hallucinations and/or delusions
- Emotional lability
- Tremors and asterixis
- Subtypes based on level of consciousness:
- Hyperactive delirium (15%): Patients are loud, rambunctious, and disruptive
- Hypoactive delirium (20%): Quietly confused; may sit and not eat, drink, or move
- Mixed delirium (50%): Features of both hyperactive and hypoactive delirium
- Normal consciousness delirium (15%): Still display disorganized thinking, along with acute onset, inattention, and fluctuation
- Current consensus is to consistently use the overall term delirium and subcategorize according to psychomotor symptoms (hyper-/hypoactive, or mixed).
- Hyperactive delirium, in the past referred to as ICU psychosis, is rare in the pure form and is associated with a better overall prognosis.
- It is characterized by agitation, restlessness, attempting to remove catheters, and emotional lability.
- Hypoactive delirium is very common and more damaging to the patient in the long term, goes unrecognized in 66–84% of hospitalized patients as the lack of activity does not appear problematic.
- Subtype is characterized by withdrawal, flat affect, apathy, lethargy, and decreased responsiveness.
- Some refer to hypoactive delirium as encephalopathy, restricting "delirium" to hyperactive patients.

PHYSICAL EXAM
- Focal neurologic signs are usually absent.
- Mini Mental Status Exam is helpful as structured interview, and followed over time.

DIAGNOSTIC TESTS & INTERPRETATION
Lab
Initial lab tests
- CBC
- Electrolytes, BUN, creatinine
- Urinalysis and urine culture
- Medication levels where applicable

Follow-Up & Special Considerations
Vigilant and frequent assessment with CAM-ICU

Imaging
Initial approach
- No specific exams
- Guided by clinical indications of underlying illness

Follow-Up & Special Considerations
Noncontrast head CT scan if:
- Unclear diagnosis
- Recent fall or trauma
- Anticoagulant use
- New focal neurologic signs

Diagnostic Procedures/Other
- Lumbar puncture:
  - Rarely necessary
  - Perform if clinical suspicion for CNS bleed or infection is substantial
- EEG:
  - Rarely necessary; consider after above evaluation if diagnosis remains unclear
  - Suspicion of seizure activity; nonconvulsive status epilepticus

DIFFERENTIAL DIAGNOSIS
- Depression
- Dementia
- Psychosis

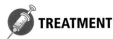

TREATMENT

MEDICATION
First Line
- There are currently no drugs with regulatory approval for the treatment of delirium.
- SCCM Recommendation: Haloperidol is the preferred agent for the treatment of delirium in critically ill patients (recommendation grade C).
- Patients should be monitored for ECG changes (QT interval prolongation and arrhythmias) when receiving haloperidol (B)

Second Line
- The atypical antipsychotics (e.g., aripiprazole, olanzapine, quetiapine, and ziprasidone) may also be helpful.
- MOA similar to haloperidol, but, in addition to dopamine, they affect a multiple neurotransmitters, including norepinephrine, serotonin, histamine, and acetylcholine.

ADDITIONAL TREATMENT
General Measures
- Nonpharmacologic prevention and treatment: In the non-ICU setting, risk factor modification has resulted in a 40% relative reduction in the development of delirium:
  - Repeated reorientation of patients
  - Repetitive cognitive stimulation
  - Nonpharmacologic sleep protocol
  - Early mobilization
  - Range-of-motion exercises
  - Timely removal of catheters and physical restraints
  - Use of eyeglasses and magnifying lenses
  - Hearing aids and earwax disimpaction
  - Adequate hydration
  - Use of scheduled pain protocol, and minimization of unnecessary noise/stimuli.
  - Delirium-specific multidisciplinary education and nurse-led intervention programs
- SCCM Recommendation: Sleep promotion should include optimization of environment and nonpharmacologic methods to promote relaxation with adjunctive use of hypnotics (B).
- Some emerging evidence that use of dexmedetomidine (Precedex), given beyond its approved 24-hour use, may equal benzodiazepines for sedation in the ICU and with less delirium
- Daily interruption of sedatives in mechanically ventilated patients

IN-PATIENT CONSIDERATIONS
Admission Criteria
ICU delirium develops in patients previously admitted to the ICU.

IV Fluids
As needed for dehydration or treatment of underlying conditions

Nursing
- Skin care program incontinent patients
- Turning regimen if at risk for pressure ulcers
- Soft restraints acceptable for short periods if needed for protection of patient and others
- Nursing protocols to better manage pain demonstrated to reduce severity and duration, but not incidence, of delirium.

Discharge Criteria
- Resolution of precipitating factor(s)
- Safe discharge site if still delirious

 ONGOING CARE

FOLLOW-UP RECOMMENDATIONS
- Delirium at hospital discharge usually requires continued care in post-acute facility.
- If no delirium at hospital discharge, follow-up with primary care physician in 1–2 weeks

Patient Monitoring
- Evaluate and assess mental status daily.
- Level and methods of monitoring based on underlying medical conditions requiring ICU care

DIET
- Dentures used properly
- Proper positioning for meals
- Assistance with meals when necessary
- Nutritional supplements if poor intake
- Temporary NG tube if functional GI tract and unable to eat

COMPLICATIONS
- Falls
- Pressure ulcers
- Malnutrition
- Functional decline
- Oversedation
- Polypharmacy
- Prolonged mechanical ventilation
- Self-extubation
- Patient injury
- Respiratory complications
- Longstanding neuropsychological deficits
- Prolonged length of stay
- Death

ADDITIONAL READING
- Francis J, Jr. Prevention and treatment of delirium and confusional states. UpToDate 2009
- Jacobi J, et al. Clinical practice guidelines for the sustained use of sedatives and analgesics in the critically ill adult. Clinical Investigations. *Crit Care Med*. 2002;30(1):119–41.
- Pun BT, et al. The importance of diagnosing and managing ICU delirium. *Chest*. 2007;132(2): 624–36.
- Wesley EE. The delirium dilemma: Advances in thinking about diagnosis, management, and importance of ICU delirium. *Clinical Web Journal*. Jan 2006;21(6).
- Wesley EE. Delirium in the intensive care unit: An under-recognized syndrome of organ dysfunction. *Semin Resp Crit Care Med*. 2001;22(2):115–26.

CODES

ICD9
- 292.81 Drug-induced delirium
- 293.0 Delirium due to conditions classified elsewhere
- 780.09 Alteration of consciousness, other

CLINICAL PEARLS
- Someone who is attentive is not delirious. Inattention is pivotal in the diagnosis of delirium.
- Those meeting some features but not full criteria may have subsyndromal delirium.
- Most delirium is hypoactive and will be missed if not actively looked for.
- Delirium may not resolve as soon as the treatable contributors are fixed; resolution may take weeks or months. Rarely will become chronic.
- Avoid diphenhydramine in older patients.
- Nonpharmacologic measures are preferable as a sleep aid, but if needed:
  - Zolpidem 5 mg h.s.
  - Trazodone 25 mg h.s.

DIABETES INSIPIDUS

Joseph Ng
Roopa Kohli-Seth

 BASICS

DESCRIPTION
- Polyuric disorder resulting from insufficient production of antidiuretic hormone (ADH) (central DI) or unresponsiveness of the renal tubules to ADH (nephrogenic DI)
  - Both can be hereditary or acquired
  - Inadequate secretion of vasopressin may be due to the loss or dysfunction of neurosecretory neurons of the posterior pituitary
  - Vasopressin insensitivity leads to failure to reabsorb water
- System(s) affected: Renal, Endocrine/Metabolic

EPIDEMIOLOGY
Incidence
- Central DI affects 1 out of every 25,000
- Central DI occurs in 15.4% of all patients with severe head trauma
- 33% of Central DI occur without an identifiable lesion
- Medications cause 12–30% of Nephrogenic DI

Prevalence
- Central DI affects men and women equally
- DI can occur in any age group

RISK FACTORS
- Central DI:
  - Neoplastic disease: Craniopharyngioma, lymphoma, meningioma, metastatic carcinoma
  - Ischemic or hypoxic disorder
  - Head trauma or surgery
  - Viral encephalitis
  - Bacterial meningitis
  - Autoimmune disorders
- Nephrogenic DI:
  - Hyperkalemia, hypercalcemia
  - Postrenal obstruction
  - Drugs: Lithium, demeclocycline, methoxyflurane
  - Sickle cell
  - Amyloidosis
  - Pregnancy

Genetics
- About 90% of patients with congenital nephrogenic DI are males with the X-linked recessive form of the disease who have mutations in the arginine vasopressin receptor 2 gene (AVPR2)
- Familial cases of DI have been reported in Wolfram syndrome, a rare autosomal recessive disorder

PATHOPHYSIOLOGY
- Central DI can be either permanent or transient, reflecting the natural history of the underlying disorder.
- Destruction of the hypothalamus or at least some of the supraoptic-hypophysial tract, rather than just posterior pituitary for permanent DI and <15% of the vasopressin-secreting cells of the hypothalamus are intact.
- Cessation of vasopressin secretion resulting from acute injury with neuronal shock and edema in transient DI
- Familial nephrogenic DI is the result of a generalized defect in either the V2 class of vasopressin receptors or the aquaporin-2 water channel of the renal collecting ducts.
- Drug-induced nephrogenic DI appears to result from sensitivity of the vasopressin receptor to lithium, fluoride, and other salts.

ETIOLOGY
- Diseases of the CNS (central DI), affecting the synthesis or secretion of vasopressin
- Diseases of the kidney (nephrogenic DI), with loss of the kidney's ability to respond to circulating vasopressin with inability to retain water
- In pregnancy, probable increased metabolic clearance of vasopressin

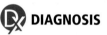 **DIAGNOSIS**

SIGNS AND SYMPTOMS
- Thirst/polydipsia
- Polyuria
- Nocturia
- Hypernatremia
- Dehydration
- Headache

DIAGNOSTIC TESTS & INTERPRETATION
Lab
Initial lab tests
- Urinary response to exogenous vasopressin is used to differentiate between nephrogenic DI and central DI. (Increases vol. in CDI) (1)[A]
- Urine osmolality <200 mOsmol/kg in the presence of polyuria (2)[A]
- Urine electrolytes
- Serum electrolytes (hypernatremia)
- Low urine osmolality with relatively elevated plasma osmolarity
- Urine glucose (rule out diabetes mellitus)

Follow-Up & Special Considerations
- Drugs that may alter lab results: Lithium, demeclocycline, methoxyflurane
- Coexistence of glucocorticoid deficiency may "mask" the presence of central DI. The development of polyuria with the initiation of glucocorticoid replacement should alert the clinician to the possible presence of DI.

Imaging
MRI of the pituitary and hypothalamus and of the skull is done to look for mass lesions

Diagnostic Procedures/Other
- Vasopressin challenge test
- Desmopressin acetate is given in an initial dose of 0.05–0.1 mL (5–10 mcg) intranasally (or 1 mcg SC or IV), with measurement of urine volume for 12 hours before and 12 hours after administration.
- The dosage of desmopressin is doubled if the response is marginal.
- Plasma vasopressin or urinary vasopressin following osmotic stimulus, such as fluid restriction or administration of hypertonic saline

Pathological Findings
Degeneration of neurosecretory neurons in the neurohypophysis

DIFFERENTIAL DIAGNOSIS
- Diabetes mellitus
- Cushing syndrome
- Corticosteroid treatment
- Nocturnal polyuria of Parkinson disease
- Psychogenic polydipsia
- Central nervous system sarcoidosis
- Iatrogenic fluid administration
- Cerebral salt wasting

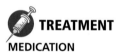 **TREATMENT**

MEDICATION
Central DI

- DDAVP (desmopressin) (3)[A]

  - Oral starting dose of 0.05 mg b.i.d. and increased to a maximum of 0.4 mg q8h as needed
  - Nasal preparation (100 mcg/mL solution) is given q12–24h as needed for thirst and polyuria. It may be administered via metered-dose nasal inhaler containing 0.1 mL/spray or via a plastic calibrated tube. Patients are started with 0.05–0.1 mL q12–24h, and the dose is then individualized according to response

- Hypotonic fluid to hydrate and correct osmolarity
- Clofibrate
- Carbamazepine
- Thiazide diuretics

Nephrogenic DI
- Cyclooxygenase inhibitors (e.g., indomethacin, 100 mg/d in divided doses)
- Thiazide diuretics
- Correcting electrolyte disturbance (K^+, Ca^{++})
- Stopping offending medication

Contraindications
Desmopressin should be used with caution in the immediate postoperative period for intracranial lesions because of possible cerebral edema

Precautions
Overdose of desmopressin may produce water intoxication in patients with excessive water intake

ADDITIONAL TREATMENT
Issues for Referral
- Chronic DI can lead to renal dysfunction
- Complications of the primary disease
- Neurosurgical intervention for tumor

Additional Therapies
- Chlorpropamide 250–500 mg/day reduces polyuria and polydipsia
- Clofibrate at a maximum dose of 1 g t.i.d. also has an antidiuretic effect

IN-PATIENT CONSIDERATIONS
Initial Stabilization
- Control fluid balance and prevent dehydration
- Check weight daily
- Provide good skin and mouth care

Admission Criteria
Initial diagnosis and management may be serious enough to require hospitalization.

IV Fluids
Rehydration with hypotonic fluids can help with water deficit as well as correcting osmolarity.

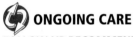

ONGOING CARE

FOLLOW-UP RECOMMENDATIONS
Regular follow-ups, at two weeks initially and then 3 to 4 months afterwards

Patient Monitoring
- Electrolytes and renal function should be monitored carefully to avoid further complications
- Normal diet with free access to fluids

PATIENT EDUCATION
- Satiation of thirst as needed.
- Medical alert bracelets or tags may help notify first responders of condition and appropriate treatment.

PROGNOSIS
- Central DI appearing after pituitary surgery or trauma may be permanent if the upper pituitary stalk is cut. However, it usually remits after days to weeks.
- Treatment with desmopressin allows normal sleep and activity.
- Hypernatremia can occur, but DI does not otherwise reduce life expectancy, and the prognosis is that of the underlying disorder.

COMPLICATIONS
- If left untreated, polyuria secondary to DI can lead to dilation of the collecting system, hydronephrosis, and renal dysfunction.
- Complications of primary disease should be anticipated.
- Mental and growth retardation may be associated with some patients who have nephrogenic DI.
- Overly rapid correction of the hyperosmolarity can result in cerebral edema.
  - Careful correction of water deficit can avoid this deadly complication.

Pediatric Considerations
Nephrogenic DI usually manifest in infancy

REFERENCES
1. Singer I, et al. The management of diabetes insipidus in adults. *Arch Intern Med*. 1997; 157:1293–1301.
2. Makaryus AN, et al. Diabetes insipidus: Diagnosis and treatment of a complex disease. *Clev Clin J Med*. 2006;731:65–71.
3. Lam KS, et al. Pharmacokinetics, pharmacodynamics, long-term efficacy, and safety of oral 1-deamino-8-D-arginine vasopressin in adult patients with central diabetes insipidus. *Br J Clin Pharmacol*. 1996;42:379–385

ADDITIONAL READING
- The Diabetes Insipidus Foundation: "What is Diabetes Insipidus?"
- Hadjizacharia P, et al. Acute diabetes insipidus in severe head injury: A prospective study. *J Am Coll Surg*. 2008;207(4):477–84.
- Morello JP, et al. Nephrogenic diabetes insipidus. *Annu Rev Physiol*. 2001;63:607–30.

CODES

ICD9
- 253.5 Diabetes insipidus
- 588.1 Nephrogenic diabetes insipidus

CLINICAL PEARLS
- Decreased uOsm and sOsm suggests psychogenic polydipsia
- Demeclocycline and other tetracyclines cause permanent if subtle nephrogenic DI; be cautious using them for acne during puberty
- Water deprivation test:
  - Baseline uOsm and sOsm
  - No further water intake: For mild cases may need to withhold water overnight
  - Measure hourly uOsm and weight
  - When uOsm stabilizes (but change <30 mmol/kg over 2 consecutive measures or loss of 3–5% of body weight), give 5 U aqueous vasopressin SC
  - Repeat uOsm 1 hour later
- Interpretation:
  - Normal: uOsm rises to 2–4 times that of plasma osmolarity, and <9% further increase with DDAVP
  - Polydipsia: Washed out concentration gradient, <9% increase with DDAVP
  - Central DI: uOsm does not increase over plasma osmolarity, >50% increase with DDAVP
  - Nephrogenic DI: no increase in uOsm; no response to DDAVP

D

DIABETIC KETOACIDOSIS

Tajender S. Vasu
Paul Marik

BASICS

DESCRIPTION
- Diabetic ketoacidosis (DKA) is a potentially life threatening hyperglycemic complication of diabetes mellitus (DM).
- It is characterized by a triad of hyperglycemia, ketosis, and metabolic acidosis.
- It most commonly occurs in patients with type 1 DM, although it may occasionally occur in type 2 DM.

EPIDEMIOLOGY
Incidence
- The annual incidence of DKA varies from 4.6–8 episodes per 1000 patients with DM.
- In 20–30% of patients, DKA is the presenting feature of new-onset diabetes.

Prevalence
The prevalence of DKA decreases significantly with age from 36% in children <5 years of age to 16% in those >14 years.

RISK FACTORS
- Noncompliance or inadequate insulin treatment
- New onset DM
- Infections (commonly urinary tract infection, pneumonia or sepsis)
- Pregnancy
- Myocardial infarction
- Stroke
- Acute pancreatitis
- Pulmonary embolism
- Protracted vomiting
- Drugs such as corticosteroids, pentamidine, sympathomimetic agents, α- and β-adrenergic blockers, and excessive use of diuretics
- In 2–10% of cases, no risk factor is identified.

GENERAL PREVENTION
- Patient diabetic education
- Assessment and maintenance of compliance to treatment

PATHOPHYSIOLOGY
- DKA commonly results from an absolute or relative deficiency of insulin in combination with increased level of stress hormones (glucagon, cortisol, growth hormone, and catecholamines).
- Most of the pathophysiologic changes occur in liver, adipose tissue, peripheral tissue, and kidney.

- Liver:
  - Lack of insulin in combination with increased level of stress hormones causes increased hepatic glycolysis and gluconeogenesis.
  - This hormonal imbalance also increases the fatty acid oxidation in the liver, which leads to increased production of ketone bodies (acetoacetate, β-hydroxybutyrate, and acetone)
- Adipose tissue:
  - Insulin deficiency stimulates the tissue lipase, which promotes lipolysis in adipose tissue and release of free fatty acids.
- Peripheral tissues:
  - Decreased glucose utilization by peripheral tissues and insulin resistance result in hyperglycemia.
- Kidneys:
  - The normal renal threshold for glucose reabsorption is >240 mg/dL.
  - Increased glucose level causes osmotic diuresis, leading to hypovolemia.
  - The glucosuria-induced osmotic diuresis also results in total body sodium and potassium deficiency.

DIAGNOSIS

HISTORY
- Patients with DKA may present with any of the following symptoms:
  - Polyuria, polydipsia, or weight loss
  - Nausea, vomiting, or abdominal pain
  - Confusion
  - Coma (presenting feature in 10%)
  - Fatigue, or malaise
  - Shortness of breath

PHYSICAL EXAM
- Hypotension, tachycardia, or dry mucus membrane due to volume depletion
- Kussmaul breathing (very rapid and deep respiration)
- Fruity odor to the breath due to the presence of acetone
- Hypothermia

DIAGNOSTIC TESTS & INTERPRETATION
Lab
- Initial lab test should include serum glucose, sodium, potassium, chloride, creatinine, BUN, ABG, and urinary ketones
- CBC with differentials, EKG, urine analysis and culture, and blood culture should also be obtained.
- The following laboratory findings may help in making the diagnosis:
  - Blood glucose (BG) >250 mg/dL
  - pH <7.30 (high anion gap metabolic acidosis)
  - Serum bicarbonate of <15 mEq/L
  - Urinary ketones of greater than 3+
  - Positive serum ketones (i.e., β-hydroxybutyrate and acetoacetate >3 mmol/L)

- β-hydroxybutyrate is the predominant ketone body that contributes to acidosis in DKA
- Euglycemic DKA:
  - In a small percentage of cases of DKA, the glucose levels are not elevated at presentation.
  - It is usually seen in patients with excessive vomiting and continued insulin administration.
  - β-hydroxybutyrate is very useful for monitoring these patients.
- Elevated serum transaminases are seen in 25–50% of cases.
- Serum creatine kinase is elevated in 25–40% of cases in the absence of MI.
- Amylase and lipase levels are elevated in 16–25% of cases in the absence of acute pancreatitis.

Imaging
Chest radiograph should be obtained to rule out pneumonia as a precipitating factor.

DIFFERENTIAL DIAGNOSIS
- Alcoholic ketoacidosis
- Hyperglycemic hyperosmolar syndrome
- Starvation ketosis
- Lactic acidosis
- Poisoning (salicylate, ethylene glycol, paraldehyde, and methanol)

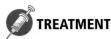

TREATMENT

MEDICATION
First Line
- The cause of DKA should be identified and treated.
- Aggressive fluid replacement (C) is the priority in the treatment of DKA because patients are usually 5–8 L fluid deficient:
  - Give 1 L of 0.9% NaCl over 30–60 minutes. Give an additional 1–2 L q30–60min until hemodynamically stable and urine output is increased.
  - Change to 0.45% NaCl and infuse at 150–500 mL/hr.
  - When BG <250 mg/dL, add dextrose 5% at 100–200 mL/hr.
  - Continue D5 $\frac{1}{2}$ NS until ketosis clears and patient is able to take fluids orally.
- Insulin treatment (B):
  - Bolus of 0.1–0.15 U/kg of regular insulin intravenously
  - Begin continuous IV infusion of regular insulin at 0.1 U/kg/hr.
  - Check BG q1H and, once stable, change BG monitoring to q2h
  - Keep the goal to decrease BG by 50–75 mg/dL/hr.
  - Decrease insulin infusion by 50%/hr if BG decreases by >100 mg/dL/hr in any 1 hour period.
  - Increase insulin infusion by 50%/hr if change in blood glucose is <50 mg/dL/hr.

- Add dextrose 5% to IV fluids when BG <250 mg/dL, and keep the goal BG 150–200 mg/dL until anion gap closed.
- Stop the insulin drip once anion gap is closed, serum bicarbonate is >15 mEq/L, and patient is able to eat.
- Before stopping the insulin infusion, administer short-acting insulin (Aspart or Lispro) SC at twice the hourly IV rate (e.g., if IV rate is 5 U/hr, give 10 U short-acting insulin SC) and also give long-acting insulin (regular, NPH or glargine) SC at 0.2–0.3 U/kg, or home insulin dose.
- To prevent relapse of DKA, the IV insulin infusion should be continued for 30 minutes after the 1st subcutaneous dose of regular insulin has been given.
- Potassium (K$^+$) replacement:
  - In general, 100–200 mEq of K$^+$ will be required in the first 24–36 hours.
  - If initial K$^+$ is <3.3 mEq/L, hold IV insulin and give 40 mEq of K$^+$ until serum K$^+$ is >3.3 mEq/L.
  - If serum K$^+$ ≥ 5.5 mEq/L, do not give K$^+$ but check it q2h.
  - If K$^+$ is 4–5.4 mEq/L; add 20 mEq KCl/L to IVF.
  - If K$^+$ is 3–3.9 mEq/L; add 40 mEq KCl/L to IVF.

Second Line
- Bicarbonate replacement is usually not necessary. (C)
- Consider bicarbonate replacement in following conditions:
  - Severe acidosis with pH <7 (stop it once the pH is >7.1)
  - Acidosis-induced cardiac or respiratory distress
  - Severe loss of buffering capacity when serum bicarbonate is <5–10 mEq/L
  - Severe hyperkalemia
  - Give sodium bicarbonate as 1–2 ampules (total of 44–88 mEq) in 1L of 0.45% NS per hour
- Routine phosphate replacement is not necessary (C):
  - Consider replacement if serum phosphate is <1 mg/dL
  - Give 30–60 mM potassium phosphate over 24 hours
  - Potential complications of phosphate treatment include hypocalcemia, hypomagnesemia, and metastatic soft-tissue calcifications.

ADDITIONAL TREATMENT
Additional Therapies
- Adjunctive therapies are used according to clinical indications.
- Broad-spectrum antibiotics may be used to treat underlying infections.
- Low-molecular-weight heparin or unfractionated heparin may be used for DVT prophylaxis.

IN-PATIENT CONSIDERATIONS
Initial Stabilization
- Stabilization of hemodynamic parameters
- Aggressive fluid replacement

Admission Criteria
- Hemodynamic instability
- Obtundation
- Inability to defend the airway
- Presence of abdominal distension
- If insulin infusion cannot be administered on the floor
- If frequent monitoring of fingerstick glucose and laboratory testing cannot be provided on the floor

IV Fluids
Aggressive volume resuscitation is required because patients are usually 5–8 L fluid deficient.

Nursing
- Frequent or continuous monitoring of heart rate, blood pressure, respiratory rate, and urine output
- Monitoring of serum glucose should be done q1–2h during treatment.
- Serum electrolytes, phosphate, and pH should be checked q2–6h, depending on the clinical response.

Discharge Criteria
- Hemodynamic stability
- Resolving electrolyte abnormalities
- Patient is alert and able to eat

 ONGOING CARE

FOLLOW-UP RECOMMENDATIONS
- Patients should have follow-up with their primary care physicians (PCP) upon discharge.
- Prevention of recurrence should be the goal.

Patient Monitoring
- Monitoring of HbA1C, foot exam, and ophthalmology exam, as per recommendations of PCP
- Assessment of adherence to treatment
- Assessment of psychosocial or family problems, including depression, eating disorder, or medical neglect

DIET
Diabetic diet

PATIENT EDUCATION
Patients should receive diabetic education including the use of short-acting insulin, blood glucose, and urinary ketone monitoring

PROGNOSIS
- It is a potentially life-threatening disorder with mortality rate of 2–5%.
- The mortality rate varies depending on:
  - Age
  - Severity of DKA
  - Presence of concomitant illnesses

COMPLICATIONS
- Cerebral edema
- Venous thromboembolism
- ARDS
- Aspiration pneumonia
- Rhinocerebral mucormycosis
- Hypoglycemia
- Acute gastric dilatation
- Electrolyte imbalance (hypokalemia, hypophosphatemia)
- Hyperchloremic normal anion gap metabolic acidosis
- Cardiac arrhythmia
- Fluid overload
- Rhabdomyolysis with or without malignant hyperthermia

ADDITIONAL READING
- Kitabchi AE, et al. Management of hyperglycemic crises in patients with diabetes. *Diabetes Care.* 2001;24(1):131–53.
- Lebovitz HE. Diabetic ketoacidosis. *Lancet.* 1995; 345:767–72.
- Magee MF, et al. Management of decompensated diabetes. Diabetic ketoacidosis and hyperglycemic hyperosmolar syndrome. *Crit Care Clin.* 2001; 17(1):75–106.
- Sharma V, et al. Diabetic ketoacidosis: Principles of management. *Br J Hosp Med.* 2007;68(4):184–9.

 CODES

ICD9
- 250.10 Diabetes mellitus with ketoacidosis type ii or unspecified type, not stated as uncontrolled
- 250.11 Diabetes mellitus with ketoacidosis, type I (juvenile type) not stated as uncontrolled

CLINICAL PEARLS
- Diabetic ketoacidosis is characterized by a triad of hyperglycemia, ketosis, and metabolic acidosis.
- It results from relative or absolute deficiency of insulin in combination with increased levels of stress hormones.
- Aggressive fluid and electrolyte replacement along with insulin are very important steps in its management.
- It is a potentially life-threatening condition, and patient education may help prevent its recurrence.

DIARRHEA IN THE ICU
Oveys Mansuri

 BASICS

DESCRIPTION
- Diarrhea can be generally defined as alterations in bowel movements resulting in increased frequency and abnormally loose or watery consistency. Clinically, it has been more specifically defined as >3 bowel movements per day, or volume >300–500 g.
- The most concerning form of diarrhea is *Clostridium difficile* toxin-induced diarrhea, which occurs in patients with exposure to broad-spectrum antibiotics and can lead to rapid development of toxic megacolon and septic shock.

EPIDEMIOLOGY
Incidence
One 12-month prospective study of ICU patients admitted for >48 hours demonstrated a 41% incidence of diarrhea.

RISK FACTORS
- ICU admission
- Enteral feeding following long-term NPO status
- Hyperosmolar enteric feed
- Exposure to broad-spectrum antibiotics (may lead to *C. difficile* diarrhea)

Geriatric Considerations
Increased concern for fecal impaction or tumor

Pediatric Considerations
Rotavirus is most common cause of viral diarrhea.

Pregnancy Considerations
- Close monitoring of fetus; consider Ob-Gyn consult if indicated
- Ensure adequate volume resuscitation.
- Optimize medical management to minimize risk to fetus (i.e., contraindicated medications in pregnant patients).

GENERAL PREVENTION
- Hand hygiene, including washing hands with soap for spore-forming bacterial (i.e., *C. diff*), and routine use of gloves
- Development of protocols involving infection control, health care workers, pharmaceutical intervention

PATHOPHYSIOLOGY
- Secretory: Mediated by increased cyclic adenosine monophosphate inhibiting absorption of sodium and promoting secretion of fluids into bowel lumen
- Infection: Increased mucous secretions from large bowel as seen with *C. diff* colitis
- Osmotic load: Increased osmotic load from medications, incomplete digestion and malabsorption (common in ICU setting)
- Medication: Promotility agents and antibiotic-related alteration of gut flora

ETIOLOGY
- Noninfectious: Bacterial overgrowth, enteral feeding, fecal impaction, inflammatory bowel disease, intestinal ischemia, malabsorption, medications, psychological stress, tumors
- Infectious:
  – *Clostridium difficile*
  – *Salmonella*
  – Rotavirus
  – Norovirus

COMMONLY ASSOCIATED CONDITIONS
Exposure to broad-spectrum antibiotics (for *C. diff* colitis)

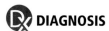 **DIAGNOSIS**

HISTORY
- May be difficult to obtain in some ICU patients
- Onset, duration, frequency, and character
- Enteral intake
- Antibiotic history
- Associated symptoms: i.e., abdominal pain, bloody diarrhea

PHYSICAL EXAM
- Abdominal distension and tenderness
- Fever
- Rectal exam

DIAGNOSTIC TESTS & INTERPRETATION
Lab
- CBC: Increased WBC may indicate infectious process; bandemia indicates bacterial infection.
- Serum chemistry panel: Hypernatremia from volume loss, hypokalemia from diarrhea, increased BUN/Cr from dehydration
- Stool sample: Occult blood, fecal leukocytes, cultures, ova/parasites, *C. difficile* toxin test

Imaging
- Abdominal x-ray in cases involving abdominal pain and/or concern for obstruction
- CT scan of abdomen/pelvis if abdominal x-ray inconclusive/nondiagnostic, persistent/worsening symptoms, concern for colitis

Diagnostic Procedures/Other
Colonoscopy for evaluation of bloody diarrhea or concern for colitis

DIFFERENTIAL DIAGNOSIS
- Medications
- Enteral feeding
- Colitis
- Ischemic bowel disease
- GI bleeding
- Postsurgical diarrhea
- Fecal impaction
- Opiate withdrawal
- Inflammatory bowel disease
- Celiac sprue

TREATMENT

MEDICATION
First Line
- Stop any medications that may be causing the diarrhea (i.e., antibiotics, pro-motility agents)
- Loperamide 4 mg initially, followed by 2 mg q30min (max 8 doses). [should not be used if any suspicion of infectious etiology, i.e., *C. diff* colitis]
- Antibiotics: Specific treatment protocols by infectious disease guidelines for specific organisms or parasites
- As severe *C. diff* colitis has a high mortality, it is advisable to treat patients with IV/PO Flagyl 500 mg t.i.d. until toxin tests are negative as long as the clinical scenario and symptoms suggest *C. diff* colitis.

ADDITIONAL TREATMENT
General Measures
- Appropriate fluid resuscitation and electrolyte replacement
- Identify any underlying causes and eliminate or modify (i.e., medications, enteral feeds)

Issues for Referral
Early surgical consult is advised if severe *C. diff* colitis is suspected and if the development of toxic megacolon is suspected and the patient's condition is rapidly deteriorating.

COMPLEMENTARY & ALTERNATIVE THERAPIES
- Bulk-forming agents in appropriate dosage for benign diarrhea
- Prebiotic and probiotic administration

SURGERY/OTHER PROCEDURES
As indicated by surgical consultation for ischemic bowel, toxic megacolon, persistent bowel obstruction, or other surgical indication

IN-PATIENT CONSIDERATIONS
Initial Stabilization
Fluid and electrolyte replacement

Admission Criteria
ICU admission should be considered for extremes of age, hemodynamic instability, severe infection, marked electrolyte abnormality, and/or need for close and constant monitoring.

IV Fluids
- Adequate fluid resuscitation with crystalloid replacement (i.e., 0.9% NS or LR)
- Ensure appropriate access and consider central venous access if inadequate access or need for monitoring volume status (CVP).

Nursing
- Patient comfort
- Frequent and routine hygiene for diarrhea symptoms, with special attention to open wounds or pressure ulcers in ICU patient population

Discharge Criteria
Resolution or significant improvement in the clinical signs

 ONGOING CARE

FOLLOW-UP RECOMMENDATIONS
At discharge from ICU, generated detailed sign-out assuring safe and seamless transfer of care to floor or for discharge to home and follow-up with primary care physician.

Patient Monitoring
Follow-up labs as appropriate, including but not limited to monitoring WBC, continued *C. diff* precautions in accordance with infection control policy, and antibiotic levels as required

DIET
May range from NPO to regular or modified diet depending on underlying cause of diarrhea

PROGNOSIS
Generally very good for benign diarrhea, variable (depending on comorbidities and severity if colitis) for *C. diff* colitis-related diarrhea

COMPLICATIONS
- Severe and/or persistent diarrhea may lead to electrolyte abnormalities, hypovolemia, renal failure, malnutrition.
- Uncontrolled infection may result in sepsis, bowel ischemia/perforation, toxic megacolon requiring emergent surgical intervention.
- Death

ADDITIONAL READING
- Bobo L, et al. Recognition and prevention of hospital-associated enteric infections in the intensive care unit. *Crit Care Med*. 2010;38:S324–34.
- Kelly TWJ, et al. Study of diarrhea in critically ill patients. *Crit Care Med*. 1983;11:7–9.
- Kim JH, et al. *Clostridium difficile* enteritis: A review and pooled analysis of the cases. *Anaerobe*. 2011; doi:10.1016/j.anaerobe.2011.02.002.

CODES
ICD9
- 557.9 Unspecified vascular insufficiency of intestine
- 558.9 Other and unspecified noninfectious gastroenteritis and colitis
- 787.91 Diarrhea

CLINICAL PEARLS
- Maybe benign or related to infections
- Poorly studied in ICU setting (except for *C. diff* colitis)
- Most worrisome is *C. diff* colitis, particularly its rapidly advancing, severe form
- Variable definitions
- Resuscitate patient appropriately.
- Identify underlying cause and remove, modify, or treat.
- Maintain close follow-up and retest as needed.
- Careful use of medications in cases of antiperistalsis agents as well as antibiotics
- Follow infectious control guidelines for *C. diff* colitis cases or epidemic diarrhea.

DIGOXIN TOXICITY

M. Kamran Athar

 BASICS

DESCRIPTION
Potentially life-threatening intoxication

EPIDEMIOLOGY
Incidence
- ~50% cases occur in patients receiving long-term digoxin therapy (1)
- 10%: Accidental overdose
- 40%: Suicidal ingestion
- Reported mortality 3–50% (2,3)

RISK FACTORS
- Any condition that increases total body levels or modifies cardiac sensitivity to the drug.
- Include:
  - Renal insufficiency
  - Advanced age
  - Cardiac diseases (active ischemia, myocarditis, cardiomyopathy, cardiac amyloidosis, cor pulmonale)
  - Metabolic factors (hypokalemia, hypomagnesemia, hypoxemia, hypernatremia, hypercalcemia, and acid–base disturbances)
  - Drugs (quinidine, verapamil, diltiazem, amiodarone, cyclosporine, tetracycline, erythromycin, paroxetine)

PATHOPHYSIOLOGY
- Inhibits Na-K-ATPase, ↑ intracellular Na and Ca.
- In toxic doses:
  - ↓ SA node automaticity
  - ↓ AV node conduction
  - ↑ Automaticity in cardiac muscle, AN node, and conduction cells

ETIOLOGY
Occurs most often during:
- Therapeutic use (chronic)
- Suicidal ingestion (acute)

COMMONLY ASSOCIATED CONDITIONS
- Hypokalemia
- Hyperkalemia
- Renal insufficiency
- Cardiomyopathy
- Myocarditis

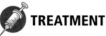 **DIAGNOSIS**

HISTORY
- Careful history to determine any change in digoxin dosing or evidence of acute ingestion
- Addition of medications that increase digoxin levels
- Symptoms are nonspecific and include anorexia, nausea, vomiting (the most common initial presentation)
- Blurred vision, photophobia, scotomata, chromatopsia (altered color perception),
- Confusion, dizziness, delirium, and occasionally hallucinations

PHYSICAL EXAM
- Bradycardia is the most common vital sign abnormality.
- Rest of physical exam is usually unremarkable.

DIAGNOSTIC TESTS & INTERPRETATION
Lab
Initial lab tests
- Serum digoxin levels must be measured at least 6 hours after last dose.
- Chem basic and Mg levels

Follow-Up & Special Considerations
- Serum digoxin levels used only as a guide to indicate toxicity
- Lowered K levels can predispose to toxicity
- Some patients are asymptomatic despite increased levels (4)
- Acute vs. chronic toxicity:
  - Acute is associated with hyperkalemia, tachyarrhythmias, and markedly elevated digoxin levels:
    ○ Hyperkalemia: Predictor of morbidity and mortality in acute poisoning, as it reflects very high tissue levels of digoxin (5)
  - Chronic is associated with hypokalemia, bradyarrhythmias, and minimally elevated or even therapeutic digoxin levels.

Imaging
No imaging studies are needed

Diagnostic Procedures/Other
- All patients should have a 12-lead EKG
- At therapeutic levels prolongation of PR interval and scooping of ST segment can be seen
- Toxic doses: Myriad EKG changes seen
- Ventricular ectopy (PVCs and bigeminy)
- Atrial tachycardias with high-degree AV block
- Ventricular arrhythmias, including ventricular tachycardia and ventricular fibrillation
- Accelerated junctional rhythm and bidirectional ventricular tachycardia: Two rhythms are highly suggestive of digoxin toxicity

DIFFERENTIAL DIAGNOSIS
- Intrinsic cardiac conduction abnormalities (sick sinus syndrome and AV node dysfunction)
- Calcium channel and β-blocker poisoning
- Electrolyte disorders especially hyperkalemia, which can also produce bradycardia

TREATMENT

MEDICATION
- Correct K and Mg abnormalities.
- Digoxin-specific Fab antibody fragments:
  - Binds intravascular digoxin
  - Diffuses into interstitial space and binds digoxin in tissues
- Indications for digoxin-specific Fab (antibody-binding) fragments:
  - Hemodynamic instability due to digoxin toxicity
  - Potentially life-threatening arrhythmias
  - Severe symptomatic bradycardia
  - Serum K >5 mEq/L following acute overdose regardless of clinical status or EKG findings
  - Consider with plasma digoxin concentration >10 ng/mL, regardless of clinical status or EKG findings
  - Altered mental status attributed to digoxin toxicity
  - Presence of a rhythm consistent with digoxin effect in setting of an elevated digoxin level
  - Consider with ingestion of >10 mg in adults or >4 mg in children
  - Effects are usually apparent within an hour.
  - The drug–antibody complexes are excreted in urine.
- Side effects include:
  - Exacerbation of CHF
  - Increased ventricular response in patients with atrial fibrillation
  - Hypokalemia due to movement of K into cells
  - Idiosyncratic allergic reactions (rare)

- Dosing regimen:
  - Digoxin-specific Fab given IV over 15–30 minutes
  - In case of cardiac arrest, give as bolus
  - Simplified calculation of the amount of digoxin needed to treat is: Vials of Fab = [digoxin level (ng/mL) × Mass (Kg)]/100. The results should be rounded up.
  - Each vial (40 mg) can neutralize 0.6 mg of digoxin.
  - If serum drug level or the amounts ingested are unknown, give digoxin-specific Fab empirically according to the following regimen:
    ○ For acute overdose in adults: Give 10 vials
    ○ For chronic toxicity: Give 6 vials to an adult and 1 vial to a child.

ADDITIONAL TREATMENT
General Measures
- GI decontamination with activated charcoal
- Repeated doses may be required because of the enterohepatic circulation of the digoxin metabolites.
- Correct K, Mg, and Ca abnormalities and hypoxemia.

Issues for Referral
In life-threatening cases with hemodynamic instability, emergent consultation with a medical toxicologist may be useful.

Additional Therapies
- Symptomatic bradycardia and 2nd- and 3rd-degree heart block: Atropine, dopamine, epinephrine, isoproterenol
- Electrical pacing may be needed, although pacing wires may precipitate ventricular arrhythmias (6)
- Ventricular arrhythmias: Magnesium sulfate, phenytoin, lidocaine, and amiodarone

IN-PATIENT CONSIDERATIONS
Initial Stabilization
- Serious cases with hemodynamic instability will require admission to ICU.
- In such cases, prepare immediately to infuse digoxin-specific Fab.
- Ensure proper IV access.
- In acute poisoning:
  - Hyperkalemia may normalize after digoxin-specific Fab administration.
  - If hyperkalemia is associated with EKG changes, treat aggressively with the exception that calcium should NOT be administered.
- In chronic toxicity: Correct hypokalemia and hypomagnesemia aggressively, as both potentiate digoxin toxicity.

 ## ONGOING CARE
FOLLOW-UP RECOMMENDATIONS
Patient Monitoring
- Monitor serum K levels in patients receiving digoxin-specific Fab therapy, as these levels fall rapidly after administration.
- Serum digoxin levels are not useful after digoxin-specific Fab therapy, as routine digoxin assays do not differentiate between bound and unbound drug.

PATIENT EDUCATION
- Reassurance of good prognosis
- Monitor medications, especially those that interact with digoxin.

PROGNOSIS
- Excellent, with prompt recognition and treatment
- Mortality rates, previously reported to be as high as 50%, (2) have declined significantly with the introduction of digoxin-specific Fab antibodies.
- A recent retrospective study reported a mortality rate of 6% (3).

COMPLICATIONS
- Life-threatening arrhythmias
- Hyperkalemia in acute poisoning, which can also be life-threatening

Pediatric Considerations
False-positive elevations of serum digoxin can occur in newborns and children, due to increased levels of endogenous digoxin-like substances.

Pregnancy Considerations
Similar false-positive elevations of serum digoxin can occur in pregnant women.

REFERENCES
1. Antman EM, et al. Treatment of 150 cases of life-threatening digitalis intoxication with digoxin-specific Fab antibody fragments. Final report of a multicenter study. Circulation 1990;81:1744.
2. Dick M, et al. Digitalis Intoxication: Recognition and treatment. J Clin Pharmacol. 1991;31:444.
3. Barrueto F Jr, et al. Cardioactive steroid poisoning: A comparison of plant- and animal-derived compounds. J Med Toxicol. 2006;2:152–5.
4. Doherty JE. Digitalis glycosides. Pharmacokinetics and their clinical Implications. Ann Intern Med. 1973;79:229.
5. Bismuth C, et al. Hyperkalemia in acute digitalis poisoning: Prognostic significance and therapeutic implications. Clin Toxicol. 1973;6:153.
6. Taboulet P, et al. Acute digitalis intoxication—is pacing still appropriate? J Toxicil Clin Toxicol. 1993;31:261.

ADDITIONAL READING
- Eddleston M, et al. Anti-digoxin Fab fragments in cardiotoxicity induced by ingestion of yellow oleander: A randomized controlled trial. Lancet. 2000;355:967.
- Williamson KM, et al. Digoxin toxicity: An evaluation in current clinical practice. Arch Intern Med. 1998;158:2444.

CODES

ICD9
972.1 Poisoning by cardiotonic glycosides and drugs of similar action

CLINICAL PEARLS
- In patients taking digoxin, suspect poisoning when a normal or fast heart rate becomes slow or the rhythm becomes regularly irregular.
- Do not treat bradycardia of unknown etiology with calcium until digoxin toxicity is excluded.

DIVERTICULITIS

Oveys Mansuri

 BASICS

DESCRIPTION
Inflammation of 1 or more diverticula (small mucosal herniations forming pouches, usually found in the colon)

EPIDEMIOLOGY
Incidence
Increases with age

Geriatric Considerations
More common in this population

Pediatric Considerations
Rare in this patient population

Prevalence
- <5% before age 40, >65% by age 85
- Male = Female

RISK FACTORS
- Increasing age
- Low-fiber diet
- Lack of exercise
- Previous episode of diverticulitis
- Obesity

GENERAL PREVENTION
- Diet with appropriate fiber
- Exercise
- Keep BMI in normal range

PATHOPHYSIOLOGY
- Fecalith formation in diverticulum eventually leads to inflammation.
- Contained inflammation is considered uncomplicated diverticulitis.
- Complicated diverticulitis arises from serosal perforation with either localized (abscess) or generalized (peritonitis) inflammation.

ETIOLOGY
Diverticulitis occurs in the presence of diverticula that have the following etiology:
- Increased intraluminal pressure in colon
- Congenital weakness of colon wall
- Acquired weakness of colon wall by age or connective tissue abnormalities

COMMONLY ASSOCIATED CONDITIONS
Diverticulosis

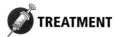 **DIAGNOSIS**

HISTORY
- Left LQ abdominal pain is most common (70%).
- Associated symptoms: Nausea, vomiting, diarrhea, constipation, fevers/chills
- Bowel movement history
- Urinary symptoms, vaginal symptoms
- Prior abdominal surgery, prior colonoscopy and findings
- Dietary history

PHYSICAL EXAM
- Vital signs: Temperature, BP, heart rate
- Localized abdominal tenderness at location of affected diverticula (LLQ most common; evaluate RLQ tenderness carefully to differentiate appendicitis from diverticulitis)
- 20% with palpable mass on abdominal, pelvic, or rectal exam notable for abscess
- Free perforation may cause generalized peritonitis.
- Colovesicular and/or colovaginal fistula formation is seen in severe cases.
- Abdominal exam may be unreliable in patient on steroids or immunosuppression.

DIAGNOSTIC TESTS & INTERPRETATION
Lab
- Elevated WBC (bandemia on differential)
- Decreased hemoglobin if diverticular bleeding
- Chemistry for electrolyte abnormalities (diarrhea)
- Liver panel and lipase for biliary issues and/or pancreatitis
- Consider blood and urine cultures for bacteremia and colovesicular fistulas, respectively.
- Pregnancy test in woman of childbearing age

Imaging
- CT abdomen/pelvis: Pericolic fat stranding, diverticula, bowel wall thickening, phlegmon/abscess
- Plain film x-rays: Not always helpful; may assist with identifying bowel obstruction or bowel perforation by the presence of free air

Diagnostic Procedures/Other
- In acute phase, lower endoscopy is *NOT* recommended given increased risk of perforation.
- Colonoscopy can be used after resolution of acute episode.

Pathological Findings
Diverticulum, inflammation, perforation

DIFFERENTIAL DIAGNOSIS
- Appendicitis
- Cholecystitis
- Chronic mesenteric ischemia
- Colonic obstruction
- Gastric/duodenal ulcers
- Gastroenteritis
- Bowel perforation
- IBS
- Inflammatory bowel disease
- Nephrolithiasis
- Pancreatitis
- Pelvic inflammatory disease
- UTI

Pregnancy Considerations
Consider differential diagnosis (i.e., pelvic inflammatory disease, ectopic pregnancy).

TREATMENT

MEDICATION
First Line
- Ciprofloxacin 500 mg q12h
- Metronidazole 500 mg q8h

Second Line
- Piperacillin/tazobactam 3.375 g IV q6h or 4.5 g IV q8h
- Ampicillin/sulbactam 3.0 g IV q6h

ADDITIONAL TREATMENT
General Measures
- Mild uncomplicated diverticulitis: Clear liquid diet and 7–10 days of oral broad-spectrum antibiotics (ciprofloxacin/metronidazole)
- Complicated/severe diverticulitis: Bowel rest (NPO), volume resuscitation, broad-spectrum intravenous antibiotics (piperacillin/tazobactam or ampicillin/sulbactam)
- Pain control with narcotics as appropriate

Issues for Referral
- Surgical consult in case perforation is suspected or proven
- Interventional radiology consult if abscess requires image-guided percutaneous drainage

SURGERY/OTHER PROCEDURES
- Surgical evaluation is warranted for worsening clinical condition, generalized peritonitis, sepsis
- Interventional radiology for image-guided percutaneous drainage of abscess

IN-PATIENT CONSIDERATIONS
Initial Stabilization
- Determine severity of diverticulitis and consider need for resuscitation
- Surgical evaluation
- Antibiotic and medical management

Admission Criteria
ICU admission should be considered for elderly, hemodynamic instability, severe infection, marked electrolyte abnormality, and/or need for close and constant monitoring.

IV Fluids
- Adequate fluid resuscitation with use of crystalloid replacement (i.e., 0.9% NS or LR)
- Ensure appropriate access and consider central venous access if inadequate access or need for monitoring volume status (CVP).

Nursing
- Patient comfort
- Stoma care and teaching if patient underwent surgery resulting in colostomy

Discharge Criteria
- Resolution of acute episode: Normalization of WBC, tolerating diet, abdominal pain resolved
- If severe and requiring intervention and/or surgery, once patient has recovered from postsurgical state

 ONGOING CARE

FOLLOW-UP RECOMMENDATIONS
Colonoscopy is advised after the acute episode has resolved to evaluate for other diagnosis (i.e., cancer, inflammatory bowel disease).

Patient Monitoring
Once stabilized medically or postsurgically, may be safe for transfer to floor

DIET
Nutrition consultation for high-fiber diet

PATIENT EDUCATION
Lifestyle modification as related to diet and exercise

PROGNOSIS
- Uncomplicated diverticulitis: 85% respond to medical management
  - Of these 85%, 1/3 will remain asymptomatic, 1/3 will have recurrent symptoms without acute diverticulitis, and 1/3 will have a 2nd episode of acute diverticulitis.
- 15–20% with acute diverticulitis will need surgery.
- Diverticulitis recurrence and indication for elective surgical resection remains controversial.

COMPLICATIONS
- Abscess
- Fistula
- Perforation
- Peritonitis
- Sepsis

ADDITIONAL READING
- Etzioni D, et al. Diverticulitis in the United States: 1998-2005, changing patterns of disease and treatment. *Ann Surg.* 2009;249:210–7.
- Marshall JC, Innes M. Intensive care unit management of intra-abdominal infection. *Crit Care Med.* 2003;31:2228–37.
- Nguyen GC, et al. Epidemiological trends and geographic variation in hospital admissions for diverticulitis in the United States. *World J Gastroenterol.* 2011;17(12):1600–5.
- Stocchi L. Current indications and role of surgery in the management of sigmoid diverticulitis. *World J Gastroenterol.* 2010;16(7):804–17.
- Unlu C, et al. A multicenter randomized clinical trial investigating the cost-effectiveness of treatment strategies with or without antibiotics for uncomplicated acute diverticulitis (DIABLO trial). *BMC Surg.* 2010;10:23.

 CODES

ICD9
- 562.11 Diverticulitis of colon (without mention of hemorrhage)
- 562.13 Diverticulitis of colon with hemorrhage

CLINICAL PEARLS
- Rapid diagnosis and stratification of severity of diverticulitis is important in determining its management; consider early surgical consultation.
- Outpatient and inpatient medical management is successful in large majority of patients.
- Patients refractory to medical management or those with hemodynamic instability, peritonitis, or worsening clinical picture warrant surgical evaluation.
- Follow-up with colonoscopy and diet/lifestyle modifications is key.
- Recurrence and indication for surgical intervention should be discussed with patient and surgeon for risk–benefit optimization.

D

ECHOCARDIOGRAPHY

Paul H. Mayo

 BASICS

DESCRIPTION

- Echocardiography is an effective means of directly assessing cardiac anatomy and function, and so is a valuable tool for the front-line intensivist. Standard cardiology-style echocardiography has several drawbacks in the ICU: time delay, offline interpretation, and an approach that discourages goal-directed or repeated examinations. In comparison, the intensivist who performs echocardiography personally acquires and interprets the image while using the information to make immediate, clinically relevant decisions.
- The exam may be limited in scope and repeated whenever clinically indicated.
- Skill at basic critical care echocardiography, which emphasizes qualitative assessment of cardiac anatomy and function, is a key skill for the front-line all intensivists. Basic skill level is straightforward to learn. Skill at advanced critical care echocardiography requires a major course of study, and is not needed for effective bedside clinical work. Only a limited number of intensivists will have the time or interest required for advanced training. This discussion focuses on basic critical care echocardiography, in the form of goal-directed echocardiography (GDE).

- The main indication for GDE is for rapid assessment of hemodynamic failure. It should be regarded as a routine and important component of the initial and ongoing assessment of any patient in shock. The results of the GDE examination may be productively combined with other aspects of critical care ultrasonography, in particular lung and vascular ultrasonography.

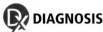 **DIAGNOSIS**

DIAGNOSTIC TESTS & INTERPRETATION
Imaging

- GDE uses a limited number of standard cardiac views that typically include the parasternal long and short axis (PSL/PSS), the apical 4-chamber (AP4), the subcostal long-axis (SCL), and the inferior vena cava (IVC) long-axis views.
- In performing GDE, the examiner should always attempt to acquire all 5 views as frequently, in the critically patient, not all may be of acceptable image quality. A key aspect to training is that the intensivist be skilled at obtaining good quality on axis views of the heart. This requires mastery of transducer manipulation and machine controls. Off-axis images and poor machine control may obscure important findings or result in factitious abnormality.

- Each view is analyzed by the bedside clinician who has full knowledge of all aspects of the case; the results are immediately integrated into the diagnostic impression and used to guide hemodynamic management of the case.
- The intensivist seeks to categorize the shock state (e.g., obstructive, hypovolemic, cardiogenic, or distributive and their respective subcategories). Using this information, the front-line intensivist develops the management plan. Subsequently, the study may be repeated as needed to look for response to therapy, additional diagnosis, or progression/regression of disease. During the course of critical illness, echocardiographic findings may change rapidly and result in change of management strategy.
- The PSL view is used to assess left ventricular (LV) size and function, right ventricular (RV) outflow tract size, septal dynamics, aortic/mitral valvular morphology, and for pericardial fluid.
- The PSS view is use to assess LV size and function, septal dynamics, RV size, and for pericardial fluid.
- The AP4 view is used to assess for RV enlargement. The RV size is compared to LV size. RV >100% of LV size indicates severe enlargement; RV >60% of LV size but <100% of LV size indicates moderate enlargement. No other information needs to be derived from the AP4 view during GDE.

- The SCL view, which is often the best quality in the critically ill, is used to assess LV/RV size and function and for pericardial effusion.
- The IVC view is used to identify preload sensitivity. Size variation of the IVC during respiratory cycle has value only if the patient is on mechanical ventilatory support and completely passive. In patients who are breathing actively, the size of the IVC may be used to identify preload sensitivity in shock cases; if the IVC is <1 cm in size, preload sensitivity is very likely; if the IVC is >3 cm is size, preload sensitivity is very unlikely. Between the 2 values, alternative methods must be used to identify preload sensitivity.
- Doppler examination of cardiac function is not part of GDE, with the exception of the use of color Doppler, which may be used to identify severe left-sided valvular regurgitation.

- Although GDE exam is a useful diagnostic tool, the intensivist must have a clear understanding of the limitations of the technique:
  - GDE is not a complete echocardiographic study. The intensivist must understand the limitations of the basic training level, and call for full echocardiogram as needed. For example, comprehensive evaluation of valve function, detailed analysis of segmental wall function, quantitative analysis of cardiac pressures and flows, or evaluation of prosthetic valve function require the services of a fully trained echocardiographer.
  - Training in image interpretation is a key skill for the intensivist engaged in GDE. This includes the ability to recognize normal anatomy and function vs. definite abnormality; as well as the ability to notice ambiguous findings that require referral to a fully trained echocardiographer.

  - Frequently, image quality may be challenging in ICU patient. The clinician must be skilled at image acquisition and persistent in her effort to obtain good quality images, as well as able to work with limited results. Image interpretation requires dedicated training. Poor transthoracic images can be resolved with transesophageal echocardiography, but this requires specific training.
  - The intensivist must have the cognitive background to integrate the GDE findings into a complex clinical picture. Multiple causes for shock may be present in any given patient, so that the intensivist must be proficient in integrating the echocardiographic findings into a sophisticated management strategy.

 CODES

ICD9
- 785.50 Shock, unspecified
- 785.59 Other shock without mention of trauma
- 785.9 Other symptoms involving cardiovascular system

ECLAMPSIA

Cynthia Chazotte
Dena Goffman

 BASICS

DESCRIPTION
Seizures during pregnancy or postpartum in patients with signs and symptoms of preeclampsia

EPIDEMIOLOGY
Incidence
- 0.04–0.1% of pregnancies in developed countries
- Approximate timing: 50% antepartum, 20% intrapartum, 30% postpartum
- Postpartum occurs usually within 48 hours of delivery but can be as late as 4 weeks

RISK FACTORS
- Nulliparity
- Chronic hypertension
- Pregestational diabetes
- Sickle cell disease
- Chronic renal disease
- Thrombophilia
- Antiphospholipid antibody syndrome
- Connective tissue disease
- Obesity
- Maternal age >40 or <18
- Personal history/1st-degree relative with PEC
- Multifetal gestation
- Hydrops fetalis
- Gestational trophoblastic disease
- Untreated preeclampsia
- No prenatal care

Genetics
- Role of genetic risk is unclear, but a possible genetic basis exists.
- Women with thrombophilias may have a genetic predisposition.

GENERAL PREVENTION
- Early recognition of symptoms of impending seizure
- Seizure prophylaxis with magnesium sulfate in women with preeclampsia

PATHOPHYSIOLOGY
Possible mechanisms:
- Cerebral vasoconstriction or vasospasm
- Loss of cerebrovascular autoregulation
- Hypertensive encephalopathy
- Cerebral edema

ETIOLOGY
No conclusive etiology

COMMONLY ASSOCIATED CONDITIONS
- Preeclampsia
- Chronic hypertension
- Renal disease
- Diabetes
- Thrombophilias
- SLE or other connective tissue diseases

DIAGNOSIS

HISTORY
- Hypertension, proteinuria, generalized edema, seizure
- Symptoms preceding eclampsia include:
  - Headache, occipital or frontal: 50–75%
  - Visual changes (scotomata, blurry vision, cortical blindness): 20–30%
  - Mental status changes
  - Epigastric pain (may herald liver rupture)

PHYSICAL EXAM
- BP >140/90
- Generalized edema
- Hyperreflexia

DIAGNOSTIC TESTS & INTERPRETATION
Lab
Initial lab tests
- CBC: May reveal hemoconcentration, thrombocytopenia, or hemolysis
- Comprehensive metabolic panel: May reveal elevated transaminases and/or BUN/creatinine
- LDH: Significant elevation suggests hemolysis.
- Uric acid: Elevation has prognostic significance for fetus.

Follow-Up & Special Considerations
Check serial laboratory values for signs of HELLP (see HELLP chapter), renal insufficiency

Imaging
Initial approach (1)[C]
- Routine imaging with CT/MRI not necessary except if:
  - Focal deficits
  - Prolonged coma
  - Seizures before 20 weeks of gestation or >48 hours after delivery
  - Diagnosis uncertain

Follow-Up & Special Considerations (2)[C]
- Fetal bradycardia occurs frequently during eclamptic seizure.
- Management is maternal treatment and stabilization.
- Immediate cesarean delivery is not necessary and may be harmful to mother.

Diagnostic Procedures/Other
- Classic imaging findings: Cerebral edema, posterior reversible leukoencephalopathy
- Bilateral symmetrical edema in posterior cerebral hemispheres, especially in the parieto-occipital regions

Pathological Findings
Autopsy findings: Edema, infarction, and hemorrhage (microhemorrhage and intracerebral parenchymal hemorrhage) in cortical and subcortical white matter

DIFFERENTIAL DIAGNOSIS
- Cerebrovascular accidents from:
  - Intracranial hemorrhage
  - Ruptured aneurysm or malformation
  - Cerebral venous thrombosis
  - Hypoxic ischemic encephalopathy
  - Angiomas
- Hypertensive encephalopathy
- Seizure disorder
- Undiagnosed brain tumor
- Hypoglycemia, hyponatremia
- Posterior reversible encephalopathy syndrome (PRES)
- Thrombophilia
- Thrombotic thrombocytopenic purpura
- Postdural puncture syndrome
- Cerebral vasculitis

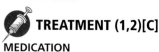 **TREATMENT (1,2)[C]**

MEDICATION
First Line
- IV Magnesium sulfate: 4–6 g loading dose in 100 mL D5W over 20–30 minutes followed by 20 g in 500 mL D5W at 50 mL/hr (2)[A] *OR*
- Intramuscular magnesium sulfate may be used if no immediate IV access: 10 g of 50% magnesium sulfate administered as 5 g in each buttock, followed by 5 g q4h (2)[A]
- BP control as described for preeclampsia

Second Line
- For recurrent seizure (10% of patients), an additional 2–4 g of magnesium sulfate may be infused over 5–10 minutes (2)[A].
- Eclamptic seizures are usually self-limited but diazepam or lorazepam can be used to break prolonged seizure activity.
- Phenytoin for seizure prophylaxis if contraindications to magnesium (myasthenia gravis, pulmonary edema, cardiac conduction defects)
- Status eclampticus: Anesthesiologist, intubation, and IV barbiturates (2)[C]

ADDITIONAL TREATMENT

General Measures
- Assure open airway
- Position on side to prevent aspiration
- Bedrails elevated and padded
- Maternal oxygen by face mask at 8–10 L/min
- Pulse oximetry
- Foley catheter to monitor urinary output
- Serial laboratory evaluation q4–6h, as in severe preeclampsia
- Continue magnesium sulfate until 24 hours postpartum or longer if no diuresis

Issues for Referral
- Maternal fetal medicine specialist
- Anesthesiologist
- Neurology consultation and imaging if focal findings, prolonged coma, uncertain diagnosis

ALERT
- Discontinue magnesium after loading dose if no urine output occurs.
- Monitor DTRs and magnesium level for toxicity (therapeutic level, 4–8 mEq/L).
- Treatment of respiratory depression from magnesium toxicity: Stop magnesium, start mechanical ventilation, and 10 mL of 10% calcium gluconate IV over 3 minutes

SURGERY/OTHER PROCEDURES
- Delivery mode is based on gestational age, fetal condition, presence of labor, and cervical Bishop score (2)[C].
- Regional anesthesia is recommended in the absence of a coagulopathy or thrombocytopenia.
- Eclampsia alone is not an indication for cesarean delivery.
- Patients with eclampsia often have laryngeal edema, making intubation difficult.

IN-PATIENT CONSIDERATIONS

Admission Criteria
- Depends on resources of obstetrical service and ICU, and condition of patient
- Must provide ICU setting for all women with eclampsia for 24 hours
- If patient is laboring, an ICU must gather needed delivery equipment (delivery set and neonatal resuscitation equipment), staff (OB MD, RN, pediatrician), proximity to an OR
- If patient is on OB unit, critical care resources should come to the OB unit.

IV Fluids
- Careful evaluation of intake and output.
- At risk for pulmonary edema

Nursing
- Vital signs q15min
- Fetal heart rate monitoring
- Hourly intake and output

Discharge Criteria
No headache, stable BP, significantly improved laboratory values, no coagulopathy, adequate urine output

ONGOING CARE

FOLLOW-UP RECOMMENDATIONS

Patient Monitoring
- Home visiting nurse to assess symptoms and BP
- Outpatient physician visit within 1 week of discharge

PATIENT EDUCATION
All pregnant and postpartum women educated about signs of impending eclampsia: Headache, visual changes

PROGNOSIS
- Can cause maternal death
- Acute neurological changes generally reversible
- Long-term effects unclear:
  - Increased rate of chronic hypertension
  - Increased risk of preeclampsia in subsequent pregnancies (25%)
  - Risk of recurrent eclampsia (2%)

COMPLICATIONS
- Maternal death
- Hypertensive crisis
- Pulmonary edema
- HELLP syndrome
- Renal failure
- Liver rupture
- Intrauterine fetal demise
- Intracranial hemorrhage
- Abruptio placenta

REFERENCES

1. Karnad DR, et al. Neurologic disorders in pregnancy. *Crit Care Med*. 2005;33(Suppl.): S362–71.
2. Sibai BM. Diagnosis, prevention and management of eclampsia. *Obstet Gynecol*. 2005;105:402–10.

ADDITIONAL READING

- American College of Obstetricians and Gynecologists. Medical emergency preparedness. ACOG Committee Opinion No 353. *Obstet Gynecol*. 2006;108:1597–99.
- American College of Obstetricians and Gynecologists. Critical care in pregnancy. ACOG Practice Bulletin No 100. *Obstet Gynecol*. 2009;113:443–50.
- American College of Obstetricians and Gynecologists. Diagnosis and Management of Preeclampsia and Eclampsia. ACOG Practice Bulletin No. 33. *Obstet Gynecol*. 2002, Reaffirmed 2008.

CODES

ICD9
- 642.60 Eclampsia complicating pregnancy, childbirth or the puerperium, unspecified as to episode of care
- 642.61 Eclampsia, with delivery
- 642.62 Eclampsia, with delivery, with mention of postpartum complication

CLINICAL PEARLS
- Eclampsia a rare event and requires emergency preparedness.
- Delivery is required; however, eclampsia alone is not an indication for cesarean delivery: Assess gestational age, fetal status, presence of labor, and state of the cervix to determine delivery mode.
- Eclampsia commonly presents in the postpartum period.
- Magnesium sulfate is the first-line treatment for eclamptic seizures.
- Appropriate dose, route, and patient monitoring are crucial for safe magnesium sulfate administration.
- Use caution on extubation of patient with eclampsia; airway edema may be severe.

E

ELECTROLYTES, OTHER

Sindhura Gogineni
Aditya Uppalapati
Roopa Kohli-Seth

 BASICS

DESCRIPTION
- Magnesium (Mg):
  - Normal: 1.7–2.4 mg/dL
  - Hypomagnesemia: Serum Mg <1.7 mg/dL
  - Hypermagnesemia: Serum Mg >2.4 mg/dL
- Phosphorus (PO_4):
  - Normal: 2.5–4.5 mg/dL
  - Hypophosphatemia: Serum PO4 <2.5 mg/dL
  - Hyperphosphatemia: Serum PO4 >4.5 mg/dL

EPIDEMIOLOGY
Incidence
- Hypomagnesemia: 60–65% in ICU
- Hypophosphatemia: 35–70%

Prevalence
- Hypomagnesemia occurs in ∼12% of hospitalized patients.
- Hypophosphatemia: 60–80% of ICU patients

RISK FACTORS
- Renal failure: Hypermagnesemia, hyperphosphatemia
- Hypophosphatemia: Sepsis, trauma

Genetics
- Hypomagnesemia: Inborn error of metabolism characterized by a selective defect in magnesium absorption; linked or autosomal recessive
- Hypophosphatemia: Primary renal phosphate wasting syndromes; X-linked hypophosphatemic rickets, autosomal dominant and recessive hypophosphatemic rickets, McCune-Albright syndrome

GENERAL PREVENTION
- In patients with renal failure, electrolytes must be frequently monitored.
- Measure serum electrolytes, PO_4, magnesium, and calcium at least once daily.

PATHOPHYSIOLOGY
- Hypomagnesemia:
  - GI:
    - Normally, small amounts of magnesium are lost by GI secretions. Marked dietary depletion and increased secretions from GI tract can cause hypomagnesemia.
  - Renal causes:
    - Primary defect in absorption
    - Inhibition of sodium reabsorption in segments where magnesium passively follows sodium
- Hypermagnesemia:
  - Overreplacement
  - Renal failure
- Hypophosphatemia:
  - Decreased intestinal absorption
  - Increased urinary excretion
  - Excessive internal redistribution
- Hyperphosphatemia: Massive acute phosphate load, renal failure, increased tubular reabsorption of phosphate

ETIOLOGY
- Hypomagnesemia:
  - GI:
    - Disorders of the small bowel, including acute or chronic diarrhea, malabsorption and steatorrhea, and small bowel bypass surgery
    - Acute pancreatitis
  - Renal:
    - Primary renal magnesium wasting,
    - Loop and thiazide diuretics,
    - Volume expansion (decrease passive magnesium transport),
    - Nephrotoxins: Amphotericin B, gentamicin, cisplatin, cyclosporine, tacrolimus (increase urinary magnesium wasting)
    - Proton pump inhibitors (impaired intestinal absorption of magnesium),
    - Alcohol (increased urinary excretion)
    - Acute tubular necrosis
    - Renal, liver transplantation
    - Bartter or Gitelman syndromes
    - Following surgery (chelation by circulating free fatty acids)
    - Others: Diabetes mellitus, massive transfusion, hungry bone syndrome
- Hypermagnesemia:
  - Renal failure
  - Others: IV magnesium infusion, oral ingestion, magnesium enema, lithium toxicity
- Hypophosphatemia:
  - Excessive internal redistribution (due to stimulation of glycolysis): Acute respiratory alkalosis, hungry bone syndrome, refeeding
  - Decreased intestinal absorption: Antacids containing aluminium, magnesium, diarrhea, malabsorption, vitamin D deficiency or resistance, small bowel resection (70–80% of dietary PO_4 is absorbed in small bowel), inadequate intake
  - Increased urinary excretion: Primary and secondary hyperparathyroidism, hypothermia, osmotic diuresis, acetazolamide, vitamin D deficiency or resistance, kidney transplantation (tertiary hyperparathyroidism)
- Hyperphosphatemia:
  - Massive acute phosphate load:
    - Rhabdomyolysis, tumor lysis syndrome, lactic and ketoacidosis, iatrogenic overreplacement of phosphate
  - Renal failure
  - Increased tubular reabsorption of phosphate:
    - Hypoparathyroidism, acromegaly, vitamin D toxicity, bisphosphonates, familial tumor calcinosis

COMMONLY ASSOCIATED CONDITIONS
- Hypomagnesemia: Hypokalemia, hypocalcemia, metabolic alkalosis
- Hypophosphatemia: Fanconi syndrome

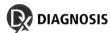 **DIAGNOSIS**

HISTORY
- Hypomagnesemia:
  - Confusion, irritability, delirium, seizures, weakness, lethargy, palpitations.
- Hypermagnesemia:
  - Most patients with levels of <3.6 mg/dL are mild and asymptomatic.
  - 4.8–7.2 mg/dL: Nausea, flushing, headache, lethargy, drowsiness
  - 7.3–12 mg/dL: Somnolence, hypocalcemia, hypotension, bradycardia, EKG changes (increase PR and QRS interval)
  - >12 mg/dL: Muscle paralysis, respiratory paralysis, complete heart block cardiac arrest
- Hypophosphatemia:
  - Muscle weakness, inability to wean from ventilator, rhabdomyolysis, paresthesias, hemolysis, cardiac failure, platelet dysfunction
- Hyperphosphatemia:
  - Associated with symptoms of hypocalcemia

PHYSICAL EXAM
- Hypomagnesemia, hyperphosphatemia
  - Positive Chvostek's and Trousseau's signs, tetany (when associated with hypocalcemia)
- Hypermagnesemia:
  - 4.8–7.2 mg/dL: Deep tendon reflexes (DTR) are diminished; >7.3 mg/dL, DTR are absent

DIAGNOSTIC TESTS & INTERPRETATION
Lab
Initial lab tests
- Serum magnesium, serum chemistry
- Total and ionized calcium, serum phosphorus
- ABG for pH, albumin

Follow-Up & Special Considerations
- Repeat labs q4–6h until patient's electrolytes are stable.
- The product of serum calcium and phosphate (>60 mg^2/dL^2; increased risk of calcium phosphate crystals)

Imaging
Hypomagnesemia: Flat plate abdomen; ileus

Diagnostic Procedures/Other
ECG:
- Hypomagnesemia:
  - Modest hypomagnesemia: Widening of QRS complex, peaking of T waves
  - Severe hypomagnesemia: Prolongation of PR, progression of QRS complex, Torsade de pointes
- Hypermagnesemia: Complete heart block

DIFFERENTIAL DIAGNOSIS
Hypocalcemia, hypercalcemia

TREATMENT

MEDICATION

First Line

- Hypomagnesemia:
  - Magnesium sulfate most commonly used IV (1–2 g over 1–2 hours)
  - Magnesium oxide most common, PO 400 mg b.i.d.
    - Torsade de pointes: 1–2 g over 5–20 minutes (1,2,3)[A].
    - Atrial fibrillation: 1–2 g over 1–2 hours (1,2,3)[A]
- Hypermagnesemia (2,3)[C]:
  - IV Calcium: 100–200 mg of elemental calcium over 5–10 minutes:
    - Calcium chloride 1 g = 13.6 meq; 270 mg of elemental calcium, calcium gluconate: 1 g = 4.65 meq; 90 mg of elemental calcium
- Hypophosphatemia (3,4)[C]:
  - Generally 20–40 mmol of sodium or potassium phosphate is given IV over 6 hours.
  - Oral 250–500 mg phosphate can be given. Maximum 2.5 g/d in divided doses
  - In normal renal function patients for phosphate levels of:
    - 2.3–2.7 mg/dL: IV PO_4, 0.08–0.16 mmol/Kg
    - 1.5–2.2 mg/dL: IV PO_4, 0.16–0.32 mmol/Kg
    - <1.5 mg/dL: IV PO_4, 0.32–0.64 mmol/Kg
- Hyperphosphatemia (3)[C]:
  - Oral phosphate binders: Calcium carbonate (667 mg), aluminium hydroxide (300–600 mg), magnesium hydroxide (400–800 mg), Sevelamer (400–800 mg) can be used 2–3 times a day.

Second Line

Replete calcium as needed

ADDITIONAL TREATMENT

General Measures

- Caution should be used in renal failure patients while replacing phosphate and magnesium.
- Hypophospatemia: Replace with potassium phosphate or sodium phosphate. Potassium phosphate has 1.5 meq of potassium for each mmol of phosphate. Sodium phosphate has 1.33 meq of sodium for each mmol of phosphate.
- Hypomagnesemia: Replace other electrolytes also, especially calcium and potassium.
- Hypermagnesemia: Discontinue magnesium replacements
- Dialysis: CRRT if patient is hemodynamically unstable.
- Hyperphosphatemia:
  - CRRT with hemofiltration is preferred over hemodialysis. PO_4 in solution acts as a larger molecule and is more difficult to remove with diffusion (dialysis) than convection (filtration).

Issues for Referral

Nephrology for hemodialysis

Additional Therapies

Treat the underlying etiology.

COMPLEMENTARY & ALTERNATIVE THERAPIES

- Eclampsia and preeclampsia: 1–2 g/hr of magnesium sulfate (1)[A]
- Severe acute asthma: Magnesium supplementation, 1.2–2 g IV over 20 minutes (1)[B]
- Subarachnoid hemorrhage: IV magnesium drip, 0.5–1 g/hr to maintain serum magnesium levels 2–3 mg/dL

SURGERY/OTHER PROCEDURES

Central venous access may be required in treatment of severe hypomagnesemia and hypophosphatemia.

IN-PATIENT CONSIDERATIONS

Initial Stabilization

- ABC
- Treat arrhythmias as per ACLS, and correct underlying electrolyte abnormalities.

Admission Criteria

Symptomatic electrolyte imbalance; some examples include:

- Cardiac arrhythmias: Torsades de pointes, cardiac arrest, rapid atrial fibrillation, bradycardia
- Respiratory failure, paralysis
- Neurological: Lethargy, paralysis, altered mental status

IV Fluids

- Hypomagnesemia: Can use Isolyte/Plasmalyte.
- NS may be used for resuscitation in hyperphosphatemia patients.

Nursing

- Neuro exam in symptomatic patients
- Draw repeat levels about an hour after the infusions (replacement).

Discharge Criteria

When electrolytes are stable and underlying etiology has been treated

ONGOING CARE

FOLLOW-UP RECOMMENDATIONS

If severe electrolyte imbalance occurs despite aggressive correction consult and follow with endocrinology and nephrology.

Patient Monitoring

ECG, neuro exam, respiratory status

DIET

- Hypomagnesemia: Halibut, almonds, cashews, spinach, cereal
- Hyperphosphatemia: Avoid foods containing high phosphorus.

PATIENT EDUCATION

Dietary education

COMPLICATIONS

- Overaggressive replacement of magnesium: Nausea, vomiting, diarrhea; overdose may lead to hypotension, muscle weakness, and coma.
- Potassium phosphate replacement has to be done over 4–6 hours to prevent thrombophlebitis and calcium-phosphate precipitation.

REFERENCES

1. Guerrera, et al. Therapeutic uses of magnesium. *Am Fam Physician*. 2009;80(2):157–62.
2. Tong GM, et al. Magnesium deficiency in critical illness. *J Intensive Care Med*. 2005;20(1):3–17.
3. Kraft, et al. Treatment of electrolyte disorders in adult patients in the intensive care unit. *Am J Health-Syst Pharm*. 2005;62:1663–82.
4. Geerse DA, et al. Treatment of hypophosphatemia in the intensive care unit. A review. *Critical Care*. 2010;14:R147.

ADDITIONAL READING

Dube, et al. The therapeutic use of magnesium in anesthesiology, intensive care and emergency medicine. *Can J Anesth*. 2003;50(7):732–46.

See Also (Topic, Algorithm, Electronic Media Element)

Hypocalcemia, Hypercalcemia, Alkalosis and Acidosis

CODES

ICD9

- 275.2 Disorders of magnesium metabolism
- 275.3 Disorders of phosphorus metabolism

CLINICAL PEARLS

- In the critically ill patient, replete hypomagnesemia and hypophosphatemia aggressively; maintain magnesium ≥2 mg/dL, phosphate, 3–4 mg/dL.
- Along with the treatment of primary electrolyte imbalance, treat the underlying etiology and other associated electrolyte imbalances.
- Treat torsade de pointes with magnesium sulfate in spite of normal magnesium levels.

E

ENCEPHALITIS
Luciano Lemos-Filho

BASICS

DESCRIPTION
Encephalitis is defined as an inflammation of the brain matter. Syndromically, it may include the meninges and be then described as meningoencephalitis. This chapter focuses on infectious causes of encephalitis.

RISK FACTORS
Pathogen-specific risk factors include arthropod vectors (e.g., arboviruses, Rickettsiae, and related pathogens), immunosuppression (e.g., JC-virus/PML, toxoplasma encephalitis, organ transplant, transfusions), extremes of age, travel to certain areas (e.g., African sleeping sickness, Japanese encephalitis), and exposure to infected animals (e.g., rabies virus, herpes B virus).

GENERAL PREVENTION
No general preventative measures, given myriad of causes

PATHOPHYSIOLOGY
Infection of brain tissue usually occurs hematogenously, in some cases via axonal transport of pathogens into the CNS.

ETIOLOGY
- In California Encephalitis Project: Viral (9%), bacterial (3%), parasitic (1%), noninfectious (10%), unexplained (62%)
- Infectious causes:
- Most common as a group are viruses.
- Herpes simplex (up to 10% of cases), West Nile Virus, Japanese encephalitis virus, St Louis encephalitis virus, adenovirus, La Crosse virus, Varicella-zoster virus, measles virus, mumps virus, poliovirus, HIV, Eastern equine encephalitis virus, rabies virus among others
  - Bacterial causes: *Mycoplasma pneumoniae, Listeria, Brucella* spp., *Bartonella* spp., *Borrelia burgdorferi, T. whipplei, Mycobacterium tuberculosis*

  - Rickettsiae and related: *R. rickettsii, Ehrlichia* spp., *Anaplasma, Coxiella*
  - Fungi: *Cryptococcus neoformans, Coccidioides* spp., *Histoplasma capsulatum*
  - Parasites: *Toxoplasma gondii, Plasmodium falciparum, Trypanosoma brucei,* cysticercosis, *Naegleria fowleri*
  - Postinfectious: Acute disseminated encephalomyelitis
  - Noninfectious: Lupus cerebritis, vasculitides, metabolic encephalopathies, drug reactions, malignancies, multiple sclerosis, among others

COMMONLY ASSOCIATED CONDITIONS
Meningitis

DIAGNOSIS

HISTORY
In encephalitis, altered mental status, more than expected with a pure meningitis, is the distinguishing factor. However, often patients present with features of both. Behavioral changes, and/or sensory/motor complaints suggest the diagnosis.

PHYSICAL EXAM
- Cerebral dysfunction on detailed neurological exam
- Possible increased intracranial pressure
- Oculomasticatory myorhythmia (a unique pendular vergence oscillation of the eyes and concurrent contractions of the masticatory muscles), strongly suggestive of, if not pathognomic for, Whipple disease

DIAGNOSTIC TESTS & INTERPRETATION
Lab
Initial lab tests
- CSF exam, if not contraindicated, should be performed and can help narrow the differential. In viral causes with accompanying meningitis, typically one sees a lymphocytic predominance with elevated protein. Nucleic acid and immunoglobulin tests should be sent in the correct clinical scenarios (e.g., IgM for West Nile virus, PCR for HSV).
- Blood cultures

- Viral DFA and antigenic tests on nasopharyngeal secretions
- Biopsy, DFA, and PCR for skin rash (e.g., Rickettsial diseases)
- Blood smear (e.g., malaria and ehrlichia diseases)
- Hyponatremia secondary to SIADH is common.

Follow-Up & Special Considerations
Despite extensive diagnostic workup, etiology often not elucidated (in one series 62% of cases remained unexplained) (1).

Imaging
Initial approach
MRI of the brain (and spinal cord in certain cases) is the test of choice. CT scan is suboptimal. Both can be unrevealing early in course.

Follow-Up & Special Considerations
Consider care in a monitored setting.

Diagnostic Procedures/Other
- Brain biopsy rarely used but maybe necessary in certain cases
- Biopsy of nape of neck in suspected rabies

Pathological Findings
Depends on etiology; brain can have findings of inflammatory necrosis, vasculitis, infarction, and demyelination

DIFFERENTIAL DIAGNOSIS
- Encephalopathy
- Subarachnoid hemorrhage
- Status epilepticus
- Stroke
- Thyroid disease
- Paraneoplastic syndrome
- CNS neoplasm
- Poisonings
- Psychiatric disease

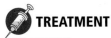

TREATMENT

MEDICATION
First Line

- Empiric IV acyclovir (adult dose 10 mg/kg q8h) is recommended for all patients with encephalitis due to the increased morbidity and mortality of untreated herpes simplex encephalitis (2)[A-I].
- Consider empiric doxycycline in patients with suspected rickettsial or ehrlichial diseases.
- 4-antimycobacterial drug therapy for suspected tuberculous meningitis, plus steroids.
- Other treatments, empiric and pathogen-specific, depend on clinical presentation and diagnostic testing.

Second Line
N/A; steroids not recommended empirically unless tuberculosis or acute bacterial meningitis due to *S. pneumoniae* is suspected.

ADDITIONAL TREATMENT
General Measures
Evaluation of airway protection and intubation if needed

Issues for Referral
Neurology and infectious diseases consultations are strongly recommended.

SURGERY/OTHER PROCEDURES
Brain biopsy in selected cases. Neuroimaging is necessary to guide surgeon to affected area.

IN-PATIENT CONSIDERATIONS
Initial Stabilization
- Airway protection, intubation if needed
- Seizure treatment

Admission Criteria
Recommend admission for diagnostic workup and serial neurological evaluations.

IV Fluids
As per protocol if patient is not taking PO adequately.

Nursing
Consider neurologic monitored nursing unit.

Discharge Criteria
Case-dependent

ONGOING CARE

FOLLOW-UP RECOMMENDATIONS
- With subspecialists
- Repeat PCR of CSF for herpes simplex recommended in patients not responding to acyclovir

Patient Monitoring
As above

DIET
Case-dependent on ability to take PO

PATIENT EDUCATION
Several resources available online; many are pathogen-specific.

PROGNOSIS
- Untreated herpes simplex encephalitis has a high morbidity and mortality (>90%). If treated within 4 days of symptoms, mortality decreases to 8% (2).
- Neurologic sequelae unfortunately are common with several pathogens.

COMPLICATIONS
- Seizures
- Permanent neurologic deficits
- Death

REFERENCES

1. Glaser CA, et al. In search of encephalitis etiologies: Diagnostic challenges in the California Encephalitis Project 1998–2000. *CID*. 2003;36(6):731–42.
2. Tunkel AR, et al. The management of encephalitis: Clinical practice guidelines by the Infectious Disease Society of America. *CID*. 2008;47:303–27.

CODES

ICD9
- 049.8 Other specified non-arthropod-borne viral diseases of central nervous system
- 322.9 Meningitis, unspecified
- 323.9 Unspecified cause of encephalitis, myelitis, and encephalomyelitis

CLINICAL PEARLS

Consider ADEM if patient is recently postinfectious disease or vaccination.

E

ENDOCARDITIS

Joanne K. Mazzarelli

BASICS

DESCRIPTION
- Infection of the endocardial surface of the heart; vegetations, composed of a collection of platelets, fibrin, microorganisms, and inflammatory cells, are usually present.
- Most commonly involves heart valves but may also occur at the site of a septal defect, on the chordae tendineae, or on the mural endocardium (1)

EPIDEMIOLOGY
Incidence
- The age-specific incidence increases from 5 cases/100,000 person-years among persons <50 years of age to 15–30 cases per 100,000 person-years in the 6th–8th decades of life.
- >50% of patients are >50.
- Male > Female (1.7:1)
- Mitral valves are affected most commonly (86%), followed by aortic (55%), tricuspid (19.6%), and pulmonic (1.1%)

Prevalence
Prevalence ranges between 1.7 and 4 per 100,000 persons.

RISK FACTORS
- Mitral valve prolapse in developed countries (20–22%)
- Rheumatic heart disease in developing countries
- Congenital heart disease (10–20%)
- Bicuspid AV, PDA, VSD, coarctation of the aorta, and tetralogy of Fallot
- Hypertrophy cardiomyopathy with outflow obstruction
- Prosthetic valve
- History of infective endocarditis
- IV drug use
- Long-term indwelling devices

GENERAL PREVENTION
- Prophylactic antibiotics for patients with the following conditions:
  - Prosthetic cardiac valve, previous infective endocarditis, unrepaired cyanotic CHD, repaired CHD with prosthetic material during first 6 months of procedure, cardiac transplantation recipients who develop cardiac valvulopathy (4)[B]
  - These criteria were recently revised, and prophylaxis is now recommended in fewer patients than before.

PATHOPHYSIOLOGY
- Initially, alteration of valve surface creates a suitable environment for microorganism attachment.
- Deposition of platelets and fibrin on the valve surface forms nonbacterial thrombotic endocarditis (NBTE).
- Bacteremia results in colonization of the altered valve.
- Microbial growth results in the secondary accumulation of more platelets and fibrin.

ETIOLOGY
- Most endocarditis occurs on damaged valves, but aggressive organisms may invade structurally normal valves.

- Acute endocarditis:
  - Gram-positive organisms: *Staphylococcus aureus*, *Streptococcus* groups A, B, C, G, *Streptococcus pneumoniae*, *Staphylococcus lugdunensis*, *Enterococcus* spp. (*E. faecalis*, *E. faecium*, *E. durans*)
  - Gram-negative: *Haemophilus influenzae* or *parainfluenzae*, *Neisseria gonorrhoeae*
- Subacute endocarditis:
  - Gram-positive: Viridans Group *Streptococcus*, *Streptococcus bovis*, *Enterococcus* spp
  - HACEK organisms (*Haemophilus parainfluenzae*, *Haemophilus aphrophilus*, *Actinobacillus actinomycetemcomitans*, *Cardiobacterium hominis*, *Eikenella corrodens*, *Kingella kingae*)
- IV drug users:
  - Gram-positive: *S. aureus*, *Enterococcus* ssp
  - Gram-negative: *P. aeruginosa*
  - *Candida* spp.
- Prosthetic valve endocarditis
  - Early: *S. aureus*, *S. epidermidis*, gram-negative bacilli, *Candida* spp. and *Aspergillus* spp.
  - Late: Viridans Group *Streptococcus*, *Enterococcus* ssp., *S. epidermidis*, *Candida* spp., and *Aspergillus* spp.

DIAGNOSIS

HISTORY
- Modified Duke Criteria (5):
  - Sensitivity is 92% and specificity 99% for the diagnosis of IE (6)
  - A definite diagnosis requires the presence of 2 major criteria, 1 major criterion and 3 minor criteria, or 5 minor criteria
  - Possible infective endocarditis requires 1 major criterion and 1 minor criterion or 3 minor criteria.
  - Major criteria:
    ○ Positive blood culture
    ○ Evidence of endocardial involvement with either echocardiogram or new valvular regurgitation
  - Minor criteria:
    ○ Predisposing heart condition or injection drug use.
    ○ Fever (>100.4°F)
    ○ Vascular phenomena: Major arterial emboli, septic pulmonary infarct, mycotic aneurysm, intracranial hemorrhage, Janeway lesions
    ○ Immunologic phenomena: Glomerulonephritis, Osler's nodes, Roth's spots
    ○ Microbiologic evidence: Positive blood cultures without meeting major criteria.
- Multiple positive blood cultures plus echocardiogram revealing vegetation, a new heart murmur, or embolic phenomena
- Interval between the initiating bacteremia and the onset of symptoms is estimated to be <2 weeks in >80% of patients.
- Native valve endocarditis:
  - Acute with high fevers and sepsis may occur more commonly with *Staphylococcus* infection.
  - Subacute with constitutional symptoms over weeks:
    ○ Fever, chills, sweats, anorexia, malaise, weight loss
    ○ Dyspnea, cough, myalgia
    ○ Nonspecific back and abdominal pain
    ○ Confusion or change in mental status

- Prosthetic valve endocarditis:
  - Early: >12 months after surgery
  - Late: >12 months after surgery
- IE in IV drug users
- Nosocomial IE is becomingly exceedingly more common.

PHYSICAL EXAM
- Fever (80–90%)
- Murmur (80–85%): <10% are known to be new.
- Peripheral manifestations are often absent particularly in IE restricted to the tricuspid valve but include:
  - Osler nodes: Painful indurated nodules on the palms and soles
  - Splinter hemorrhage
  - Petechiae
  - Janeway lesions: Painless, flat red macules on the palms and soles
  - Roth spots: Visualized near the optic disc as a pale retinal patch with surrounding area of hemorrhage that represents vasculitis of small retinal arteries with or without retinal infarction
- Splenomegaly (15–50%)
- Embolic events (20–40%):
  - Infrequent after 2 weeks of therapy
- Congestive heart failure with mitral or aortic valve endocarditis
- Renal insufficiency (<15%)

DIAGNOSTIC TESTS & INTERPRETATION
Lab
Initial lab tests
- At least 3 blood culture sets should be obtained in the first 24 hours.
- CBC, chem 7, LFTs, and urinalysis

Follow-Up & Special Considerations
- Blood cultures fail to isolate an etiologic agent in 3–23% of cases:
  - Most often due to antibiotic use in the previous 2 weeks
  - Cultures should be held for at least 3 weeks.

Imaging
- Electrocardiogram to assess for new conduction system abnormalities
- Transthoracic echocardiography (TTE) should be performed in all patient in whom IE is reasonably suspected:
  - Sensitivity for detection of vegetation varies between 65% and 85%
  - Sensitivity is highest in right-sided IE
  - Unable to resolve vegetations <2 mm in diameter
  - Poor quality in evaluating prosthetic valve endocarditis due to acoustic shadowing
  - Must be able to acquire adequate windows

Diagnostic Procedures/Other
- Transesophageal echocardiography (TEE) is ~90–95% sensitive
- A negative TEE has a negative predictive value for IE of >92% (7)
- TEE is recommended as a first-line diagnostic study to diagnose prosthetic valve endocarditis (8)[C].
- Indications for TEE include:
  - Negative TTE but high clinical suspicion for IE (9)[A]
  - Prosthetic valves or intracardiac devices
  - Perivalvular abscess (sensitivity 80%, specificity 95%)

DIFFERENTIAL DIAGNOSIS

- Atrial myxoma
- Carcinoid tumors
- Infected aneurysm
- Libman-Sach endocarditis
- Thrombotic nonbacterial endocarditis
- Antiphospholipid antibody syndrome
- SLE

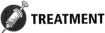 **TREATMENT**

MEDICATION

First Line

- The duration of antimicrobial therapy is counted from the 1st day of sustained blood culture negativity.
- In general, duration of therapy is 4–6 weeks for native valves and 6–8 weeks for prosthetic valves.
- Penicillin-sensitive strains of *S. viridans* and non-enterococcal streptococci (MIC <0.2 μg/mL):
  - Penicillin G 12–18 million units IV daily in 6 divided doses with gentamicin 1 mg/kg IV or IM q8h for 2 weeks
  - Penicillin G 12–18 million units IV daily in 6 divided doses for 4 weeks
  - Ceftriaxone 2 g IV daily for 4 weeks
- Relatively penicillin-resistant streptococci (MIC >0.1–0.5 μg/mL):
  - Penicillin G 24 million U/24 h IV with gentamicin 1 mg/kg q8h OR ceftriaxone 2 g IV q.d. with gentamicin 1 mg/kg q8h for 4–6 weeks
- Staphylococcus, methicillin sensitive:
  - Nafcillin or oxacillin 2 g IV q4h for 4–6 weeks and gentamicin 1.0 mg/kg q8h for first 3–5 days
- Staphylococcus, methicillin resistant:
  - 30 mg/kg/24 h IV in 2 equally divided doses for 4–6 weeks
- HACEK organisms:
  - Ceftriaxone 2 g/d IV for 4 weeks

Second Line

Patients allergic to β-lactams can be treated with vancomycin 30 mg/kg/24 h IV in 2 equally divided doses, not to exceed 2 g in 24 hours unless serum levels are monitored.

SURGERY/OTHER PROCEDURES

- Surgery consultation should be obtained immediately in hemodynamically unstable patients. Delays in surgical intervention can result in increased mortality.
- Urgent indications for surgery:
  - Valve stenosis or regurgitation resulting in refractory heart failure (8)[B]
  - Failure to clear bacteremia (8)[C]
  - Evidence of conduction disturbance, such as heart block, annular or aortic abscess, or destructive penetrating lesion (8)[B]
  - Recurrent emboli (8)[C]
  - Rupture into the pericardium (11)[A]
- Elective indication for surgery:
  - Staphylococcal prosthetic valve endocarditis (11)[B]
  - Early prosthetic valve endocarditis (11)[B]
  - Evidence of progressive perivalvular prosthetic leak (11)[A]
  - Fungal endocarditis due to mold (11)[A]
  - Fungal endocarditis due to yeast (11)[B]

IN-PATIENT CONSIDERATIONS

Initial Stabilization

- Management of sepsis
- Hemodynamic support and/or mechanical ventilation as indicated for severe respiratory distress due to either congestive heart failure or acute valvular disruption, particularly with aortic valve involvement

Admission Criteria

All patients diagnosed with endocarditis should be admitted for monitoring and further management.

 ONGOING CARE

FOLLOW-UP RECOMMENDATIONS

- Consider repeating TTE or TEE at 7–10 days into therapy, to look for enlarging vegetations or other complications (10)[B].
- TTE should be performed at completion of therapy to establish a new baseline (10)[C].

Patient Monitoring

- Frequent and close monitoring for resolution of symptoms
- Monitoring for emerging indications for surgical interventions
- Repeat blood cultures should be obtained q48h until they are repeatedly sterile.
- Daily electrocardiogram to assess for conduction disturbance

PROGNOSIS

- Major CNS complications, uncontrolled infection, especially abscess formation
- Staphylococcal etiology and mold-related endocarditis are associated with increased mortality. (10)
- Overall survival for patients with infective endocarditis is ~75–80% (12).

COMPLICATIONS

- See indications for surgical intervention regarding cardiac complications.
- Systemic embolization occurs in 22–50% of cases of IE (12).
- Splenic abscess
- Infarction of renal, splenic, and pulmonary beds
- Intracranial and extracranial mycotic aneurysms
- Antibiotic toxicity

REFERENCES

1. Mylonakis E, et al. Infective endocarditis in adults. *N Engl J Med.* 2001;345(18):1318–30.
2. Michel PL, et al. Native cardiac disease predisposing to infective endocarditis. *Eur Heart J.* 1995;16:2–6.
3. Moreillon P, et al. Infective endocarditis. *Lancet.* 2004;363:139.
4. Nishimura RA, et al. ACC/AHA 2008 Guideline update on valvular heart disease: Focused update on infective endocarditis. *J Am Coll Cardiol.* 2008;52:676–85.
5. Hasbun R, et al. Complicated left-sided native valve endocarditis in adults: Risk classification for mortality. *JAMA.* 2003;289:1933.
6. Li JS, et al. Proposed modifications to the Duke criteria for the diagnosis of infective endocarditis. *Clin Infect Dis.* 2000;30:633–8.
7. Lowry, RW et al. Clinical impact of transesophageal echocardiography in the diagnosis and management of infective endocarditis. *Am J Cardiol.* 1994;73:1089–91.
8. Bonow RO, et al. Focused Update Incorporated in the ACC/AHA 2006 Guidelines for the Management of Patients with Valvular Heart Disease. *Circulation.* 2008;118:e523–661.
9. Horstkotte D, et al. Guidelines on prevention, diagnosis and treatment of infective endocarditis. Full text. The Task Force on Infective Endocarditis of the European Society of Cardiology, access at www.escardio.org. Executive summary. *Eur Heart J.* 2004;25:267.
10. Baddour LM, et al. Infective endocarditis: Diagnosis, antimicrobial therapy, and management of complications. A statement for healthcare professionals from the Committee on Rheumatic Fever, Endocarditis, and Kawasaki Disease, Council on Cardiovascular Disease in the Young, and the Councils on Clinical Cardiology, Stroke, and Cardiovascular Surgery and Anesthesia, American Heart Association: Endorsed by the Infectious Diseases Society of America. *Circulation.* 2005;111:e394–434.
11. Olaison L, Pettersson G. Current best practices and guidelines: Indications for surgical intervention in infective endocarditis. *Infect Dis Clin North Am.* 2002;16:453,1992.
12. Hasbun R, et al. Complicated left-sided native valve endocarditis in adults: Risk classification for mortality. *JAMA.* 2003;289:1933.

 CODES

ICD9

- 421.0 Acute and subacute bacterial endocarditis
- 424.90 Endocarditis, valve unspecified, unspecified cause
- 996.61 Infection and inflammatory reaction due to cardiac device, implant, and graft

CLINICAL PEARLS

- Most endocarditis occurs on damaged valves, but aggressive organisms may invade structurally normal valves.
- 80–95% of patients with endocarditis will present with fever and murmur. However, <10% of murmurs will be detected as a new murmur.
- Peripheral manifestation of endocarditis are often absent on physical exam.
- Early referral to surgery for complications associated with endocarditis may reduce mortality in a subpopulation of patients.

E

ENTEROCUTANEOUS FISTULA (ECF)

Amy Rezak
Reza Askari

 BASICS

DESCRIPTION
- A fistula is an abnormal connection between 2 epithelialized surfaces.
- An enterocutaneous fistula (ECF) or external fistula involves a connection between the intestine and the skin.
- ECFs are classified according to their location (duodenum, jejunum, or ileum), etiology (iatrogenic, Crohn's), and volume (low-output fistulas <200 mL/day and high-output fistulas >500 mL/day).

RISK FACTORS
- Previous radiation therapy
- Inflammatory bowel disease
- Malnutrition
- Anemia
- Hypothermia
- Intra-abdominal infection
- Emergency procedures with associated hypotension (1).

GENERAL PREVENTION
During an emergency procedure, generally meticulous surgical technique, use of healthy bowel with adequate blood supply for anastomosis, avoiding tension and thorough hemostasis may minimize the risk for the development of ECF (1).

PATHOPHYSIOLOGY
Patients with ECF often exhibit dehydration, electrolyte abnormalities, and malnutrition.

ETIOLOGY
The majority of ECFs are iatrogenic. Some other causes include trauma, erosion from catheters, inflammatory bowel disease, or foreign bodies. Previous radiation therapy, malignancy, and infectious disease may contribute to the formation of ECFs.

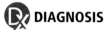 DIAGNOSIS

HISTORY
- Fevers, prolonged ileus, and wound or abdominal wall erythema
- Postoperative ECFs will usually manifest between 7 and 10 days following surgery.

PHYSICAL EXAM
Wound or erythematous skin opening draining enteric contents

DIAGNOSTIC TESTS & INTERPRETATION
Lab
Initial lab tests
- Check chemistry including serum electrolytes
- WBC in CBC maybe elevated
- Albumin

Follow-Up & Special Considerations
It is important to continue to follow electrolytes and nutrition parameters

Imaging
Initial approach
- CT scan with enteral contrast to diagnose and locate the fistula.
- Fistulogram

Follow-Up & Special Considerations
If an intra-abdominal collection has not yet fistulized to the skin, then IR percutaneous drain may be used to control the fistula to the skin.

Diagnostic Procedures/Other
Placing an ostomy appliance over the fistula to determine daily volume.

DIFFERENTIAL DIAGNOSIS
- Intra-abdominal abscess collection
- Necrotizing fasciitis

 TREATMENT

MEDICATION
First Line
Octreotide/somatostatin (octreotide has been shown to reduce GI secretions and reduce fistula output; however, there have been no prospective randomized studies to date) (2).

Second Line
Infliximab (if ECF is result of Crohn's disease)

ADDITIONAL TREATMENT
General Measures
- Phase 1: Stabilize, hydrate, correct electrolyte abnormalities, control fistula drainage, begin nutritional support, and protect the skin. Reduction of fistula output may also be attempted.
- Phase 2: Delineate the fistula anatomy.
- Phase 3: Determine the likelihood that the fistula will close with conservative nonoperative management (90% of fistulas that will close with conservative treatment close within 5 weeks) (3)
- Factors preventing spontaneous fistula closure
- The mnemonic "FRIEND" (Foreign body within the fistula tract, Radiation enteritis, Infection/Inflammation at fistula origin, Epithelialization of the fistula tract, Neoplasm at the fistula origin, Distal intestinal obstruction)
- Phase 4: Plan the definitive operative therapy.

Issues for Referral
General surgery consult, in addition to metabolic support, nutrition, and enterostomal nursing consults are strongly recommended.

Additional Therapies
- PT
- Supplemental IV fluid for high-output EC fistula is sometimes necessary

COMPLEMENTARY & ALTERNATIVE THERAPIES

Vacuum-assisted wound management may also be used with fistulas not amendable to an ostomy appliance.

SURGERY/OTHER PROCEDURES

- Most surgeons will trial conservative management for 4–6 months before contemplating surgery.
- Once the patient is optimized nutritionally, resection of the ECF and establishing continuity of the GI tract is the definitive therapy.

IN-PATIENT CONSIDERATIONS

Initial Stabilization

Immediate concerns include correction of fluid and electrolyte imbalance, treatment of sepsis, source control (drainage of abscesses), control of drainage and protection of the skin.

Admission Criteria

- Newly diagnosed or suspected ECFs, chronic ECFs with sudden change in output
- Dehydration secondary to high-output fistula

IV Fluids

Aggressive IV fluid resuscitation with NS and the addition of HCO_3^- and electrolytes (this may vary depending on the location of the fistula).

Nursing

- Meticulous skin care
- Emotional support
- Wound care (often with the assistance of an enterostomal nurse)

Discharge Criteria

Patients with an ECF typically require skilled nursing facility upon discharge. This is due to the often complex wound care, physical deconditioning and nutritional support required (supplemental enteral or parenteral).

 ## ONGOING CARE

FOLLOW-UP RECOMMENDATIONS

Patient Monitoring

It is important to follow the fistula output and nutritional parameters as an outpatient. This should be done on a regular basis to determine if the fistula is likely to close, and if not, when the patient is nutritionally optimized for surgery.

DIET

This is often a case by case determination, however if enteral feeding is not an option then these patients are typically NPO, and on TPN. If enteral nutrition is possible, then this may be accomplished via tube feeds or by mouth.

PATIENT EDUCATION

Patients with an ECF should be educated that their illness is physically and emotionally demanding (wound care, metabolic challenges, and extended rehabilitation).

PROGNOSIS

50% of all intestinal fistulas will close spontaneously. ECFs are associated with a 10–15% mortality rate primarily due to infection or sepsis. If the patient undergoes surgery for the fistula, there is a >50% mortality rate with 10% chance of recurrence (3).

COMPLICATIONS

- Recurrent or persistent fistula
- Sepsis
- Death

REFERENCES

1. Fischer J, et al. Gastro-cutaneous fistulae. In Fischer JE, et al., eds. *Mastery of Surgery*, 5th ed. Philadelphia: Lippincott Williams & Wilkins.
2. Schecter W, et al. Enteric fistulas: Principles of management. *J Am Coll Surg.* 2009;209(4): 484–91.
3. Tavakkolizadeh A, et al. Small intestine. In Brunicardi FC, et al., eds. *Schwartz's Principles of Surgery*, 9th ed. New York: McGraw-Hill.

 ## CODES

ICD9

- 537.4 Fistula of stomach or duodenum
- 569.81 Fistula of intestine, excluding rectum and anus

CLINICAL PEARLS

- Rule out factors ("FRIEND") that inhibit ECF closure prior to initiating definitive surgical therapy.
- Key principles: early recognition, promoting fistula formation of abscesses, long term nutritional and management plans, management of associated malnutrition and electrolyte abnormalities

E

EHRLICHIA BABESIA

Parul Kaushik

 BASICS

DESCRIPTION
- Human ehrlichiosis, such as human monocytic ehrlichiosis (HME), human granulocytic anaplasmosis (HGA), and human ewingii ehrlichiosis (HEE), along with the protozoal disease babesiosis, are tick-borne diseases.
- They cause nonspecific febrile illness with various cytopenias, biochemical abnormalities, and different organ involvement.

EPIDEMIOLOGY
Incidence
- The average incidence of HME in the US is estimated at 0.7 cases per million and of HGA is 1.6 cases per million population; however, it is believed the true incidence of these diseases is much higher owing to subclinical infections in endemic areas.
- The cases tend to occur in late spring and summer for HME, and peak in June and July for HGA.
- Babesiosis is considered an emerging infectious disease in US, as the number of cases has steadily been climbing, with over 1,500 cases notified from New York State alone since 1986.
- Babesiosis is mainly seen May–September.

Prevalence
- HME is seen primarily in southeastern, midwestern, and south central states.
- Babesiosis and HGA follow the same geographic distribution as Lyme disease, and are found in northeastern and upper midwestern states.
- Based on the seroprevalence studies done in endemic areas, there is a much higher prevalence of these diseases than deduced from clinical practice.

RISK FACTORS
- Residence in or travel to endemic area
- Most cases of these diseases tend to occur when tick, deer, rodents, and humans are outdoors in close proximity to each other.
- HEE tends to occur in immunocompromised patients.

GENERAL PREVENTION
- Wearing light colored clothes
- Regular tick checks when visiting outdoors in endemic region in spring and summer months
- Applying chemoprophylactic agents, such as DEET to exposed skin

PATHOPHYSIOLOGY
- Following tick bite, ehrlichia and anaplasma enter the circulation and multiply within their target cells (monocytes/macrophages and neutrophils, respectively), where they appear as clustered intracytoplasmic inclusions known as *morulae*.
- Host response plays an important role in the pathogenesis of HME and HGA. Ehrlichia and anaplasma are believed to exert their pathogenic effect through a series of proinflammatory cytokines.

- Babesia species have a complex life cycle, with asexual reproduction occurring in the erythrocytes of mammalian hosts and sexual reproduction in tick vector. After the sporozoites are deposited in the dermis of the human host, they enter the erythrocytes and become trophozoites. A trophozoite divides by binary fission into either 2 or 4 merozoites. A tetrad of merozoites is called "Maltese cross." Egress of merozoites lead to red cell hemolysis.
- Babesiosis has also been transmitted by blood transfusion.

ETIOLOGY
- Ehrlichia and anaplasma are small obligate intracellular gram-negative bacteria.
- HME is caused by *E. chaffeensis*, which is spread by the lone star tick, *Amblyomma americanum*.
- *E. ewingii* causes HEE and is also transmitted by the lone star tick.
- HGA, previously known as human granulocytic ehrlichiosis (HGE), is caused by *Anaplasma phagocytophilum*.
- Babesiosis is caused by different *Babesia* spp. with *B. microti* being the most common in the US.
- The blacklegged tick, *Ixodes scapularis,* that also transmits agents that causes Lyme disease, transmits HGA and babesiosis.
- The reservoir for HME is white-tailed deer, and for HGA are small rodents such as white-footed mice.
- The life cycle of *Babesia* involves two hosts, tick and white-footed mouse, with humans entering as an accidental host when bitten by an infected tick.

COMMONLY ASSOCIATED CONDITIONS
Owing to their common vector, *Ixodes* spp., and similar geographic distribution, approximately 10% of patients with HGA have serologic evidence of coinfection with Lyme disease or babesiosis.

DIAGNOSIS

HISTORY
- A nonspecific febrile illness characterized by fever, chills, headache, myalgia, malaise, and arthralgia is seen.
- GI symptoms such as nausea, vomiting, and abdominal pain are variably present.

PHYSICAL EXAM
- Often unremarkable except for fever
- Rash, maculopapular or petechial, is more commonly seen in HME, occurring in 66% of pediatric patients, whereas in HGA, <10% of patients have rash. Rash is rare in babesiosis.
- Mild splenomegaly and hepatomegaly can be found.

DIAGNOSTIC TESTS & INTERPRETATION
Lab
Initial lab tests
- CBC, CMP, peripheral smear
- Leukopenia, thrombocytopenia, elevated liver enzymes are seen in ehrlichia diseases and babesiosis. Elevated creatinine may also occur. In children, mild hyponatremia may be seen.
- Morulae are seen in 7% of the cases of HME and 25–75% of the cases of HGE in peripheral smear stained with Giemsa or Wright stain in the 1st week of illness.
- Hemolytic anemia with indirect hyperbilirubinemia and elevated lactate dehydrogenase may occur in babesiosis.
- Peripheral smear can identify round, oval, piriform shaped intraerythrocytic parasites in babesiosis with Giemsa and Wright stains.Maltese crosses (rarely seen) are pathognomic of this disease.
- Detection of DNA by PCR is a rapid diagnostic test with high sensitivity and specificity but is not widely available.

Follow-Up & Special Considerations
- Paired serologic testing of IgM and IgG antibodies collected during a 3–6-week interval specific to *E. chaffeensis* and *A. phagocytophilum* is the most frequently used confirmatory test.
- A single IgG antibody titer of at least 256 or seroconversion from negative to positive titers with a minimum titer of 64, and a 4-fold increase in titer when acute or convalescent sera are compared indicate HME infection.
- Babesial IgM and IgG could be used to confirm the diagnosis of *Babesia*. A titer of ≥1:1024 signifies active or recent infection.
- Specific antibodies may be negative initially.
- No specific serologic testing is available for *E. ewingii*.

Imaging
Initial approach
- Chest x-ray
- Head CT or brain MRI as needed

Follow-Up & Special Considerations
Based on the abnormality of initial Imaging

Diagnostic Procedures/Other
- Lumbar puncture: CSF pleocytosis with elevated protein is seen in HME. Morulae are rarely seen in CSF monocytes by Giemsa stain.
- Bone marrow biopsy may be done.

Pathological Findings
When bone marrow biopsy is done in HME, granuloma formation, myeloid hyperplasia, and megakaryocytes are seen.

DIFFERENTIAL DIAGNOSIS

- Often HME and HGA are hard to distinguish from each other and from babesiosis.
- Other differential diagnosis include other tick-borne diseases such as Rocky Mountain spotted fever, relapsing fever, tularemia, Colorado tick fever, Lyme disease; viral syndromes, bacterial sepsis, Kawasaki disease, collagen-vascular disease, and immune thrombocytopenic purpura
- Babesiosis should be distinguished from malaria.

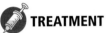 TREATMENT

MEDICATION

First Line

- Doxycycline 100 mg PO or IV b.i.d. for a total of 7–10 days is single preferred agent for HME and HGA.
- Atovaquone and azithromycin for 7–10 days for mild-moderate disease and clindamycin and quinine for 7–10 days for severe babesiosis are the treatment of choice.

Second Line

Rifampin (300 mg b.i.d. or in children weighing <45.4 kg: 10 mg/kg b.i.d.) can be used in cases of contraindication to doxycycline.

ADDITIONAL TREATMENT

General Measures

Airway protection and hemodynamic stability

Pregnancy Considerations

Rifampin can be used in pregnant patients for HME and HGA as doxycycline is contraindicated.

Pediatric Considerations

Doxycycline remains the drug of choice in this population despite the risk of dental discoloration.

Issues for Referral

Infectious diseases consult is strongly recommended.

Additional Therapies

Exchange red cell transfusion is indicated in babesiosis if parasitemia exceeds 10% or patient develops renal, hepatic, or pulmonary failure.

IN-PATIENT CONSIDERATIONS

Initial Stabilization

- Airway protection, circulatory support
- Institution of appropriate antibiotics as soon as possible

Admission Criteria

Severe disease, biochemical abnormalities, and complications warranting close monitoring

IV Fluids

As per protocol if patient does not tolerate PO

Nursing

Can be monitored in general wards; if complications develop, may need ICU monitoring

Discharge Criteria

- Resolution of constitutional symptoms
- Healthy appearance

 ONGOING CARE

FOLLOW-UP RECOMMENDATIONS

Patient may be followed-up for convalescence sera testing.

DIET

Continued nutrition is essential to promote recovery.

PATIENT EDUCATION

- Reduce further tick exposure by taking appropriate precautions if patient continues to reside in or travel to endemic area.
- See General Prevention

PROGNOSIS

- Variable
- HME tends to have worse outcome in immunocompromised patients such as with HIV, on steroids, and in transplant recipients.
- In addition to immunocompromised state and old age, asplenism is also a risk factor for developing severe babesiosis.

COMPLICATIONS

- ARDS
- Acute renal insufficiency
- Meningitis and meningoencephalitis with HME may occur in 20 % of patients; rare with HGA.
- Coagulopathy
- GI hemorrhage
- Hepatic failure

ADDITIONAL READING

- Dumler JS, et al. *Ehrlichia chaffeensis, Anaplasma phagocytophilum* and other Anaplasmataceae. In: Mandell GL, et al., eds. *Mandell, Douglas, and Bennett's principles and practice of infectious diseases*, 7th ed. Philadelphia: Elsevier, 2010; 2531–8.
- Gelfand JA, et al. Babesia species. In: Mandell GL et al., eds. *Mandell, Douglas, and Bennett's principles and practice of infectious diseases*, 7th ed. Philadelphia: Elsevier, 2010;3539–46.
- Ismail N, et al. Human ehlichiosis and anaplasmosis. *Clin Lab Med*. 2010;30(1):261–92.
- Vannier EG, et al. Human babesiosis. *Infect Dis Clin N Am*. 2008;22:469–88.
- http://www.cdc.gov/ehrlichiosis
- http://www.cdc.gov/parasites/babesiosis

 See Also (Topic, Algorithm, Electronic Media Element)

Tick diseases

CODES

ICD9

- 082.40 Unspecified ehrlichiosis
- 082.49 Other ehrlichiosis
- 088.82 Babesiosis

CLINICAL PEARLS

- If a patient with HGA does not improve clinically in 72 hours with doxycycline, *Babesia* coinfection should be suspected.

E

EXTENDED SPECTRUM β-LACTAMASES (ESBL)

Miguel Angel Russo

BASICS

DESCRIPTION
- β-Lactamases are a group of enzymes capable of hydrolyzing the 4-membered β-lactam ring of β-lactam antibiotics (penicillins, cephalosporins, monobactams, and carbapenems). They are the most important mechanism of resistance to β-lactam antibiotics.
- The extended spectrum β-lactamases (ESBLs) are mutated enzymes of β-lactamases, forms of enzymes that are capable of destroying monobactams and 3rd-generation cephalosporin and enzymes that are resistant to β-lactamases inhibitors.
- These enzymes emerged soon after the introduction of the extended-spectrum cephalosporins and were first reported in Europe in the early 1980s.

EPIDEMIOLOGY
A surveillance study conducted across the U.S. indicated that 15% of *E. coli* and 24% of *Klebsiella pneumoniae* have elevated MICs of 2 μg/mL or more to ceftazidime, consistent with an ESBL phenotype among selected isolates.

RISK FACTORS
- Device-related (arterial catheters, central venous catheters, urinary tract catheters, gastrostomy or jejunostomy tube)
- Surgical-related (abdominal surgery, emergency laparotomy)
- Antibiotic exposure (3rd-generation cephalosporin, fluoroquinolones, trimethoprim-sulfamethoxazole)
- Previous nursing home residence
- Prolonged duration of hospital or ICU stay (longer stay is associated with more severe underlying disease, with invasive procedures, and with antibiotic administration)
- Severity of illness (APACHE III score)

GENERAL PREVENTION
- Surveillance: Laboratory-based surveillance should be conducted on a continuous basis to detect ESBL producing gram-negative bacteria among patients who have had cultures obtained for clinical reasons.
- Prevent cross-infections.
- Control antimicrobial pressure.
- Hand-washing by health care workers
- Use of appropriate aseptic techniques and bundles during insertion of indwelling catheters

PATHOPHYSIOLOGY
- Extended-spectrum β-lactamases are primarily plasmid-mediated enzymes that are frequently derived from either a TEM- or SHV-related enzyme. Both TEM-1 and SHV-1 are parent enzymes that confer resistance to ampicillin.
- Resistance determinants encoding ESBLs are found on mobile genetic elements, facilitating the spread among Enterobacteriaceae.
- *K. pneumoniae* and *E. coli* are most commonly cited in the literature as harboring such resistance determinants.

ETIOLOGY
ESBL enzymes are most commonly produced by 3 bacteria: *E. coli*, *K. pneumoniae*, and *Proteus mirabilis*.

COMMONLY ASSOCIATED CONDITIONS
Infections caused by ESBL-producing bacteria can be subdivided according to the various organs/systems as follows:
- Urinary tract infection
- Bacteremia (primary or secondary)
- Respiratory tract infection (nosocomial pneumonia, ventilator associated pneumonia)
- GI tract infection (intra-abdominal abscess, peritonitis, cholangitis)
- Skin and soft tissue infection
- Catheter- or device-related infection
- Sinusitis
- Neurosurgical meningitis, related to ventricular drainage catheters

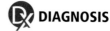

DIAGNOSIS

PHYSICAL EXAM
- Urinary tract: Pain and burning when urinating, the need to urinate more often, fever
- Intestine: Diarrhea (may be bloody), pain in the abdomen, stomach cramps, gas, fever, loss of appetite
- Skin wound: Redness of the skin around the wound and oozing of fluid from the wound
- Blood: High fever, chills, nausea and vomiting, shortness of breath, confusion
- In nosocomial pneumonia due to an ESBL-producing organism the diagnosis can be problematic. The isolation of an ESBL-producing organism from a sputum sample or an endotracheal aspirate does not necessarily indicate that it is the cause of the pneumonia. In the absence of clinical signs such as fever, signs of consolidation, or radiological changes, a positive culture may indicate colonization and not require any antibiotic therapy.

DIAGNOSTIC TESTS & INTERPRETATION
Lab
All clinically significant isolates of *E. coli* or *K. pneumoniae* should be tested against β-lactam drugs either using a disc diffusion method or the minimum inhibition concentration (MIC) method (as advocated by the revised NCCLS interpretive criteria). Any decrease in the zone sizes or MIC <2 mg/L for the 3rd-generation cephalosporins should be used as a criterion to test for ESBLs.

Diagnostic Procedures/Other
- Aspiration of potentially infected body fluids (pleural, peritoneal, CSF) when appropriate
- Drainage of potentially infected tissues (abscess, biliary tree, ulcers, others) when appropriate

TREATMENT

MEDICATION
- Empirical therapy:
  - If gram-negative sepsis and the suspected cause is Enterobacteriaceae, avoid ceftazidime and aztreonam and empirically select an agent based on institutional antibiogram:
    - β-lactam–β-lactamase inhibitors
    - Non-ceftazidime cephalosporins (e.g., cefotaxime)
    - Fluoroquinolones
    - Aminoglycosides
- Direct therapy:
  - Against culture-confirmed gram-negative bacteria, if ESBL positive:
  - Life-threatening: Change empirical therapy to carbapenem.
  - Non–life-threatening: Streamline therapy based on initial response and sensitivity result (β-lactam therapy except ceftazidime and aztreonam, fluoroquinolones, aminoglycosides, TMP-SMX.

ADDITIONAL TREATMENT
- DVT prophylaxis:
  - Prophylaxis with either low-dose unfractionated heparin or low-molecular-weight heparin should be used, unless contraindicated.
  - Very high-risk patients should receive combination of mechanical and pharmacological therapy.
- Stress ulcer prophylaxis:
  - H_2 blocker or proton pump inhibitors should be used.

 ONGOING CARE

DIET
- NPO initially
- Enteral feeds when possible

PATIENT EDUCATION
Medline Plus. At: http://www.nlm.nih.gov/medlineplus/

PROGNOSIS
Following factors have been associated with worse prognosis: Extreme ages, neutropenia, diabetes mellitus, alcoholism, renal failure

COMPLICATIONS
- Bacteremia
- Sepsis
- ARDS
- DIC
- Death

ADDITIONAL READING

- Jones RN, et al. Antimicrobial activity and spectrum investigation of eight broad-spectrum β-lactam drugs: A 1997 surveillance trial in 102 medical centers in the United States. *Diagn Microbiol Infect Dis.* 1998;30:215–28.
- National Committee for Clinical Laboratory Standards. Performance standards for antimicrobial susceptibility testing. 13th informational supplement. M1000-S12. Wayne PA, 2003.
- Oteoa J, et al. What is new in bacterial resistance to antimicrobials? *Enferm Infec Microbiol Clin.* 2002;20:28–33.
- Paterson DL, et al. Epidemiology of ciprofloxacin resistance and its relationship to extended spectrum β-lactamase production in *Klebsiella pneumoniae* isolates causing bacteremia. *Clin Infect Dis.* 2000;30:473–8.
- Paterson DL. Extended-spectrum β-lactamases: The European experience. *Curr Opin Infect Dis.* 2001;14:697–701.
- Winokur PL, et al. Variations in the prevalence of strains expressing an extended-spectrum β-lactamasas phenotype and characterization of isolates from Europe, the Americas, and the Western Pacific Region. *Clin Infect Dis.* 2001;32(Suppl 2): S94–S103.

CODES

ICD9
- V09.70 Infection with microorganisms resistant to other specified antimycobacterial agents without mention of resistance to multiple antimycobacterial agents
- 041.4 Escherichia coli (e. coli) infection in conditions classified elsewhere and of unspecified site
- 041.89 Other specified bacterial infections in conditions classified elsewhere and of unspecified site, other specified bacteria

E

FATTY LIVER OF PREGNANCY, ACUTE

Nelli Fisher
Dena Goffman

 BASICS

DESCRIPTION
- Form of hepatic microvesicular steatosis associated with mitochondrial dysfunction
- Presents late in pregnancy, often as fulminant hepatic failure with sudden onset of coagulopathy and encephalopathy in a woman without a prior history of liver disease
- Historically, thought to be universally fatal but early recognition, aggressive stabilization of the mother, and prompt delivery have improved prognosis.

EPIDEMIOLOGY
Incidence
- 1 in 6,659 births
- 12.5% maternal mortality
- 15% fetal mortality (1)[C]

Prevalence
Similar across populations

RISK FACTORS
- Nulliparity
- Multiple pregnancy
- Male fetus
- Preeclampsia
- Mother heterozygous for long-chain 3-hydroxyacyl coenzyme A dehydrogenase (LCHAD) deficiency

Genetics
- Autosomally inherited mutation that causes deficiency of the LCHAD, a fatty acid β-oxidation enzyme
- Single point mutation of a guanine to cytosine at base pair 1528 (G1528C)
- LCHAD deficiency in affected fetus is associated with AFLP in a mother (2)[C].

PATHOPHYSIOLOGY
- Nonoxidized long-chain fatty acids accumulate in LCHAD deficient fetus.
- Excess fatty acids are produced by placenta.
- Excess of hepatotoxic long-chain fatty acids enter maternal serum.

ETIOLOGY
Fetal fatty acid accumulation leads to maternal hepatotoxicity.

COMMONLY ASSOCIATED CONDITIONS
- Preeclampsia
- DIC
- Hemorrhagic shock
- Pancreatitis
- Diabetes insipidus
- Renal failure
- ARDS
- Pulmonary edema

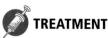 DIAGNOSIS

HISTORY
- Nausea (2)[C]
- Malaise
- Jaundice
- Anorexia
- Vomiting
- Abdominal pain
- Polydipsia
- Polyuria
- Headache
- Altered mentation

PHYSICAL EXAM
- Ill-appearing (2)[C]
- Jaundice
- Low-grade fever
- Hypertension
- Bleeding
- Neurologic exam from normal to lethargy, agitation, confusion, and coma

DIAGNOSTIC TESTS & INTERPRETATION
Lab
Initial lab tests
- Elevated conjugated bilirubin—distinguishing feature from HELLP and PEC
- Prolonged PT
- Hypofibrinogenemia
- Increased serum ammonia
- Elevated uric acid
- Elevated blood urea nitrogen and creatinine
- Elevated WBC
- Platelets from low to normal
- Acidosis
- Hypoglycemia; variable
- Hyperglycemia if associated pancreatitis
- Decreased antithrombin III
- ALT, AST from barely elevated to 1000 (2)[C]

Follow-Up & Special Considerations
- Quick progression to:
- DIC
- Diabetes insipidus (DI)
- Pancreatitis
- ARDS
- Renal failure
- Hepatic encephalopathy

Imaging
- US: Increased echogenicity, poor specificity
- CT scan: Decreased or diffuse attenuation in the liver; more sensitive (2)[C]

Diagnostic Procedures/Other
Liver biopsy rarely done

Pathological Findings
- Frozen section liver biopsy with oil red O stain
- Swollen, pale hepatocytes with central nuclei
- Periportal fibrin deposition
- Hemorrhagic cell necrosis
- Intracytoplasmic microsteatosis

DIFFERENTIAL DIAGNOSIS
- HELLP
- Preeclampsia
- Cholestasis of pregnancy
- Budd-Chiari syndrome
- Adult-onset Reye syndrome
- Acetaminophen overdose
- Tetracycline-induced toxicity
- Anticonvulsant drugs hypersensitivity
- Methyldopa hepatitis

TREATMENT

MEDICATION
First Line
- Stabilize the mother (2)[C].
- Therapy depends on complication:
  - Administer IV dextrose to correct hypoglycemia.
  - Correct electrolytes.
  - Maintain ventilatory support if ARDS.
  - Correct coagulopathy if DIC.
  - Remove ammonia.
  - Institute dialysis if renal failure.
  - Administer desmopressin if DI:
    ○ DDAVP, a derivative of vasopressin, is available PO, nasal spray, parenterally
    ○ 0.2–0.6 mg at bedtime
- Labor induction: Expeditious delivery within 24 hours is the ultimate treatment.

ADDITIONAL TREATMENT
General Measures
Monitor for:
- Progressive hepatic failure
- Coagulopathy
- Hypoglycemia
- CBC, PT, PTT, fibrinogen, chemistry, liver function tests q6h
- Postpartum acute refractory hypotensive shock
- Worsening laboratory values postpartum
- Strict I/O (3)[C]

Issues for Referral
- GI follow-up
- Genetics
- Maternal fetal medicine specialist for:
  - Preconception counseling
  - Management of future pregnancies

Additional Therapies
- Fetal assessment
- Avoid drugs requiring hepatic metabolism:
  - Facilitate colonic emptying with enemas, magnesium citrate
  - Neomycin, 6–12 g PO qd to reduce ammonia production by colonic bacteria
  - H2 blockers, GI prophylaxis

SURGERY/OTHER PROCEDURES
- Cesarean delivery (CD) decision is based on obstetrical indications.
- Avoid epidural analgesia.
- General anesthesia if CD
- Exchange transfusion
- Hemodialysis
- Plasmapheresis
- Liver transplantation

IN-PATIENT CONSIDERATIONS
Initial Stabilization
Immediate hospitalization on labor and delivery with critical care backup:
- Confirm diagnosis.
- Obtain and correct glucose, electrolytes.
- Correct coagulopathy.
- Initiate delivery.

Admission Criteria
- Immediate admission to L&D with available ICU setting and critical care involvement
- ICU postpartum

IV Fluids
IV Dextrose (5–25%)

Nursing
- Frequent VS
- Observe for bleeding
- Strict I/O
- Frequent neurological exam

Discharge Criteria
- Resolution may occur 3 days after delivery.
- Normalization of all laboratory values
- Evidence of absence of hemorrhagic complications after delivery
- Absence of associated complications

 ONGOING CARE

FOLLOW-UP RECOMMENDATIONS
- Mother, father, and child should be tested for the G1528C LCHAD mutation.
- Home care nursing for the 1st week to assure BP control, stable symptoms, appropriate healing.
- High risk follow-up
- Contraception discussion
- Preconception counseling

Patient Monitoring
Follow-up 1–2 weeks and then 6 weeks postpartum

DIET
- Goal is to reduce nitrogenous waste and to prevent or treat hypoglycemia.
- 2000–2500 calories a day:
  - Primarily in the form of glucose
  - Dextrose can be administered via NG tube.
  - Exclude protein during acute phase of illness.

PATIENT EDUCATION
The risk of recurrence is increased in carriers for the LCHAD mutation.

PROGNOSIS
- Improvement in 2–3 days postpartum
- Some may take 1–4 weeks postpartum to improve.
- Improved survival is reported with prompt diagnosis, delivery of the infant, and intensive care.
- 12.5% maternal mortality rate
- 15 % perinatal mortality rate

COMPLICATIONS
- Fulminant hepatic failure
- Hepatic encephalopathy
- Pulmonary edema
- Pancreatitis
- DI
- Infection
- DIC
- Seizures
- Coma
- Liver transplantation

ADDITIONAL READING
- Castro MA, et al. Reversible peripartum liver failure: A new perspective on the diagnosis, treatment, and cause of acute fatty liver of pregnancy based on 28 cases. *Am J Obstet Gynecol*. 2000;181:389–95.
- Fesenmeier MF et al. Acute fatty liver of pregnancy in 3 tertiary care centers. *Am J Obstet Gynecol*. 2005;192:1416–9.
- Guntupalli SR, et al. Hepatic disease and pregnancy: An overview of diagnosis and management. *Crit Care Med*. 2005;33[Suppl]:S332–S9.
- Ibdah JA. Acute fatty liver of pregnancy: An update on pathogenesis and clinical implications. *World J Gastroenterol*. 2006;12:7397–404.
- Sibai BM. Immitators of severe preeclampsia. *Obstet Gynecol*. 2007;109:956–66.

CODES
ICD9
- 570 Acute and subacute necrosis of liver
- 646.73 Antepartum liver disorders

F

CLINICAL PEARLS
- Early diagnosis and aggressive multidisciplinary management drastically improves prognosis for mother and fetus.
- Hyperbilirubinemia and progressive jaundice with only mildly elevated liver transaminases may be the important early distinguishing sign from preeclampsia and HELLP. Progression to coagulopathy, hypoglycemia, and altered mentation will follow.
- After initial stabilization, prompt delivery within 24 hours is the ultimate treatment.
- Postpartum recovery requires ICU management because of worsening laboratory and clinical parameters.

FEVER, NEUTROPENIC

Negia E. Lalane

 BASICS

DESCRIPTION
- Neutropenia is defined as an absolute neutrophil count of (ANC) <500 or <1000 cells/μL
- ANC = WBC × % bands
- Neutropenic fever is defined as a single temperature of >101°F (38.3°C) or a sustained temperature of >100.4°F (38°C).

ALERT
Patients on corticosteroids might not mount a fever; in fact fever could manifest as hypotension and hypothermia, so a low threshold of suspicion should be maintained for this type of patients.

PATHOPHYSIOLOGY
- In the neutropenic host, several factors conjugate to make the patient prone to infection. Defense mechanisms are usually altered, making the host susceptible to a wide range of infections.
- Predisposing factors:
  - Oral mucositis associated with increasingly potent chemotherapeutic agents
  - Profound and prolonged neutropenia
  - increasing use of indwelling intravascular catheters
  - Fluoroquinolone and trimethoprim-sulfamethoxazole prophylaxis;
  - Use of antacids and histamine blockers

ETIOLOGY
- The etiology of neutropenic fever has changed over the decades. In 1950s, the major etiologic agent among febrile neutropenic patients was *Staphylococcus aureus*. During the subsequent 2 decades, gram-negative bacteria such as *Pseudomonas* emerged as the main group. By the 1980s and during the 1990s, gram-positive bacteria reemerged as the principal causative agents.
- The most common infective currently still is gram-negative bacteria, but now coagulase-negative staphylococci, considered traditionally as a contaminant, and fungal infections have also emerged.
- Bacterial etiology: See Table in Guidelines
- Fungal etiology: *Candida* spp. cause infections ranging from superficial lesions to organ involvement and severe systemic candidiasis.
  - *Aspergillus* spp. produce mainly invasive pulmonary aspergillosis; primary cutaneous aspergillosis is associated with the use of IV catheters.
  - *Fusarium* spp. cause disseminated infection with involvement of noble organs and invasion of blood vessels, leading to thrombosis and infarction.
  - *Trichosporon beigelii, Blastoschizomyces capitatus, Scedosporium apiospermum,* and *Scedosporium prolificans*
  - *Candida krusei, C. lusitaniae, C. utilis, C. dubliniensis,* and *C. guillermondii*

- Viral etiology: Viral infection, reinfection, or reactivation can occur:
  - CMV, human metapneumovirus, herpesvirus.
- Parasites: *Toxoplasma gondii* can cause cerebral abscesses, *Cryptosporidium* spp. can cause enteropathy, and *Strongyloides stercoralis* can cause diarrhea.

COMMONLY ASSOCIATED CONDITIONS
- Patients who have received courses of broad-spectrum antibiotics are predisposed to fungal infections.
- Insertion of intravascular device (central lines, pacemakers)

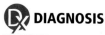 **DIAGNOSIS**

HISTORY
Thorough history

PHYSICAL EXAM
A search should be undertaken in the sites most commonly infected, including the periodontium, pharynx, lower esophagus, lung, perineum, eyes(including the fundus), and skin, including bone marrow aspiration sites, vascular catheter access sites, and tissue around the nails.

DIAGNOSTIC TESTS & INTERPRETATION
- CBC serum creatinine, BUN, transaminases, C-reactive protein
- Blood cultures × 2 (samples from a peripheral vein and/or catheter)
- UA, urine culture (signs or symptoms of UTI, urinary catheter in place)

Imaging
- Chest radiography is indicated for patients with respiratory signs or symptoms.
- CSF if an infection of the CNS is suspected and thrombocytopenia is absent or manageable
- CT scan to look for source of infections

Diagnostic Procedures/Other
- Aspiration or biopsy of skin lesions suspected of being infected should be done for cytological testing.
- Gram stain and culture

 TREATMENT

- See Table for bacteria in guidelines.
- Antiviral drugs are indicated only if there is clinical or laboratory evidence of viral disease; in cases such as skin infections with herpes simplex or varicella zoster virus without fever, treatment is acyclovir.
- colony-stimulating factors, although not recommended on a routine basis, can be give in situations in which worsening of the course is predicted or there is an expected delay in recovery.

ADDITIONAL TREATMENT
General Measures
Antibiotic prophylaxisfor afebrile neutropenic patients:
- TMP-SMZ
- Quinolones
- Vancomycin
- Fluconazole and itraconazole

 ONGOING CARE

DIET
Neutropenic diet:
- Avoid all fresh fruits and vegetables; raw or rare-cooked meat, fish, and eggs; raw nuts; dairy products must be pasteurized. Avoid yogurt and yogurt products with live and active cultures.
- Wash your hands before handling food. Wash all surfaces, cutting boards, and cutting utensils thoroughly. Keep hot food hot and cold food cold.

ADDITIONAL READING
- Hughes WT, et al. 2002 guidelines for the use of antimicrobial agents in neutropenic patients with cancer. *Clin Infect Dis*. 2002;34(6):730–51.
- Kanamuru A, et al. Microbiological data for patients with febrile neutropenia. *Clin Infect Dis*. 2004; 39:(Suppl 1):S7–S10.
- Picazo JJ. Management of the febrile neutropenic patient: A consensus conference. *Clin Infect Dis*. 2004;39: (Suppl 1):S1–S6.
- Urabe A. Clinical features of the neutropenic host: Definitions and initial evaluation. *Clin Infect Dis*. 2004;39: (Suppl 1):S53–S55.

 CODES

ICD9
- 288.00 Neutropenia, unspecified
- 780.60 Fever, unspecified

F

FOURNIER'S GANGRENE

Rafael Alba Yunen

 BASICS

DESCRIPTION
- Necrotizing fasciitis an infectious disease emergency with high mortality manifested by extensive soft tissue infection and thrombosis of the microcirculation with resultant necrosis.
- Fournier's gangrene, a type of necrotizing fasciitis of the perineum, is a rare, life-threatening emergency. The necrotizing localized infection affects the genital and perineal area and may occasionally extend to the abdominal wall. People of all ages may suffer from this disease, but men are more likely to be affected than women.

EPIDEMIOLOGY
Incidence
- 0.4/100,000 adults
- 0.08/100,000 children
- Male > Female (10:1)

Prevalence
- 1 case in 7500 persons
- No seasonal variation, and is not indigenous to any region of the world

RISK FACTORS
- Diabetes mellitus
- Cirrhosis
- Morbid obesity
- Vascular disease of the pelvis
- Chronic alcoholism
- Injuries to the genital area
- Immunosuppression, chemotherapy
- AIDS
- Malignancies

PATHOPHYSIOLOGY
- Trivial infections of the perianal region or lower urogenital tract may develop into an aggressive, soft tissue infection.
- Etiologic factors allow the portal of entry of microorganism into the perineum, the compromised immunity provides a favorable environment to initiate infection, and the virulence of the microorganism promotes its rapid spread.

ETIOLOGY
- Necrotizing process commonly originates from an infection in the anorectum, the urogenital tract, or the skin of the genitalia.
- Usually polymicrobial, causative agents include a synergistic relationship between the streptococcal, staphylococcal, Enterobacteriaceae species, fungi, and anaerobic organisms. Portal of entry most commonly occurs from trauma to the genital area.

COMMONLY ASSOCIATED CONDITIONS
- DIC
- Renal failure
- Sepsis
- Ketoacidosis
- Multiple organ failure

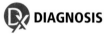 DIAGNOSIS

- Mostly clinical
- Anatomy: Fournier's involves the superficial and deep fascial planes of the genitalia.

HISTORY
- Review all systems for history of:
  - Diabetes
  - Alcohol abuse
  - Colorectal or urogenital disease or surgery
  - Steroid use
  - Sexual history
  - HIV status

PHYSICAL EXAM
- Pain disproportional to visible signs, and tenderness in genitalia is the "hallmark."
- Fever
- Rapid, widespread edema of surrounding tissue
- Erythema of overlaying skin
- Loss of sensation
- Skin darkens to maroon, blue, black color
- Bullae may be present
- Thin, clear discharge ("dirty dishwater")
- Presence of sweet, sickly odor
- Soft tissue crepitus or fluctuance

DIAGNOSTIC TESTS & INTERPRETATION
Lab
Initial lab tests
- CBC (to look for evidence of sepsis-induced thrombocytopenia and leukocytosis)
- Basic metabolic panel (to look for electrolytes abnormalities, glucose impairment, and dehydration)
- LFTs
- Coagulation profile (to look for evidence of sepsis-induced coagulopathy)
- ABGs
- Pan culture (blood, urine, stool)
- Wound culture

Imaging
Initial approach
- X-ray may show soft tissue edema and subcutaneous emphysema
- Ultrasound: For hyperechoic foci, thickening of and gas within scrotal wall
- CT may show the extent of soft tissue gas and fascial edema, identify site of entry
- MRI: For definition of soft tissue pathology

Diagnostic Procedures/Other
Incisional biopsy (allows pathological distinction of necrotizing infection from severecellulitis)

Pathological Findings
- Pathognomonic findings upon pathologic evaluation:
- Necrosis of the superficial and deep fascial planes
- Fibrinoid coagulation of the nutrient arterioles, polymorphonuclear cell infiltration, and microorganisms identified within the involved tissues.

DIFFERENTIAL DIAGNOSIS
- Testicular trauma
- Testicular torsion
- Balanitis
- Hernias
- Hydrocele
- Orchitis
- Acute epididymo-orchitis

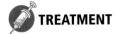

TREATMENT

Successful treatment depends on early diagnosis, fluid and electrolyte replacement, aggressive radical debridement of all areas of subcutaneous necrosis, and prompt institution of broad-spectrum IV antibiotics. Diverting colostomy may be necessary.

MEDICATION
First Line
- Upon suspicion of Fournier's gangrene, a broad-spectrum antibiotic should be initiated immediately.
- Initial empiric antibiotic therapy should include a combination of cephalosporins or aminoglycosides and penicillins, and metronidazole or clindamycin.
- Clindamycin is particularly useful in the treatment of necrotizing soft-tissue infections because of its gram-positive and anaerobic spectrum of activity.
- Also, if Gram stain or culture suggests mixed infection, consider imipenem; vancomycin if MRSA.
- For gram-negative, use gentamicin instead of cephalosporins.
- Use vancomycin and gentamicin for patients with penicillin allergy.

Second Line
Antifungal therapy if underlying infection present

ADDITIONAL TREATMENT
Additional Therapies
- Volume support
- Tetanus prophylaxis

COMPLEMENTARY & ALTERNATIVE THERAPIES
- Hyperbaric oxygen
- Unprocessed honey, applied directly to the surface of the wounds, has been reported to enzymatically débride, sterilize, and dehydrate wounds and to improve local tissue oxygenation and re-epithelialization. Controversial; no current studies support this practice.

SURGERY/OTHER PROCEDURES
- Aggressive surgical debridement of necrotic tissue to the level of viable tissue
- Occasionally including excision of scrotal skin and sometimes diverting colostomy
- 2–4 surgeries may be necessary

ONGOING CARE

FOLLOW-UP RECOMMENDATIONS
Psychology consult

DIET
Normal, unless patient is diabetic

PATIENT EDUCATION
Potential disfigurement and dysfunction after debridement

PROGNOSIS
- 4–75% mortality reported, but 25–35% is average range.
- The mortality risk may be directly proportional to the age of the patient, extent of systemic toxicity upon admission, and extent of the local tissue involvement.

COMPLICATIONS
- Ongoing pain
- Sexual dysfunction
- Loss of sensitivity
- Pain during erection
- Unresolved sepsis leading to septic shock

ADDITIONAL READING
- Clayton MD, et al. Causes, presentation and survival of fifty-seven patients with necrotizing fasciitis of the male genitalia. *Surg Gynecol Obstet.* 1990;170(1): 49–55.
- http://www.medscape.com/viewarticle/563170_4
- http://www.ncbi.nlm.nih.gov/pmc/articles/PMC2890137/?tool=pubmed
- http://emedicine.medscape.com/article/778866-overview
- http://radiology.rsna.org/content/226/1/115.full.pdf
- http://emedicine.medscape.com/article/438994-diagnosis
- Norton KS, et al. Management of Fournier's gangrene: An eleven year retrospective analysis of early recognition, diagnosis, and treatment. *Am Surg.* 2002;68(8):709–13.
- Paty R, Smith AD. Gangrene and Fournier's gangrene. *Urol Clin North Am.* 1992;19(1):149–62.

CODES

ICD9
608.83 Vascular disorders of male genital organs

CLINICAL PEARLS
- Fournier gangrene is a necrotizing soft tissue infection of the perineum or genitalia that is rapidly progressive, potentially lethal, and is a true surgical emergency.
- Once recognized, prep for surgery, fluid resuscitate, and administer IV Abx.
- It can affect all age groups and both sexes. Most common predisposing condition is diabetes.
- Even with urgent surgical debridement, the mortality rate is as high as 10–30%.

F

FRACTIONAL EXCRETION: SODIUM, UREA, AND MAGNESIUM

Holly Llobet
John Oropello

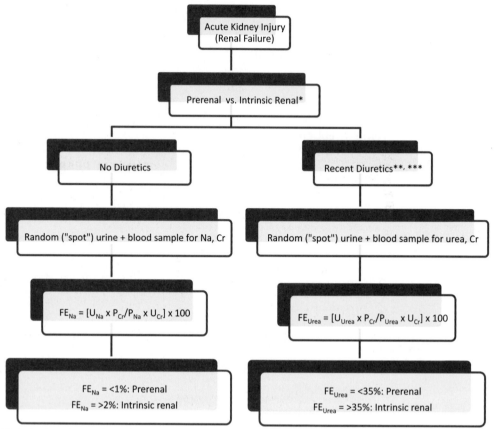

FE, fractional excretion; U, urine; P, plasma; Na, sodium (mEq/L); Cr, creatinine (mg/dL). *Kidney failure may be intrinsic (e.g., acute tubular necrosis, acute glomerulonephritis, interstitial nephritis, vascular disease) or extrinsic (decreased renal perfusion [prerenal] or obstructive [postrenal]). To the extent that they may cause intrinsic renal tubular damage, prerenal and postrenal states may also lead to increased FE_{Na}.

**The duration of the naturetic affect of diuretics on the FE_{Na} (increase followed by decrease) is variable and may last beyond 6–8 hours after the last diuretic dose.

***The fractional excretion of urea (FE_{urea}) may be more accurate after recent diuretics; however, the data published thus far are not conclusive.

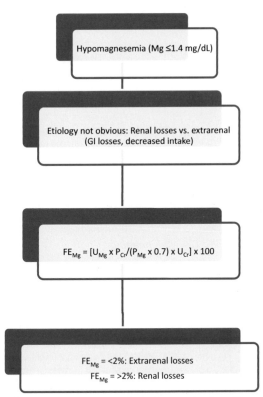

Hypomagnesemia (Mg ≤1.4 mg/dL)

Etiology not obvious: Renal losses vs. extrarenal (GI losses, decreased intake)

$FE_{Mg} = [U_{Mg} \times P_{Cr}/(P_{Mg} \times 0.7) \times U_{Cr}] \times 100$

FE_{Mg} = <2%: Extrarenal losses
FE_{Mg} = >2%: Renal losses

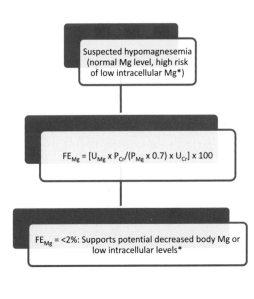

Suspected hypomagnesemia (normal Mg level, high risk of low intracellular Mg*)

$FE_{Mg} = [U_{Mg} \times P_{Cr}/(P_{Mg} \times 0.7) \times U_{Cr}] \times 100$

FE_{Mg} = <2%: Supports potential decreased body Mg or low intracellular levels*

F

FE, fractional excretion; U, urine; P, plasma; Mg, magnesium (in mg/dL or mEq/L) Normal serum Mg: 1.5–2.5 mg/dL. Risk factors for hypomagnesemia include malnutrition, use of TPN, malabsorption, prolonged use of nasal gastric tube suction, chronic diarrhea, laxative abuse, alcoholism, diabetic ketoacidosis, osmotic diuresis, diuretic phase of ATN, renal tubular acidosis, hypercalcemia, hypoparathyroidism, medications (e.g., diuretics, cisplatinum, amphotericin, aminoglycosides, cyclosporine, tacrolimus), and hyperthyroidism. Symptoms of hypomagnesemia may include neurologic symptoms (e.g., weakness, tetany, seizures) or cardiac arrhythmias (e.g., ventricular fibrillation, ventricular tachycardia, torsades de pointes).

REFERENCES

1. Tong GM, et al. Magnesium deficiency in critical illness. *J Intensive Care Med* 2005;20:3–17.
2. Bagshaw SM, et al. Urinary biochemistry and microscopy in septic acute renal failure: a systematic review. *Am J Kidney Dis* 2006;48: 695–705.
3. Bagshaw SM, et al. A systematic review of urinary findings in experimental septic acute renal failure. *Crit Care Med* 2007;35:1592–1598.
4. Carvounis CP, et al. Significance of the fractional excretion of urea in the differential diagnosis of acute renal failure. *Kidney Int* 2002;62:2223–2229.
5. Elisaf M, et al. Fractional excretion of magnesium in normal subjects and in patients with hypomagnesemia. *Magnes Res* 1997;10:315–320.
6. Espinel CH. The FENa test. Use in the differential diagnosis of acute renal failure. *JAMA* 1976;236: 579–581.
7. Steiner RW. Interpreting the fractional excretion of sodium. *Am J Med* 1984;77:699–702.

ADDITIONAL READING

• Cogan MG. *Fluid & Electrolytes Pathology & Pathophysiology*. Connecticut, California: Appelton & Lange; 1991.
• Reilly RF, et al. *Instant Access: Acid-Base, Fluids, and Electrolytes*. New York: McGraw-Hill; 2007:496.
• Schrier RW, ed. *Renal and Electrolyte Disorders*, 7th ed. Philadelphia, Lippincott Williams & Wilkins; 2010:631.

CODES

ICD9
• NA

CLINICAL PEARLS

• Fe$_{Na}$ is used to differentiate between prerenal and intrinsic (ATN) renal disease. The 2 most common causes of acute kidney injury.
• FE_{Na} is superior to simple urine Na because it minimizes the effect of changes in the rate of water reabsorption and directly measure sodium handling.
• Fe$_{Urea}$ may be more useful than Fe$_{Na}$ if diuretics have been given.
• The history, physical exam, and overall clinical assessment are more important in clinical decision making than FE measurements.
• Hypovolemia with FE_{Na} >1–2 may occur with tubular damage, chronic renal failure, diuretics, osmotic diuresis from mannitol or glycosuria (e.g., uncontrolled diabetes), hypoaldosteronism, increased physiologic ADH release.
• Limitations of Fe$_{Na}$:
  – Fe$_{Na}$ is less reliable after diuretic use.
  – FE_{Na} and FEurea are not great discriminators of extrinsic vs. intrinsic renal disorders in critically ill patients with sepsis and multiple systemic organ dysfunction receiving vasopressors and massive fluid resuscitation.
  – The FE_{Na} is unreliable when acute renal failure is superimposed on chronic renal failure or in acute kidney injury associated with sepsis
  – FE_{Na} <1 may occur in the setting of intrinsic renal disease caused by contrast induced nephropathy and heme pigment nephropathy (hemolysis or rhabdomyolysis), or glomerular diseases, while tubular function is still intact.
  – Clinical studies in resuscitated septic patients reveal a hyperdynamic state with increased renal perfusion in the setting of acute kidney injury; however, decreased FE_{Na} (<1%) is found in resuscitated septic animals with AKI and increased renal blood flow.
  – Metabolic alkalosis with bicarbonate diuresis or diuresis of ketoanions may increase urinary sodium excretion, elevating the FE_{Na} in the setting of hypovolemia. The FE of chloride may be more reflective of effective circulating volume in this setting.
• Hypomagnesemia is common in critically ill patients.
• The cause of hypomagnesemia can usually be determined from the history and physical exam.

FUNGI
Sophia Koo

BASICS

DESCRIPTION
Invasive candidiasis and invasive aspergillosis are the most common fungal infections in the ICU setting, although invasive infections by less common mold (*Mucorales*, *Fusarium*, and *Scedosporium*) and yeast (*Trichosporon*, *Blastoschizomyces*) species may be rising in incidence. Diagnosis of these infections is challenging, and invasive fungal infections carry substantial morbidity and mortality.

EPIDEMIOLOGY
Incidence
Highly dependent on local epidemiology and risk factors of the population of interest: ICU patients are at increased risk of invasive candidiasis by definition, and often have many additional risk factors for candidiasis (as outlined below); many patients in the ICU also have risk factors for invasive mold infections.

Prevalence
Also highly dependent on local epidemiology and the host: *Candida* is the 4th most common bloodstream isolate in hospitalized patients (12% of hospital-acquired bloodstream infections).

RISK FACTORS
- For invasive candidiasis: ICU hospitalization, receipt of TPN, central venous catheters, prior exposure to broad-spectrum antibiotics, high APACHE scores, abdominal surgery, enteric perforations/anastomotic leaks, receipt of hemodialysis, hematologic malignancy, solid organ transplantation, hematopoietic stem cell transplantation, mucositis
- For invasive aspergillosis and other invasive mold infections: Corticosteroid exposure, treatment with T-cell immunosuppressants, prolonged neutropenia, allogeneic stem cell transplantation, grade III–IV graft-vs.-host disease

Genetics
Certain defects in innate immunity (mannose binding lectin and dectin-1 deficiencies, TLR4 polymorphisms) may increase the risk of invasive fungal infections.

GENERAL PREVENTION
- Difficult, given the ubiquity of fungal spores in the environment, but environmental control measures (e.g., HEPA filters, masks) and avoidance of high spore inocula (construction sites, gardening) may abate the risk of invasive mold infections.
- Data exists to support use of posaconazole prophylaxis in certain populations at high risk of developing invasive fungal infections (patients with grade III–IV graft-vs.-host disease, patients receiving chemotherapy for acute leukemia).

PATHOPHYSIOLOGY
Aspergillus and other mold spores are ubiquitous in the environment and frequently inhaled; *Candida* and other yeasts are common commensals. In a compromised host (impaired cellular immunity, loss of normal anatomic barriers), these fungi can germinate, invade blood vessels, and disseminate to multiple end organs.

ETIOLOGY
- *Candida*: *C. albicans* (>50% of invasive isolates in the ICU setting), *C. glabrata*, *C. parapsilosis*, *C. tropicalis*, *C. krusei*, *C. lusitaniae*; reports of rising incidence of non-*C. albicans* species at some centers
- *Aspergillus*: *A. fumigatus* (70–90% of invasive isolates), *A. flavus*, *A. terreus*, *A. niger*
- Other yeasts: *Cryptococcus neoformans*, *Trichosporon asahii*, *Saccharomyces cerevisiae*, *Blastoschizomyces capitatus*
- Other molds: Mucorales (*Rhizopus*, *Mucor*), *Fusarium*, *Scedosporium*, dematiaceous fungi, dermatophytes
- Dimorphic fungi: Yeasts at body temperature, molds at ambient temperature: *Penicillium marneffei*, *Histoplasma*, *Blastomyces*, *Coccidioides*

COMMONLY ASSOCIATED CONDITIONS
Patients immunocompromised enough to develop invasive fungal infections are also often at high risk for other opportunistic infections, such as CMV and *Pneumocystis jirovecii* pneumonia.

DIAGNOSIS

HISTORY
- Nonspecific symptoms for both invasive candidiasis (fevers, hemodynamic instability, rash) and aspergillosis (fevers, cough, hemoptysis, dyspnea, chest pain, sinusitis, rash)
- Assessment of host risk factors for invasive candidiasis and invasive aspergillosis
- Recent exposure to antifungal therapy: Chronic fluconazole exposure increases risk of azole-resistant yeast species, risk of breakthrough invasive zygomycosis, and other resistant mold infections with chronic voriconazole exposure.

PHYSICAL EXAM
- Vital signs: Fevers, hemodynamics, tachypnea, hypoxia
- Sinuses: Cranial nerve exam, eye exam to assess for evidence of invasive fungal sinusitis
- Lung exam: Crackles, effusions
- Cardiovascular exam: Murmurs, rubs
- Assessment for rashes: Invasive candidiasis and invasive aspergillosis (and many other invasive fungal infections, including classically, fusariosis) can disseminate to the skin and cause deep nodular lesions, pustular lesions, and necrotic eschars.

DIAGNOSTIC TESTS & INTERPRETATION
Lab
Initial lab tests
- Blood cultures (*Candida* sp. and other yeasts grow well in routine blood cultures; fungal isolator cultures add little sensitivity to routine blood cultures for recovery of most yeasts and molds.)
- Deep respiratory tract cultures (although often lack sensitivity and specificity for invasive aspergillosis)
- Serum galactomannan (89% specificity for invasive aspergillosis, sensitivity 71% at a cutoff of 0.5 units; most sensitive in hematologic malignancy patients, lower in solid organ transplant recipients, patients receiving antifungal therapy active against *Aspergillus*; false-positives in patients receiving IV piperacillin-tazobactam, IV amoxicillin-clavulanate (not available in the US)
- Serum $(1\rightarrow3)\beta$-D-glucan (sensitivity 70–80%, specificity 80–90% for invasive fungal infections: Elevated in most invasive fungal infections (not cryptococcosis or zygomycosis); many ICU patients have factors that may cause false-positive assays (extensive exposure to surgical gauze and packings, hemodialysis with cellulose-containing membranes, IVIG or albumin therapy)

- BAL galactomannan: At a cutoff of 0.7–1.0 units, comparable to slightly increased sensitivity for invasive aspergillosis compared to serum galactomannan, lower specificity
- Blood/serum PCR for invasive candidiasis and invasive aspergillosis is not well-standardized or widely available for clinical use.

Follow-Up & Special Considerations
- In patients with elevated serum galactomannan in the setting of invasive aspergillosis, serial measurements every 2–3 days are helpful to assess response to antifungal therapy; initial height of galactomannan and rate of decline have prognostic value.
- Important to document clearance of candidemia with serial blood cultures

Imaging
- As directed by history and exam findings
- Chest CT to assess for nodules (classic "halo" sign is a transient early finding in invasive aspergillosis, "air-crescent sign" with cavitation of nodular lesions is a later radiographic finding in patients with invasive aspergillosis; both lack sensitivity and specificity)
- Sinus CT to assess for invasive fungal sinusitis
- Brain MRI if any suspicion of CNS involvement
- Abdominal MRI to assess for hepatosplenic candidiasis in patients with prolonged neutropenia, fevers, elevated LFTs

Diagnostic Procedures/Other
- Consider BAL/transbronchial or percutaneous biopsy and culture of suspicious pulmonary nodules to increase the likelihood of microbiological diagnosis, particularly if galactomannan, cultures, and β-glucan are negative. Invasive fungal infections have clinically overlapping manifestations, and susceptibility to antifungal drugs varies widely between species. It is very helpful to isolate the causative organism and obtain formal antifungal drug susceptibility testing to guide therapy.
- Biopsy and culture of suspicious skin lesions
- Biopsy and culture of other lesions, as guided by history, exam, and radiology

Pathological Findings
- In invasive candidiasis: Yeast forms with hyphae and pseudohyphae
- In invasive aspergillosis: Tissue-invasive septate hyphal forms with acute angle branching in the setting of acute/chronic inflammation; several other fungi (*Fusarium*, *Scedosporium*) are often morphologically indistinguishable from *Aspergillus*, and definitive diagnosis requires growth on culture.
  - Immunohistochemistry and tissue PCR assays for *Aspergillus* are available if biopsy specimens do not grow in culture, but these can lack sensitivity and cross-react with other fungal species.
- Broad aseptate/pauciseptate hyphal "ribbons" with right-angle branching are suggestive of invasive zygomycosis.

DIFFERENTIAL DIAGNOSIS
- Candidiasis: Other invasive yeast infections, bacterial infections
- Aspergillosis: Bacterial pneumonia, septic pulmonary emboli, malignancy, other invasive mold infections

TREATMENT

MEDICATION

First Line

- For candidiasis: In the ICU setting, an echinocandin (micafungin 100 mg/d IV, caspofungin 70 mg × 1, then 50 mg/d, or anidulafungin 200 mg × 1, then 100 mg/d) should generally be first-line therapy, particularly in patients with any clinical instability, prior azole exposure, or in institutions with a high proportion of *C. glabrata* or *C. krusei* isolates.
- If isolate turns out to be sensitive to fluconazole, can switch to fluconazole 800 mg × 1, then 400 mg/d
  - PO and IV have equivalent bioavailability; use oral fluconazole if possible.
- In clinically stable patients without prior azole exposure at institutions with a low rate of *C. glabrata* and *C. krusei*, can consider first-line therapy with fluconazole 800 mg × 1, then 400 mg/d.
- Consider empiric therapy in ICU patients with persistent fevers of unknown source despite broad-spectrum antibiotics, risk factors for candidiasis, positive serum β-glucan, and the isolation of *Candida* species from multiple nonsterile sites.
- For aspergillosis: Voriconazole (6 mg/kg IV b.i.d. × 2 doses, then 4 mg/kg IV b.i.d. or 200–300 mg b.i.d.) is the treatment of choice for confirmed invasive aspergillosis.
- Empiric therapy is recommended in certain subpopulations (e.g., patients with persistent chemotherapy-associated febrile neutropenia despite broad-spectrum antibiotic therapy).
- For other invasive fungal infections: If patient is suspected to have an invasive mold infection but the causative species is unknown, amphotericin B has the broadest antifungal spectrum and is the treatment of choice for invasive zygomycosis and severe infections with the endemic fungi:
  - Reasonable to treat with amphotericin B while attempting to identify the etiologic species.

Second Line

- For invasive candidiasis: Amphotericin B; amph voriconazole, posaconazole
- For invasive aspergillosis: Amphotericin B, echinocandins, itraconazole, posaconazole

ADDITIONAL TREATMENT

General Measures

Supportive care of shock, respiratory failure, multiorgan failure

Issues for Referral

- Infectious diseases consultation is strongly recommended.
- Ophthalmology consultation in patients with candidemia to assess for *Candida* endophthalmitis
- Dermatology consultation in patients with rashes that suggest disseminated candidiasis or aspergillosis
- Consider surgical consultation to consider resection of infarcted lung from zygomycosis, mold infections in critical/sheltered locations outlined below.

Additional Therapies

Removal of indwelling intravascular catheters in patients with candidemia

SURGERY/OTHER PROCEDURES

- Surgical resection improves clinical outcome in invasive zygomycosis, which is associated with lung infarcts and infected, devitalized tissue and can be difficult to treat with medical therapy alone.
- Consider surgical debridement of invasive aspergillosis if it involves certain areas (pericardium, great vessels, valvular vegetations, CNS, osteomyelitis).

IN-PATIENT CONSIDERATIONS

Initial Stabilization

Supportive care if hemodynamic instability, respiratory failure, or multiorgan dysfunction are present

Admission Criteria

Most patients with newly suspected invasive aspergillosis or invasive candidiasis should be hospitalized for a diagnostic workup and initiation of antifungal therapy. Early initiation of therapy is critical, and patients can deteriorate rapidly if treatment is delayed or ineffective against the causative organism.

IV Fluids

As per protocol, if patients not taking PO adequately

Nursing

No special considerations; consider ICU care if any hemodynamic instability, respiratory failure, or severe end-organ dysfunction is present.

Discharge Criteria

- Resolution of fevers, hemodynamic issues, respiratory failure
- Clearance of *Candida* from blood cultures
- In patients with an initial positive galactomannan, a decrease in their galactomannan EIA with antifungal therapy
- Receipt of definitive antifungal therapy without any intolerable side effects

ONGOING CARE

FOLLOW-UP RECOMMENDATIONS

- Infectious diseases follow-up to ensure the patient is improving clinically and tolerating antifungal therapy without any untoward side effects or major drug interactions
- Voriconazole is associated with several important drug interactions, visual disturbances, prolonged QTc, hepatotoxicity, phototoxicity, increased risk of squamous cell carcinoma of the skin, and periostitis, particularly with chronic exposure.
- Consider monitoring of trough voriconazole levels in patients with aspergillosis, particularly if the patient is not improving with what should be adequate therapy; pharmacokinetics can be unpredictable and highly variable.
- Amphotericin therapy is associated with nephrotoxicity and electrolyte wasting (potassium and magnesium), and patients receiving long-term treatment should be followed closely.

DIET

No special restrictions

PATIENT EDUCATION

- Long-term voriconazole use has many side-effects, including phototoxicity and an increased risk of squamous cell carcinoma of the skin; patients should be advised to avoid sun exposure and wear protective clothing and sunblock with high SPF if they spend time outdoors. Patients should be warned that voriconazole is associated with transient hallucinations and visual disturbances (often flashes of light) that often improve over time. Patients should be instructed to take their voriconazole on an empty stomach to maximize absorption.
- Patients receiving posaconazole should be instructed to take their medication with a fat-containing meal or with an acidic beverage (such as Coca-Cola); these conditions are critical for adequate absorption of this medication.

PROGNOSIS

Historically associated with high mortality, although widely varying estimates (30–90%). With recent advances in diagnostic methods (serum galactomannan, β-glucan, high-resolution imaging) and antifungal therapeutic options, mortality related to invasive aspergillosis and invasive candidiasis has probably declined over the past decade. Mortality related to emerging and resistant fungal species such as the Mucorales, *Scedosporium*, *Fusarium*, and some yeast species remains extremely high.

COMPLICATIONS

- Respiratory failure
- Shock
- Multiorgan failure
- Death

ADDITIONAL READING

- Limper AH, et al. An official American Thoracic Society statement: Treatment of fungal infections in adult pulmonary and critical care patients. *Am J Respir Crit Care Med*. 2011;183:96–128.
- Pappas PG, et al. Clinical practice guidelines for the management of candidiasis. *Clin Infect Dis*. 2009; 48:503–35.
- Walsh TJ, et al. Treatment of aspergillosis: Clinical practice guidelines of the Infectious Disease Society of America. *Clin Infect Dis*. 2008;46:327–60.
- http://www.aspergillus.org.uk
- http://www.doctorfungus.org

 CODES

ICD9

- 112.9 Candidiasis of unspecified site
- 117.3 Aspergillosis
- 117.9 Other and unspecified mycoses

CLINICAL PEARLS

- Early recognition of invasive fungal infections and initiation of antifungal therapy are critical. Delays in appropriate treatment of invasive candidiasis and invasive aspergillosis are associated with increased mortality. Entertain a high index of suspicion in patients with risk factors, and pursue diagnostic testing aggressively.

F

FUNGI, ENDEMIC

Sophia Koo

BASICS

DESCRIPTION
The endemic fungi (*Histoplasma*, *Coccidioides*, and *Blastomyces*) and *Cryptococcus* are acquired via inhalation of aerosolized spores in endemic areas. These infections can have a wide range of clinical manifestations, from fully asymptomatic to disseminated disease with multiple organ system involvement to fulminant ARDS.

EPIDEMIOLOGY
Incidence
- Varies highly according to exposure and host
- 6–15% of patients with HIV/AIDS have been reported to develop cryptococcal infections.
- Annual incidence of histoplasmosis is about 1–6% in endemic areas.
- In healthy military recruits performing desert exercises in Coccidioides-endemic areas, annual incidence was 6–32%, but no severe infections were reported.
- Blastomycosis is relatively rare; only 1–2 cases per 100,000 people per year.

Prevalence
- Also varies highly according to exposure and host
- In highly endemic areas, up to 80% of people show evidence of *Histoplasma capsulatum* infection by age 20. 75–90% of people in *Coccidioides*-endemic areas show evidence of cell-mediated immunity to *Coccidioides*.

RISK FACTORS
- Generally a function of the degree of exposure to spores and defects in host cell-mediated immunity: TNF-α inhibitors, HIV/AIDS, solid organ and hematopoietic stem cell transplantation, hematologic malignancy, corticosteroid therapy, sarcoidosis, exposure to aerosolized conidia in an endemic area (archaeologists, farmers, construction workers, military, spelunkers)
- Pregnant women in their 2nd or 3rd trimester, African Americans, and Filipino Americans are at higher risk for severe coccidioidomycosis.

GENERAL PREVENTION
Difficult; avoidance of areas likely to have high concentrations of aerosolized conidia (e.g., construction sites)

PATHOPHYSIOLOGY
Endemic fungi are generally acquired via inhalation of conidia aerosolized from the soil, with the development of a localized pneumonia/pneumonitis; in hosts with impaired T-cell immunity or patients exposed to a large inoculums of spores, these fungi can disseminate to multiple organs and cause a wide array of symptoms.

ETIOLOGY
- *Cryptococcus neoformans* and *C. gatii*: *C. neoformans* is found worldwide, particularly in pigeon roosts, soil contaminated with bird droppings; *C. gatii* is endemic in the Pacific Northwest and Vancouver Island, parts of Papua New Guinea and Northern Australia; *C. neoformans* generally causes disease only in immunocompromised hosts; *C. gatii* usually infects hosts with normal immune systems

- *Histoplasma capsulatum*: Endemic to Ohio, Missouri, Mississippi River valleys, and some parts of Central America, but has a worldwide distribution
- *Blastomyces dermatitidis*: Endemic in the central and southeastern US
- *Coccidioides immitis* and *C. posadasii*: Most endemic in the San Joaquin Valley (California) and the Sonoran desert area of Arizona and Mexico, but cases occur from the southwestern US to South America

COMMONLY ASSOCIATED CONDITIONS
Patients immunocompromised enough to develop severe, disseminated endemic fungal infections are also often at risk for other opportunistic infections, such as other invasive fungal infections (e.g., aspergillosis), *Pneumocystis jirovecii* pneumonia, and CMV.

DIAGNOSIS

HISTORY
- Multiple organ systems may be involved, and symptoms are often nonspecific: Fevers, malaise, weight loss, fatigue, headache, altered mental status, cranial nerve abnormalities, cough, chest pain, dyspnea, nausea, vomiting, diarrhea, nodular/pustular rash, erythema nodosum, arthralgias/arthritis.
- Assessment of host risk factors for disseminated endemic fungal infection
- Travel/exposure history: Many of the endemic fungi are geographically restricted.

PHYSICAL EXAM
- Vital signs: Fevers, hemodynamics, tachypnea, hypoxia
- Funduscopic exam: Papilledema, endophthalmitis
- Lung exam: Crackles, effusions
- Cardiovascular exam: Murmurs, rubs
- CNS: Cranial nerve exam, assessment for meningeal signs (nuchal rigidity, altered mental status), assessment for any focal neurologic deficits
- GI: Hepatosplenomegaly
- Assessment for rashes: Pustular, nodular, ulcerative, verrucous, or plaque lesions; secondary erythema nodosum on the lower extremities
- Assessment for signs of adrenal insufficiency from primary destruction of adrenal cortex: Orthostasis, skin hyperpigmentation
- Lymph node exam: lymphadenitis, lymphadenopathy
- Joints: Effusions, soft-tissue swelling

DIAGNOSTIC TESTS & INTERPRETATION
Lab
Initial lab tests
- CBC (may show pancytopenia in patients with bone marrow involvement), basic chemistries (hypernatremia, hypokalemia with adrenal insufficiency, renal function), LFTs
- Blood and urine cultures
- Fungal isolator blood cultures
- Serum cryptococcal antigen (high sensitivity for cryptococcosis)

- Urine histoplasma antigen (positive in ~90% of patients with disseminated histoplasmosis and a large burden of organisms; may also be positive in patients with certain other fungal infections, such as blastomycosis, coccidioidomycosis, paracoccidioidomycosis, penicilliosis)
- Deep respiratory tract cultures in patients with suspected pulmonary involvement
- CSF studies in patients with clinical evidence of meningitis: Culture, India ink stain, CSF cryptococcal antigen; CSF protein may be elevated and CSF glucose low; may show a lymphocytic pleocytosis; eosinophils may be elevated in patients with *Coccidioides* meningitis
- Serologies for *Histoplasma*, *Coccidioides*, *Blastomycosis* (useful to document prior exposure, high titers are often suggestive of active infection)
- Serum *Histoplasma* antigen (lower sensitivity than urine histoplasma antigen, only about 50%)
- Urine *Coccidioides* antigen (sensitivity ~70% in patients with moderate-severe coccidioidomycosis)
- Urine *Blastomyces* antigen (sensitivity reported as 90% in patients with disseminated blastomycosis, although small series; cross-reactivity with histoplasmosis, paracoccidioidomycosis, penicilliosis)
- Serum $(1\rightarrow 3)$ β-D-glucan (sensitivity 70–80%, specificity 80–90% for invasive fungal infections; can be elevated in patients with histoplasmosis, blastomycosis, coccidioidomycosis; not elevated in patients with cryptococcosis)

Follow-Up & Special Considerations
Patients should be followed by an infectious disease consultant through their treatment course, and to determine the need for secondary prophylaxis or surveillance after the initial treatment course ends.

Imaging
- Chest imaging (X-ray, CT) may show a wide array of findings: Calcified pulmonary nodules from prior exposure to endemic fungi; patchy infiltrates; mediastinal/hilar adenopathy; dense lobar infiltrates; diffuse, widespread infiltrates
- Brain CT/MRI: In patients with meningeal signs, consider performing head imaging prior to LP to assess for mass lesions, particularly if focal neurologic deficits on exam.

Diagnostic Procedures/Other
- Lumbar puncture in patients with symptoms and signs of meningitis: Measurement of opening pressures (high pressures of >25 cm H_2O are associated with poor prognosis in cryptococcal meningitis and may require repeated drainage of CSF); if endemic fungal infection is a concern, send CSF for routine cell counts (percentage of eosinophils may be elevated with meningitis from *Coccidioides*), protein, glucose, India ink stain, cryptococcal antigen, fungal cultures
- Consider BAL/transbronchial or percutaneous biopsy and culture of suspicious pulmonary nodules.
- Biopsy and culture of suspicious skin lesions
- Biopsy and culture of other lesions as guided by history, exam, and radiology

Pathological Findings

- In cryptococcosis: Round yeast forms surrounded by a thick polysaccharide capsule; some cells may show a single budding daughter cell; in fixed tissue samples, mucicarmine stains can delineate the capsule of *C. neoformans,* and Fontana-Masson stains highlight melanin in the cell wall (not present in other yeasts)
- In histoplasmosis: Oval, heterogeneously sized, narrow-based budding yeast forms in areas of caseating necrosis/granulomatous inflammation
- In coccidioidomycosis: Large, thick-walled spherules containing endospores in a background of inflammation/necrosis
- In blastomycosis: Broad-based budding yeast forms with thick cell walls in a background of inflammation/necrosis

DIFFERENTIAL DIAGNOSIS

- Tuberculosis
- Sarcoidosis
- Malignancy (lung cancer, lymphoma)
- Other invasive fungal infections

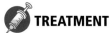 TREATMENT

MEDICATION

First Line

- For cryptococcosis: Fluconazole 400 mg/d or itraconazole 400 mg/d; initial therapy for cryptococcal meningitis or disseminated disease is amphotericin B deoxycholate 0.7–1.0 mg/kg/d IV or liposomal amphotericin B 3–6 mg/kg/d IV, with or without flucytosine 100 mg/kg/d
- For histoplasmosis: For severe, disseminated disease, CNS involvement, or immunocompromised hosts, initial therapy with amphotericin B deoxycholate 0.7–1.0 mg/kg/d IV or liposomal amphotericin B 3–5 mg/kg/d IV; for mild-moderate disease, itraconazole 200 mg b.i.d.
- For blastomycosis: Itraconazole 200 mg b.i.d. for 6 months for mild-moderate infections (longer in immunosuppressed patients and patients with bony involvement); for severe, life-threatening disease or CNS involvement, amphotericin B deoxycholate 0.7–1.0 mg/kg/d IV or liposomal amphotericin 5 mg/kg/d IV
- For coccidioidomycosis: Fluconazole 400 mg/d or itraconazole 400 mg/d; for meningitis, fluconazole 400–1000 mg/d or itraconazole 400–600 mg/d; for severe infections or diffuse pulmonary disease, initial therapy with liposomal amphotericin B 3–5 mg/kg/d IV or amphotericin B deoxycholate 0.7–1.0 mg/kg/d IV

Second Line

- For histoplasmosis, blastomycosis: Voriconazole, posaconazole, and fluconazole can be considered if the patient tolerates itraconazole poorly.
- For coccidioidomycosis: Voriconazole, posaconazole
- Prednisone 40–60 mg/d for 1–2 weeks can be considered in patients with hypoxemia and diffuse lung disease, in combination with antifungal therapy. Steroids can also be considered in HIV patients with cryptococcosis who develop an immune reconstitution syndrome with the initiation of antiretroviral therapy.

ADDITIONAL TREATMENT

General Measures

- In patients with cryptococcal meningitis and persistently elevated opening pressures, it is important to keep intracranial pressure under control by repeated removal of CSF.
- Supportive care of shock, respiratory failure/ARDS, multiorgan failure.

Issues for Referral

- Infectious diseases consultation is strongly recommended.
- Dermatology consultation in patients with nodular/pustular/ulcerating rashes suggestive of a disseminated endemic fungal infection or erythema nodosum without a clear etiology
- Neurosurgical consultation in patients with CNS mass lesions, persistently elevated opening pressures

SURGERY/OTHER PROCEDURES

Neurosurgical evaluation for consideration of shunt placement in cryptococcosis patients with persistently elevated CSF opening pressures

IN-PATIENT CONSIDERATIONS

Initial Stabilization

Supportive care if hemodynamic instability, respiratory failure/ARDS, or multiorgan dysfunction are present.

Admission Criteria

Patients with systematic, respiratory, or CNS symptoms suspicious for an endemic fungal infection should be hospitalized for a diagnostic workup and initiation of antifungal therapy.

IV Fluids

As per protocol if patients not taking PO adequately

Nursing

No special considerations; consider ICU care if any hemodynamic instability, respiratory failure, or severe end-organ dysfunction.

Discharge Criteria

- Resolution of fevers, hemodynamic issues, respiratory failure
- Receipt of antifungal therapy without any intolerable side effects

 ONGOING CARE

FOLLOW-UP RECOMMENDATIONS

- Infectious diseases follow-up to ensure the patient is improving clinically and tolerating antifungal therapy without any untoward side effects or major drug interactions; also, to determine duration of therapy and need for further secondary prophylaxis
- Consider monitoring of trough itraconazole levels; can have considerable pharmacokinetic variability.

DIET

No special restrictions

PATIENT EDUCATION

Long-term itraconazole use has some side effects, including elevated LFTs, nausea, vomiting, fatigue, jaundice, and a risk of developing congestive heart failure. Patients should be instructed to take itraconazole with a meal to increase absorption.

PROGNOSIS

With effective antifungal therapy, mortality rates for most endemic fungal infections are relatively low, in the 10–20% range, although infections can still be fulminant and fatal in patients with poor cellular immunity and widely disseminated disease.

COMPLICATIONS

- Respiratory failure/ARDS
- Shock
- Multiorgan failure
- Death

ADDITIONAL READING

- Chapman SW, et al. Clinical practice guidelines for the management of blastomycosis: 2008 Update by the Infectious Diseases Society of America. *Clin Infect Dis.* 2008;46:1801–12.
- Galgani JN, et al. Coccidioidomycosis. *Clin Infect Dis.*2005;41:1217–23.
- Limper AH, et al. An official American Thoracic Society statement: Treatment of fungal infections in adult pulmonary and critical care patients. *Am J Respir Crit Care Med.* 2011;183:96–128.
- Perfect JR, et al. Clinical practice guidelines for the management of cryptococcal disease: 2010 Update by the Infectious Diseases Society of America. *Clin Infect Dis.* 2010;50:291–322.
- Wheat J, et al. Practice guidelines for the management of patients with histoplasmosis. *Clin Infect Dis.* 2000;30:688–95.
- http://www.doctorfungus.org

CODES

ICD9

- 114.9 Coccidioidomycosis, unspecified
- 115.90 Histoplasmosis, unspecified without mention of manifestation
- 116.0 Blastomycosis

CLINICAL PEARLS

- Endemic fungal infections and cryptococcosis can be difficult to diagnose. Consider endemic fungal infections in patients with potential epidemiologic exposures and a compatible clinical syndrome. In patients with infections severe enough to require ICU-level care, it is reasonable to use amphotericin B deoxycholate or liposomal amphotericin empirically while a diagnostic workup is ongoing.

F

GASTROINTESTINAL BLEEDING, LOWER
Ofer Ben-Bassat

 BASICS

DESCRIPTION
- Lower GI bleeding (LGIB) refers to blood loss of recent onset originating from a site distal to the ligament of Treitz.
- Most instances of LGIB are self-limited.
- Encompasses a wide spectrum that ranges from trivial hematochezia to massive hemorrhage with shock
- LGIB in elderly patients is commonly caused by colonic diverticula or vascular ectasias, whereas in young patients, infectious or inflammatory conditions are more likely.

EPIDEMIOLOGY
The mortality rate is ~4% in 1 large series. Mortality was more likely in older adults, those with intestinal ischemia, and comorbid illnesses.

Incidence
- ~21 per 10,000 adults in the U.S. require hospitalization each year for severe LGIB.
- In a survey by the American College of Gastroenterology, LGIB accounted for 24% of all GI bleeding events.

PATHOPHYSIOLOGY
- The 2 major causes of significant LGIB are colonic diverticula and vascular ectasia.
- Hemodynamically insignificant bleeding is frequently caused by hemorrhoids and neoplasms.

ETIOLOGY
- Common:
  - Colonic diverticula
  - Angiectasia
- Less common:
  - Colonic neoplasms (including post-polypectomy bleeding)
  - Inflammatory bowel disease
  - Colitis: Ischemic, radiation, unspecified (infectious or nonspecific)
  - Hemorrhoids
  - Small bowel source
  - Upper GI source
- Rare:
  - Dieulafoy lesion (rupture of a large arteriole into the lumen)
  - Colonic ulcerations
  - Rectal varices

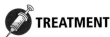 **DIAGNOSIS**

HISTORY
- Blood originating from the left colon typically is bright red. In comparison, blood from the right side of the colon usually appears dark or maroon-colored and may be mixed with stool.
- Rapid transit of blood from the right side of the colon or massive upper GI bleeding (UGIB) can appear bright red.
- Melena suggests UGIB, although bleeding from the cecum may present in this manner.
- In patients with apparent massive LGIB, it is important to exclude upper GI bleeding by examining an aspirate from a nasogastric tube.
- Visible rectal bleeding occurring in adults warrants an evaluation in all cases.
- Patients should be categorized as either low- or high-risk for complications based upon their clinical presentation and hemodynamic status:
  - Low-risk patients: For example, a young otherwise healthy patient with self-limited rectal bleeding that is most likely due to an internal hemorrhoid may be evaluated in the outpatient setting.
  - High-risk patients, including those with hemodynamic instability, serious comorbid diseases, persistent bleeding, the need for multiple blood transfusions, or evidence of an acute abdomen, should be promptly resuscitated and hospitalized, with early involvement of a gastroenterologist and general surgeon.

DIAGNOSTIC TESTS & INTERPRETATION
- Once the bleeding is suspected to be coming from a lower GI source, colonoscopy is the initial exam of choice for diagnosis and treatment.
- In massive bleeding: Perform an upper GI endoscopy; if negative perform an urgent colonoscopy or a tagged-RBC scintigraphy ± angiography.
- In slow or intermittent bleeding: Assess for anorectal source; urgent colonoscopy. If negative consider tagged-RBC scintigraphy, angiography, capsule endoscopy, enteroscopy. CT, Meckel's scan, provocative angiography.
- A number of reports have shown that urgent colonoscopy is safe and yields a specific diagnosis in a high proportion of patients with LGIB.
- Bowel preparation can be administered by mouth or a nasogastric tube. It does not reactivate bleeding.
- Barium studies have no role in the evaluation of LGIB.

Lab
- CBC
- Chemistries (including renal and liver functions tests)
- Coagulation profile
- Cross-matching for blood transfusions

TREATMENT

ADDITIONAL TREATMENT
General Measures
Resuscitation: All patients with hemodynamic instability (shock, orthostatic hypotension), those with evidence of severe bleeding (a hematocrit decrease of at least 6%, or transfusion requirement of greater than 2 units of packed RBCs), or continuous active bleeding should be admitted to an ICU for resuscitation and close observation.
- 2 large-caliber (≥18-gauge) peripheral catheters or a central venous line should be inserted.

- Patients with congestive heart failure or valvular disease may benefit from pulmonary catheter monitoring, to minimize the risk of fluid overload.
- Review laboratory data and correct:
  - Coagulopathy: INR >1.5 or thrombocytopenia (<50,000).
  - Keep hematocrit 20–25 for young patients without significant medical problems and 30 for high-risk patients.

Additional Therapies
- Endoscopic therapy:
  - Methods of hemostatic therapy include: Injection, laser therapy, heater probe, monopolar and multipolar electrocoagulation, and argon plasma coagulation (APC).
  - Many lesions can be treated, most commonly:
    - Actively bleeding diverticula
    - Nonbleeding visible vessels
    - Adherent clots
    - Angiectasias
- Angiographic therapy:
  - When a bleeding site is identified by angiography, hemostasis can be achieved by intra-arterial infusion of vasopressin or superselective embolization:
    - Ischemia is an important potential complication.
    - The risk of ischemic complication of angiography is higher when performed for colonic hemorrhage than for UGIB!
    - Local expertise will determine priority and effectiveness among the therapeutic options.
    - Currently, it is reserved for patients who are poor surgical candidates.

SURGERY/OTHER PROCEDURES
- May be necessary for continuing or recurrent LGIB
- Has been carried out in 15–25% of patients
- Recommended for patients with acute LGIB with a high transfusion requirement (generally >4 units within a 24-hour period or >10 units overall) and for those with recurrent bleeding.
- Accurate preoperative localization, particularly by angiography, helps minimize surgical morbidity and mortality.
- The role of surgery includes:
  - Elective resection of:
    - A known bleeding source, such as a carcinoma
    - Meckel's diverticulum
    - Rebleeding colonic diverticula
  - Emergency surgery for an actively bleeding lesion that has been localized by colonoscopy or angiography
  - Blind subtotal colectomy for presumably colonic hemorrhage that cannot be localized. Associated with high morbidity and mortality; used only as a last resort

ADDITIONAL READING

Feldman M, et al., eds. *Sleisenger and Fordtran's gastrointestinal and liver disease*, 8th edition. Philadelphia: Saunders, 2006.

 ## CODES

ICD9
- 562.12 Diverticulosis of colon with hemorrhage
- 569.85 Angiodysplasia of intestine with hemorrhage
- 578.9 Hemorrhage of gastrointestinal tract, unspecified

CLINICAL PEARLS
- Most instances of LGIB are self-limited.
- LGIB in elderly patients is commonly caused by colonic diverticula or vascular ectasias, whereas in young patients, infectious or inflammatory conditions are more likely.
- Rapid transit of blood from the right side of the colon or massive UGIB can appear bright red.
- Patients who are hemodynamically unstable or massively bleeding should be admitted to an ICU for resuscitation and close monitoring.
- Melena suggests UGIB, although bleeding from the cecum may present in this manner.
- Colonoscopy is the initial exam of choice for diagnosis and treatment.
- Ischemia is an important potential complication of therapeutic angiography.
- Accurate preoperative localization, particularly by angiography, helps minimize surgical morbidity and mortality.
- Blind subtotal colectomy is performed only as a last resort.

G

GASTROINTESTINAL BLEEDING, UPPER

Ofer Ben-Bassat

 BASICS

DESCRIPTION
- Bleeding from the upper GI tract (UGIB) is ~5 × more common than bleeding from the lower GI tract.
- GI bleeding is more common in men and elderly persons.
- The risk of UGIB appears to be increased in certain groups of patients, particularly those with underlying cardiovascular disease, chronic renal failure, and perhaps those >65.
- Historically, the most common cause of UGIB has been gastroduodenal ulcer disease. Other mucosal lesions account for substantial proportion of cases.

EPIDEMIOLOGY
UGIB has been estimated to account for up to 20,000 deaths annually in the U.S.

Incidence
- Overall incidence is estimated at 50–100 per 100,000 persons per year.
- Annual hospitalization rate of ~100 per 100,000 hospital admissions

PATHOPHYSIOLOGY
UGIB), most commonly arises from mucosal erosive disease.

ETIOLOGY
- Common:
  – Gastric ulcer
  – Duodenal ulcer
  – Esophageal varices
  – Mallory-Weiss tear
- Less common:
  – Gastric erosions/gastropathy
  – Esophagitis
  – Cameron lesions (erosions at diaphragmatic hernia margins)
  – Dieulafoy lesions
  – Telangiectasias
  – Portal hypertensive gastropathy
  – Gastric antral vascular ectasia (watermelon stomach)
  – Gastric varices
  – Neoplasms
- Rare:
  – Esophageal ulcer
  – Erosive duodenitis
  – Aortoenteric fistula (after surgical graft for Aortic aneurysm)
  – Hemobilia
  – Pancreatic disease
  – Crohn disease

 DIAGNOSIS

HISTORY
- UGIB commonly presents with hematemesis (fresh blood or coffee-ground like material).
- Ask about the use of aspirin, other NSAIDs, alcohol, history of liver disease or variceal bleeding, history of weight loss, dysphagia, heartburn, an abdominal aortic aneurysm (AAA), or an abdominal aortic graft.

DIAGNOSTIC TESTS & INTERPRETATION
- Nasogastric or orogastric tube lavage should be performed to remove particulate matter, fresh blood, and clots to facilitate endoscopy and confirm an upper source of bleeding.
- Lavage may not be positive if bleeding has ceased or arises beyond a closed pylorus.
- Stool color is not a reliable indicator of the location of bleeding.
- Esophagogastroduodenoscopy (EGD) is the diagnostic modality of choice for UGIB.

Lab
- CBC
- Chemistries (including renal and liver functions tests)
- Coagulation profile
- Cross-matching for blood transfusions

Diagnostic Procedures/Other
- The stomach should be lavaged via a large-bore orogastric tube for a clearer endoscopic view.
- Gastric lavage does not slow or stop the bleeding.

 TREATMENT

- Patients with significant bleeding should undergo an EGD as soon as possible.
- EGD should be performed only when it can be accomplished safely and effectively:
  – Aggressive ICU monitoring and resuscitation
  – Adequate resuscitation prior to endoscopy
  – Airway protection during the procedure
  – Patient should be intubated in the setting of aggressive bleeding or altered mental status.
  – With continued bleeding: Give continuous transfusion, with a target hematocrit value of:
    ○ Elderly patients: 30%.
    ○ In younger, otherwise healthy patients: 20–25% may be satisfactory
    ○ In patients with portal hypertension: Do not exceed 27–28%.

MEDICATION

- For ulcer bleeding:
  - Proton pump inhibitors (PPIs), particularly at high doses: More effective than H_2-receptor antagonists
  - Give IV pantoprazole 80 mg in bolus, followed by 8 mg/hr infusion. If no rebleeding within 24 hours, may switch to PO pantoprazole 40 mg/d or omeprazole 20 mg/d.
- If stigmata of liver disease:
  - Administer IV octreotide or vasopressin + nitroglycerin (or terlipressin).

ADDITIONAL TREATMENT

General Measures

- Erythromycin: 3 mg/kg, over 30 minutes, given IV, can help clear the stomach of blood.
- Ulcer bleeding:
  - Thermal coagulation, injection (epinephrine) therapy, hemostatic clips, fibrin sealant (or glue), argon plasma coagulation, and combination therapy
  - Combination therapy is more effective than either epinephrine injection or mechanical methods alone.
- Esophageal varices:
  - Endoscopic therapy: Band ligation (EBL) or sclerotherapy with secondary prophylaxis (EBL $\pm$ β-blocker).

Issues for Referral

Upper GI endoscopy can identify patients who can be immediately discharged.

SURGERY/OTHER PROCEDURES

- Endoscopy is the best initial diagnostic and therapeutic procedure.
- Surgery and transcatheter arteriography/intervention (TAI) are equally effective following failed therapeutic endoscopy, but TAI should be considered particularly in patients at high risk for surgery.
- TAI is less likely to be successful in patients with impaired coagulation.

IN-PATIENT CONSIDERATIONS

Initial Stabilization

- Resuscitate and stabilize.
- Assess onset and severity of bleeding.
- Diagnostic endoscopy: Prepare for emergent endoscopy, localize and identify bleeding site, stratify the risk for rebleeding.
- Therapeutic endoscopy: Control active bleeding or high-risk lesions, minimize treatment-related complications, treats persistent or recurrent bleeding.

 ONGOING CARE

FOLLOW-UP RECOMMENDATIONS

- Ulcer bleeding:
  - If rebleeding occurs: Repeat endoscopic therapy or surgery
  - If no rebleeding: Give further ulcer therapy: PO PPIs, cease NSAID therapy, and consider necessity for further aspirin therapy, give eradication therapy if positive urease test or biopsy for *Helicobacter pylori*.
- Bleeding from esophageal varices:
  - If rebleeding occurs: Endoscopic therapy or transjugular intrahepatic portosystemic shunt (TIPS).
  - If no rebleeding: Secondary prophylaxis (EBL $\pm$ β-blocker).
- Other causes of bleeding (Mallory Weiss tear, Dieulafoy lesion etc):
  - If rebleeding occurs: Endoscopic therapy or surgery.

PROGNOSIS

Rebleeding rate, the need for surgery, and mortality rates vary according to the ulcer endoscopic appearance.

ADDITIONAL READING

- Feldman M, et al., eds. *Sleisenger and Fordtran's Gastrointestinal and Liver Disease*, 8th ed. Philadelphia: Saunders, 2010.

CODES

ICD9

- 531.40 Chronic or unspecified gastric ulcer with hemorrhage, without mention of obstruction
- 578.9 533.40 Chronic or unspecified peptic ulcer of unspecified site with hemorrhage, without mention of obstruction

CLINICAL PEARLS

- UGIB most commonly arises from mucosal erosive disease.
- Most common causes are gastric and duodenal ulcers, bleeding esophageal varices, and Mallory-Weiss tears.
- Upon admission, rapid initial assessment and resuscitation is needed.
- Patients should receive aggressive ICU monitoring and resuscitation.
- A therapeutic endoscopy should be performed immediately once the patient has been hemodynamically stabilized.
- Medical treatment should include IV PPIs and terlipressin/octreotide (in the case if bleeding esophageal varices).
- If rebleeding occurs, a repeat endoscopic therapy should be attempted.

G

GLOMERULONEPHRITIS

Brian Sherman
Roopa Kohli-Seth

BASICS

DESCRIPTION
- Glomerulonephritis is characterized by an inflammatory process causing renal dysfunction with damage to the basement membrane, mesangium, or capillary endothelium. This can occur within days to weeks. Diagnosis essentials are findings of hematuria, dysmorphic red cells, red cell casts, and proteinuria.
- It may present as nephritic or nephrotic syndrome, acute renal insufficiency with possible dependant edema, and hypertension. However, hypertension may not be observed depending on other clinical problems.

EPIDEMIOLOGY
Incidence
- The reported biopsy-proven glomerulonephritis incidence varies according to population characteristics.
- Glomerulonephritis represents 10–15% of glomerular diseases.
- Variable incidence due to subclinical presentation
- The incidence of any glomerulonephritis is 17.6 per 10^5 population.

Prevalence
- A relatively uncommon cause of acute kidney injury, ~5% of cases of hospitalized intrinsic renal failure
- Male > Female (2:1)

RISK FACTORS
Risk factors for glomerulonephritis include:
- Family history of glomerulonephritis
- The presence of a known cause of glomerulonephritis
- Behaviors that increase exposure to infectious diseases such as HIV, Hep B and C, IVDU

Genetics
- Over the past 2 decades, the study of knockout and transgenic mice has provided tremendous insight into kidney development; however, there is still much progress needed.
- Congenital nephrotic syndrome from mutations in NPHS1 (nephrin) and NPHS2 (podocin) affect the slit-pore membrane at birth, and TRPC6 cation channel mutations in adulthood produce focal segmental glomerulosclerosis (FSGS).
- Partial lipodystrophy from mutations in genes encoding lamin A/C or PPAR cause a metabolic syndrome that can be associated with membranoproliferative glomerulonephritis (MPGN), which is sometimes accompanied by dense deposits and C3 nephritic factor.

- Pathogenesis of minimal-change glomerulopathy remains unclear; this disorder is most likely a consequence of abnormal regulation of T-cell subset and pathologic elaboration of circulating permeability factor; whether there is a genetic cause is unknown.
- Alport syndrome is most often an X-linked disorder in which affected male patients have hematuria from infancy. Female carriers have hematuria from birth but are generally not subject to renal failure. The disease is attributed to mutations in the genes encoding for the chains of type IV collagen.

GENERAL PREVENTION
- In the ICU environment, it is difficult prevent; however, a general approach to screening and decreasing exacerbating factors for AKI is essential.
- A complete medical history of the patient, with focused attention on preexisting renal disease and specifically for prior diagnosis of inflammatory renal disease.
- Screen ICU patients for risks of viral infections, including HIV, specific high-risk medications, and IV drugs.
- Diabetes or high blood pressure should be recognized and treated aggressively.
- Prompt nephrology referral when a disease that can cause glomerulonephritis is present

PATHOPHYSIOLOGY
- Immune complex deposition leading to glomerular injury usually occurs when moderate antigen excess over antibody production occurs.
- Pauci-immune acute glomerulonephritis is a form of small-vessel vasculitis associated with ANCA, causing primary and secondary renal diseases that do not have direct immune complex deposition or antibody binding.
- Pathologically, inflammatory glomerular lesions are seen. These include mesangioproliferative, focal, and diffuse proliferative, and crescentic lesions.

ETIOLOGY
- Immune complex:
  – IgA nephropathy
  – Endocarditis
  – SLE
  – Cryoglobulinemia
  – Postinfectious
  – Membranoproliferative
  – Henoch-Schönlein purpura
- Pauci-immune (ANCA+):
  – Wegener's granulomatosis
  – Churg-Strauss syndrome
  – Microscopic polyarteritis
- Anti-GBM:
  – Goodpasture syndrome
  – Anti-GBM glomerulonephritis
- Other:
  – Malignant hypertension
  – Thrombotic thrombocytopenic purpura
  – Sclerodermal renal crisis
  – Preeclampsia/eclampsia

COMMONLY ASSOCIATED CONDITIONS
- Vasculitis:
  – Thrombotic microangiopathy
  – Antiphospholipid syndrome
- Systemic disease:
  – Atherosclerosis
  – Cholesterol emboli
  – Hypertension
  – Sickle cell anemia
  – Autoimmunity
- Infectious diseases-associated syndrome:
  – Subacute bacterial endocarditis
  – Malaria
  – Schistosomiasis
  – HIV
  – Chronic hepatitis B and C
  – Strep pharyngitis

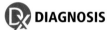

DIAGNOSIS

HISTORY
- History is important to elicit PMH, risk factors.
- Symptoms vary depending on whether the glomerulonephritis is acute or chronic.
- Patient may report fatigue, weight gain, s.o.b., nausea and vomiting, and lack of appetite

PHYSICAL EXAM
- Edema; periorbital and scrotal regions usually affected first
- Dark urine
- Hypertension
- Other physical findings will vary according to underlying disease.
- Articular pain, hemoptysis/cough, rash

DIAGNOSTIC TESTS & INTERPRETATION
Urine dipstick and microscopic evaluation:
- Hematuria, lipiduria
- Moderate proteinuria (usually <2 g/d), and
- Cellular elements such as red cells, red cell casts, and white cells:
  – Red cell casts are specific for glomerulonephritis

Lab
Initial lab tests
- These initial studies help frame further diagnostic workup that typically involves some testing of the serum for the presence of various proteins:
  – HIV and hepatitis B and C antigens
- Antibodies:
  – Anti-GBM, antiphospholipid, ASO, anti-DNAse, antihyaluronidase, ANCA, anti-DNA, cryoglobulins, anti-HIV, and antihepatitis B and C antibodies
- Depletion of complement components:
  – C3 and C4

Follow-Up & Special Considerations
- Follow-up by a kidney specialist and possible co-management with rheumatologist
- Microscopic urine analysis and serial measurements of level of proteinuria for tracking of resolution of disease

Imaging
- US can identify the thickness and echogenicity of the renal cortex, medulla, and pyramids, and a distended urinary collecting system.
- Other imaging modalities include CT, MRI, nuclear scan.

Diagnostic Procedures/Other
Renal biopsy: Type of glomerulonephritis can be categorized according to the light microscopy immunofluorescence pattern and electron microscopy appearance.

DIFFERENTIAL DIAGNOSIS
- Acute interstitial nephritis
- Acute tubular necrosis
- Hemorrhagic cystitis
- Benign causes of mild proteinuria

 # TREATMENT
MEDICATION
First Line

- Depending on the nature and severity of disease, treatment can consist of high-dose corticosteroids and cytotoxic agents such as cyclophosphamide (2)[A]
- Plasma exchange can be used in Goodpasture disease as a temporizing measure until chemotherapy can take effect.
- Antihypertensive agents for membranoproliferative steroids (1)[B]
- Diuretics and restriction of salt and water for fluid overload
- ACE inhibitors and angiotensin II receptor blockers for scleroderma renal crisis (3)[A]

Second Line
- Renal replacement therapy
- Kidney transplantation

ADDITIONAL TREATMENT
General Measures
- Electrolytes monitoring
- Daily weight
- Follow albumin and patients edema

Issues for Referral
- Timely referral to specialists is essential for a good outcome.
- Consider nephrology and rheumatology.

Additional Therapies
Dictated by the specific underlying disease process causing the glomerulonephritis

SURGERY/OTHER PROCEDURES
- There is no role for surgery in glomerulonephritis.
- Renal biopsy

IN-PATIENT CONSIDERATIONS
Initial Stabilization
- Control blood pressure.
- Immediately treat underlying cause for glomerulonephritis.

Admission Criteria
- Deteriorating kidney function
- Severe electrolytes imbalances
- Significant fluid overload
- Need for kidney biopsy or plasmapheresis
- Primary cause manifesting severe systemic multiorgan dysfunction:
  – TTP, PRES, serositis, anemia

IV Fluids
IV fluids should be used with caution when warranted to prevent fluid overload:
- Hypotonic solution may be preferred if sodium overload is an issue.
- Consider third spacing issues with hypotonic solutions.

Nursing
- Strict I&O, daily weight, monitor salt intake.
- Follow vital signs and medication contraindications.
- Follow patients for severe edema.

Discharge Criteria
- Depends on the severity of systemic disease
- Reversal or control of primary process

 # ONGOING CARE

FOLLOW-UP RECOMMENDATIONS
Regular follow-up with nephrologists and other specialist as dictated by underlying disease state

Patient Monitoring
Clinical picture, complement levels, and urine protein levels

DIET
Low-salt diet, water restriction in some cases

PATIENT EDUCATION
Should have education on specific disease and nutrition consult

PROGNOSIS
- Depends on etiology and response to treatment
- Glomerular disease dependant on severity of system disease

COMPLICATIONS
ESRD requiring dialysis:
- Complications related to primary disease process
- Complication related to specific treatment (cytotoxic drugs)

REFERENCES
1. Levine A. Management of membrano-proliferative glomerulonephritis: EBM recommendations. *Kidney Int*. 1999;55(Suppl 70):41–46.
2. Ponticelli C, et al. A randomized pilot trial comparing methylprednisolone plus a cytotoxic agent versus synthetic adrenocorticotropic hormone in idiopathic membranous nephropathy. *Am J Kidney Dis*. 2006;47:233–40.
3. Teixeira L, et al. Group Français de Recherche sur le Sclérodermie (GFRS). Mortality and risk factors of scleroderma renal crisis: A French retrospective study of 50 patients. *Ann Rheum Dis*. 2008;67(1): 110–6.

ADDITIONAL READING
- Brenner BM. *Brenners & Rector's the kidney*, 8th ed. New York: Elsevier Saunders, 2007.
- Jennette JC. *Heptinstall's pathology of the kidney*, 6th ed. Philadelphia: Wolter Kluwer Lippincott Williams & Wilkins, 2007.

CODES

ICD9
- 583.0 Nephritis and nephropathy, not specified as acute or chronic, with lesion of proliferative glomerulonephritis
- 583.9 Nephritis and nephropathy, not specified as acute or chronic, with unspecified pathological lesion in kidney
- 759.89 Other specified congenital anomalies

CLINICAL PEARLS

- In progressive renal failure with dysmorphic red cells, hypertension; consider acute GN
- Pulmonary etiology present with renal failure; consider acute glomerulonephritis due to autoimmune-related disease.

G

GRAFT-VERSUS-HOST DISEASE (GVHD)

Stephen M. Pastores
Ann A. Jakubowski

 BASICS

DESCRIPTION
- GVHD is the most frequent complication of allogeneic hematopoietic stem cell transplantation (HSCT).
- Clinicopathologic syndrome is caused by an immunologic reaction of donor lymphocytes to "foreign" antigens present on the surface of host (recipient) cells.
- Can affect liver, GI tract, skin and mucosa, eye, lung
- Grading systems for severity: Scoring of involvement or symptoms of each organ; stage 0–4 for acute and 0–3 for chronic:
  - Stage of each organ involved is combined to determine an overall grade: Grade 1–4 for acute; mild, moderate, and severe for chronic.

EPIDEMIOLOGY
Incidence
- Acute GVHD: Within 100 days post HSCT 10–60% using histocompatible leukocyte antigen (HLA)-matched sibling donors; up to 80% with nonidentical or unrelated donors. Can be seen as persistent, recurrent, or late acute after the first 100 days, often with tapering of immunosuppression
- Chronic GVHD: Within 2–3 years post HSCT 10–50% in HLA-identical sibling donor, up to 50–70% in unrelated donor HSCT
- Combined acute + chronic = overlapping features of both

Prevalence
- Acute and chronic GvHD: More common in unrelated and mismatched donor HSCT, lowest in patients receiving T-cell depleted grafts; more acute following myeloablative vs. nonmyeloablative conditioning
- Chronic: More common after acute GvHD; and after peripheral blood vs bone marrow HSCT
- Occurs in a small proportion of autologous HSCT patients and rarely with transfusion

RISK FACTORS
- HLA, donor/host gender disparity
- Increasing age of patient/donor
- Intensity of the conditioning
- Intensity and duration of immunosuppression
- Stem cell source: PBSC vs. BM vs. cord blood
- Allosensitization of donor
- Unmodified vs. T cell depleted graft
- Development of acute GvHD

Genetics
- HLA-A, -B, -C, -DR, -DQ, and -DP control T-cell recognition and determine histocompatibility.
- Polymorphism of portions of the killer immunoglobulin-like receptor (KIR) affect allorecognition of donor natural killer (NK) cells.
- Genetic polymorphisms in patient and donor are both implicated in "cytokine storm" of GvHD.

GENERAL PREVENTION
- Optimize choice of donor and stem cell source
- T-cell depletion of the donor graft
- Maximize posttransplant immunosuppression for T-replete grafts

PATHOPHYSIOLOGY
- Requirements for GVHD:
  - Graft must contain immunocompetent cells (T lymphocytes).
  - Immunosuppressed host is unable to reject the transplanted cells.
  - Host tissue expresses antigens not present in the donor.

ETIOLOGY
- Reaction of donor T lymphocytes against nonshared recipient antigens
- No consensus on the etiology of chronic GvHD

COMMONLY ASSOCIATED CONDITIONS
- Infection
- Ileus, dehydration, hemorrhage
- Wasting syndrome
- Cytopenias
- Myopathy
- Respiratory compromise
- Renal insufficiency

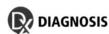 **DIAGNOSIS**

HISTORY
- Acute GVHD:
  - Maculopapular rash, abdominal cramping, voluminous watery or bloody diarrhea jaundice, anorexia, nausea, vomiting
  - Weight loss, oral ulcers, mouth pain (1)
- Chronic GVHD:
  - Eye irritation, dryness, photophobia
  - Mucosal dryness, sensitivity, pain
  - Weight loss
  - Wheezing, dyspnea and chronic cough
  - Neuropathic pain, weakness/muscle cramps
  - Skin: Lichen planus–like, sclerotic changes
  - Musculoskeletal: Joint stiffness, reduced range of motion, cramping
  - GI: Anorexia, nausea/vomiting, weight loss, malabsorption
  - Liver: Jaundice

PHYSICAL EXAM
- Skin: Maculopapular rash, jaundice, rarely bullous lesions/toxic epidermal necrolysis; lichenoid and sclerotic changes with chronic GVHD; thinned or absent hair growth.
- Mucosa: Ulcerations, lichenoid changes
- Eye: Icteric, injected, dry
- Lung: Rales or wheezing
- Abdomen: Hyperactive/hypoactive bowel sounds, diffuse abdominal or RUQ tenderness, hepatomegaly
- Musculoskeletal: Weakness, limited range of motion of joints associated +/– contractures

DIAGNOSTIC TESTS & INTERPRETATION
Lab
Initial lab tests
- Chemistry panel: Electrolyte abnormalities, abnormal liver transaminases; elevated bilirubin and alkaline phosphatase, renal function.
- CBC: Anemia, thrombocytopenia, leukopenia/leukocytosis eosinophilia
- Stool studies: Infection, blood
- CMV PCR
- Immunosuppressive drug levels

Follow-Up & Special Considerations
- Chemistry panel and CBC after fluid and electrolyte repletion
- Follow immunosuppressive drug levels.

Imaging
Initial approach
- Hepatic Doppler sonography to rule out other diagnoses
- CAT scan of chest

Diagnostic Procedures/Other
- Skin/mucosal/liver or lung biopsy
- Upper and lower GI endoscopy with biopsy
- Pulmonary function tests to identify obliterative bronchiolitis
- Assess joint range of motion.

Pathological Findings
- **Acute:** Epithelial damage, usually apoptotic in target organs (1)
  - GI: Crypt destruction and mucosal ulceration, lymphocyte apoptosis at base of crypts
  - Skin: Epidermal and basal cell degeneration, disorganized epidermal cell maturation, dermal perivascular lymphocytic infiltration
  - Liver: Periductal epithelial injury, bile duct atypia/cellular degeneration, segmental disruption small ducts with lymphocytic infiltration
  - Disparity between lymphocytic infiltration and severity of tissue destruction.
- Chronic:
  - Skin: Epidermal atrophy, dermal fibrosis/sclerosis
  - Liver: Hyalinization portal triad, fibrosis, bile duct obliteration
  - GI: Inflammation, destruction of centrally draining ducts

DIFFERENTIAL DIAGNOSIS
- Drug toxicity
- Viral hepatitis
- Hepatic veno-occlusive disease
- Viral/bacterial gastroenteritis
- Erythema multiforme
- Malabsorption
- Autoimmune disease

TREATMENT

MEDICATION

First Line

- Depends on the type of graft, acute vs. chronic and ongoing prophylactic therapy
- Acute: Add topical or systemic corticosteroids
- Calcineurin inhibitor for T-cell depleted grafts
- All chronic: Generally combinations
- Topical steroids or calcineurin inhibitor for skin and eye, Decadron mouth rinses
- Systemic calcineurin inhibitor
- Systemic steroids (2)

Second, Third and Fourth Line

- Acute:
  − Antithymocyte globulin
  − Mycophenolate mofetil 2 g/d: Also for steroid-refractory chronic GVHD (2)
  − Sirolimus
  − Antibody therapy: Daclizumab, infliximab, etanercept, rituximab
- Chronic: Combinations
  − Pentostatin
  − Psoralen and ultraviolet A irradiation (PUVA) - cutaneous
  − Antimetabolites: Azathioprine
  − Hydroxychloroquine
  − Imatinib
  − Extracorporeal photopheresis
  − Rituximab

ADDITIONAL TREATMENT

General Measures

- Venous access
- Hydration and electrolyte replacement for diarrhea
- Analgesics for pain
- Antimotility agents for diarrhea
- Transfusions and growth factor for cytopenias
- IV administration of medications for concerns about absorption
- Adjust medications and dosing for toxicity
- Monitoring for infection
- Prophylaxis for viral, bacterial, and fungal infections
- Monitoring of drug levels

Issues for Referral

- Dental: mucosal biopsy
- GI: Endoscopy or liver biopsy
- Interventional radiology: Transjugular liver biopsy
- Dermatology: Skin biopsy
- Pulmonary: PFTs and bronchoscopy and biopsy
- Thoracic surgery: Lung biopsy
- Ophthalmology
- Nutrition: Adequate caloric intake, appropriate diet
- Burn ICU: Stage IV skin GVHD

Additional Therapies

- Psychosocial support
- Nutrition: TPN
- Clonazepam for neuromuscular symptoms
- Ursodeoxycholic acid for hepatic chronic GVHD
- Physical therapy

SURGERY/OTHER PROCEDURES

- Skin debriding bullous or ulcerated lesions
- Venous access

IN-PATIENT CONSIDERATIONS

Initial Stabilization

- Hydration and electrolyte replacement for diarrhea
- Antimotility agents
- Cultures and imaging studies to rule out infection; antibiotics
- Transfusion and growth factor support for cytopenia

Admission Criteria

- Hypotension
- Inability to take medications or concerns about absorption
- Suspected infection
- Dehydration/electrolyte imbalance
- Hemorrhagic diarrhea

IV Fluids

- Initially, standard D5NS + electrolytes; replete and then ongoing replacement of losses
- TPN as indicated

Nursing

- Skin and wound care
- Monitoring I and O
- Assist in pain management
- Encourage physical therapy
- Monitor for sites of infection
- Psychological support

Discharge Criteria

- GvHD controlled and improving
- Able to maintain hydration and nutrition intake orally
- Absorbing oral medications
- Therapeutic medication levels

ONGOING CARE

FOLLOW-UP RECOMMENDATIONS

- Close outpatient clinical monitoring
- Physical therapy
- Evaluate any fever or sign of infection

Patient Monitoring

- Chemistry and hematology labs
- Drug levels of immunosuppressives.

DIET

- Acute GI GVHD: Keep NPO and use TPN
- Advance to bland diet or BRAT diet as tolerated
- Protein-containing dietary supplements when tolerated

PATIENT EDUCATION

- Nutrition
- Skin care
- Exercise
- Protection from infections.

PROGNOSIS

- Acute GVHD: Overall grade correlates well with outcome and response to treatment
- 20–25% mortality rate in patients achieving complete response compared to >75% mortality rate in those with no response or with progression
- Chronic GVHD: 42% 6-year survival rate; 10% in patients with progressive onset
- Poor prognostic factors: Inability to taper immunosuppressives without flare:
  − Serum bilirubin >2 mg/dL
  − Early time to onset and treatment of GVHD
  − Extensive disease
  − Thrombocytopenia

COMPLICATIONS

- Hepatitis
- Desquamative dermatitis
- Infection
- GI hemorrhage
- Malnutrition
- Renal insufficiency

REFERENCES

1. Deeg HJ, et al. The clinical spectrum of acute graft-versus-host disease. *Semin Hematol*. 2006;43:24–31.
2. Couriel D, et al. Acute graft-versus-host disease: Pathophysiology, clinical manifestations, and management. *Cancer*. 2004;101:1936–46.

ADDITIONAL READING

- Pene F, et al. Outcome of critically ill allogeneic hematopoietic stem-cell transplantation recipients: A reappraisal of indications for organ failure supports. *J Clin Oncol*. 2006;24(4):643–9.

 See Also (Topic, Algorithm, Electronic Media Element)

http://www.marrow.org

CODES

ICD9

- 279.50 Graft-versus-host disease, unspecified
- 279.51 Acute graft-versus-host disease
- 279.52 Chronic graft-versus-host disease

CLINICAL PEARLS

- GVHD is a common clinicopathologic syndrome involving the skin, liver, and GI tract after allogeneic HSCT.
- HLA disparity, older age, intensity of transplant conditioning chemotherapy, number of T cells transplanted, and some gender disparities are major risk factors.
- Treatment for GVHD involves treatment with additional immunosuppression depending on severity of GVHD.
- Acute grade IV GVHD has a high mortality rate.

G

GUILLAIN-BARRÉ SYNDROME

Alina Dulu

 BASICS

DESCRIPTION
- Acute inflammatory demyelinating polyneuropathy (AIDP) known as Guillain-Barré syndrome is an acute immune-mediated polyradiculopathy predominantly affecting motor function.
- Guillain-Barré syndrome variants:
  – Acute motor-sensory axonal neuropathy is usually severe with poor recovery.
  – Acute motor axonal neuropathy has been described in northern China.
  – The Miller-Fisher syndrome (5% of cases) of ophthalmoplegia, ataxia, and areflexia
  – Acute pandysautonomia characterized by sympathetic and parasympathetic failure

EPIDEMIOLOGY
Incidence
- Bimodal peaks of occurrence at 15–35 and 50–75 years:
  – Older age is associated with poor prognosis.
- 0.6–1.9 cases/100,000 persons annually without geographic variation
- Incidence increases with age: 0.8 cases per 100,000 at 18 years, 3.2 cases at 100,000 at 60 years

Prevalence
The most common cause of acute flaccid paralysis in the Western hemisphere and probably worldwide

RISK FACTORS
- Infections: Viral (HIV, CMV, EBV, influenza, hepatitis B), bacterial (*Campylobacter jejuni*, Lyme disease, *Mycoplasma pneumonia*), toxoplasmosis:
  – *C. jejuni* infection is associated with severe disease.
- Systemic illness: Lymphoma, SLE
- Immunizations (influenza vaccination)

PATHOPHYSIOLOGY
- Immune-mediated disorder caused by a synergistic interaction of cell-mediated and humoral immune responses to still incompletely characterized peripheral nerve antigens
- Inflammatory demyelination starts at the level of the nerve roots.
- Followed by multifocal, patchy, widespread peripheral nerve demyelination
- Peripheral nerve remyelination occurs over several weeks to months.

ETIOLOGY
- A preceding infection may trigger an autoimmune response through molecular mimicry.
- The infectious organism shares epitopes with the host's peripheral nerves.

COMMONLY ASSOCIATED CONDITIONS
60% of patients have a history of respiratory or GI illness or surgery within 30 days of onset symptoms.

 DIAGNOSIS

HISTORY
- Paresthesias is initial symptom.
- Rapid progression of acute symmetric weakness:
  – Weakness usually starts in the proximal legs.
  – Progresses upward, involving the arms, respiratory, facial, and bulbar muscles
  – Weakness is more severe distally than proximally.
  – Weakness is worse in the legs than the arms.
  – Difficulty in ambulating, getting up from a chair, or climbing stairs
  – Maximal clinical weakness within 4 week of disease onset and then plateaus
- Sensory loss is predominantly of position and vibration senses; this is variable and usually mild.
- Pain occurs in 50% of patients and is most severe in the shoulder girdle, back, and posterior thighs; may be accompanied by muscle cramps.

PHYSICAL EXAM
- Symmetric weakness:
  – Initially involving proximal muscles, subsequently involving both proximal and distal muscles
- Depressed or absent reflexes bilaterally
- Sensory loss limited to the distal impairment of vibration sense:
  – Glove and stocking anesthesia/paresthesias
- Cranial nerve involvement:
  – Facial paresis, difficulty swallowing
- Ataxia and pain in a segmental distribution caused by involvement of posterior nerve roots
- Autonomic abnormalities: Cardiac dysrhythmias and blood pressure abnormalities, urinary retention, GI atony, anhidrosis or episodic diaphoresis, and thermoregulation problems
  – Severe autonomic dysfunction is occasionally associated with sudden death.
- Respiratory insufficiency caused by weakness of intercostal muscles necessitates mechanical ventilation in 30% of patients.

DIAGNOSTIC TESTS & INTERPRETATION
Lab
- CSF exam shows albumino-cytological dissociation:
  – Elevated CSF protein (especially IgG)
  – Few mononuclear leukocytes, usually <10 cells/mL
- CBC leukocytosis with left shift
- Antibodies against GQ1b (a ganglioside component of nerve) are found in 90% of patients with Miller-Fisher syndrome.
- Antibodies to GM1, GD1a, GalNac-GD1a, GD1b are mostly associated with axonal variants.
- To exclude other causes of weakness:
  – Electrolytes
  – Heavy metal testing
  – Urine porphyria screen
  – Creatine kinase
  – HIV titers

Imaging
Initial approach
Lumbosacral spinal MRI may demonstrate gadolinium enhancement of lumbar roots.
Follow-Up & Special Considerations
- Repeat lumbar puncture:
  – In the 1st week of neurological symptoms, the CSF protein may be normal.

Diagnostic Procedures/Other
- Needle electromyography (EMG) and nerve conduction studies (NCS):
  – Evaluation of sensory and motor nerves in the upper and lower extremities, including proximal stimulation of motor nerves and F wave studies
  – Slowed conduction velocities
  – Prolonged motor, sensory, F-wave latencies, andabsent H reflexes
  – Increased distal latencies and conduction blocks with temporal dispersion of motor responses
  – EMG of weak muscles shows reduced recruitment.
  – NCS can be normal at the beginning and progress over time, so frequent serial testing might be necessary.
- ECG: T-wave abnormalities, ST-segment depression, QRS widening, QT prolongation, and various forms of heart block

Pathological Findings
- Multifocal inflammatory demyelination of spinal roots and peripheral nerves:
  – Endoneurial perivascular mononuclear cell infiltration and multifocal demyelination
  – Intense inflammation may lead to axonal degeneration.

DIFFERENTIAL DIAGNOSIS
- Toxic peripheral neuropathies: Heavy metal poisoning (lead, thallium, arsenic), medications (vincristine, disulfiram), organophosphate poisoning, hexacarbon (glue sniffer's neuropathy)
- Nontoxic peripheral neuropathies: Acute intermittent porphyria, vasculitic polyneuropathy, infectious (poliomyelitis, diphtheria, Lyme disease), tick paralysis
- Neuromuscular junction disorders: Myasthenia gravis, botulism, snake envenomations
- Myopathies such as polymyositis
- Severe electrolyte abnormalities: Hypokalemia, hypophosphatemia
- Acute central nervous system disorders basilar artery thrombosis, brainstem encephalomyelitis, transverse myelitis, or spinal cord compression
- Hysterical paralysis or malingering

TREATMENT

MEDICATION
First Line
- Infusion of IV immunoglobulin 0.4 g/kg/d for 5 days:
  - Check serum IgA levels before infusion to prevent anaphylaxis in deficient patients.
  - Adverse reactions: Aseptic meningitis, congestive heart failure, thrombotic complications (strokes and myocardial infarction), and renal failure
- Early therapeutic plasma exchange 50 mL/kg over 5 sessions q.o.d.), started within 7 days of onset of symptoms:
  - Use cautiously in patients with cardiovascular disease, sepsis, and autonomic dysfunction.
- IVIg and PE are equally effective
- Efficacy of PE and IVIg are established for patients who have lost the ability to walk, to shorten recovery time.

Second Line
Corticosteroids cannot be recommended.

Pediatric Considerations
IVIG seems to be of similar efficacy as in adults.

ADDITIONAL TREATMENT
Issues for Referral
- Cardiology consult for 2nd- or 3rd-degree atrioventricular blocks, for which a temporary pacemaker insertion is needed
- Physical and occupational therapy for rehabilitation, including supportive devices:
  - Physical therapy started early prevents contractures, joint immobilization, and venous stasis.

SURGERY/OTHER PROCEDURES
- ENT for tracheotomy, if prolonged ventilatory support is required
- Surgery for percutaneous endoscopic gastrostomy (PEG), if temporary nutritional support is required

IN-PATIENT CONSIDERATIONS
Initial Stabilization
- Never give primary treatment in the outpatient setting.
- Patients with rapidly worsening GBS should be observed in ICU until the maximum extent of progression has been established.
- Supportive care is the backbone of therapy.

Admission Criteria
- Close monitoring ICU for respiratory, cardiac, and hemodynamic function
- Respiratory monitoring: Bedside measurements of forced vital capacity (FVC) and negative inspiratory force (NIF)

- Close monitoring in ICU if:
  - Rapid disease progression (onset to admission in <7 days)
  - Bulbar dysfunction
  - Autonomic dysfunction
  - Bilateral facial palsies
  - FVC >20 mL/kg
  - NIF ≤30 cm H_2O
- Mechanical ventilation may be needed if:
  - FVC is <12–15 mL/kg
  - FVC declines by 30% from baseline
  - FVC is rapidly decreasing
  - NIF ≤20 cm H_2O
  - PaO_2 is <70
- Early signs of respiratory fatigue
  - Increased respiratory secretions
  - Difficulty clearing respiratory secretions
- Monitoring and treatment of autonomic dysfunction:
  - Bradyarrhythmias; might need pacemaker
  - Unstable tachyarrhythmias with cardioversion
  - Hypotension is best managed by the rapid infusion of fluid, and sympathomimetics usually are not needed.
  - Hypertension should not be treated unless severe and persistent.
  - Altered sweating with cooling blanket
- Mildly affected patients can be admitted on telemetry ward with monitoring of blood pressure and vital capacity q4h.

Nursing
- Frequent repositioning of patient minimizes formation of pressure sores.
- Chest physical therapy and frequent oral suctioning aid in preventing atelectasis.
- Pressure-induced ulnar or fibular nerve palsies are prevented by proper positioning and padding.
- Prevent exposure keratitis in cases of facial plegia by using artificial tears and by taping the eyelids closed at night.
- Laxative, enema to avoid fecal impactions
- Foley catheter for urine retention
- Tracheal suctioning may induce " vagal spells" with bradycardia and asystole.
- Prophylaxis for deep vein thrombosis

Discharge Criteria
Neurologically stable

 ONGOING CARE

FOLLOW-UP RECOMMENDATIONS
Weakness reaches its maximum within 14 days.

PROGNOSIS
- Mortality is approximately 5–10%:
  - Causes of death include cardiac arrest, pulmonary embolism, sepsis.
- Prognosis for full recovery is very good.
- A spontaneous recovery generally occurs after 6 weeks to 6 months.
- There is mild residual weakness in 15%, moderately severe residual weakness in 10%, and 5% may remain in bed 1 year after the onset of symptoms.
- Recurrence may occur in >5% of patients following full recovery.

COMPLICATIONS
Respiratory failure requiring mechanical ventilation develops in up to 30%.

REFERENCES
1. Hughes RAC, et al: Intravenous immunoglobulin for Guillain-Barré syndrome. *Cochrane Database Syst Rev.* 2006;1:CD002063.
2. Rapha'l JC, et al. Plasma exchange for Guillain-Barré syndrome. *Cochrane Database Syst Rev.* 2002;2:CD001798.

ADDITIONAL READING
- Daroff RB, Bradley WG eds. *Neurology in clinical practice*, 5th ed. Boston: Butterworth, 2007.

 CODES

ICD9
357.0 Acute infective polyneuritis

CLINICAL PEARLS
- When performing endotracheal intubation, avoid the use of paralyzing agents (e.g., succinylcholine) due to increased risk for life-threatening hyperkalemia.
- ABGs are poor indicators of impending respiratory failure.

HELLP SYNDROME

Shilpi Mehta-Lee
Ellen J. Landsberger

 BASICS

DESCRIPTION
- A recognized complication of preeclampsia (PEC)-eclampsia that involves **H**emolysis, **E**levated **L**iver enzymes, and **L**ow **P**latelets
- Can occur in the absence of hypertension and proteinuria
- Systems affected: Hepatic, Hematologic, Cardiovascular, CNS

EPIDEMIOLOGY
Incidence
- 1–5/1000 of pregnancies
- 4–20% of patients with comorbid PEC

RISK FACTORS
- PEC (especially severe)
- Caucasian
- Maternal age >25
- Multifetal gestation
- Personal/1st-degree relative with history of HELLP/PEC
- Chronic hypertension
- Antiphospholipid syndrome
- Inherited thrombophilias

Genetics
- Family history of PEC/HELLP is a risk factor.
- No clear genetic etiology has been described.
- Increased risk of HELLP with inherited thrombophilias such as factor V Leiden mutation, antithrombin III, prothrombin gene mutation

GENERAL PREVENTION
- No preventative therapy has been shown to be effective in the overall pregnant population.
- Appropriate prenatal care can facilitate early recognition and appropriate treatment of PEC.

PATHOPHYSIOLOGY
- Exact cause of HELLP is unknown.
- General activation of the coagulation cascade is the main underlying problem.
- Fibrin forms cross-linked networks in small blood vessels, leading to microangiopathic hemolytic anemia.
- Platelet consumption coagulopathy occurs.
- As the liver appears to be the main site of this process, downstream liver cells suffer ischemia, leading to periportal necrosis.

ETIOLOGY
The exact cause of HELLP is unknown.

COMMONLY ASSOCIATED CONDITIONS
- Acute or chronic HTN, renal disease, diabetes, obesity
- PEC, eclampsia
- Acute renal failure
- DIC, which complicates emergency surgery
- May have evidence of subcapsular hematoma that can result in acute liver rupture
- Intracranial hemorrhage: Combination of hypertension, coagulopathy, thrombocytopenia increases risk

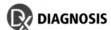 **DIAGNOSIS**

HISTORY
- Symptoms may include malaise, headache, visual disturbances (scotomata and blurry vision), epigastric pain, nausea/vomiting, shortness of breath, decreased urine output, or altered mental status (1)[C].
- History specific to HELLP syndrome: RUQ pain, petechiae and ecchymoses, hematuria, or bleeding from mucosal surfaces

PHYSICAL EXAM
- Mild PEC: BP >140/90, twice, 6 hours apart
- Severe PEC: BP >160/110, twice, 6 hours apart
- Hyperreflexia, epigastric tenderness, rales, peripheral edema, jaundice
- Petechiae or ecchymoses, papilledema/retinal hemorrhages possible

DIAGNOSTIC TESTS & INTERPRETATION
Lab
Initial lab tests
- All labs as described in section on PEC
- Abnormal peripheral smear (burr cells, schistocytes, echinocytes)
- Hemolysis as indicated by elevated indirect bilirubin and LDH (>600 IU/L), and low serum haptoglobin (2)[C]
- Elevation of liver transaminases
- Thrombocytopenia (platelets <100 K)

Follow-Up & Special Considerations
- Although most abnormal lab values will resolve in 48 hours, platelet values may nadir postpartum, and liver function/hemolysis may continue to worsen for several days (2)[C].
- Labs q4–6h postpartum until evidence of resolving disease
- Platelets can fall rapidly in HELLP syndrome.
- HELLP syndrome may develop in the postpartum period (30%) (1)[C].

Imaging
- Chest x-ray if shortness of breath or pulmonary findings
- Head CT if neurologic changes
- Abdominal CT/RUQ US, if severe RUQ pain and suspected subcapsular liver hematoma

ALERT
If liver rupture is suspected, do not delay surgery to obtain imaging studies; this is a surgical emergency.

Pathological Findings
- Gross autopsy of liver shows rigid consistency, yellow-brown cut surface and hemorrhagic foci
- Histopathologic liver findings: Periportal hepatocellular necrosis

DIFFERENTIAL DIAGNOSIS
- Acute fatty liver of pregnancy
- Thrombotic thrombocytopenic purpura
- Hemolytic uremic syndrome
- Immune thrombocytopenic purpura
- SLE
- Antiphospholipid syndrome
- Cholestasis
- Fulminant viral hepatitis
- Acute pancreatitis
- Disseminated herpes simplex
- Hemorrhagic or septic shock

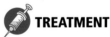 **TREATMENT**

MEDICATION
First Line

IV magnesium sulfate as described in section on PEC to prevent seizures (1,2)[A]

ALERT
Magnesium sulfate is contraindicated in patients with pulmonary edema. In patients with renal dysfunction or oliguria, magnesium levels must be followed and dose adjusted to avoid toxicity.

- Aggressive blood pressure control (2)[C]
- Antenatal corticosteroids for fetal lung maturity at <34 weeks' gestation are desired, but patients with HELLP syndrome may deteriorate rapidly and delivery must not be delayed (1)[C].

Second Line
IV corticosteroids may improve platelet count but have not been shown to improve maternal morbidity (4)[C].

ADDITIONAL TREATMENT
General Measures
- Expeditious delivery is the cure for HELLP syndrome.
- Expectant management of HELLP syndrome is controversial and should involve a maternal fetal medicine specialist (1)[C].
- Trial of labor may be appropriate in select patients with mild to moderate HELLP syndrome in whom imminent vaginal delivery is anticipated.
- Cesarean delivery may be indicated after maternal stabilization if remote from vaginal delivery.
- Control of hypertension is crucial (5)[C].
- Scrupulous fluid management as outlined in General Measures in PEC chapter.
- Judicious use of blood products (RBCs, platelets, fresh frozen plasma, cryoprecipitate) is warranted in patients with DIC.
- Observation for evidence of bleeding, including close attention to neurologic exam

Issues for Referral
- Patients with subcapsular liver hematoma should have general surgery consultation.
- Surgeon and OR should be immediately available in case of suspected liver rupture.
- Neurology/neurosurgical consultation if any suspicion of neurologic changes or evidence of intracranial hemorrhage

Additional Therapies
Plasma exchange has been used in a select subset of postpartum women who continue to deteriorate 4 days postpartum (4)[C].

SURGERY/OTHER PROCEDURES
- Surgical intervention may be required in patients with subcapsular hepatic hematoma.
- Patients with PEC/HELLP often have laryngeal edema, making intubation and extubation challenging.

IN-PATIENT CONSIDERATIONS
Initial Stabilization
- See Preeclampsia topic
- With fulminant DIC, fluid resuscitation and blood component therapy as needed
- Maternal stabilization is of paramount importance.
- Fetal status must then be considered.

Admission Criteria
- All patients with HELLP syndrome should be admitted to a tertiary care center.
- Admission to the ICU is based upon evidence of DIC, subcapsular hematoma, hypertensive crisis, evidence of stroke or intracranial hemorrhage.

IV Fluids
- See Preeclampsia topic.
- When platelets <50,000/mm^2, initiate platelet transfusion prior to surgical intervention, such as cesarean section.

Nursing
- Tertiary care environment with ICU nursing should be available at all times.
- See Preeclampsia topic for requirements.

Discharge Criteria
- Status post delivery of infant
- Evidence of resolving HELLP, such as improvement in liver function tests, platelets, and indicators of hemolysis
- Stable BP, adequate urine output

 ONGOING CARE

FOLLOW-UP RECOMMENDATIONS
- Close monitoring for 48 hours postpartum with labs, nursing care
- Lab parameters should be improving prior to discharge.
- Close outpatient follow-up in the first 2 weeks after discharge
- In future pregnancies, patients have a 2–19% recurrence rate.

Patient Monitoring
- Disease can rarely worsen in the postpartum period, so patients must know signs and symptoms that require immediate medical attention.
- Patients should have blood pressure check within a week after discharge.

DIET
If renal dysfunction, recommend renal-specific diet with low salt and low potassium.

PATIENT EDUCATION
- Disease can worsen in the postpartum period.
- Patients must know signs and symptoms that require immediate medical attention.
- Patients are at increased risk of developing HELLP or PEC in a subsequent pregnancy.

PROGNOSIS
- HELLP syndrome is associated with increased risk of maternal death (1%).
- Increased rates of maternal morbidities: Pulmonary edema (8%), acute renal failure (3%), DIC (15%), placental abruption (9%), liver hemorrhage/failure (1%), ARDS, sepsis, and stroke (<1%).
- Development of HELLP postpartum increases the risk of renal failure and pulmonary edema.
- Placental abruption increases the risk of DIC, pulmonary edema, and renal failure.
- Large-volume ascites indicates a high rate of cardiopulmonary complications.
- Patients who meet all criteria have greater rates of maternal complications than do those who have partial HELLP.
- Perinatal mortality and morbidity is increased.
- Perinatal death rate 7.4–20.4%.
- Preterm delivery in ~70%, with 15% occurring before 28 weeks of gestation.

COMPLICATIONS
- Maternal death
- Maternal morbidity as listed above.
- Wound hematomas
- Perinatal morbidity and mortality

REFERENCES
1. Sibai BM. Imitators of severe preeclampsia. *Obstet Gynecol.* 2007;109(4):956–66.
2. Guntupalli SR, et al. Hepatic disease and pregnancy: An overview of diagnosis and management. *Crit Care Med.* 2005;33(10 Suppl): S332–9.
3. Vinnars MT, et al. Severe PEC with and without HELLP differ with regard to placental pathology. *Hypertension.* 2008;51(5):1295–9.
4. Sibai BM, et al. Dexamethasone to improve maternal outcome in women with hemolysis, elevated liver enzymes and low platelets. *Am J Obstet Gynecol.* 2005;193(5):1587–90.
5. Osmanagaoglu MA, et al. Maternal outcome in HELLP syndrome requiring intensive care management in a Turkish Hospital. *Sao Paulo Med J.* 2006;124(2):85–9.

ADDITIONAL READING
- Barton JR, et al. Diagnosis and management of hemolysis, elevated liver enzymes, and low platelets syndrome. *Clin Perinatol.* 2004;31(4):807–33, vii.
- Matchaba P, et al. Corticosteroids for HELLP syndrome in pregnancy. *Cochrane Database Syst Rev.* 2004.
- Weinstein L. Syndrome of hemolysis, elevated liver enzymes, and low platelet count: a severe consequence of hypertension in pregnancy. *Am J Obstet Gynecol.* 1982;142:159–67.

See Also (Topic, Algorithm, Electronic Media Element)
- Preeclampsia
- Eclampsia

 CODES

ICD9
- 642.50 Severe pre-eclampsia, unspecified as to episode of care
- 642.51 Severe pre-eclampsia, with delivery
- 642.52 Severe pre-eclampsia, with delivery, with mention of postpartum complication

CLINICAL PEARLS
- Patients with HELLP do not always present with proteinuria or blood pressure elevation.
- HELLP can present in the postpartum period.
- Platelets can fall rapidly in HELLP syndrome and should be followed closely.
- Epigastric pain can herald liver rupture, which is a surgical emergency.

H

HEMATOMA, EPIDURAL

Merritt D. Kinon
Nrupen Baxi

 BASICS

DESCRIPTION
- Collection of blood between the dura mater and skull caused by a ruptured blood vessel (usually meningeal arterial vessels) in the epidural space
- Usually caused by trauma (i.e., skull fracture) but can be caused by coagulopathies, medical or surgically lowered ICP, or rapid correction of shock (i.e., hemodynamic "surge")

EPIDEMIOLOGY
Incidence
- 2.7–4% of traumatic brain injuries (TBI)
- Up to 9% of coma patients with TBI
Prevalence
- Male >Female (4:1)
- Peak incidence in 2nd decade (age 20–30)
- Rare in children <2 or adults >60
- Pediatric Prevalence Age 6–10

RISK FACTORS
- High speed/high impact head trauma usually with skull fracture (traffic-related accidents 53%, falls 30%, and assaults 8%)
- Coagulopathies
- Aggressive ICP management
- Postop craniotomy
Genetics
- No specific mutation is associated with EDH.
- Increased risk of coagulopathies, collagen vascular disorders, osteogenesis imperfecta

GENERAL PREVENTION
Trauma prevention

PATHOPHYSIOLOGY
Temporal skull fracture usually causes a tear in a meningeal artery (36% middle meningeal artery) or vein, which causes bleeding that dissects the dura mater from the inner table.

ETIOLOGY
- Head trauma with skull fracture (seen in 70–95% of epidural hematomas)
- Coagulopathies
- ICP management (shearing force on meningeal vessels as dura is pulled away from the inner table of the skull):
  – Medically with osmotic diuretics and/or surgically with craniotomy reduces "tamponading" effect
- Collagen vascular disorders

COMMONLY ASSOCIATED CONDITIONS
- Can be associated with other traumatic intracranial injuries (2–5% of patients have bilateral epidural hematomas), 30% have intraparenchymal lesions.
- Other bodily traumatic injuries

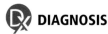 **DIAGNOSIS**

HISTORY
Brief loss of consciousness after trauma followed by recovery then progressive deterioration of neurologic exam (lucid interval):
- Decreased level of consciousness
- Hemiparesis (usually contralateral)
- Pupillary dilation (usually ipsilateral)
- Seizures
- Headache
- Nausea
- Vomiting

PHYSICAL EXAM
Neurologic exam with attention to mental status with Glasgow Coma Scores (GCS) (best predictor of outcome), presence of flexor or extensor posturing, pupillary exam (fixed and dilated in about 30% of surgical patients), cranial nerves, and motor exam, presence or absence of cushing reflex (bradycardia and hypertension)

DIAGNOSTIC TESTS & INTERPRETATION
Lab
- Important to order routine preop labs because treatment is usually surgical
- Check for coagulopathies and correct.

Initial lab tests
Chemistry, CBC, coags, type and screen, toxicology screen

Imaging
Noncontrast head CT:
- High density biconvex lens-shaped hematoma adjacent to the skull usually confined to a small area, frequently with mass effect

Pathological Findings
- Clot
- Torn meningeal artery or vein

DIFFERENTIAL DIAGNOSIS
- Epidural hematoma
- Subdural hematoma
- Infection
- Abscess
- Mass

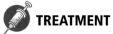 **TREATMENT**

MEDICATION
- An epidural hematoma <30 cm³ in volume, and <15-mm thickness, and with a <5-mm midline shift on CT scan in patients with a GCS score >8 without focal deficit can be managed nonoperatively (1)[C].
- Small (<1 cm) epidural hematomas with minimal neurological signs/symptoms not in the posterior fossa may be managed medically:
  – Admitted to monitored setting with close neurological observation and repeat imaging
  – Medical management of ICP (i.e., head elevation, osmotic diuresis, hyperventilation)
  – Load fosphenytoin (15–20 mg/kg) and continue therapeutic levels for 7 days for seizure prophylaxis. Alternatives that can be used include carbamazepine, valproate, and levetiracetam (2)[A].

SURGERY/OTHER PROCEDURES

- Any symptomatic epidural hematoma
- Acute asymptomatic epidural hematoma >30 cm³ or >5 mm midline shift, or >15 mm thickness
- Epidural hematomas in pediatric patients are more likely to be surgically managed because of the decreased space.
- Surgical treatment involves a generous craniotomy that exposes the clot in its entirety so that complete evacuation and hemostasis can be achieved, with placement of dural tack-up sutures to prevent reaccumulation.
- Emergent decompression with placement of a burr hole may be necessary when neurosurgical consultation is unavailable. For patients showing rapid deterioration with clinical signs of impending herniation, place a burr hole on the side of the dilating pupil. In the absence of a CT scan, place the burr hole 2 finger-widths anterior to the tragus of the ear and 3 finger-widths above the tragus of the ear.

IN-PATIENT CONSIDERATIONS

Initial Stabilization

Cardiopulmonary stabilization, neurologic exam, check labs, and STAT head CT

Admission Criteria

All patients with intracranial blood and/or neurologic symptoms should be admitted for observation and repeat imaging (2).

Nursing

- Admit to monitored setting
- Vitals q1hr
- Neuro checks q1hr (3)
- Strict in/out (with Foley)
- Head of bed >30 degrees
- NPO
- Routine labs

Discharge Criteria

Neurologic exam back to baseline with stable repeat imaging

 ONGOING CARE

FOLLOW-UP RECOMMENDATIONS

- Repeat CT scan of head 2–4 weeks after discharge to document resolution
- Follow-up as directed by neurosurgeon

Patient Monitoring

Go to ER if experiencing headache, nausea, vomiting, seizure, loss of consciousness, change in mental status, or development of neurologic deficit.

DIET

NPO unless no plan for surgery

PATIENT EDUCATION

Trauma prevention

PROGNOSIS

- GCS (3–5 associated with 36% mortality), age, pupillary abnormalities, associated intracranial lesions, time between neurological deterioration and surgery, and ICP have been identified as important factors determining outcome from EDH (1).
- 10% mortality in adult populations, 5% in pediatrics

COMPLICATIONS

- Death from cardiopulmonary arrest secondary to brainstem compression
- Seizures
- Sequelae of traumatic brain injury
- Sustained increased ICP after decompression
- Temperature dysregulation
- Behavior and cognitive changes

REFERENCES

1. Bullock MR, et al. Surgical management of acute epidural hematomas. *Neurosurgery*. 2006; 58(3 Suppl):S7–15; discussion Si–iv.
2. Ling GS, et al. Management of traumatic brain injury in the intensive care unit. *Neurol Clin*. 2008;26(2):409–26, viii.
3. Servadei F, et al. The role of surgery in traumatic brain injury. *Curr Opin Crit Care*. 2007;13(2): 163–8.

ADDITIONAL READING

- Greenberg MS. *Handbook of neurosurgery*, 6th ed. New York: Thieme, 2006.
- Lui JT, et al. Emergency management of epidural haematoma through burr hole evacuation and drainage. A preliminary report. *Acta Neurochir (Wien)*. 2006;148(3):313–7.
- Rengachary SS, et al. *Principles of neurosurgery*, 2nd ed. New York: Elsevier Mosby, 2005.
- Winn HR, et al. *Youmans neurological surgery*, 5th ed. New York: Elsevier, 2003.

 CODES

ICD9

- 432.0 Nontraumatic extradural hemorrhage
- 852.40 Extradural hemorrhage following injury, without mention of open intracranial wound, with state of consciousness unspecified

CLINICAL PEARLS

- Lenticular-shaped hyperdensity on CT following a traumatic brain injury
- Caused by tearing of a meningeal vessel
- Immediate neurosurgical intervention for epidural hematoma meeting criteria for evacuation
- Exam on presentation a good predictor of outcome

H

HEMATOMA, SUBDURAL

Oren N. Gottfried
Martin E. Weinand

 BASICS

DESCRIPTION
- Accumulation of blood in subdural space:
  - Acute: Most severe form, usually result of trauma involving acceleration or deceleration head injury and commonly associated with parenchymal brain injury. Hematoma age is ≤3 days.
  - Chronic: Often result of trivial head injury in older patients; 25–50% have no history of head trauma. Hematoma is classically >3 weeks and associated with encapsulating membrane.
  - Subacute: Appearing 4–21 days from maturation of acute subdural hematoma.
- System(s) affected: Cardiovascular; Nervous
- Synonym(s): Subdural hemorrhage

EPIDEMIOLOGY
Incidence
- Predominant age:
  - Acute: <60 years. Relatively infrequent in newborns and children, occurring 25% as often as in adults.
  - Chronic: >50 years. Occurs in children of all ages.
- Males > Females

Prevalence
- Acute: 1–2/100,000:
  - Present with 5–22% of episodes of severe head trauma
- Chronic: 1–2/100,000

RISK FACTORS
- Acute:
  - Severe head trauma
  - High-velocity acceleration or deceleration head injury (motor vehicle accidents, falls, blunt head trauma)
  - Suspected nonaccidental trauma in infants
- Chronic:
  - Chronic alcoholism
  - Epilepsy
  - Coagulopathy/anticoagulation therapy
  - CSF shunt for hydrocephalus
  - Rarely, metastatic carcinoma to subdural space

ALERT
Cerebral atrophy is common and predisposes to subdural hematomas.

GENERAL PREVENTION
- Acute: Trauma-prevention programs
- Chronic:
  - Alcoholism prevention
  - Medical and surgical management of epilepsy
  - Conservative use of anticoagulation therapy
- Medium- or high-pressure ventriculoperitoneal shunt valves in at-risk patients with hydrocephalus

ETIOLOGY
- Acute:
  - High-velocity acceleration or deceleration head injury resulting in tearing of bridging veins between cerebral cortex and dural venous sinuses.
  - Injury to surface of brain with bleeding from injured cortical vessels
- Chronic:
  - Adults: Often from trivial head injury
  - Children: May be caused by unrecognized/unreported trauma, abuse, or, rarely, birth trauma
  - Balance between recurrent bleeding from hematoma membrane and resorption determines ultimate size of hematoma.

COMMONLY ASSOCIATED CONDITIONS
- Acute:
  - Multisystem trauma
  - Cervical spinal cord injury
  - Injury to the thoracic, lumbar, or sacral spine
  - DIC
- Chronic:
  - Alcoholism
  - Epilepsy
  - Coagulopathy
  - CSF shunt
  - Birth trauma
  - Child abuse
  - Rarely, metastatic carcinoma

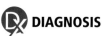 DIAGNOSIS

PHYSICAL EXAM
- Acute:
  - Altered level of consciousness: 99%
  - Pupillary irregularity (usually unilateral to hematoma): 47–53%
  - Hemiparesis (usually contralateral to hematoma): 34–47%
  - Decerebrate posturing or flaccid motor exam: 47%
  - Papilledema: 16%
  - Cranial nerve VI palsy: 5%
- Chronic:
  - Impaired consciousness: 53%
  - Hemiparesis: 45%
  - Papilledema: 24%
  - Cranial nerve III abnormality: 11%
  - Hemianopsia: 7%
  - Infants often with accelerated increase in head size with or without irritability, poor feeding, occasional vomiting, or tension of anterior fontanelle (60% of cases), and may present with seizures.

DIAGNOSTIC TESTS & INTERPRETATION
Lab
Initial lab tests
- Acute: Consumptive coagulopathy due to underlying parenchymal injury diagnosed with:
  - Elevated PT and PTT
  - Elevated fibrin degradation products
  - Decreased fibrinogen
  - Decreased platelet level
  - Extended bleeding time
- Chronic:
  - Bleeding time or coagulation parameters: Appropriate abnormalities produced by predisposing factors such as coagulopathy or anticoagulation therapy
  - Subtherapeutic anticonvulsant levels in patients with epilepsy
  - Serum ethanol level in alcoholics

Follow-Up & Special Considerations
- Drugs that may alter lab results: Anticoagulants (e.g., warfarin)
- Disorders that may alter lab results: DIC and other coagulopathies (e.g., hemophilia)

Imaging
- Acute:
  - Imaging study of choice: CT head scan (without intravascular contrast)
  - Axial view demonstrates hyperdense, cresenteric, extra-axial collection usually adjacent to inner table.
- Chronic:
  - Imaging study of choice: CT head scan
  - Hematomas usually evolve from isodense to hypodense by 3 weeks.
  - MRI brain: May aid in diagnosis for hematomas isodense with brain due to mixture of chronic hematoma with recurrent hemorrhage

Diagnostic Procedures/Other
- EEG for seizures
- ICU: Continuous cardiac, intra-arterial pressure, and intracranial pressure monitoring if acute subdural hematoma and decreased mental status (with ventriculostomy or intraparenchymal or subdural pressure-monitoring probe)

Pathological Findings
- Acute: Fresh hemorrhage
- Chronic:
  - Liquefied hematoma
  - Outer membrane beneath dura after 1 week
  - Inner membrane between hematoma and arachnoid after 3 weeks
  - On rare occasions, cytology exam may reveal association between metastatic carcinoma cells and hemorrhage.

DIFFERENTIAL DIAGNOSIS
- Acute vs. chronic
- Other forms of intracranial hematoma (e.g., epidural hematoma, cerebral contusion/hematoma)
- Dementia
- Stroke
- Transient ischemic attack
- Brain tumor
- Subdural empyema
- Meningitis

ALERT
The insidious onset of symptoms may lead to misdiagnosis of dementia, tumor, or depression.

 TREATMENT

MEDICATION
- Acute:
  - Before surgery, management of cerebral edema and elevated intracranial pressure may require mannitol 20% solution 0.5–1.0 g/kg followed by 0.25–0.75 g/kg q4–6h. If loop diuretic used in conjunction with mannitol, administer furosemide (Lasix) 0.5 mg/kg IV. Check serum osmolality q8h and serum electrolytes at least daily. A 5% or 25% albumin preparation (Plasmanate) may be used either as continuous or intermittent infusion to augment osmotherapy as needed.
  - Seizure prophylaxis includes phenytoin (Dilantin) 1000 mg load (50 mg/min IV) with ECG monitoring, followed by 100 mg IV q8h or as needed to maintain therapeutic blood levels (10–20 μg/mL [40–79 μmol/L]). Convert Dilantin therapy to oral route as soon as possible to avoid cardiovascular complications of IV Dilantin administration.
  - 3% saline bolus or as maintenance fluid is used in patients with hyponatremia (Na <135) or to supplement medical treatment with diuretics in patients with significant cerebral edema or mass effect.
- Chronic:
  - Medical management alone for large subdural hematomas or in patients with significant neurologic signs is frequently unsuccessful and entails risks of neurological deterioration.
  - However, when small and asymptomatic or mildly symptomatic (i.e., headache), may be appropriate to treat conservatively with observation, as some chronic subdural hematomas have been known to resolve spontaneously:
    o Steroids may be helpful for symptomatic treatment in these patients, if not otherwise contraindicated.

ADDITIONAL TREATMENT
General Measures
- Inpatient
- Acute: Medical management:
  - Maintain adequate airway and ventilation and support of cardiovascular system to promote normal cerebral perfusion.
  - Treat elevated intracranial pressure with osmotic and loop diuretics.
  - Elevate head of bed to reduce intracranial pressure.

- Hyperventilate to induce hypocapnia ($PaCO_2$ of <35 mm Hg)
- Treat multisystem traumatic injury.
- Spine precautions:
  o Maintain patient in rigid cervical collar until cervical spine is cleared clinically and by imaging.
  o Avoid flexion of lower body until thoracic, lumbar, or sacral spine injuries are ruled out.
- Subacute and chronic:
  - Spinal precautions: Same as for acute if signs of elevated intracranial pressure

SURGERY/OTHER PROCEDURES
- Acute: Emergent craniotomy indicated for evacuation of hematomas causing significant mass effect.
- Subacute:
  - If patient is neurologically stable, surgery may be delayed until hematoma matures and becomes chronic, at which time a burr hole drainage can be performed.
  - If causing significant mass effect, neurologic deficit, and solid (nonliquified) clot, may require craniotomy for complete evacuation
- Chronic: Burr hole drainage (2 approaches):
  - Bedside twist drill vs. operation with burr holes and irrigation: Both effective in a prospective randomized trial (1)[B] and a prospective, nonrandomized series (2)[C]:
    o Bedside twist drill with placement of subdural drain with or without suction reservoir
    o Operative drainage with 1–2 burr holes, irrigation of collection with or without placement of subdural drain
    o Drain is removed after either treatment when output is clear (~24–72 hours) and confirmed improvement on CT.

IN-PATIENT CONSIDERATIONS
Initial Stabilization
As explained above

IV Fluids
NS with 20 mEq/L KCl as needed; refrain from hypotonic fluids or fluids with glucose

 ONGOING CARE

FOLLOW-UP RECOMMENDATIONS
- Patients with chronic subdural hematomas should have a follow-up CT scan 1–2 months after surgery to confirm interval improvement.
- Patients requiring anticoagulation should resume this medical treatment when risk of hemorrhage is low; this decision is made on an individualized patient basis.

DIET
- Acute: Most patients require enteral or total parenteral nutrition initially if decreased mental status.
- Chronic: Depending on the level of consciousness, patients can usually have diet advanced to regular food as tolerated.

PATIENT EDUCATION
The National Institute of Neurological and Communicative Disorders and Stroke (NINDS), the National Institutes of Health, Bethesda, MD 20892

PROGNOSIS
The prognosis varies widely depending on the size of the blood collection, the location and type of head injury, and how quickly treatment is placed.

- **DISPOSITION**
- Outcome is highly dependent on presurgical neurologic status.
- Acute:
  - Mortality >50%; lower in patients <40 than in those >40
  - Significant neurologic disability and impairment of function is seen in most surviving patients.
  - Although the literature supports the benefit of seizure prophylaxis in the period immediately after acute head trauma (7 days), there is no proven benefit for long-term seizure prophylaxis.
- Chronic:
  - Mortality <10%
  - Most patients resume preoperative functional status.
  - Seizure prophylaxis:
    o Recent Cochrane Review identified no randomized, controlled trials and, thus, no formal recommendations could be made about the use of prophylactic anticonvulsants in patients with chronic subdural hematoma (3).

COMPLICATIONS
- Immediate postoperative complications:
  - Elevated intracranial pressure and brain edema
  - New or recurrent hematoma
  - Seizures (in ~1/3 of cases)
- Chronic:
  - Recurrent hematoma in up to 50% of cases (reduced with use of drainage catheter)
  - Infection (subdural empyema, wound)
  - Seizures in up to 10% of cases

REFERENCES
1. Muzii VF, et al. Chronic subdural hematoma: Comparison of two surgical techniques. Preliminary results of a prospective randomized study. *J Neurosurg Sci.* 2005;49:41–6; discussion 46–7.
2. Horn EM, et al. Bedside twist drill craniotomy for chronic subdural hematoma: A comparative study. *Surg Neurol.* 2006;65:150–3; discussion 153–4.
3. Ratital B, et al. Anticonvulsants for preventing seizures in patients with chronic subdural haematoma. *Cochrane Database Syst Rev.* 2005;.

 CODES

ICD9
- 432.1 Subdural hemorrhage
- 852.20 Subdural hemorrhage following injury, without mention of open intracranial wound, with state of consciousness unspecified

H

HEMODIALYSIS, INTERMITTENT

Tzvi Y. Neuman
Roopa Kohli-Seth

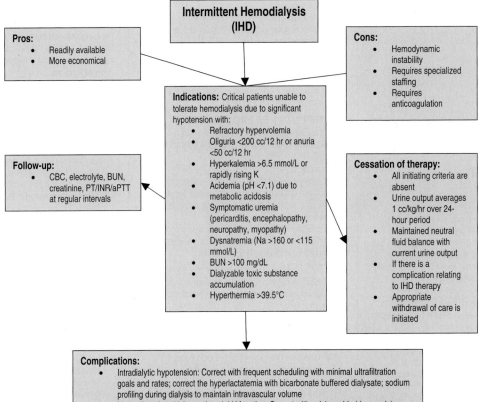

Intermittent Hemodialysis (IHD)

Pros:
- Readily available
- More economical

Cons:
- Hemodynamic instability
- Requires specialized staffing
- Requires anticoagulation

Indications: Critical patients unable to tolerate hemodialysis due to significant hypotension with:
- Refractory hypervolemia
- Oliguria <200 cc/12 hr or anuria <50 cc/12 hr
- Hyperkalemia >6.5 mmol/L or rapidly rising K
- Acidemia (pH <7.1) due to metabolic acidosis
- Symptomatic uremia (pericarditis, encephalopathy, neuropathy, myopathy)
- Dysnatremia (Na >160 or <115 mmol/L)
- BUN >100 mg/dL
- Dialyzable toxic substance accumulation
- Hyperthermia >39.5°C

Follow-up:
- CBC, electrolyte, BUN, creatinine, PT/INR/aPTT at regular intervals

Cessation of therapy:
- All initiating criteria are absent
- Urine output averages 1 cc/kg/hr over 24-hour period
- Maintained neutral fluid balance with current urine output
- If there is a complication relating to IHD therapy
- Appropriate withdrawal of care is initiated

Complications:
- Intradialytic hypotension: Correct with frequent scheduling with minimal ultrafiltration goals and rates; correct the hyperlactatemia with bicarbonate buffered dialysate; sodium profiling during dialysis to maintain intravascular volume
- Hypocalcemia, which may impair LV function: Correct with calcium chloride or calcium gluconate accordingly
- Hypothermia may lead to depressed myocardial function, decreased perfusion, blood clotting and poor renal recovery: Use appropriate warming modalities
- Thrombosis/clotted circuits or access: Use standard dose unfractionated heparin; use oh LMWH has no clinical advantage; in cases of HIT type II use danaparoid, hirudin or argatroban
- Other associated complications: Hypoglycemia, arrhythmia, infection, thrombocytopenia, leucopenia, increased risk of bleeding

Evidence-based guidelines:
- IHD is equivalent to continuous venovenous hemodialysis (CVVH) in patients with severe sepsis and acute renal failure **(2B)**, regarding mortality, renal recovery, and risk of hemodynamic instability or hypotensive events
- However, CVVH may better facilitate management of fluid balance in hemodynamically unstable patients **(2D),** and may be better in patients suffering from elevated ICP (such as neurosurgical, TBI, or liver patients).

References:
1) Dellinger RP, et al. Surviving Sepsis Campaign: International guidelines for management of severe sepsis and septic shock: 2008. *Int Care Med* 2008;34:17–60.
2) Rabindranath KS, et al. Intermittent versus continuous renal replacement therapy for acute renal failure in adults (review). *Cochrane Database Syst Rev* 2007;3:CD003773. DOI: 10.1002/14651858.CD—3773.pub3.

I. Intermittent Hemodialysis (IHD)
  A. **Indications:**
    1. Refractory hypervolemia
    2. Oliguria <200 cc/12 hr or anuria <50 cc/12 hr
    3. Hyperkalemia >6.5 mmol/L or rapidly rising K
    4. Acidemia (pH <7.1) due to metabolic acidosis
    5. Symptomatic uremia (pericarditis, encephalopathy, neuropathy, myopathy)
    6. Dysnatremia (Na >160 or <115 mmol/L)
    7. BUN >100 mg/dL
    8. Dialyzable toxic substance accumulation
  B. **Cessation of therapy:**
    1. All initiating criteria are absent
    2. Urine output averages 1 cc/kg/hr over 24-hour period
    3. Maintained neutral fluid balance with current urine output
    4. If there is a complication relating to IHD therapy
    5. Appropriate withdrawal of care is initiated

  C. **Complications:**
    1. Intradialytic hypotension: Correct with frequent scheduling with minimal ultrafiltration goals and rates; correct the hyperlactatemia with bicarbonate buffered dialysate; sodium profiling during dialysis to maintain intravascular volume
    2. Hypocalcemia, which may impair LV function: Correct with calcium chloride or calcium gluconate accordingly
    3. Hypothermia may lead to depressed myocardial function, decreased perfusion, blood clotting and poor renal recovery: Use appropriate warming modalities
    4. Thrombosis/clotted circuits or access: Use standard dose unfractionated heparin; use oh LMWH has no clinical advantage; in cases of HIT type II use danaparoid, hirudin, or argatroban

    5. Other associated complications: hypoglycemia, arrhythmia, infection, thrombocytopenia, leucopenia, and increased risk of bleeding
  D. **Evidence-Based Guidelines:**
    1. IHD is equivalent to continuous venovenous hemodialysis(CVVH) in patients with severe sepsis and acute renal failure **(2B)**, regarding mortality, renal recovery, and risk of hemodynamic instability or hypotensive events
    2. However, CVVH may better facilitate management of fluid balance in hemodynamically unstable patients **(2D)**, and may be better in patients suffering from elevated ICP (such as neurosurgical, TBI, or liver patients).

 CODES

ICD9
- 276.52 Hypovolemia
- 276.7 Hyperpotassemia
- 788.5 Oliguria and anuria

H

HEMODYNAMIC MONITORING, INVASIVE

Catherine Porter

BASICS

DESCRIPTION
- Monitoring of intravascular and intracardiac pressures, flow, and oxygen saturation to assess volume status and cardiac output
- Force created by pressure waves from the cardiac chambers is transmitted through a closed system to transducers.
- The central venous compartment is monitored by catheterizing the vena cava to give a description of right-sided filling pressure (central line).
- The right heart can be catheterized and monitored to measure pressures of the vena cava, right atrium, right ventricle, and pulmonary capillary wedge pressure. Left heart filling pressures and cardiac output may be obtained from indirect calculations as well (Swan-Ganz catheterization).

EPIDEMIOLOGY
Incidence
PA catheter insertion reported to decrease from 5.66 per 1000 medical admissions in 1993 to 1.99 per 1000 medical admissions in 2004.

PATHOPHYSIOLOGY
- Arterial blood pressure reflects cardiac pump function, peripheral vascular compliance, peripheral vascular resistance, and intravascular blood volume.
- Central venous pressure reflects the intravascular blood volume and assesses right ventricular preload, assuming a normal tricuspid valve.
- Normal RA pressure: 0–8 mean
  - RA pressure $\approx$ CVP $\approx$ RV end diastolic pressure
- Normal RV pressure: 16–30/0–8 (systolic/diastolic)
- Normal PA pressure: 10–16 mm Hg
- Normal PCWP: 1–10 mean
- PCWP $\approx$ left atrial pressure $\approx$ LV end diastolic pressure:
  - This assumes catheter is appropriately positioned, and that mitral valve and pulmonary venous vasculature are normal
- Normal SVR: 770–1500 dynes/s/cm:
  - SVRI = (MAP-RAP) $\times$ 80/CI
- Normal cardiac index: 2.6–4.2 L/min:
  - CI = CO/BSA
- CO can be measured by comparing the difference in saturated oxygen before and after the lungs (Fick method) or the indicator dilution method, which determines volume by adding a known volume of indicator and measures the concentration of the indicator over time.

COMMONLY ASSOCIATED CONDITIONS
- Hemodynamic monitoring may be used as a diagnostic tool in any disease state that alters normal hemodynamic physiology. Some examples are:
  - Shock: Hypovolemic, cardiogenic, hemorrhagic, neurogenic, septic
  - Intravascular volume assessment
  - Poor LV function
  - Complications of MI (mitral insufficiency, VSD, ventricular aneurysm)
- Indications (2)[A]:
  - Cardiogenic shock
  - Discordant right and left ventricular failure
  - Severe chronic heart failure requiring inotropic, vasopressor and vasodilator therapy
  - Reversible systolic heart failure
  - To help establish the differential diagnosis of pulmonary hypertension
  - To assess response to therapy for pulmonary hypertension

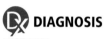

DIAGNOSIS

HISTORY
- Patients who may benefit from hemodynamic monitoring may have a history of MI, infection (1)[A], or trauma (3)[A].
- Intravascular volume status may prove difficult to assess in times of stress in patients with oliguric or anuric renal failure, and additional information may be derived from invasive hemodynamic monitoring.

PHYSICAL EXAM
- Patients in need of hemodynamic monitoring may show clinical indices of inadequate perfusion, including:
  - Hypotension
  - Tachycardia or bradycardia
  - Cool, mottled skin
  - Decreased mentation
  - Oliguria or anuria

DIAGNOSTIC TESTS & INTERPRETATION
Lab
Initial lab tests
- Lactate: In instances of inadequate perfusion, lactate levels may be elevated (>2 mEq/L).
- SvO_2 (mixed venous oxygen saturation) or $ScvO_2$ (central venous oxygen saturation) decrease below 70% indicates impaired tissue oxygen delivery due to low cardiac output, anemia, or hypoxemia
- Although measurement of SVO_2 is the most reliable measurement of oxygen supply, $ScvO_2$ has been shown to be a reliable and less invasive indicator as well (9)[A].

Follow-Up & Special Considerations
- Placement of central venous catheter for hemodynamic monitoring
- Right heart catheterization (pulmonary artery catheter; PAC)

Imaging
- CXR confirms position of catheter.
- Subclavian or internal jugular catheter: Tip should be at or above the 3rd intercostal space.
- PAC: Tip should be positioned in zone 3 of the lung, no more than 2–3 cm from the heart border and below the level of the left atrium.
- CXR also will detect complications: Pneumothorax, hemothorax

Diagnostic Procedures/Other
- Hemodynamic profiles of shock:
- Cardiogenic: CVP, SVR increased; CI, SVO_2, decreased
- Hypovolemic: SVR increased; CVP, CI, SVO_2 decreased
- Septic:
  - Hyperdynamic: CI, SVO_2 increased; SVR decreased; CVP variable
  - Hypodynamic: SVR increased; CI decreased; CVP, SVO_2 variable
- Neurogenic: CI, CVP, SVR, SVO_2 all decreased

TREATMENT

- The use of PAC is somewhat controversial:
  - RCT with 1994 elderly high-risk surgical patients showed no benefit observed to therapy directed by PAC (4)[A].
  - An RCT with 676 patients with shock, ARDS, or both showed no benefit to morbidity or mortality (5)[A].
  - The 2005 PAC-man trial with 1014 patients in the UK showed no difference in hospital mortality among those patients who did and did not have a PAC and showed no clear benefit or harm (6)[A].
  - The 2005 ESCAPE trial with 433 patients in congestive heart failure used as endpoints days alive out of the hospital during the first 6 months, exercise, quality of life, biochemical and echocardiographic changes. The use of PAC did not affect days alive and out of the hospital the first 6 months, mortality or the number of days hospitalized. PAC did not affect mortality and hospitalization, but did increase adverse events (7)[A].
  - 2006 ARDS CVP vs. PAC trial covered 1000 patients with acute lung injury, comparing hemodynamic management guided by central venous catheter verses PAC; PAC-guided therapy did not improve survival or organ function (8)[A].
- However, proponents of PAC-directed therapy state that the misuse of information collected from the PAC is responsible for the lack of improvement in mortality, not the catheter itself. And the PA catheter is most often useful in settings outside of those tested in clinical trials.

IN-PATIENT CONSIDERATIONS

Initial Stabilization
Hemodynamic monitoring should be performed in a critical care setting.

Nursing
- Catheters should be covered with a clean, dry dressing.
- Local wound care has a role in preventing catheter-associated infections.
- Catheters must be flushed periodically to prevent thrombotic obstruction, unless filled with heparinized saline or used for infusions.
- PA catheters should have the balloons deflated, unless obtaining a wedge pressure, to prevent infarction or rupture of the PA.

Discharge Criteria
When removing a central venous catheter, pressure must be applied to the catheter site to prevent hematoma formation and air embolization.

ONGOING CARE

COMPLICATIONS

- Complications of central catheter placement include: Pneumothorax, hemorrhage, pseudoaneurysm, arteriovenous fistulization, air/catheter embolization, dysrhythmias, arterial puncture, and dissection
- In addition, complications of PAC placement include: Arrhythmias, conduction defects, pulmonary infarction, PA rupture, valvular damage, catheter entrapment
- In the Sandham study, PAC placement was associated with hemothorax, pulmonary artery hemorrhage, pulmonary infarction, arterial puncture, pneumothorax in 1.5% vs. central venous catheter placement associated with arterial puncture and pneumothorax in 0.7% (4)[A].
- Both the PAC-man and ARDS trial found the rate of complications to be 10–14% (6,8)[A].

REFERENCES

1. Chatterjee K. The Swan-Ganz catheters: Past, present, and future. A viewpoint. *Circulation.* 2009;119(1):147–52.
2. Rivers E, et al. Early goal-directed therapy in the treatment of severe sepsis and septic shock. *N Engl J Med.* 20001;345(19):1368–77.
3. McKinley BA, et al. Central venous pressure vs pulmonary artery catheter: Directed shock resuscitation. *Shock.* 2009.
4. Reinhart K, et al. Continuous central venous and pulmonary artery oxygen saturation monitoring in the critically ill. *Intensive Care Med.* 2004;30(8):1572–8.
5. Sandham JD, et al. A randomized, controlled trial of the use of pulmonary-artery catheters in high-risk surgical patients. *N Engl J Med.* 2003;348(1):5–14.
6. Richard C, et al. Early use of the pulmonary artery catheter and outcomes in patients with shock and acute respiratory distress syndrome: A randomized controlled trial. *JAMA.* 2003;290(20):2713–20.
7. Harvey S, et al. Assessment of the clinical effectiveness of pulmonary artery catheters in management of patients in intensive care (PAC-Man): A randomized controlled trial. *Lancet.* 2005;366(9484):472–7.
8. Binanay C, et al. Evaluation study of congestive heart failure and pulmonary artery catheterization effectiveness: The ESCAPE trial. *JAMA.* 2005; 294(13):1625–33.
9. Wheeler AP, et al. Pulmonary-artery versus central venous catheter to guide treatment of acute lung injury. *N Engl J Med.* 2006;354(21):2213–24.

ADDITIONAL READING

- Marino PL. *The ICU book*. Philadelphia: Lippincott Williams and Wilkins, 2007.
- Townsend CM, et al., eds. *Sabiston textbook of surgery*. Philadelphia: Saunders Elsevier, 2008.

CODES

ICD9
- 785.50 Shock, unspecified
- 785.51 Cardiogenic shock
- 785.59 Other shock without mention of trauma

CLINICAL PEARLS

- Hemodynamic measurement provides important information about intravascular volume and cardiovascular pathophysiology.
- Hemodynamic monitoring is an important tool for resuscitation.
- Although PACs provide a wealth of information, they should be used judiciously as a diagnostic tool.

H

HEMOPERFUSION

Nirav Mistry
Roopa Kohli-Seth

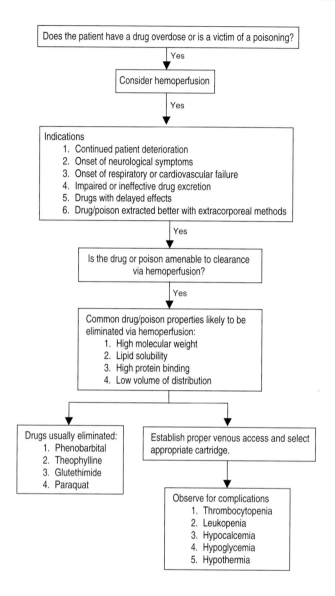

Does the patient have a drug overdose or is a victim of a poisoning?

↓ Yes

Consider hemoperfusion

↓ Yes

Indications
1. Continued patient deterioration
2. Onset of neurological symptoms
3. Onset of respiratory or cardiovascular failure
4. Impaired or ineffective drug excretion
5. Drugs with delayed effects
6. Drug/poison extracted better with extracorporeal methods

↓ Yes

Is the drug or poison amenable to clearance via hemoperfusion?

↓ Yes

Common drug/poison properties likely to be eliminated via hemoperfusion:
1. High molecular weight
2. Lipid solubility
3. High protein binding
4. Low volume of distribution

Drugs usually eliminated:
1. Phenobarbital
2. Theophylline
3. Glutethimide
4. Paraquat

Establish proper venous access and select appropriate cartridge.

↓

Observe for complications
1. Thrombocytopenia
2. Leukopenia
3. Hypocalcemia
4. Hypoglycemia
5. Hypothermia

BACKGROUND

The extracorporeal methods for elimination of drugs and poisons have many rationales. Continued exposure to toxic compounds will lead to serious clinical consequences. Prompt initiation of therapy can preserve organ function and prevent crucial organ failure. Such therapies have been shown to be more efficient in their ability to enhance the elimination of the offending agent, leading to less exposure to the body and thus fewer morbidities and mortalities. Hemoperfusion is an extracorporeal technique, similar to hemodialysis, utilized primarily in the management of drug overdose and poisoning.

METHOD

The initial step is to obtain vascular access via a dual lumen large bore catheter either in the internal jugular or femoral vein. Once access is confirmed, the patient is attached to the system and his/her blood is passed through a cartridge containing specific sorbents. As the blood passes, adsorption occurs secondary to the hydrophobic properties of the cartridge contents. Depending on the type of cartridge used (charcoal, nonionic resin, etc), specific types of drugs and poisons can be effectively extracted from the patient's blood.

INDICATIONS FOR HEMOPERFUSION

In general, the indications for hemoperfusion remain the same as hemodialysis for the removal of poisoning/drug overdose. If the patient has concurrent renal failure, hemodialysis is a better option. As always, clinical judgment should be used prior to initiating such invasive therapies.

1. Progressive deterioration of the patient's condition that is thought to be related to the offending drug such as hypoventilation, hypothermia, and hypotension
2. Development of coma, sepsis, or pneumonia
3. Blood levels that indicate the quantity of the drug ingested can lead to severe morbidity or mortality
4. Impairment of drug excretion by the concomitant presence of:
   a. Renal or liver failure for drugs eliminated by the kidney or the liver, respectively
   b. Ingestion or administration of "slow-release" drugs
   c. Nausea or vomiting that prevents the administration of charcoal to effect drug removal from the gastrointestinal tract
5. The drug has been shown to be removed efficiently by the currently available extracorporeal techniques
6. The volume of distribution (VD) of the drug is relatively small
7. No effective and specific antidotes are available to reverse the effects of the toxin

Figure 1 When to start hemoperfusion? Adapted from Quinibi W. Extracorporeal treatment of poisoning and drug overdose. In Henrich WL, ed. *Principles and Practice of Dialysis,* 4th ed. Philadelphia: Lippincott Williams & Williams; 2009.

DRUGS ELIMINATED

As indicated above, properties that make the drug more amenable to elimination via hemoperfusion include low volume of distribution, high molecular weight, lipid solubility, and high protein binding. The technique has been used more frequently in the extraction of theophylline, phenobarbital, and glutethimide. Alcohols, on the other hand, do not effectively bind to the cartridges and as such, hemoperfusion cannot be used for the clearance of ethylene glycol, methanol, or isopropyl alcohol (1)[A].

COMPLICATIONS

As with hemodialysis, thrombocytopenia and leucopenia are common. Additional complications include hypocalcemia, hypoglycemia, and hypothermia.

FUTURE CONSIDERATION

Recently, much data has been published as to the utility of hemoperfusion using polymyxin b resins in patients with gram-negative intra-abdominal sepsis and septic shock. A Cochrane review concluded that this method was associated with improved outcomes including better mean arterial pressures, less vasopressor use, improved oxygenation, and improved overall mortality. However, the authors also commented that the studies were questionable in their design and that the results may not be reliable. Further investigation with better study methods and improved power are needed (2)[B]. The EUPHAS trial showed that outcomes (hemodynamics, organ dysfunction, and 28-day mortality) were improved when patients received hemoperfusion versus conventional therapy (3)[C].

REFERENCES

1. De Pont A. Extracorporeal treatment of intoxications. *Curr Opin Crit Care.* 2007;13: 668–73.
2. Cruz DN, et al. Effectiveness of polymyxin B-immobilized fiber column in sepsis: A systematic review. *Critical Care.* 2007;11(2):R47.
3. Cruz DN, et al. Early use of polymyxin B hemoperfusion in abdominal septic shock: The EUPHAS randomized controlled trial. *JAMA.* 2009;301(23):2445–52.

ADDITIONAL READING

• Quinibi W. Extracorporeal treatment of poisoning and drug overdose. In Henrich WL, ed. *Principles and Practice of Dialysis,* 4th ed. Philadelphia: Lippincott Williams & Williams; 2009.
• Winchester J, et al. Use of dialysis and hemoperfusion in the treatment of poisoning. In Daugirdas JT, et al., eds. *Handbook of Dialysis,* 4th ed. Philadelphia: Lippincott Williams & Williams; 2007.

 CODES

ICD9
977.9 Poisoning by unspecified drug or medicinal substance

H

HEMOPHILIA

Alina Dulu
Stephen M. Pastores

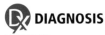 **BASICS**

DESCRIPTION
Hereditary bleeding disorder caused by deficiency of factor VIII in hemophilia A or factor IX in hemophilia B

EPIDEMIOLOGY
Incidence
1:5,000 males, with 85% having FVIII deficiency and 10–15% having FIX deficiency

Prevalence
Affects all races and ethnic groups

RISK FACTORS
Family history of hemophilia

Genetics
- Congenital X-linked recessive mutations (1)
- 30% of hemophilia A cases arise from spontaneous mutations.
- Factor VIII gene F8 located on the X chromosome at band q28:
  - 50% of severe cases have spontaneous homologous recombination resulting in "inversion" involving F8 intron 22.
  - Other large gene rearrangements, insertions, and deletions, or small mutations affecting only a small number of nucleotides
- Factor IX gene located on the X chromosome comprising 34 kb, 8 exons, and 7 introns

GENERAL PREVENTION
- Carrier detection and antenatal diagnosis
- Genetic counseling

PATHOPHYSIOLOGY
- Factors VIII and IX with phospholipids and calcium form a complex required for the activation of factor X in the coagulation cascade.
- Deficiency of FVIII or F IX results in inefficient generation of thrombin with delay in formation of an unstable clot.
- Deficiency of FVIII or IX is also associated with the development of allo-antibodies to the factors introduced via replacement therapy.

ETIOLOGY
Absence of functional FVIII or IX in plasma results in serious bleeding.

 DIAGNOSIS

HISTORY
- Clinical features of hemophilia A and B are generally indistinguishable from each other.
- Characteristic is bleeding in a closed space, such as a joint, that stops by tamponade.
- Open wounds can produce profuse bleeding with significant blood loss.
- Frequent rebleeding, spontaneously or with minimal new trauma

PHYSICAL EXAM
- Hemarthroses (bleeding into a joint):
  - Hot, swollen, painful joints (ankle, knees, and elbows)
  - Spontaneously or by minor trauma
  - Subsequent crippling joint deformity
- Soft tissue hematomas including bleeding into muscles with localized pain and swelling
- Easy bruising, epistaxis
- Bleeding in the GI or genitourinary tract.
- Poor wound healing
- Excessive bleeding with surgery, trauma, dental extraction; particularly following trauma
- Compartment syndrome with nerve damage and/or ischemia

Pediatric Considerations
- Bleeding can appear from birth, umbilical stump bleeding, or may occur in the fetus.
- Easy bruising, intramuscular hematomas, and hemarthroses begin when the child "begins to cruise."
- Factor IX activity levels during childhood remain at ~75% of adult levels.
- Hemophilia B Leyden: Rare form of factor IX deficiency that undergoes postpubertal phenotypic resolution

DIAGNOSTIC TESTS & INTERPRETATION
Lab
- Prolonged aPTT, usually 2–3 times the upper limit of normal
- Platelet count, bleeding time, PT, thrombin time, and von Willebrand factor are normal.
- Specific assays for FVIII and IX confirm the diagnosis.
- Baseline level of Factors VIII or IX:
  - 1 IU of each factor is defined as that amount in 1 mL of normal plasma.
  - Severe deficiency (50–70%): <1% activity, spontaneous bleeding 2–4 times per month
  - Moderate deficiency (10%): 1–5% activity, bleeding with mild trauma
  - Mild (30%): >5% activity, bleeding with significant trauma

Imaging
- X-ray and MRI of the affected joints: Erosive and degenerative changes
- Early CT of head for head trauma
- CT of the abdomen and pelvis for suspected retroperitoneal bleeding and compartment syndrome

Diagnostic Procedures/Other
Molecular genetic testing may be useful to confirm diagnosis in any patient with low circulating levels of factor VIII or factor IX.

Pathological Findings
- Synovial hemosiderosis and articular cartilage degeneration
- Bony hypertrophy
- Tissue hematomas with calcification, pseudotumor syndrome

DIFFERENTIAL DIAGNOSIS
- Von Willebrand disease
- Vitamin K deficiency

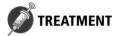 **TREATMENT**

MEDICATION
First Line
- For mild cases: Desmopressin acetate (DDAVP) 0.3–0.4 μg/kg
- For moderate to severe bleeding cases: F VIII and IX replacement using plasma-derived or recombinant factor products
- Recombinant factors cost 2–3 times more than plasma-derived factors with limited availability.
- Amount and duration of factor replacement depends on the indication and nature of bleeding.
- Levels of FVIII or IX must be raised at least to hemostatic level, 35–50% range.
- 1 U/kg of recombinant F VIII raises the plasma F VIII activity by 2%, and 1 U/kg of recombinant factor IX raises the plasma factor IX activity by about 1%.
- Plasma half-life of F VIII is about 12 hours and F IX is 24 hours.
- Life-threatening hemorrhages require replacement therapy to achieve a level equal to that of normal plasma (100 IU/dL, or 100%) and for longer duration, up to 2 weeks.
- After major surgery, factor levels should be kept around 50% for 2–3 weeks.

Second Line
- For acquired inhibitors:
  - Induction of immune tolerance through frequent administration of F VIII eliminates inhibitors in 80% of patients.
  - Recombinant activated F VII
  - Immunosuppressive therapy with daily administration of PO cyclophosphamide 1–2 mg/kg/d and prednisone or rituximab
  - Exchange plasmapheresis
  - Very high doses of FVIII in patients with very low titer inhibitors and in settings where there is rapid availability of F VIII level monitoring
  - Recombinant porcine F VIII has less cross-reactivity with the human product.
- ε-Aminocaproic acid: 4 g PO q4h may be use in cases of mucosal bleeding.

Pediatric Considerations
Lifelong prophylaxis replacement of factors to prevent spontaneous joint bleeding and deformities (1):
- Initiated with the first joint hemorrhage
- 3 times a week intensive home therapy
- Goal is to maintain measurable plasma level of clotting factor (1–2%) when assayed just before the next infusion (trough level).
- Indwelling catheters are required.

Pregnancy Considerations
Carrier detection and antenatal diagnosis:

- Gene deletion, rearrangements, or identifiable restriction fragment length polymorphism analysis from DNA extracted from the cells in the amniocentesis fluid or from a chorionic villus sample taken at 12 weeks of gestation.
- Before 12 weeks' gestation, determining whether the conceptus is female is possible by noninvasive testing of maternal blood Y chromosome DNA at ~10 weeks.

ADDITIONAL TREATMENT
General Measures
- Goal is reversal and prevention of acute bleeding.
- For urgent treatment of bleeding, the choice of hemostatic agent depends primarily on the inhibitor titer and to a lesser extent on the severity of bleeding (2).
- Admitting physician and hematology consultant should know:
  – Patient's FVIII or IX activity level
  – Blood type
  – Presence of antihemophilic factor
  – Time of last hospitalization

Issues for Referral
- Appropriate referral to a hemophilia center if locally available
- Orthopedic evaluation and physical therapy evaluation in patients with joint involvement

Additional Therapies
Patients with fever or who fail to respond to factor replacement need joint aspiration to rule out septic arthritis.

COMPLEMENTARY & ALTERNATIVE THERAPIES
- Immunoadsorption may be considered in patients who continue to bleed despite optimal therapy with factor concentrates.
- IV immunoglobulin

SURGERY/OTHER PROCEDURES
- Arthrocentesis, within 24 hours (after factor replacement), may be symptomatically beneficial but can introduce infection.
- Brief joint immobilization for no more than 2 days often aids in pain control.
- Correction of flexion contractures by wedging casts, night splints, or judicious use of traction
- Synovectomy for persistent hemarthroses
- Total joint replacements in end-stage arthropathy.

IN-PATIENT CONSIDERATIONS
Initial Stabilization
- Pain control
- Severe bleeding:
  – Suitable peripheral or central IV access
  – Type and cross
  – Fluid resuscitation
  – Packed RBC transfusion
  – Constant-infusion techniques for administering factor concentrate
- Early endotracheal intubation for bleeding involving the tongue or the retropharyngeal space that can rapidly compromise the airways

Admission Criteria
- Patients with moderate bleeding need hospitalization.
- Admit to ICU for management of hemorrhagic shock, or after major surgery.

IV Fluids
NS resuscitation for severe bleeding

Nursing
The patient should not receive intramuscular injections or unnecessary venipunctures.

Discharge Criteria
- Controlled bleeding
- Response to therapy monitored by:
  – Clinical improvement
  – Decreasing aPTT
  – Serial F VIII activity levels

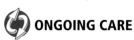 ONGOING CARE

FOLLOW-UP RECOMMENDATIONS
Regular evaluations every 6–12 months to include evaluation of musculoskeletal function, liver function, and tests for antibodies to hepatitis viruses and HIV.

Patient Monitoring
MRI is the best method of detecting progressive arthropathy.

DIET
No restrictions.

PATIENT EDUCATION
- Avoid contact sports.
- Avoid aspirin and other NSAIDs that affect platelet function.
- Initiate intensive physical therapy for muscle building and increased joint stability.

PROGNOSIS
Life expectancy of patients with severe hemophilia may be up to 60 years, and for mild or moderate disease, is closer to that for the normal population.

COMPLICATIONS
- Arthropathy: Chronic synovial hypertrophy and damage to the cartilage, with subchondral bone cyst formation, bony erosion, and flexion contractures
- Development of inhibitor to either FVIII or IX
- Intracranial bleeding is a common cause of death.
- Transfusion-transmitted diseases are no longer a risk with recombinant factors:
  – 20% of hemophiliacs are HIV-seropositive.

REFERENCES
1. Mannucci PM, et al. The hemophiliac: From royal genes to gene therapy. *N Engl J Med.* 2001;344: 1773–9.
2. Barnett B, et al. Current management of acquired factor VIII inhibitors. *Curr Opin Hematol.* 2008;15: 451–5.

ADDITIONAL READING
- Rodriguez NI. Advances in hemophilia: Experimental aspects and therapy. *Pediatr Clin North Am.* 2008; 55(2):357–76.

 CODES

ICD9
- 286.0 Congenital factor viii disorder
- 286.1 Congenital factor ix disorder

CLINICAL PEARLS
- Hemophilia A and B are hereditary bleeding disorders caused by deficiencies of factors VIII and IX, respectively.
- Clinical features include hemarthroses, epistaxis, GI bleeding, and excessive bleeding with surgery, trauma, or dental extraction, particularly following trauma.
- Laboratory criteria include prolonged aPTT but normal PT, von Willebrand factor, and platelet count.
- Treatment of critically ill patients involves factor VIII or IX replacement to raise levels to hemostatic levels.

H

HEMOPTYSIS

Moses Bachan
John Oropello

 BASICS

DESCRIPTION

- Hemoptysis describes expectoration of blood from the lower respiratory tract. It is a complication of numerous diseases, the most common of which are: Bronchiectasis (20%), lung cancer (19%), bronchitis (18%), and pneumonia (16%) (1)[A].
- In HIV patients, the most common cause of hemoptysis is pneumonia, not Kaposi's sarcoma. Based on the amount and duration of the bleeding it is described as either mild hemoptysis (nonmassive) or massive hemoptysis.
- Mild hemoptysis is usually benign and more common than massive hemoptysis.
- Massive hemoptysis is life threatening and commonly leads to death by asphyxiation. The mortality rate is 38%. It refers to the loss of $\geq$200 mL of blood within 24 hours or blood loss resulting in hemodynamic or respiratory compromise:
  - Patients with massive hemoptysis must be treated in the ICU, whereas those with mild hemoptysis may be treated on the general floor.
  - As hemoptysis is a complication of many diseases, therapy involves treating the diseases; however, the patient must first be stabilized.

PATHOPHYSIOLOGY

- Hemoptysis results from complications of diseases affecting the blood supply to the lungs. The lungs receive about 95% of blood flow via deoxygenated blood from the lower-pressure pulmonary arteries. The bronchial arteries, from the systemic circulation, supply 5% of the blood flow (oxygenated blood) at higher pressures and also supply the airways. Therefore, bleeding from the bronchial arteries may lead to massive hemoptysis, and bleeding from the pulmonary artery tends to be milder. The blood vessels can become inflamed and eroded in inflammatory diseases, trauma, or tumor, resulting in hemoptysis.
- In neoplastic diseases, there is increased cell mass and angiogenesis. Necrosis of the cells and ulceration of the blood vessels leads to bleeding.

ETIOLOGY

The most common etiologies of massive hemoptysis are (2)[A]:
- Neoplasm: Bronchial carcinoma, adenoma and metastatic lung cancer.
- Bronchiectasis
- Infections: Mycobacteria especially TB, fungal infections, lung abscess, necrotizing pneumonia, paragonimiasis and hydatid cysts.
- Vascular: Pulmonary infarction, mitral stenosis.

- Iatrogenic rupture of the pulmonary artery by balloon-tipped catheter, broncho-arterial fistula, ruptured thoracic aneurysm, arteriovenous malformation.
- Vasculitis: Behçet disease, Wegener's granulomatosis.
- Miscellaneous: Anticoagulant therapy, coagulopathies (von Willebrand disease, hemophilia, thrombocytopenia), Goodpasture syndrome, trauma, lymphangioleiomyomatosis.

COMMONLY ASSOCIATED CONDITIONS

- Hereditary telangiectasia (Osler-Weber-Rendu syndrome)
- Cystic fibrosis (CF)
- Pulmonary renal syndrome:
  - Wegener's granulomatosis
  - Goodpasture syndrome
  - Systemic lupus erythematosus
  - Behçet syndrome
  - Henoch-Schönlein purpura

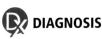 **DIAGNOSIS**

HISTORY

- Age: Cancer in older smokers, CF in younger patients
- Travel history: Rule out TB, parasitic, fungal infections.
- Prior hemoptysis
- Bleeding diathesis
- Anticoagulant treatment, ASA, NSAIDs
- Work history: Asbestos exposure
- Heart lung or kidney disease
- Smoking exposure: Cancer
- GI complaints: Hematemesis
- Family history: Hemoptysis, HHT

PHYSICAL EXAM

- General appearance
- Vital signs, skin (rashes, telangiectasia)
- Face (saddle nose, Wegener's), mucous membrane, oral cavity and gum, nasopharynx, larynx
- Neck for lymph node enlargement and jugular venous distention (JVD)
- Chest and lungs for deformities, signs of trauma, rales, wheezing, dullness
- Abnormal heart sounds of valvular stenosis
- Abdomen for hepatic congestion or masses
- Extremities for clubbing or cyanosis, vessel grafts or fistulas, dialysis catheter

DIAGNOSTIC TESTS & INTERPRETATION
Lab
Initial lab tests

- CBC with differential: Increased WBC, infections; decreased H/H, anemia; decreased platelets, thrombocytopenia
- Chem 7: Elevated BUN, upper GI bleeding, renal failure; elevated creatinine, renal failure
- LFT: Elevated, liver failure, coagulopathic
- PT, PTT, INR: Elevated, coagulopathic
- ABG: Respiratory failure
- D-dimer: Elevated, DVT/pulmonary embolism
- Sputum: Source of bleeding; food material or acidic pH indicate GI source, alveolar macrophage and alkalotic pH lung source, stain and culture for AFB
- PPD skin test, TB
- HIV viral test

Follow-Up & Special Considerations

- CBC: Decreased H/H, transfuse blood; decreased platelets, transfuse platelets; elevated WBC, evaluate for infection and give empiric antibiotics. Frequent CBC until bleeding stops.
- Pulmonary and thoracic surgery consults for massive hemoptysis.
- PT/PTT/INR: Elevated, give FFP and vitamin K.
- Chem 7: Replete electrolytes.
- ABG: Ventilator management

Imaging
Initial approach

- CXR: Infiltrate, cavity, abscess, effusions, atelectasis, cardiomegaly, mass lesions
- Flexible (to determine bleeding site) and rigid bronchoscopy (for massive bleeding and to suction out the blood/clots)
- CT scan of chest: More sensitive than CXR; localizes the bleeding site

Follow-Up & Special Considerations

- Antibiotics for pneumonia and TB
- Antifungals for fungal infections
- Isolation for suspected TB
- Bronchoscopy and biopsy for mass lesions
- Cardiac echo and possible right-heart catheter for pulmonary HTN

Diagnostic Procedures/Other
- Fiberoptic bronchoscopy: If source of bleed cannot be located
- Bleeding scan: The source of bleed cannot be located with other methods.
- High-resolution CT scan gives better resolution of lung abnormalities:
  - Source of bleed cannot be located with other methods.

Pathological Findings
- Cancer
- Bronchiectasis

DIFFERENTIAL DIAGNOSIS
- Hematemesis
- Epistaxis
- Oral bleeding

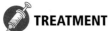 TREATMENT

MEDICATION
First Line
- Varies with the cause of the hemoptysis. Treat the disease that caused the hemorrhage.
- Cough suppressant: Codeine sulfate (10–20 mg) PO q4–6h.

> **ALERT**
> Codeine may weaken the cough reflex, causing aspiration in the nonintubated patient.

Second Line
- Varies with the cause of the hemoptysis:
- Acute on chronic bronchitis: Treat with any of the following antibiotics:
  - Bactrim 15–20 mg/kg/d IV divided q6–8h × 14 days
  - Doxycycline 100 mg IV q12h.
  - Amoxicillin/clavulanate 500 mg PO q8h.
  - Gatifloxacin 400 mg PO/IV q12h.
  - Azithromycin 500 mg IV q.d.
- Tuberculosis:
  - Isoniazid (INH) 300 mg PO q.d.
  - Rifampin (RIF) 600 mg PO q.d.
  - Pyrazinamide (PZA) 2 g PO q.d.
  - Ethambutol (ETB) 2 g PO q.d.

ADDITIONAL TREATMENT
General Measures
- Codeine or morphine to prevent coughing
- Large-bore intravascular access

Additional Therapies
- Influenza vaccine as per CDC guidelines
- Pneumovax as per CDC

SURGERY/OTHER PROCEDURES
- Surgical consultation for resection of the bleeding lobe or segment in patients who have high lung reserve and persistent bleeding after embolization
- Interventional radiology consultation for embolization of the bleeding vessel

IN-PATIENT CONSIDERATIONS
Initial Stabilization
- Airway management
- If massive hemorrhage is localized to one lung, intubate the corresponding main bronchus to prevent the blood from being aspirated into the normal lung.
- Place the patient in the lateral decubitus position on the side of the bleeding lung (i.e., the bleeding lung down.) This prevents blood from moving over to the nonbleeding lung.
- Maintain oxygenation.
- Control bleeding:
  - Flexible bronchoscopy to localize the bleeding source. If the bleeding is brisk, use rigid bronchoscopy to suction out the blood and blood clots. Use sclerosing agents (cold water or epinephrine) to control the bleeding. If the bleeding is still not controlled, transfer to interventional radiology to embolize the vessel. Bronchial artery embolization is the most effective nonsurgical treatment in massive hemoptysis.
  - If bleeding is still not controlled, obtain a thoracic surgery consultation for possible resection of the bleeding segment or lobe of the lung.
- Control coughing:
  - Codeine or morphine sulfate
- Calm the patient.
- Maintain BP:
  - IV fluids or blood
- Correct coagulopathy:
  - Fresh frozen plasma to correct the INR to near normal values
  - Platelet replacement for platelet count ≤50 with renal failure; ≤15 without renal failure

IV Fluids
- Isotonic fluids
- Treat dehydration and shock with crystalloids.
- If anemic, transfuse packed red blood cells.

 ONGOING CARE

DIET
NPO until stabilized

PROGNOSIS
- Varies with the type of hemoptysis and the cause of the hemoptysis
- Mild hemoptysis: Generally good prognosis; mortality rate 2.5%.
- Massive hemoptysis: High mortality rate, 38% (1)[A]

COMPLICATIONS
- Asphyxiation
- Accidental embolization of the spinal artery (prevalence <1%) (3)[A]

REFERENCES
1. Hirshberg B, et al. Hemoptysis: Etiology, evaluation, and outcome in a tertiary referral hospital. *Chest.* 1997;112:440–44.
2. Jean-Baptiste E. Clinical assessment and management of massive hemoptysis. *Crit Care Med.* 2000;28(5):1642–7.
3. Zhang JS, et al. Bronchial arteriography and transcatheter embolization in the management of hemoptysis. *Cardiovasc Intervent Radiol.* 1994; 17:276–9.

ADDITIONAL READING
- Bidwell JL, et al. Hemoptysis: Diagnosis and management. *Am Fam Physician.* 2005;72:1253–60.

CODES

ICD9
- 486 Pneumonia, organism unspecified
- 494.0 Bronchiectasis without acute exacerbation
- 786.30 Hemoptysis, unspecified

CLINICAL PEARLS
- Position patient with the bleeding lung down.
- Err on the side of early intubation and mechanical ventilation if hemoptysis is significant or if patient is hemodynamically unstable.
- Anticipate the need for consultations early on: (pulmonary, anesthesiology (directed intubation/lung isolation) and thoracic surgery.

H

HEMORRHAGE, INTRACEREBRAL

Javed Iqbal
Raghad Said

 BASICS

DESCRIPTION
- Intracerebral hemorrhage (ICH) is focal bleeding from a blood vessel in the brain parenchyma.
- Predilection sites for ICH include:
  - Basal ganglia (40–50%)
  - Lobar regions (20–50%)
  - Thalamus (10–15%)
  - Pons (5–12%)
  - Cerebellum (5–10%)
  - Other brainstem sites (1–5%)

EPIDEMIOLOGY
Incidence
- ICH accounts for only 15% of all strokes but it is one of the most disabling forms of stroke.
- Each year, ICH affects ~12–15 per 100,000 individuals, including 350 hypertensive hemorrhages per 100,000 elderly individuals.

RISK FACTORS
- Older age
- Male sex
- Hypertension
- Increased alcohol intake
- Drug abuse
- Trauma

Genetics
Independent risk factors for lobar ICH includes the presence of an apolipoprotein E2 or E4 allele and 1st-degree relative with history of ICH.

GENERAL PREVENTION
- Prevention and treatment of hypertension
- Avoidance of drugs (cocaine)/alcohol/ sympathomimetic agents.

PATHOPHYSIOLOGY
- ICH and accompanying edema may disrupt or compress adjacent brain tissue, leading to neurological dysfunction.
- Substantial displacement of brain parenchyma may cause elevation of intracranial pressure (ICP) and potentially fatal herniation syndromes (1).
- Growth of the volume of ICH was associated with early neurological deterioration, poor outcome, and death (2).

ETIOLOGY
- Hypertensive damage to blood vessel walls
- Arteriopathy (e.g., cerebral amyloid angiopathy, Moyamoya)
- Trauma
- Rupture of an aneurysm

- Arteriovenous malformation (AVM)
- Excessive cerebral blood flow (reperfusion injury)
- Altered hemostasis (e.g., thrombolysis, anticoagulation, bleeding diathesis)
- Hemorrhagic necrosis (e.g. tumor, infection)
- Venous outflow obstruction (e.g. cerebral venous thrombosis)

COMMONLY ASSOCIATED CONDITIONS
- Acute ischemic stroke
- Subarachnoid hemorrhage

 DIAGNOSIS

HISTORY
- The classic presentation of ICH is sudden onset of a focal neurological deficit that progresses over minutes to hours with accompanying headache, nausea, vomiting, decreased consciousness, and elevated BP (1)
- Important parts of the history are:
  - Age >70
  - Time of onset of symptoms
  - Trauma
  - Seizures
  - PMHx: Previous CVA, HTN, dementia, liver disease, cancer, bleeding diathesis,
  - Medications: Heparin, antiplatelet, anticoagulant use
  - History of tobacco, cocaine, amphetamines

PHYSICAL EXAM
- Neurologic deficits are related to the site of parenchymal hemorrhage:
  - Large hemorrhages, when located in the hemispheres, cause hemiparesis.
  - When located in the posterior fossa, they cause cerebellar or brainstem deficits (e.g., conjugate eye deviation or ophthalmoplegia, pinpoint pupils, coma).
  - Ataxia is the initial deficit noted in cerebellar hemorrhage.

DIAGNOSTIC TESTS & INTERPRETATION
Lab
- CBC, PT/PTT, INR, chem-7, serum magnesium, LFTs, CPK, troponin, D-dimer, serum fibrinogen, urine and/or blood toxicology
- Type and cross blood products
- Others: EKG, CXR, ABG

Imaging
Initial approach

- STAT CT of the head without contrast: Determine location, volume of blood, hydrocephalus, midline shift, evidence of trauma. (3)[A]
- MRI is superior at detecting underlying structural lesions(e.g., tumor) and delineating the amount of perihematomal edema and herniation. (3)[A]

Follow-Up & Special Considerations
CT angiogram/cerebral angiogram/MRA in cases of SAH or AVM

Pathological Findings
- Collection of platelets surrounded by fibrin with adjacent destruction of parenchyma
- Charcot-Bouchard microaneurysms may be seen at bifurcations of distal lateral lenticulostriate vessels in hypertensive ICH.
- Lobar hemorrhages of cerebral amyloid angiopathy may reveal pathological deposition of β-amyloid protein within the media of small cortical and meningeal vessels (1).

DIFFERENTIAL DIAGNOSIS
- Venous infarct
- Hemorrhagic transformation of Ischemic stroke
- Hemorrhagic leukoencephalopathy

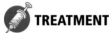 **TREATMENT**

MEDICATION
First Line
- Reversal of coagulopathy:
  - Patient on warfarin: Administer vitamin K 10 mg IVPB over 10 minutes and give FFP 10–15 mL/kg body weight; repeat INR after FFP and after 6–8 hours, if INR is still >1.5, consider more FFP.
  - For patient on heparin and LMWH, consider protamine as per protocol based on last heparin dose.
  - For patients previously on antiplatelet agents, there is no evidence that platelet transfusion improves outcomes in ICH.
- For thrombolytic related-coagulopathy:
  - Stop thrombolytic agent and transfuse 6–8 units of cryoprecipitate containing factor VIII and 6–8 units of platelets
  - rFVIIa reduced growth of the hematoma but did not improve survival or functional outcome after ICH, and it increases risk of thrombosis, especially with high doses (4).
  - Prothrombin complex concentrate (PCC) is not widely available in the U.S.

Second Line
- BP control
- Target BP on the basis of individual patient factors, such as baseline BP, presumed cause of hemorrhage, age, and elevated ICP.
- Most hospital protocols will target a MAP of >75 and <130.

- Hypertension: Maintain SBP 160–180 and MAP <130 with labetalol 5–20 mg bolus and infusion at 2 mg/min (maximum 300 mg) or nicardipine 5–15 mg/hr (3)[B].

- Hypotension: SBP <90, begin isotonic saline, consider phenylephrine drip at 2–10 mg/kg/min.

ADDITIONAL TREATMENT
Steroids are not helpful and might increase infectious complications (3).

General Measures
- Seizure management: IV Ativan 0.1 mg/kg
- Blood sugar control (insulin drip if blood glucose >185)
- Fever is associated with worse outcome and should be treated with Tylenol and other measures.

Issues for Referral
- After stabilization, patient is moved to ICU and a center with neurosurgical facilities.
- Neurosurgery consult if:
  – Intraparenchymal hemorrhage >3 cm
  – Intraventricular hemorrhage
  – Hydrocephalus
  – Signs of increased ICP
  – Rapid deterioration despite maximum medical management
- Neurosurgery and or neuroradiology consult for suspected SAH aneurysmal bleed

Additional Therapies
Seizure prophylaxis for lobar bleeds: IV Dilantin or Keppra can be used (3)[B]

SURGERY/OTHER PROCEDURES
- The routine evacuation of supratentorial ICH by standard craniotomy is not recommended.
- Surgical removal of the hemorrhage should occur as soon as possible for patients with cerebellar hemorrhage >3 cm who are deteriorating neurologically or who have brainstem compression and/or hydrocephalus; these patients should have decompressive suboccipital craniectomy to evacuate the hematoma (3)[A].
- Other surgical options include:
  – Evacuation of supratentorial ICH by standard craniotomy for lobar clots within 1 cm of the surface only might improve function (3)[B].
  – Stereotactic infusion of urokinase into the clot cavity and aspiration might help but it increases bleeding risk.
  – Endoscopic hematoma evacuation needs further studies.
  – Ventriculostomy may be needed in patients with increased ICP and intraventricular extension.
  – Intraventricular fibrinolysis for acute obstructive hydrocephalus followed by lumbar drain for late communicating hydrocephalus may decrease the need for permanent shunt.

IN-PATIENT CONSIDERATIONS
Initial Stabilization
- Assess for ABC:
  – Intubation for airway protection, impending ventilatory failure
- Assess for signs of increased ICP and treat if present:
  – For increased ICP, the head should be elevated to 30 degrees, 1.0–1.5 g/kg of 20% mannitol should be given by a rapid infusion, and the patient should be hyperventilated to a PCO_2 of 30–35 mm Hg
- Activate stroke team beeper.

Admission Criteria
Admit to ICU or stroke unit.

IV Fluids
- Isotonic saline or hypertonic saline to prevent cerebral edema (keep sodium to 145–155)
- Watch for cerebral salt wasting and diabetes insipidus.

Nursing
- Head of bed elevation
- Caution when using of sedatives
- DVT prophylaxis with pneumatic compression devices, SC heparin may be started in high-risk patient day 3 post ICH if no evidence of further bleed (3)[B]
- Early mobilization

Discharge Criteria
- Stable neurological status
- Controlled BP
- Airway protection and stable respiratory status

 ## ONGOING CARE

FOLLOW-UP RECOMMENDATIONS
- Occupational and speech therapy
- BP control
- The decision torestart antithrombotic therapy after ICH:
  – Antiplatelet agents: For patients with lower risk of cerebral infarction and a higher risk of amyloid angiopathy or with very poor overall neurological function
  – Warfarin: In patients with a very high risk of thromboembolism, may be restarted at 7–10 days after onset of the original ICH (3)[B]

Patient Monitoring
- Serial neurological exam every hour in the first 24 hours
- Repeat CT scan in 6–24 hours and earlier if any sign of clinical deterioration

DIET
- Aspiration precautions:
  – NGT feeding as early as possible
  – Speech and swallow evaluation with regular feeding when stabilized
- GI prophylaxis in all patients is a must.

PATIENT EDUCATION
- Hypertension control
- Avoidance of alcohol/drugs
- Warning signs of stroke

PROGNOSIS
- Prognosis depends on size of bleed, level of consciousness (GCS) at presentation
- 30-day mortality rate of 35–52%; 1/2 of the deaths occur in the 1st 2 days
- Death at 1 year for ICH varies by location of ICH: 51% for deep hemorrhage, 57% for lobar, 42% for cerebellar, and 65% for brainstem bleeds
- Hydrocephalus carries a poor prognosis.
- Only 20% are expected to be functionally independent at 6 months.
- The use of early DNR is associated with worse outcome than it would if full care was provided, although physicians may concur on the appropriate circumstances for DNR use in ICH (3).

COMPLICATIONS
- Brainstem herniation
- Brain death
- Neurological deficit/spasticity/disability
- Seizures
- Aspiration pneumonia and respiratory failure
- DVT/PE
- UTI

REFERENCES
1. Manno EM, et al. Emerging medical and surgical management strategies in the evaluation and treatment of intracerebral hemorrhage. *Mayo Clin Proc.* 2005;80:420–33.
2. Brott T, et al. Early hemorrhage growth in patients with intracerebral hemorrhage. *Stroke.* 1997;28:1–5.
3. Broderick J, et al., American Heart Association, American Stroke Association Stroke Council, High Blood Pressure Research Council, Quality of Care and Outcomes in Research Interdisciplinary Working Group. Guidelines for the management of spontaneous intracerebral hemorrhage in adults: 2007 update. *Stroke.* 2007;38(6):2001–23.
4. Mayer SA, et al. Efficacy and safety of recombinant activated factor VII for acute intracerebral hemorrhage. *N Engl J Med.* 2008;358(20):2127–37.

ADDITIONAL READING
- http://www.guideline.gov/summary/summary.aspx?doc_id=10867

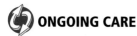 ## CODES

ICD9
- 430 Subarachnoid hemorrhage
- 431 Intracerebral hemorrhage
- 853.00 Other and unspecified intracranial hemorrhage following injury, without mention of open intracranial wound, with state of consciousness unspecified

CLINICAL PEARLS

Steroids are not helpful and might increase infectious complications.

H

HEMORRHAGE, POSTPARTUM (PPH)

Ashlesha K. Dayal
Dena Goffman

BASICS

DESCRIPTION
- Excess of 500 cc blood loss for vaginal and 1000 cc blood loss for cesarean delivery
- Estimates of blood loss are notoriously underreported.
- Hypotension, pallor, and oliguria occurs after loss of at least 10% of total blood volume
- Classified as primary hemorrhage or secondary hemorrhage depending on timing of bleeding:
  - Primary: Within 24 hours of delivery
  - Secondary: After 24 hours, within 6–12 weeks

EPIDEMIOLOGY
- Prevalence: PPH occurs in up 18% births worldwide (WHO) and 4–6% in US
- Leading cause of maternal mortality worldwide
- Mortality often preventable

RISK FACTORS
- History of PPH
- Prolonged labor
- Precipitous labor
- Grand multiparity
- Prior cesarean delivery
- Episiotomy/laceration
- Overdistended uterus (twin gestation, polyhydramnios, large fetus)

Genetics
A variety of genetic disorders can predispose to bleeding but no specific genetic etiology for PPH is noted.

GENERAL PREVENTION
- Minimize obstetric risk factors
- Bimanual massage after placental delivery
- Active management of 3rd stage of labor (start IV oxytocin at delivery of anterior shoulder)
- Continue oxytocin in IV solution after placental delivery (40 units into 1 L NS)

PATHOPHYSIOLOGY
- Atony: Myometrial muscle fibers fatigue and remain elongated. Spiral arterioles, which travel in the myometrium, are then open to the endometrial cavity, resulting in excessive bleeding.
- Pregnancy increases plasma volume by 40% and red cell mass by 25% as an adaptation to prepare for delivery.
- Excessive blood loss supersedes this physiologic accommodation, resulting in hypovolemia and progressively, shock.

ETIOLOGY
- Atonic uterus
- Lacerations to genital tract:
  - Can be anywhere along the pelvic outlet
- Retained products of conception:
  - May be associated with abnormal placentation (placenta accreta, increta, percreta)
- Coagulopathy

COMMONLY ASSOCIATED CONDITIONS
- Placental abruption
- Placenta previa
- Placenta accreta, increta, percreta
- Placental abruption
- Uterine inversion

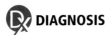

DIAGNOSIS

HISTORY (1)[C]
- Previous history of PPH
- Heavy bleeding with menses
- Prolonged labor with or without chorioamnionitis
- Twin gestation
- Increased amniotic fluid volume

PHYSICAL EXAM
- Brisk vaginal bleeding after delivery of the fetus
- Uterine atony:
  - Boggy, soft uterus.
  - Bladder may be distended and palpable.
  - Cavity and lower uterine segment may be filled with clot.
- Lacerations: Anatomic defect in integrity of cervix corpus, vaginal mucosa (sulcus most common site), or perineal body possible
- Adherent placenta: Placenta imbeds into myometrium and fails to separate
- Uterine inversion: Bluish reddish mass protruding from vagina; often placenta is still attached
- Coagulation disorder: No response to usual measures for PPH or bleeding from puncture sites
- Hypovolemia: Orthostatic vital signs, pallor, tachycardia, decreased urine output, hypotension. May see rapid hemodynamic deterioration soon after tachycardia.

ALERT
Aggressive early resuscitation with IV fluids and blood products is advised.

DIAGNOSTIC TESTS & INTERPRETATION
Lab
Initial lab tests
Initial studies: CBC (10% decrease in HCT indicative of significant hemorrhage), coagulation profile, fibrinogen, clot test, type and cross-match

ALERT
Coagulation profile in pregnancy differs from nonpregnant adults due to increases in multiple clotting factors: Fibrinogen is increased (680 mg/dL) and PTT is decreased (24 seconds). Therefore, coagulopathy may appear at values different from nonpregnant adults.

Follow-Up & Special Considerations
- CBC post transfusion, coagulation profile after replacement products
- Then serially to assure stable and bleeding has ceased

Imaging
Initial approach
- US of uterus: Retained products of conception diagnosed by hyperechoic areas in place of endometrial stripe (3)[C]
- May require CT imaging to appreciate the extent and course of genital tract hematoma

Follow-Up & Special Considerations
Interventional radiology may be able to localize and treat persistent bleeding in a stable patient.

Diagnostic Procedures/Other
Dilation and curettage with wide banjo curette may diagnose retained products

Pathological Findings
Products of conception (membranes, placenta)

DIFFERENTIAL DIAGNOSIS
- Atony
- Trauma
- Retained products
- Coagulopathy

TREATMENT (4)[C]

MEDICATION

First Line
- Oxytocin (Pitocin) 20–40 units in 1 L IV solution NS (active management 3rd stage: NNT18), 200 cc/hour
- Empty bladder and bimanual massage of uterus
- Ergot alkaloid (Methergine) 0.2 mg IM/SC, can be repeated q2–4h
  – Contraindication: Preeclampsia, hypertension
- Methyl-prostaglandin f2-α (Hemabate/Carboprost) 250 mcg IM or intramyometrial q15min until 2 mg (8 doses)
  – Contraindication: Hypersensitivity
  – Relative contraindication: Asthma, hypertension

Second Line
Misoprostol (Cytotec) 1000 mcg PR (NNT18). Although used, is not FDA approved for this indication.

Third Line
Recombinant activated factor VIIa is an option. IV doses vary by case; however, concern is for risk of subsequent thromboembolic event in the hypercoagulable obstetric patient

ADDITIONAL TREATMENT
General Measures
- Call for Help
- 2 large-bore IVs
- Communication with anesthesia, nursing, operating room, interventional radiology
- Notify blood bank of potential needs

Issues for Referral
- Persistent vaginal bleeding, dropping blood count despite resuscitation, see Surgery
- End-organ malperfusion (shock)

Additional Therapies
Surgical team may be able to temporize with packing or balloon tamponade. Prompt communication with ob-gyn or surgeon is crucial.

SURGERY/OTHER PROCEDURES (4)[C]
- May require hysterectomy to preserve life: Notify ob-gyn or surgeon
- May need incision and drainage in cases of genital tract hematoma: Notify ob-gyn or surgeon
- Interventional radiology is useful in cases where patient is stable and future fertility is desired.

IN-PATIENT CONSIDERATIONS
Initial Stabilization
- Fluid resuscitation
- Blood product resuscitation
- Uterotonics

Admission Criteria
- Brisk vaginal bleeding
- Change in vital signs
- Coagulation derangements

IV Fluids
20–40 units oxytocin in 1 L NS at 200 cc/hr

Nursing
- q15min VS
- Monitor vaginal bleeding
- Monitor fundal height (should remain at level of umbilicus) a rising fundus may indicate bleeding into the uterine cavity

Discharge Criteria
- Vaginal bleeding less than menses
- Normal vital signs
- Stable hemoglobin/hematocrit × 2
- Correction of coagulation abnormalities

 ONGOING CARE

FOLLOW-UP RECOMMENDATIONS
2-week follow-up in office to assess uterine size and bleeding

Patient Monitoring
Monitor vaginal bleeding; delayed PPH can occur.

DIET
Regular

PATIENT EDUCATION
- Signs of secondary postpartum hemorrhage
- Symptoms and signs of hypovolemia

PROGNOSIS
Good overall, with rapid management

COMPLICATIONS
- Maternal death with late recognition, inadequate resuscitation, or treatment delay
- Post shock metabolic or organ derangements
- Sheehan syndrome (panhypopituitarism)

REFERENCES

1. ACOG Clinical Management Guidelines for Obstetrician-Gynecologists. #76. October 2006.
2. Anderson JM, et al. Prevention and management of postpartum hemorrhage. *Am Fam Physician.* 2007;75:875–82
3. Hertzberg BS, et al. Ultrasound of the postpartum uterus: Prediction of retained placenta tissue. *J Ultrasound Med.* 1991;10:451–6 (level III).
4. Mousa HA, et al. Treatment for primary postpartum hemorrhage. *Cochrane Database Syst Rev.* 2003; (1):CS003249.

 See Also (Topic, Algorithm, Electronic Media Element)

- Placenta Previa
- Placental Abruption

 CODES

ICD9
- 666.10 Other immediate postpartum hemorrhage, unspecified as to episode of care
- 666.12 Other immediate postpartum hemorrhage, with delivery
- 666.14 Other immediate postpartum hemorrhage

CLINICAL PEARLS

- Postpartum hemorrhage is a leading preventable cause of maternal mortality.
- Obstetric hemorrhage can rapidly lead to shock and death.
- Pregnant patients are young, have fewer comorbidities, and the physiologic changes of pregnancy can allow the patient to appear well when in impending shock.
- Life-saving measures in PPH include prompt recognition, aggressive resuscitation, and often surgical intervention.

H

HEMORRHAGE, SUBARACHNOID

Raghad Said
Zaid Said

 BASICS

DESCRIPTION
Bleeding into the space between the arachnoid and the pia mater, which is filled with cerebrospinal fluid

EPIDEMIOLOGY
Incidence
Nontraumatic SAH occurs in 10/100,000 of U.S. population yearly
Prevalence
More prevalent in:
- Females, especially postmenopausal
- Age >50 years (1)
- African Americans and Mexican Americans

RISK FACTORS
- Personal and/or family history of SAH
- Illicit drug use (especially cocaine)
- Smoking
- Moderate-heavy alcohol use
- Hypertension
Genetics
APOE4 allele may increase the risk of a negative outcome in patients with SAH (2).

GENERAL PREVENTION
- Smoking cessation (3)[B]
- Blood pressure (BP) control (3)[A]
- Follow-up imaging for SAH patients (3)[A]
- Screening asymptomatic relatives should be considered on individual basis (3)[B].
- Screening high-risk population is of uncertain value (3)[B].

PATHOPHYSIOLOGY
SAH decreases cerebral perfusion pressure and microvascular perfusion by:
- Increasing intracranial pressure (ICP)
- Altering cerebral autoregulation
- Decreasing nitric oxide availability
- Microvascular collagenases and platelets activation

ETIOLOGY
- Ruptured saccular aneurysm (20% multiple)
- Trauma
- Arteriovenous malformations
- Vasculitides
- Intracranial arterial dissections
- Amyloid angiopathy
- Benign perimesencephalic SAH
- Anticoagulation therapy

COMMONLY ASSOCIATED CONDITIONS
- Familial intracranial aneurysm syndrome
- Polycystic kidney disease
- Type IV Ehlers-Danlos disease
- Fibromuscular dysplasia
- Marfan syndrome

DIAGNOSIS

HISTORY
- Severe headache: Described by the patient as the "worst headache in my life" in 80%
- Nausea and vomiting: 77%
- Loss of consciousness: 53%
- New-onset seizure: 6–20%
- Meningismus symptoms: 35% (1)
- Sentinel headache occurring days-weeks prior to presentation due to aneurysmal expansion: 5–43%
- Diplopia usually seen with PCOMM aneurysm

PHYSICAL EXAM
- Could be normal
- Altered mental status and confusion
- Focal neurological signs
- Papilledema
- Subhyaloid retinal hemorrhage
- Signs of increased ICP
- Initial physical exam correlates with survival
- Grading systems in SAH:
  - Hunt and Hess Score:
    - **1** Minimal headache and slight neck stiffness
    - **2** Moderate to severe headache; neck stiffness; no neurologic deficit except cranial nerve palsy
    - **3** Drowsy; mild neurologic deficit
    - **4** Stuporous; moderate to severe hemiparesis
    - **5** Deep coma: Decerebrate
  - World Federation of Neurological Surgeons Grade (5 grades) incorporates the Glasgow Coma Scale (GCS) and the presence or absence of a focal deficit

DIAGNOSTIC TESTS & INTERPRETATION
Lab
Initial lab tests
- CBC
- Chem 7, LFT, and serum magnesium
- PT/INR and PTT
- Urine or serum toxicology
- Troponin-I
- ECG and chest x-ray
- EEG for poor-grade patients or in presence of deterioration in mental status that cannot be explained

Follow-Up & Special Considerations
- Correct coagulopathy and thrombocytopenia
- Anemia, hyperglycemia, hypomagnesemia, and elevated troponin I are associated with bad outcome.
- ECG changes are common and correlate with cardiopulmonary complications, arrhythmias, and true MI do occur due to high catecholamine surge.

Imaging
Initial approach
- CT scan of the head without contrast (3)[A]:
  - Sensitivity 98% in first 12 hours, 90% after 24 hours, 50% after 1 week
  - Also identify hydrocephalus, intraventricular bleed, and intracranial bleeds
  - Amount of blood on initial head CT has strong correlation with the risk for vasospasm.
  - The Fisher Grade: Classifies the appearance of subarachnoid hemorrhage on CT scan:
    - 1: None evident
    - 2: <1 mm thick
    - 3: >1 mm thick
    - 4: Any thickness with intraventricular hemorrhage or parenchymal extension
- Lumbar puncture: Identifies clearing blood or xanthochromia in patient with negative head CT

Follow-Up & Special Considerations
- MRI and MRA are used to diagnose delayed SAH presentation (3)[B].
- MRI is the initial test in pregnant women.

Diagnostic Procedures/Other
- Catheter angiography (gold standard) (3)[A]:
  - Define operative planning (coiling vs. clipping)
  - 20% of patients with clinically diagnosed SAH have negative angiographic findings. A repeat angiogram is needed in 1–3 weeks.
  - Complication rate <1%
  - Bed rest for 6 hours after to prevent bleeding
- CT and MR angiography:
  - Noninvasive
  - Used for screening and presurgical planning in unstable patients
  - Might play a role in follow-up after clipping
  - Sensitivity compared to conventional angiography is 95% when the aneurysm is >5 mm and 60% when it is <5 mm in size
- Echocardiogram and/or PA catheter if patient is hypoxic or hypotensive or prior to starting HHH therapy in a patient with preexisting cardiopulmonary disease.

Pathological Findings
- Aneurysms form because of thinning of arterial tunica media.
- Aneurysms occur usually at the bifurcations of the basal cerebral arteries, implying a shear stress effect on the vessel wall.
- 20% of cases have ≥1 aneurysm.

DIFFERENTIAL DIAGNOSIS
- Migraine
- Tension headache

TREATMENT

MEDICATION
First Line

- Nimodipine: For vasospasm prophylaxis, dose is 60 mg PO q4h for 14–21 days (1)[A]
- Symptomatic vasospasm is currently treated with HHH therapy: **H**ypervolemia (CVP 8–12 mm Hg, PCWP 12–16 mm Hg) and induced **H**ypertension (using phenylephrine, norepinephrine)+/ − **H**emodilution to Hct ≤30
- Inotropic support with dobutamine or milrinone in patients with depressed myocardial function

Second Line
Glucocorticoid use is controversial (3)[C].

ADDITIONAL TREATMENT
General Measures
- BP management (with nicardipine, esmolol, or labetalol IV drips):
  - Prerepair procedure: Lower SBP to <150 mm Hg (lower the risk of rebleeding) (3)[A]
  - Postrepair procedure: Tolerate SBP to 200
  - The patient's cognitive status may be a useful guide to target BP (awake patients have adequate CPP).
- Hyperglycemia (requiring insulin drip)
  - Optimal blood sugar level remains unknown
- Seizures:
  - 7 days prophylactic therapy with Dilantin or Keppra may be considered in patients with prior seizures, MCA aneurysms, parenchymal hematoma and infarct, and postcraniotomy (3)[B].
  - For seizures after SAH, treat for 6 months
- Hyponatremia (cerebral salt-wasting or SIADH):
  - More common in poor-grade SAH, ACA aneurysms, and hydrocephalus
  - Fluid restriction is associated with delayed ischemic deficits.
  - 3% hypertonic saline and fludrocortisones improve Na level (3)[B].
- Stool softener to avoid straining
- Fever is associated with worse outcome; maintain core body temperature ≤37.2°C using APAP 325–650 mg PO q4–6h; cooling devices may be used.
- DVT prophylaxis with compressive devices and heparin SC after definite treatment of the aneurysm
- Analgesia for headache

Issues for Referral
Early referral to a high-volume center that has both experienced endovascular specialist and neurosurgeons is reasonable (3)[B].

Additional Therapies
Intraoperative hypothermia has no benefit.

COMPLEMENTARY & ALTERNATIVE THERAPIES
Antifibrinolytic prior to coiling or clipping:

- Recent evidence suggests that a short course of tranexamic acid given immediately after diagnosis decreases rebleeding without increasing delayed ischemia risk (4)[B].

- Routine use is not recommended because of delayed ischemia risk.
- Might have a role in decreasing risk of rebleed during hospital transfers

SURGERY/OTHER PROCEDURES
- Early intervention (within 72 hours of SAH) decreases the risk for rebleeding; achieved by:
  - Endovascular coiling of the aneurysm
  - Neurosurgical clipping when aneurysm are not amenable for coiling, typically for large aneurysms and/or those with wide necks
- Presence of edema renders surgery technically challenging, especially in high-grade SAH for which coiling is preferred.
- Rebleeding risk is greater after coiling.
- Functional dependence is similar for clipping and coiling after 5 years (5).
- 5-year mortality is significantly higher with clipping (5).
- Hydrocephalus: Requires a ventriculostomy or a lumbar drain and a shunt placement if persistent
- Arteriovenous malformations may be obliterated with embolization and surgery.

IN-PATIENT CONSIDERATIONS
Initial Stabilization
- Maintain ABCs:
  - Rapid sequence intubation
  - Avoid hyperventilation unless high ICP signs.
  - Avoid BP fluctuation during intubation.
- Interventions to decrease ICP if signs and symptoms of intracranial hypertension are present
- Emergent ventriculostomy is indicated in comatose patients and in lethargic patients with hydrocephalus.

Admission Criteria
All patients with SAH are admitted to ICU.

IV Fluids
- Hypovolemia increases vasospasm risk.
- Avoid hypotonic solution.
- Hypertonic saline of ≥3% concentration is used in cases of increased ICP and/or severe hyponatremia.

Nursing
Strict bed rest

Discharge Criteria
Clinical stability and no complications

 ONGOING CARE

FOLLOW-UP RECOMMENDATIONS
Digital subtraction angiography at 3 months

Patient Monitoring
- CVP and arterial BP for patients on HHH
- Daily transcranial Doppler to diagnose and to follow vasospasm

DIET
NPO pending angiography

PATIENT EDUCATION
Risk of recurrence and need for follow-up

PROGNOSIS
- SAH is associated with a 45% mortality rate.
- Prognosis depends on patient's age and neurological grade on admission and the amount of blood on initial head CT.
- Only 30% of patients who survive report no major disability.

COMPLICATIONS
- Vasospasm: See vasospasm chapter
- Delayed ischemic deficits
- Rebleeding:
  - Mortality 70%
  - Preventable by early treatment
  - Incidence: 4% within the 1st 24 hours, 20% within 2 weeks, and 50% within 1 month
- Myocardial stunning (reversible)
- Pulmonary edema (neurogenic or cardiac)

REFERENCES

1. van Gijn J, et al. Subarachnoid haemorrhage: Diagnosis, causes, and management. *Brain*. 2001;124:249–78.
2. Lanterna LA, et al. Meta-analysis of APOE genotype and SAH: Clinical outcome and delayed ischemia. *Neurology*. 2007:69(8):766–75.
3. Bederson JB, et al. Guidelines for the management of aneurysmal subarachnoid hemorrhage: A statement for healthcare professionals from a special writing group of the Stroke Council, American Heart Association. *Stroke*. 2009; 40(3):994–1025.
4. Hillman J, et al. Immediate administration of tranexamic acid and reduced incidence of early rebleeding after aneurismal SAH. *J Neurosurg*. 2002;97:771–8.
5. Molyneux AJ, et al. Risk of recurrent subarachnoid haemorrhage, death, or dependence and standardised mortality ratios after clipping or coiling of an intracranial aneurysm in the International Subarachnoid Aneurysm Trial (ISAT): Long-term follow up. *Lancet Neurol*. 2009;8(5): 427–33.

 See Also (Topic, Algorithm, Electronic Media Element)

- Aneurysm
- Cerebral Salt-wasting
- Vasospasm

CODES

ICD9
- 430 Subarachnoid hemorrhage
- 852.01 Subarachnoid hemorrhage following injury, without mention of open intracranial wound, with no loss of consciousness

CLINICAL PEARLS

- Early intervention decreases mortality
- Treatment in high-volume centers improves outcome.

H

HEPATITIS, FULMINANT

David Dahan

BASICS

DESCRIPTION
- Fulminant hepatitis (FHF) is a condition in which rapid deterioration of liver function results in mental alteration (encephalopathy) and coagulation abnormality (INR >1.5) within 26 weeks of jaundice in a patient without preexisting liver disease.
- Patients with Wilson disease, vertically acquired HBV, or autoimmune hepatitis may be included in spite of the possibility of cirrhosis, if their disease has only been recognized for <26 weeks.

EPIDEMIOLOGY
- FHF is a rare condition and often affects young persons.
- Male < Female (75%)
- Incidence: Approximately 2000 deaths occur annually from acute viral hepatitis. In addition, if "hepatic coma" without any mention of chronic liver disease, alcoholism, or cancer is used to uncover cases, then almost 7500 deaths were caused by FHF from 1980–1988. This corresponds to 3.5 deaths per million people.

Prevalence
2000 cases per year in the U.S.

RISK FACTORS
Genetics
Wilson disease is an autosomal recessive disorder caused by mutations in the ATP7B gene, a membrane-bound copper-transporting ATPase.

PATHOPHYSIOLOGY
- Confluent necrosis with cell dropout and parenchymal collapse in either zonal or a nonzonal distribution:
  - Activated sinusoidal-lining cells, including Kupffer cells, stellate cells, and endothelial cells
- Microvesicular steatosis in cases due to AFLP or mitochondrial toxins
- Malignant infiltration

ETIOLOGY
- The most common causes of FHF are acetaminophen overdose (39%), cryptogenic (17%), drug toxicity (13%), and viral hepatitis A or B (12%).
- Viral hepatitis: HAV, HBV, HDV (coinfection with B), HEV, HGV, EBV, HSV
- Drug toxicity (e.g., acetaminophen)
- Toxins (*Amanita phalloides*)
- Miscellaneous:
  - Wilson disease
  - Acute Budd Chiari
  - Acute fatty liver of pregnancy/HELLP
  - Ischemic hepatitis
  - Heat stroke
  - Autoimmune hepatitis
  - Reyes syndrome
- Cryptogenic

DIAGNOSIS

HISTORY
- Review of possible exposures to viral infection, drugs, or other toxins (1).
- If severe encephalopathy is present, the history may be provided entirely by the family or may be unavailable.

PHYSICAL EXAM
- Assess and document mental status and search for stigmata of chronic liver disease (1).
- Jaundice is often but not always seen at presentation.
- Right upper quadrant tenderness
- Palpation of liver:
  - Inability to palpate the liver may suggest decreased liver volume due to massive hepatocyte loss.
  - An enlarged liver may be seen early in viral hepatitis or with malignant infiltration, CHF, or acute Budd-Chiari syndrome.
- Absent signs of cirrhosis

DIAGNOSTIC TESTS & INTERPRETATION
Lab
Initial laboratory exam must be extensive to evaluate both the etiology and severity of ALF (1).

Initial lab tests
- CBC
- PT/PTT
- Chemistries:
  - Sodium, potassium, chloride, bicarbonate, calcium, magnesium, phosphate, glucose, AST, ALT, ALP, GGT, total bilirubin, albumin, creatinine, BUN, ABG, arterial lactate, ammonia, amylase, and lipase.
- Blood type and screen
- Acetaminophen level
- Toxicology screen
- Diagnostic tests for Wilson disease:
  - Ceruloplasmin, serum and urinary copper levels, total bilirubin/alkaline phosphatase ratio, slit lamp exam for Kayser-Fleischer rings
- Pregnancy test (females)
- Serology:
  - ANA, ASMA, immunoglobulin levels, HIV status, anti-HAV IgM, HBSAg, anti-HBc IgM, anti-HEV, anti-HCV.

Follow-Up & Special Considerations
- The etiology of the insult must be determined; a disease-specific therapy may be available and ameliorate or reverse liver failure.
- Early identification of patients who are unlikely to survive with supportive treatment should be made, to enable successful liver transplantation.

Imaging
- Abdominal US
- In cases of suspected Budd Chiari or SOL, the diagnosis should be confirmed with CT, Doppler US, venography, magnetic resonance venography.
- In grade I/II encephalopathy consider brain CT to rule out other causes of decreased mental status.

Diagnostic Procedures/Other
- Liver biopsy:
  - Most often done via the transjugular route because of coagulopathy
  - May be indicated when certain conditions, such as autoimmune hepatitis, metastatic liver disease, lymphoma, or herpes simplex hepatitis, are suspected
  - Hepatic copper levels

TREATMENT

MEDICATION
- N-acetylcysteine (NAC) is recommended for the treatment of acetaminophen overdose, even if the ingestion was 48–72 hours before presentation (4):
  - For patients with known or suspected acetaminophen overdose within 4 hours of presentation, give activated charcoal just prior to starting NAC.
  - NAC may be used in cases of acute liver failure in which acetaminophen ingestion is possible or when knowledge of circumstances surrounding admission is inadequate.
- In patients with known or suspected mushroom poisoning, consider administration of penicillin G and silymarin.
- In patients with acute hepatitis B virus infection, consider treatment with lamivudine (100–150 mg/d PO) (3).
- Patients with known or suspected herpes virus or varicella zoster as the cause of acute liver failure should be treated with acyclovir (IV 30 mg/kg/d).
- Patients with autoimmune hepatitis should be treated with corticosteroids (prednisone, 40–60 mg/d).
- Close monitoring and prevention of infectious complications and aggressive treatment of organ dysfunction may successfully bridge patients and allow time for the liver to recover (1,2).
- Consider treatment of hyperammonia (arterial ammonia level >200 mcg/dL being strongly associated with cerebral herniation):
  - Lactulose may be used, but concern has been raised about increasing bowel distention during the subsequent transplant procedure.
  - Neomycin as a nonabsorbable antibiotic carries the risk of nephrotoxicity.
- Seizure activity should be treated with phenytoin and low-dose benzodiazepines.
- Mannitol is recommended as 1st-line therapy for intracranial hypertension. Should be administered when ICP is >25 mm Hg (0.25–1 g IV boluses):
  - Hypertonic saline boluses have been used increasingly with efficacy similar or superior to mannitol.
- Barbiturate coma, induced by pentobarbital (3–5 mg/kg IV loading bolus followed by 1–3 mg/kg/hr IV infusion) has been advocated in patients with ALF refractory to mannitol.
- Hyperventilation may be considered to temporarily reduce the ICP but not as a prophylactic treatment.
- Maintenance of euthermia (36.5–37.5°C) is recommended.
- Adequate analgesia and judicious sedation is required in patients who progress to stage III/IV hepatic encephalopathy (3):
  - No standard agent for sedation; however, both propofol and benzodiazepines are the most commonly used sedatives.
  - An opiate infusion is recommended to prevent or treat discomfort. Agents with shorter half-life, such as fentanyl, are preferred.
- Replacement therapy for thrombocytopenia and/or prolonged prothrombin time is recommended only in the setting of hemorrhage or prior to invasive procedures:

– Administration of vitamin K empirically in all patient (parenteral vitamin K 10 mg)
- Prophylaxis with H_2 blocking agents or PPIs (or sucralfate as a 2nd-line agent) for acid-related GI bleeding associated with stress
- Periodic surveillance cultures should be performed to detect bacterial and fungal infections as early as possible.
- Empirical administration of antibiotics is recommended when infection or the likelihood of impending sepsis is high:
  – When surveillance cultures reveal significant isolates, progression of or advanced stage (III/IV) hepatic encephalopathy, refractory hypotension, presence of SIRS, patients are listed for OLT.
  – Provide broad-spectrum coverage for gram-positive and gram-negative bacteria and antifungal agent in any patient without prompt improvement in signs of infection after institution of antibacterial agents.
- A trial of hydrocortisone should be considered in patients with persistent hypotension despite a volume challenge and norepinephrine.
- Systemic vasopressor support with agents such as epinephrine, norepinephrine, or dopamine but not vasopressin should be used if fluid replacement fails to maintain MAP of 50–60 mm Hg:
  – Norepinephrine is preferred, because it may provide a more consistent and predictable increase in cerebral perfusion than the latter.
- Management of renal failure requires appropriate volume resuscitation and treatment of hypotension:
  – Continuous forms of hemofiltration or dialysis are preferred over intermittent hemodialysis

ADDITIONAL TREATMENT
General Measures
- Hospital admission.
- The precise etiology should be sought to guide further management decisions.
- ICP monitor placement should be considered in all patients listed for OLT with stage III/IV hepatic encephalopathy:
  – Treatment of the bleeding diathesis before insertion is recommended:
    ○ Consider administering recombinant factor VIIa (rFVIIa) in circumstances where FFP has failed to correct PT/PTT to an acceptable level.

Issues for Referral
- Planning for transfer to a transplant
- center should begin in patients with grade I or II encephalopathy (1).
- For patients with acetaminophen-related ALF in particular, an arterial pH of 7.3 should prompt immediate consideration for transfer to a transplant center and placement on a transplant list.
- Patients with poor prognosis (cryptogenic, Wilson, autoimmune, Budd Chiari, mushroom poisoning, acute HBV) must be immediately placed on the liver transplant list.

SURGERY/OTHER PROCEDURES
- Orthotopic liver transplantation remains the only effective therapy:
  – ABO-identical grafts are preferred, but ABO-compatible grafts also can be used.
- Currently available liver support systems are not recommended outside of clinical trials.

IN-PATIENT CONSIDERATIONS
Initial Stabilization
- Patients with progressive encephalopathy, grade III or IV, should be intubated and sedated; elevate head of bed (30 degrees).
- Analgesia and sedation is required in patients who progress to stage III/IV hepatic encephalopathy.
- Careful attention must be paid to fluid resuscitation and maintenance of adequate intravascular volume in patients with FHF.

Admission Criteria
- Patients with FHF should be admitted and monitored frequently.
- Those with altered mentation should preferably be monitored in an ICU.

IV Fluids
- The use of Hartmann's or LR solution must be discouraged.
- Use crystalloids with glucose.
- Can use also albumin solutions.

Nursing
- Patients with only grade I encephalopathy may sometimes be safely managed on a medicine ward with skilled nursing in a quiet environment to minimize agitation.
- Frequent mental status checks should be performed, with transfer to an ICU if level of consciousness declines.

 ONGOING CARE

FOLLOW-UP RECOMMENDATIONS
- Assessment regarding transplant candidacy should be made on admission to the ICU by the transplant and intensive care teams, with specific consideration of poor prognostic factors included in the King's College criteria (PT, creatinine, pH, encephalopathy grade, age, BR).
- The etiology and rapidity of evolution also must be considered.
- Metabolic homeostasis must be maintained. Overall nutritional status, as well as glucose, phosphate, potassium, and magnesium levels should be monitored frequently.

DIET
- Feeding is usually commenced within 24 hours following ICU admission with a target caloric aim of 25–30 kcal/kg/d (2).
- Prefer the enteral over the parenteral route.
- If enteral nutrition is poorly tolerated, parenteral nutrition is a reasonable alternative.
- No evidence suggesting that normal protein intake of 1 g/kg/d worsens hyperammonemia and hepatic encephalopathy.

PROGNOSIS
- The prognosis of patients with ALF varies depending on etiology, patient age, and the length of time over which the illness evolves.
- Prior to transplantation, most series suggested <15% survival.
- Overall short-term survival with transplantation is >65%.

COMPLICATIONS
- Encephalopathy
- Cerebral edema:
  – Intracranial hypertension
- Bacterial and fungal infection
- Bleeding diathesis
- Upper GI bleeding

- Circulatory dysfunction
- Relative adrenal insufficiency
- Hypoglycemia
- Renal failure

Pregnancy Considerations
- Hepatitis E is a significant cause of liver failure in countries where it is endemic, and it tends to be more severe in pregnant women.
- Acute fatty liver of pregnancy/HELLP (hemolysis, elevated liver enzymes, low platelets) syndrome: A small number of women near the end of pregnancy will develop rapidly progressive hepatocyte failure:
  – Associated with increased fetal or maternal mortality
  – Early recognition of these syndromes and prompt delivery are critical in achieving good outcomes.
  – Recovery is typically rapid after delivery, and supportive care is the only other treatment required.
- Postpartum transplantation has occasionally been necessary.
- Pregnancy (especially in the 3rd trimester) appears to increase the risk of FHF due to herpes virus, which should be treated with acyclovir.

REFERENCES

1. Polson J, Lee WM. AASLD Position Paper: The management of acute liver failure. *Hepatology.* 2005;41(5):1179–97(A).
2. Keays R, et al. IV Acetylcysteine in paracetamol induced fulminant hepatic failure: A prospective controlled trial. *BMJ.* 1991;303:1026–9(B).
3. Stravitz RT, et al. Intensive care of patients with acute liver failure: Recommendation of the U.S Acute Liver Failure Study Group. *Crit Care Med.* 2007;35(11):2498–25089(A).
4. Auzinger G, Wendon J. Intensive care management of acute liver failure. *Curr Opin Crit Care.* 2008;14:179–88(A).

CODES

ICD9
- 070.6 Unspecified viral hepatitis with hepatic coma
- 070.9 Unspecified viral hepatitis without mention of hepatic coma

CLINICAL PEARLS
- FHF is an unpredictable and often rapidly progressing disease complicated by multiple organ failure (MOF) resulting from massive liver injury.
- The defining clinical symptoms are coagulopathy and encephalopathy occurring within days or weeks of the primary insult in patients without preexisting liver injury.
- The etiology of the insult must be determined, as disease-specific therapy may be available to ameliorate or reverse liver failure.
- Close monitoring and prevention of infectious complications and aggressive treatment of organ dysfunction may successfully bridge patients through this phase and allow time for the liver to recover.
- Despite significant improvement in survival over time, in part due to better intensive care management, mortality exceeds 90% in the most severe cases, and emergency liver transplantation remains the only effective treatment option.

HEPATITIS, HYPOXIC

Marius Braun

 BASICS

DESCRIPTION
- Massive increase in ALT, AST, and LDH in a patient with cardiac, circulatory, or respiratory failure
- Rapidly reversible upon correction of underlying cause
- Toxic injury should be ruled out.

EPIDEMIOLOGY
- Incidence is from 0.9% in general ICU to 22% in patients admitted to cardiac units with decreased cardiac output.
- Patients with chronic liver disease are more prone to ischemic damage.

PATHOPHYSIOLOGY
- Most damage occurs in zone 3 of the liver lobule, which is most sensitive to ischemia- hepatocellular necrosis.
- Liver congestion renders the liver highly sensitive to reduction in perfusion even if systemic hypotension is not noticed.
- In sepsis, there are both circulatory dysfunctions, the direct effects of bacterial translocation, endotoxin, and activation of the innate immune system and increased metabolic demands.
- Respiratory failure may cause hypoxemia and right-heart failure and liver congestion, particularly when using CPAP or high PEEP.

ETIOLOGY
- Congested liver is an important predisposing factor:
  – Right heart failure
  – Hepatic outflow obstruction
- Low hepatic perfusion:
  – Hepatic artery thrombosis
  – Portal vein thrombosis
  – Hypotension
  – Cardiogenic or circulatory shock
  – Sepsis
  – Heat stroke
  – Ergotamine poisoning
- Hypoxia:
  – Chronic respiratory failure
  – High PEEP
  – Obstructive sleep apnea
  – CO poisoning

DIAGNOSIS

DIAGNOSTIC TESTS & INTERPRETATION
- Increase in ALT, AST >20 times the upper limit of normal in a patient with predisposing factors; see etiology
- Rule out toxins, viral hepatitis, and liver trauma

Lab
- ALT, AST, LDH, bilirubin, alkaline phosphatase
- Albumin, prothrombin time
- ABGs
- Arterial lactate
- Glucose
- Anti-HAV IgM, Anti-HBcAb IgM, Anti-HSV, Anti-HEV, Anti-HCV
- Paracetamol serum levels
- Blood cultures

Imaging
Abdominal US

Diagnostic Procedures/Other
- Doppler US to rule out hepatic outflow obstruction, hepatic artery or portal vein thrombosis
- Cardiac echocardiogram
- EKG
- CXR

DIFFERENTIAL DIAGNOSIS
- Toxic injury
- Acute viral infection
- Liver trauma

TREATMENT

ADDITIONAL TREATMENT
General Measures
- Treat the underlying condition:
  – Improve oxygenation
  – Reverse hypotension
  – Increase cardiac output
  – Treat sepsis
  – Decrease liver congestion:
    ○ Avoid high CPAP or PEEP
- Liver-directed therapy:
  – No proven therapy
  – N-acetyl-cysteine 140 mg/kg 1st dose, followed by 16 doses of 70 mg/kg q4h may be tried based on case reports.

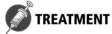 **ONGOING CARE**

FOLLOW-UP RECOMMENDATIONS
Patient Monitoring
- Serum glucose, frequently
- Standard ICU monitoring:
  – Oxygenation
  – Hemodynamic: HR, BP, CVP
  – Acid–base status
  – Urine output

DIET
- Maintain enteral nutrition, avoid protein malnutrition; at least 1 g/kg protein
- Glucose infusion if hypoglycemic

PROGNOSIS
- Depends on adequate control of the initial insult
- If the initial insult is removed, the liver enzymes decrease by 50% by 72 hours, and the liver function usually recovers.
- Predicted by SOFA score, INR, and the duration of liver dysfunction.

ADDITIONAL READING

- Assy N, et al. The beneficial effect of N-acetylcysteine and ciprofloxacin therapy on the outcome of ischemic fulminant hepatic failure. *Dig Dis Sci*. 2007;52:3507–10.
- Birrer R, et al. Hypoxic hepatopathy: Pathophysiology and prognosis. *Intern Med*. 2007;46(14):1063–70.

- Ebert EC. Hypoxic liver injury. *Mayo Clin Proc*. 2006;81(9):1232–6.
- Fuhrmann V, et al. Hypoxic hepatitis: Underlying conditions and risk factors for mortality in critically ill patients. *Intensive Care Med*. 2009;35(8): 1397–405.
- Henrion J. Hypoxic hepatitis: Clinical and hemodynamic study in 142 consecutive cases. *Medicine (Balt)*. 2003;82(6):392–406.

 CODES

ICD9
- 573.3 Hepatitis, unspecified
- 573.8 Other specified disorders of liver

H

HEPATORENAL SYNDROME
Kagan Ilya

 BASICS

DESCRIPTION
- Functional renal failure that frequently develops in patients with advanced cirrhosis and severe circulatory dysfunction
- System(s) affected: Renal/Liver/Cardiovascular
- Classification:
  - Type-1 HRS: Severe and rapidly progressive renal failure that has been defined as doubling of serum creatinine reaching a level >2.5 mg/dL in <2 weeks
  - Type-2 HRS: Moderate and slowly progressive renal failure (serum creatinine <2.5 mg/dL

EPIDEMIOLOGY
Incidence
- 18% after 1 year of liver cirrhosis, 39% after 5 years (2)
- 20% of all renal failure in cirrhotic patients

RISK FACTORS
- Bacterial infections, especially spontaneous bacterial peritonitis (SBP)
- GI hemorrhage
- Large-volume paracentesis
- Major surgical procedure
- Acute hepatitis superimposed on cirrhosis

GENERAL PREVENTION
- Prevention of bacterial infections, particular of SBP
- Albumin (1.5 mg/kg IV at infection diagnosis and 1 g/kg IV 48 hours later) for patients with cirrhosis and SBP
- Primary SBP prophylaxis by oral norfloxacin
- Tumor necrosis factor inhibitor pentoxifylline (400 mg t.i.d.) for patients with severe alcoholic hepatitis

PATHOPHYSIOLOGY
- Portal hypertension/liver failure
- Splanchnic vasodilatation
- Reduction of effective circulating volume
- Stimulation of the renin-angiotensin system, sympathetic system and antidiuretic hormone
- Reduction in renal blood flow and GFR
- Intense sodium and dilutional hyponatremia
- Recent data indicate that a reduction in cardiac output plays a significant role.

ETIOLOGY
- Liver cirrhosis
- Acute alcoholic hepatitis

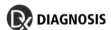 **DIAGNOSIS**

HISTORY
- Demonstration of reduced GFR (not easy in advance cirrhosis)
- Based on the exclusion of other disorder that can cause renal failure in cirrhosis
- Diagnostic criteria (International Ascites Club):
  - Cirrhosis with ascites
  - Serum creatinine >133 μmol/L (1.5 mg/dL)
  - No improvement of serum creatinine (decrease to level of <133μmol/L) after at least 2 days with diuretic withdrawal and volume expansion with albumin; recommended dose of albumin is 1 g/kg of body weight per day up to maximum of 100 g/d
  - Absence of shock
  - No current of recent treatment with nephrotoxic drugs.
  - Absence of parenchymal kidney disease as indicated by proteinuria >500 mg/d, microhematuria (>50 RBS per high-power field), and/or abnormal renal ultrasonography

PHYSICAL EXAM
- Type-1 HRS:
  - Severe and rapidly progressive renal failure
  - May arise spontaneously or in relationship with precipitating factors (especially patients with spontaneous bacterial peritonitis).
  - Type-1 HRS induced by SBP shows symptoms of rapid and severe deterioration of liver function (jaundice, coagulopathy, and hepatic encephalopathy)
  - Circulatory dysfunction (hypotension, very high level of plasma renin and norepinephrine)
- Type-2 HRS:
  - Moderate and slowly progressive renal failure
  - Severe refractory ascites is the dominant clinical feature.
  - Signs of liver failure and hypotension to lesser extent than in type-1 HRS

DIAGNOSTIC TESTS & INTERPRETATION
Diagnostic Procedures/Other
Lack of specific tests

Pathological Findings
No pathological changes in the renal tissue

DIFFERENTIAL DIAGNOSIS
- Prerenal renal failure: Diuretics or external fluid loss (renal function improves after volume expansion)
- Acute tubular necrosis (medical history of shock before the onset of renal failure, improvement of renal failure following antibiotic administration, or resolution of infection)
- Drug induced: Aminoglycosides, NSAIDs, vasodilators (rennin-angiotensin system inhibitors, prazosin, nitrates)
- Glomerulonephritis: Deposition of immunocomplexes in patients with hepatitis B and C, deposition of IgA in patients with alcoholic hepatitis (presents with proteinuria, hematuria, abnormal renal US: Small irregular kidney with abnormal echostructure).

TREATMENT

MEDICATION

- Type-1 HRS:
  - IV vasoconstrictors and albumin:
    - Type-1 HRS is reversible after treatment with IV albumin and vasoconstrictors
    - Terlipressin is the most widely used vasoconstrictor agent in type-1 HRS.
    - Terlipressin dosage should be progressive, starting with 0.5–1 mg q4–6h. If serum creatinine does not decrease by >30% in 3 days, the dose should be doubled.
    - The maximal dose of terlipressin has not been defined (patients who are not responding to 12 mg/d will not respond to higher dose)
    - Albumin should be given starting with a priming dose of 1 g/kg of body weight followed by 20–40 g/d.
    - Other options: Vasopressin, ornipressin, noradrenaline, combination of PO midodrine and IV or SC octreotide
    - In patients responding to therapy, treatment should be continued until normalization of serum creatinine (<1.5 mg/dL)
  - Extracorporeal albumin dialysis:
    - Molecular absorbents recirculating system (MARS) is a modified dialysis method using an albumin-containing dialysate that is recirculated and perfused online through serial charcoal anion exchanger columns.
    - When MARS was applied to the treatment of type-1 HRS, a possible benefit from this treatment was suggested as a consequence of removal of albumin-driven vasoactive substance such as nitric oxide, TNF, and other proinflammatory cytokines (2)
  - Transjugular intrahepatic portasystemic shunt.

- Type-2 HRS:
  - Treatment of this type of HRS should consider not only survival but also the control of ascites.
  - Transjugular intrahepatic portasystemic shunt
  - The current state of knowledge on vasoconstrictor therapy in type-2 HRS is very poor.
  - Hemodialysis

SURGERY/OTHER PROCEDURES

Orthotopic liver transplantation is the treatment of choice for any patient with advanced cirrhosis, including those with type-1 and type-2 HRS.

IN-PATIENT CONSIDERATIONS

Initial Stabilization

- Diagnosis and management of type-1 HRS require hospitalization.
- Patients with HRS respond poorly to diuretics.

 ONGOING CARE

PROGNOSIS

- Median survival in type-1 HRS without treatment is 2 weeks.
- Median survival of patients with type-2 HRS (6 months) is worse than that of patients with nonazotemic cirrhosis with ascites.
- 3-year survival of patients who undergo liver transplantation is 60%.

REFERENCES

1. Arroyo V, et al. Pathogenesis and treatment of hepatorenal syndrome. Review. *Semin Liver Dis*. 2008;28(1):81–95.
2. Angeli P, et al. Pathogenesis and management of hepatorenal syndrome. Review. *J Hepatol*. 2008;(Suppl 1):S93–103.

CODES

ICD9

- 572.4 Hepatorenal syndrome
- 997.4 Digestive system complications, not elsewhere classified

CLINICAL PEARLS

- There are 2 types of HRS: Type-1, severe and rapidly progressive renal failure, and type-2, moderate and steady development of renal failure.
- Orthotopic liver transplantation is the treatment of choice for any patient with advanced cirrhosis, including those with type-1 and type-2 HRS.

HERPES SIMPLEX VIRUS (HSV)

Francisco Bautista

 BASICS

DESCRIPTION
- HSV a very common viral infection caused by 2 DNA virus, HSV-1, HSV-2. This virus causes acute infections on the skin, invading and replicating itself in the neurons, as well as in epidermal and dermal cells. It usually manifested as a group of painful vesicles with an erythematous base.
- The most common is oral herpes, primarily caused by HSV-1.
- Genital herpes is usually caused by HSV-2; however, each type may cause infection in all areas.
- There are other conditions in which HSV manifests: Herpetic whitlow, herpes gladiatorum, ocular herpes, cerebral herpes infection, neonatal herpes, and possibly associated with Bell's palsy

EPIDEMIOLOGY
- Evidence suggests that infection with HSV-1 is more common and earlier than with HSV-2. By the 5th decade, 90% of people have antibodies against HSV-1.
- Only ~30% of individuals with HSV-1 have clinically apparent outbreaks. Even though the incidence of HSV-2 is much lower, the chances of manifesting the disease is higher.
- The lifetime seroprevalence can be 20–80% (1)

RISK FACTORS
- Everyone is at risk for oral herpes from HSV-1, which is easily transmitted. Most people with HSV-1 infection were first infected during childhood.
- All sexually active people are at risk for genital herpes.
- Women have a greater risk of being infected after sex with an unprotected partner than men do. Men, however, have twice the recurrences of women.
- People with compromised immune systems are at increased risk for severe form of the disease.

GENERAL PREVENTION
- Barrier methods, such as condoms, even when lesions are not visible. Condoms offer protection against genital herpes. However, it is limited because it does not prevent skin or bodily fluid contact.
- Vaccines for HSV are undergoing trials for the prevention and the treatment of existing infections. The NIH is conducting phase III clinical trial with Herpevac, which seems to be promising so far (2).
- Avoidance of known triggers for diminishing flare-ups like UV light or stressful situations may diminish the number of outbreaks.

Pregnancy Considerations
- During the last trimester of pregnancy, seronegative women should avoid sexual contact with a seropositive partner. If HSV lesions are suspected during labor, C-section is a must.
- Avoidance of known triggers of HSV recurrences such as UV light or stress may diminish the number of outbreaks.

PATHOPHYSIOLOGY
- HSV is double-stranded DNA virus that belongs to the Herpesviridae family.
- Both have latency and reactivation properties
- Infection occurs when a susceptible host is exposed to the virus and it penetrates through abraded skin or mucosal surfaces. During the 1st phase of infection, the virus replicates in the ganglia and nearby neuronal tissue. After that, virions can migrate fallowing the peripheral sensitive nerves (centrifuge migratory capacity).
- Histopathologic changes are due to cell necrosis, due to the inflammatory response this cytolytic virus produces.
- Most cellular changes include cell edema, inclusion internuclear bodies (Cowdry type A), chromatin marginalization, and the formation of multinucleated giant cells.

ETIOLOGY
- HSV-1 is transmitted through saliva while sharing personal items, kissing, and receiving oral sex from someone who has the infection. HSV-2 is sexually transmitted. Either type can be found in either the oral or genital area, and at other sites.
- The virus must get into the body through broken skin or a mucous membrane, but can also be carried in bodily fluids such as saliva, semen, and fluid in the female genital tract. Both can be contagious even if the infected person does not have active lesions.
- During pregnancy, a mother can pass the infection to the baby as it passes through the birth canal, especially if there is active infection at the time of delivery.

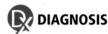 DIAGNOSIS

HISTORY
- Oral herpes:
  - Primary infection:
    - Prodrome of fever
    - Sore throat
    - Cervical or mandibular lymphadenopathy
    - Painful erythematous vesicles develop on the lips, gums, palate, or the tongue.
    - Duration: 2–3 weeks.
  - Recurrences:
    - Reactivation of HSV-1 occurs.
    - Preceded by pain, burning, itching sensation
    - Small, painful blisters filled with fluid around the lips or edge of the mouth
    - Last ~1 week
    - Common to see a gradual decrease in the recurrence rate, accompanied by a decrease in the clinic severity

- Genital herpes:
  - Primary infection:
    - Occurs within 2 days to 2 weeks after exposure
    - Men: Painful, erythematous, vesicular lesions that ulcerate most commonly occur on the penis, but can also occur on the anus and perineum
    - Women: Vesicular lesion that ulcerate on the cervix and painful vesicles on the external genitalia bilaterally, but can also occur on the vagina, perineum, buttocks, and legs in a sacral nerve distribution
    - Associated symptoms: Fever, malaise, edema, inguinal lymphadenopathy, dysuria, and vaginal or penile discharge
    - Duration: 2–3 weeks
  - Recurrences:
    - May be latent for months to years
    - Reactivation of HSV-2 in the lumbosacral ganglia leads to recurrences below the waist.
    - Recurrences are usually preceded by a prodrome of pain, itching, tingling, burning, or paresthesia on genitalia, buttocks, and thighs.

PHYSICAL EXAM
- Clinical infections appear as erythematous vesicles that often will progress to an ulcer that finally will form a crust. The lesions tend to recur at or near the same location within the distribution of a sensory nerve.
- In the 1st infection, systemic symptoms usually accompany the lesions.

DIFFERENTIAL DIAGNOSIS
- Aphthous stomatitis
- Chancroid
- Chicken pox
- Erythema multiforme
- Hand-foot-and-mouth disease
- Herpes zoster
- Syphilis

 ## TREATMENT

- There is no cure for herpes. Most infections are self-limited; however, antiviral medications can shorten and prevent outbreaks and transmission. It's very important to stat the treatment a soon as possible for it to be effective.
- Oral and genital herpes require episodic courses of oral antiviral medications such as acyclovir, valacyclovir, and famciclovir.
  - 1st episode mucocutaneous herpes simplex: 200 mg PO 5 times daily or 400 mg t.i.d. for 7–10 days or until clinical resolution occurs
  - Complicated HSV infections such as disseminated, neonatal HSV, or patients who are immunocompromised, require IV acyclovir.
  - Acyclovir-resistant HSV strains: IV foscarnet or cidofovir.

 ## ONGOING CARE

PROGNOSIS
Most people with HSV have acute infections that are temporary and resolve without sequelae, but these people are never completely rid of the virus.

COMPLICATIONS
- Long-term sequelae, such as visceral and CNS dissemination, are more common with neonatal HSV infection and in patients who are immunocompromised.
- Other complications include: Herpetic keratitis, persistent herpes infection, herpes infection in the esophagus, liver cirrhosis, encephalitis, and/or meningitis.

REFERENCES

1. Fleming DT, et al. Herpes simplex virus type 2 in the United States, 1976 to 1994. *N Engl J Med*. 1997;337(16):1105–11.
2. ClinicalTrials.gov. HerpeVac Trial for Young Women. Bethesda, MD: U.S. National Library of Medicine; retrieved 2008 Feb 25. Available from: http://clinicaltrials.gov/ct/show/NCT00057330.

 ## CODES

ICD9
- 054.6 Herpetic whitlow
- 054.9 Herpes simplex without mention of complication
- 054.10 Genital herpes, unspecified

H

HIGH-FREQUENCY OSILLATORY VENTILATION (HFOV)

Aly Hemdan Abdalla
Stephen M. Pastores

 BASICS

DESCRIPTION

- Unconventional mode of ventilation characterized by rapid delivery of small tidal volumes of gas and application of higher mean airway pressures than usually used in conventional mechanical ventilation
- May be used as rescue therapy in patients with acute respiratory distress syndrome (ARDS) when conventional mechanical ventilation (CMV) fails
- Use of HFOV has been associated with improvement in oxygenation but no survival benefit in adult ARDS patients (1)

PHYSIOLOGY

Mechanism of gas transport

Because tidal volumes (Vt) delivered by HFOV are often below the volume of dead space, mechanisms other than convectional bulk flow transport are invoked:

- Bulk flow of gas limited to large alveolar units close to proximal airways
- Augmented mixing of gas within the airway secondary to radial mixing of gas and difference in velocity profiles
- Asynchronous filling of adjacent alveolar spaces due to difference in alveolar emptying times, collateral ventilation, and pumping action of the heart
- Passive molecular diffusion of gas

Rationale for use

- Improve oxygenation while using less toxic levels of oxygen
- Maintain high mean airway pressures to help achieve and maintain lung recruitment
- Delivering small tidal volumes at a high rate helps avoiding cyclical lung recruitment and derecruitment

TECHNIQUE

- A piston pump oscillates at frequency of 180–600 breaths per minute (3–10 Hz)
- An inspiratory bias flow of fresh gas and a resistance valve are used to control mean airway pressure

Control of oxygenation

- Fraction of inspired oxygen (FIO_2)
- Mean air way pressure (Paw)

Control of ventilation

- Pressure amplitude (D P) of oscillation, which is a measurement created by the force that the piston moves and is controlled by adjusting the Power setting (increasing power will increase D P leading to increase in Vt)
- Respiratory frequency measured in Hertz (Hz) which is inversely related to tidal volumes (lower frequency result in higher Vt by increasing cycle time)
- Percentage inspiratory time (% I time) which if increased will result in longer time in forward motion and consequently increase tidal volumes

CLINICAL USE

Patient Selection

Consider HFOV in patients with ARDS who have failed CMV (low tidal volume ventilation according to the ARDS network protocol) as evident by either:

- Oxygenation failure: $FIO_2 \geq 0.7$ and positive end-expiratory pressure (PEEP) >14 cm H_2O or
- Ventilation failure: pH <7.25 with tidal volumes ≥ 6 mL/kg predicted ideal body weight and plateau airway pressure ≥ 30 cm H_2O

CONTRAINDICATIONS

- Severe air flow obstruction (e.g., severe asthma or chronic obstructive pulmonary disease)
- Intracranial hypertension
- HFOV may fail to improve oxygenation in burn patients with ARDS who have had smoke inhalation injury

INITIAL SETTINGS

- $FIO_2 = 1.0$
- Paw = 34 cm H_2O (or 3–5 cm H_2O higher than Paw on CMV)
- Bias flow = 30 (20–40 L/min)
- Amplitude (D P) = 60–90 cm H_2O, which correspond to Power setting of 4.0–6.0 (start lower and increase until you observe adequate chest wiggle from patient's clavicles to the mid-thighs)
- Frequency = 5 Hz (range of 3–7 Hz can be used according to the pH)
- % I time = 33%
- Increase Paw until you are able to decrease FIO_2 to 0.6 while maintaining oxygen saturation $>88\%$

RECRUITMENT MANEUVERS (RM)

Technique

- On initiation of HFOV and after each ventilator disconnect consider using RM to rapidly expand the lung and optimize oxygenation
- After turning off the piston and while closely monitoring patient's blood pressure and pulse oximetry apply Paw of 40 cm H_2O for 40 seconds

Contraindication

- Pneumothorax, hypotension, or active air leak

Precautions

- Terminate RM in case of hypotension or desaturation
- Do not repeat RM for 24 hours if previous attempt was terminated

GOALS

- Oxygen saturation = 88–94% on FIO_2 of <0.6
- pH = 7.25–7.35
- Avoid lung hyperinflation and hypotension.

ADJUSTING SETTINGS

Hypoxemia

- If FIO_2 of >0.6 is required to maintain oxygen saturation $>88\%$, consider the following:
  - Increase Paw in increments of 2–3 cm H_2O waiting 30 minutes between changes
  - Perform RM

Hypercapnia

- While frequency set at 5 Hz and adequate chest wiggle is present, increase D P by increasing the Power setting incrementally.
- If maximum Power settings are reached and hypercapnia persists, decrease frequency by 1 Hz decrements to a minimum of 3 Hz.
- Increase % I time toward 50%.
- Deflate endotracheal tube (ETT) cuff.
- Allow permissive hypercapnia.
- Consider bicarbonate infusion.

ROLE OF ADJUNCTIVE THERAPIES

If patients remain hypoxemic during HFOV, one or more of the following measures can improve oxygenation:

- Nitric oxide (NO)
  - Inhaled NO applied at a rate of 5–20 parts per minute
- Prone positioning
- Recruitment maneuvers (RM)

FAILURE OF HFOV

Criteria

- Inability to decrease FIO_2 by 10% within the first 24 hours using maximum settings
- Inability to improve or maintain ventilation and pH at safe levels after optimizing both amplitude and frequency

Action

- Use adjuvant therapies for oxygenation failure.
- Return to CMV.

WEANING AND TRANSITION TO CMV

Criteria

- Stable FIO_2 of <0.6.
- Stable arterial blood gases

Action

- Gradually decrease Paw by 2 cm H_2O decrements until reaching a stable level of 22 cm H_2O or less while maintaining $FIO_2 <0.5$.
- Assess patient for tolerance of suctioning, changes in position and manual ventilation
- Switch to CMV (e.g., tidal volume 6 mL/kg, PEEP of 10 cm H_2O).

ONGOING CARE

MONITORING
- Oxygen saturation should be closely monitored especially initially and when FIO_2 is changed.
- Heart rate and blood pressure should be monitored for any hemodynamic compromise.
- Chest wiggle should be closely monitored at initiation and thereafter.
  - Absent or diminished chest wiggle bilaterally is a sign of airway or ETT obstruction.
  - Absent chest wiggle on one side only is an indication that the ETT has moved into a main bronchus or pneumothorax has occurred.
- Auscultation is challenging due to continuous chest wall movement and the noise produced by the ventilator:
  - Stop the piston while maintaining Paw and listen for heart sounds.
  - Disconnection from the ventilator should be avoided as it may result in loss of lung volume and desaturation.
  - Assess breath sounds by listening to the intensity of the sound produced by the piston throughout the chest as it should be equal.
- ABG should be obtained 30–60 minutes after initiation of HFOV and after any change in Paw, amplitude, or frequency.
- Chest x-rays should be obtained 1 hour after initiation of HFOV to evaluate the level of lung inflation.

PATIENT CARE
Suctioning
- Use of closed in-line suctioning is recommended to avoid disconnection and de-recruitment
- Suctioning should be performed if there is decrease in chest wiggle, desaturation or change in delta P

Positioning
- Repositioning of the patient should be minimized during the first 24 hours of HFOV
- Head of bed should be elevated to 30 degrees
- Prone position is possible if indicated
- Following repositioning, patient should be assessed regarding oxygen saturation, chest wiggle, ETT position, and ventilator parameters.

Sedation and NM Blockade
- Deep sedation or paralysis (only if deep sedation fails) may be needed to avoid discomfort resulting from inadequate bias flow to meet the demands of a spontaneously breathing ARDS patient.
- Spontaneous respiratory efforts during HFOV may result in large pressure swings which may be sensed by the ventilator as circuit disconnect resulting in oscillation cessation.

Transport
- Transporting a patient on HFOV is challenging and should be avoided unless it is critically needed for ongoing management
- Transport on HFOV can be achieved using a battery transport system and a compressed gas system
- Switching to CMV or manual resuscitation bag is an alternative that can be achieved by clamping the ETT while on HFOV, attaching the bag or the transport ventilator to the ETT, and then removing the clamp to maintain alveolar recruitment.

Procedures
- Central venous catheterization:
  - Femoral vein is the preferred site
  - Subclavian or internal jugular vein catheterization, if necessary, can be attempted after stopping the piston to discontinue oscillation while maintaining Paw and consequently oxygenation
- Fiberoptic bronchoscopy is problematic and require HFOV removal and manual ventilation

Aerosol Medication Delivery
- Metered-dose inhalers are ineffective during HFOV but can be administrated via manual bag ventilation
- Flow-driven nebulizers may be more effective but require titration of Paw and delta P owing to the additional flow
- IV terbutaline is an alternative

Infection Control
- Higher infection control risk than CMV due to dispersal of vented gas from the Paw control diaphragm
- According to diagnosis, negative pressure room or personal protective equipment may be required

TECHNICAL ASPECTS
Alarms
- Visual and auditory alarms:
  - If Paw exceeds 60 or drops below 5 cm H_2O which prompt the oscillator to stop
  - If Paw falls outside a set minimum and maximum limit (usually set 5 cm H_2O above and below the selected Paw)
  - Power failure
- Visual alarm only:
  - Oscillator overheated
  - Low battery
  - Low gas source

Circuit Changes
Regular circuit changes are not needed as it requires temporary disconnection

Humidification
- Achieved by passing bias flow over a conventional heated humidifier
- Confirmed by observing condensation in the ETT and inspiratory tubing

COMPLICATIONS
Hypotension
- Secondary to decrease venous return due to increase Paw
- Can be exacerbated by presence of hypovolemia
- Administer fluid boluses and vasopressors if necessary

Pneumothorax
- Can manifest classically with hypotension, tachycardia, desaturation, tracheal deviation, and asymmetry of chest wall
- Acute asymmetry of chest wiggle and acute changes in Paw may indicate a pneumothorax

Endotrachial tube obstruction or migration
- Migration to the mainstem bronchus should be suspected if chest wiggle decreased unilaterally
- Bilateral cessation or decrease in chest wiggle may indicate ETT obstruction and need for suctioning

REFERENCES

1. Wunsch H, et al. High-frequency ventilation versus conventional ventilation for the treatment of acute respiratory distress syndrome: a systematic review and Cochrane analysis. *Anesth Analg.* 2005;100(6): 1765–72.
2. Mehta S, et al. Implementing and troubleshooting high-frequency oscillatory ventilation in adults in the intensive care unit. *Respir Care Clin N Am.* 2001;7:683–95.
3. Chan K, et al. High-frequency oscillatory ventilation for adult patients with ARDS. *Chest.* 2007;131: 1907–16.
4. Rose L. High-frequency oscillatory ventilation in adults, clinical considerations and management priorities. *AACN Adv Crit Care.* 2008;19(4): 412–20.
5. Fessler HE, et al. A protocol for high-frequency oscillatory ventilation in adults: results from a roundtable discussion. *Crit Care Med.* 2007; 35(7):1649–54.

 ## CODES

ICD9
518.5 Pulmonary insufficiency following trauma and surgery

H

CLINICAL PEARLS

- HFOV is a lung-protective ventilatory strategy that is being increasingly used for adult patients with ARDS who remain hypoxemic during conventional ventilation.
- HFOV delivers small tidal volumes at very high respiratory rates and utilizes higher mean airway pressures to facilitate lung recruitment and prevent derecruitment.
- Familiarity with the equipment and its unique features is mandatory for successful implementation and troubleshooting.
- Future trials are needed to determine whether earlier initiation of HFOV might improve outcomes and which subgroups of ARDS patients might derive greater benefit.

HIV IN THE ICU

Parul Kaushik

 BASICS

DESCRIPTION

- Human immunodeficiency virus (HIV) weakens cell-mediated immunity by decreasing CD4 + helper T cells.
- HIV patients are admitted to ICU for the management of either opportunistic infections (OI) such as *Pneumocystis* pneumonia (PCP), cryptococcal meningitis, and toxoplasmosis; adverse effects of highly active antiretroviral therapy (HAART) or as a result of medical or surgical conditions unrelated to HIV.
- Management of antiretroviral drugs could be challenging in ICU due to their numerous side effects and drug–drug interactions.
- Respiratory failure, bacterial pneumonia, and sepsis are the leading causes of ICU admission in this population.

EPIDEMIOLOGY
Incidence
- ~4–5 % of hospitalized HIV-positive patients are admitted to the ICU.
- 40% of HIV-positive patients admitted to the ICU are unaware of their diagnosis.
- With the widespread use of HAART, ICU mortality in HIV patients has improved significantly in the last 2 decades.
- The incidence of Kaposi sarcoma and CNS lymphoma has decreased in the HAART era, but the incidence of non-CNS B-cell lymphoma, unusual tumors related to human herpes virus 8 and other solid tumors are increasing in this population.
- There is an increased incidence of cardiovascular disease and osteoporosis in HIV patients.
- Blacks and Hispanics have the highest incidence of HIV in the U.S.

Prevalence
With ~1.2 million people living with HIV/AIDS in North America, ICUs in the U.S. see a considerably large number of HIV patients.

RISK FACTORS
- Men who have sex with men
- IV drug users
- Sex workers
- Children born to HIV positive mothers

GENERAL PREVENTION
- Awareness
- Avoiding unprotected sex
- Antiretroviral use
- Timely OI chemoprophylaxis

PATHOPHYSIOLOGY
- Following infection, HIV is localized in the lymphoid organs where it attacks CD4-positive helper T lymphocytes.
- The envelope of HIV contains glycoprotein spikes gp120 and gp41 that bind with the host surface receptors CD4, CCR5, and CXCR4.
- After entering the host cell, HIV produces enzyme reverse transcriptase that enables transcription of genomic RNA to proviral DNA that integrates into the host cell DNA.
- Viremia is seen soon after contracting HIV infection followed by a progressive depletion of CD4 + T cells with continuous viral replication.

ETIOLOGY
- HIV is an enveloped single-stranded RNA virus.
- There are 2 HIV viruses: HIV 1 and HIV 2. HIV 1 is found globally, and HIV 2 is mainly confined to Western Africa.
- *Streptococcus pneumoniae* is overall the most common cause of bacterial pneumonia in HIV patients.
- Depending on the geographical location and CD4 count, disseminated *Histoplasma capsulatum* and *Coccidioides immitis* can be seen.
- *Mycobacterium avium-intracellulare* (MAI) is seen with CD4 counts <50.

COMMONLY ASSOCIATED CONDITIONS
- HIV patients may be co-infected with hepatitis B or C due to their common risk factors.
- HIV patients with hep B co-infection on therapy should have their treatment continued in the ICU as severe flare due to hep B are seen if treatment is stopped abruptly.

DIAGNOSIS

HISTORY
- Depending on the illness, HIV patients can present with variable clinical signs and symptoms.
- Knowing the recent CD4 count may aid in making the diagnosis, as most of the OIs occur with lower CD4 counts.
- PCP presents with a subacute illness characterized by dry cough, fever, and shortness of breath.
- Cryptococcal meningitis presents with long-standing headaches and fever.
- CNS toxoplasmosis and primary CNS lymphoma presents with headache and focal sensory or motor deficit.
- Disseminated MAI infection presents with fever, weight loss, and chronic diarrhea.
- Some older nucleoside reverse transcriptase inhibitors (NRTI) may present with abdominal pain, nausea, vomiting, myalgia, and peripheral neuropathies due to lactic acidosis.
- Abacavir can cause a nonspecific hypersensitivity reaction presenting with fever, abdominal pain, nausea, and vomiting.

PHYSICAL EXAM
- Molluscoid skin lesions in cryptococcosis.
- Meningeal signs are often absent in cryptococcal meningitis.
- Rash may be seen with abacavir and some nonnucleoside reverse transcriptase inhibitors (NNRTI).
- Lymphadenopathy and hepatosplenomegaly is seen with MAI.

DIAGNOSTIC TESTS & INTERPRETATION
Lab
Initial lab tests
- CBC: Pancytopenia may be seen in advanced HIV disease. Zidovudine causes anemia.
- CMP: Elevated BUN/creatinine may be due to HIV associated nephropathy, co-morbidities such as hypertension, diabetes, or drugs such as tenofovir. Elevated liver enzymes may be seen with hep B or hep C co-infection.
- High LDH and hypoxemia on arterial blood gas is seen with PCP.
- High serum lactate is seen with some NRTIs such as stavudine and didanosine.
- Serum toxoplasma IgG antibody and serum cryptococcal antigen as clinically indicated.
- High amylase and lipase may be seen with didanosine, stavudine, and zalcitabine.

Follow-Up & Special Considerations
- Nevirapine can cause fulminant liver failure in patients with higher CD4 count.
- Stavudine can cause acute liver failure with high mortality.

Imaging
Initial approach
- Chest x-ray: diffuse bilateral infiltrates in PCP.
- Head CT or brain MRI may show ring-enhancing lesions suggestive of CNS toxoplasmosis or primary CNS lymphoma.
- Brain MRI may show white matter lesions in Progressive multifocal leukoencephalopathy (PML).

Follow-Up & Special Considerations
Based on the abnormality of initial Imaging

Diagnostic Procedures/Other
- Bronchoalveolar lavage for PCP.
- Lumbar puncture (LP): A high opening pressure, low glucose, high protein, and positive CSF cryptococcal antigen in cryptococcal meningitis.
- Stereotactic brain biopsy for CNS lymphoma.
- Funduscopy for cytomegalovirus (CMV) retinitis: perivascular fluffy infiltrates with hemorrhages.

Pathological Findings
Pneumocystis jiroveci may be seen with Gomori methenamine silver or Giemsa stain on Bronchoalveolar lavage.

DIFFERENTIAL DIAGNOSIS
- CNS toxoplasmosis may be difficult to distinguish from primary CNS lymphoma.
- PCP and atypical bacterial pneumonia may present similarly.
- Both MAI and CMV colitis may present with diarrhea.

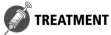 **TREATMENT**

MEDICATION
First Line
- Trimethoprim-sulfamethoxazole, PO or IV with or without steroids for PCP.
- Amphotericin B deoxycholate and flucytosine for cryptococcal meningitis.
- Pyrimethamine/sulfamethoxazole for CNS toxoplasmosis.
- Clarithromycin, ethambutol, and rifabutin for MAI.
- Intraocular or IV ganciclovir for CMV.

Second Line
- IV pentamidine or clindamycin and Primaquine or Atovaquone for PCP.
- Fluconazole for cryptococcal meningitis.
- Fluoroquinolone for MAI.

ADDITIONAL TREATMENT
General Measures
Airway protection and hemodynamic stability.

Pregnancy Considerations
- Pregnant women should be on HAART irrespective of their CD4 count to prevent perinatal transmission.
- Efavirenz, a NNRTI is a class D pregnancy drug.

Issues for Referral
- Infectious Diseases consult is recommended.
- When in doubt, ART should be stopped and HIV specialist or pharmacist should be consulted.

Additional Therapies
- Persistence of symptoms in cryptococcal meningitis requires frequent or daily LPs.
- Corticosteroids may be used for HIV associated nephropathy.
- Riboflavin, thiamine, and L-carnitine may reverse toxicity of lactic acidosis associated with some NRTIs.
- Early institution of HAART may reverse HIV associated nephropathy.

COMPLEMENTARY & ALTERNATIVE THERAPIES
- HIV/hep C co-infected patients with liver failure may be candidates for orthotropic liver transplant.
- End-stage renal disease patients with HIV may need dialysis or renal transplant.

IN-PATIENT CONSIDERATIONS
Initial Stabilization
Airway protection, circulatory support.

Admission Criteria
Severe symptoms, biochemical abnormalities, and advanced HIV disease

IV Fluids
As per protocol if patient does not tolerate PO

Nursing
Mild disease from OI's can be monitored in general wards. If complications or worsening of symptoms leading to organ failure develops, intensive care monitoring may be needed.

Discharge Criteria
Resolution of symptoms

 ONGOING CARE

FOLLOW-UP RECOMMENDATIONS
- Patients need to follow up with HIV specialist for further care.
- Patient with CMV retinitis should follow with an ophthalmologist.

DIET
Continued nutrition is essential to promote recovery.

PATIENT EDUCATION
- Consistent condom use
- Adherence to ART (see General Prevention)

PROGNOSIS
Admission to ICU due to non–AIDS-related diagnosis has better prognosis than those with HIV-/AIDS-related illness

COMPLICATIONS
- ARDS and pneumothorax with PCP.
- Bacteremia due to *Streptococcus pneumoniae*.
- Cranial nerve deficit and hydrocephalus with cryptococcal meningitis.
- Focal neurological deficit and coma with CNS toxoplasmosis.
- Blindness can occur with CMV retinitis.

REFERENCES
1. Corona A, et al. Caring for HIV-infected patients in the ICU in the highly active antiretroviral therapy era. *Curr HIV Res*. 2009;7(6):569–79.
2. Sharma SK, et al. Management of the patient with HIV disease. *Disease-a-Month*. 2008;54(3): 162–95.
3. Henry M. Management of patients with HIV in the intensive care unit. *Proc Am Thorac Soc*. 2006;3(1): 96–102.

ADDITIONAL READING
- http://www.cdc.gov/hiv
- http://aidsinfo.nih.gov

 CODES

ICD9
- 042 Human immunodeficiency virus (hiv) disease
- 136.3 Pneumocystosis
- 321.0 Cryptococcal meningitis

CLINICAL PEARLS
- All NRTIs except abacavir require dose adjustment with renal failure.
- Protease inhibitors and NNRTIs are metabolized by the cytochrome p-450 enzyme system.
- Immune Reconstitution Syndrome (IRIS) is paradoxical worsening of symptoms or new OIs few days after the initiation of HAART and may require treatment with steroids.
- The decision to continue HAART in the ICU patients should be made after assessing their risks and benefits in a particular case.
- Early initiation of HAART in case of PCP pneumonia has shown to decrease mortality.

H

HYPERCALCEMIA

Tzvi Y. Neuman
Roopa Kohli-Seth

 BASICS

DESCRIPTION
Elevated serum calcium level of >10.5 mg/dL due to disordered calcium flux into the extracellular compartment or because of hyperparathyroidism:
- Mild or chronic: Serum calcium level <12 mg/dL
- Moderate to severe: Serum calcium level 12–14 mg/dL
- Severe: Serum calcium levels >14 mg/dL

PATHOPHYSIOLOGY
- Normal calcium homeostasis is under control of parathyroid hormone (PTH), leading to bone resorption, increased renal reabsorption or decreased renal excretion of calcium, increased gut uptake of calcium, synthesis of calcitriol (1,25-dihydroxyvitamin D), and conversion of 25-hydroxyvitamin D to calcitriol.
- Disordered flux of calcium into the extracellular compartment when normal calcium homeostasis is disrupted via:
  - Increased calcitriol: Granulomatous disorders despite low PTH levels
  - Increased bone resorption:
    ○ Metastasis mediated local osteolytic damage
    ○ Humoral hypercalcemia due to tumor secreted parathyroid hormone-related peptide (PTH-rP), or via tumor related hydroxylation of 25-hydroxyvitamin D to calcitriol
- Hyperparathyroidism: Elevated PTH leading to hypercalcemia and hypophosphatemia:
  - Primary: Single functional adenoma, 4-gland hyperplasia, or parathyroid cancer
  - Tertiary: Seen in chronic kidney disease with chronic PTH stimulation due to low serum calcium or decreased calcitriol via negative feedback

ETIOLOGY
- Increased bone resorption:
  - Hyperparathyroidism
    ○ Primary: Adenoma, hyperplasia, or cancer
    ○ Tertiary
  - Multiple endocrine neoplasia (MEN) type I or IIA
  - Malignancy related: Squamous cell cancer via PTH-rP secretion
  - Metastatic disease to bone in breast or prostate cancer
  - Hyperthyroidism
  - Immobilization
  - Paget disease
  - Pregnancy or lactation-mediated release of PTH-rP
- Decreased renal excretion:
  - Thiazide diuretics
  - Familial hypocalciuric hypercalcemia

- Increased gut absorption:
  - Increased PO intake of calcium:
    ○ Milk alkali syndrome
  - Renal failure patients taking vitamin D supplements
  - Granulomatous disease:
    ○ Sarcoidosis
    ○ Leprosy
    ○ Tuberculosis
    ○ Berylliosis
    ○ Histoplasmosis
    ○ Silicosis
    ○ Disseminated candidiasis
    ○ Wegener, brucellosis
    ○ Cat-scratch disease
    ○ Talc granulomatosis
    ○ Hodgkin disease or non-Hodgkin's lymphoma
  - Pharmaceutically induced:
    ○ Thiazide diuretics
    ○ Estrogen or antiestrogen therapy in breast cancer
    ○ Use of topical calcipotriol
    ○ Hypervitaminosis A
    ○ Hypervitaminosis D
- May also be associated with:
  - Pheochromocytoma
  - Adrenal insufficiency
  - Rhabdomyolysis
  - Coccidiomycosis

COMMONLY ASSOCIATED CONDITIONS
Primary hyperparathyroidism, ESRD, granulomatous disease or malignancy:
- Most common outpatient cause is primary hyperparathyroidism
- Most common inpatient cause is malignancy-related (breast cancer, lung cancer, or multiple myeloma are most common)

℞ DIAGNOSIS

HISTORY
May complain of different symptoms
- CNS: Malaise, fatigue, depression, confusion, coma, sweating, tremors or decreased pain threshold
- Cardiovascular: Palpitations
- Pulmonary: Cough
- GI: Nausea, vomiting, anorexia, constipation, or recent weight loss
- Heme: Easy bruising
- Renal: Increased thirst, polyuria, nocturia, hematuria, or flank pain
- Musculoskeletal: Bone pain

PHYSICAL EXAM
- Neuro: Depression, confusion, poor cognition, or coma
- Cardiovascular: Hypertension, arrhythmia
- GI: Abdominal tenderness, distended abdomen, hematemesis, melena or evidence of visceral perforation
- Renal: Costovertebral tenderness, hematuria secondary to stones, or dilute urine
- Oncology: Masses or lymphadenopathy
- Musculoskeletal: Bone tenderness or pathologic fractures
- Skin: Erythema nodosum (suggestive of sarcoidosis or tuberculosis)

DIAGNOSTIC TESTS & INTERPRETATION
Lab
Initial lab tests
- Repeat serum calcium level to confirm
- Check serum albumin to correct the calcium:
  - [Measured total Ca mg/dL] + 0.8 (4.0 − [serum albumin g/dL])
- Measure intact PTH level:
  - Elevated in hyperparathyroidism; decreased in other pathology
- Check 24-hour urine for calcium excretion:
  - High in primary hyperparathyroidism, malignancy-related, or excess vitamin D; low in diuretic-related, milk alkali syndrome, or familial hypocalciuric hypercalcemia
- Need to check age- and sex-appropriate malignancy screen; check PTH-rP
- May need to rule out sarcoidosis, tuberculosis, or other granulomatous disease
- If PTH and PTH-rP are low, check 25-hydroxyvitamin D and 1,25-dihydroxyvitamin D levels.
- Check CBC, serum electrolytes, serum phosphate, BUN and creatinine, serum alkaline phosphatase.
- Thyroid function studies
- Check serum electrophoresis.
- Check urine for protein spillage; consider checking for Bence-Jones proteins.

Follow-Up & Special Considerations
- Follow-up with specialist for the underlying pathology (endocrinology, oncology, or nephrology, and possibly surgery)
- Avoid thiazide diuretics.

Imaging
Initial approach
- Chest x-ray
- ECG: Check for shortened QT interval.
- Skeletal survey
- Bone scan
- Consider DEXA scan

Follow-Up & Special Considerations
- Sestamibi scan or US to localize isolated adenoma
- May consider CT or MRI to localize parathyroid adenomas
- Other malignancy-appropriate workup as needed

Diagnostic Procedures/Other
May require tissue biopsy of underlying pathologic organ

Pathological Findings
Tissue biopsy may show malignancy (solid organ or blood related), parathyroid disease (adenoma, hyperplasia or cancer), or granulomatous disease.

DIFFERENTIAL DIAGNOSIS
- Malignancy
- Hyperparathyroidism (primary or tertiary)
- Thyrotoxicosis
- Granulomatous disease
- Immobilization
- Use of TPN
- Chronic kidney disease
- Medication induced

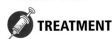 TREATMENT

Urgent treatment is required if serum calcium is >14 mg/dL or if patient is symptomatic with serum calcium >12 mg/dL.

MEDICATION
First Line

Bisphosphonate therapy (1)[A], to block bone resorption; most effective in malignancy-related hypercalcemia:

- Pamidronate, single infusion: 30 mg for calcium <12 mg/dL; 60 mg for calcium 12–13.5 mg/dL; 90 mg for calcium >13.5 mg/dL
- Zoledronate: 4 mg IV or 8 mg IV for relapse or refractory hypercalcemia, or for use in patients with bone metastases (2)[A]
- Side effects include fever, arthralgia, myalgia, fatigue, bone pain, uveitis, hypocalcemia, hypophosphatemia, impaired renal function, nephrotic syndrome, or osteonecrosis of the jaw.

Second Line

- Calcitonin 200 IU SQ or IV q8–12h for up to 2 days (1)[A]:
  - Rapidly decreases serum calcium by inhibiting osteoclast mediated bone resorption; may result in tachyphylaxis.
- Hydrocortisone: 100 mg q8–12h (1)[A]:
  - Decreases gut absorption and reduces extrarenal calcitriol
- Plicamycin (mithramycin): 25 mcg/kg IV over 4–6 hours daily
- Gallium nitrate may be used to inhibit osteoclastic bone resorption and PTH secretion:
  - Works for PTH-rP and non-PTH-rP hypercalcemia

ADDITIONAL TREATMENT
Additional Therapies
- Hemodialysis with low calcium dialysate may be necessary in severe symptomatic hypercalcemia unresponsive to pharmacotherapy.
- Chloroquine 250 mg q12h for sarcoidosis-related hypercalcemia; blocks peripheral production of calcitriol
- Ketoconazole can be used for calcitriol-induced hypercalcemia.
- Cinacalcet is a calcimimetic that mimics high levels of calcium and acts on calcium-sensitive receptors to decrease PTH secretion; it may be used in patients with primary hyperparathyroidism and symptomatic hypercalcemia who are unable to go to surgery (1)[B].

SURGERY/OTHER PROCEDURES
May require removal of parathyroid adenoma or hyperplastic parathyroid glands (1)[A]:

- Criteria for removal:
  - Age <50 years
  - Symptomatic primary hyperparathyroidism: Nephrolithiasis, lethargy, and fatigue
  - Serum calcium 1 mg/dL greater than the upper limits of normal
  - Urine calcium excretion >400 mg/d
  - Creatinine clearance reduction by >30%
  - DEXA scan T-score -2.5 at any major site

IN-PATIENT CONSIDERATIONS
Initial Stabilization

- Saline infusion to maintain urine output 250–300 cc/hr and restore euvolemia (1)[B]:
  - Calcium is resorbed together with sodium in the kidney; by decreasing sodium resorption, more calcium will be cleared.
  - Must monitor patient's volume and electrolyte status
  - Only effective for short-term treatment
- Stop all calcium and vitamin D preparations.
- Correct the underlying pathology.

IV Fluids

- Saline to maintain intravascular volume (1)[B]
- Furosemide to induce kaliuresis; its use in conjunction with saline therapy is controversial (3,4)[C], but may be considered after adequate volume expansion.

 ONGOING CARE

DIET
- Ensure adequate PO hydration.
- Calcium intake may need to be limited in milk alkali syndrome and hypervitaminosis D; avoid low-calcium diet in primary hyperparathyroidism.
- Vitamin D may need to be restricted.
- Avoid excessive vitamin A.
- Adequate phosphate intake is necessary.

PROGNOSIS
Depends on the underlying pathology; very poor when associated with malignancy

COMPLICATIONS
- Osteoporosis
- Nephrolithiasis
- Renal failure
- CNS dysfunction which may result in confusion, dementia or coma
- Arrhythmia

REFERENCES
1. Kahn A. Hypercalcemia. Physicians' Information and Educational Resource 2009. Retrieved from http://pier.acponline.org/physicians/diseases
2. Berenson JR. Recommendations for zoledronic acid treatment of patients with bone metastases. *Oncologist*. 2005;10:52–62.
3. LeGrand SB, et al. Narrative review: Furosemide for hypercalcemia: An unproven yet common practice. *Ann Intern Med*. 2008;149:259–63.
4. Stewart AF. Clinical practice. Hypercalcemia associated with cancer. *N Engl J Med*. 2005;352: 373–9.

ADDITIONAL READING
- Carrol MF, et al. A practical approach to hypercalcemia. *Am Fam Phys*. 2003;67:1959–66.
- Moe SM. Disorders involving calcium, phosphorus, and magnesium. *Prim Care Clin Office Pract*. 2008;35:215–37.
- Ralston SH, et al. Medical management of hypercalcemia: Review. *Calcif Tissue Int*. 2004;74:1–11.

 CODES

ICD9
- 252.00 Hyperparathyroidism, unspecified
- 275.42 Hypercalcemia

CLINICAL PEARLS
- Initiate treatment with large-volume saline infusion to ensure adequate intravascular volume.
- Use bisphosphonate therapy to decrease serum calcium; may need to add 2nd-line therapy.
- Correctly diagnose and treat the underlying pathology.

H

HYPERCALCEMIA, ACUTE

Urvashi Vaid
Paul E. Marik

 BASICS

DESCRIPTION
Hypercalcemia is defined as an increase in serum calcium >1 mg/mL above the normal range (8.5–10.2 mg/dL or 2.2–2.5 mmol/L):
- Mild hypercalcemia: 10.2–11.9 mg/dL
- Moderate hypercalcemia: 12–13.9 mg/dL
- Severe hypercalcemia: ≥14 mg/dL

EPIDEMIOLOGY
Incidence
- The most common cause of asymptomatic hypercalcemia in an outpatient setting is primary hyperparathyroidism.
- The most common cause of inpatient hypercalcemia is malignancy.
- 20–30% of patients with cancer have hypercalcemia at some point in the course of their disease.

Prevalence
Primary hyperparathyroidism and malignancy associated hypercalcemia account for >90% of causes.

RISK FACTORS
- Malignancy is the single most important risk factor.
- Primary hyperparathyroidism can coexist with cancer in up to 15%.
- The most common cancers associated with hypercalcemia are:
  - Breast
  - Squamous-cell cancer (head and neck, esophagus, cervix, or lung)
  - Renal
  - Ovarian/endometrial
  - HTLV-associated lymphoma
  - Multiple myeloma
  - Lymphoma

Genetics
- Familial hypocalciuric hypercalcemia:
  - Autosomal dominant
  - Loss-of-function mutation in calcium-sensing receptor in parathyroid and renal cells resulting in insensitivity to calcium levels
- MEN I and IIA
- Metaphyseal chondrodysplasia:
  - Dwarfism with hypercalcemia and hyperphosphatemia
  - Mutation in parathyroid hormone (PTH)-related protein receptor gene

GENERAL PREVENTION
- With the advent of outpatient chemistry panels measuring calcium levels routinely, patients with mild hypercalcemia are being detected more frequently.
- The presence of a malignancy should trigger monitoring of calcium levels.

PATHOPHYSIOLOGY
- Calcium exists as 3 forms in plasma: Biologically inert bound to albumin (55%) or to other proteins/nonproteins and the biologically active ionized form (45%).
- Calcium concentrations are regulated by the interplay among PTH, calcitonin, and vitamin D:
  - PTH increases serum calcium by increasing bone resorption, decreasing renal excretion, and increasing renal production of 1,25-dihydroxyvitamin D.
  - 1,25-dihydroxyvitamin D in turn increases intestinal calcium and phosphate absorption.
  - PTH also decreases serum phosphate concentrations by increasing its renal excretion.
  - A calcium-sensing receptor on the parathyroid gland provides a negative feedback loop.
  - Calcitonin secreted by parafollicular thyroid cells opposes the actions of PTH.
- Hypercalcemia can thus result from increased PTH secretion, increased vitamin D levels, insensitivity of the calcium-sensing receptor, or rarely, decreased calcitonin.
- Malignancy associated hypercalcemia results from any of four mechanisms:
  - Local osteolytic hypercalcemia from increased osteoclastic resorption of bone surrounding malignant cells in the bone marrow
  - Humoral hypercalcemia of malignancy (HHM) caused by secretion of PTH-related protein (PTHrP) from the cancer cells
  - Secretion of the active form of vitamin D
  - Ectopic secretion of PTH, which is very rare

ETIOLOGY
- Hyperparathyroidism:
  - Primary: Most common cause is a parathyroid adenoma (85%)
  - Tertiary: From autonomous parathyroid glands in end-stage renal disease
- Genetic syndromes as outlined above
- Hypercalcemia of malignancy
- Chronic granulomatous disease from increased production of active vitamin D
- Drug-induced:
  - Vitamin D intoxication
  - Lithium
  - Thiazide diuretics
  - Vitamin A toxicity
  - Theophylline
- Others:
  - Endocrine disorders (hyperthyroidism, acromegaly, adrenal insufficiency, phaeochromocytoma)
  - Immobilization
  - TPN
  - Milk-alkali syndrome (from excess calcium carbonate ingestion)

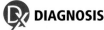 **DIAGNOSIS**

HISTORY
- Mild hypercalcemia may be asymptomatic or have nonspecific symptoms like constipation, fatigue, or depression.
- The rate of rise of serum calcium, as well as the level it rises to, is important.
- Neuropsychiatric symptoms:
  - Range from cognitive dysfunction to lethargy, confusion, stupor, and coma
  - More severe if the rate of rise of serum calcium is higher and in elderly patients
- GI symptoms:
  - Anorexia, nausea, and constipation
  - Peptic ulcer disease from calcium-mediated increase in gastrin secretion
  - Pancreatitis from deposition of calcium in ducts
- Cardiovascular symptoms:
  - Arrhythmias are rare.
  - Chronic hypercalcemia can cause hypertension and cardiomyopathy
- Renal symptoms:
  - Polyuria from a defect in concentration at the tubular level (nephrogenic diabetes insipidus) resulting in increased thirst and then dehydration
  - Pain from nephrolithiasis
- Musculoskeletal symptoms:
  - Weakness
  - Bone pain

PHYSICAL EXAM
- The physical exam may be nonspecific and related to the underling diagnosis rather than hypercalcemia.
- Acute hypercalcemia usually presents with signs of dehydration and alteration of mental status.

DIAGNOSTIC TESTS & INTERPRETATION
Lab
Initial lab tests
- Hypercalcemia must be confirmed by ionized calcium measurements as albumin affects values of total but not ionized calcium (total serum calcium falls 0.8 mg/dL for every 1 g/dL reduction in serum albumin).
- Intact PTH levels help aid in the diagnosis, with high levels indicating primary hyperparathyroidism and low levels indicating other causes.
- Levels of PTHrP can be measured but are usually unnecessary in the clinical scenario of malignancy.
- Plasma 1,25 dihydroxyvitamin D levels may be useful in sarcoidosis or other granulomatous disorders.
- An EKG may show shortened QTc from shortening of the myocardial action potential, and there have been reports of ST segment elevation and arrhythmias, although uncommon.

Follow-Up & Special Considerations
Acid–base status should be assessed as acidosis increases ionized calcium levels.

Imaging
- CT brain or MRI for alteration of mental status
- Renal imaging with US or CT scan for nephrolithiasis
- Sestamibi scan with technetium-99m with SPECT scanning to localize parathyroid adenomas in primary hyperparathyroidism
- Bone scan for metastatic disease causing hypercalcemia

 TREATMENT
MEDICATION
First Line
- Rehydration and calciuresis:
  - Normal saline 200–500 mL/hour
  - Guided clinically by volume status and evidence of fluid overload and cardiovascular status
  - Use of loop diuretics is controversial and should not be used until volume resuscitation is complete.
- IV bisphosphonates:
  - Block osteoclastic bone resorption
  - Superior to all other modes of treatment
  - Pamidronate 60–90 mg IV over 2 hours in 50–200 mL of saline or 5% dextrose in water
  - Zoledronate 4 mg IV over 15 min in 50 mL saline or 5% dextrose in water
  - Both drugs are associated with renal failure, flu-like symptoms, chills, and fever, a response requires 2–4 days with the nadir in serum calcium occurring in 4–7 days.
  - Lasts for 1–3 weeks

Second Line
- Glucocorticoids:
  - In lymphomas with elevated levels of active vitamin D
  - 60 mg of prednisone for 10 days
- Calcitonin:
  - Maximal response occurs in 12–24 hours
  - Reductions in serum calcium are small and transient (1 mg/dL)
  - Can cause flushing and nausea
- Mithramycin:
  - Effective but limited by adverse effects like thrombocytopenia, anemia, leucopenia, hepatitis, and renal failure
- Gallium nitrate:
  - 100–200 mg/m^2 body surface area IV continuously over 24 hours for 5 days
  - Can cause renal failure

ADDITIONAL TREATMENT
General Measures
- Remove calcium fromenteral feeding solutions.
- Discontinue medications like calcium, lithium, calcitriol, vitamin D, and thiazides
- Discontinue sedatives.
- Replace phosphate if necessary orally to maintain levels in the range 2.5–3.0 mg/dL, keeping the calcium-phosphate product below 40 to prevent severe hypocalcemia and metastatic deposition.

Additional Therapies
- Hemodialysis:
  - In patients with acute or chronic renal failure who cannot be hydrated safely and in whom bisphosphonates may not be safe
  - The dialysate contains little or no calcium.
  - Especially when the GFR is <10–20 mL/min
- New therapies:
  - Receptor activator of nuclear factor-κB ligand (RANKL) is involved in osteoclast-mediated bone resorption in cancer.
  - Osteoprotegerin and antibodies against RANKL and PTHrP are being proposed.

SURGERY/OTHER PROCEDURES
Parathyroidectomy in patients with primary hyperparathyroidism indicated if:
- Serum calcium 1 mg/dL above the accepted range
- 24-hour urinary calcium >400 mg
- >30% reduction in creatinine clearance
- Bone density <2.5 SD below *t* score
- Age <50
- Symptomatic (nephrolithiasis, pathologic fractures, pancreatitis)

IN-PATIENT CONSIDERATIONS
Initial Stabilization
- Assess ABCs
- Hydrate with IV saline
- Confirm diagnosis by ionized calcium levels

Admission Criteria
Acute hypercalcemia warrants inpatient treatment and cardiac monitoring.

IV Fluids
Normal saline at 200–500 mL/hr depending on volume and cardiac status

Nursing
- Aspiration and seizure precautions
- Frequent vital sign monitoring

Discharge Criteria
Once the diagnosis of hypercalcemia is confirmed and its etiology determined and the calcium level stabilized

 ONGOING CARE
FOLLOW-UP RECOMMENDATIONS
Follow-up with endocrinology and/or oncology to address the underlying cause of hypercalcemia
PROGNOSIS
- Hypercalcemia in a patient with cancer portends a poor prognosis.
- 50% of patients die within 30 days.

COMPLICATIONS
- Seizures
- Cardiomyopathy
- Renal failure
- Nephrolithiasis
- Pancreatitis

ADDITIONAL READING
- Stewart AF. Hypercalcemia associated with cancer. *N Engl J Med*. 2005;352:373–9.
- Ariyan CE, et al. Assessment and management of patients with abnormal calcium. *Crit Care Med*. 2004;32(4):S146–54.
- Legrand SB, et al. Narrative review: Furosemide for hypercalcemia: An unproven yet common practice. *Ann Intern Med*. 2008;149(4):259–63.
- Conroy S, et al. Hypercalcemia in cancer. *BMJ*. 2005;331:954.

 CODES
ICD9
- 252.00 Hyperparathyroidism, unspecified
- 252.01 Primary hyperparathyroidism
- 275.42 Hypercalcemia

CLINICAL PEARLS
- Primary hyperparathyroidism and malignancy are the most common causes of hypercalcemia.
- The rate of rise of ionized calcium as well as the level it rises to, determines symptoms.
- Frequently presents as dehydration and alteration of mental status
- Saline hydration and bisphosphonates are the mainstay of treatment.
- 50% of patients with cancer and hypercalcemia die within 30 days.

HYPERGLYCEMIA, STRESS

Paul E. Marik

 BASICS

DESCRIPTION
- Stress hyperglycemia is common in critically ill and injured patients and is a component of the "fight and flight" response.
- Until recently, stress hyperglycemia was considered a beneficial adaptive response, with the raised blood glucose providing a ready source of fuel for the brain, skeletal muscle, heart, and other vital organs at a time of increased metabolic demand.
- However, retrospective studies in patients undergoing cardiac surgery suggested that perioperative hyperglycemia was associated with an increased risk of postoperative infections and increased mortality (1–3).
- Furthermore, these studies suggested that control of blood glucose reduced these complications.
- Following the First Leuven Intensive Insulin Therapy Trial in 2001, "tight glucose control" became regarded as the worldwide standard of care in all ICU patients (4).

EPIDEMIOLOGY
- Stress hyperglycemia is considered in any critically ill patient with a blood glucose in >110 mg/dL (5).
- In the Leuven Intensive Insulin Therapy Trial, 12% of patients had a baseline blood glucose >200 mg/dL on the day following ICU admission. However, 74.5% of patients had a baseline blood glucose >110 mg/dL, with 97.5% having a recorded blood glucose level >110 mg/dL at some time during their ICU stay (4).

RISK FACTORS
- Activation of the stress response
- Hypotension
- Hypoxia
- Sepsis
- Trauma
- Surgery
- Burns
- Myocardial infarction
- IV glucose (especially TPN)
- Glucocorticoids
- Exogenous catecholamines
- Enteral formula high in glucose

PATHOPHYSIOLOGY
- Activation of the stress response with the production of glucagon, epinephrine, cortisol, growth hormone, as well as proinflammatory cytokines (IL-1, IL-6, TNF-α), results in increased gluconeogenesis, glycogenolysis, and insulin resistance, resulting in increased blood glucose levels.
- Increased hepatic gluconeogenesis appears central to the pathogenesis of stress hypoglycemia.
- Both acute and chronic hyperglycemia have been demonstrated to have adverse effects, most notably:
  – Increases oxidative injury
  – Potentiates the proinflammatory response
  – Promotes clotting
  – Causes abnormal vascular reactivity
  – Impairs leukocyte and mononuclear cell immune responsiveness

 DIAGNOSIS

- Most ICUs in the world (and in the U.S. in particular) use bedside capillary blood glucose measurements to monitor blood glucose levels.
- However, multiple studies have shown that these devices are inaccurate and tend to overestimate "true" plasma glucose levels (6,7).
- A number of factors may lead to inaccurate capillary blood glucose measurements, including:
  – Poor peripheral perfusion (shock)
  – Peripheral edema
  – Use of vasopressors
  – Low hemoglobin
  – Single-channel "glucometers"
  – Poor technique
- Using bedside capillary blood glucose measurements to manage insulin infusions is likely to lead to an unacceptably high rate of hypoglycemia.
- It is therefore suggested that arterial/venous, rather than capillary blood, be used for the bedside "measurement" of blood glucose and that these values be correlated with the blood glucose measured at the central laboratory (at least q12h).

 TREATMENT

- Initially, a study demonstrated that tight glycemic control using intensive insulin therapy improved the outcome of critically ill surgical patients (4).
- This study was rapidly adopted as the standard of care in ICUs worldwide and endorsed by many national organizations.
- The same clinical researchers repeated the study in medical ICU patients (8). A reduction in morbidity was seen in medical ICU with tight glycemic control. A reduction in mortality was seen in the subset of patients with an ICU stay of $\geq$3 days, yet not for the entire set of patients.
- Several studies were discontinued due to an alarmingly high rate of hypoglycemia in the "tight glycemic control" arm with no mortality benefit (9,10).
- The summary data of multiple studies, including the recent NICE-SUGAR study, demonstrates an absolute increase in 90-day mortality in patients randomized to tight glucose control.
- The findings of some of the studies may be explained by high rate of use of parenteral nutrition (TPN).
- Parenteral glucose load may be an independent predictor of organ failure and death.
- Multiple studies clearly demonstrate that tight glycemic control (70–110 mg/dL) has no role in the management of general ICU patients, yet it may improve outcomes in patients undergoing cardiac surgery, with a glucose target probably between 100 and 140 mg/dL.
- It seems reasonable to maintain blood glucose concentration between 140 and 200 mg/dL for all ICU patients, except those undergoing cardiac surgery.

- The methods to achieve the glucose goals are unclear, but the options are:
  - Insulin infusion could be administered if blood glucose level exceeds 180 mg/dL, and discontinued if the blood glucose level drops below 144 mg/dL.
  - In patients with enteral tube feeds, a 6-hourly, subcutaneous, regular insulin sliding scale is preferred when the blood glucose exceeds 160 mg/dL, followed by a twice daily NPH-intermediate acting insulin regimen (together with the regular insulin sliding scale).
  - NPH should be limited to a maximum of 20 units q12h. Insulin infusion should be started if this approach does not adequately control blood glucose (<200 mg/dL).
  - Although the absorption of SC insulin may be impaired, sliding scales are still considered adequate to control blood glucose in the critically ill.

ADDITIONAL TREATMENT
General Measures
- Avoid TPN at all costs.
- Limit the amount of IV dextrose.
- Use a low-carbohydrate enteral formula.
- Avoid high-dose corticosteroids.

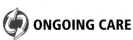 ONGOING CARE

COMPLICATIONS
- Tight glycemic control is associated with significant hazards.
- Severe hypoglycemia occurs in up to 18% of treated patients, with these patients being at an increased risk of death.
- Hypoglycemia is particularly hazardous in ICU patients who are frequently intubated and sedated and therefore unable to respond appropriately (masked hypoglycemia).

- Using cerebral microdialysis in patients following severe brain injury, Oddo and colleagues demonstrated that tight glycemic control is associated with a greater risk of brain energy crisis and death (14). These data suggest that tight glycemic control may result in neuroglycopenia at a time of increased cerebral metabolic demand.

ALERT
- Avoid long-acting insulin in the ICU (glargine, etc.).
- Avoid PO hypoglycemic agents in the ICU (these agents can be restarted on discharge from the ICU).

REFERENCES
1. Furnary AP, et al. Clinical effects of hyperglycemia in the cardiac surgery population: The Portland Diabetic Project. *Endocrine Pract*. 2006;12(Suppl 3):22–26.
2. Furnary AP, et al. Eliminating the diabetic disadvantage: The Portland Diabetic Project. *Semin Thorac Cardiovasc Surg*. 2006;18:302–8.
3. Zerr KJ, et al. Glucose control lowers the risk of wound infection in diabetics after open heart operations. *Ann Thorac Surg*. 1997;63:356–61.
4. van den Berghe G, et al. Intensive insulin therapy in critically ill patients. *N Engl J Med*. 2001; 345:1359–67.
5. Garber AJ, et al. American College of Endocrinology position statement on inpatient diabetes and metabolic control. *Endocrine Pract*. 2004;10:77–82.
6. Critchell C, et al. Accuracy of bedside capillary blood glucose measurements in critically ill patients. *Intensive Care Med*. 2007;33:2079–84.
7. Kanji S, et al. Reliability of point-of-care testing for glucose measurement in critically ill adults. *Crit Care Med*. 2005;33:2778–85.
8. van den Berghe G, et al. Intensive insulin therapy in the medical ICU. *N Engl J Med*. 2006;354: 449–61.
9. Devos P, et al. Impact of tight glucose control by intensive insulin therapy on ICU mortality and the rate of hypoglycaemia: Final results of Glucotrol (European society of Intensive Care Medicine 20th Annual Congress abstract 0735). *Intensive Care Med*. 2007;33(Suppl 2):S189.
10. Brunkhorst FM, et al. Intensive insulin therapy and pentastarch resuscitation in severe sepsis. *N Engl J Med*. 2008;358:125–39.
11. De La Rosa GD, et al. Strict glycemic control in patients hospitalized in a mixed medical and surgical intensive care unit: A randomized clinical trial. *Crit Care*. 2008;12:R120.
12. Arabi Y, et al. Intensive versus conventional insulin therapy: A randomized controlled trial in medical and surgical critically ill patients. *Crit Care Med*. 2008;36:3190–7.
13. Intensive versus conventional glucose control in critically ill patients. The NICE-Sugar Study Investigators. *N Engl J Med*. 2009;360:1283–97.
14. Oddo M, et al. Impact of tight glycemic control on cerebral glucose metabolism after severe brain injury: A microdialysis study. *Crit Care Med*. 2008;36:33233–3238.

 CODES

ICD9
790.29 Other abnormal glucose

CLINICAL PEARLS
- Hypoglycemia is much worse than hyperglycemia in ICU patients.
- Tight glycemic control increases mortality in ICU patients.
- Insulin should only be used when the blood glucose exceeds 180–200 mg/dL.
- Limit the IV glucose load (i.e., no TPN).

H

HYPERGLYCEMIC HYPEROSMOLAR NONKETOTIC ACIDOSIS (HONK)

Amyn Hirani
Paul E. Marik

 BASICS

DESCRIPTION
- A complication of type 2 diabetes mellitus (DM) that results in extremely high sugars and low to absent ketones
- Ketones are low to absent, as there is no fat breakdown.
- This metabolic derangement can be life-threatening.
- It is characterized by hyperglycemia, hyperosmolarity, and dehydration.
- Features that suggest HONK include:
  – Plasma glucose of $\geq$600 mg/dL
  – Serum osmolality of at least 320 mg/kg
  – Dehydration resulting in elevation of serum urea-to-creatinine ratio.
  – Low to absent ketones.
  – Serum bicarbonate concentration usually >15 mEq/L
  – Alteration in mental status
- Alterative name is nonketotic hyperglycemic hyperosmolar coma (NKHHC).

EPIDEMIOLOGY
Incidence
- The incidence of HONK is less than diabetic ketoacidosis but has a higher mortality rate of up to 11%.
- The incidence is 1 case per 1000 person years
- The mean age of onset is in the 6th and 7th decades of life; slight increase in female predominance.
- Demented nursing home residents have the highest incidence.

RISK FACTORS
- Relative insulin deficiency
- Undiagnosed DM
- Noncompliance to medications
- Infection:
  – UTI
  – PNA
  – Cellulitis
  – Dental infections
- Volume depletion from any cause
- Pancreatitis
- Myocardial injury
- Pulmonary embolism
- Cerebrovascular accident
- Cushing syndrome
- GI bleeding
- Cocaine use
- Rhabdomyolysis
- Acromegaly
- Drugs: Diuretics, β-blockers, antipsychotics, alcohol, parental nutrition, steroids, and immunosuppressant medications.
- Postoperative from neurosurgery, coronary artery bypass graft.

GENERAL PREVENTION
- Screen for DM in patients with family history.
- Screen all nursing home residents.
- Continue insulin in patients with known diabetes and seek medical help when sick.

PATHOPHYSIOLOGY
- Reduced effective action of insulin, but enough available insulin to prevent lipolysis. (It takes only 10% of insulin to prevent lipolysis)
- Increased levels of counter-regulatory hormones like glucagon, catecholamine, cortisol, and growth hormones, but at a lower level than DKA
- Failure of glucose to enter insulin-sensitive cells like liver, muscle, and fat cells
- Glycosuric diuresis impairing kidneys concentrating ability and worsening water loss
- Loss of more water than sodium leads to increased serum osmolarity.
- Intracellular dehydration

ETIOLOGY
- Related to type 2 diabetes:
  – Can be seen new undiagnosed type 2 diabetes
  – Noncompliant type 2 diabetics

COMMONLY ASSOCIATED CONDITIONS
- Old age
- Nursing home residents
- Dementia
- Underhydration

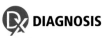 **DIAGNOSIS**

HISTORY
- Insidious onset over days or weeks
- Altered sensorium that can lead to coma
- Focal neurological weakness or seizures
- Polyuria
- Polydipsia
- Polyphagia

PHYSICAL EXAM
- Vitals signs will show features of dehydration like tachycardia, hypotension, loss of skin turgor, dry mucus membranes.
- Hypothermia; normal temperature should suggest infection.
- Increased respiratory rate may be seen to compensate for acidosis.
- Serum osmolarity >330 mOsm/kg is associated with neurological changes like seizures, strokes, and focal weakness.

DIAGNOSTIC TESTS & INTERPRETATION
Lab
Initial lab tests
- High glucose Accu-Chek
- Serum osmolarity >320 mOsm/kg
- ABG with mild acidosis: pH >7.30; if less, other causes of acidosis should be checked.
- Leukocytosis is commonly seen, but a level >25,000 cells/uL should initiate an infection workup.
- Metabolic panel that shows hypernatremia or hyponatremia; always look for pseudohyponatremia in patients with hyperglycemia.
- Elevated serum potassium due to shifts secondary to insulin deficiency and hypomagnesemia
- Anion gap is usually $\leq$12.
- Elevated BUN and creatinine
- Mild ketosis
- Elevated creatinine phosphokinase because of underlying rhabdomyolysis, or myocardial injury.
- Always obtain blood cultures, urine cultures to look for occult infection.
- Urinalysis shows increased specific gravity, glucose, and signs of infection. Ketones are rare.
- Acute renal failure may also occur in the setting of volume depletion and rhabdomyolysis.
- Metabolic panel and electrolytes monitoring q4h

Follow-Up & Special Considerations
- The basic metabolic panel should be followed q4–6h, along with renal function, CPK.
- Obtain a hemoglobin A1c level as this may help to determine patient's glucose management.

Imaging
- Radiological studies may be used to look for infection (e.g., chest radiograph).
- CT scan of head may be useful in patients with mental status changes.

Diagnostic Procedures/Other
- Diagnostic procedure such as lumbar puncture may be required to eliminate diagnosis like meningitis.
- Procedures like central venous catheter and arterial catheter placement may be necessary to obtain and monitor hemodynamic stability

DIFFERENTIAL DIAGNOSIS
- Diabetic ketoacidosis
- Alcoholic ketoacidosis
- Starvation ketoacidosis
- Lactic acidosis
- Uremic acidosis
- Rhabdomyolysis
- Methanol or ethylene glycol ingestion
- Isopropyl alcohol ingestion
- Dementia
- Drug overdose (salicylates)
- Meningitis/encephalitis

TREATMENT

MEDICATION

First Line

- If patient is in coma or unresponsive, obtaining an airway and venous access, and optimizing hemodynamics with fluids is of utmost importance.

- The fluid requirement in HONK is immense (can be 10 liters or more in severe cases) (4)[A]:
  - Initial administration of 1–2 liters of isotonic fluids is recommended in first hour (15–20 mL/kg/hr for initial resuscitation phase) if underlying poor cardiac or renal status replete at slower rate (4)[A].
  - This should be followed by 0.45% or normal saline at 250–500 mL/hr. If serum sodium is low, NS should be continued.
  - If blood glucose concentration falls below 200 mg/dL, change to fluids containing dextrose.

Second Line

- Insulin should be started after adequate fluid resuscitation. A initial bolus of 0.15 U/kg followed by 0.1 U/kg/hr infusion (4)[A]:
  - An hourly fall of 50–70 mg/dL of blood glucose is recommended; may need to double infusion rate until steady decline achieved.

- Potassium: After establishment of urine output of at least 50 mL/hr (4)[A]:
  - If serum potassium is low (3.3 mEq/L), then replete before initiating insulin.
  - If serum potassium >5.0 mEq/L, start insulin and check serum potassium q2h.
  - If serum potassium is between 3.3–5.0 mEq/L, then replete 20–30 meq in each liter of fluid to maintain potassium >4.0 mEq/L but keep <5.0 mEq/L

ADDITIONAL TREATMENT

Additional Therapies

- Replete other electrolytes, especially phosphates if <1.0 mg/dL (4)[A].

- Transition to subcutaneous low-dose sliding-scale insulin should occur when patient is alert and blood glucose is <300 mg/dL and serum osmolarity is normal.

- Look and treat precipitating causes (4,6)[C].

- Treat with antibiotics until cultures return to cover for underlying infection in severe cases.

- Look for myocardial injury, rhabdomyolysis, medications as a precipitating factor (4,6)[C].

IN-PATIENT CONSIDERATIONS

Initial Stabilization

- Should include basic ABC assessment

- Patients may present with coma and in cardiogenic or hypovolumic shock; treatment is supportive.

- Further stabilization includes correction of volume deficits and any major electrolyte abnormalities.

Admission Criteria

All cases of HONK should be monitored as an inpatient and admitted to ICU.

IV Fluids

- Aggressive volume resuscitation is often required secondary to volume deficit.

- May need to monitor for signs of volume overload in patients with underlying poor renal and cardiac function

Nursing

- Frequent or continuous monitoring of heart rate, blood pressure, mental status, and respiratory status may be necessary.

- Monitoring of hourly urine output

- Hourly Accu-Chek and titration of insulin infusion.

- Teach use of SC insulin to patient when patient improves.

- Lab draws q4–6h for 1st 24–48 hours

- Aspiration precautions

Discharge Criteria

- Resolving electrolyte abnormalities, improved mental status

- SC insulin administration technique teaching

- Social work consult for need of placement

ONGOING CARE

FOLLOW-UP RECOMMENDATIONS

- A follow-up with primary care physician and endocrinologist for diabetic teaching is necessary to prevent recurrence.

- Further nursing care may be needed at home to improve compliance.

- Check Hb A1c q3mon.

PATIENT EDUCATION

Explain to patient and caregivers the life-threatening implications of missing insulin doses.

PROGNOSIS

- If recognized early and treated, outcomes are good.

- Development of renal failure and further multiorgan failure are predictive of increased mortality.

COMPLICATIONS

- Myocardial infarction
- Mesenteric Ischemia
- DIC
- Rhabdomyolysis
- Cerebral edema
- Respiratory failure
- Hypoglycemia due to excess insulin use
- Aspiration pneumonitis/pneumonia
- Venous thromboembolism
- Multisystem organ failure; death
- If insulin is given before adequate fluid resuscitation, it may lead to further hypotension as insulin moves water and electrolytes intracellularly.

REFERENCES

1. Chiasson JL, et al. Diagnosis and treatment of diabetic ketoacidosis and the hyperglycemic hyperosmolar state. *CMAJ.* 2003;168:859–66.
2. De Beer K, et al. Diabetic ketoacidosis and hyperglycaemic hyperosmolar syndrome: Clinical guidelines. *Nurs Crit Care.* 2008;13:5–11.
3. Kitabchi AE, et al. Hyperglycemic crises in adult patients with diabetes: A consensus statement from the American Diabetes Association. *Diabetes Care.* 2006;29:2739–48.
4. Kitabchi AE, et al. Hyperglycemic crises in diabetes. *Diabetes Care.* 2004;27(Suppl 1):S94–102
5. Nugent BW. Hyperosmolar hyperglycemic state. *Emerg Med Clin North Am.* 2005;23:629–48, vii.
6. Stoner GD. Hyperosmolar hyperglycemic state. *Am Fam Physician.* 2005;71:1723–30.

ADDITIONAL READING

- http://www.diabetes.org/type-2 diabetes/ treatment-conditions/hhns.jsp

CODES

ICD9

250.20 Diabetes mellitus with hyperosmolarity, type ii or unspecified type, not stated as uncontrolled

CLINICAL PEARLS

- Maintain a high clinical suspicion for hyperosmolar hyperglycemic coma as it can be life-threatening.
- Low to absent ketones with hyperglycemia should raise a suspicion.
- Serum osmolarity >330 mOsm/Kg is associated with worse outcomes.
- Adequate fluid resuscitation is key to treatment.
- Insulin should begin after initial fluid resuscitation.
- Frequent electrolyte monitoring is required.
- Check Hb A1C q3-4mon in known diabetics.

H

HYPERKALEMIA

Sindhura Gogineni
Aditya Uppalapati
Roopa Kohli-Seth

 BASICS

DESCRIPTION
Life-threatening metabolic abnormality with plasma potassium level >5.5 mEq/L (5 mmol/L)

EPIDEMIOLOGY
Prevalence
1–10% in hospitalized patients

RISK FACTORS
- Renal failure
- Acidemia
- Massive cell breakdown
- Use of potassium-sparing diuretic
- Excess potassium supplementation

Genetics
- Familial hyperkalemic periodic paralysis
- Congenital adrenal hyperplasia

GENERAL PREVENTION
- Low-potassium diet in renal failure patients
- Monitoring electrolytes on patient with diuretics and potassium supplementation

PATHOPHYSIOLOGY
- Total body potassium is 50 mmol/Kg body weight
- Potassium distribution:
  - Extracellular space: 1–2%
  - Intracellular space: 98–99%
- Concentration gradient is a key factor in regulating the resting membrane potential.
- Potassium homeostasis:
  - External balance:
    ◦ Intake-diet: 50–150 mmol/d, salt substitutes, Iatrogenic administration
    ◦ Excretion, renal: 90%; extrarenal, feces (5–15 mmol/d)
    ◦ Cutaneous (insensible, burns), 5–10 mmol/d
  - Regulation of renal potassium secretion:
    ◦ Peritubular factors: Serum potassium concentration, aldosterone
    ◦ Extracellular pH: Luminal factors, distal tubular flow rate, sodium delivery, anion composition

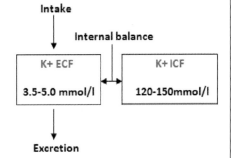

ETIOLOGY
- Increased potassium release from cells:
  - Metabolic acidosis:
    ◦ Buffering of hydrogen ions in to the cells. To maintain electro neutrality potassium moves in to the ECF.
  - Diabetes ketoacidosis and hyperosmolar nonketotic coma (HONK):
    ◦ Insulin promotes the entry of potassium into the cells. In deficiency, hyperglycemia causes increase in serum osmolarity leading to hyperkalemia by solvent drag, water efflux into ECF, followed by potassium.
- Increased tissue catabolism:
  - Tumor lysis syndrome: Massive tumor lysis leading to hyperkalemia, hyperphosphatemia, and hyperuricemia. Most cases are associated with initiation of chemotherapy.
  - Traumatic rhabdomyolysis is associated with AKI.
  - Burns
- β-adrenergic blockade:
  - Impairs potassium entry in to cells. Most cases associated with nonselective β blockers.
- Exercise:
  - Delay in K^+ efflux and reuptake; depletion of ATP and loss of inhibitory action of K^+ channels leading to increased efflux.
- Mannitol: Hyperosmolarity, transcellular shift
- Digoxin toxicity: Inhibition of NA^+ K^+ ATPase, increase in ECF K^+.
- Succinylcholine: Occurs when given in conditions that cause up-regulation and widespread distribution of acetylcholine receptors throughout the muscle membrane (e.g., burns, extensive trauma).
- Hyperkalemic periodic paralysis:
  - Autosomal dominant, precipitated by cold, ingestion of small dose of potassium
- Reduced urinary potassium excretion:
  - Hypoaldosteronism:
    ◦ Primary deficiency
    ◦ Hyporeninemic hypoaldosteronism
    ◦ Drugs: Heparin, triamterene, ACE inhibitors, ARBs, spironolactone
    ◦ Type 4 RTA
  - Renal failure
- Decreased effective circulating volume:
  - Cirrhosis, heart failure, salt-wasting nephropathy
- Medications:
  - Calcineurin inhibitors: Cyclosporine, tacrolimus; decrease the activity of rennin-angiotensin-aldosterone system and impair tubular responsiveness to aldosterone
  - Potassium penicillin G, NSAIDs.
- Ureterojejunostomy: Due to absorption of urinary K^+ by the jejunum

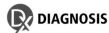 **DIAGNOSIS**

HISTORY
- Nausea, vomiting, palpitations, abdominal pain, diarrhea, weakness in extremities, dizziness
- History regarding fluid intake, diabetes
- History regarding hemodialysis and if patient missed any hemodialysis
- Medications

PHYSICAL EXAM
- CNS: Assess mental status, muscle strength (rule out flaccid paralysis).
- Reflexes: decreased deep tendon reflex
- Abdominal exam: Skin (ecchymosis), palpation (mass; rule out hematoma), postoperative (JP drains, output to rule out bleeding, NG output to rule out UGI bleeding)
- Extremities: Rule out compartment syndrome

DIAGNOSTIC TESTS & INTERPRETATION
Lab
- Serum electrolytes (including magnesium and phosphorus)
- Renal function: BUN, creatinine
- ABG: Increased K, hyponatremia, calcemia, acidosis
- Urine for pH, K, creatinine, and osmolality
- Fractional excretion of potassium (FEK) (3):
  - (Urine K × Serum Creatinine)
    (Serum K × Urine Creatinine):
    ◦ FEK gradient <10% renal etiology
    ◦ FEK gradient >10% extra renal cause
- Transtubular potassium gradient (TTKG):
  - (Urine K × Serum Osmolality)
    (Serum K × Urine Osmolality)
    ◦ With potassium intake, the normal TTKG is 8-11; if TTKG <5 and hyperkalemia is present, then it indicates inappropriate renal response to high potassium.
    ◦ Gradient <6–8 indicates renal causes.
    ◦ Gradient >8 indicates extrarenal causes.
    ◦ Serum cortisol and aldosterone

Imaging
US to rule out obstruction; CT scan of abdomen if retroperitoneal hematoma, bleeding is suspected.

Diagnostic Procedures/Other
- EKG: Progression of hyperkalemia:

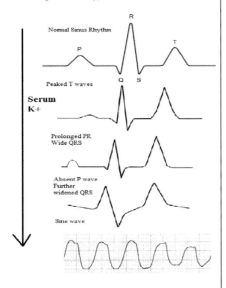

- Sinus rhythm can be normal with hyperkalemia.
- Ventricular fibrillation itself might also be a common 1st manifestation of hyperkalemia.

DIFFERENTIAL DIAGNOSIS
- Pseudohyperkalemia:
  - Traumatic vein puncture with hemolysis
  - Drawing blood sample from the same line (e.g., triple-lumen catheter) infusing potassium
- Rule out lab error.

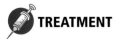 TREATMENT

MEDICATION (1,2,3)[C]
First Line
- Membrane stabilization:
  - IV calcium:
    ○ Calcium chloride or calcium gluconate (10%)
    ○ 10 mL IV over 10 minutes
    ○ Onset is immediate, duration is 30–60 minutes
- Internal redistribution:
  - Insulin (short acting):
    ○ 10 units IV with 25–40 g dextrose (50% solution)
    ○ Onset, 20 minutes; duration, 4–6 hours
  - β-adrenergic agonists (Albuterol):
    ○ 20 mg in 4 mL NS solution, nebulized over 10 minutes
    ○ Onset, 30 minutes; duration, 2 hours
- Elimination:
  - Loop diuretics:
    ○ Furosemide (40–80 mg) or bumetanide (1–2 mg IV)
    ○ Onset, 15 minutes; duration, 2–3 hours

Second Line
- Elimination:
  - Sodium polystyrene sulfonate (Kayexalate):
    ○ 15–30 g in 15–30 mL
    ○ Can be given orally (as sorbitol solution) or as retention enema
    ○ Onset, >2 hours; duration, 4–6 hours

ADDITIONAL TREATMENT
General Measures
- Assess ABCs.
- IV access, triple-lumen catheter, especially if patient is hemodynamically unstable
- Cardiac monitor

Issues for Referral
- Nephrology for emergent dialysis:
  - Onset, immediate; duration 2–3 hours, after which rebound may occur
  - Magnitude of post-rebound plasma K is proportional to predialysis plasma K.

Additional Therapies
- Sodium bicarbonate: Dose, 150 mmol/L IV; onset, hours. Not routinely recommended as initial or monotherapy to treat life-threatening hyperkalemia. Its use is probably best reserved for patients who also have a severe metabolic acidosis.
- Discontinue any medications that contain potassium or might impair potassium excretion.

SURGERY/OTHER PROCEDURES
- Hematoma and bleeding: Evacuation and stabilization of bleeding
- Compartment syndrome: Decompression/fasciotomy

IN-PATIENT CONSIDERATIONS
Initial Stabilization
- Follow ACLS for treatment of arrhythmias and cardiac arrest.
- Treat hyperkalemia emergently for plasma K of >6.5 mmol/L or EKG manifestations regardless of plasma K levels (1,2)[C].

Admission Criteria
- Emergent hemodialysis
- Patients with cardiac arrhythmias secondary to hyperkalemia
- Acute Kidney injury with AKI
- Metabolic acidosis with hyperkalemia
- Hyperkalemia >6.5 mmol/L

IV Fluids
- NS
- Avoid Plasmalyte and LR (they contain potassium):
  - 5% or 25% albumin can also be used.

Nursing
- Monitor EKG changes.
- Make sure blood samples are drawn after the line is flushed and the minimal requirement of blood wasted. Do not draw it from the line infusing any fluids containing potassium.
- When hyperkalemia or a trend with increased potassium is noted, hold any IV fluids, feeds, or TPN with potassium and inform doctor.

Discharge Criteria
Stabilization of potassium levels and treating the etiology of hyperkalemia

 ONGOING CARE

FOLLOW-UP RECOMMENDATIONS
Patient Monitoring
- Following initial treatment for unstable arrhythmias or potassium of >6.5 mmol/L, check plasma potassium on an ICU panel or chemistry as frequently as needed (15 minutes-1 hour) and repeat treatment and recheck until potassium starts trending down and has stabilized.

- Once stabilized or after emergent hemodialysis for hyperkalemia, check potassium levels q2–4h to make sure no rebound hyperkalemia occurs

DIET
- Low-potassium diet
- Avoid potassium in TPN and feeds.

PATIENT EDUCATION
Consult with dietician about low-K diet

PROGNOSIS
Varies from cardiac arrest, death, to response to treatment. Depends on associated morbidities and etiology.

COMPLICATIONS
Life-threatening cardiac arrhythmias (cardiac arrest)

REFERENCES
1. Weisberg LS. Management of severe hyperkalemia. *Crit Care Med*. 2008;36:3246–51.
2. Evans KJ, Greenberg A. Hyperkalemia: A review. *J Intensive Care Med*. 2005;20:272–90.
3. Hollander-Rodriguez JC, Calvert JF. Hyperkalemia. *Am Fam Phys*. 2006;73:283–90.

ADDITIONAL READING
- Advanced cardiac life support (ACLS), AHA. http://www.heart.org/HEARTORG/
- Desai AS. Hyperkalemia in patients with heart failure: Incidence, prevalence and management. *Curr Heart Fail Rep*. 2009;6(4):272–80.

 See Also (Topic, Algorithm, Electronic Media Element)

- Renal Tubular Acidosis
- Renal Failure

 CODES

ICD9
- 276.2 Acidosis
- 276.7 Hyperpotassemia

CLINICAL PEARLS
- Emergency treatment of hyperkalemia for plasma levels of >6.5 mmol/L or for EKG manifestations of hyperkalemia.
- Follow-up potassium levels closely with frequent monitoring until it reaches normal level, as plasma K can bounce back after treatment (including dialysis).
- ACLS protocol can be used in treating arrhythmias, in addition to treatment of hyperkalemia.

H

HYPERNATREMIA

Rakesh Sinha
Roopa Kohli-Seth

 BASICS

DESCRIPTION
- Hypernatremia is defined as serum sodium (Na^+) concentration >145 mmol/L
- Common electrolyte disorder due to water homeostasis imbalance
- System(s) affected: Endocrine/Metabolic

EPIDEMIOLOGY
Incidence
- Incidence of hypernatremia among patients admitted to hospital is 1%.
- Incidence of hypernatremia among patients admitted to ICU is 26%.
- Incidence density of hypernatremia in ICU is 7.4 per 100 ICU days.

Prevalence
- Daily prevalence of hypernatremia among inpatients is 0.8%.
- Prevalence of hypernatremia in ICU patients is 15%.

RISK FACTORS
- Age: Infants and elderly
- Neurologic disease
- Impaired mental status
- Intubation and mechanical ventilation

Geriatric Considerations
Increasing age associated with diminished osmotic stimulation of thirst via an unknown mechanism, therefore increased risk

Genetics
- Central diabetes insipidus (DI):
  - Autosomal dominant and recessive: Arginine vasopressin-neurophysin gene mutation
  - X-linked recessive gene mutation
- Congenital nephrogenic DI:
  - X-linked recessive: Defect in the renal V_2 receptors for anti-diuretic hormone (ADH)
  - Autosomal dominant and recessive: Defect in the ADH sensitive water channel (aquaporin 2 gene)

GENERAL PREVENTION
- Replace water loss and prevent dehydration, especially in nephrogenic DI.
- Avoid excessive sodium load in IV infusions.

PATHOPHYSIOLOGY
- Hypernatremia is almost always caused by loss of free water.
- Persistent hypernatremia does not occur in healthy subjects because rising plasma osmolality stimulates thirst and release of ADH.
- Thirst leads to water intake, and ADH minimizes water loss thereby normalizing the serum sodium concentration.
- Hypernatremia occurs primarily in patients who cannot express thirst normally or do not have access to free water.
- Administration of hypertonic sodium solutions can sometimes also be a cause of hypernatremia.

ETIOLOGY
- Unreplaced water loss
- Insensible and sweat losses:
  - Fever
  - Exercise
  - Exposure to high temperature
- GI losses:
  - Vomiting
  - Nasogastric drainage
  - Enterocutaneous fistula
  - Diarrhea
  - Osmotic cathartic agents (lactulose)
- Central DI:
  - Congenital
  - Idiopathic (autoimmune injury)
  - Head trauma
  - Neurosurgery (pituitary surgery)
  - Tumors (craniopharyngioma, lymphoma, leukemia, metastasis)
  - Granulomatous diseases (histiocytosis, tuberculosis, sarcoidosis)
  - Infections (meningitis, encephalitis, abscess)
  - Vascular disorder (aneurysms)
  - Miscellaneous (cysts, Guillain-Barré syndrome, hypoxic or ischemic encephalopathy, ethanol ingestion)
- Nephrogenic DI:
  - Congenital
  - Acquired metabolic aberrations:
    ○ Hypercalcemia
    ○ Hypokalemia
    ○ Drugs: Lithium, demeclocycline, foscarnet, methoxyflurane, amphotericin B, vasopressin V receptor antagonists
  - Medullary damage:
    ○ Chronic pyelonephritis
    ○ Infiltrative disease (leukemia, lymphoma, amyloidosis)
    ○ Sickle cell disease
    ○ Cystinosis
    ○ Obstructive uropathy
    ○ Other forms of chronic renal failure
- Renal loss:
  - Loop diuretics
  - Osmotic diuresis (glucose, urea, mannitol)
  - Postobstructive diuresis
  - Polyuric phase of acute tubular necrosis
  - Intrinsic renal disease
- Cutaneous loss (burns)
- Hypothalamic lesions affecting thirst or osmoreceptor function:
  - Primary hypodipsia
  - Essential hypernatremia
  - Reset osmostat in mineralocorticoid excess
- Hypertonic sodium gain:
  - Hypertonic sodium bicarbonate infusion
  - Hypertonic feeding preparation
  - Ingestion of sodium chloride
  - Ingestion of sea water
  - Sodium chloride–rich emetics
  - Hypertonic saline enemas
  - Intrauterine injection of hypertonic saline
  - Hypertonic sodium chloride infusion
  - Hypertonic dialysis
- Water loss into cells: Severe exercise and seizures may lead to transient hypernatremia

COMMONLY ASSOCIATED CONDITIONS
- Impaired mental status
- Other conditions mentioned under etiology

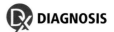 **DIAGNOSIS**

HISTORY
- Polyuria or oliguria
- Nausea, vomiting or diarrhea
- Excessive sweating
- Intense thirst initially which wanes
- Lethargy and weakness
- Neuromuscular irritability
- Seizures and coma
- Severity of clinical symptoms is related to acuity and magnitude of rise of serum Na^+ concentration.
- Most symptoms arise when serum Na^+ concentration >160 mmol/L.
- Chronic hypernatremia is less symptomatic
- Infants may also have hyperpnea and a characteristic high-pitched cry even at lower sodium concentrations.
- Review medication list

PHYSICAL EXAM
- Cool skin with decreased skin turgor
- Sunken eyes
- Hypotension and tachycardia may be present reflecting marked hypovolemia
- Focal neurological deficit may be noted

DIAGNOSTIC TESTS & INTERPRETATION
Lab
Initial lab tests
- Cause is usually evident from history
- Check serum BUN, creatinine, electrolytes, and glucose
- Check urine volume to assess polyuria
- Check plasma osmolality: Usually >295 mOsmol/kg in hypernatremia
- Check urine osmolality
- Urine osmolality >800 mOsmol/kg:
  - Check urine sodium
    ○ <20 mEq/L → unreplaced insensible or GI loss
    ○ >100 mEq/L → sodium overload
- Urine osmolality < plasma osmolality:
  - Administer extrinsic ADH (desmopressin 10 μg nasal or vasopressin 5 units SC)
    ○ Urine osmolality rises ≥50% → central DI
    ○ No change → nephrogenic DI
- Urine osmolality 300–800 mOsmol/kg:
  - Relatively severe central DI
  - Partial central or nephrogenic DI:
    ○ To distinguish the type of DI, perform water deprivation test
    ○ Check ADH level and then administer ADH
  - Osmotic diuresis:
    ○ Measure urine glucose or urea
    ○ Confirm by measuring total solute excretion

Follow-Up & Special Considerations
Serum electrolytes should be measured frequently (q4–6h) during treatment of severe hypernatremia with IV fluids.

Imaging
Initial approach
- Chest x-ray may show evidence of sarcoidosis, tuberculosis, and histiocytosis.
- Low threshold for obtaining head CT in severely hypernatremic patients

Follow-Up & Special Considerations
If central DI is diagnosed, brain imaging including MRI may be indicated.

 TREATMENT

MEDICATION
First Line
- Treatment for central DI (1)[B]:
  - Desmopressin 1–2 μg q.d.–b.i.d. SC or IV
  - Desmopressin intranasal 10–20 μg b.i.d.–t.i.d. nasal spray
  - Desmopressin 100–400 μg b.i.d.–t.i.d. PO
- Treatment for nephrogenic DI (1)[C]:
  - Hydrochlorothiazide 25 mg q.d.–b.i.d. PO
  - Amiloride 5–10 mg b.i.d. PO

Second Line
Treatment for nephrogenic DI (1)[C]: NSAIDs

ADDITIONAL TREATMENT
General Measures
Calculate water deficit (2)[B]:
- Water deficit = total body water $\times$ {1–[140 ÷ serum sodium concentration]}
  - Total body water = 0.6 $\times$ weight (kg)
  - Use factor 0.5 for younger females and elderly men and 0.45 for elderly females
- This formula provides an adequate estimate of water deficit caused by pure water loss but does not incorporate ongoing water losses.

ALERT
- Rate of correction (2,3,4)[B]:
  - Water deficit should be slowly corrected over 48–72 hours with no more than 1/2 during the first 24 hours.
  - The plasma sodium concentration should be lowered by $\leq$0.5 mmol/L/hr and no more than 10 mmol/L/d.
  - Overly rapid correction can cause cerebral edema if rate exceeds 0.7 mmol/L/hr.
  - In patients with hypernatremia that has developed over a period of hours, rapid correction at the rate of 1 mmol/L/hr improves the prognosis without increasing the risk of cerebral edema.
  - The goal of treatment is to reduce the serum concentration to 145 mmol/L.
- Water can be given orally if patient condition permits.

Issues for Referral
- Nephrology evaluation for patients with renal failure and need for dialysis
- Endocrinology referral important for patients with DI
- Neurosurgery referral for patients with brain tumors, aneurysms, cysts

Additional Therapies
- Discontinue offending drugs in nephrogenic DI.
- Correct hypercalcemia and hypokalemia in nephrogenic DI.

IN-PATIENT CONSIDERATIONS
Initial Stabilization
Treat hypotension and hypovolemia with isotonic fluid.

Admission Criteria
- Symptomatic patients, usually with serum sodium concentration >155 mmol/L
- IV fluid therapy required

IV Fluids
- Isotonic fluid (normal saline, plasmalyte or LR) IV bolus till hemodynamically stable
- 5% D5W or D2.5W to correct serum Na^+ concentration
- Check serum sodium frequently during correction with IV fluids, q4–6h.
- Sodium, potassium, calcium, phosphate, magnesium, bicarbonate may be added to IV fluids as indicated.

Nursing
Bed rest until hemodynamically stable

Discharge Criteria
Asymptomatic with normal serum sodium

 ONGOING CARE

DIET
Low-sodium, low-protein diet in nephrogenic DI can diminish urine output.

PATIENT EDUCATION
In central DI, educate patient not to drink water for reasons other than thirst as it may lead to water intoxication, leading to hyponatremia if patient is being treated with desmopressin.

PROGNOSIS
ICU-acquired hypernatremia is associated with increased risk of hospital mortality; the more severe the hypernatremia, the higher the mortality.

COMPLICATIONS
Neurologic injury:
- Focal intracerebral hemorrhage
- Sub cortical and subarachnoid hemorrhage
- Subdural hematoma
- Venous sinus thrombosis
- Cerebral edema (treatment related)

REFERENCES
1. Makaryus AN, et al. Diabetes insipidus: Diagnosis and treatment of a complex disease. *Cleve Clin J Med*. 2006;73:65–71.
2. Lin M, et al. Disorders of water balance. *Emerg Med Clin N Am*. 2005;23:749–70.
3. Adler SM, et al. Disorders of body water homeostasis in critical illness. *Endocrinol Metab Clin N Am*. 2006;35:873–94.
4. Andogue HJ, et al. Hypernatremia. *N Eng J Med*. 2000;342:1493–9.

 See Also (Topic, Algorithm, Electronic Media Element)

Diabetes insipidus

 CODES

ICD9
- 253.5 Diabetes insipidus
- 276.0 Hyperosmolality and/or hypernatremia

CLINICAL PEARLS
- In hypernatremia, first treat hypotension and hypovolemia with isotonic fluid (NS, Plasmalyte, LR)
- Water deficit = total body water $\times$ {1–[140 ÷ serum sodium concentration]}
- Water deficit should be slowly corrected over 48–72 hours with no more than 1/2 during the first 24 hours.
- The plasma sodium concentration should be checked frequently and lowered by $\leq$0.5 mmol/L/hr and no more than 10 mmol/L/d.

H

HYPERTENSION

John C. D'Ambrosio

 BASICS

DESCRIPTION
- Defined as the elevation of blood pressure (BP) on average of ≥ 2 BP on ≥ 2 visits
- Prehypertension: Systolic 120–139 mm Hg or diastolic 80–89 mm Hg
- Hypertension:
  - Stage 1: Systolic 140–159 mm Hg or diastolic 90–99 mm Hg
  - Stage 2: Systolic ≥ 160 mm Hg or diastolic ≥ 100 mm Hg
- Hypertensive crisis:
  - Terms such as malignant hypertension, accelerated hypertension can be confusing and are not used. Current terminology includes hyptensive crisis, which includes both hyptensive emergencies and urgencies
- JNC VII has defined *hypertensive emergencies* as those with severe elevations of BP, usually >180/120 (could be lower depending on the chronicity of hypertension) complicated by impending or progressive end-organ damage. These cases require immediate BP reduction to prevent or limit further organ damage:
  - Examples of end organ damage: Hypertensive encephalopathy, intracerebral hemorrhage, acute MI, acute left ventricular failure, dissecting aortic aneurysm or eclampsia
- Hypertensive urgencies are those with severe elevations of BP in the upper levels of stage II hypertension without end organ damage:
  - Symptoms such as headaches, epistaxis, shortness of breath, or anxiety can occur

EPIDEMIOLOGY
Incidence
- 30% or 50 million Americans have high BP. 1/3 of these patients don't know they have high BP and only 1/3 of those who are diagnosed have BP controlled
- Estimated worldwide to be ≥ 1 billion
- 7.1 million deaths per year are attributable to hypertension
- Severe hypertension occurs in ~1% of those with chronic hypertension

Prevalence
- ~50% of patients aged 60–69 are affected.
- ~75% of patients older >70 are affected.
- Lifetime risk for normotensive patients aged 55–65 who live to 80 is ~90%.

RISK FACTORS
- Age
- Diabetes
- Renal insufficiency
- Hyperlipidemia
- Abdominal obesity
- Proteinuria
- Smoking
- Family history
- Excess sodium intake
- Lack of fruits and vegetables
- Excess alcohol
- Physical inactivity
- Medications: NSAID use

Genetics
- Mineralocorticoid excess states
- Liddle syndrome
- Cushing syndrome
- 11-β and 17-α hydroxylase deficiency
- Pseudohypoaldosteronism type 2

GENERAL PREVENTION
Diet, exercise

PATHOPHYSIOLOGY
BP is determined by the product of cardiac output (CO) and systemic vascular resistance (SVR). In most hypertensive crises, the initial rise in BP results from increased SVR. This increase causes mechanical stress on the walls of arteriolar walls, leading to endothelial damage and potential fibrinoid necrosis.

ETIOLOGY
Secondary causes are uncommon in the general hypertensive populations (5–10%), but 20–50% of those with hypertensive emergencies will have a secondary cause.

COMMONLY ASSOCIATED CONDITIONS
- Renal insufficiency
- Diabetes
- Hyperlipidemia
- Abdominal obesity
- Sleep apnea
- Thyroid or parathyroid disease

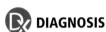 **DIAGNOSIS**

HISTORY
- Most people are asymptomatic.
- Any history of chest pain, shortness of breath, orthopnea, abdominal pain, changes in vision, headaches, or any neurological changes
- History of hypertension before the age of 30 without family history, new-onset renal failure precipitated by ACE inhibitors (ACEI) or angiotensin receptor blockers (ARBs) and controlled HTN that becomes difficult to control, could indicate renal vascular hypertension.
- Use of steroids, NSAIDs, cocaine, amphetamines, decongestants, monoamine oxidase uptake inhibitors, selective serotonin reuptake inhibitors
- Cessation of antihypertensives

PHYSICAL EXAM
- Accurate measurement of BP with verification in contralateral arm
- Exam of optic fundi for papilledema or retinopathy
- Calculation of the body mass index
- Auscultation for femoral, carotid, and abdominal bruits
- Thorough exam of the heart and lungs
- Palpation of the thyroid gland
- Palpation of the lower extremities to assess for edema and evaluate pulses

DIAGNOSTIC TESTS & INTERPRETATION
- Assess lifestyle and identify other cardiovascular risk factors that may guide treatment.
- Reveal identifiable causes of high BP
  - Chronic kidney disease
  - Coarctation of the aorta
  - Cushing syndrome
  - Chronic steroid therapy
  - Drug-induced obstructive uropathy
  - Pheochromocytoma
  - Primary aldosteronism
  - Renovascular hypertension
  - Sleep apnea
  - Thyroid or parathyroid disease
- Assess the presence or absence of target organ damage and CVD
- Classification:
  - Prehypertension
  - Stage I
  - Stage II
- Obtain initial blood work, EKG

Lab
- Glucose
- Potassium
- Creatinine with calculation of estimated GFR
- Fasting lipid profile
- Urinalysis

Imaging
- Chest x-ray
- CT scan of head for patients with hypertensive encephalopathy, eclampsia, or suspected stroke
- CT scan of chest if aortic dissection or coarctation is suspected

Diagnostic Procedures/Other
Echocardiogram is useful to assess left ventricular function, segmental abnormalities, and left ventricular wall thickness (remodeling)

Pathological Findings
- Retinopathy
- Pathological murmur
- Edema
- Rales
- S3, S4

DIFFERENTIAL DIAGNOSIS
- Chronic kidney disease
- Coarctation of the aorta
- Cushing syndrome
- Chronic steroid therapy
- Drug-induced obstructive uropathy
- Pheochromocytoma
- Primary aldosteronism
- Renovascular hypertension
- Sleep apnea
- Thyroid or parathyroid disease

TREATMENT

Lifestyle changes:
- Weight loss
- Diet
- Sodium reduction
- Physical activity
- Alcohol reduction

MEDICATION

Goal is systolic ≤140 mm Hg and diastolic ≤90 mm Hg unless other cardiovascular risk factors, such as renal disease and diabetes, are present. Then the goal is systolic ≤130 mm Hg and diastolic ≤80 mm Hg.

First Line
- Essential hypertension
- Stage I:
  - Thiazide-type diuretics, ACEI, β-blockers (BB), ARBs, calcium channel blockers (CCB)
- Stage II:
  - Two drug combination, usually thiazide-type diuretic combined with ACE-I, ARB, BB, or CCB
- Hypertensive emergency:
- IV (bolus and continuous infusion):
  - Nitroprusside, initial dose 0.25 mcg/kg/min, maximum dose 8–10 mcg/kg/min
  - Labetalol bolus; start at 10–20 mg bolus q10min to maximum dose 300 mg. Continuous infusion at 0.5 to 2 mg/min
  - Nicardipine start at 5 mg/hr to maximum dose 15 mg/hr
  - Esmolol 50 mcg/kg/min bolus, then infuse 50–300 mcg/kg/min
  - Fenoldopam initial dose 0.1 mcg/kg/min with titration every 15 minutes, no bolus
  - Clevidipine initial dose 1–2 mg/hr, titrate every 5–10 minutes to maximum dose 16 mg/hr
  - Nitroglycerin initial infuse at 5–20 mcg/min to maximum 200 mcg/min

Second Line
- Consists of adding a 2nd first–line drug in hypertensive emergencies either by continuous infusion or IV bolus
- Some other drugs to consider:
  - Hydralazine, IV 10–20 mg/dose q4–6h as needed, may increase to 40 mg/dose
  - Enalaprilat, IV 1.25 mg q6h to a max dose of 5 mg q6h
  - Phentolamine 0.05–0.1 mg/kg/dose, maximum single dose 5 mg

ADDITIONAL TREATMENT
General Measures
- Hypertensive emergencies warrant arterial line insertion and continuous infusion of antihypertensive medications.
- Autoregulation in hypertensive emergencies is often impaired. The goal is to lower BP by no more than 15–25% over a period of minutes to hours for most situations. Some exceptions may include hemorrhagic stroke and ischemic stroke patients being considered for thrombolytic therapy:
  - Ischemic stroke patients who are eligible for thrombolytics require BP of <185/110 mm Hg and should be maintained after thrombolytics. Otherwise, only patients with systolic of >220 or diastolic >120 should be considered for treatment.

- Intracerebral hemorrhage (ICH) patients with systolic >200 mm Hg or MAP of >150 mm Hg require aggressive reduction; patients with systolic >180 mm Hg or MAP >130 mm Hg with signs of elevated intracranial pressure require monitoring of intracranial pressure; BP goal is to maintain cerebral perfusion pressure between 60 and 80 mm Hg.
- ICH with systolic >180 mm Hg or MAP >130 mm Hg and no signs of raised ICP: Goal is MAP of 110 mm Hg or BP ~160/90 mm Hg

Issues for Referral
- Critical care for hypertensive emergencies
- Nephrology for possible renal vascular hypertension
- Cardiology for any signs of myocardial ischemia

Additional Therapies
Anxiolytics, analgesics, relieve obstructive uropathy

SURGERY/OTHER PROCEDURES
Postoperative hypertension:
- Think about pain or urinary retention as possible cause of hypertension

IN-PATIENT CONSIDERATIONS
Admission Criteria
- Hypertensive emergencies
- Hypertensive urgencies with symptoms or with poor follow-up

IV Fluids
Hypertension can cause a pressure natriuresis and therefore some patients may require IV fluids.

Nursing
- When monitoring BP via arterial line, MAP is preferred for titrating drugs.
- When monitoring cuff pressures, a systolic pressure is preferred for titrating medications.
- Hypertensive emergency patients should have frequent neurological exams, close monitoring of urine output, and frequent vital signs (at least every hour).

Discharge Criteria
Hypertensive emergency has resolved, no further progression of end organ disease, and BP is stable.

ONGOING CARE

FOLLOW-UP RECOMMENDATIONS
Patient Monitoring
- Hypertensive urgency can be monitored as an outpatient.
- Stage I and II can be followed in office, usually q3–6mon. Frequency is determined by stability of BP and comorbidities

DIET
- Low-sodium diet
- Reduced alcohol intake

PATIENT EDUCATION
Lifestyle changes including:
- Low-sodium diet
- Regular aerobic exercise
- Avoidance of excess alcohol
- Smoking cessation

PROGNOSIS
Excellent, if compliant with treatment program

COMPLICATIONS
- Heart disease
- Stroke
- Renal disease

ADDITIONAL READING
- Adams HP Jr., et al. Guidelines for the early management of adults with ischemic stroke. *Stroke.* 2007;38:1655.
- Broderick J, et al. Guidelines for the management of spontaneous intracerebral hemorrhage in adults, 2007 update. *Stroke.* 2007;38:2001–23.
- Chobanian AV, et al. The Seventh Report of the Joint National Committee on Prevention, Detection, Evaluation, and Treatment of High Blood Pressure: The JNC 7 Report. *JAMA.* 2003;289:2560.
- Zanotti-Cavazzoni SL. *Hypertensive crises: Critical care medicine principles diagnosis and management in the adult.* 2008;723–4.

CODES

ICD9
- 401.9 Unspecified essential hypertension
- 437.2 Hypertensive encephalopathy

CLINICAL PEARLS

Lowering the BP too quickly can compromise cerebral blood flow.

H

HYPERTHERMIA

Sreedhar Chintala

 BASICS

DESCRIPTION

- Hyperthermia is elevation in core body temperature beyond the normal range of 36–37.5°C.
- Due to failure of thermoregulatory center in anterior hypothalamus
- Core temperature ≥40°C is a life-threatening emergency.
- Neuroleptic malignant syndrome (NMS) is an idiosyncratic disorder associated with use of neuroleptic medication, due to dopamine receptor blockade in brain
- Malignant hyperthermia: Hypermetabolic response to potent inhalation agents, depolarizing muscle relaxant, and rarely to stress, such as vigorous exercise and heat.
- Heat stroke: A form of hyperthermia with abnormally elevated temperatures associated with physical and neurological symptoms. It is a medical emergency.

EPIDEMIOLOGY

Incidence

- Heat stroke: During 1979–2002, 4780 deaths were classified as heat related.
- Off the 4686 (98%), 260 (6%) in children <15 years, 2356 (50%) in 15–64, 2070 (44%) among persons aged >65.
- The incidence is 3–7 times greater in Arizona compared to U.S. overall.
- NMS: 0.02–3% among patients taking neuroleptic agents
- Malignant hyperthermia: Anywhere from 1:60,000 anesthetics to suspected in 1:4000
- Mortality:
  - Heat stroke: Will decrease from 80% to 10% if treatment is started immediately.
  - NMS: Average about 10%
  - Malignant hyperthermia: Dropped from 80% 30 years ago to <5%

RISK FACTORS

- Heat stroke:
  - Socially isolated
  - History of psychiatric illness
  - Unable to care for self
  - Use of diuretics
- NMS:
  - Dehydration
  - Electrolyte abnormalities
  - Concurrent use of lithium
- Malignant hyperthermia:
  - Genetically susceptible people exposed to inhalation anesthetics and succinylcholine

Genetics

Malignant hyperthermia:

- Autosomal dominant pattern of inheritance
- Due to mutation in gene for skeletal muscle Ryanodine receptor (RyR1) on 19q13

PATHOPHYSIOLOGY

- Heat stroke:
  - Ineffective heat dissipation mechanisms when environmental temperature exceeds skin temperature.
  - Uncoupling of oxidative phosphorylation and inactivation of enzymes.
- NMS: Due to dopamine receptor blockade
- Malignant hyperthermia: In susceptible people, an increase in intracytoplasmic calcium leading to muscle rigidity, then to hypermetabolism and cell death.

ETIOLOGY

- Heat stroke: Exposure to extreme hot environment
- NMS: Idiosyncratic reaction to neuroleptic drugs and antiemetic, commonly haloperidol, chlorpromazine, metoclopramide, domperidone
- Malignant hyperthermia: Following treatment with inhalation anesthetics and succinylcholine

COMMONLY ASSOCIATED CONDITIONS

- Malignant hyperthermia:
  - Duchenne muscular dystrophy
  - Becker muscular dystrophy
  - Periodic paralysis
- NMS:
  - Drug intoxication with cocaine, ecstasy, phencyclidine
  - Rapid removal of dopaminergic medication
- Heat stroke:
  - Chronic medical conditions
  - Psychiatric illness

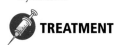 **DIAGNOSIS**

HISTORY

- Use of inhalation anesthetics
- Use of succinylcholine
- Use of atypical and typical neuroleptics
- Use of antiemetic
- Substance abuse
- Exposure to hot environment

PHYSICAL EXAM

- Heat stroke:
  - Marked temperature elevation
  - Altered level of consciousness
  - Excessive bleeding due to DIC
- NMS:
  - Markedly elevated temperature >38°C
  - Muscle rigidity; lead pipe rigidity
  - Altered LOC—Agitated, delirious
  - Autonomic instability

- Malignant hyperthermia:
  - Muscle rigidity: Masseter muscle
  - Increase in end tidal CO_2
  - Marked elevation in temperature
  - Hyperkalemia, acidosis

DIAGNOSTIC TESTS & INTERPRETATION

Lab

Initial lab tests

- CBC, Chem10, LFT, CPK
- PT, PTT, Fibrinogen
- Urine for myoglobin, heme, RBC sediments
- Urine for toxic screen

Follow-Up & Special Considerations

ECG to rule out arrhythmias and conduction abnormalities

Imaging

Initial approach

CXR to rule out pulmonary edema

Follow-Up & Special Considerations

- Head CT, noncontrast, to rule out CVA
- EEG to rule out seizure

Diagnostic Procedures/Other

- Lumbar puncture to rule out infectious etiology
- Muscle biopsy
- Caffeine halothane contracture test

DIFFERENTIAL DIAGNOSIS

- Heat stroke
- Neuroleptic malignant syndrome
- Malignant hyperthermia
- Serotonin syndrome
- Cocaine use
- Delirium tremors
- Thyroid storm

TREATMENT

- Heat stroke:
  - Move patient to cool area.
  - Continuous core temperature monitoring
  - Use cooling blanket and ice water gastric lavage.
  - Remove clothing to promote heat loss.
  - Cold compresses to torso, head, neck, and groin
  - Fan may be used to help in evaporation.
  - Adequate hydration, IV and orally
- NMS:
  - Discontinue any neuroleptic medication.
  - Fluid resuscitation
  - Use cooling blankets and ice pack application.
  - Use benzodiazepines for seizure.
  - Bromocriptine, a dopamine agonist is well tolerated.

- Malignant hyperthermia:
  – Stop the triggering anesthetics.
  – Give 100% oxygen.
  – Cold IV fluids
  – Dantrolene 2.5 mg/kg bolus and repeat until symptoms disappear or to a maximum of 10 mg/kg

MEDICATION
Side effects:

- Bromocriptine
  – Palpitations
  – Swelling of feet and ankle
  – Confusion
  – Headache, nausea, and vomiting
  – Watery discharge from nose
- Dantrolene:
  – Insomnia
  – Speech disturbance
  – Visual disturbance
  – Constipation
  – Urinary incontinence
  – Abnormal hair growth

ADDITIONAL TREATMENT
General Measures
- Monitor ABCs
- Continuous core temperature monitoring
- Fluid resuscitation with cold IV fluids
- Monitor urine output and color
- Monitor electrolytes, especially potassium and calcium

Issues for Referral
- Airway compromise
- Acute renal failure due to rhabdomyolysis
- Dysrhythmias, DIC
- Electrolyte abnormalities

Additional Therapies
- **A**lkalinize urine and diuresis for myoglobinuric renal failure.
- **B**icarbonate infusion is given for acidosis, **b**enzodiazepines for seizures.
- **C**ompartment syndrome is rare, but monitor extremities and bladder pressure after initial insult.
- **D**ysrhythmias are treated with amiodarone, lidocaine, and adenosine.
- **E**lectrolyte abnormalities: If hyperkalemic, treat with bicarbonate, glucose/insulin, calcium

 ONGOING CARE

FOLLOW-UP RECOMMENDATIONS
Patient Monitoring
- ABCs
- Continuous core temperature measurement
- Serial CPK, electrolytes, liver function test, ABG, and coagulation profile
- Urine color and output monitoring
- Neurological assessment

PATIENT EDUCATION
- Avoid exposure to hot environment.
- Adequately hydrate.
- Wear light, loose-fitting clothing.
- Avoid polypharmacy.
- Avoid alcohol, caffeinated drinks.
- Know heat-related signs and symptoms.

PROGNOSIS
- Most episodes resolve within 2 weeks.
- Increased mortality in those >65, with chronic medical conditions, psychiatric illness

COMPLICATIONS
- Anoxic injury
- Acute renal failure
- Respiratory failure requiring mechanical ventilation
- Dysrhythmias
- Seizures
- Hypotension
- Rhabdomyolysis

REFERENCES

1. Den borough. *lancet*. 19983;352(9142).
2. Shalev A, Hermesh. *J Clin Psychiatry*. 1989;50.
3. Malignant Hyperthermia association of United States.

ADDITIONAL READING
- www.mhuas.org
- www.anes.ucla.edu
- www.nmsis.org

 CODES

ICD9
- 333.92 Neuroleptic malignant syndrome
- 780.60 Fever, unspecified
- 995.86 Malignant hyperthermia

CLINICAL PEARLS
- It is important to identify the cause of hyperthermia.
- Cool rapidly with cooling blanket, cold IV fluids, cold water gastric lavage.
- Provide supportive therapy for heat stroke, give dantrolene for malignant hyperthermia, and bromocriptine for NMS.
- Monitor electrolytes, CPK, LFTs, and coags, and correct them.

H

HYPERTHERMIA, MALIGNANT

Monvasi Pachinburavan
Paul E. Marik

BASICS

DESCRIPTION
An inherited disorder of the skeletal muscle membrane that presents as a hypermetabolic response to depolarizing muscle relaxants and inhalational anesthetic agents

EPIDEMIOLOGY
Incidence
Incidence during anesthesia is estimated to be between 1:5,000 and 1:50,000 anesthesias.

Prevalence
- Prevalence in the general population is unknown.
- MH can be found in all ethnic groups.

RISK FACTORS
Genetics
MH is an autosomal dominant condition. In the majority of patients, mutations are found in the ryanodine receptor (RYR1) gene.

GENERAL PREVENTION
- Genetic testing and muscle contracture test in high-risk patients, such as patients with a family history of MH or patients with suspected MH.
- For known MH-susceptible patients, surgery should be done under regional or local anesthesia if possible. Use nontriggering agents for general anesthesia, such as nonpolarizing neuromuscular blockers, benzodiazepines, opiates, and nitrous oxide.

PATHOPHYSIOLOGY
In most cases, likely to be secondary to a defective calcium channel in the sarcoplasmic reticulum causing increased intracellular calcium. Prolonged muscle contractions leads to increased metabolism.

COMMONLY ASSOCIATED CONDITIONS
- Strong association with central core disease (CCD), which is a hereditary myopathy. Also associated with multi-mini core disease (MmCD)
- In the pediatric population, MH is associated with succinylcholine-induced masseter muscle rigidity.
- MH may be associated with an increased risk of heat stroke.

DIAGNOSIS

HISTORY
MH is a clinical diagnosis. Patient may have a previous history of MH or adverse reaction to general anesthesia. Previous uncomplicated exposure to anesthetic agents does not preclude diagnosis, as patients may require several anesthesias to trigger. Family history of MH in a 1st-degree relative warrants screening measures prior to elective procedures.

PHYSICAL EXAM
- Early findings can be subtle: Unexplained sinus tachycardia, hypertension, increased minute ventilation during spontaneous ventilation. An unexplained increase in end-tidal CO_2 is an important hallmark of early MH.
- Late findings include generalized muscle rigidity, hyperthermia, dark urine, bleeding, and tachyarrhythmias.

DIAGNOSTIC TESTS & INTERPRETATION
Lab
Initial lab tests
- Increased $PaCO_2$, metabolic acidosis
- Hyperkalemia, elevated CPK, myoglobinuria from rhabdomyolysis
- Coagulopathy from DIC

Follow-Up & Special Considerations
- Gold standard for diagnosis is the caffeine halothane muscle contracture test (CHCT) used in the U.S. or the in vitro muscle contracture test (IVCT) used in Europe.
- RYR1 gene sequencing is also available: Sensitivity is near 100%, specificity is ~80%.

DIFFERENTIAL DIAGNOSIS
Other causes of end tidal PO elevation and hyperthermia, such as sepsis, pheochromocytoma, should be considered.

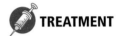

TREATMENT

MEDICATION
Give dantrolene starting at 2.5 mg/kg. Give repeated doses until vital signs stabilize.

ADDITIONAL TREATMENT
General Measures
- Stop surgery and triggering agent immediately upon clinical suspicion.
- Hyperventilate with 100% oxygen.
- Start aggressive cooling measures, such as cooling blankets, cold saline irrigation, etc.

Issues for Referral

Patient should be referred for muscle contracture test and genetic testing. If patient is MH-susceptible, patient should undergo genetic counseling, and screening test should be performed on 1st-degree relatives.

IN-PATIENT CONSIDERATIONS

Initial Stabilization

- Dantrolene should be given at a dose of 2.5 mg/kg IV until patient is stabilized. Repeated doses can be given up to a total of 10 mg/kg.
- In the post acute phase, dantrolene should be continued at a dose of 1 mg/kg IV q4–6h for the first 24–48 hours.
- Patients should be admitted and monitored for possible rhabdomyolysis, acute renal failure, hyperkalemia, and DIC.

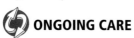 ONGOING CARE

FOLLOW-UP RECOMMENDATIONS

- Send patients for definite diagnostic testing and genetic counseling.
- Report to the North American Registry of Malignant Hyperthermia.

PATIENT EDUCATION

- Patients should be advised to undergo diagnostic testing.
- MH-susceptible patients should be educated on triggering medications and informed that alternative methods of anesthesia are available.
- MH-susceptible patient should be educated on the autosomal dominant inheritance pattern of MH.
- MH-susceptible patients should be advised of the possible increased risk of heat stroke. It is not necessary to limit exercise.

PROGNOSIS

Since the introduction of dantrolene, mortality has decreased from ~70% to 5%. Survival is excellent with early detection and treatment.

ADDITIONAL READING

- http://www.mhaus.org/
- Rosenberg H, et al. Malignant hyperthermia Orphanet. *J Rare Dis*. 2007;2:21.
- Urwyler A, et al. Guidelines for molecular genetic detection of susceptibility to malignant hyperthermia. *Brit J Anaesth*. 2001;86(2):283–7.

 CODES

ICD9
995.86 Malignant hyperthermia

CLINICAL PEARLS

- MH is a autosomal dominant disorder of the skeletal muscle that causes a severe hypermetabolic reaction to inhalation anesthetic agents.
- An early hallmark is unexplained elevated end tidal CO_2.
- Treated with dantrolene.

H

HYPOCALCEMIA

Adel Bassily-Marcus
Roopa Kohli-Seth

 BASICS

DESCRIPTION

Hypocalcemia is defined as a serum calcium level of <2.0 mmol/L (<8 mg/dL) or an ionized calcium level of >1.0 mmol/L (<4 mg/dL).

EPIDEMIOLOGY

Incidence

Found in 26% of hospital admissions and 88% of ICU admissions. In a series of 500 postsurgical patients operated on for hyperparathyroidism, 2% had permanent hypocalcemia.

Prevalence

Reported to be 60–85% among medical, surgical, and trauma ICU patients. Prevalence of ionized hypocalcemia is 15–20% in the critically ill.

RISK FACTORS

- Advanced age
- Sepsis, shock
- Acute renal failure
- Multiple blood transfusions
- Malnutrition
- Magnesium deficiency
- Colloid volume resuscitation

Genetics

- Autosomal recessive, autosomal dominant in familial hypoparathyroidism
- 22q11.2 deletion in DiGeorge Syndrome

GENERAL PREVENTION

- Adequate nutrition
- Sunlight exposure
- Treatment with calcium (Ca) and vitamin D for 1–2 days prior to parathyroid surgery
- Check calcium levels in patients on drugs that may cause hypocalcemia.

PATHOPHYSIOLOGY

- Approximately 99% of the total body calcium is deposited in the skeleton; 0.9% is intracellular, and 0.1% is extracellular. In the extracellular fluid, 50% of the calcium is bound (mostly to albumin, with a smaller fraction to phosphorus and citrate) and 50% is free or ionized.
- 2 hormones (PTH, vitamin D) and 3 organs (bone, kidney, small intestine) are involved in calcium homeostasis.
- A slight decrease in calcium stimulates the calcium-sensing receptors present on chief cells of the parathyroid gland to secrete PTH. In bone, PTH increases the resorption of Ca and phosphate; in kidney, it increases reabsorption of Ca and inhibits reabsorption of phosphates, as well as enhances the hydroxylation of 25 [OH] D_3 to the activated form. Vitamin D stimulates intestinal absorption of calcium and phosphate, decreases real Ca reabsorption, and activates osteoclasts in concert with PTH to promote Ca release by bone resorption.

ETIOLOGY

- Hypoparathyroidism:
  - Acquired:
    - Parathyroidectomy (most common cause)
  - Hungry bone syndrome may develop after profound longstanding hypocalcemia in which Ca is sequestered into the remineralizing bone; magnesium uptake occurs, leading to hypomagnesemia as well:
    - Infiltrative or malignant disease
  - Congenital (rare)
  - Idiopathic
- Vitamin D deficiency:
  - Common in elderly, institutionalized patients, poor PO intake, inadequate sun exposure
  - Malnutrition: Leads to Ca and vitamin D deficiency
  - Malabsorption: Postgastrectomy, small bowel disease, laxatives abuse, phenytoin
  - Liver disease
  - Kidney disease:
    - Decreased vitamin D_3 synthesis
    - Increased phosphate

- Redistribution:
  - Tissue sequestration:
    - Acute pancreatitis: Unclear etiology. Hypocalcemia is present in 85% of patients with acute severe pancreatitis. Ca accumulates in pancreas, liver, and skeletal muscle in animal models.
    - Rhabdomyolysis: Multifactorial Ca deposition in skeletal muscle in presence of hyperphosphatemia forms Ca-phosphate complex, decreases synthesis of vitamin D
  - Complexation:
    - Complexation with alkali: Citrates and bicarbonates:
  - Citrate: After massive blood transfusion, citrate chelates Ca and forms Ca citrate complex to cause transient hypocalcemia. The Ca citrate complex is metabolized in liver, where it is converted into bicarbonate and ionized Ca, which is then released into the circulation. Citrate may also be used for anticoagulation of the CVVH plasmapheresis circuit, causing same effect. In liver failure, total Ca maybe misleadingly normal, but ionized Ca is low.
  - Bicarbonate: The use of sodium bicarbonate to treat metabolic acidosis leads to Ca binding to albumin and formation of carbonate complexes:
    - Complexation with phosphate: Any condition that causes an acute rise of phosphate levels can cause complexation and resultant ionized hypocalcemia by forming insoluble Ca-phosphate complexes (e.g., tumor-lysis syndrome, phosphate-containing laxatives/Fleet enemas and in rhabdomyolysis).
  - Ethylenediamine tetra-acetic acid
- Drugs:
  - Cis-platinum, plicamycin
  - Bisphosphonates: By impairing osteoclasts function and number.
  - Colchicine
  - Calcitonin
  - Phenytoin
  - Foscarnet

- Miscellaneous:
  - Systemic inflammatory response syndrome
  - Sepsis: Unclear mechanisms, proposed:
    - Ca sequestration
    - Effect on inflammatory cytokines
    - Calcitonin precursors
    - Hypomagnesemia with hypoparathyroidism
    - PTH resistance
    - Vitamin D deficiency from coexisting liver and kidney dysfunction
  - Hypomagnesemia:
    - Impairs PTH secretion
    - Causes PTH resistance
    - Reduced bone calcium release
  - Acute renal failure
  - Impaired 1α-hydroxylation

COMMONLY ASSOCIATED CONDITIONS
- Factitious hypocalcemia
- Medications and toxins
- Critical illness or chronic illness
- Thyroid or parathyroid surgery
- Vitamin D disorders
- Developmental disorders of parathyroid gland

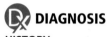

DIAGNOSIS

HISTORY
- Muscle cramping/tetanic contractions
- Shortness of breath secondary to bronchospasm
- Angina
- Dysphagia
- Diarrhea
- Chronic pruritus

PHYSICAL EXAM
- Neuromuscular inability:
  - Chvostek's sign (negative in 30% of cases): Contraction of the ipsilateral facial muscles elicited by tapping the facial nerve just anterior to the ear.
  - Trousseau's sign (94% sensitive, more specific): Induction of carpopedal spasm which is adduction of the thumb, flexion of the metacarpophalangeal joints, extension of the interphalangeal joints, and flexion of the wrist by inflation of a sphygmomanometer above systolic blood pressure for 3 minutes
  - Paresthesias
  - Tetany/seizures (focal, petit mal, grand mal)
  - Polymyositis
  - Laryngeal spasms/bronchial spasms

- Neurological signs and symptoms:
  - Extrapyramidal signs due to calcification of basal ganglia
  - Increased intracranial pressure
  - Choreoathetosis/dystonic spasms
- Mental status:
  - Confusion/disorientation, psychosis
- Ectodermal changes:
  - Coarse hair, brittle nails
  - Enamel hypoplasia/delayed tooth eruption
  - Psoriasis
  - Impetigo herpetiformis
- Smooth muscle involvement:
  - Biliary colic, preterm labor, detrusor dysfunction
- Ophthalmologic manifestations:
  - Subcapsular cataracts, papilledema
- Cardiac
  - Congestive heart failure, cardiomyopathy

DIAGNOSTIC TESTS & INTERPRETATION
Lab
Initial lab tests
- A total or ionized serum calcium level (blood should be drawn in an unheparinized syringe for best results)
- Serum albumin level:
  - Corrected serum Ca = total Ca +(0.8 × [4- Albumin])
- Serum magnesium, phosphorus
- Serum intact PTH level (an antibody-mediated radioimmunoassay)
- Vitamin D metabolites levels:
  - 25-hydroxyvitamin D and $1,25(OH)2D_3$, the active vitamin D hormone
- Urinary cAMP may help to differentiate hypoparathyroidism from pseudohypoparathyroidism types I and II.
- 24-hour urinary excretion of calcium and magnesium
- Liver function test
- ABG for acid–base status assessment
- Test results:
  - High PTH, normal or high phosphorus, normal magnesium, high creatinine: Renal failure/pseudohypoparathyroidism
  - High PTH, normal or low phosphorus, normal magnesium, normal creatinine: Vitamin D deficiency
  - Low PTH, normal or high phosphorus, normal creatinine: Hypoparathyroidism or hypomagnesemia
  - Alkalosis: Tends to decrease ionized calcium levels due to increased binding to albumin.

- ECG:
  - Prolonged QTc interval (>0.4 s)
  - ST segment shortened or absent 50% of patients
  - Ventricular arrhythmias; torsades de pointes

Follow-Up & Special Considerations
- In life-threatening condition, ICU admission
- Endocrinology follow-up

Imaging
Initial approach
- Skeletal x-rays:
  - Manifestation of rickets
  - Osteoblastic metastases from certain tumors (e.g., breast, prostate, lung) can cause hypocalcemia.
- CT scan of the head:
  - Basal ganglia calcification and extrapyramidal neurologic symptoms (in idiopathic hypoparathyroidism)

Follow-Up & Special Considerations
Severe ionized hypocalcemia (<0.8 mmol/L) requires urgent treatment.

Diagnostic Procedures/Other
Hemodialysis for patient with hyperphosphatemia and symptomatic hypocalcemia

Pathological Findings
Osteitis fibrosis cystica and osteomalacia occur in patients with hypercalcemia and secondary hyperparathyroidism.

DIFFERENTIAL DIAGNOSIS
- Hypercalcemia
- Hypermagnesemia
- Hyperosmolar hyperglycemic nonketotic coma
- Hyperparathyroidism
- Hyperphosphatemia

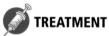

TREATMENT

MEDICATION
First Line

- There is no clear evidence that parenteral calcium supplementation impacts the outcome of critically ill patients (1)[A].

- Hypocalcemia accompanied with serious cardiovascular or neuromuscular signs should be treated urgently.

- For ionized Ca of 1–1.12 mmol/L: 2 g of calcium gluconate in 50–150 mL of D5W or 0.9% NaCl over 2 hours

H

- For ionized Ca of <1 mmol/L: Recommend 4 g of calcium gluconate in 50–150 mL of D5W or 0.9 % NaCl over 4 hours (2)[C]:
  - IV calcium gluconate: 10% 10 mL contains 90 mg elemental calcium
  - IV calcium chloride: 10% 10 mLcontains 272 mg elemental calcium
  - Calcium infusion drips should be started at 0.5 mg/kg/h and increased to 2 mg/kg/h as needed.
  - For mild, asymptomatic, or chronic hypocalcemia, treatment with oral supplementation of 1000–2600 mg/d is adequate (3)[C].

Pediatric Considerations
IV 10–20 mg/kg elemental calcium (1–2 mL calcium gluconate/kg) slowly over 5–10 minutes to control seizures; may be continued as IV infusion at 50–75 mg/kg/d over 24 hours

Pregnancy Considerations
- Category B; usually safe but benefits must outweigh the risks
- Correction of electrolytes abnormalities: Correct hypomagnesemia as it impairs PTH release and end organ response, also directly reduce Ca release from the bone. It may restore normal Ca levels without Ca supplementation.
  - Patients with hypocalcemia and hyperphosphatemia need to have hyperphosphatemia corrected first to avoid complexation. Hemodialysis is often indicated in patients who have symptomatic hypocalcemia.
  - Correction of severe metabolic acidosis should await correction of hypocalcemia, as correction of acidosis worsens the ionized hypocalcemia and precipitates tetany.

- Contraindications of calcium replacement:
  - Renal calculi, hypercalcemia, hypophosphatemia, renal or cardiac disease, digitalis toxicity
- Interactions:
  - Calcium supplements may decrease effects of tetracyclines, atenolol, salicylates, iron salts, and fluoroquinolones; when administered IV, antagonizes effects of calcium channel blockers.
- Precautions:
  - Caution with patients on digoxin, respiratory failure, acidosis, severe hyperphosphatemia; closely monitor IV calcium supplementation because it can cause cardiac arrhythmias.

Second Line
- Start PO calcium and vitamin D treatment early:
  - Calcium carbonate 500 mg chewable tabs (Tums) 200 mg
  - Calcium carbonate 250 mg + Vitamin D 125 IU/tablet (OsCal 250+D) 100 mg

ADDITIONAL TREATMENT
General Measures
- Identify and treat the causes of hypocalcemia.
- During replacement, the ionized calcium level rises to 0.5–1.5 mmol and should last 1–2 hours.
- Determine Ca $\times$ PO$_4$ product in mg/dL before administering calcium. If product is greater than 60 mg/dL, there is an increased risk of calcium phosphate precipitation in the cornea, lung, kidney, cardiac conduction system, and blood vessels.
- Determine potassium, phosphorus, and magnesium levels. Correct abnormalities.
- For each 5 units of packed RBCs transfused, administer 1–2 g (1–2 amps) of calcium gluconate.
- Patients who develop acute hypocalcemia after parathyroidectomy may require up to 10 g of calcium gluconate intravenously in 1000 mL fluid at a rate of 1 g/hr (100 mL/hr).

Issues for Referral
Care is determined by the probable underlying etiology of hypocalcemia.

Additional Therapies
- In hypothyroidism:
  - Calcium: 1.0–1.5 g/d elemental (total diet + supplement) in divided doses
  - Vitamin D: Ergocalciferol (D$_2$)/cholecalciferol (D$_3$) 25,000–100,000 IU/d
- Pediatric dose:
  - Ergocalciferol 50,000–200,000 IU/d PO
- Contraindications:
  - Hypercalcemia or malabsorption syndrome
- Interactions:
  - Colestipol, mineral oil, and cholestyramine may decrease absorption from small intestine; thiazide diuretics increase effects of vitamin D
- Pregnancy:
  - Category A; safe in pregnancy
- Precautions:
  - Caution in impaired renal function, renal stones, heart disease, or arteriosclerosis
- In renal failure:
  - Phosphate binders:
    - Sevelamer 800–1600 mg PO t.i.d. with meal

SURGERY/OTHER PROCEDURES

Parathyroidectomy (subtotal or total) may be indicated in patients with severe secondary hyperparathyroidism and renal osteodystrophy.

IN-PATIENT CONSIDERATIONS

Initial Stabilization
- Adequate oxygenation/airway protection
- Homodynamic monitoring and ECG

Admission Criteria
Severe or symptomatic hypocalcemia

IV Fluids
Isotonic crystalloids

Nursing
- Monitor for ECG changes, notify the physician if ventricular arrhythmia develops.
- When giving calcium supplements, frequently check the patient's pH because a pH >7.45 inhibits calcium ionization.
- Focus on IV site for signs of infiltration because calcium can cause tissue sloughing.

Discharge Criteria
Patient in stable condition with corrected electrolytes abnormalities that do not require IV calcium replacement

 ONGOING CARE

FOLLOW-UP RECOMMENDATIONS

Patients with calcium supplementation can have hypercalciuria as earliest sign of toxicity, and this can develop in the absence of hypercalcemia.

Patient Monitoring
- If low albumin is also present, ionized calcium should be monitored q4–6h.
- Measure serum calcium q4–6h to maintain serum calcium levels at 8–9 mg/dL

DIET
- Supplementation with dietary calcium to >1 g/d.
- In chronic renal failure-associated hypocalcemia, dietary intake of phosphate should be decreased to 400–800 mg/d to prevent hyperphosphatemia and require phosphate binders and vitamin D supplementation.

PATIENT EDUCATION
Teaching regarding drug interaction with potassium supplements and regular follow-up are necessary.

PROGNOSIS
- Mortality is higher in hypocalcemic patients but is not an independent risk factor (3)[B].
- There is no clear evidence that parenteral calcium supplementation impacts the outcome of critically ill patients (1)[A].

COMPLICATIONS
- Complications of chronic hypocalcemia predominantly are those of bone disease.
- Osteomalacia and rickets result from vitamin D deficiency.

REFERENCES

1. Forsythe RM, et al. Parenteral calcium for intensive care unit patients. *Cochrane Database Syst Rev.* 2008(4):CD006163.
2. Dickerson RN. Treatment of hypocalcemia in critical illness: Part 2. *Nutrition.* 2007;23(5):436–7.
3. Hastbacka J, et al. Prevalence and predictive value of ionized hypocalcemia among critically ill patients. *Acta Anaesthesiol Scand.* 2003;47(10):1264–9.

ADDITIONAL READING

- Marx SJ. Hyperparathyroid and hypoparathyroid disorders. *N Engl J Med.* 2000;343(25):1863–75.

 CODES

ICD9
- 275.41 Hypocalcemia
- 781.7 Tetany

CLINICAL PEARLS

- Hypocalcemia results from parathyroid gland insufficiency and calcium precipitation/chelation.
- Rapid infusion of large quantities of calcium-free fluid, albumin, citrated blood, and sodium bicarbonate can contribute to hypocalcemia.

H

HYPOCALCEMIA, ACUTE

Urvashi Vaid
Paul E. Marik

 BASICS

DESCRIPTION
- Hypocalcemia is a potentially life-threatening electrolyte abnormality frequently found in critically ill patients.
- Defined as an ionized calcium <4.65 mg/dL (1.16 mmol/L) or a total calcium <8.5 mg/dL (2.12 mmol/L)

EPIDEMIOLOGY
Incidence
- In critically ill patients, the incidence is as high as 88%.
- Can occur in 20% of post thyroid surgery patients transiently.

Prevalence
- 18% in the general population
- 85% in the ICU population

RISK FACTORS
- Severity of illness: Patients with higher APACHE scores are more likely to be hypocalcemic.
- Concomitant hypomagnesemia
- Number of packed red cell transfusions
- Development of acute renal failure
- Recent neck/thyroid/parathyroid surgery

Genetics
A number of genetic syndromes are associated with hypoparathyroidism and resultant hypocalcemia:
- Polyglandular autoimmune syndrome type 1
- X-linked or AR hypoparathyroidism
- DiGeorge syndrome
- Activating mutations of the calcium sensing receptor of the parathyroid gland

GENERAL PREVENTION
Ionized calcium levels are checked frequently in critically ill patients, but it is unclear if correcting hypocalcemia is beneficial.

PATHOPHYSIOLOGY
- The concentration of serum calcium is regulated by the action of parathyroid hormone (PTH) and vitamin D on the kidney, bones, and GI tract:
  - Normally, PTH stimulates calcium resorption in the kidney and from bone and encourages renal conversion of 25-hydroxyvitamin D to its active form 1,25-dihyroxyvitamin D, which then increases GI absorption of calcium.
  - Hence low levels of PTH or vitamin D or insensitivity of tissue receptors to PTH (also called pseudohypoparathyroidism) can result in hypocalcemia.
- In critically ill patients, multiple mechanisms have been proposed: Complex formation with lactate/citrate, tissue precipitation, PTH suppression by inflammatory mediators, depressed renal calcitriol production, or tissue resistance.
- Calcium has been implicated in cell death and injury in animal models of sepsis. It has been hypothesized that hypocalcemia may be a protective mechanism in critical illness.

ETIOLOGY
- Hypocalcemia with low PTH (hypoparathyroidism):

  - Autoimmune
  - Neck/thyroid/parathyroid surgery and hungry bone syndrome
  - Irradiation or infiltration of the parathyroid glands
  - Genetic mutations as outlined above
  - Hypomagnesemia (<0.8 meq/L or 1 mg/dL)- causing PTH resistance or decreasing PTH secretion
- Hypocalcemia with high PTH concentrations:
  - Vitamin D deficiency or resistance
  - Hypomagnesemia
  - Pseudohypoparathyroidism
  - Renal disease
  - Loss of circulatory calcium due to deposition in tissue, as in hyperphosphatemia, tumor lysis, acute pancreatitis, osteoblastic metastases, and acute severe illness
- Drug-induced hypocalcemia:
  - Calcium chelators (citrate, EDTA, phosphate)
  - Bisphosphonates in conjunction with vitamin D deficiency
  - Fluoride poisoning
  - Foscarnet (complexes with calcium)
- Spurious hypocalcemia:
  - Gadolinium contrast agents interfere with colorimetric assays for calcium but not ionized calcium.
  - Hypoalbuminemia reduces total serum calcium but not ionized calcium (total serum calcium falls 0.8 mg/dL for every 1 g/dL reduction in serum albumin).
- Acid–base disturbances:
  - Acute respiratory alkalosis enhances the binding of calcium to albumin, thus decreasing levels of ionized calcium.

 DIAGNOSIS

HISTORY
- A history of neck surgery, alcoholism resulting in hypomagnesemia, chronic kidney disease, recent bisphosphonate use, or a family history of hypocalcemia may be elicited.
- Most patients are asymptomatic, but large and abrupt changes in ionized calcium leads to symptoms.
- Tetany is the classic presentation of acute hypocalcemia.
- Characterized by neuromuscular irritability
- Mild symptoms include paresthesias, muscle cramps, and perioral numbness.
- Severe symptoms include carpopedal spasm (Chvostek's and Trousseau's signs), laryngospasm, and seizures.

PHYSICAL EXAM
- Chvostek's sign is ipsilateral facial muscle contraction elicited by tapping the facial nerve anterior to the ear (occurs in 10% of normal people).
- Trousseau's sign is carpopedal spasm developing from mild hypoxemia induced by blood pressure cuff inflation (specificity, 94%).
- Hypotension may develop with a rapid fall in serum calcium.
- Papilledema and rarely optic neuritis

DIAGNOSTIC TESTS & INTERPRETATION
Lab
Initial lab tests
- Ionized calcium should be measured to confirm hypocalcemia, especially in critically ill patients.
- Measuring magnesium, creatinine, phosphate vitamin D levels, amylase, lipase, and CPK will help determine the etiology of hypocalcemia.
- Serum intact PTH is the most valuable test as an inappropriately normal or low level in the face of hypocalcemia confirms hypoparathyroidism.
- The QT interval may be prolonged on the EKG and rarely torsades de pointes may be triggered.

Follow-Up & Special Considerations
Intact PTH levels must have concomitant ionized calcium measurements as hypocalcemia is the most potent stimulant for PTH production.

Imaging
- In case of alteration of mental status and seizures, a noncontrast CT or MRI of the brain is advisable.
- Renal failure may necessitate an US of the kidneys.

TREATMENT

- Correction of hypocalcemia in the critically ill patient is controversial as hypocalcemia may be an adaptive response to severe stress. Calcium is a vital intracellular messenger and regulates cell function. It is essential for various processes including excitation-contraction coupling in muscle, neurotransmission, protein secretion, hormonal release, phagocytosis, and much more. It also regulates injurious processes such as cytokine release, free radical production, and vasoconstriction, which may be detrimental in critical illness. Studies have failed to show a beneficial effect of calcium administration in septic patients.
- Acute symptomatic hypocalcemia warrants specific treatment. Few studies address the optimal treatment of hypocalcemia. Most recommendations are based on expert opinion.

MEDICATION
First Line
- IV calcium gluconate is indicated for acutely symptomatic patients, an acute fall in serum calcium, or patients unable to take oral supplements.
- 1–2 g (90–180 mg of elemental calcium) injected in 50 mL of 5% dextrose slowly over 10–20 minutes with EKG monitoring
- Giving it at a faster rate may precipitate cardiac arrest in systole.
- It is contraindicated in concomitant hyperphosphatemia for fear of precipitation of the calcium-phosphate product.
- Should be followed by a slow infusion of calcium in dextrose or saline if hypocalcemia persists (10 × 10 mL ampoules in 1 L of 5% dextrose or normal saline at a rate of 50 mL/hr)

Second Line
- 10% calcium chloride (270 mg elemental calcium per 10 mL) may also be used.
- Extravasation may cause tissue necrosis, hence calcium gluconate is preferred.

ADDITIONAL TREATMENT
General Measures
- Correct hypomagnesemia if present.
- Prescribe oral calcium and vitamin D supplements when necessary.

Issues for Referral
An endocrinology referral and outpatient follow-up may be indicated.

IN-PATIENT CONSIDERATIONS
Initial Stabilization
- Secure the airway and maintain adequate circulation.
- Establish the diagnosis of hypocalcemia by checking serum ionized calcium.
- Cardiac monitoring for arrhythmias should be in place.

Admission Criteria
- Acute symptomatic hypocalcemia warrants inpatient monitored care.
- Chronic hypocalcemia may well be managed as an outpatient.

Nursing
Frequent monitoring of vital signs, continuous EKG monitoring, aspiration and seizure precautions should be in effect.

Discharge Criteria
- Resolution of hypocalcemia and other electrolyte abnormalities
- Correction of the underlying etiology

 # ONGOING CARE
COMPLICATIONS
- Seizures
- Hypotension
- QT prolongation
- Heart block
- Torsades de pointes

ADDITIONAL READING
- Cooper MS, et al. Diagnosis and management of hypocalcemia. *BMJ*. 2008;336:1298–1302.
- Moe SM. Disorders involving calcium, phosphorus, and magnesium. *Prim Care Clin Office Pract*. 2008;35:215–37.
- Williams SF, et al. Spurious hypocalcemia after gadolinium administration. *Mayo Clin Proc*. 2005;80:1655–7.
- Zaloga G. Ionized hypocalcemia during sepsis. *Crit Care Med*. 2000;28(1):266–8.
- Zivin JR, et al. Hypocalcemia: A pervasive metabolic abnormality in the critically ill. *Am J Kidney Dis*. 2001;37(4):689–98.

 # CODES
ICD9
- 252.1 Hypoparathyroidism
- 258.8 Other specified polyglandular dysfunction
- 275.41 Hypocalcemia

CLINICAL PEARLS
- Defined as an ionized calcium <4.65 mg/dL (1.16 mmol/L) or a total calcium <8.5 mg/dL (2.12 mmol/L)
- Incidence as high as 88% in critically ill patients
- Hypomagnesemia is an important underlying correctable cause.
- Serum intact PTH levels are vital to establishing etiology.
- Symptomatic patients with tetany require IV calcium gluconate.

HYPOGLYCEMIA

Vinia Mendoza
Paul Marik

 BASICS

DESCRIPTION

- Hypoglycemia is a condition characterized by low plasma glucose leading to autonomic and neurologic symptoms.
- True hypoglycemia is defined as low plasma glucose level accompanied by the usual signs and symptoms, and resolution of symptoms and signs once normal glucose level is restored (Whipple's triad).
- Most cases of hypoglycemia are drug-induced or iatrogenic, particularly in persons with diabetes mellitus or hospitalized individuals.
- Drug-induced hypoglycemia accounts for almost 1/4 of hospital admissions for adverse drug reactions.
- Hypoglycemia is usually secondary to aggressive attempts to tightly control glucose levels using insulin, usually given as continuous infusion, or due to errors in monitoring.
- The incidence of hypoglycemia in the ICU is between 20% and 30%.
- Hypoglycemia is associated with worse outcomes in critically ill patients based on several studies.
- Recent evidence shows that wide fluctuations in blood sugar levels may be more deleterious than actual levels.

PATHOPHYSIOLOGY

- Glucose level in the blood is tightly regulated to maintain a level of 60–100 mg/dL or 3.3–5.5 mmol/L.
- Because food intake is intermittent, a complex mechanism that involves a number of hormones keeps the blood glucose level at this tight range.
- Insulin is the hormone that promotes utilization and storage of glucose after a meal. Thus, insulin prevents hyperglycemia.
- When plasma glucose level starts to fall, counterregulatory hormones are released to stimulate production of glucose or release of stored glucose.

- The hormones that counteract the effects of insulin are:
  - Glucagon
  - Cortisol
  - Epinephrine
  - Growth hormone
- Glucagon is the primary hormone that prevents hypoglycemia. The others play a minor role when glucagon is available but play a substantial role in its absence or deficiency.
- Studies have demonstrated that these counterregulatory hormones are released into the circulation at a higher glucose level than that at which symptoms usually begin to occur.

ETIOLOGY

- Drugs:
  - Dispensing error
  - Exogenous insulin
  - Sulfonylureas
  - Meglitinides
  - Disopyramide
  - ACE-I
  - Propoxyphene
  - Quinine
  - Trimethoprim-Sulfamethoxazole
  - Pentamidine
  - Alcohol
  - Salicylates
  - Haloperidol
- Neoplasms:
  - Insulinoma
  - Large mesenchymal tumors (fibroma, sarcoma, small-cell carcinoma, mesothelioma)
- Miscellaneous:
  - Insulin autoimmune hypoglycemia
  - Islet hypertrophy/nesidioblastosis
  - Ketotic hypoglycemia
  - Total parenteral nutrition and insulin therapy
  - Shock
  - Sepsis
  - Starvation (eating disorders)
  - Severe liver disease
  - Chronic renal failure
  - Ackee-fruit poisoning and undernutrition
  - Adrenal insufficiency
  - Addison disease
  - Growth hormone deficiency
  - Hypopituitarism
  - Carnitine deficiency

 DIAGNOSIS

- Symptoms of hypoglycemia have traditionally been categorized into autonomic, or those thought to be a result of activation of the autonomic nervous system, and neuroglycopenic, or those that arise from low glucose supply to the brain.
- Patients with hypoglycemia usually experience the following:
  - Sweating
  - Trembling
  - A warm feeling
  - Nausea
  - Anxiety
  - Dizziness
  - Confusion
  - Blurred vision
  - Headache
  - Difficulty concentrating
  - Weakness
  - Tingling
  - Chest pounding
  - Fatigue
- Different people will experience different symptoms, but symptoms are generally consistent with every episode for any single person.
- The blood glucose level at which people experience symptoms also may vary.
- Individuals who have had episodes of hypoglycemia in the past may tolerate lower glucose levels before developing symptoms.
- Some patients with very profound hypoglycemia may be found to have behavioral changes, unresponsive, be in a coma, or having seizures.

DIAGNOSTIC TESTS & INTERPRETATION

- The diagnostic pathway for hypoglycemia will depend on whether a person is healthy-appearing or if he is ill.
- Healthy person:
  - The first step in the evaluation of a patient for hypoglycemia is to confirm that the patient's symptoms are related to low blood glucose levels (≤40 mg/dL).
  - It is often difficult to ascertain the relationship between the 2 as glucometers that patients usually use at home are not very reliable.

- It is difficult to ensure that the timing of symptoms coincides with the blood sugar determination.
- It is recommended that confirmation of hypoglycemia be done in a controlled setting such as a 72-hour fast.
- This test should be done in the hospital setting. Levels of plasma glucose, insulin, proinsulin, C-peptide, and B-hydroxybutyrate are measured before the fast, at specific intervals after the start, and at the end of the test.
- The test is ended when plasma glucose level is <45 and patient has symptoms of hypoglycemia.
- If a person does not develop symptoms or signs of hypoglycemia during the 72-hour period, then hypoglycemic disorder is rules out.
- High insulin, pro-insulin, and C-peptide levels point to an insulinoma or sulfonylurea-induced hypoglycemia.
- Checking for sulfonylurea level may differentiate the two.
- Factitious hypoglycemia is characterized by high insulin, but C-peptide and pro-insulin levels are low.
- Other tests that may aid in the diagnosis are the mixed meal, C-peptide suppression, and tolbutamide tests.
- Mixed-meal test is used for individuals who develop postprandial symptoms.
- The C-peptide suppression test may help look for insulinoma as cause of hypoglycemia and uses normative data for interpretation.
- Checking for insulin antibodies may lead to a diagnosis of autoimmune hypoglycemia, though persons with insulinoma, and some persons without hypoglycemia have detectable insulin antibodies.
- Ill patient:
  - Patients with conditions known to be at risk for hypoglycemia who have symptoms or signs of hypoglycemia may not need extensive evaluation.
  - Identification of the underlying disease is important.
  - Patients with renal disease, liver dysfunction, adrenal insufficiency, malnutrition, and shock are all at high risk for hypoglycemia.

- Hospitalized patients are at risk for developing hypoglycemia because of an underlying disease or from iatrogenic causes.
- About 1–2% of hospitalized patients have an episode of hypoglycemia.
- Common causes include too aggressive measures for correcting hyperglycemia with insulin, erratic oral food intake, and failure to reduce or discontinue hypoglycemic medications when patient's oral food intake is not possible or is being withheld for a purpose.
- Workup for hypoglycemia in a hospitalized patient should start with reviewing records and history.

 TREATMENT

MEDICATION
- Oral simple sugar (e.g., juice or candy) for mild hypoglycemia and mild symptoms.
- IV glucose in the form of 50% dextrose for more symptomatic patients or those who cannot tolerate oral intake.
- Glucagon by IV or intramuscular route for more profound hypoglycemia, or if signs and symptoms are refractory to IV glucose.
- 5–10% dextrose continuous infusion may be necessary until a stable plasma glucose level is attained.

ADDITIONAL TREATMENT
General Measures
- Identification of the cause of hypoglycemic episode is important.
- In the hospital setting, hypoglycemic agents including insulin should be withheld or reduced in dose until a regular pattern of oral intake is assured.
- The patient's medication list should be reviewed for other drugs that can cause hypoglycemia.
- For factitious hypoglycemia, confronting the patient usually makes him admit to the activity and stop.

Additional Therapies
Controversy regarding the management of insulinoma:
- The mass is usually difficult to localize within the pancreas.

- Intraoperative US, octreotide scanning, and transhepatic portal vein sampling for insulin have all been done to localize insulinomas.
- For unlocalized mass, treatment with diazoxide, verapamil, octreotide, propranolol, or phenytoin could be considered.

ADDITIONAL READING
- Cryer PE, et al. Evaluation and management of adult hypoglycemic disorders: An Endocrine Society clinical practice guideline. *J Clin Endocrinol Metab*. 2009;93:709–28.
- Fahy BG, et al. Glucose control in the intensive care unit. *Crit Care Med*. 2009;37:1–8.
- Murad MH, et al. Drug-induced hypoglycemia: a: A systematic review. *J Clin Endocrinol Metab*. 2009; 94:741–5.
- Service FJ. Hypoglycemic disorders. *N Engl J Med*. 1995;332:1144–52.

 CODES

ICD9
- 250.00 Diabetes mellitus without mention of complication, type ii or unspecified type, not stated as uncontrolled
- 251.2 Hypoglycemia, unspecified

CLINICAL PEARLS
- Hypoglycemia is characterized by Whipple's triad: Low plasma glucose level accompanied by the usual signs and symptoms, and resolution of symptoms and signs once normal glucose level is restored.
- High insulin, pro-insulin, and C-peptide levels point to an insulinoma or sulfonylurea-induced hypoglycemia; sulfonylurea level may differentiate the two.
- Factitious hypoglycemia is characterized by high insulin, but C-peptide and pro-insulin levels are low.

H

HYPOKALEMIA

Adel Bassily-Marcus
Roopa Kohli-Seth

BASICS

DESCRIPTION
- Hypokalemia is defined as a potassium level of <3.5 mEq/L
- Moderate hypokalemia is a serum level of 2.5–3 mEq/L.
- Severe hypokalemia is defined as a level <2.5 mEq/L.

EPIDEMIOLOGY
Incidence
- The most common electrolyte abnormality encountered in clinical practice
- Up to 21% of hospitalized patients are hypokalemic
- Up to 48% of patients who are receiving diuretics become hypokalemic

Prevalence
Occurs in 2.6 % of the yearly hospitalizations

RISK FACTORS
- Inadequate potassium (K^+) intake
- Excessive GI loss
- Excessive renal loss

Genetics
- Familial hypokalemic periodic paralysis
- Congenital adrenogenital syndromes
- Bartter, Liddle, and Gitelman syndromes: Autosomal recessive
- Familial interstitial nephritis

GENERAL PREVENTION
- Adequate potassium (K) supplementation
- Early detection of the cause of hypokalemia

PATHOPHYSIOLOGY
- Total body K^+ is 50 mEq/kg, about 3500 mmol, of which only 2% is extracellular.
- The large K^+ concentration gradient between the intracellular (Ki =140 mmol/L) and extracellular (Ke = 4.5 mmol/L) space is maintained by Na-K ATPase, Na-K pum, Na-H exchanger, and Na-K-Cl cotransporter to maintain electroneutrality.
- Hypokalemia increases the resting membrane potentials of neural and muscular tissues, reducing excitability and impairing muscle contractility.
- The resting membrane potential (Em) is calculated according to the Nernst Equation:

$$Em\ (mV) = -61 \log (Intracellular K^+ / Extracellular K^+).$$

- The normal ratio of intracellular K^+ to extracellular K^+ is about 30, and therefore normal Em is −90 mV.
- The membrane potential tends to increase with hypokalemia, where both intra- and extracellular K^+ tend to decrease, but the extracellular concentration tends to decrease proportionately more than the intracellular concentration. Hence, the ratio of intracellular K^+ to extracellular K^+ tends to increase.
- Alkalosis, insulin, and β_2-agonists can cause hypokalemia by stimulating $Na^+- K^+$ ATPase activity.
- On average, a reduction of serum potassium by 0.3 mmol/L suggests a total body deficit of 100 mmol.
- Hypokalemia increases the risk for cardiac arrhythmias, including ventricular fibrillation.
- Muscle hyperpolarization leads to weakness, fatigue, cramping, myalgia, paralysis, rhabdomyolysis, and decreased gut motility, leading to constipation and paralytic ileus.
- Stimulation of proximal tubules to increase ammoniagenesis can predispose encephalopathy.
- Hypokalemia can cause polyuria due to increased thirst and by inducing a mild and reversible renal concentrating defect that represents decreased renal response to antidiuretic hormone (ADH).

ETIOLOGY
- Hypokalemia occurs by 1 of 3 main mechanisms: Intracellular shift, reduced intake, or increased loss.
- Malnutrition:
  - Decreased dietary intake
  - Parenteral nutrition
  - Refeeding syndrome
- GI losses:
  - Vomiting or nasogastric suctioning: Through renal K^+ wasting as a result of volume depletion and hypochloremic metabolic alkalosis
  - Diarrhea
  - Enemas or laxative use
  - Uretero-sigmoidostomy: Urine rich Na and Cl entering the sigmoid will be altered by addition of the secreted colonic K^+ and HCO_3 with reabsorption of NaCl into the blood.
  - Geophagia: Potassium-binding clay soil ingestion
- Drug-induced:
  - Transcellular shift:
    - B_2 adrenergic agonist: Epinephrine
    - Bronchodilators: Albuterol, terbutaline, isoproterenol
    - Tocolytics: Ritodrine, nylidrin
    - Theophylline
    - Caffeine
    - Insulin
    - Verapamil intoxication
    - Barium toxicity: Blocks K^+ exit from cells, causing ascending paralysis that could result in death, termed Pa Ping.

- Renal K^+ loss:
  - Diuretics (most common cause): Acetazolamide, furosemide, bumetanide, torsemide, metolazone
  - Mineralocorticoids: Fludrocortisone
  - Mineralocorticoids effect: Licorice, carbenoxolone, gossypol
  - High-dose glucocorticoids
  - High-dose antibiotics: Penicillin, nafcillin, carbicillin, ampicillin
  - Drugs with magnesium depletion: Foscarnet, aminoglycosides, cisplatin
  - Amphotericin B
  - Excess K^+ loss in stool: Sodium polystyrene sulfonate, phenolphthalein
- Renal losses:
  - Renal tubular acidosis
  - Hyperaldosteronism
  - Magnesium depletion
  - Leukemia (mechanism uncertain)
  - Salt-wasting nephropathies
  - High urinary concentrations of anions (e.g., penicillin)
  - Intrinsic renal transport defects (Bartter, Liddle, and Gitelman syndromes)
  - Post-obstructive diuresis
- Hypokalemic periodic paralysis:
  - Unknown etiology; these episodes of muscle weakness or paralysis can affect the respiratory muscles.
- Thyrotoxic periodic paralysis:
  - Acquired form of hypokalemic periodic paralysis
  - Most common in Asian males
  - Increased Na-K-ATPase activity
- Hypothermia:
  - Involves K^+ shift from the extracellular space to the interstitial or intracellular space with a reverse shift upon rewarming.
- Alkalosis, correction of acidosis:
  - Metabolic alkalosis drives K^+ to enter cells in exchange for H^+. (K^+ levels decline 0.1–0.4 mEq/L for each 0.1-unit increase in pH)
  - In turn, hypokalemia increases renal HCO_3^+ absorption, perpetuating the alkalosis.
  - Hypokalemia during acidosis suggests an even larger total-body deficit.
  - Correction of acidosis aggravates the hypokalemia and often requires very aggressive K^+ administration.
- Renal replacement therapies:
  - Dialysis, continuous renal replacement therapy, peritoneal dialysis can cause K losses.
- Plasmapheresis:
  - Albumin replacement leads to dilutional hypokalemia.

- Spurious hypokalemia:
  - Delayed sample analysis is a well-recognized cause of spurious hypokalemia, due to increased cellular uptake.
  - Clinically relevant if ambient temperature is increased; rarely in acute leukemia.
- Rapid cell growth in acute anabolic states:
  - Acute leukemia, high-grade lymphoma, following administration of granulocyte-macrophage colony-stimulating factor to a patient with refractory anemia and excess blast cells
- Hypomagnesemia:
  - Magnesium is a cofactor for the enzyme Na^+–K^+ ATPase, which may be a partial explanation for high renal K^+ losses observed in patients with hypomagnesemia.
  - Hypomagnesemia aggravates the physiologic effects of hypokalemia and renders deficit correction difficult.
- Syndromes:
  - Bartter syndrome: Defective NaCl reabsorption in the thick ascending limb of Henle
  - Gitelman syndrome: Defect in thiazide-sensitive NaCl transporter in distal tubules
  - Liddle syndrome: Mutation in the epithelial sodium channel leading to excessive sodium reabsorption and K excretion

COMMONLY ASSOCIATED CONDITIONS
- Diuretics use, hypokalemic drugs
- Acute GI losses with severe vomiting or diarrhea

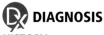 **DIAGNOSIS**

HISTORY
- Psychosis, depression, delirium or hallucinations
- Skeletal muscle weakness or cramping
- Paralysis, paresthesias
- Palpitations
- Constipation, nausea, vomiting, diarrhea
- Polyuria
- Concurrent medication evaluation

PHYSICAL EXAM
- Hypertension may be a clue to primary hyperaldosteronism, renal artery stenosis, licorice ingestion.
- Most patients are asymptomatic, and hypokalemia is incidentally found on serum electrolyte testing.
- Moderate-severe hypokalemia can produce generalized lassitude, muscle weakness and fasciculation, restless legs, paresthesias, depressed deep tendon reflexes, paralysis, and ileus.
- If serum K^+ <2 mEq/L) or if the decrease in serum K^+ is rapid, premature atrial or ventricular beats, hypoventilation, respiratory failure, lethargy, sudden death may develop.

DIAGNOSTIC TESTS & INTERPRETATION
Lab
Initial lab tests
- Serum K^+ is not always an accurate indicator of total body potassium.
- Serum level of sodium, chloride (CL), bicarbonate, magnesium, BUN, and creatinine performed in addition to the serum potassium
- Serum digoxin level
- ABG
- Serum aldosterone and plasma rennin in unexplained or persistent hypokalemia
- Urine analysis for potassium (Uk) and chloride:
  - Low Uk: If the urine potassium <20 mEq/L, this suggests a nonrenal cause with proper renal K conservation:
    ○ Diarrhea, poor intake, or skin losses
    ○ A low urinary potassium + low urinary chloride suggests GI losses.
    ○ A low urinary potassium and normal urinary chloride suggests laxative abuse.
  - High Uk: If the urinary K^+ concentration is high (>20 mEq/L), this suggests an adrenal or renal disease with inadequate K^+ conservation:
    ○ If hypertension: Check plasma aldosterone level: High (>22 ng/dL): Hyperaldosteronism Low (<22 ng/dL): Cushing syndrome, mineralocorticoid excess, Liddle syndrome
    ○ If acidemia (HCO_3 <22 mmol/L): RTA types I and II
    ○ A high urinary potassium + low urinary chloride (<15 mEq/L): Alkalosis, NG tube drainage
    ○ A high urinary potassium + high urinary chloride (>25 mEq/L): Diuretic use, Mg depletion, Bartter syndrome, Gitelman syndrome
- ECG:
- ST segment depression
- T-wave flattening or inverted T waves
- Prominent U wave, appears as QT prolongation
- Increase in P wave amplitude, PR interval, QRS duration.
- Ventricular arrhythmias (e.g., premature ventricular contractions, torsade de pointes, ventricular fibrillation)
- Atrial arrhythmias (e.g., premature atrial contractions, atrial fibrillation)

Follow-Up & Special Considerations
- Potassium replacement therapy is immediately indicated for severe hypokalemia (<2.5 mEq/L) or if the hypokalemia is causing muscle paralysis or malignant cardiac arrhythmias.
- Geriatric consideration: Cardiac arrhythmias are uncommon in healthy patients with hypokalemia, but are far more common and significant in elderly patients with underlying heart disease.

- Hypokalemia enhances the risk of digitalis toxicity, which may occur despite normal digitalis levels in the presence of modest hypokalemia.
- Hypokalemia in a context of metabolic acidosis or serum hypertonicity often indicates K^+ deficits.
- Treating underlying hyperthyroidism is the key to treating the hypokalemia in thyrotoxic hypokalemic periodic paralysis.

Imaging
Pituitary, adrenal imaging to assess for adenoma, Cushing

Initial approach
The goals of therapy in hypokalemia are to prevent life-threatening conditions (diaphragmatic weakness, rhabdomyolysis, and cardiac arrhythmias), to replace any K^+ deficit, and to diagnose and correct the underlying cause.

Pathological Findings
In severe hypokalemia, necrosis of cardiac and skeletal muscle

DIFFERENTIAL DIAGNOSIS
- Cushing syndrome
- Renal tubular acidosis
- Thyrotoxicosis
- Hypomagnesemia
- Hypocalcemia

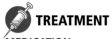 **TREATMENT**

MEDICATION
First Line
- Potassium chloride (KCL) should be the default salt of choice in most patients. Other forms of K^+ includes K phosphate, K bicarbonate or its precursors (K citrate, K acetate), and potassium gluconate.
- KCL raises serum K^+ at a faster rate because Cl^- does not enter cells to the same extent as bicarbonate, keeping the administered K^+ in the extracellular fluid compartment.
- PO supplementation is possible and may be faster than IV K^+ supplementation, due to limitations in the rapidity of IV K^+ infusion.
- KCl, 20–40 mEq PO b.i.d./q.i.d.; not to exceed 40 mEq PO/dose is suitable for most forms of hypokalemia.

Second Line
- KCL 10–20 mEq/h IV via peripheral or central line:
  - Potassium carbonate (or citrate) should only be used in patients with renal tubular acidosis and an associated metabolic acidosis.
  - Potassium phosphate can be used in patients with associated phosphate deficiency.

H

ADDITIONAL TREATMENT
General Measures
- In asymptomatic patient with mild hypokalemia, start oral replacement.
- Rapid IV bolus administration of potassium is usually contraindicated; it can cause lethal cardiac arrhythmias and respiratory muscle paralysis.
- Hypomagnesemia should be suspected if hypokalemia is refractory to supplementation.
- Concomitant administration of potassium-sparing diuretics (spironolactone, triamterene, amiloride, ACE inhibitors) magnify the risk of hyperkalemia.
- Cautions with potassium replacement in hypokalemic periodic paralysis; rebound hyperkalemia may occur.
- In patients receiving digitalis or with acute myocardial ischemia, hypokalemia should be treated urgently because of risk of ventricular arrhythmias.

Issues for Referral
ICU admission for supervised IV administration of potassium especially in severe hypokalemia

Additional Therapies
Strategies to minimize K^+ losses should be considered.

COMPLEMENTARY & ALTERNATIVE THERAPIES
Increase dietary intake of potassium-rich foods.

IN-PATIENT CONSIDERATIONS
Initial Stabilization
- Assess respiratory status
- Continues cardiac monitoring
- Establish proper IV access
- Stop offending drug if drug induced.

- Indication for IV K supplementation:
  - Cardiac arrhythmias, digoxin toxicity
  - Severe myopathy, paralysis
  - Severe diarrhea
  - Plasma K^+ <3 mEq/L in high-risk patients
- Asymptomatic, K^+ >3 mEq/L:
  - In the absence of ongoing losses, PO potassium chloride 10–20 mEq given b.i.d.–q.i.d./d
  - 5–10 mEq/L can be given IV without cardiac monitoring in a stable patient.
- Mild to moderate symptoms, or K^+ <3.0 mEq/L:
  - PO potassium chloride (40–60 mEq t.i.d.–q.i.d., total 120–240 mEq), until the plasma serum potassium concentration remains above 3.0–3.5 mEq/L and symptoms resolve.
  - IV KCL is commonly given at 10–20 mEq in 100 mL of normal saline over 1 hour with continuous cardiac monitoring and 1 hour postdose check.
- Severe symptoms or unable to take oral meds:
  - 5–10 mEq/hr is standard IV replacement rate
  - 20–40 mEq/hr if serum potassium <2.5 mEq/L or moderate-severe symptoms
  - Up to 40 mEq in 100 mL over 1 hour can be safely given through a central venous line.
- IV magnesium replacement therapy:
  - Coexisting magnesium and potassium depletion could lead to refractory potassium repletion (1)[B].

Admission Criteria
- Severe or symptomatic hypokalemia
- IV potassium is going to be rapidly administered

IV Fluids
- IV 0.9% sodium chloride
- Dextrose-containing vehicles may worsen the hypokalemia by stimulating insulin release that will cause intracellular shifting.

Nursing
- Cardiac monitoring with frequent and on time vital signs and lab checks
- Serum K^+ should be checked more frequently in groups at higher risk: Elderly, diabetics, and patients with renal insufficiency.

Discharge Criteria
Patient in stable condition with corrected electrolytes abnormality

ONGOING CARE

FOLLOW-UP RECOMMENDATIONS
- Be aware that serum potassium concentration can rise acutely by as much as 1–1.5 mEq/L after an oral dose of 40–60 mEq, and by 2.5–3.5 mEq/L after 135–160 mEq.
- Caution should be taken in K replacement in patients on ACE inhibitors, angiotensin receptor blockers (ARB), spironolactone, and in patient with underlying kidney disease.

Patient Monitoring
- If an infusion rate >10 mEq/hr is needed, continuous cardiac monitoring is recommended to detect any signs of hyperkalemia.
- For severe hypokalemia, continuous ECG monitoring is required; the infusion is stopped immediately if signs of hyperkalemia develop.

DIET
- Increase intake of bananas, tomatoes, oranges, peaches, squash, potatoes, beans, prunes, spinach.
- In patients on a low-salt diet, hypokalemic hypochloremic alkalosis is a possibility that may require chloride as well as potassium supplementation.

PATIENT EDUCATION
Teaching regarding K^+ supplements, potassium-rich foods, and regular follow-up is necessary.

PROGNOSIS
Hypokalemia per se can increase in-hospital mortality rate up to 10-fold likely due to the cardiovascular morbidity (2)[C].

COMPLICATIONS
- Hyperkalemia
- Digitalis toxicity

REFERENCES

1. Cohn JN, et al. New guidelines for potassium replacement in clinical practice: A contemporary review by the National Council on Potassium in Clinical Practice. *Arch Intern Med*. 2000;160(16): 2429–36.
2. Paltiel O, et al. Management of severe hypokalemia in hospitalized patients: A study of quality of care based on computerized databases. *Arch Intern Med*. 2001;161(8):1089–95.

ADDITIONAL READING

- Gennari FJ. Hypokalemia. *N Engl J Med*. 1998; 339(7):451–8.

CODES

ICD9
- 255.8 Other specified disorders of adrenal glands
- 276.8 Hypopotassemia
- 359.3 Periodic paralysis

CLINICAL PEARLS
- Determining serum K^+ alone is not sufficient to justify replacement. Clinical context dictates the need for therapy.
- The risk of arrhythmia from hypokalemia is highest in older patients, patients with evidence of organic heart disease, and patients on digoxin or antiarrhythmic drugs
- Treatment should be followed by serial K^+ measurements.
- A decrease in plasma K from 4 mEq/L to 3 mEq/L represents 100–200 mEq decline in total body K; below 3 mEq/L, every 1 mEq/L fall reflects a 200–400 mEq decline in total body K.
- Assess and correct acid–base and extracellular fluid volume abnormalities.
- In presence of hypomagnesemia, successful K^+ replacement depends on management of the hypomagnesemia.

H

HYPONATREMIA

Rakesh Sinha
Roopa Kohli-Seth

 BASICS

DESCRIPTION
- Hyponatremia is defined as serum sodium (Na^+) concentration ≤ 135 mmol/L
- System(s) affected: Endocrine/Metabolic

EPIDEMIOLOGY
Incidence
- Incidence of hyponatremia among ICU patients is 11%.
- Incidence density of hyponatremia in ICU is 3.1 per 100 ICU days.

Prevalence
- Prevalence of hyponatremia in ICU patients is 15%.
- Prevalence of hyponatremia among in-patients 6.2%.

RISK FACTORS
- Hospitalization
- Thiazide diuretics
- Post operative state
- Polydipsia in psychiatric patients
- Transurethral prostatectomy

Geriatric Considerations
Elderly are more than twice at risk for hyponatremia as compared to younger patients.

GENERAL PREVENTION
Exercise-associated hyponatremia can be prevented by appropriate fluid intake.

PATHOPHYSIOLOGY
- Hypotonic hyponatremia, the most common form of the hyponatremia, is caused by excess water retention in relation to existing Na^+ stores, which can be decreased, normal, or increased.
- Retention of water occurs most commonly because of impaired renal excretion of water but is sometimes due to excessive water intake and normal excretory capacity.
- Hypertonic (translocational) hyponatremia results from a shift of water from cells to the extracellular compartment because of solutes confined in the extracellular compartment.

ETIOLOGY
Hypotonic hyponatremia with impaired capacity of renal water excretion:
- Decreased extracellular fluid (ECF) volume:
  - Renal sodium loss:
    - Diuretic agents
    - Osmotic diuresis: Glucose, urea, mannitol
    - Adrenal insufficiency
    - Salt-wasting nephropathy
    - Cerebral salt wasting
    - Bicarbonaturia: Renal tubular acidosis, disequilibrium stage of vomiting
    - Ketonuria
  - Extrarenal sodium loss:
    - Diarrhea
    - Vomiting
    - Blood loss
    - Excessive sweating (endurance exercise)
    - Fluid sequestration in "third space": Bowel obstruction, peritonitis, pancreatitis, muscle trauma, burns

- Increased ECF volume:
  - Congestive heart failure (CHF)
  - Cirrhosis
  - Nephrotic syndrome
  - Advanced renal failure
  - Pregnancy
- Normal ECF volume:
  - Thiazide diuretics
  - Hypothyroidism
  - Adrenal insufficiency
  - Syndrome of inappropriate secretion of antidiuretic hormone (SIADH):
    - Cancer: Pulmonary, mediastinal, or extrathoracic tumor
    - CNS disorders: Acute psychosis, mass lesion, inflammatory and demyelinating diseases, stroke, hemorrhage, trauma
    - Drugs:
      - Desmopressin
      - Oxytocin
      - Prostaglandin-synthesis inhibitors
      - Nicotine
      - Phenothiazines
      - Tricyclics
      - Serotonin-reuptake inhibitors
      - Opiate derivatives
      - Chlorpropamide
      - Clofibrate
      - Carbamazepine
      - Cyclophosphamide
      - Vincristine
    - Pulmonary conditions: Infections, acute respiratory failure, positive-pressure ventilation
    - Miscellaneous: Postoperative state, pain, severe nausea, HIV infection
  - Decreased intake of solutes:
    - Beer potomania
    - Tea-and-toast diet
- Hypotonic hyponatremia with excessive water intake:
  - Primary polydipsia
  - Dilute infant formula
  - Sodium-free irrigant solutions (hysteroscopy, laparoscopy, transurethral resection of prostate)
  - Accidental intake of large amounts of water (e.g., during swimming lessons)
  - Fresh water drowning
  - Multiple tap-water enemas
- Nonhypotonic hyponatremia
- Hypertonic hyponatremia:
  - Hyperglycemia
  - Mannitol, sorbitol, glycerol, maltose
  - Radiocontrast
- Isotonic (pseudohyponatremia) hyponatremia:
  - Hyperlipidemia
  - Hyperproteinemia

COMMONLY ASSOCIATED CONDITIONS
- CHF
- Cirrhosis
- Pneumonia
- CNS disease
- Renal failure
- Lung cancer

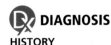 **DIAGNOSIS**

HISTORY
- Severity of clinical symptoms related to acuity and magnitude of decrease in serum Na^+
- Neurologic symptoms caused by brain edema when serum Na^+ <125 mmol/L
- Nausea and malaise
- Headache
- Lethargy and disorientation
- Seizure and coma
- Respiratory arrest
- Slowly developing hyponatremia over >2–3 days has fewer neurologic symptoms, even when serum Na^+ as low as 115 mmol/L
- Nonspecific symptoms seen with chronic hyponatremia include fatigue, dizziness, gait disturbances, falls, confusion, and muscle cramps.
- Medication list should be reviewed in all cases.

PHYSICAL EXAM
- Neurological signs: Depressed deep-tendon reflexes, positive Babinski sign, cranial nerve palsies, Cheyne-Stokes breathing
- Signs of hypovolemia: Tachycardia, orthostatic hypotension, dry mucous membrane, decreased skin turgor, and sunken eyes
- Signs of hypervolemia: Jugular venous distension, ascites, edema, and pulmonary rales

DIAGNOSTIC TESTS & INTERPRETATION
Lab
Initial lab tests
- Serum electrolytes, glucose, and renal function
- Serum and urine osmolality
- Urine sodium and potassium

Follow-Up & Special Considerations
- Thyroid function test
- Cortisol level and cosyntropin test

Imaging
Initial approach
Chest x-ray may show pulmonary disease.

Follow-Up & Special Considerations
CT of brain may be indicated in SIADH.

TREATMENT

ALERT
- The serum Na^+ concentration should not be raised by $>10-12$ mmol/L in the first 24 hours and by >18 mmol/L in the first 48 hours.
- Rapid correction of serum Na^+ (>20 mmol/L in the first 24 hours) can cause osmotic demyelination syndrome (ODS) leading to irreversible brain damage.
- ODS may presents as flaccid paralysis, dysarthria, dysphagia, behavioral disturbance, seizures, coma, and death.
- Symptoms may be delayed by 2–6 days.
- CT scan or MRI can detect demyelinating lesions but may take up to 4 weeks to be positive.
- No effective therapy; prevention is key.
- Hepatic failure, hypokalemia, malnutrition, premenopausal women have increased risk.
- Rapid Na^+ correction can occur with administration of hypertonic saline OR with isotonic saline in hypovolemia, cortisol in adrenal insufficiency, and cessation of thiazides.

MEDICATION
First Line
- Hypertonic (3%) saline in patients with acute hyponatremia ($\leq$48–hour duration) with neurologic symptoms usually with serum Na^+ concentration $<120-125$ mmol/L (1,2,3,4)[B]:
  - An initial infusion rate is estimated by multiplying patient's body weight (in kilograms) by the desired rate of increase in serum Na^+ (in mmol/L) per hour.
  - Aggressive institute initial correction of 2–4 mmol/L over 2–4 hours in severe symptoms.
  - Stop when symptoms resolve or serum Na^+ concentration reaches safe range ($\sim$120–125 mmol/L).
  - Monitor serum Na^+ q2h.
- Isotonic saline in hypovolemic hyponatremia (1)[B]
- Conivaptan (vasopressin receptor antagonist) in euvolemic and hypervolemic hyponatremia (1)[B]:
  - 20 mg loading dose over 30 minutes
  - 20 mg/d continuous infusion for up to 4 days

Pediatric Considerations
Caution in children when using Conivaptan

Second Line
- Demeclocycline 300–600 mg b.i.d. in SIADH
- Urea 15–60 g/d in SIADH
- Clozapine in primary polydipsia

ADDITIONAL TREATMENT
General Measures
- Fluid restriction in advanced renal failure, SIADH, and primary polydipsia
- Fluid restriction in increased ECF volume (heart failure, cirrhosis) to achieve negative solute-free water balance
- Discontinue thiazides, replete potassium
- Loop diuretics in CHF and cirrhosis
- Correct hyperglycemia, adrenal insufficiency, hypothyroidism, and underlying cause of SIADH

Issues for Referral
- Nephrology consult in severe symptomatic, refractory, or complicated cases with need for demeclocycline, conivaptan, or dialysis
- Cardiology, hepatology, and endocrinology in difficult to manage CHF, cirrhosis, hypothyroidism, and adrenal insufficiency

IN-PATIENT CONSIDERATIONS
Initial Stabilization
Isotonic saline in patients with hypotension and hyponatremia to correct volume deficit

Admission Criteria
Symptomatic patients, usually with serum sodium concentration <125 mmol/L

IV Fluids
- Isotonic saline in hypovolemia initially then switch to hypotonic when volume is restored
- Hypertonic (3%) as indicated

Nursing
- Bed rest until hemodynamically stable
- Input/output recording
- Seizure precaution

Discharge Criteria
Asymptomatic with normal Na^+ concentration

ONGOING CARE

FOLLOW-UP RECOMMENDATIONS
Do not rechallenge with thiazides if hyponatremia was caused by thiazides.

Patient Monitoring
Follow serum Na^+ concentration in patients initiated on loop diuretics following cessation of thiazides for thiazide-induced hyponatremia.

DIET
- Dietary sodium restriction in hyponatremia with hypervolemia
- Proper nutrition with adequate solutes and protein in beer potomania and tea-and-toast diet

PATIENT EDUCATION
Behavior modification in primary polydipsia

PROGNOSIS
Mortality is increased in patients with hyponatremia.

COMPLICATIONS
Cerebral edema leading to irreversible brain damage, brain herniation, and death

REFERENCES
1. Verbalis JG, et al. Hyponatremia treatment guidelines 2007: Expert panel recommendations. *Am J Med*. 2007;120:S1–S21.
2. Lin M, et al. Disorders of water balance. *Emerg Med Clin N Am*. 2005;23:749–70.
3. Ellison DH, et al. Clinical practice. The syndrome of inappropriate antidiuresis. *N Engl J Med*. 2007; 356:2064–72.
4. Andogue HJ, et al. Hyponatremia. *N Engl J Med*. 2000;342:1581–9.

See Also (Topic, Algorithm, Electronic Media Element)
Evaluation of Hyponatremia
I. Serum osmolality
  A. Normal
    (280–295 mOsm/kg)
    Isotonic hyponatremia
    1. Hyperlipidemia
    2. Hyperproteinemia
  B. Low
    (<280 mOsm/kg)
    Hypotonic hyponatremia
    ECF Volume status
    1. Hypovolemic
      Urine sodium
      a. <10 mmol/L
        Extrarenal salt loss
        (1) Diarrhea
        (2) Vomiting
        (3) Dehydration
        (4) Third spacing
      b. >20 mmol/L
        Renal salt loss
        (1) Diuretics
        (2) Nephropathy
        (3) Adrenal insufficiency
        (4) Cerebral salt wasting
    2. Euvolemic
      a. SIADH
      b. Adrenal insufficiency
      c. Hypothyroidism
      d. Thiazides
      e. Decreased intake of solutes
    3. Hypervolemic
      a. CHF
      b. Cirrhosis
      c. Nephrotic syndrome
      d. Advanced renal failure
  C. High
    (>295 mOsm/kg)
    Hypertonic hypernatremia
    1. Hyperglycemia
    2. Mannitol

CODES

ICD9
276.1 Hyposmolality and/or hyponatremia

CLINICAL PEARLS
- Hypotonic hyponatremia, the most common form of the hyponatremia, is caused by excess water retention in relation to existing Na^+ stores, which can be decreased, normal, or increased.
- Use isotonic saline in patients with hypotension to correct volume deficit.
- Hypertonic saline initial infusion rate is estimated by multiplying patient's body weight (in kilograms) by the desired rate of increase in serum Na^+ (in mmol/L) per hour.
- The serum Na^+ concentration should not be raised by $>10-12$ mmol/L in the first 24 hours and by >18 mmol/L in the first 48 hours.

H

HYPOTHERMIA, ACCIDENTAL

Hayder Said

 BASICS

DESCRIPTION
- An unintentional decline in core temperature below 35°C (95°F).
- Primary hypothermia is due to accidental exposure to cold.
- Secondary hypothermia is due to failure of thermoregulatory function (1).
- Hypothermia is classified according to severity:
  - Mild: 32–35°C (90–95°F)
  - Moderate: 28–32°C (82–90°F
  - Severe: Below 28°C (82°F)
  - System(s) affected: All

EPIDEMIOLOGY
Incidence
- Uncommon condition
- Race: Hypothermia affects all racial groups.
- Sex: Males and females are equally susceptible to hypothermia (2).

Geriatric Considerations
- The elderly are at increased risk of developing hypothermia and its complications (3,4).
- Decreased physiologic reserve and social isolation are the predisposing factors.
- In elderly patients, sepsis can manifest as hypothermia (5).
- Empiric, broad-spectrum antibiotics should be administered if there is an obvious source of infection, aspiration, failure to rewarm, or other signs suggestive of sepsis.
- Older persons with preexisting medical conditions such as congestive heart failure, diabetes, or gait disturbance also are at increased risk for hypothermia (6).

RISK FACTORS
- Old age
- Recreational exposure to a cold
- Cold water submersion
- Medical conditions (e.g., hypothyroidism, sepsis).
- Toxins (e.g., ethanol abuse).
- Medications (e.g., oral antihyperglycemics, sedatives-hypnotics).

GENERAL PREVENTION
- Wear appropriate clothing to the weather.
- Travel with a partner.
- Carry survival bags with space blankets.
- Drink cold water rather than ice or snow.
- Stay dry.
- Keep the homes of the elderly heated to at least 70°F (21.1°C).

PATHOPHYSIOLOGY
- Body temperature reflects the balance between heat production and heat loss.
- Heat is generated by cellular metabolism.
- Heat is lost by the skin and lungs via evaporation, radiation, conduction, and convection.
- Convective heat loss to cold air and conductive heat loss to water are the most common mechanisms of accidental hypothermia (1).
- Hypothermia alters cell membrane function, efflux of intracellular fluid, enzymatic dysfunction, and electrolyte imbalances (including prominent hyperkalemia).
- The hypothalamus stimulates heat production through shivering and increased thyroid, catecholamine, and adrenal activity.
- Sympathetically mediated vasoconstriction minimizes heat loss by reducing blood flow to peripheral tissues, where cooling is greatest (1,2).

ETIOLOGY
- Hypothermia is more frequent among persons who are elderly, homeless, mentally ill, trauma victims, outdoor workers, and children.
- Causes of hypothermia can be divided into the following 3 categories:
  - Decreased heat production
  - Increased heat loss
  - Impaired thermoregulation

COMMONLY ASSOCIATED CONDITIONS
- Hypothyroidism
- Sepsis
- CNS dysfunction
- Drug intoxication
- Alcoholism
- Malnutrition
- Ketoacidosis
- Burns
- Addison's disease

DIAGNOSIS

HISTORY
- History of exposure to cold environment
- Symptoms are vague and nonspecific.
- Patients may complain of stiffness, weakness, shivering, dizziness, and dyspnea.
- Clinical manifestations depend on the severity of the temperature reduction and the patient's premorbid condition.

PHYSICAL EXAM
- A rectal probe thermometer is practical in most cases.
- In patients with endotracheal intubation, an esophageal probe is used.
- The reliability of tympanic thermometers in the setting of significant hypothermia has NOT been established (5).

- A total body survey should be conducted in all hypothermic patients:
  - Mild hypothermia: Tachypnea, tachycardia, increased BP, impaired judgement; suspect CNS pathology if patient is comatose
  - Moderate hypothermia: Expect bradycardia; hypotension, hypoventilation, cyanosis, arrhythmias, semicoma, and muscular rigidity
  - Severe hypothermia: Hypotension, no pulse; ventricular fibrillation or asystole, apnea, fixed pupil, areflexia, coma

DIAGNOSTIC TESTS & INTERPRETATION
Lab
- Fingerstick glucose
- Coagulation studies: Clinical coagulopathy may be present despite normal measured coagulation times.
- Fibrinogen level
- CBC: Increased hematocrit may reflect hemoconcentration.
- Basic electrolytes
- BUN and creatinine
- Creatine phosphokinase
- Sodium. bicarbonate: Low bicarbonate suggests anion-gap acidosis; if so, obtain ABG, UNCORRECTED for temperature.

Imaging
Chest radiograph (care must be taken to avoid jostling the patient)

Diagnostic Procedures/Other
- Toxicologic screen if altered mental status
- Serum cortisol
- Thyroid function
- ECG:
  - Rhythm abnormalities (atrial fibrillation, sinus bradycardia) may be present.
  - Intervals (PR, QRS, and QTc) may be prolonged.
  - Osborn J waves characteristic of hypothermia; occurs at junction of QRS and ST segments, most prominent in V2–V5
  - Distortion of the earliest phase of membrane depolarization could be misinterpreted as ischemic injury pattern.

DIFFERENTIAL DIAGNOSIS
- Increased heat loss:
  - Induced vasodilation (drugs, alcohol, toxins)
  - Skin disorders (burns, psoriasis, exfoliative dermatitis)
  - Iatrogenic (cold infusion, emergent deliveries, cardiopulmonary bypass, continuous renal replacement therapy)
- Decreased heat production:
  - Endocrinologic disease (hypopituitarism, hypoadrenalism, hypothyroidism)
  - Insufficient fuel (hypoglycemia, malnutrition)
  - Neuromuscular inefficiency (extremes of age, impaired shivering, inactivity)

- Impaired regulation:
  - Peripheral: Spinal-cord transection, neuropathies, diabetes mellitus
  - Central: Cerebrovascular accident, subarachnoid hemorrhage, parkinsonism, hypothalamic dysfunction, multiple sclerosis, anorexia nervosa
  - Drugs: Intoxicants, anxiolytics, antidepressants, antimanic agents, antipsychotics, opioids, oral hypoglycemic agents, β blockers
- Other:
  - Sepsis
  - Pancreatitis
  - Carcinomatosis
  - Uremia
  - Vascular insufficiency
  - Trauma
  - Psychiatric illness, including attempted suicide

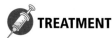

TREATMENT

- Initiate rewarming, monitor core temperature. "Rewarming techniques are based on degree of hypothermia:
  - Mild hypothermia: Passive external rewarming, remove wet clothing, cover with blankets
  - Moderate hypothermia: Active external and internal rewarming:
    ○ Warmed humidified oxygen, forced air warming systems
    ○ Beware of initial paradoxical drop in core temperature due to return of cold blood from extremities to core circulation.
    ○ Rewarm trunk first to minimize risk of core temperature afterdrop.
  - Severe hypothermia: Active internal rewarming (active core rewarming) and active external rewarming:
    ○ Warmed humidified oxygen, warmed IV fluids (42°C)
    ○ Pleural and peritoneal irrigation with warm saline (40–42°C)
    ○ Extracorporeal options: Continuous venovenous rewarming, hemodialysis, continuous arteriovenous rewarming, and cardiopulmonary bypass
- Identify and treat complications:
  - Treatment of arrhythmias:
    ○ Arrhythmias may persist until patient rewarmed
    ○ Ignore atrial arrhythmias with slow ventricular response
    ○ Ventricular fibrillation is a common rhythm; may be precipitated by physical jostling, manage according to ACLS protocol, electrical defibrillation may be attempted but is rarely successful until core temperature is above 30°C.

MEDICATION

- Drug metabolism and excretion are reduced in patients with hypothermia.
- Hypothermia compromises host defenses and predisposes to sepsis.
- Consider empiric antibiotics in pediatric, geriatric patients.
- For patients with altered mental status, consider IV thiamine, 100 mg; dextrose, 25 g; naloxone, 0.8–2.0 mg.

IN-PATIENT CONSIDERATIONS
Initial Stabilization
- Stabilize airway, breathing, and circulation
- Avoid rough movements and activity, which may induce ventricular fibrillation.
- Consider endotracheal intubation;may be necessary in obtunded patients and those with bronchorrhea.
- Crystalloid or dopamine for BP support; treat hypotension with warmed crystalloid (42°C) initially, dopamine if necessary.

 ONGOING CARE

FOLLOW-UP RECOMMENDATIONS
Patient Monitoring
- During acute episode:
  - Monitor electrolytes and glucose frequently.
  - Monitor urinary output.
  - Follow blood gases.
- Following acute episode:
  - Continued therapy for any underlying disorder

DIET
Alcohol intake increases risk of becoming hypothermic in cold conditions.

PATIENT EDUCATION
- Patient education centers on prevention of the causative factors.
- People who participate in outdoor recreation should become familiar with weather patterns, qualities of outdoor clothing, and sensible precautions to take prior to undertaking the activity.

PROGNOSIS
- Depends on etiology, comorbidities, and complications, and possibly influenced by treatment and rewarming strategies
- The mortality rate varies by location.
- Mortality is 0.49 persons per 100,000 population in southern states.
- Mortality is 4.64 persons per 100,000 population in Alaska (6).
- Males have higher mortality rates.

COMPLICATIONS
- Arrhythmias
- Lactic acidosis
- Rhabdomyolysis
- Bleeding diathesis and DIC
- Infection, sepsis
- Medication toxicity

REFERENCES

1. Jolly BT, et al. Accidental hypothermia. *Emerg Med Clin North Am.* 1992;10:311
2. Lee-Chiong TL, et al. Disorders of temperature regulation. *Compr Ther.* 1995;21:697.
3. Ranhoff AH. Accidental hypothermia in the elderly. *Int J Circumpolar Health.* 2000;59:255.
4. Ballester JM, et al. Hypothermia: An easy-to-miss, dangerous disorder in winter weather. *Geriatrics.* 1999;54:51.
5. Danzl DF, et al. Accidental hypothermia. *N Engl J Med.* 1994;331:1756.
6. DeGroot DW, et al. Epidemiology of U.S. Army cold weather injuries, 1980–1999. *Aviat Space Environ Med.* 2003;74(5):564–70.[Medline].

 See Also (Topic, Algorithm, Electronic Media Element)

See chapter on Therapeutic Hypothermia

CODES

ICD9
- 780.65 Hypothermia not associated with low environmental temperature
- 991.6 Hypothermia

CLINICAL PEARLS

- Hypothermia during anesthesia:
  - Due to anesthetic-induced inhibition of thermoregulation combined with cold operating room environment.
  - Volatile anesthetics cause vasodilation through a direct peripheral action and inhibit tonic thermoregulatory vasoconstriction, leading to increase in cutaneous heat loss.
- Major outcome studies proved that mild hypothermia during surgery:
  - Triples the incidence of morbid cardiac outcomes
  - Triples the incidence of surgical wound infections and prolongs hospitalization by 20%
  - Significantly increases surgical blood loss and the need for allogeneic transfusion

H

HYPOTHROIDISM, SEVERE/MYXEDEMA COMA

Amyn Hirani
Paul E. Marik

 BASICS

DESCRIPTION
- The most severe form of hypothyroidism
- A severe decompensated state of hypothyroidism that, if unrecognized, can have a high mortality
- First described in 1879
- The main distinguishing signs differentiating severe hypothyroidism from myxedema coma are hypothermia and hemodynamic instability with poor mentation leading to coma.
- The clinical severity cannot be assessed by thyrotropin (TSH) levels.
- Mortality has improved over years from 60% to 25% due to advances in supportive care.

EPIDEMIOLOGY
Incidence
- The occurrence of myxedema coma is rare.
- It usually occurs in elderly, during the winter months.
- Incidence of overt hypothyroidism is 0.3% in general population, which can rise to 1.7% in patients >65 years.
- Males < Females (1:8)
- Precipitating factors:
  - Hypothermia
  - Neurological events, cerebrovascular event
  - Cardiac: Congestive heart failure
  - Drugs: Anesthetics, narcotics, sedative agents, amiodarone, lithium carbonate
  - Metabolic: Hypoglycemia, hyponatremia, hypoxemia, hypercapnia, acidosis, hypercalcemia.
  - Infection:
    - UTI
    - PNA
  - Trauma
  - GI bleeding
  - Noncompliance

GENERAL PREVENTION
- Past medical history can sometimes be the key to diagnosis.
- Routine screening can prevent this life-threatening complication.

PATHOPHYSIOLOGY
- Hypothyroidism can be primarily of thyroid origin or secondary from pituitary failure.
- Primary hypothyroidism is the main offender: It results from a primary defect in thyroid gland with subsequent decrease in synthesis of the hormone.
- Causes of primary hypothyroidism include:
  - Hashimoto's thyroiditis (chronic autoimmune) with or without goiter, and with cell-mediated and antibody damage of the gland.
  - Iodine deficiency is one of the most common causes.
  - Iodine excess can briefly result in hypothyroidism. Known to also occur with iodine dye injection or amiodarone (Wolff-Chaikoff effect)

- Postablative hypothyroidism after radioactive iodine therapy or radiation
- Partial or total thyroidectomy
- Drugs: Amiodarone, lithium, ethionamide
- Infiltrative diseases like Riedel disease, sarcoid, hemochromatosis, leukemia, and scleroderma
- Infection: *Mycobacteriumtuberculosis, Pneumocystis carinii*
- Central hypothyroidism:
  - Due to decreased or defective function of pituitary or hypothalamus resulting in decreased TSH or TRH, respectively.
  - Secondarily from pituitary etiologies like tumors, hemorrhage, necrosis, infiltrative disorders, and pituitary apoplexy
  - Tertiary causes are hypothalamic.

DIAGNOSIS

- Given that thyroid receptors are present in the vast majority of organ systems, deficiency results in malfunction of these organs. Reduced metabolism elucidates the major mechanism.
- The deposition of protein matrix glycosaminoglycan in various tissues:
  - CNS: Diminished cognitive state, delayed relaxation phase of deep-tendon reflexes, lethargy, decreased mentation and coma; seizures can also occur
  - Metabolic: Hypothermia, hyponatremia, hypoglycemia
  - Respiratory System: Hypoxia, hypercapnia, carbon dioxide narcosis, decreased respiratory drive, and reduced muscle function may lead to transient mechanical ventilation in severe cases. Pleural effusion may lead to restriction of lung, and macroglossia causes obstruction of airway and can worsen underlying sleep apnea.
  - Cardiovascular system: Bradycardia, diastolic hypertension, decreased pulse pressure, pericardial effusion with or without pericardial rub; cardiomegaly, prolonged QT interval, dilated cardiomyopathy, and hypotension may occur in severe cases.
  - GI system: Decreased gluconeogenesis, constipation, decreased motility, gastric atony, nausea, fecal impaction. Ileus and megacolon may occur in severe cases.
  - Renal system: Decreased GFR, decreased free water clearance. Severe cases can have acute renal failure.
  - Endocrine system: Excess vasopressin release leading to water retention. Adrenal insufficiency in some cases; more likely in central causes
  - Integumentary system: Coarse hair, dry skin, nonpitting edema, macroglossia

DIAGNOSTIC TESTS & INTERPRETATION
The diagnosis is usually suspected with the clinical presentation, history, and physical exam. If the likelihood appears high, treatment is begun without confirmatory testing.

Lab
Initial lab tests
- Routine initial lab tests are often abnormal but rarely diagnostic alone.
- Mild anemia: Normocytic normochromic
- Hyponatremia, hypoglycemia, hypochloremia, and rising creatinine
- Increased serum vasopressin levels
- Elevated creatinine phosphokinase and lactate dehydrogenase levels
- Increased serum cholesterol.
- ABG may show respiratory acidosis and hypoxia.
- Thyroid function test: Elevated TSH, and low T3 and T4 are diagnostic. TSH may be normal or mildly elevated in cases of central hypothyroidism.
- Use of vasopressor (dopamine) and steroids may also inaccurately show normal TSH with low T4.

Follow-Up & Special Considerations
Repeat thyroid function test in 4– 6 weeks is recommended.

Imaging
Radiological studies may be used to rule out other disorders contributing to or worsening the disease process.

Diagnostic Procedures/Other
- No specific diagnostic procedure is needed.
- Procedures such as central venous access, mechanical ventilation, arterial access for hemodynamic monitoring are needed for supportive care.

DIFFERENTIAL DIAGNOSIS
- Encephalopathy from various causes
- Septic shock
- Hypothermia
- Heart failure
- Amyloid

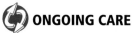 TREATMENT

MEDICATION
- Administration of thyroid replacement hormone can be life-saving (5)[C].
- T3 is the active hormone.
- T4 converts to T3 in the peripheral tissue by enzyme deiodinase. The enzyme function may be reduced in severe hypothyroidism.
- If T4 is used, IV a loading dose of 250–500 mcg is recommended, followed by 50–100 mcg IV until patient can take oral medications (3,5)[B].
- T3 can be used with T4 or alone.
- Its usual dose is 10 mcg q8h for the first 24 hours or until patient can take oral medications (3,5)[C].
- Watch for cardiac complications and manifestations of underlying coronary artery disease; more likely with T3 than T4 (2)[B].

ADDITIONAL TREATMENT
Additional Therapies
- Hypotension: Treat with fluids and vasopressors if needed. Watch for arrhythmia if vasopressor is used.
- Mechanical ventilation for hypercapnia and hypoxia
- Workup for underlying occult infection with blood cultures, chest radiograph, etc.
- Hydrocortisone 100 mg q8h until adrenal insufficiency is proven or excluded [C].
- Correct electrolyte abnormalities.
- Hypothermia should be treated with passive rewarming as active rewarming may worsen hypotension by vasodilatation effect.

SURGERY/OTHER PROCEDURES
If any emergent surgery is needed, Thyroid supplement along with hydrocortisone should be continued.

IN-PATIENT CONSIDERATIONS
Initial Stabilization
- Should include basic ABC assessment
- Patients may present with respiratory failure, hypotension, hypothermia; treatment is supportive.
- Further stabilization includes correction of volume deficits and any major electrolyte abnormalities.
- Early intubation in patients with hypercapnia, hypoxia, or who are unable to protect the airway

Admission Criteria
All cases of suspected severe hypothyroidism or myxedema coma should be monitored as an inpatient, likely in the ICU.

IV Fluids
- Aggressive volume resuscitation along with vasopressor agents is often required secondary to hypotension and poor perfusion.
- May need to monitor for signs of cardiac arrhythmias and ischemia in older patients

Nursing
- Continuous monitoring of heart rate, blood pressure, mental status, and respiratory status is necessary.
- Frequent turning to prevent bedsores as patients are sometimes comatose and intubated
- Aspiration precautions

Discharge Criteria
- Resolving electrolyte abnormalities and improved cognition
- Underlying cardiac and adrenal diseases have been excluded.
- Many patients need short-term rehabilitation or long-term nursing home care.

 ONGOING CARE

FOLLOW-UP RECOMMENDATIONS
- Follow-up with thyroid function test in 4–6 weeks is required.
- Normality of serum cholesterol is usually reached in 3–6 months.
- Precipitating cause needs to be identified and treated.

PATIENT EDUCATION
- Patient and family members should be educated about importance of compliance.
- Treatment is lifelong in most cases.
- Watch for symptoms, along with the signs of thyrotoxicosis or infection.

PROGNOSIS
- Good, if recognized early. In the stage of myxedema coma, mortality is usually >20%.
- Patients with higher APACHE II, worse Glasgow coma scale, cardiac comorbidities have worse outcomes.
- Predictors of worse outcomes:
  – Old age
  – Underlying cardiovascular disease
  – Diminished consciousness

COMPLICATIONS
- Congestive heart failure
- Respiratory failure
- Ileus
- Hyponatremia
- Hypothermia
- Infection and sepsis
- Adrenal insufficiency
- Coagulopathy
- Increased sensitivity to medications, sedatives, and narcotics
- Multisystem organ failure; death

REFERENCES
1. Devdhar M, et al. Hypothyroidism. *Endocrinol Metab Clin North Am.* 2007;36(3):595–615, v.
2. Fliers E, et al. Myxedema coma. *Rev Endocr Metab Disord.* 2003;4(2):137–41.
3. Kwaku MP, et al. Myxedema coma. *J Intensive Care Med.* 2007;22(4):224–31.
4. Roberts CG, et al. Hypothyroidism. *Lancet.* 2004; 363(9411):793–803.
5. Wartofsky L. Myxedema coma. *Endocrinol Metab Clin North Am.* 2006;35(4):687–98, vii–viii.

ADDITIONAL READING
- www.endocrine.niddk.nih.gov/pubs/Hypothyroidism/

CODES

ICD9
- 244.8 Other specified acquired hypothyroidism
- 244.9 Unspecified acquired hypothyroidism

H

CLINICAL PEARLS
- Maintain a high clinical suspicion for myxedema coma as it can present with mental status change and can lead to death.
- It should always be in the differential diagnosis of hypothermia and bradycardia.
- More atypical presentations are common.
- Compliance to medication is the key factor to prevent reoccurrences.
- Treat for underlying infection and adrenal insufficiency unless excluded.
- Arrange for follow-up thyroid function test in 4–6 weeks.

IDIOPATHIC SYSTEMIC CAPILLARY LEAK SYNDROME (CLARKSON DISEASE)

Omar Rahman

BASICS

DESCRIPTION
- Uncommon life-threatening disorder characterized by acute massive extravasation of plasma due to increased capillary permeability
- Chronic disease with cyclical acute recurrences at unpredictable and variable time intervals
- Acute attack can be divided into 2 distinct phases:
  - Capillary leak phase: Leakage of plasma from systemic capillary beds in large amounts occurs rapidly. Hemoconcentration, tachycardia, hypotension, and edema formation occur within a few hours. Clinical manifestations depend on individual organ system involved. Compartment syndromes of extremities, rhabdomyolysis, pulmonary edema, ascites, and airway edema have been described. Consequences of shock such as acute renal failure, lactic acidosis, ischemic hepatitis, and ultimately multiple organ failure can be seen.
  - Recruitment or resolution phase: Active plasma extravasation resolves with persistent slowly resolving tissue edema. Acute intravascular volume overload has been described with consequent acute lung injury.

EPIDEMIOLOGY
Incidence
Rare. Exact incidence unknown. >100 case reports since 1960.

Prevalence
- Mostly reported in Caucasian adults
- Male = Female

RISK FACTORS
- Viral illnesses:
  - Upper respiratory tract infections
  - GI viral disorders
- Physical stress
- Menstruation

Genetics
Unknown genetic predisposition

GENERAL PREVENTION
- Avoid precipitants of attacks.
- Education of patient and local health care professionals due to rare nature of illness
- Prophylactic therapy

PATHOPHYSIOLOGY
- Exact pathogenesis is unknown.
- IL-2, IFN-β 1b, CD 8+ lymphocytes, and 5-lipoxygenase metabolite activation implicated
- Endothelial apoptosis demonstrated in vitro
- Hypoalbuminemia occurs due to leakage of albumin.
- Monoclonal gammopathy is a frequent finding (~70%).

ETIOLOGY
Primary etiology is unknown.

COMMONLY ASSOCIATED CONDITIONS
- Monoclonal gammopathy of undetermined significance (MGUS)
- Other paraproteinemia
- Deep venous thrombosis

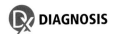

DIAGNOSIS

ALERT
Patient's condition deteriorates very rapidly despite initial apparently stable picture. Rising hematocrit precedes change in hemodynamics.

HISTORY
- Flu-like illness or GI prodrome
- Symptoms of acute attack:
  - Dizziness
  - Shortness of breath
  - Swelling of limbs (1)[C]
- Prior similar episodes

PHYSICAL EXAM
- Tachycardia and hypotension
- Tachypnea
- Decreased level of consciousness
- Weight gain
- Limb edema that may be associated with tenderness, loss of distal pulses, and paresthesias
- Poor capillary refill and cyanosis
- Cold extremities
- Diaphoresis
- Decreased breath sounds, rales and rhonchi
- Abdominal distension and fluid thrill
- Decreased CVP (during the leak phase)
- Elevated limb compartment pressure
- Elevated intra-abdominal pressure

DIAGNOSTIC TESTS & INTERPRETATION
Lab
Initial lab tests
- CBC:
  - Hemoglobin/hematocrit are elevated (2)[C]
  - Leucocytosis
- CPK elevated with rhabdomyolysis and compartment syndrome
- BUN, creatinine, LFT, urinalysis
- ABG, CO_2, lactic acid, and LDH
- Albumin and total protein levels

Follow-Up & Special Considerations
- Serum protein and immune electrophoresis (2)[C]
- Bence-Jones protein

Imaging
- CXR
- Vascular Doppler US

Diagnostic Procedures/Other
- CVP monitoring:
  - Decreased CVP during active leak phase; fluid response can be gauged.
- Echocardiography or other hemodynamic monitoring
- Compartment pressure measurements at frequent intervals starting soon after presentation
- Intra-abdominal pressure monitoring to detect intra-abdominal hypertension and abdominal compartment syndrome (ACS)

DIFFERENTIAL DIAGNOSIS
- Septic shock
- Anaphylaxis
- Polycythemia
- Hantavirus infection with pulmonary involvement
- Hyperviscosity syndromes (e.g., associated with Waldenström's macroglobulinemia, multiple myeloma)

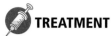

TREATMENT

MEDICATION

First Line
Corticosteroids:
- Hydrocortisone (300 mg/d IV in divided doses) or methylprednisolone (up to 500 mg/d IV in divided doses) (2)[C]
- Administer early in acute phase.

Second Line
Vasoactive agents:
- Start early for hypotension as IV fluids rapidly leak from vascular compartment.
- Phenylephrine (40–200 mcg/min infusion), norepinephrine (5–20 mcg/min infusion)
- Other agents such as vasopressin, dopamine, or dobutamine may be required

ADDITIONAL TREATMENT

General Measures
- ABCs
- Oxygen, monitoring
- Large-bore IVs, central venous catheter

Additional Therapies
- Aminophylline and theophylline
- Leukotriene antagonists
- Terbutaline (2)[C]
- Plasmapheresis
- IV immunoglobulins (IVIg) (3)[C]
- Furosemide (in recruitment phase)

COMPLEMENTARY & ALTERNATIVE THERAPIES
- Thalidomide
- Endothelial growth factors

SURGERY/OTHER PROCEDURES
- Early or preemptive limb fasciotomies
- Exploratory laparotomy for ACS
- Hemodynamic and other monitoring:
  – Central venous or pulmonary artery catheter
  – Arterial catheter
  – Foley catheter

IN-PATIENT CONSIDERATIONS

Initial Stabilization
- Early endotracheal intubation and mechanical ventilation
- Bolus and continuous IV crystalloids and colloids (judicious and cautious use)
- Pharmacologic venous thromboembolism prophylaxis (enoxaparin, heparin, fondaparinux)
- Therapeutic anticoagulation if VTE present

Admission Criteria
ICU admission even if initially stable

IV Fluids
- 0.9% saline
- 5% albumin
- 25% albumin
- Hetastarch 6% and pentastarch 10%

Nursing
Standard ICU nursing care

Discharge Criteria
Clinical and biochemical resolution of acute attack

ONGOING CARE

FOLLOW-UP RECOMMENDATIONS
- Primary care, hematology
- Rehabilitation, physical and occupational therapy

Patient Monitoring
- Initial ICU care
- Hemoglobin
- Serum protein and immune electrophoresis

DIET
Restrictions only if organ system failure persists (renal, hepatic)

PATIENT EDUCATION
- Goal is to seek medical attention early.
- Risk factor avoidance methods

PROGNOSIS
- Statistical data scant
- High morbidity and mortality due to recurrent acute attacks

COMPLICATIONS
- Permanent disability
- Limb contractures
- Amputation
- ARDS
- Chronic renal failure
- ICU and hospital stay-related complications
- Progression to bone marrow malignancies

REFERENCES

1. Clarkson B, et al. Cyclical edema and shock due to increased capillary permeability. *Am J Med*. 1960;29:193–216.
2. Dhir V, et al. Idiopathic systemic capillary leak syndrome (SCLS): Case report and systemic review of cases reported in the last 16 years. *Intern Med*. 2007;46(12):899–904.
3. Lambert M, et al. High dose IV immunoglobulins dramatically reverse systemic capillary leak syndrome. *Crit Care Med*. 2008;36(7):2184–7.

ADDITIONAL READING
- Kawabe S, et al. Systemic capillary leak syndrome. *Intern Med*. 2002;41(3):211–5.
- Tahirkheli NK, et al. Treatment of the systemic capillary leak syndrome with terbutaline and theophylline. A case series. *Ann Intern Med*. 1999;130:905–9.

CODES

ICD9
448.9 Other and unspecified capillary diseases

CLINICAL PEARLS
- Although described as rare, this condition may be underrecognized.
- In acute attacks, patients initially may be deceptively stable but rapidly decompensate.
- Plasma leakage causes shock, hemoconcentration, and compartment syndromes.
- Acute management is largely supportive, with cautious IV fluid use and volume status monitoring.
- Corticosteroids, IVIg, and plasmapheresis may attenuate the severity of the acute event.

I

ILEUS
Oveys Mansuri

 BASICS

DESCRIPTION
- Ileus can be defined as absence of motility or hypomotility of the GI tract when bowel obstruction has been ruled out.
- The form of ileus (acute colonic pseudo-obstruction) that presents with signs of a bowel obstruction in the absence of mechanical obstruction is known as *Ogilvie syndrome*.
- Paralytic ileus (pseudo-obstruction) is most common in infants and children and can be due to viral or bacterial infection or food poisoning.

EPIDEMIOLOGY
Incidence
- ~50% of patients have postoperative ileus following major abdominal surgery.
- Drug-induced megacolon can lead to high mortality (10–20%)
- Ogilvie syndrome may have 30% mortality (usually a disease of critically ill patients).

RISK FACTORS
- Abdominal surgery or GI procedures
- Use of narcotics
- Pancreatitis
- Abdominal infections or injury
- Electrolyte imbalance
- Diabetic ketoacidosis (DKA) (6) and other causes of metabolic acidosis
- Hypothyroidism
- Critical illness (inflammation with peritonitis)
- Spinal cord injury, usually above T5 level

Geriatric Considerations
Ogilvie pseudo-obstruction is more common in elderly and critically ill patients.

GENERAL PREVENTION
- Minimize the use of narcotics following abdominal surgery.
- Use of epidural analgesia postoperatively has been shown to reduce the incidence of postoperative ileus.

PATHOPHYSIOLOGY
- Inhibitory spinal reflex arcs
- Endocrine and inflammatory mediators
- Motilin, gastrin, cholecystokinin increase GI motility.
- Somatostatin and glucagon decrease GI motility.

ETIOLOGY
- Abdominal surgery
- Electrolyte abnormalities
- Hypothyroidism
- Intra-abdominal infection/inflammation
- Medications (narcotics)
- Severe illness

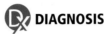 **DIAGNOSIS**

HISTORY
- Abdominal pain or discomfort
- Associated symptoms: Nausea, vomiting, and/or poor oral intake
- May not be passing flatus or stool
- Belching

PHYSICAL EXAM
- Abdominal distension, possible tenderness
- Minimal to absent bowel sounds

DIAGNOSTIC TESTS & INTERPRETATION
Lab
- Electrolytes
- CBC

Imaging
Plain abdominal x-rays demonstrate gas dilatation of small bowel and colon, scattered air-fluid levels, or nonspecific bowel gas patterns.

Diagnostic Procedures/Other
Small bowel radiographic contrast follow-through

DIFFERENTIAL DIAGNOSIS
- Mechanical bowel obstruction
- Pseudo-obstruction

 TREATMENT

MEDICATION
- Only ileus related to the use of narcotics can be treated with medications (opioid antagonists), although the reduction of the dose of narcotics is often sufficient to improve the symptoms.
- Acute colonic obstruction (Ogilvie syndrome) can be treated with IV neostigmine.

ADDITIONAL TREATMENT
General Measures
- Colonoscopic decompression for Ogilvie syndrome
- Treatment of the underlying causes
- Appropriate volume resuscitation
- Electrolyte replacement
- Limiting use of opioids
- Although most physicians treat ileus by keeping the patients NPO, there is some evidence that small amounts of enteric feeds may promote its resolution.

Issues for Referral
Surgical consultation is advised for severe bowel distention that may lead to bowel ischemia.

Additional Therapies
- Peripherally selective opioid antagonists (i.e., methylnaltrexone, alvimopan) for postoperative ileus
- Prokinetic medications (erythromycin, metoclopramide); but no strong evidence in support of these

COMPLEMENTARY & ALTERNATIVE THERAPIES
Chewing gum may stimulate GI motility in the postoperative patient.

SURGERY/OTHER PROCEDURES
- Surgery not indicated for true ileus
- Thoracic epidurals may improve postoperative ileus.

IN-PATIENT CONSIDERATIONS
Initial Stabilization
- Appropriate fluid resuscitation
- Electrolyte replacement
- Symptomatic use of nasogastric decompression; no evidence for ileus treatment
- Must verify the absence of mechanical bowel obstruction

Admission Criteria
- ICU admission may be considered for elderly patients, hemodynamic instability, marked electrolyte abnormality, and/or need for close and constant monitoring.
- Ileus by itself is not an indication for ICU admission.

IV Fluids
Adequate fluid resuscitation with use of crystalloid replacement (i.e., 0.9% NS or LR)

Nursing
- Patient comfort
- Assistance with ambulation
- Optimization of nonopioid pain control

Discharge Criteria
- Patients can often be discharged from the ICU before the full resolution of ileus as indicated by tolerance of diet, passing of flatus, and bowel movement.
- Resolution and/or recovery from underlying cause of ileus (i.e., surgery, electrolyte abnormality)

 ONGOING CARE

FOLLOW-UP RECOMMENDATIONS
Patient Monitoring
Once stabilized medically or postsurgically, may be safe for transfer to floor

DIET
- NPO initially
- Early enteral feeding is encouraged
- Avoid TPN unless absolutely necessary

PATIENT EDUCATION
Transition from opioid to nonopioid pain medication if ileus secondary to narcotic use

PROGNOSIS
Often good for postoperative ileus; less so for Ogilvie syndrome

COMPLICATIONS
- Missed diagnosis of mechanical bowel obstruction
- Bowel ischemia due to extreme dilation, hypoperfusion

ADDITIONAL READING

- Akca O. Use of selective opiate receptor inhibitors to prevent postoperative ileus. *Minerva Anestesiol*. 2002;68:162–5.
- Fruhwald S, et al. Gastrointestinal motility in acute illness. *Wien Klin Wochenschr*. 2008;120(1–2): 6–17.
- Hiranyakas A, et al. Epidemiology, pathophysiology and medical management of postoperative ileus in the elderly. *Drugs Aging*. 2011;28(2):107–18.
- Kurz A, Sessler DI. Opioid-induced bowel dysfunction: Pathophysiology and potential new therapies. *Drugs*. 2003; 63(7):649–71.

 CODES

ICD9
- 560.1 Paralytic ileus
- 560.89 Other specified intestinal obstruction
- 997.4 Digestive system complications, not elsewhere classified

CLINICAL PEARLS
- Ileus is extremely common after abdominal surgery.
- Diagnosis must exclude mechanical bowel obstruction.
- While bowel rest, nasogastric decompression, ambulation, and prokinetic medications are commonly utilized, no definitive data supports this.
- Epidural analgesia, peripherally acting opioid antagonists, and use of NSAIDs in lieu of narcotics have shown some benefit.
- Ogilvie syndrome has a poorer prognosis but often responds to neostigmine treatment (be aware of possible bradycardia in response to neostigmine and be prepared to treat it promptly with atropine).

I

INFECTIONS, SURGICAL SITE

Sharon S. Leung

 BASICS

DESCRIPTION
- Defined as infections occurring within 30 days after a surgical operation (or within 1 year in the presence of prosthetic materials) and affecting either the incision or deep tissue at the surgical site
- The clinical criteria used to define a surgical site infection (SSI) include any of the following:
  - Purulent exudate draining from a surgical site
  - Positive fluid culture obtained from a surgical site
  - Surgeon's diagnosis
  - A surgical site that requires reopening
- SSIs are classified as follows:
  - Superficial incisional (involving only skin or subcutaneous tissue of the incision)
  - Deep incisional (involving fascia and/or muscular layers)
  - Organ/space
- Rates of SSIs for individual procedures vary depending upon patient population, size of hospital, experience of the surgeon, and methods used for surveillance.

EPIDEMIOLOGY
Prevalence
- 2nd most common health care-associated infection (HAI), 17% with hospitalized patients.
- Among surgical patients, SSIs are the most common HAI.
- ~2% following operative procedures

RISK FACTORS
- Surgical environment and procedure-related:
  - Preoperative shaving of hair (clipping preferred)
  - Excessive personnel traffic during an operation
  - Excessive use of electrosurgical cautery units.
  - Presence of a prosthesis or other foreign body
  - Prolonged duration of surgery
  - Duration of preoperative hospitalization
  - Need for blood transfusion
- Patient-related:
  - Extremes of age
  - Diabetes
  - Obesity
  - Malnutrition
  - Cigarette smoking
  - Cancer
  - Immunosuppressive state
  - Preoperative nasal carriage or colonization with *Staphylococcus aureus*
  - Preoperative severity of illness
  - History of infection

GENERAL PREVENTION
- Strict hand washing
- Preoperative skin washing with chlorhexidine-alcohol scrub
- Preoperative use of intranasal mupirocin
- Remote site infection/colonization control
- Preoperative hair removal using electric clippers
- Antimicrobial prophylaxis
- Surgical attire and drapes
- Stop tobacco use prior to procedure (use nicotine patch)
- Blood sugar control

PATHOPHYSIOLOGY
- Most SSIs are acquired at the time of surgery.
- Most common source is direct inoculation of endogenous patient flora at the time of the surgery.
- For clean procedures, the most common pathogens are normal skin flora.
- For procedure involving viscus opening, the infections are typically polymicrobial.
- Although the species of microorganisms isolated from SSIs have not changed markedly over decades, the percentage caused by antibiotic-resistant pathogens and fungi has increased.
- Exogenous sources of infection include contamination of the surgical site by flora from the operating room environment or personnel.
- Common pathogens include:
  - *S. aureus*
  - Gram-negative bacilli
  - Coagulase-negative *Staphylococcus*

COMMONLY ASSOCIATED CONDITIONS
- Abscess
- Hematoma

DIAGNOSIS

HISTORY
- Fever or chills
- Pain
- Tenderness
- Localized swelling
- Erythema

PHYSICAL EXAM
- Erythema
- Tenderness and warm
- Bleeding at surgical site
- Increased discharge
- Foul-smelling discharge
- Increased tightness of the sutures
- Increased swelling beyond surgical site
- Fever or hypothermia
- Tachycardia
- Tachypnea
- Altered mental status

DIAGNOSTIC TESTS & INTERPRETATION
Lab
Initial lab tests
- CBC with differential
- Serum electrolytes
- ABGs
- Serum lactate
- BUN and creatinine
- CPK
- Blood cultures
- Wound culture and Gram stain may not be helpful and only identify colonizing organisms.

Follow-Up & Special Considerations
Tissue biopsy

Imaging
CT scan/MRI

TREATMENT
- Antibiotics
- Initial broad coverage for HAIs
- Coverage should include gram-negative and anaerobic organisms for perforated visci.
- Consider local resistance patterns and results of microbiological tests in choosing an antibiotic.
- Removal of prosthetic material
- Debridement

 # ONGOING CARE

PROGNOSIS
- Despite advances in infection control practices, SSIs still cause a substantial amount of morbidity and mortality.
- Postoperative length of hospital stay increased by 7–10 days.
- Mortality is >8%.
- Hospital charges increase by $2,000–4,500.

COMPLICATIONS
- Abscess
- Necrotizing fasciitis
- Gangrene
- Severe sepsis/septic shock
- Acute respiratory failure
- ARDS
- Acute renal failure
- Multisystem organ dysfunction

ADDITIONAL READING

- Anderson DJ, et al. Strategies to prevent surgical site infections in acute care hospitals. *Infect Control Hosp Epidemiol*. 2008;29:S51–S61.
- Mangram AJ, et al. Guideline for prevention of surgical site infection. *Infect Control Hosp Epidemiol*. 1999;20:247–78.
- Surgical site infection prevention and treatment of surgical site infection. Accessed at www.nice.org.uk

CODES

ICD9
998.59 Other postoperative infection

CLINICAL PEARLS

SSIs are often HAIs.

I

INTRA-AORTIC BALLOON PUMP (IABP)

Hady Lichaa
Isaac Halickman

BASICS

DESCRIPTION
- Mechanical device consisting of a cylindrical balloon placed in the aorta, which inflates at the onset of diastole and deflates at the onset of systole. Used to decrease myocardial oxygen demand while increasing myocardial oxygen supply.
- Most commonly triggered by ECG signals. The balloon starts inflating in the middle of the T wave and starts deflating prior to the end of the QRS complex. This is performed by a computer program that controls the flow of helium from a pressurized gas reservoir into and out of the balloon.
- Arterial waveform is used as a trigger in the case of tachyarrhythmias, paced rhythm, and poor ECG signals.
- Balloon usually inflated on each cardiac cycle, but can be inflated every 2nd or 3rd beat, depending on the level of hemodynamic support required.
- Mechanism of action:
  - Diastolic inflation increases coronary perfusion pressure.
  - By deflating in systole, IABP decreases left ventricular (LV) afterload and improves forward blood flow. The end result is decreased myocardial work and modest increase in cardiac output, depending on the underlying contractility reserve of the ventricular myocardium.
  - Therefore, IABP decreases myocardial oxygen demand and increases coronary blood supply.
- Indications:
  - Cardiogenic shock secondary to acute myocardial infarction (AMI) (1)[B]
  - Refractory post-AMI angina as a bridge to angiography and revascularization (1)[B]
  - Acute mitral regurgitation or ventricular septal defect, complicating AMI as a bridge to repair/revascularization (1)[B]
  - Recurrent intractable ventricular arrhythmias with hemodynamic instability (2)[B]
  - Severe multivessel or left main CAD requiring urgent noncardiac surgery (3)[B]

- High-risk PTCA owing to LV dysfunction and/or large territory at risk (4)[C]
  - Preoperative IABP use in CABG patients with ejection fraction <25% who are undergoing nonelective operation or reoperation, or who have New York Heart Association class III–IV symptoms (5)[B]
  - Inability to wean from bypass after cardiac surgery (5)[C]
- Contraindications:
  - Significant aortic regurgitation
  - Abdominal aortic aneurysm
  - Aortic dissection
  - Uncontrolled septicemia
  - Uncontrolled bleeding disorder
  - Severe bilateral peripheral vascular disease not correctable by peripheral angioplasty or cross-femoral surgery
  - Bilateral femoral-popliteal bypass grafts for severe peripheral vascular disease

EPIDEMIOLOGY
In patients with AMI, the prevalence of IABP utilization in decreasing order of frequency:
- Cardiogenic shock: 27.3%
- Hemodynamic support during catheterization and/or angioplasty: 27.2%
- Prior to high-risk surgery: 11.2%
- Mechanical complications of AMI: 11.7%
- Refractory post-MI unstable angina: 10.0% (6)

ONGOING CARE

FOLLOW-UP RECOMMENDATIONS
- Verify timing and effectiveness of arterial augmentation:
  - Mean arterial BP >60–70 mm Hg.
  - Inflation occurring at the dicrotic notch
  - Optimal diastolic augmentation
  - Deflation at end-diastole with a drop in pressure of at least 8–10 mm Hg below unassisted end-diastole.
  - Decreasing requirements for inotropic support over the course of IABP assistance.

- Examples of incorrect inflation/deflation timing and appropriate rectification:

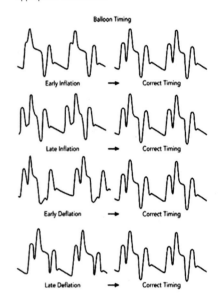

- Check for IABP failure:
  - IABP leak
  - Poor inflation
  - Difficult insertion
  - Poor augmentation

Patient Monitoring
- Avoid complications:
  - Maintain cannulated extremity in a straight position and avoid hip flexion.
  - Keep head of bed at a 15-degree backrest position or lower. If the head of the bed needs to be elevated, change to reverse Trendelenburg position.
  - Check peripheral pulses, capillary refill, cannulated extremity skin color and temperature on hourly basis.
  - Maintain anticoagulation at prescribed range.

- Early IABP discontinuation is required in only 2.1% of patients (6).
- Removal technique:
  - Check for balloon dependence by adjusting the frequency of balloon inflation (1:1–1:2).
  - Prior to balloon removal, normalize coagulation status and platelet count if necessary.
  - Discontinue balloon inflation.
  - Hold pressure on the distal femoral artery and remove the balloon and sheath.
  - Allow the proximal femoral artery to exsanguinate for 2–4 seconds to flush out any debris.
  - Transfer pressure to the proximal artery for a few seconds so that the distal artery clears its debris.
  - Hold pressure on the insertion site for at least 30 minutes.

PROGNOSIS

- In patients with AMI and secondary cardiogenic shock, IABP in conjunction with revascularization by percutaneous intervention or CABG is associated with lower in-hospital mortality rates than standard medical treatment (7).
- Early IABP insertion (<24 hours) in patients presenting with AMI and cardiogenic shock tends to lower mortality at 1 month and 1 year (8).
- Mortality rates for patients requiring IABP in the setting of AMI depend on indication for insertion (6):
  - Refractory angina: 6.4 %
  - Preoperative for high risk surgery: 7.3%
  - Intraoperative support: 7.7 %
  - Support for high-risk percutaneous coronary intervention: 9.6%
  - Refractory LV failure: 21.2%
  - Mechanical complications of AMI: 22.4%
  - Weaning from cardiopulmonary bypass:25.9%
  - Cardiogenic shock (without percutaneous or operative intervention): 38.7% (6)

COMPLICATIONS

- Major IABP complications occur in 2.7% and range between 1% and 14% (6):
  - Access-site bleeding
  - Retroperitoneal bleeding
  - Transfusion
  - Limb ischemia
  - Femoral artery pseudo-aneurysm
  - Arterial thrombosis
  - Amputation
  - Infection

- Deep or superficial venous thrombosis
- Stroke
- Bowel, renal, or spinal cord infarction
- Aortic dissection
- Aortoiliac laceration
- Myocardial ischemia from asynchronous timing of balloon augmentation
- Peripheral vascular disease (PVD), female sex and small body surface area are independent risk factors of major complications (9).

REFERENCES

1. Ryan TJ, et al. 1999 Update: ACC/AHA guidelines for the management of patients with acute myocardial infarction: A report of the American College of Cardiology/American Heart Association Task Force on Practice Guidelines (Committee on Management of Acute Myocardial Infarction). *J Am Coll Cardiol*. 1999;34:890–911.
2. Fotopoulos GD, et al. Stabilization of medically refractory ventricular arrhythmia by intra-aortic balloon counterpulsation. *Heart*. 1999;82:96–100.
3. Georgeson S, et al. Prophylactic use of the intra-aortic balloon pump in high-risk cardiac patients undergoing noncardiac surgery: A decision analytic view. Review. *Am J Med*. 1992;92(6):665–78.
4. Mishra S, et al. Role of prophylactic intra-aortic balloon pump in high-risk patients undergoing percutaneous coronary intervention. *Am J Cardiol*. 2006;98(5):608–12.
5. Baskett RJ, et al. The intraaortic balloon pump in cardiac surgery. *Ann Thorac Surg*. 2002;74(4):1276–87.
6. Stone GW, et al. Contemporary utilization and outcomes of intra-aortic balloon counterpulsation in acute myocardial infarction. *J Am Coll Cardiol*. 2003;41:1940.
7. Sanborn TA, et al. Impact of thrombolysis, intra-aortic balloon pump counterpulsation, and their combination in cardiogenic shock complicating acute myocardial infarction: A report from the SHOCK trial registry. *J Am Coll Cardiol*. 2000;36:1123–9.
8. Anderson RD, et al. Use of intraaortic balloon counterpulsation in patients presenting with cardiogenic shock: Observations from the GUSTO-I Study. *J Am Coll Cardiol*. 1997;30(3):708–15.
9. Cohen M, et al. Sex and other predictors of intra-aortic balloon counter pulsation-related complications: Prospective study of 1119 consecutive patients. *Am Heart J*. 2000;139:282–7.

ADDITIONAL READING

- Weber KT, et al. Intraaortic balloon counterpulsation: A review of physiologic principles, clinical results and device safety. *Ann Thorac Surg*. 1994; 17:602–36.
- Williams DO, et al. The effect of intraaortic balloon counterpulsation on regional myocardial blood flow and oxygen consumption in the presence of coronary artery stenosis in patients with unstable angina. *Circulation*. 1982;66:593–7.

 CODES

ICD9

- 413.9 Other and unspecified angina pectoris
- 427.9 Cardiac dysrhythmia, unspecified
- 785.51 Cardiogenic shock

CLINICAL PEARLS

- IABP decreases myocardial demand while increasing coronary blood supply.
- IABP may be inserted for the prevention or treatment of cardiogenic shock and/or large MI.
- IABP should be avoided in severe PVD, aortic aneurysm/dissection, and significant aortic regurgitation.
- Effectiveness of arterial pressure augmentation and timing should be monitored carefully, although new balloons are self-timed and manual adjustment is rarely necessary.
- Close clinical follow-up should be performed to avoid serious complications.

I

INTRACEREBRAL PRESSURE

Raghad Said
Graciela J. Soto

BASICS

DESCRIPTION
- Normal intracranial pressure (ICP) is $\leq$15 mm Hg in adults.
- Intracranial hypertension (ICH) occurs if pressure is $\geq$20 mm Hg.
- ICH complicates many conditions, compromises cerebral blood flow (CBF), and can lead to cerebral ischemia.

EPIDEMIOLOGY
Incidence
- Elevated ICP occurs in 53–63% of patients with severe traumatic brain injury (TBI) and Glasgow Coma Scale (GCS) of 3–8 (1).
- 10–50% of strokes are complicated by elevated ICP in the U.S.

PATHOPHYSIOLOGY
- ICP depends on the volume of its 3 components: Brain parenchyma (80%), cerebrospinal fluid (CSF) (10%), and blood (10%)
- As per the Monroe-Kellie doctrine, if the volume in 1 component increases, ICP is maintained by a decrease of 1 or both of the other compartments
- Changes in ICP are related to changes in intracerebral volume: As cerebral edema increases, ICP rises and CBF decreases with development of cerebral ischemia.
- CBF is maintained at a wide range of mean arterial pressures (MAPs) by cerebral vasculature autoregulation. It is difficult to measure clinically, therefore, cerebral perfusion pressure (CPP) is used as a surrogate for CBF.
- CPP is the pressure causing blood flow to the brain and is usually maintained between 50 and 150 mm Hg by cerebral autoregulation.
- CPP is indirectly measured as = MAP – ICP.
- Optimal CPP is 50–60 mm Hg.
- CPP decreases as ICP increases. To increase blood flow to the brain, MAP will increase and cerebral vasculatures will vasodilate (hyperemia). This will ultimately further elevate ICP and compromise CPP.

ETIOLOGY
- Many local, systemic, and metabolic conditions can elevate ICP and reduce CPP.
- Brain injury impairs cerebral vasculature autoregulation.

COMMONLY ASSOCIATED CONDITIONS
- TBI
- Brain tumors
- Hydrocephalus
- Seizures
- Hepatic encephalopathy
- Impaired CNS venous outflow
- Intracranial hemorrhage (IH)
- Subarachnoid hemorrhage (SAH)
- Infectious processes (e.g., meningitis)
- Benign ICH (pseudotumor cerebri)
- Stroke (CVA)
- Global ischemia after cardiac arrest
- Metabolic (e.g., hypercapnia, hypoxemia, hyponatremia, hyperthermia)

DIAGNOSIS

- Clinical findings are due to cerebral edema, ischemia, and/or herniation.
- The severity of ICP elevation does not correlate with clinical findings.

HISTORY
- Head trauma
- Liver disease
- Coagulopathy
- Use of anticoagulants
- Drug overdose
- Malignancy
- Fever
- Neurological deficits
- Nuchal rigidity
- Headache
- Depressed mental status
- Nausea, vomiting

PHYSICAL EXAM
- Vital signs: Blood pressure (hypotension or SBP <90, and hypertension), temperature, hypoxemia, heart rate (bradycardia), respiratory rate (Cheyne-Stokes breathing)
- Pupillary exam: Fixed and dilated pupil(s)
- Funduscopic exam: Papilledema, retinal hemorrhages
- CN III and VI palsies
- Cushing's reflex (bradycardia, respiratory depression, and hypertension)
- In trauma patients: Careful inspection for craniofacial injuries, periorbital bruising
- GCS: Aids in risk stratification and prognostication
- Decerebrate or decorticate posturing

DIAGNOSTIC TESTS & INTERPRETATION
Lab
Initial lab tests
- CBC, BUN, creatinine, sodium, glucose, serum osmolarity (sOsm)
- Liver function tests
- Coagulation panel
- Toxicology screen
- Blood cultures, CSF cultures

Follow-Up & Special Considerations
Frequent neurological assessment, including pupillary exam is imperative to identify patients at risk of herniation.

Imaging
Initial approach
Gold standard: Head CT, MRI/MRA of brain as per etiology of high ICP

Follow-Up & Special Considerations
Chest x-ray: To evaluate for aspiration and pneumothorax (from hyperventilation)

Diagnostic Procedures/Other
- EEG: Rule out seizures
- Lumbar puncture: Rule out meningitis

Pathological Findings
- Head CT: Tumor, mass effect, midline shift, herniation, effacement of basilar cisterns, SAH, stroke, IH
- EEG: Seizures, encephalopathy, or brain death

DIFFERENTIAL DIAGNOSIS
According to the primary condition

TREATMENT

- Therapy should be individualized according to patient's history, clinical findings, and etiology of ICH.
- ICP control requires invasive pressure measurement and treatment is indicated if >20 mm Hg.
- Goal is to decrease ICP without affecting CPP.
- Use a stepwise approach with an institutional algorithm to limit complications from harmful therapies.
- Prognosis is related to the underlying cause of elevated ICP: ICP control in TBI patients is associated with improved survival.
- Sustained ICH is associated with poor outcomes (2).

MEDICATION
First Line
- Treat the underlying condition.
- Correct any hemodynamic instability.
- Osmotic diuretics: Mannitol (20% solution):
  - Give 1 g/kg bolus and then 0.25–0.5 g/kg q6–8h until ICP is controlled or sOsm reaches 320 mOsm/kg H_2O.

Second Line
- Therapies to decrease metabolic demand:
  - Barbiturates ("pentobarb coma"): Pentobarbital loading dose of 5–20 mg/kg and followed by 1–4 mg/kg/hr targeted to burst suppression on continuous EEG. ICP monitoring is required. Use sodium thiopental as alternative.
  - Sedation and analgesia: Short-acting and reversible medications preferred. Propofol recommended due to its short half-life and antiseizure effects.
  - Diuretics: Furosemide can be given with mannitol to potentiate its effect.
- Hypertonic saline (3%, 7.5%): Used to acutely decrease ICP. Its long-term clinical outcomes are not well established.

ADDITIONAL TREATMENT
General Measures
- Keep head elevated at 30 degrees and in neutral position.
- Temperature control: Avoid fever and maintain normothermia (<37°C).
- Blood pressure control: Avoid hypotension (keep SBP >90), and treat hypertension when CPP >120 mm Hg and ICP >20 mm Hg.
- Avoid hypoxemia (keep PO_2 >60 mm Hg) since it increases ICP.
- Correct any existing metabolic abnormalities.
- Rapid sequence intubation (e.g., lidocaine, fentanyl) if possible to avoid increased ICP during intubation

Issues for Referral
Neurosurgery: Mass removal, invasive ICP monitor placement, hematoma or IH drainage, decompressive craniectomy (DC)

Additional Therapies
- Hyperventilation: Goal PCO_2 is 25–30 mm Hg; short effect, used to control ICH within the first 24 hours, contraindicated in TBI or acute CVA (risk of further neurological injury from vasoconstriction)
  - "Rebound effect" after several hours, may be life-saving during impending herniation while more definitive treatment is instituted.

- Anticonvulsants: Use prophylactically in conditions at risk (e.g., TBI, SAH, SDH).

COMPLEMENTARY & ALTERNATIVE THERAPIES
- Therapeutic hypothermia: Goal is core temperature of 32–34°C; there may be some decreased mortality and improved neurological outcomes (3,4); use is limited to elevated ICP refractory to conventional therapies.
- Glucocorticoids: Indicated for elevated ICP from brain tumors or infections (e.g., meningitis). Not indicated in head injury, and is associated with increased mortality (MRC CRASH trial) (5)

SURGERY/OTHER PROCEDURES
- Mass removal (e.g., tumor, hematoma) if amenable to neurosurgical intervention (6)
- DC: Used in medically refractory ICH from TBI, SAH, and middle cerebral artery (MCA) stroke; however, no Class I evidence is available for SAH and TBI (7). DC may be effective in patients with TBI and is recommended by the American Brain Trauma Foundation guidelines within 48 hours of head injury (6,8).
  - Await results of DECRA and RESCUE ICP studies in severe head injury patients.
  - Lobectomy may also be performed.
- Ventriculostomy: Allows removal of CSF if hydrocephalus is diagnosed in imaging studies

IN-PATIENT CONSIDERATIONS
Initial Stabilization
- ABCD: Evaluate patient for airway, breathing, circulation, and disability
- These patients need ICU-level care for:
  - Depressed mental status
  - Frequent neurological assessment
  - Airway management and mechanical ventilation
  - Hemodynamic instability
  - ICP monitoring, which is indicated for:
    ○ Patients with closed head injury and GCS of 3–8 plus abnormal head CT
    ○ Patients with GCS = 3–8 but normal head CT plus ≥2 of the following: Age >40 years, posturing, or SBP <90 mm Hg

IV Fluids
- Goal is euvolemia.
- Give isotonic fluids without dextrose.
- Crystalloids = colloids

Nursing
- Control fever aggressively with antipyretics, cooling blankets, and cold IV fluids.
- Minimize patient stimulation and endotracheal suctioning, which elevates ICP.
- Remove any devices that constrict the neck.
- Both MAP and ICP are transduced at the level of the ear (correlate with the Circle of Willis).
- Change dry sterile dressing on ICP device every 3 days or if it becomes wet or soiled.

Discharge Criteria
Some of these patients may have a poor prognosis, and goals of care must be discussed with family and patient, including placement in long-term facility, tracheostomy, and feeding tube.

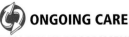

ONGOING CARE

FOLLOW-UP RECOMMENDATIONS
- Physical exam: Frequent neurological exams q1–2h.
- Diagnostic procedures:

  - Repeat head CT if worsening mental status or new neurological deficits
  - Follow-up EEG in the first 2 days after TBI can help in prognostication
- Metabolic abnormalities:
  - Monitor serum Na and sOsm.
  - Patients are at risk for hyponatremia and serum Na goal is 145–150 mEq/L
  - sOsm goal is 280–320 mOsm/Kg H_2O
  - Serum glucose control as per institution protocol to prevent further neurological injury from hypo- or hyperglycemia
- Medications:
  - Avoid vasodilators (e.g., nitroprusside, hydralazine) which may increase ICP.

Patient Monitoring
- ICP monitoring:
  - Confirms a clinical suspicion of ICH
  - Recommended for all TBI with GCS ≤8
  - Decreases mortality in TBI (5)
  - Goal ICP is <20 mm Hg.
  - Goal CPP is 60–75 mm Hg.
  - Both MAP and ICP need to be invasively monitored with an arterial line and ICP device
- Invasive ICP monitoring:
  - Intraventricular (gold standard):
    ○ Higher rate of infectious complications and some risk of hemorrhage
    ○ Allows CSF drainage to reduce ICP.
  - Intraparenchymal (e.g., Camino catheter):
    ○ Transducer cannot be recalibrated after placement
    ○ Low risk of infection and hemorrhage
  - Subarachnoid (e.g., Richmond bolt):
    ○ Low risk of infection and hemorrhage
    ○ Unreliable due to debris
  - Epidural:
    ○ Useful in coagulopathic patients
- Noninvasive ICP monitoring:
  - Jugular venous oxygen saturation (SjO$_2$):
    ○ Normal SjO$_2$ is 55–75%. If <50%, implies decreased CBF from cerebral ischemia and correlates with elevated ICP
  - Transcutaneous Doppler (TCD): Operator dependent, useful for vasospasm in SAH
  - Other methods: Tissue resonance analysis, intraocular pressure measurement, tympanic membrane displacement, brain tissue oximetry

DIET
- Monitor for risk of aspiration.
- Enteral feeding should be started as soon as possible in intubated patients, or if aspiration occurs.
- Avoid free water, hypotonic and dextrose-containing fluids.
- Frequently monitor serum glucose.
- Provide stress ulcer prophylaxis.

PATIENT EDUCATION
- Educate patient on the etiology of ICH, the possibility of permanent deficits (cognitive, motor, or sensory), alternative means of oxygenation and feeding (e.g., tracheostomy, gastrostomy tube).
- Patients should be informed of the common complications of critical illness (e.g., infections, decubitus ulcers, deep venous thrombosis).

COMPLICATIONS
- Renal failure: Due to dehydration from diuretics (e.g., mannitol, furosemide)
- Hemodynamic instability: From the side-effects of sedative agents, paralytics, and diuretics

---

- Respiratory failure: Due to aspiration pneumonia, loss of protective airway reflexes, herniation, or neurogenic pulmonary edema
- Neurological complications: Herniation (mass effect of cerebral edema), coma, persistent vegetative state, brain death
- ICU-related: Nosocomial pneumonia, UTIs, catheter-related infections, deep venous thrombosis, pulmonary embolism, malnutrition, decubitus ulcers

REFERENCES
1. Bullock MR (for the Task Force): Indications for intracranial pressure monitoring. Management and prognosis of severe traumatic brain injury Part 1: Guidelines for the management of severe traumatic brain injury. *J Neurotrauma*. 2000;17:479–91.
2. Rosner MJ, et al. Cerebral perfusion pressure: Management protocol and clinical results. *J Neurosurg*. 1995;83:949–62.
3. McIntyre LA, et al. Prolonged therapeutic hypothermia after traumatic brain injury in adults. A systematic review. *JAMA*. 2003;289:2992.
4. Alderson P, et al. Therapeutic hypothermia for head injury. *Cochrane Database Syst Rev*. 2004; CD001048.
5. Edwards P, et al. Final results of MRC CRASH: A randomized placebo-controlled trial of IV corticosteroid in adults with head injury-outcomes at 6 months. *Lancet*. 2005;365:1957.
6. Lane PL, et al. Intracranial pressure monitoring and outcomes after traumatic brain injury. *Can J Surg*. 2000;43:442–8.
7. Schirmer CM, et al. Decompressive craniectomy. *Neurocrit Care*. 2009;8:456–70.
8. Bullock R, et al. Guidelines for the management of severe head injury. Brain Trauma Foundation. *Eur J Emerg Med*. 1996;3(2):109–27.

 ## CODES

ICD9
- 348.2 Benign intracranial hypertension
- 430 Subarachnoid hemorrhage
- 431 Intracerebral hemorrhage

CLINICAL PEARLS
- ICH may be suspected from clinical findings and symptoms; however, an ICP monitor is needed to confirm the diagnosis.
- Initial resuscitation starts with A, B, C, D.
- 1st line of therapy is to treat the underlying condition and start osmotic diuresis.
- Agents used to treat ICH depend on the response to therapy to achieve ICP control.
- ICP elevation for a prolonged period is associated with poor outcomes.
- A brief period of hyperventilation can decrease cerebral edema acutely and allow time for more definitive therapies.
- Each institution should use a step-wise algorithm to guide clinicians in the management of ICH and prevent the use of harmful therapies.
- DC may be a salvage therapy in medically refractory ICH due to large MCA stroke. Its role in TBI and SAH needs to be established with Class I evidence.

ISCHEMIA, MESENTERIC

Elad S. Grozovski

BASICS

DESCRIPTION
- Ischemia of either large or small bowel caused by:
  - Occlusion of the superior or inferior mesenteric arteries (MI)
  - Nonocclusive mesenteric ischemia (NOMI)
  - Mesenteric vein thrombosis (MVT)
- May be:
  - Symptomatic or nonspecific symptomatics
  - 30–50% due to arterial occlusion, 15–30% due to thromboembolism
- Difficult to diagnose
- Common endpoint: Bowel ischemia or necrosis
- High mortality (60–80%)
- Survival approaches 50% if diagnosed within 24 hours after symptoms onset

EPIDEMIOLOGY
Predominant in elderly, multimorbid patients

Prevalence
Adults >50 years

RISK FACTORS
- For either NOMI or MI:
  - Low cardiac output
  - Congestive heart failure
  - Sepsis and/or septic shock
  - Hypotension
  - Hypovolemia
- Mainly for MI:
  - General chronic atherosclerotic disease
  - Cardiac arrhythmia (atrial fibrillation)
  - Diabetes mellitus
  - Recent myocardial infarction
  - Arterial stenosis
  - Cardiac valve disease

- Mainly for MVT:
  - Primary clotting disorder
  - Previous abdominal surgery
  - Hypercoagulable state
  - Previous MVT
  - Smoking
  - Alcohol abuse
  - Malignant tumors
  - Cirrhosis
  - Oral contraceptives

ETIOLOGY
- Cessation of blood flow to the dependant bowel region resulting in ischemia (MI)
- Low-flow state resulting in critical underperfusion to dependent bowel region (NOMI)

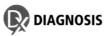

DIAGNOSIS

HISTORY
- Sudden onset of severe abdominal pain
- High index of suspicion
- Postprandial abdominal pain
- Weight loss
- Sickness and vomiting
- Diarrhea (in some cases bloody)
- Previous arterial or cerebral embolism
- Other potential sources for an embolus
- Periarteritis nodosa
- Intra-abdominal tumors
- Discrepancy between subjective pain and physical findings
- Shock (MI, NOMI)
- Sepsis (MI, NOMI)
- Dehydration (MI, NOMI)
- Bleeding (MI, NOMI)
- Diuretics (MI, NOMI)
- Bloody diarrhea (MI, NOMI)
- Medications: (digoxin, catecholamines, angiotensin II, vasopressin, β-blocker [NOMI])

PHYSICAL EXAM
- Abdominal tenderness
- Abdominal distention
- Decreased bowel sounds
- Peritonitic signs
- Temperature >38°C

DIAGNOSTIC TESTS & INTERPRETATION
Lab
- No specific tests
- Limited value:
  - Leucocytes count (elevated)
  - Platelets count (low)
  - Serum lactate
  - Blood gases
  - Urea and creatinine
  - Basic coagulation

Imaging
Initial approach
- Gold standard is abdominal angiogram (may be used as port for therapy)
- Dynamic CT scan
- Colonoscopy
- Sigmoidoscopy (NOMI)
- CT (for MVT, sensitivity 90–100%)

Follow-Up & Special Considerations
- Resuscitation and correction of predisposing factors
- Plain film (ruling out other causes)
- Abdominal US (thickening of bowel walls, signs of ileus)
- Duplex US of the splanchnic arteries (highly operator dependent)
- If no peritoneal findings, then abdominal angiogram (intra-arterial digital subtraction)
- If history of DVT or hypercoagulable state, dynamic CT scan
- Endoscopy (detection of ischemic mucosa)

Diagnostic Procedures/Other
- Tonometry
- Intra-abdominal pressure measurement (nonspecific)

TREATMENT

MEDICATION

- Crystalloids
- Broad-spectrum antibiotics (levofloxacin + metronidazole or piperacillin-tazobactam)
- Heparin: Goal is APTT of 50–70 seconds
- Selective papaverine infusion (via angiography catheter)
- NOMI:
  – Selective application of papaverine into the SMA via the angiographic catheter 30–60 mg/h (caution in hypotension or hypovolemia). Usual infusion is for 24 hours.
- MVT:
  – Anticoagulation with heparin
- Reducing mesenteric vasospasm:
  – IV infusion of glucagon: 1–10 μg/kg/min
- Reduce reperfusion syndrome:
  – Allopurinol (cost effectiveness is unclear)
  – ACE inhibitors (cost effectiveness is unclear)

SURGERY/OTHER PROCEDURES

- Nasogastric tube
- If stable and without peritoneal signs, angiography should be performed. In cases of positive findings, the catheter can be used for local application of therapy (embolectomy, thrombolysis, etc.)
- For mesenteric arterial occlusion: Rapid operative disobliteration of the obstruction
- NOMI: Surgical exploration only in patients with peritoneal signs.
- Selective thrombolysis (alteplase, urokinase)

 ONGOING CARE

FOLLOW-UP RECOMMENDATIONS
Liberal use of "second-look" laparotomy

PROGNOSIS
- Generally, if diagnosis is delayed, the condition is almost always fatal.
- Once signs of peritonitis or bloody diarrhea are present, shock, sepsis, and death are almost always inevitable.

COMPLICATIONS
Very often survivors, mainly those after surgical therapy, will remain with "short-bowel syndrome."

ADDITIONAL READING

- American gastroenterological association medical position statement on intestinal ischemia. *Gastroenterology*. 2000;118:951–3.
- Guntram L. Acute intestinal ischemia. *Best Pract Res Clin Gastroenterol*. 2001;15(1):83–98.
- Kolkman JJ, et al. Splancnic ischemia in
- Mansour MA. Management of acute mesenteric ischemia. *Arch Surg*.1999;134–330.
- Schoots IG, et al. Thrombolytic therapy for acute superior mesenteric artery occlusion. *J Vasc Radiol*. 2005;16:317–3297.
- Todd B, et al. Acute mesenteric ischemia. *Curr Gastroenterol Rep*. 2008;10:341–6.

 CODES

ICD9
- 557.0 Acute vascular insufficiency of intestine
- 557.1 Chronic vascular insufficiency of intestine

CLINICAL PEARLS

- Entertain a high index of suspicion for high-risk patients (cardiac dysfunction, diffuse atherosclerosis, following cardiac surgery or arterial catheterization).
- Mesenteric angiography is the investigation of choice.
- Treatment is mostly surgical, through arterial reconstruction with bypass or embolectomy, or resection of nonviable bowel.
- NOMI is treated by volume resuscitation and avoidance of α-adrenergic drugs.
- Enteral nutrition should be used cautiously.
- Colonoscopy is investigation of choice for mucosal ischemic colitis.

IVC FILTER

Rakesh Sinha
John Oropello

Indications of IVC filter placement for VTE treatment and prophylaxis

I. Contraindication to anticoagulation for VTE treatment (1)[B]
   Or
   Complication on anticoagulation during VTE treatment (1)[B]

A. No
   Failure with adequate anticoagulation for VTE treatment[#] (1)[C]
   Or
   Patient with chronic thromboembolic pulmonary hypertension undergoing pulmonary thromboendarterectomy (1,2)[C]
   Or
   Preoperative patient with VTE within 1 month in whom anticoagulation needs to be interrupted (1)[C]
   Or
   Pregnant patient with VTE within 2 weeks prior to delivery (1)[C]
   1. Yes
      Place IVC filter*
   2. No
      No indication for IVC filter[+]

B. Yes
   Place IVC filter*
   [#] High-intensity anticoagulation (target INR 3–5) or low-molecular-weight heparin should be considered before placing filter (1)[C]
   * Place retrievable filter if short-term contraindication exists (1)[C].
   *Resume or start anticoagulation as soon as contraindication resolves (1,2)[C].
   [+] IVC filter is not indicated as additional therapy along with anticoagulation for VTE with:

   ○ Free-floating thrombus (1)[B]

   ○ Thrombolysis (1)[C]
   [+] IVC filter is not indicated for:
   ○ Trauma VTE prophylaxis (1)[C]
   ○ Spinal cord injury VTE prophylaxis (1)[C]

REFERENCES

1. British Committee for Standards in Haematology Writing Group, et al. Guidelines on use of vena cava filters. *Br J Haematol*. 2006;134:590–95.
2. Hirsh J, et al. Executive summary: American College of Chest Physicians Evidence-Based Clinical Practice Guidelines (8th Edition). *Chest*. 2008;133(6 Suppl):71S–109S.

ADDITIONAL READING

• Young T, et al. Vena caval filters for the prevention of pulmonary embolism. *Cochrane Database Sys Rev*. 2007;17;(4):CD006212.

 CODES

ICD9
453.9 Embolism and thrombosis of unspecified site

I

LEMIERRE SYNDROME

Raghu Seethala

 BASICS

DESCRIPTION
Lemierre syndrome is a rare condition characterized by septic thrombophlebitis of the internal jugular vein caused by oropharyngeal or odontogenic infections.

EPIDEMIOLOGY
Incidence
- The incidence of Lemierre syndrome has been reported between 0.6 and 2.3 per million persons per year (1).
- Typically affects young healthy adults:
  - In 1 study, 89% of patients were between 10 and 35 years (2).

RISK FACTORS
- Male sex
- Late adolescent to early adult age

GENERAL PREVENTION
Currently, no general preventative measures are known.

PATHOPHYSIOLOGY
Infection progresses from the oropharynx to the parapharyngeal space with subsequent invasion of the carotid sheath, leading to thrombophlebitis of the internal jugular vein. This may also occur via hematogenous or lymphatic spread from peritonsillar vessels. Infection then disseminates to other organ systems by direct extension into the bloodstream or by septic emboli.

ETIOLOGY
- Usually caused by bacteria present in the oropharynx.
- The most common pathogen by far is *Fusobacterium necrophorum* (>80% of cases).
- Can be polymicrobial 10–30%

- Other less common causes that have been reported:
  - *Fusobacterium nucleatum*, Group B *Streptococcus*, Group D *Streptococcus*, *Bacteroides fragilis*, *Bacteroides distasonis*, *Eikenella corrodens*, MRSA, *Peptostreptococcus*, *Staphylococcus epidermis*, *Streptococcus oralis*

COMMONLY ASSOCIATED CONDITIONS
- Pharyngitis
- Exudative tonsillitis
- Peritonsillar abscess

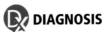 DIAGNOSIS

HISTORY
Usual presentation is a young healthy adult with an acute tonsillar infection or recent resolution of a tonsillar infection now in profound sepsis.

PHYSICAL EXAM
- Fever
- Rigors
- Acutely ill appearing
- Oropharyngeal exam can range from normal appearance to severe exudative tonsillitis with peritonsillar abscess.
- Cervical lymphadenopathy
- Tenderness and swelling over the jugular vein (over the angle of the mandible or along the sternocleidomastoid) may be present.
- Other physical findings can be present depending on the metastatic spread of septic emboli.

DIAGNOSTIC TESTS & INTERPRETATION
Lab
Initial lab tests
- CBC, electrolytes, BUN, creatinine, glucose
- Blood cultures:
  - Blood culture positive for *F. necrophorum* should be assumed to be Lemierre syndrome until proven otherwise.
- Cultures of exudate from oropharynx if present

Follow-Up & Special Considerations
Patients are usually critically ill and septic, so routine sepsis lab work should be performed.

Imaging
Initial approach
- CT scan of the neck with IV contrast is the imaging modality of choice for diagnosing internal jugular vein (IJV) thrombosis. CT will also demonstrate the anatomy of the parapharyngeal space, diagnosing any abscess that may need surgical intervention.
- US can also visualize IJV thrombosis. It has the benefit of being able to be performed at the bedside and avoid radiation. However, US cannot visualize the area under the clavicle or mandible, and can also miss fresh thrombus with low echogenicity.
- MRI of the neck is also accurate at diagnosing IJV thrombosis. In addition, MRI provides excellent visualization of surrounding soft tissues. However, this modality is not always readily available and is costly, precluding it from being the first-line study.

Follow-Up & Special Considerations
- Chest x-ray should be performed, given that septic embolization to the lungs is a common complication. X-ray may reveal ill-defined infiltrates or nonspecific abnormalities.
- CT scan of the chest should also be performed if clinically warranted to further delineate any lung abnormalities. Findings can include infiltrates, pleural effusion, cavitary lesions, or empyema.

Diagnostic Procedures/Other

Arthrocentesis of joints with culturing of joint fluid may be necessary if signs of arthritis from septic emboli are present.

DIFFERENTIAL DIAGNOSIS

- Infectious mononucleosis
- Legionnaire's disease
- Bacterial pneumonia
- Right-sided endocarditis

 TREATMENT

MEDICATION

First Line

- Most common organism is *F. necrophorum*, which is an anaerobic gram-negative rod. Traditionally, penicillin was used, but now an increasing number of *F. necrophorum* isolates are resistant to penicillin (are β-lactamase positive).
- Currently, empiric IV β-lactamase-resistant antibiotic with anaerobic coverage is recommended. Regimens include ampicillin-sulbactam (3 g q6h), piperacillin-tazobactam (4.5 g q6h), ticarcillin-clavulanate (3.1 g q6h), or monotherapy with a carbapenem.
- Metronidazole and clindamycin can be considered also if *F. necrophorum* is isolated from cultures.
- The optimal duration of treatment has not been established. The usual course of treatment is between 3 and 6 weeks (3)[C].

Second Line

Some authors recommend anticoagulation during the course of acute illness (4)[C]. The role of anticoagulation is highly controversial. Since this condition occurs so infrequently, no randomized control studies have been performed.

ADDITIONAL TREATMENT

General Measures

- Patients can present in severe sepsis. Ensure adequate fluid resuscitation and hemodynamic optimization.
- Patients can also present in frank respiratory failure from septic emboli to the lungs; those patients should be evaluated for the need for ventilatory support.

Issues for Referral

Infectious disease consultation is recommended for all patients. Surgical consultation is recommended on a case-by-case basis.

SURGERY/OTHER PROCEDURES

- Drainage of abscesses from septic emboli (lung and liver most common)
- Internal jugular ligation or excision may become necessary for patients with persistent septic emboli despite adequate antibiotic treatment (3)[C].

IN-PATIENT CONSIDERATIONS

Initial Stabilization

- Early antibiotics
- Adequate IV access
- Fluid resuscitation
- Intubation if necessary

Admission Criteria

Admission is recommended for all patients, given the severity of this illness.

IV Fluids

Crystalloid IV fluids (NS or LR) as needed for hemodynamic optimization

Nursing

Consider ICU-level monitoring if severely septic.

Discharge Criteria

Case-dependent

 ONGOING CARE

DIET

Case-dependent on ability to take PO

PROGNOSIS

Untreated Lemierre syndrome has a high mortality (90%). Treated, Lemierre syndrome has a mortality rate between 4% and 18% (2).

COMPLICATIONS

Most complications are a result of septic emboli and can include:

- Empyema
- Septic pulmonary emboli
- Septic arthritis, osteomyelitis
- Soft-tissue abscess
- Cavernous sinus thrombosis
- Meningitis
- Cerebral abscess
- Hepatic abscess
- Splenic abscess

REFERENCES

1. Ridgway JM, et al. Lemierre syndrome: A pediatric case series and review of literature. *Am J Otolaryngol.* 2010;31:38–45.
2. Riordan T. Human Infection with Fusobacterium necrophorum (Necrobacillosis), with a focus on Lemierre's syndrome. *Clin Microbiol Rev.* 2007;20: 622–59.
3. Syed MI, et al. Lemierre syndrome: Two cases and a review. *Laryngoscope.* 2007;117(9):1605–10.
4. Bondy P, et al. Lemierre's syndrome: What are the roles for anticoagulation and long-term antibiotic therapy? *Ann Otol Rhinol Laryngol.* 2008;117: 679–83.

 CODES

ICD9

- 451.89 Phlebitis and thrombophlebitis of other sites
- 463 Acute tonsillitis

CLINICAL PEARLS

- Consider this diagnosis in severely ill patients with pharyngitis or recent history of pharyngitis.
- Administer empiric IV β-lactamase-resistant antibiotics early on if Lemierre syndrome is suspected.

L

LIVER INJURY, HYPOXIC
Shaul Lev

 BASICS

DESCRIPTION
Profound and transient elevation in serum transaminase levels due to an imbalance between hepatic oxygen supply and demand in the absence of other acute causes of liver damage

EPIDEMIOLOGY
- 0.16% of all inpatient admissions
- 1% of ICU admissions
- 2.6% of cardiac care unit (CCU) admissions
- 1.5–4.6% of patients with cirrhosis
- 22% for patients admitted to the CCU with decreased cardiac output

RISK FACTORS
- Chronic liver congestion
- Congestive heart failure

PATHOPHYSIOLOGY
Flow reduction in the portal vein or the hepatic artery leads to ischemia followed by reperfusion injury to the hepatic tissue. This results in oxygen-dependent generation of superoxide free radicals and other mediators that induce Kupffer cells to produce chemokines that attract neutrophils. Toxic substances produced by both cell types promote liver injury and cause platelets to aggregate into micro thrombi.

ETIOLOGY
- Severe decrease in hepatic blood supply (i.e., focal obstruction of hepatic artery with portal vein thrombosis)
- Severe hypoxia
- Severe hypotension
- Combination of hepatic congestion and mild hypotension

COMMONLY ASSOCIATED CONDITIONS
- Profound anemia
- Obstructive sleep apnea
- Carbon monoxide poisoning
- Heat stroke
- Cocaine abuse
- Ergotamine poisoning
- Bacterial endocarditis
- Sickle cell disease

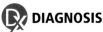 **DIAGNOSIS**

Combination of:
- Typical clinical setting of cardiac or circulatory shock
- Massive but rapidly reversible increase in serum aminotransferase levels
- The exclusion of other causes of liver damage

DIAGNOSTIC TESTS & INTERPRETATION
Diagnostic Procedures/Other
- Lactate dehydrogenase (LDH) and transaminase values increase 12–48 hours after the initiating event.
- LDH levels peak before transaminase levels.
- The transaminase value decreases by 50% within 72 hours.
- The INR may rarely increase.
- Creatinine values are often elevated.
- Clinical jaundice is unusual.

Pathological Findings
Centrilobular necrosis

DIFFERENTIAL DIAGNOSIS
- Viral hepatitis
- Toxin- or drug-induced hepatitis
- Liver trauma

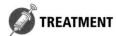 TREATMENT

MEDICATION
None has been proven

ADDITIONAL TREATMENT
General Measures
• Restore cardiac output
• Avoid hypovolemia

Additional Therapies
IV N-acetylcysteine (NAC) has been reported in case reports

 ONGOING CARE

FOLLOW-UP RECOMMENDATIONS
Patients should be monitored for other manifestations of end-organ hypoperfusion injury.

Patient Monitoring
Look for signs of decreased renal function or altered mental status.

PROGNOSIS
• Nearly always self limited in 7–10 days.
• The mortality rate in patients with hypoxic liver injury is high due to underling systemic disease, especially in patients with congestive heart failure or cirrhosis.
• Death is usually due to the underlying disease, and not the hypoxic liver failure.

COMPLICATIONS
• Rarely deteriorates into acute fulminant hepatic failure
• Multiple episodes of hypoxic liver failure may produce so-called cardiac sclerosis, with fibrous bands around the central vein and eventually cardiac cirrhosis.

ADDITIONAL READING
• Ebert EC. Review for clinicians: Hypoxic liver injury. *Mayo Clin Proc*. 2006;81(9):1232–36.

 CODES

ICD9
• 572.8 Other sequelae of chronic liver disease
• 573.0 Chronic passive congestion of liver
• 799.02 Hypoxemia

CLINICAL PEARLS
• The transaminase levels usually decrease more slowly in viral hepatitis.
• LDH level is particularly high in hypoxic liver failure.

L

LONG QT AND TORSADES DE POINTES

Peter Y. Kim

BASICS

DESCRIPTION
- Long QT syndrome (LQTS) is a hereditary disorder characterized by predisposition to ventricular arrhythmias (such as torsades de pointes) and sudden cardiac death.
- Torsades de pointes is a syndrome consisting of rapid polymorphic ventricular tachycardia characterized by "twisting" of the peaks of the QRS complexes around an isoelectric baseline in the setting of a long QT interval:
  - QTc >460 in females and >440 in males
  - Can degrade into ventricular fibrillation

EPIDEMIOLOGY
Incidence
Mutations occur in 1 in 2000 people, but most are clinically asymptomatic.

Prevalence
- Estimated prevalence is 1 in 5000 people
- More commonly found in younger individuals
  - Mean age of presentation is 12 years

RISK FACTORS
- Personal history of syncope
- Family member with LQTS
- Unexplained sudden death in a 1st-degree relative <30 years old

Genetics
- Over 10 types of inherited LQTS have been identified.
- Most common variants are LQTS 1, 2, and 3:
  - LQTS1: KCNQ1 gene mutation on Chromosome 11 involving the slow repolarizing potassium channel (IKs)
  - LQTS2: KCNH2 gene mutation on Chromosome 7 involving the fast repolarizing potassium channel (IKr)
  - LQTS3: SCN5A gene mutation on Chromosome 3 involving the late depolarizing sodium channel (INa)
- Most transmission is autosomal dominant with variable penetrance.

GENERAL PREVENTION
- Early identification of high-risk individuals with unexplained syncope
- Identification and correction of QT-prolonging conditions (e.g., metabolic abnormalities)

PATHOPHYSIOLOGY
- QT prolongation is most commonly a result of delayed repolarization (LQTS1, LQTS2).
- Less commonly a result of prolonged depolarization (LQTS3)
- 2 distinct mechanisms of ion channel dysfunction:
  - Ineffective incorporation of the mutant subunits into the cell membrane leading to loss of channel function
  - Formation of defective channels with mutant subunits leading to dysfunctional overactive channel proteins

- Channel dysfunctions lead to action potential prolongation and increased transmural repolarization gradients
- These conditions facilitate early afterdepolarization and reentry, which can lead to torsades de pointes.

ETIOLOGY
- Inherited/sporadic mutations
- Acquired/secondary causes:
  - Hypokalemia
  - Hypocalcemia
  - Hypomagnesemia
  - Hypothyroidism
  - Hypothermia
  - Medications (see www.torsades.org for full list):
    ○ Methadone
    ○ Haloperidol
    ○ Erythromycin
    ○ Antiarrhythmics, particularly class Ia and III

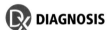

DIAGNOSIS

HISTORY
- History of presyncope, syncope, or palpitations
- Obtain a detailed family history of sudden death and other events that may be a hidden manifestation of LQTS (1)[C]:
  - Drowning
  - Motor vehicle accidents
  - Sudden infant death
  - Congenital sensorineural hearing loss seen with Jervell and Lange-Nielsen syndromes (2)[C]
- Certain clinical features may differentiate between LQTS subtypes:
  - LQTS1: Exercise-related triggers (e.g., swimming)
  - LQTS2: Loud noise triggers (e.g., alarm clock)
  - LQTS3: Onset during sleep
  - LQTS7 (Andersen-Tawil syndrome): Skeletal abnormalities (e.g., micrognathia)
  - LQTS8 (Timothy syndrome): Syndactyly of hands and feet

DIAGNOSTIC TESTS & INTERPRETATION
Lab
Initial lab tests

- ECG (3)[A]:
  - Bazett's formula for corrected QT (QTc):
    ○ $QTc = QT/RR$
- Chemistry panel
  - K^+, Mg^+, and Ca^{+2} levels
- Thyroid function tests

Follow-Up & Special Considerations
Genetic testing for common LQTS mutation subtypes is available and should be considered in borderline cases and for early identification of in family members (3)[C].

Imaging
No definitive imaging modality is indicated to confirm the diagnosis of LQTS.

Diagnostic Procedures/Other
Holter monitor and electrophysiologic testing are generally not helpful (1)[C].

Pathological Findings
- No diagnostically identifiable cardiac structural abnormalities
- Tissue specimens can demonstrate shortened sarcomeres and increased mitochondria with dense granules (4)[C].

DIFFERENTIAL DIAGNOSIS
- Vasovagal syncope and medications that can cause bradycardia and hypotension
- Hypertrophic cardiomyopathy, typically in young athletes with syncope
- Brugada syndrome
- Arrhythmogenic right ventricular dysplasia
- Anomalous coronary arteries

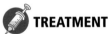

TREATMENT

MEDICATION
First Line

- β blockers (1)[A]:
  - Typically long-acting agents such as nadolol, which is available orally 20–320 mg/d
  - Most effective in LQTS1
- Magnesium sulfate (5)[B]:
  - Should be administered in the setting of torsades de pointes
  - Typical dosage is 2 g IVP

Second Line

- Isoproterenol can be used as temporary treatment for patients with torsades de pointes without LQTS (5)[B]:
  - Bolus 0.02–0.06 mg IV or infusion at 2 mg in 250 mL D5W given at 5 mcg/min
  - Pediatric doses: 0.05–2 mcg/kg/min IV
- Mexiletine (Ib), flecainide(Ic) are antiarrhythmics that can shorten the QT interval and may have some efficacy in LQTS3 (5)[C]:
  - Mexiletine starting dosage is 200 mg q8h
  - Flecainide starting dosage ranges from 50 mg q12h to 100 mg q12h.
  - Antiarrhythmic therapy should ONLY be administered under the supervision of a cardiologist.
- Ranolazine is an antianginal agent that also has effects on delayed Na current, which has been shown to shorten the QT interval (3)[C]:
  - Typical starting dosage is 500 mg b.i.d.

Geriatric Considerations
Dosing and titration of antiarrhythmic medications should be adjusted in elderly patients

ADDITIONAL TREATMENT
General Measures
- Stop QT-prolonging medications (5)[A].
- Avoid adrenergic stimuli (5)[B]:
  – Alarm clocks
  – Roller coasters
- Restrict patient's participation in competitive sports (5)[B]:
  – Particular avoidance of water sports as sudden immersion can trigger cardiac arrhythmias

Issues for Referral
- Early referral to a cardiac electrophysiologist is recommended in suspected LQTS.
- Consider genetic counseling in identified high-risk patients, particularly those considering pregnancy.

SURGERY/OTHER PROCEDURES
- Implantable cardioverter-defibrillator (ICD) (5)[A]:
  – Survived a cardiac arrest
  – Recurrent syncope despite β-blocker therapy
  – High-risk patients (i.e., LQTS with QTc >550)
- Left cervicothoracic sympathetic denervation (5)[B]:
  – Consider in patients with recurrent syncope and ventricular arrhythmias despite β-blocker and ICD therapy
- Radiofrequency ablation (2)[C]:
  – Focal ablation of triggered ventricular premature beats

IN-PATIENT CONSIDERATIONS
Initial Stabilization
- If the patient has torsades de pointes with hemodynamic compromise, DC cardioversion should be performed (5)[B].
- IV magnesium sulfate therapy should be administered for torsades de pointes in the setting of LQTS (5)[B].
- Temporary pacing should be considered for patients presenting with torsades de pointes due to heart block or bradycardia (5)[B].
- For polymorphic ventricular tachycardia, do not administer amiodarone in the setting of congenital or acquired LQTS (5)[C].

Pregnancy Considerations
- Pregnant patients with unstable ventricular arrhythmias should be electrically cardioverted or defibrillated (5)[B].
- Pregnant patients with LQTS with symptoms should continue their β blockers unless there are significant contraindications (5)[C].

Admission Criteria
- Syncope with suspicion of an arrhythmic etiology, such as prolonged QT on ECG
- Documented torsades de pointes
- Need for medical or surgical antiarrhythmic therapy

IV Fluids
Isotonic saline with appropriate electrolyte repletion

Nursing
- Staff should be comfortable in quickly administering external defibrillator therapy.
- The patient should be observed on a telemetry monitor.

Discharge Criteria
- Successful treatment of torsades de pointes
- Correction of metabolic abnormalities and removal of offending medications
- Medical or surgery therapy to prevent recurrence of refractory torsades de pointes

ONGOING CARE

FOLLOW-UP RECOMMENDATIONS
Patients with LQTS should follow closely with a cardiologist or a cardiac electrophysiologist upon discharge.

Patient Monitoring
- If patient presents with torsades de pointes, ICU monitoring is initially recommended.
- Upon discharge, follow-up should be customized to the level of clinical risk and the degree of the treatment.
- Timing of prophylactic ICD therapy is controversial in asymptomatic individuals with LQTS.

DIET
No special dietary restrictions

PATIENT EDUCATION
- Patients and family members should be well educated regarding modifiable risk factors, such as avoidance of stimuli and QT-prolonging medications.
- Genetic testing and expanded family history investigation may be beneficial in identifying other high-risk individuals.

PROGNOSIS
- Due to variable penetrance, prognosis is difficult to determine without risk stratification.
- Several factors contribute to long-term risk of sudden cardiac death:
  – Onset of syncope:
    ○ 5-fold increased risk if occurs <18 years
  – Timing:
    ○ Up to 20-fold risk if within 2 years since last syncopal episode
  – QTc interval:
    ○ 6-fold increased risk if QTc >550

REFERENCES
1. Roden D. Long-QT syndrome. *N Engl J Med.* 2008;358:169–76.
2. Goldenberg I, et al. Long QT syndrome. *J Am Coll Cardiol.* 2008;51(24):2291–300.
3. Zareba W, et al. Long QT syndrome and short QT syndrome. *Prog Cardiovasc Dis.* 2008;51(3):264–78.
4. Moothart R, et al. The heritable syndrome of prolonged QT interval, syncope and sudden death: Electron microscopic observations. *Chest.* 1976;70(2):263–6.
5. Zipes D, et al. Management of ventricular arrhythmias and the prevention of sudden cardiac death. *J Am Coll Cardiol.* 2006;48:1064–108.

ADDITIONAL READING
- Medications known to cause prolonged QT, at www.torsades.org

See Also (Topic, Algorithm, Electronic Media Element)
- Algorithm of Long QT Risk Assessment
  – Schwartz P, et al. Diagnostic criteria for the
  – Long QT syndrome: An update. *Circulation.* 1993;88:782–4.
- Ventricular Arrhythmias
- Bradyarrhythmias and Pacing indications

CODES

ICD9
- 426.82 Long qt syndrome
- 427.1 Paroxysmal ventricular tachycardia

CLINICAL PEARLS
- Risk of arrhythmias is increased with a
- QTc >460 in females and >440 in males.
- Holter monitor and electrophysiologic testing are generally not helpful in diagnosing LQTS.
- Do not administer amiodarone for polymorphic VT in the setting of prolonged QT.

L

LUMBAR PUNCTURE

Jose R. Yunen
Vicente San Martín

PROCEDURE

INDICATIONS
- Diagnosis of various central venous system infections and inflammatory diseases (i.e., encephalitis, meningitis, Guillian-Barré syndrome)
- Evaluation of CSF pressure
- Administration of medications (i.e., chemotherapeutic agents, antibiotics)

CONTRAINDICATIONS
- Skin infection
- Unequal pressures between the supratentorial and infratentorial compartments
- Increased intracraneal pressure
- Coagulopathy
- Brain abscess

TECHNIQUE
See algorithm.

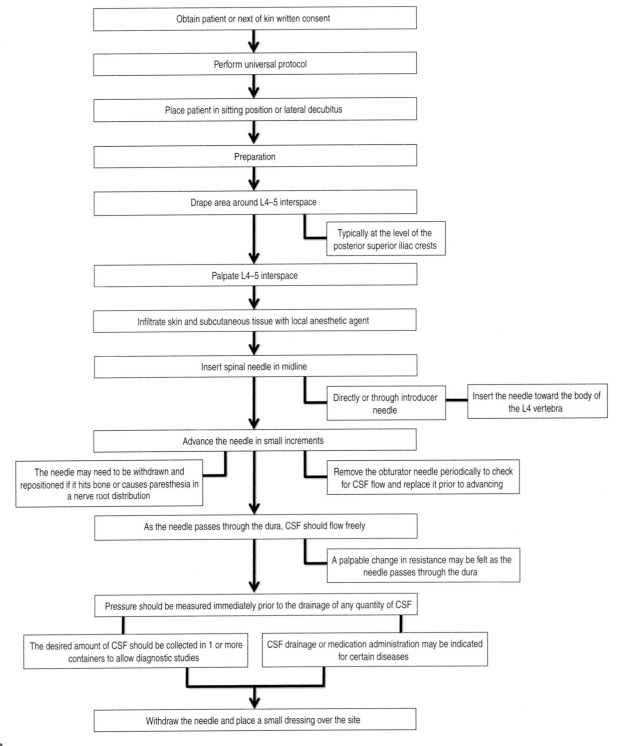

Obtain patient or next of kin written consent

Perform universal protocol

Place patient in sitting position or lateral decubitus

Preparation

Drape area around L4–5 interspace

Typically at the level of the posterior superior iliac crests

Palpate L4–5 interspace

Infiltrate skin and subcutaneous tissue with local anesthetic agent

Insert spinal needle in midline

Directly or through introducer needle

Insert the needle toward the body of the L4 vertebra

Advance the needle in small increments

The needle may need to be withdrawn and repositioned if it hits bone or causes paresthesia in a nerve root distribution

Remove the obturator needle periodically to check for CSF flow and replace it prior to advancing

As the needle passes through the dura, CSF should flow freely

A palpable change in resistance may be felt as the needle passes through the dura

Pressure should be measured immediately prior to the drainage of any quantity of CSF

The desired amount of CSF should be collected in 1 or more containers to allow diagnostic studies

CSF drainage or medication administration may be indicated for certain diseases

Withdraw the needle and place a small dressing over the site

COMPLICATIONS

Post–lumbar puncture headache (spinal headache)

- Infection
- Dysesthesia

- Postdural puncture cerebral herniation (may occur in patients with increased intracraneal pressure)

ADDITIONAL READING

- Ellenby M, et al. Lumbar puncture. *N Engl J Med*. 2006;355:e12.

L

LYME DISEASE

Eliany Mejia Lopez

 BASICS

DESCRIPTION
- Lyme disease (LD) is a multisystem bacterial infection caused by the spirochete *Borrelia burgdorferi* (Bb), the main cause in the U.S.
- In Europe, other bacteria, *B. afzelii* and *B. garinii*, also cause LD.
- Early symptoms may include fever, headache, fatigue, depression, and a characteristic target like or bull's eye skin rash called *erythema migrans*. If left untreated, later symptoms may affect the joints, heart and central nervous system.
- Transmission:
  - Lyme disease is transmitted by the bite of an infective tick.
  - Transmitters of the bacteria in North America include: The Western black-legged (*Ixodes pacificus*) tick in the West, and the black-legged tick (*Ixodes scapularis*) is the main vector on the east coast.
  - The black-legged tick was temporarily known as the "deer" tick (*Ixodes dammini*). The lone star tick (*Amblyomma americanum*) may also transmit the infection. It has been implicated in a related syndrome called Southern tick-associated rash illness, which resembles a mild form of LD.
  - The Ixodes tick can also carry and transmit several other parasites such as *Theileria microti* and *Anaplasma phagocytophilum*, which cause the diseases babesiosis and human granulocytic anaplasmosis (HGA), respectively.
  - The body does not maintain a natural immunity to the disease. A person can be reinfected with the disease on subsequent tick bites.

EPIDEMIOLOGY
Incidence
- 389,138 cases of LD have been reported to the Centers for Disease Control, 1980–2010 (05/22/10).
- 3,561 cases of LD were reported to the CDC for 2010 (05/22/10); it is estimated that only 1 in 10 cases of LD is actually reported to the CDC; therefore, there may have been at least as many as 3.89 million cases of LD since 1980 and 35,610 cases in 2010.

GENERAL PREVENTION
- Prophylaxis:
  - A single 200 mg dose of doxycycline given within 72 hours after an *I. scapularis* tick bite can prevent the development of LD.

PATHOPHYSIOLOGY
- Bb is able to move around the body through the bloodstream and between tissues, and has been found in the skin, heart, joint, peripheral nervous system, and central nervous system; this spread is aided by the attachment of the host protease plasmin to the surface of the spirochete.
- Many of the signs and symptoms of LD are a consequence of the immune response to the spirochete in those tissues. The bacteria invade tissue, replicate, and leave the cell, destroying it as it emerges.
- Sometimes, as the bacterium emerges, the cell wall collapses around the bacterium, forming a "cloaking device." This action may aid the bacteria's ability to hide from the immune system response.
- If untreated, the infection may persist for months to years, despite the production of anti-*B. burgdorferi* antibodies. Bd avoid the immune response by decreasing expression of surface proteins that, antigenic variation of the VlsE surface protein, inactivation of the complement system, and hiding in the extracellular matrix, which may interfere with the function of immune factors.

ETIOLOGY
- Caused by the bite of deer ticks (*Ixodes* ticks) which transmits *B. burgdorferi*. The disease has been reported in the Northeast, Mid-Atlantic, North Central, and Pacific coastal regions of the U.S. and in Europe.
- Most prevalent in the northeastern states of the U.S. (New York and Connecticut).
- Interestingly, LD only became apparent in 1975, in the town of Lyme, in Connecticut, where a number of cases were identified that year.
- <5% of tick bites in high-contact areas result in Lyme infections.

COMMONLY ASSOCIATED CONDITIONS
- Erythema migrans
- Arthritis
- Facial palsy
- Arrhythmias (AV block)
- Meningitis
- Encephalitis
- Polyneuropathy

 DIAGNOSIS

HISTORY
- Early localized infection:
  - The initial infection can occur with minimal or no symptoms. Many patients experience a flu-like primary illness or a characteristic erythema migrans (bull's eye rash) several days to a few weeks following a tick bite, in 80% of the patients.
  - Left untreated, symptoms of the primary illness usually will go away on their own within a few weeks although the rash may recur.
- Early disseminated infection:
  - Erythema chronicum migrans
  - Neurological problems, which appear on 15% of untreated patients
  - Meningitis
  - Facial palsy
  - Radiculoneuritis
  - Encephalitis
  - Carditis, with rhythm abnormalities and heart failure
- Late persistent Infection:
  - Also called stage 3, or tertiary, LD; occurs in 5% of untreated patients; characterized by:
    ○ Polyneuropathy
    ○ Lyme arthritis: Intermittent episodes of arthritis, polyarticular and migratory, usually involves the knee and wrist.
    ○ Chronic encephalomyelitis
    ○ Mood changes
    ○ Sleep disorder
    ○ Memory loss
  - The diagnosis of this stage is often difficult because can mimic symptoms of many other diseases. For this reason, LD is also called the new "great imitator."

PHYSICAL EXAM
- Objectives physical findings such as:
  - Erythema migrans
  - Facial palsy
  - Arthritis
  - Meningeal signs
  - AV block
- History of possible exposure to infected ticks is crucial for the diagnosis.

DIAGNOSTIC TESTS & INTERPRETATION
LD is clinical diagnosis, based on signs and symptoms, with the patients travel history to endemic areas and test results being additional pieces of information in the complete picture. No specific diagnostic test. No test can "rule-out" Lyme disease.

Lab
Initial lab tests
- ELISA
- Western blot
- Antigen detection
- PCR
- Bacterial culture:
  - Difficult and can take months.

Follow-Up & Special Considerations
- The 2 most important co-infections are ehrlichiosis (HGE) and babesiosis. Additional tests should be order to diagnose these conditions:
  - LFTs
  - CBC
  - Peripheral smear

Imaging
Initial approach
- CXR
- ECG
- Echocardiogram
- CT scan
- MRI of the brain

Follow-Up & Special Considerations
Single-photon emission CT (SPECT) has been used to detect cerebral hypoperfusion in patients with Lyme encephalitis.

Diagnostic Procedures/Other
- LP
- Arthrocentesis

DIFFERENTIAL DIAGNOSIS
- Rheumatoid arthritis
- Multiple sclerosis
- Fibromyalgia
- SLE
- Chronic fatigue syndrome
- Neurodegenerative diseases

TREATMENT

- Antibiotic therapy is the cornerstone of the LD treatment.
- Treatment varies and depends on how early a diagnosis is made and the systems involved. No definitive treatment regimens have been determined, and failures occur with all protocols.
- Oral antibiotics may be sufficient for early stages of nondisseminated infection.
- Longstanding or disseminated LD is better treated with 1 or several courses of either oral or IV antibiotics.

ADDITIONAL TREATMENT
General Measures
Hyperbaric oxygen therapy, as an adjunct to antibiotic therapy has been discussed.

SURGERY/OTHER PROCEDURES
Arthrocentesis often performed in cases of late persistent infection or stage 3 diseases for diagnosis and treatment of Lyme arthritis.

IN-PATIENT CONSIDERATIONS
Initial Stabilization
- Tick removal: The prompt removal of an infected tick, within 24 hours, reduces the risk of transmission to nearly 0; to transmit the infection the tick must be attached to the skin for at least 24 hours.

- A single dose of antibiotics may be offered to a patient soon after being bitten by a tick, if all of the following are true:
  - The person has a tick that can carry Lyme disease attached to his body.
  - The tick is thought to have been attached to the patient for at least 36 hours.
  - The person can begin taking the antibiotics within 72 hours of removing the tick.
  - The person is >8 years old and is not pregnant or breastfeeding.

MEDICATION
- Adults:
  - Doxycycline (in adults), 100 mg, PO, b.i.d. for 20–30 days
  - Amoxicillin 500 mg, PO, t.i.d. for 20–30 days.
  - Erythromycin (for pregnant women) and ceftriaxone, with treatment lasting 14–28 days
  - Alternatives in case of doxycycline or amoxicillin allergy:
    - Cefuroxime axetil, 500 mg PO b.i.d. for 20–30 days.
    - Erythromycin, 150 mg PO 4 times a day or 20 mg/kg/d in divided doses for 20–30 days.
- Children:
  - Amoxicillin 500 mg, PO, t.i.d. for 20–30 days.
  - Alternatives in case of penicillin allergy:
    - Cefuroxime axetil, 125 mg PO, b.i.d. for 20–30 days
    - Erythromycin, 250 mg PO t.i.d. or 30 mg/kg/d in divided doses for 14–20 days
- Arthritis:
  - Doxycycline 100 mg PO, b.i.d. for 30–60 days
  - Amoxicillin 500 mg PO 4 times a day for 30–60 days or ceftriaxone 2 g IV once a day for 14–39 days
  - Penicillin G, 20 million U IV in 4 divided doses daily for 30 days
- Neurologic abnormalities:
  - Ceftriaxone 2 g IV once a day for 14–30 days
  - Penicillin G, 20 million U IV in 4 divided doses for 30 days
  - Alternative in case of ceftriaxone or penicillin allergy:
    - Doxycycline, 100 mg PO t.i.d. for 30 days
- Facial palsy alone: Oral regimens may be adequate.
- Cardiac abnormalities:
  - 1st-degree AV block:
    - Oral regimens, as for early infection
  - High-degree AV block:
    - Ceftriaxone, 2 g IV once a day for 30 days
    - Penicillin G, 20 million U IV in 4 divided doses daily for 30 days
  - Once the patient has stabilized, the course may be completed with oral therapy.

Pediatric Considerations
Doxycycline should not be used in children <8 years old.

Pregnancy Considerations
Doxycycline is contraindicated in pregnant patients.

ONGOING CARE
DIET
No special diet needed
PROGNOSIS
- Most patients can be cured with a few weeks of oral antibiotics.
- Patients treated with antibiotics in the early stages of the infection usually recover rapidly and completely. A few patients, particularly those diagnosed with later stages of disease, may have persistent or recurrent symptoms. These patients may benefit from a 2nd 4-week course of therapy. Longer courses of antibiotics have been linked to serious complications, including death.
- Studies of women infected during pregnancy have found that there are no negative effects on the fetus if the mother receives appropriate antibiotic treatment for her LD.

COMPLICATIONS
Late persistent infection as explain above.

ADDITIONAL READING

- Lyme Disease Foundation, Inc.: www.lyme.org Nadelman RB, et al. Prophylaxis with single-dose doxycycline for the prevention of Lyme disease after an Ixodes scapularis tick bite. *N Engl J Med*. 2001;345:79–84.
- Pachner AR, et al. Lyme neuroborreliosis: Infection, immunity, and inflammation. *Lancet Neurol*. 2007;6(6):544–52.
- Steere AC, et al. The emergence of Lyme disease. *J Clin Invest*. 2004;113(8):1093–101.
- Steere AC, et al. Systemic symptoms without erythema migrans as the presenting picture of early Lyme disease. *Am J Med*. 2003;114(1):58–62.
- Smith RP, et al. Clinical characteristics and treatment outcome of early Lyme disease in patients with microbiologically confirmed erythema migrans. *Ann Intern Med*. 2002;136(6):421–8.

CODES

ICD9
- 088.81 Lyme disease
- 320.7 Meningitis in other bacterial diseases classified elsewhere
- 711.80 Arthropathy, site unspecified, associated with other infectious and parasitic diseases

CLINICAL PEARLS

- LD is transmitted by the bite of an infective tick, which transmit the bacteria *B. burgdorferi*.
- To transmit the infection, the tick must be attached to the skin for at least 24 hours.
- If left untreated, the symptoms of the primary illness (erythema migrans) usually will go away on their own within a few weeks; nevertheless, the patient must receive antibiotic therapy to prevent late persistent infection.

L

MALARIA
Miguel Angel Russo

 BASICS

DESCRIPTION
- Malaria is an acute systemic illness caused by infection with *Plasmodium falciparum*, *P. vivax*, *P. malariae*, or *P. ovale*, all of which are transmitted to humans by female *Anopheles* sp. mosquitoes.
- There are an estimated 300–800 million clinical cases of malaria and 1–3 million deaths due to malaria annually in the tropics and subtropics.
- Incubation:
  - The time from insect bite to the release of merozoites into the bloodstream varies:
  - *P. falciparum*: Between 5 and 15 days
  - *P. vivax*: 13.4 days
  - *P. ovale*: 14.1 days
  - *P. malariae*: 34.7 days

EPIDEMIOLOGY
Incidence
- Malaria exists in tropical locations where the anopheline mosquito is present and the pool of infected people is high.
- In parts of the U.S., the anopheline mosquito exists; however, malaria is not present, except in rare cases.
- >1 million deaths, mainly in children, occur annually in Africa.
- Malaria is so well established in Africa that adaptation with the sickle cell gene, which confers protection, is present in as many as 25% of the population.
- *P. falciparum* exists in tropical locations where mosquitos live year round. In areas where mosquitos do not live year round (dry season), *P. vivax* and *P. ovale* can persist due to the liver hypnozoite stage.
- *P. falciparum* occurs in Africa, Papua New Guinea, Haiti, and East Asia.
- *P. vivax* occurs in Central and South America, India, North Africa, and East Asia.
- *P. ovale* occurs in West Africa.
- *P. malariae* is present worldwide, but it is found mostly in Africa.

RISK FACTORS
- Immunity plays an important role in the disease that malarial infection causes. Patients with no prior immunity will often have the highest rates of parasitemia and the most complications. Risk of complications also is present in young children with little or no immunity.
- Patients who are asplenic have greater complications.
- Pregnant women have more severe disease.

GENERAL PREVENTION

PATHOPHYSIOLOGY
The pathophysiology of malaria results from destruction of erythrocytes (both infected and uninfected), the consequent liberation of parasite and erythrocyte material into the circulation, and the host reaction to these events. *P. falciparum* malaria–infected erythrocytes specifically sequester in the microcirculation of vital organs, interfering with microcirculatory flow and host tissue metabolism.

ETIOLOGY
- Malaria infects 200–300 million people per year.
- The 4 strains are *P. falciparum*, *P. vivax*, *P. malariae*, and *P. ovale*.
- *P. falciparum* can invade erythrocytes at all stages of maturation, and is responsible for severe disease with the greatest mortality. It is often drug resistant. Because of the lack of a dormant live stage, *P. falciparum* does not cause relapses.
- *P. vivax* and *P. ovale* cause acute illness, and they are also responsible for late relapse >6–11 months after acute infection.
- *P. malariae* infections may persist for decades within the bloodstream, but relapse does not occur, except under rare circumstances, such as trauma or surgery.

COMMONLY ASSOCIATED CONDITIONS
- Factors predisposing to candiduria include:
- Diabetes mellitus.
- Urinary tract abnormalities.
- Malignancy.

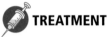 **DIAGNOSIS**

PHYSICAL EXAM
- Malaria causes fevers that, at times, are cyclic in nature.
- In patients with *P. falciparum*, fevers can be continuous, with occasional spikes.
- Patients with *P. ovale* and *P. vivax* have high fevers every 48 hours. For *P. malariae*, fevers are noted every 72 hours.
- Fevers are associated with rigors, tachycardia, and headaches. After 2–6 hours, the fevers will break and sweating occurs.
- In children and people who have no natural immunity, mental status changes, meningismus, seizures, and coma may occur.

- Patients may note shortness of breath and cough, which are harbingers of pulmonary edema.
- Renal failure due to hemoglobinuria (blackwater fever) is common in overwhelming *P. falciparum* infection.

DIAGNOSTIC TESTS & INTERPRETATION
Lab
Initial lab tests
- Thin and thick smear of blood
- Enzyme-linked immunosorbent assay for a histidine-rich *P. falciparum* antigen
- Assay for parasite lactate dehydrogenase

Follow-Up & Special Considerations
- Anemia with evidence of hemolysis (elevated LDH and decreased haptoglobin)
- Thrombocytopenia
- Renal insufficiency

DIFFERENTIAL DIAGNOSIS
- Typhoid fever
- Rheumatic fever

💉 **TREATMENT**

The mortality of untreated severe malaria is thought to approach 100%. With antimalarial treatment the mortality falls to 15–20% overall, although within the broad definition are syndromes associated with mortality rates that are lower (e.g., severe anaemia) and higher (metabolic acidosis). Death from severe malaria often occurs within hours of admission to hospital or clinic, and so it is essential that therapeutic concentrations of antimalarial are achieved as soon as possible. Clinical assessment of the patient, specific antimalarial treatment, adjunctive therapy and supportive care should be the main areas of comprises of the severe malaria management.

MEDICATION
First Line
- Chloroquine-sensitive *P. ovale*, *malariae*, *falciparum*, and *vivax*:
  - Chloroquine base 600 mg PO, followed by 300 mg PO in 6 hours and 300 mg PO on day 2 and day 3
- Chloroquine-resistant *P. falciparum*:
  - Quinine sulfate 650 mg orally q8h for 3–7 days, along with doxycycline 100 mg PO b.i.d. for 7 days, OR
  - Quinine sulfate 650 mg PO q8h for 3–7 days, followed by pyrimethamine-sulfadoxine, 3 tablets PO on the last day of quinine treatment
- For elimination of the hypnozoite stage in *P. ovale* and *P. vivax*:
  - Primaquine phosphate base 15.3 mg/d for 14 days

Second Line
- Quinine, followed by clindamycin 900 mg PO t.i.d. for 5 days
- Mefloquine 1250 mg PO as a single dose
- Atovaquone 1000 mg/d for 3 days and proguanil 400 mg/d for 3 days
- Halofantrine 500 mg q6h for 3 doses, with repeat 3 doses given in 1 week

ADDITIONAL TREATMENT
Additional Therapies
Exchange transfusion has been used in patients with malaria who have complications and high parasitemia rates.

COMPLEMENTARY & ALTERNATIVE THERAPIES
- Artemisinins:
  - This class of drug is not yet approved by the U.S. FDA. However, because of their ability to rapidly reduce levels of parasitemia (artemisinins are active against all of the erythrocytic stages of the malaria parasite, including gametocytes), tolerability, and limited resistance, artimisins are recommended by the WHO as 1st-line therapy for uncomplicated malaria. In the management of severe malaria, artesunate is easier and safer to use than quinine.

IN-PATIENT CONSIDERATIONS
Admission Criteria
- Clinical:
  - Abnormal level of consciousness
  - Cerebral malaria: Glasgow coma scale <11, Blantyre coma scale ≤3107
  - Deep coma has the worst prognosis, but delirium, obtundation, and stupor are associated with poor outcome.
  - Retinal hemorrhages
  - Repeated seizures (≥3 in 24 hours)
  - Respiratory distress (rapid, deep labored, stertorous breathing)
  - Heavy bleeding (unusual)
  - Shock
  - Jaundice with other vital organ dysfunction
- Parasitologic:
  - >500,000 parasites/μL blood (~10%)
  - >10,000 mature trophozoites and schizonts/μL blood (parasites with pigment)
  - >20% parasites with visible pigment
  - >5% neutrophils with malaria pigment

- Laboratory:
  - Elevated serum creatinine (>250 μmol/L)
  - Acidosis (plasma bicarbonate <15 mmol/L)
  - Hyperlactatemia (venous lactate >4 mmol/L)
  - Hypoglycemia (blood glucose <2.2 mmol/L)
  - Elevated liver enzymes (>3 × normal)
  - Elevated total bilirubin (>50 μmol/L)
  - Severe anemia (hematocrit <15%)
  - DIC (with bleeding)

Discharge Criteria
- Clinical improvement within 48–72 hours
- Thick and thin smears prepared q12h.
- Parasitemia reduced by 75% within 48 hours.

 ## ONGOING CARE

FOLLOW-UP RECOMMENDATIONS
Signs of malaria may start after a person leaves an endemic region. Travelers should be instructed to seek medical attention if fevers should occur.

COMPLICATIONS
- Coma due to increased vascular permeability and cerebral edema occur in patients with no immunity who have a high degree of parasitemia.
- Hypoglycemia is multifactorial in etiology. It is due to hepatic glycogen depletion, increased metabolic demands, and hyperinsulinemia.
- Oliguric renal failure can occur with massive hemolysis. This may be due to malaria itself or due to use of quinine in patients with glucose-6 phosphate deficiency.
- Pulmonary edema occurs due to the capillary leak syndrome.

Pregnancy Considerations
Chemoprophylaxis is an important issue for pregnant women because they are at increased risk of serious disease, especially primigravidas; because maternal malaria may decrease fetal survival; and because chloroquine is the only antimalarial agent known to be safe in pregnancy. This is a particularly difficult issue because of concern about teratogenicity during pregnancy. Although data suggest that mefloquine may also be safe, the number of women studied thus far is limited, and mefloquine has not yet been approved by the U.S. FDA for chemoprophylaxis during pregnancy. In contrast to the concerns about chemoprophylaxis, treatment is essential for pregnant women with symptomatic malaria to save their lives and their pregnancies. In fact, despite the known abortifacient effects of quinine at higher doses, therapeutic doses of quinine intravenously decrease both premature uterine contractions and fever in pregnant women with *P. falciparum* infection.

ADDITIONAL READING
- Breman JG, et al. The intolerable burden of malaria: A new look at the numbers. *Am J Trop Med Hyg*. 2001;64:iv–vii.
- Freedman DO, et al. Spectrum of disease and relation to place of exposure among ill returned travelers. *N Engl J Med*. 2006;354(2):119–30.
- Geosentinel. The global surveillance network of the ITSM and CDC. Available at: http://www.istm.org/geosentinel/main.html.
- Hill DR, et al. The practice of travel medicine: guidelines by the Infectious Disease Society of America. *Clin Infect Dis*. 2006;43:1499–539.
- International Society of Travel Medicine. The body of knowledge for the practice of travel medicine Available at http://www.istm.org/educational_resources-body-ed-aspx.
- Malaria Surveillance—United States, 2002. *MMWR Surveill Summ*. 2004;53:21–34.
- UN World Tourism Organization. Historical perspective of world tourism. Available at: http://unwto.org/facts/eng/historical.htm
- White NJ. The treatment of malaria. *N Engl J Med*. 1996;335:800–806.

 ## CODES

ICD9
- 084.6 Malaria, unspecified
- 647.40 Malaria of mother, complicating pregnancy, childbirth or the puerperium, unspecified as to episode of care
- 647.41 Malaria of mother, with delivery

M

MENINGITIS
Luciano Lemos-Filho

BASICS

DESCRIPTION
- Meningitis is the inflammation of the membranous layers of the CNS.
- The syndrome can be due infectious agents or be sterile, it may be acute or chronic, and it often overlaps with encephalitis. Infectious agents range from bacterial and viral, to mycobacterial, fungal, and parasitic.

EPIDEMIOLOGY
Incidence
- Acute bacterial meningitis: ~2.4 cases per 100,000 population per year in U.S. (1)
- Incidence of *Haemophilus influenzae* meningitis is declining in pediatric population, likely due to conjugate vaccine.

RISK FACTORS
- For acute bacterial meningitis: Extremes of age (though can happen at any age), immunocompromise, splenectomy, complement deficiency, CSF leak, head trauma (including neurosurgery), presence of CNS hardware
- Travel to epidemic regions (e.g., "meningitis belt" of Africa, Brazil, India, China, areas of Middle East).

Genetics
Susceptibility to pneumococcal and meningococcal meningitis is associated with several complement deficiencies and dysfunctions, including mutation of the mannose-binding lectin gene. Toll-like receptor mutations may affect susceptibility to tuberculous meningitis.

GENERAL PREVENTION
- Immunoprophylaxis with vaccination against Hib, pneumococcus, and meningococcus, depending on the age and risk factors, is recommended.
- Chemoprophylaxis is recommended for those with close contact with patients with meningococcal disease and in some cases of *H. influenzae*.

PATHOPHYSIOLOGY
In acute infectious meningitis, there is usually colonization of mucosal surfaces followed by dissemination and invasion of subarachnoid space. In turn, the host response to the microorganism leads to inflammation of the space, edema, vasculitis, oxidant stress, and loss of normal blood flow regulation. These processes can lead to a cycle of neuronal death, further inflammation, increased cerebral pressure, and death.

ETIOLOGY
- Because meningitis is an inflammation of the meningeal space, its causes are legion.
- Among viruses: Enteroviruses, mumps, HSV, HIV, measles and influenza.
- Bacterial causes: H. *influenzae, N. meningitides, S pneumoniae, Listeria monocytogenes, S. agalactiae, E. coli, M. tuberculosis, T. pallidum, Borrelia burgdorferi,* and *Rickettsial spp.*
- Fungal: *Coccidioides, Cryptococcus.*
- Parasitic causes: *Naegleria fowleri, Angiostrongylus,* and *Strongyloides.*
- Among noninfectious causes:
  - Neoplasms
  - Medications: Antibiotics, NSAIDs, and others
  - Collagen vascular diseases: SLE.

Pregnancy Considerations
Listeria monocytogenes meningitis is classically associated with meningitis in pregnancy.

COMMONLY ASSOCIATED CONDITIONS
- Paraspinal abscess
- Sinusitis
- CNS hardware

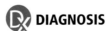

DIAGNOSIS

HISTORY
- Triad of headache, fever, and neck stiffness are the hallmarks, but may not be present in every patient (2/3 of patients present with classic triad).
- Altered sensorium is also common in bacterial meningitis (~80% of patients), as well as seizures (~30% at presentation).
- History of swimming in untreated water is a clue to amebic meningoencephalitis. A history of travel and eating snails, slugs, or crustaceans can point toward eosinophilic meningitis due to *Angiostrongylus.*

PHYSICAL EXAM
- In acute bacterial meningitis, Kerning's and Brudzinski's signs are present in > 1/2 the patients, focal cranial dysfunction in up to 20%.
- Rash is common with meningococcus (macular to petechial to purpuric).

ALERT
Immunosuppressed, neutropenic, elderly, and neonatal patients may have atypical presentations lacking classic findings. A high index of suspicion is paramount in making the diagnosis in these groups.

DIAGNOSTIC TESTS & INTERPRETATION
Lab
Initial lab tests
- CSF exam is the single most important laboratory test. Per current guidelines, lumbar puncture and blood cultures should be performed emergently in all patients with suspected acute bacterial meningitis in the absence of contraindications that could predispose to herniation from CSF removal.
- Factors that allow for delay of lumbar puncture pending neuroimagingare: Immunocompromise, history of CNS disease, new seizure, altered consciousness, papilledema, and focal neurologic deficit.
- If lumbar puncture is delayed for neuroimaging, blood cultures should be obtained emergently.
- CSF tests should include cell count, glucose, total protein, Gram stain and culture at a minimum. Classically acute bacterial meningitis is characterized by a high neutrophil content (typically 500 to >10,000 cells/mm^3), low glucose, and high protein. Interpretation of results must take into account the host status (including age) and clinical picture.
- Additional tests that can be sent depending on suspicion include bacterial antigen test, India ink stain +/− cryptococcal antigen, PCR for viruses and/or TB, and AFB culture and stain.

Follow-Up & Special Considerations
- Opening pressure of lumbar puncture should always be measured and documented. Pressures >20–25 mm can be associated with herniation and should prompt neurosurgical consultation and abortion of lumbar puncture (use sample in manometer for studies).
- Treatment should not be delayed in cases of suspected bacterial meningitis pending results.

Imaging
Initial approach
A noncontrast head CT can be obtained in certain cases prior to lumbar puncture to rule out hydrocephalus/mass lesions, as noted in the previous sections. Again, treatment should not be delayed pending imaging.

Follow-Up & Special Considerations
- Neuroimaging could be especially useful in cases of CSF leak.
- Consider follow-up neuroimaging if inadequate response to therapy suggests brain abscess or other pathology.

Diagnostic Procedures/Other
- Blood cultures should be obtained prior to antibiotic treatment.
- CSF can be sent to specialized labs for characterization of viral pathogens.
- Withdrawing and reintroducing certain drugs in the case of medication-induced aseptic meningitis can aid diagnosis.
- Cytology for suspected neoplasm-associated meningitis

Pathological Findings
- Inflammation of the meninges ranging from frank purulence to less severe changes
- Obliteration of arachnoid space seen in severe cases with hydrocephalus

DIFFERENTIAL DIAGNOSIS
- Brain abscess
- Sepsis
- Seizure disorder
- Subarachnoid hemorrhage
- Encephalitis

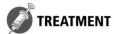 **TREATMENT**

MEDICATION
First Line

ALERT
To penetrate CSF, medication dosage is often higher. Recommended dose of antibiotic agents also varies according to age and other factors; check guidelines referenced for specific recommendations (2).

- For community-acquired acute bacterial meningitis, empiric therapy in patients between 1 month and 50 years of age guidelines recommend: Vancomycin + 3rd generation cephalosporin
- In children with suspected *H. influenzae* type b meningitis guidelines recommend: Dexamethasone (0.15 mg/kg q6h for 2–4 days) as an adjunct prior to 1st dose of antibiotics
- In adults with suspected *S. pneumoniae* meningitis: Dexamethasone (0.15 mg/kg q6h for 2–4 days) recommended prior to 1st dose of antibiotic.
- For infants <1 month: Recommendations for acute bacterial meningitis include ampicillin plus either cefotaxime or aminoglycoside
- For patients >50 years of age, guidelines suggest: Vancomycin plus ampicillin plus 3rd-generation cephalosporin
- In cases of penetrating trauma, and postneurosurgery, recommendations are to empirically start treatment with vancomycin and an antipseudomonal agent (such as cefepime, ceftazidime, or meropenem).
- Therapy in any case should be narrowed as allowed by pathogen identification and susceptibility profile.
- In case of viral meningoencephalitis due to HSV, acyclovir is the drug of choice (2).

Second Line
Patients with severe β-lactam and/or cephalosporin allergy and meningococcal disease may be treated with chloramphenicol or with a fluoroquinolone. Expert consultation is recommended.

ADDITIONAL TREATMENT
General Measures
Patients with suspected meningococcal disease should be placed on droplet isolation. Close contacts, including health care workers exposed to oral/nasal secretions, should receive postexposure prophylaxis. (See alert at end of section.)

Issues for Referral
Entertain a low threshold for expert consultation to include infectious disease, neurology, and possibly neurosurgery experts.

Additional Therapies
- Some patients with increased intracranial pressure may benefit from measures to decrease this parameter; however, expert opinion is recommended.
- Surgical correction of persistent CSF leakage
- Removal of infected hardware may be needed.

IN-PATIENT CONSIDERATIONS
Initial Stabilization
- In patients with obtundation and/or inability to protect the airway, endotracheal intubation is recommended. Attention must be paid during induction for patients with suspected increased ICP.
- Blood pressure maintenance in normal range in cases of shock is paramount to perfuse and protect at-risk brain tissue.

Admission Criteria
- Patients with acute bacterial meningitis should be admitted for treatment and observation, including ICU-level care at least initially.
- Consider ICU-level care for any patient with meningitis and neurological changes, elevated opening pressures, and/or immunosuppression.

IV Fluids
As needed for maintenance of intravascular volume in patients who cannot tolerate PO or need to be resuscitated for shock

Nursing
Per routine care to admission unit, including neuro checks and ICU-level care when appropriate

Discharge Criteria
Typically, discharge in acute bacterial meningitis is only possible after completion of course of IV antibiotics, with duration depending on pathogen and clinical course. Outpatient IV therapy after an appropriate initial course maybe an option but expert consultation is advised prior to this course of therapy.

 ONGOING CARE

FOLLOW-UP RECOMMENDATIONS
- Follow-up of CSF studies is mandatory, including some tests such as fungal or AFB cultures, which can take weeks to complete.
- Repeat CSF studies might be necessary if diagnosis not established or if clinical worsening occurs.
- Appropriate follow-up with subspecialties in case of sequelae

Patient Monitoring
ICU-level care is initially recommended for acute bacterial meningitis.

DIET
No particular restrictions

PATIENT EDUCATION
Depends on cause of meningitis

PROGNOSIS
- Acute bacterial meningitis has a case fatality rate of between 10% and 30% depending on pathogen and age group (*S. pneumoniae* and infants having the worst prognosis).
- Sequelae are seen in 20–50% of survivors of acute bacterial meningitis.

COMPLICATIONS
- Death
- Seizures
- Deafness
- Cognitive impairment
- Shock
- Amputation
- Hydrocephalus, herniation

ALERT
- For *Neisseria meningitidis* disease, chemoprophylaxis is recommended for those known to be or likely to have been exposed to nasopharyngeal secretions of patients. These include household and daycare contacts, as well as health care workers involved in intubation and respiratory care. Prophylaxis should ideally be administered within 24 hours but probably not after 14 days. Rifampin, ciprofloxacin, and ceftriaxone are the recommended agents; however, there have been recent reports of fluoroquinolone resistance.
- For *H. influenzae* disease, chemoprophylaxis is recommended for household contacts and most likely is beneficial for school contacts. Rifampin is the agent of choice.
- In either case, expert consultation, including public health authorities, is recommended in determining who should receive prophylaxis and what agent should be used.

REFERENCES

1. Schuchat A, et al. Bacterial meningitis in the U.S. in 1995. Active Surveillance Team. *N Engl J Med*. 1997;337(14):970–6.
2. Tunkel A, et al. Practice guidelines for the management of bacterial meningitis. *Clin Infect Dis*. 2004:39(9):1267–84.

CODES

ICD9
- 320.9 Meningitis due to unspecified bacterium
- 322.2 Chronic meningitis
- 322.9 Meningitis, unspecified

CLINICAL PEARLS
- Meningitis is potentially life-threatening and treatment with wide-spectrum antibiotics should not be delayed while confirmatory tests are being conducted.

M

METHEMOGLOBINEMIA

Adel Bassily-Marcus
Samir Pesh-Imam

BASICS

DESCRIPTION
- Methemoglobinemia (MetHba) is a clinical syndrome caused by an increase in the blood levels of methemoglobin (MetHb) $Hgb(Fe^{3+})$.
- This reaction impairs the ability of hemoglobin to transport oxygen and carbon dioxide, leading to tissue hypoxemia, cyanosis, metabolic acidosis, and in severe cases, death.

RISK FACTORS
- Household chemical:
  - Room deodorizer propellants
  - Aniline compounds found in inks, polishes, paints, varnishes
- Topical anesthetics:
  - Benzocaine (most common), lidocaine
  - As little as 15–25 mg/kg of topical benzocaine can induce MetHb
- Common IV medications:
  - Nitrate, nitrites, NTG, nipride, sulfonamides, pyridium, quinones, dapsone
  - Phenytoin, phenols, silver nitrate
  - Dapsone

PATHOPHYSIOLOGY
- Oxidation is the process of removal of an electron from normal ferrous (bivalent or Fe^{2+}) to the ferric (trivalent or Fe^{3+}) state. Hemoglobin in the ferric form is unable to bind oxygen and is termed methemoglobin (MetHb)

$$Hgb(Fe^{2+}) \; \blacktriangleright \text{Oxidative Stress} \; Hgb(Fe^{3+})$$

- Oxidizing agents accelerate 100–1000x the oxidation of Hgb and overwhelms the capacity of endogenous reduction capacity.
- The oxidized ferric (3+) state (methemoglobin) has an increased affinity for its bound oxygen and a decreased affinity for any unbound oxygen.
- The oxyhemoglobin dissociation curve is shifted to the left, with less oxygen being transported and released. The affinity of carbon dioxide (CO_2) is decreased, with resultant less CO_2 removed from the tissues.
- In erythrocytes, ferrous iron undergoes slow oxidation at a rate of 3% per day.

- Reduction of the MetHb to ferrous hemoglobin occurs to maintain intraerythrocytic MetHb concentration at <1%. The pathways are:
  - Nicotinamide adenine dinucleotide (NAD)-cytochrome b5 reductase:
    - Allows NADH to donate an electron to cytochrome b5, which then transfers the electron to MetHb reducing it to ferrous hemoglobin $Hgb(Fe2+)$.
    - This pathway is responsible for reducing 95% of methemoglobin.
  - NADPH MetHb reductase:
    - This pathway uses the reduced form of nicotinamide adenine dinucleotide phosphate (NADPH) and NADPH-methemoglobin reductase to affect methemoglobin reduction.
    - Responsible for <5% of total reduction
    - This enzyme is crucial for the antidote effect of methylene blue (MB).
    - Patients with glucose-6-phosphate dehydrogenase deficiency (G6PD) lack NADPH production that is required for MB reduction, causing MB treatment to be ineffective and may cause hemolysis.
  - Direct electron transfer from ascorbic acid and glutathione:
    - Much slower pathway
- Normally, MetHb fractions in circulating whole blood are <1–2%
- Functional anemia:
  - Oxy-hemoglobin dissociation curve is shifted left, impairing oxygen delivery at the tissue level.

ETIOLOGY
- Acquired:
  - By far the most common cause
  - Rate of MetHb formation exceeds the rate of reduction.
  - 2nd to drug/chemical exposure (see below)
  - Occasionally secondary to pathologic conditions (e.g., sepsis, sickle cell crisis, and GI infections in children)
- Inherited-enzyme deficiency:
  - Cytochrome b5 reductase (b5R):
    - Autosomal recessive trait
    - Type I (majority) and type II (10–15%)
    - Heterozygotes
    - Asymptomatic
    - Predisposed to met HG after exposure to oxidizing agent
  - Hemoglobin M disorder

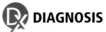

DIAGNOSIS

HISTORY
- Exposure to causative agents
- Critically ill, septic patients are more prone to MetHba due to large amount of nitric oxide released, which is converted to MetHb and nitrates.

PHYSICAL EXAM
- Altered mental status
- Dyspnea
- Headache
- Fatigue, lethargy, stupor and coma
- Tachycardia, tachypnea, hypotension, shock
- Seizure
- Pulse oximetry:
  - Utilizes 2 wavelengths of light, 660 nm and 940 nm
  - Only detects OxyHb and DeoxyHb
  - Reading usually decreased: 80–85%
- Acute cyanosis: Not correctable with oxygen therapy.
- Generalized cyanosis in the presence of a normal arterial oxygen tension is almost always present.
- Dysrhythmias and arrest (severe cases)
- Chocolate-brown colored blood
- Urine may appear black/brown
- % MetHba:
  - 10–20%: Mild cyanosis
  - 30–40%: Headache, fatigue, tachycardia, weakness, dizziness
  - 50–60%: Acidosis, arrhythmias, coma, seizures, bradycardia,
  - >70%: Fatal

DIAGNOSTIC TESTS & INTERPRETATION
Lab
Initial lab tests
- ABG:
  - Normal PaO^2
  - Paradoxical elevation of PaO_2 despite clinical cyanosis
  - Falsely normal (or elevated) SaO_2
  - Saturation gap: Oxygen saturation is significantly different between the pulse oximetry and the calculated saturation from ABG. >5% gap is a significant clue.
  - Lactic acidosis
- Arterial blood takes on a "chocolate-brown" appearance (chocolate cyanosis); unlike deoxyhemoglobin, color does not change on exposure to atmospheric oxygen.

- Bedside test (Kronenberg test): Place 1–2 drops of patients blood placed on white filter paper. The chocolate brown appearance of MetHb does not change after exposure to 100% oxygen; in contrast, deoxyhemoglobin appears dark red/violet initially but brightens with time.
- The diagnosis is confirmed by multiple-wavelength co-oximetry (test of choice):
  – Determines the amount of oxyhemoglobin, deoxyhemoglobin, carboxyhemoglobin, and MetHb
- Standard pulse oximetry neither accurately nor reliably measures percent saturation.
- G6PD deficiency level

Follow-Up & Special Considerations
- MB dye will cause a falsely increased estimation of desaturated hemoglobin by pulse oximeter.
- MB is contraindicated in patients with G6PD deficiency.

Imaging
Initial approach
To rule out other causes of hypoxic respiratory failure

Follow-Up & Special Considerations
Rebound of MetHb can occur for up to 18 hours. Monitor patient for 24 hours.

Pathological Findings
Evidence of anoxic injury

DIFFERENTIAL DIAGNOSIS
- Carbon monoxide poisoning (no cyanosis)
- Sulfhemoglobinemia
- Cyanide poisoning
- Respiratory failure
- Cardiac structural abnormalities

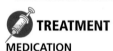 TREATMENT

MEDICATION
First Line
Remove causative agent:
- Hg will return to normal state in 48–72 hours
- Ingested: Gastric lavage/activated charcoal
- Consider hemodialysis.

Second Line
MB in symptomatic, non-G6PD deficient patients:
- Most effective antidote
- 1–2 mg/kg of 1% MB (10 mg/mL) IV over 5 min (max dose 7 mg/kg); repeat if cyanosis not corrected within 30–60 minutes
- Reduces the amount of MetHb by 50% within 1 hour

- MB (oxidized form of the dye) acts as an electron donor, NADPH is utilized by methemoglobin reductase to convert MB to leukomethylene (reduced form). This reduced form reduces the MetHb Hgb($Fe3+$) to hemoglobin Hgb($Fe2+$).
- In G6PD deficiency, there is lack of NADPH production; MB will be ineffective, but in large doses it can function as an oxidizing agent, causing hemolytic anemia and convert Hgb to MetHb, thus exacerbating the condition it used to treat.
- Co-oximetry reads MB as if it were MetHb; use Evelyn-Malloy method for determining the concentration of MetHb while receiving MB.
- Response to MB is rapid; a repeat dose may be needed in 30–60 minutes.
- ICU monitoring is usually needed in patients who require MB.

ADDITIONAL TREATMENT
General Measures
- Blood transfusion/exchange transfusion for patients in shock, G6PD-deficient patient with life-threatening MetHba if MB deemed ineffective
- Ascorbic acid:
  – 300–1000 mg/d PO in divided doses
  – High doses can cause hemolysis.
- Hyperbaric oxygen

IN-PATIENT CONSIDERATIONS
Initial Stabilization
- Prompt treatment is paramount.
- Rapid recognition coupled with immediate infusion of MB can be life-saving.
- Removal of offending agent is critical.
- Supplemental high-flow oxygen to increase plasma level of dissolved oxygen.
- Maintain an open airway; may need to assist ventilation

IV Fluids
Isotonic crystalloids in shock

 ONGOING CARE

DIET
Avoid nitrite-rich food. Nitrites are used as meat preservatives; also found in many vegetables (e.g., beets).

PROGNOSIS
- Mild-moderate cases have favorable prognosis once prompt diagnosis and early treatment is established.
- In severe cases, prognosis is determined by the degree of anoxic end-organ damage.

COMPLICATIONS
- Rebound for up to 18 hours
- Shock
- Seizures
- Anoxic end-organ damage including cardiac ischemia, anoxic brain injury.
- Death

ADDITIONAL READING
- Conkling PR. Brown blood: Understanding methemoglobinemia. *N C Med J*. 1986;47(3): 109–11.
- Mansouri A, et al. Concise review: Methemoglobinemia. *Am J Hematol*. 1993;42:7.

 CODES

ICD9
289.7 Methemoglobinemia

CLINICAL PEARLS
- The typical clinical picture includes profound cyanosis with minimal symptoms in the presence of normal/elevated PaO_2, frequently in the perioperative period.
- Central cyanosis refractory to oxygen supplementation is the main characteristic of MetHba.
- Standard pulse oximetry registers falsely high SpO_2 in patients with MetHba.
- Arterial blood gases typically demonstrate a normal PaO_2 and a normal calculated oxygen saturation; co-oximetry ABG must be ordered to calculate true SaO_2
- Treatment of MetHba consists of oxygen, MB, and exchange transfusion.
- No need to treat if patient is not symptomatic (levels <20–30%) unless other condition contribute to the clinical picture (e.g., anemia, cardiac disease, respiratory failure).
- MB is the treatment of choice unless the patient is G6PD deficient.

M

METHICILLIN-RESISTANT *STAPHYLOCOCCUS* AUREUS (MRSA)

Oveys Mansuri

BASICS

DESCRIPTION
- Methicillin-resistant *Staphylococcus aureus* (MRSA) is a strain that is resistant to methicillin, and other antibiotics in the penicillin class.
- 2 types of MRSA: Hospital-acquired (HA-MRSA) and community-acquired (CA-MRSA)
- CDC definition for CA-MRSA: Identification of MRSA in patients with signs and symptoms of infection, either outpatient or within 48 hours of admission, with no history of MRSA infection or colonization, no history of admission to hospital or nursing home in past year, and absence of dialysis, surgery, permanent indwelling catheters or medical devices passing through skin to the body

EPIDEMIOLOGY
Incidence
64% of all patients in the ICU

Prevalence
- 46 out of every 1,000 patients were either infected or colonized with MRSA according to a 2006 APIC study
- 0.8–2% of the general US population is colonized with MRSA
- Pooled MRSA colonization prevalence rate of 1.3% in the community in 1 meta-analysis.
- Colonization with CA-MRSA in toddlers attending daycare ranges from 0.6% to 23%

RISK FACTORS
- Severe asthma
- Influenza
- Leukemia
- Tumors
- Immunocompromised
- (organ transplant, HIV/AIDS)
- Burns
- Diabetes
- Surgical wounds
- Urinary catheters
- Venous access catheters including dialysis catheters
- IV drug abusers
- Sharing of personal space/products:
  - Very young and elderly
  - Higher rates of CA-MRSA in low-income families and minorities

Geriatric Considerations
- Increased risk secondary to prevalence of chronic diseases
- Exposed prosthetics or catheter infections

Pediatric Considerations
- Children in school and/or daycare
- Newborn infants
- Antibiotics being the mainstay of treatment, it is vitally important to use appropriate dosage adjustments by weight for pediatric patients
- Recently observed high mortality with CA-MRSA

Pregnancy Considerations
- Nursing newborn baby
- Important to consider pregnancy categorization of antibiotic agents before use; pharmacy consultation is recommended.

Genetics
Panton-Valentine leukocidin (PVL) genes lukF-PV and lukS-PV are commonly found in CA-MRSA.

GENERAL PREVENTION
- Hand-washing and/or approved alcohol-based antiseptic gels (universal precautions)
- CDC mandated contact precautions for MRSA

PATHOPHYSIOLOGY
- Resistance to β-lactam antibiotics
- Mediated through penicillin-binding-proteins (PBP)
- β-lactam antibiotics bind to PBP preventing cell wall construction by bacteria
- Mutation causes resistance by altering the PBPs, thereby reducing their binding of the β-lactam antibiotics.

ETIOLOGY
- Colonization of nasopharynx and/or skin
- Infection enters through breaks in skin (surgical incisions, catheter insertion sites, shaving).
- After infection has occurred, abscess cavity may form at the site and subsequently lead to hematogenous spread (bacteremia).
- Ratio of clinical infection to colonization higher for CA-MRSA then HA-MRSA
- CA-MRSA and HA-MRSA manifest differently:
  - 72–84% of patients with CA-MRSA have superficial or deep skin or soft tissue infections compared with 22–38% of HA-MRSA patients.
  - HA-MRSA is more likely to be invasive.

DIAGNOSIS

HISTORY
- Report of fever
- Localized skin infection with or without drainage and/or abscess formation
- General malaise/aches
- Recent hospitalization or surgery
- Recent pregnancy

PHYSICAL EXAM
- Localized skin infection
- Examination of surgical incisions/wounds
- Fever, hypotension
- Altered mental status

DIAGNOSTIC TESTS & INTERPRETATION
Lab
Initial lab tests
- Culture and Gram stain from wound, drainage, and blood/urine/sputum as indicated
- CBC to evaluate for elevated WBC
- Chemistry panel

Follow-Up & Special Considerations
Follow-up blood cultures are required if bacteremia is found.

Imaging
- Chest x-ray to evaluate for pneumonia
- CT may be necessary to locate abscesses.

Diagnostic Procedures/Other
Echocardiogram for patients with bacteremia to rule out endocarditis

Pathological Findings
Soft tissue abscesses, necrotizing pneumonia with cavitation, parapneumonic effusion are common (especially if antibiotic administration is delayed).

DIFFERENTIAL DIAGNOSIS
- Cellulitis
- Abscess
- Septic arthritis
- Septic shock
- UTI
- Wound infection

TREATMENT

MEDICATION
First Line
- Bacteremia: Vancomycin IV 6 mg/kg/d (duration: 2–6 weeks depending on complicated vs. uncomplicated bacteremia)
- Pneumonia: Vancomycin IV or linezolid 600 mg PO/IV b.i.d. or clindamycin 600 mg PO/IV t.i.d. (duration: 7–21 days)
- Bone and joint: IV vancomycin and daptomycin 6 mg/kg/d (duration: 8 weeks recommended for MRSA osteomyelitis)
- CA-MRSA tends to be more susceptible to most antibiotic classes except β-lactams: Empiric vancomycin is recommended until susceptibilities are available, given the challenge in differentiating CA-MRSA from HA-MRSA at presentation.

Second Line
For persistent MRSA bacteremia after vancomycin treatment: Daptomycin 10 mg/kg/d in combination with gentamicin 1 mg/kg IV q8h or rifampin 600 mg/d PO/IV or 300–450 mg PO/IV b.i.d. or linezolid 600 mg PO/IV b.i.d. or TMP-SMX 5 mg/kg IV b.i.d.

ADDITIONAL TREATMENT
General Measures
- Timely removal of foreign body, prosthetic device, or catheters as part of source control
- Timely drainage of abscess and parapneumonic effusion

Issues for Referral
- Cardiology and cardiac surgical consult may be needed if endocarditis is established.
- ID consult is advised for complex MRSA infections with poor response to initial treatment.

SURGERY/OTHER PROCEDURES
- Surgical drainage/source control of all abscesses is emergent.
- Cutaneous abscess: Incision and drainage + antibiotics in some cases (severe disease, rapid progression, difficult to drain, extremes of age)
- For complex skin/soft tissue infections antibiotic therapy can consist of vancomycin IV or PO/IV linezolid 600 mg b.i.d. or clindamycin 600 mg PO or IV t.i.d. 7–14 days of therapy.

IN-PATIENT CONSIDERATIONS
Initial Stabilization
- Identification of primary infection
- Antibiotic therapy and source control
- Hemodynamic stabilization and resuscitation

Admission Criteria
- ICU admission for those with hemodynamic instability, need for frequent monitoring, respiratory failure, and other intensive care needs
- Hospital admission is advised for all suspected MRSA infections (due to rapid progression and high mortality of recent CA-MRSA infections, in particular in the younger patient population).

IV Fluids
- Adequate fluid resuscitation with use of crystalloid replacement (i.e., 0.9% NS or LR)
- Ensure appropriate access and consider central venous access if inadequate access or need for monitoring volume status (CVP). Note prior removal of any infected lines or catheters.

Nursing
Patient comfort

Discharge Criteria
- Drainage and removal of primary infectious site/catheter
- Resolution of overt signs of infection and no need for further intervention
- Ability to deliver long-term antibiotic treatment on an outpatient bases (if required, NB: PICC lines may be necessary for outpatient antibiotic treatment)

 ONGOING CARE

FOLLOW-UP RECOMMENDATIONS
- At discharge from ICU, generate detailed sign-out assuring safe and seamless transfer of care to floor or for discharge to home and follow-up with primary care physician.
- Stabilized patients may complete course of antibiotics as outpatients. Outpatient IV antibiotics may require arrangements for temporary access and home health services.

Patient Monitoring
- Continue close monitoring while in ICU.
- Frequently examine wounds suspected of infection.

DIET
Maintain appropriate enteral feeding to optimize nutrition if no contraindications.

PATIENT EDUCATION
- Appropriate hygiene
- Hand-washing
- Contact precautions

PROGNOSIS
- MRSA accounts for almost 20,000 deaths per year in the US.
- 86% of deaths are attributed to HA-MRSA.
- 14% of deaths are attributed to CA-MRSA.
- Pneumonia and septicemia from MRSA infection have a 20% mortality rate.

COMPLICATIONS
- Sepsis
- Pneumonia
- Shock
- Long-term organ dysfunction of failure (pulmonary fibrosis, kidney failure, etc.)
- Death

ADDITIONAL READING
- Climo MW, et al. The effect of daily bathing with chlorhexidine on the acquisition of methicillin-resistant Staphylococcus aureus, vancomycin-resistant Enterococcus, and healthcare-associated bloodstream infections: Results of a quasi-experimental multicenter trial. *Crit Care Med*. 2009;37:1858–65.
- Huskins WC, et al. Intervention to reduce transmission of resistant bacteria in intensive care. *N Engl J Med*. 2011;364:1407–18.
- Jain R, et al. Veterans Affairs initiative to prevent methicillin-resistant Staphylococcus aureus infections. *N Engl J Med*. 2011;364:1419–30.
- Lin MY, et al. Methicillin-resistant Staphylococcus aureus and vancomycin-resistant enterococcus: Recognition and prevention in intensive care units. *Crit Care Med*. 2010;38(Suppl):S335–44.
- Maltezou HC, et al. Community-acquired methicillin-resistant Staphylococcus aureus infections. *Int J Antimicrob Agents*. 2006;27:87–96.
- Yamamoto T, et al. Community-acquired methicillin-resistant Staphylococcus aureus: community transmission, pathogenesis, and drug resistance. *J Infect Chemother*. 2010;16:225–54.

CODES

ICD9
- 038.12 Methicillin resistant Staphylococcus aureus septicemia
- 041.12 Methicillin resistant Staphylococcus aureus
- 482.42 Methicillin resistant pneumonia due to Staphylococcus aureus

CLINICAL PEARLS
- Stabilize patient for any acute issues.
- Identify source and site of infection; provide urgent source control.
- Physical exam is focused on soft-tissue infection, postsurgical wounds, prosthetics, and catheters.
- Fundamentals of therapy: Source control/surgical debridement, antibiotic therapy, complex management of sepsis and ARDS if disease advances to that stage.

M

MITRAL REGURGITATION, ACUTE

Jina Sohn
Isaac Halickman

 ## BASICS

DESCRIPTION
Acute occurrence of mitral valve incompetence resulting in regurgitation of the left ventricle (LV) volume into the left atrium during systole

EPIDEMIOLOGY
Incidence
- Rare, but most commonly occurs as a complication of acute myocardial infarction (AMI).
- In the era of thrombolysis, incidence of some degree of mitral regurgitation (MR) in the setting of AMI is 27%.
- Papillary muscle rupture leading to acute mitral regurgitation accounts for 6.9% of cardiogenic shock in patient with AMI.

PATHOPHYSIOLOGY
- In acute MR, there is sudden increase in left atrial volume load due to regurgitation from the LV. The left atrium cannot accommodate the sudden increase in volume, resulting in pulmonary congestion and large V waves on right heart catheterization.
- The LV does not have time to dilate to maintain forward stroke volume and cardiac output in the acute MR state. This results in decreased cardiac output and cardiogenic shock, particularly in the setting of AMI.
- Rupture of posterior leaflet chords is more common than in anterior leaflet chords.
- Acute MR is more common in inferior infarction.

ETIOLOGY
- Most often due to complication of MI, such as papillary muscle rupture.
- Spontaneous chordal rupture
- Infective endocarditis
- Rheumatic fever
- Prosthetic valve dysfunction
- Trauma

COMMONLY ASSOCIATED CONDITIONS
- MI
- Cardiogenic shock
- Pre-existing MR due to mitral valve prolapse (MVP), rheumatic heart disease, and collagen vascular disease

DIAGNOSIS

HISTORY
- Acute onset of dyspnea and tachypnea
- Pulmonary edema
- Hemodynamic instability in setting of cardiogenic shock

PHYSICAL EXAM
- Systolic murmur of mitral regurgitation heard best at the base. The murmur may not be holosystolic in the acute state, and may be absent in the setting of low cardiac output
- LV apical impulse is hyperdynamic. However, in the acute state, the LV may not be hypertrophied and the apical impulse may not be hyperdynamic.
- 3rd heart sound and early diastolic flow rumble.
- Rales in the setting of pulmonary edema.
- Increased pulmonary pressures occur, and thus increased pulmonic 2nd heart sound. Paradoxical splitting of the 2nd heart sound may occur.
- In the setting of cardiogenic shock or overt heart failure, there is rise in central venous pressure evidenced by a prominent V wave on jugular venous pulse.

DIAGNOSTIC TESTS & INTERPRETATION
Lab
- Lab tests for diagnosis of MI
- Blood cultures for the diagnosis of endocarditis.
- No specific lab tests for the diagnosis of MR.

Imaging
Initial approach
- Echocardiography is the gold standard in the evaluation of acute MR.
- Color Doppler and spectral Doppler displays can be used to assess the severity of the regurgitation.
- Transesophageal echocardiography can evaluate the severity and etiology of MR more accurately than a transthoracic echocardiogram.
- Transesophageal echocardiogram can assess valve morphology and motion, and also assess for valvular vegetations in the setting of infective endocarditis.

- Transthoracic echocardiogram can underestimate the severity of the MR by inadequate imaging of the color Doppler.
- If there is hyperdynamic systolic function of the LV in the setting of acute heart failure, severe MR should be considered.
- Ruptured papillary muscle head and flailed mitral valve leaflets are readily visualized on both transthoracic and transesophageal echocardiogram.
- Chest x-ray will show evidence of pulmonary venous congestion. There may be no evidence of left atrial enlargement in the acute setting.

Follow-Up & Special Considerations
In the setting of CAD, cardiac catheterization should be considered prior to surgery.

Diagnostic Procedures/Other
- Right heart catheterization can also be used to measure pulmonary pressure and provide a thorough hemodynamic assessment.
- By measuring oxygen saturations, acute MR and ventral septal defect (VSD) can be distinguished in the setting of AMI and new systolic murmur.

Pathological Findings
- Rupture papillary muscle
- Ischemic papillary muscle
- Chordal rupture
- Flailed mitral valve leaflets
- In the setting of endocarditis, vegetative destruction of the valve leaflets

DIFFERENTIAL DIAGNOSIS
- In the setting of myocardial infarction, other etiologies of cardiogenic shock should be considered:
  - VSD
  - Mitral annular dilation due to severe LV dysfunction
  - Free wall rupture
  - Pump failure

TREATMENT

MEDICATION

First Line

Medical therapy is not a first-line therapy in the setting of acute MR and is used primarily to stabilize the patient prior to surgery:

- In a normotensive patient, nitroprusside will aid in increasing forward output and reducing the MR.
- In a hypotensive patient, nitroprusside should be used in conjunction with an inotropic agent, such as dobutamine.

Second Line

- Diuretics, β blockers, and biventricular pacing are used for primary treatment of LV dysfunction in functional MR.
- If atrial fibrillation is encountered, maintenance of a normal ventricular response with β blockers, calcium channel blockers, and/or digitalis therapy is considered.

ADDITIONAL TREATMENT

Additional Therapies

- Intra-aortic balloon pump (IABP) can also be used in the hypotensive patient to achieve effects similar to medical therapy.
- IABP can increase forward output and increase mean arterial pressure while reducing MR volume.

SURGERY/OTHER PROCEDURES

- Surgical repair or replacement of the valve is the definitive therapy for acute MR.
- Mitral valve repair has been shown to improve outcomes with a lower operative mortality and 30% increase in 10-year survival compared to mitral valve replacement.

IN-PATIENT CONSIDERATIONS

Initial Stabilization

- Patients often present with acute pulmonary edema and usually require intubation.
- All patients will need aggressive afterload reduction with IV nitroprusside to improve forward flow and thus cardiac output.
- In patients with hypotension and shock, vasoactive agents may be needed to support blood pressure.
- IABP is an effective alternative to medical therapy to reduce afterload and improve cardiac output.

Admission Criteria

Patients are critically ill, requiring admissions to the ICU.

IV Fluids

IV fluid resuscitation is not effective in the management of acute MR and may worsen the already elevated left-sided filling pressures.

Discharge Criteria

- Resolution of cardiogenic shock. Patients often need surgical intervention for long-term stabilization.
- Patients with cardiogenic shock due to acute MR have longer length of stay. Among the survivors in the SHOCK registry, the average length of stay was 20 vs. 15 days in survivors of cardiogenic shock due to LV failure.

ONGOING CARE

PROGNOSIS

- Mortality rate is up to 60% in all cardiogenic shock patients. In patients with cardiogenic shock due to acute MR, the mortality rate was 55% in the SHOCK registry.
- Surgical repair or replacement of the mitral valve is the only definitive therapy. Mortality is significantly improved with surgical intervention; 40% for surgical vs. 71% for nonsurgical intervention in the SHOCK registry.

ADDITIONAL READING

- Bonow et al. Focused update incorporated into the ACC/AHA 2006 Guidelines for the management of patients with valvular heart disease. *JACC.* 2008;52: e55–6.
- Oh JK, et al. *The Echo Manual*, 3rd ed. Philadelphia: Lippincott, Williams, and Wilkins, 2007;158–173.
- Parrillo JE, ed. *Critical Care Medicine: Principles of Diagnosis and Management in the Adult*, 3rd ed. Philadelphia: Mosby, 2007;423–437, 689–695.
- Picard MN, et al. Echocardiographic predictors of survival and response to early revascularization in cardiogenic shock. *Circulation.* 2003;107:279–284.
- Thompson CR, et al. Cardiogenic shock due to acute severe mitral regurgitation complicating acute myocardial infarction: A report from the SHOCK Trial Registry. Should we emergently revascularize occluded coronaries in cardiogenic shock? *J Am Coll Cardiol.* 2000;36(Suppl A):1104–9.

CODES

ICD9

- 394.1 Rheumatic mitral insufficiency
- 424.0 Mitral valve insufficiency NOS
- 429.6 Rupture of papillary muscle

CLINICAL PEARLS

- In the setting of cardiogenic shock, the murmur of MR may be soft or absent.
- When there is hyperdynamic LV function in the setting of cardiogenic shock on the echocardiogram, acute MR should be ruled out.

M

MITRAL STENOSIS
Qasim Durrani

 BASICS

DESCRIPTION
- Normal area of mitral valve (MV) is 4–6 cm^2. In mitral stenosis (MS), narrowing of the MV restricts left ventricle filling during diastole.
- Most commonly caused by rheumatic heart disease; however, as the incidence of rheumatic fever is decreasing, other causes are rising proportionally.

EPIDEMIOLOGY
Incidence
- Not precisely known, but steadily decreasing
- Females > Males (2:1).

Prevalence
- Steadily decreasing in developed countries; <1 in 100,000.
- More prevalent in developing countries; 100–150/100,000 and decreasing more slowly

RISK FACTORS
- Female gender (1)
- Immigrants from countries with a higher prevalence of rheumatic fever (e.g., India), especially for juvenile MS.

Genetics
Congenital MS (usually "parachute MV," with shortened chordae, thick leaflets, and supravalvular ring) is extremely rare and associated with other cardiac defects.

GENERAL PREVENTION
- Early treatment of streptococcal throat or skin infection
- Prophylaxis against recurrence of acute rheumatic fever

PATHOPHYSIOLOGY
- As the orifice size decreases, pressure gradient across the MV increases to maintain adequate flow; Bernoulli principle.
- As the valve narrows progressively, the resting diastolic MV gradient, and hence left atrial (LA) pressure, increases.
- This leads to transudation of fluid into the lung interstitium and decreased pulmonary compliance.
- The elevated LA pressure causes LA dilatation and increases the risk of atrial fibrillation, with a risk of thromboembolism.
- Pulmonary hypertension develops because of retrograde transmission of LA pressure, pulmonary arteriolar constriction, interstitial edema, and obliterative changes in the pulmonary vascular bed.
- As pulmonary hypertension increases, right ventricular (RV) dilation occurs, which leads to tricuspid regurgitation. RV failure leads to elevated jugular venous pressure, liver congestion, ascites, and pedal edema.

ETIOLOGY
- Common antigenic features between streptococcal M protein and cardiac tissue (antigenic mimicry) in rheumatic fever leads to pancarditis (inflammation of all 3 layers of heart), most prominently with MV scarring and fusion of mitral leaflets.
- Other than rheumatic fever:
  - Hypereosinophilic syndrome
  - Endomyocardial fibrosis
  - Carcinoid syndrome (rare)
  - Mucopolysaccharidosis
  - SLE, rheumatoid arthritis (rarely)
  - Methysergide

COMMONLY ASSOCIATED CONDITIONS
- In rheumatic heart disease: Pulmonary hypertension, myocarditis, pericarditis
- Rare association with ASD is called Lutembacher syndrome: More severe LV filling defect

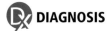 **DIAGNOSIS**

HISTORY
- After rheumatic fever, latent period of 10–20 years (asymptomatic phase)
- Once symptoms develop, severe disability occurs in 5–10 years:
  - Common symptoms include dyspnea, palpitations, fatigability, hemoptysis, recurrent cough, chest pain

PHYSICAL EXAM
- Cardiac:
  - Low-volume pulse, low pulse pressure
  - RV heave, loud S$_2$ with pulmonary hypertension
  - Loud snapping S$_1$ when leaflets are flexible due to high LV closing pressure
  - Opening snap (OS) in diastole heard best at apex.
  - S$_2$-OS interval decreases with increasing MS severity. Both loud S1 and OS disappear when increasing severity renders MV immobile.
  - Low-pitched diastolic rumble at apex, with presystolic accentuation that disappears in A-fib
- Noncardiac:
  - General: Cachexia in severe CHF
  - HEENT: Malar flush
  - Ortner syndrome: Voice change due to recurrent laryngeal nerve palsy because of enlarged LA impinging on the nerve
  - Crepitations at lung bases, cardiac asthma, hydrothorax with severe MS
  - Ascites, mild hepatomegaly
  - Sydenham's chorea with rheumatic fever

DIAGNOSTIC TESTS & INTERPRETATION
Lab
- EKG: LA hypertrophy (P mitrale), RVH
- Inflammatory markers like CRP

Imaging
- CXR: Enlarged left atrium (double balloon sign), cephalization from venous congestion, pleural effusion, etc.
- 2-D and Doppler echocardiography is considered modality of choice for diagnosis and assessment of the severity of MS:
  - 2-D echo demonstrates thickening and calcification of the leaflets, with restricted mobility of the anterior leaflet with diastolic doming and a fixed posterior leaflet.
  - LV size and function are generally normal. LA enlargement, pulmonary hypertension, and RV dysfunction can be seen depending on the severity of disease.
  - Concomitant mitral regurgitation can also be seen.
  - Rheumatic changes with resultant valvular stenosis or regurgitation can also be seen in the other valves.
  - Doppler echo can be used to estimate the mean pressure gradient between the LA and LV and the pressure half-time (time for diastolic gradient to decrease to half its original value). MV area can be estimated as 220/pressure half-time.
  - MS severity by mean gradient (mm Hg): Mild <5, moderate 6–12, severe >12. The gradient is also influenced by heart rate.
  - MS severity by pressure half time (ms): Mild 90–150, moderate 150–219, severe >220.
  - MV area may also be estimated by planimetry on transesophageal echocardiography.
  - MS severity by MVA (cm^2): Mild 1.5–2.5, moderate 1–1.5, severe <1.
  - An echo score index for mitral stenosis can be derived to assess the appropriateness for balloon valvotomy.
  - Leaflet mobility, leaflet thickening, subvalvular thickening, calcification are graded 1–4.
  - To determine the echocardiographic score, add the grades from the 4 categories. The minimum score is 4 and maximum score is 16. Patients with score <8 are more favorable candidates for balloon valvotomy (2).

Initial approach
Management according to severity of symptoms:
- Asymptomatic: Prophylaxis
- NYHA Class I/II: Add diuretics
- >Class II: Consider balloon mitral valvoplasty (BMV) or mitral valve replacement (MVR).

Follow-Up & Special Considerations
Close monitoring and referrals may be needed in following conditions:
- Respiratory tract infections
- Infective endocarditis
- Pregnancy

Pregnancy Considerations
- Increased blood volume in pregnancy can increase symptoms of MS.
- MS may present as AF or pulmonary edema.
- Warfarin should be avoided in the 1st trimester; consider using heparin.

Diagnostic Procedures/Other
Cardiac catheterization may be required for assessment of co-existing CAD or, uncommonly, for further assessment of MS severity.

Pathological Findings
Aschoff bodies in myocardium and endocardium (fibrinoid necrosis with reactive histiocytes and multinucleated giant cells)

DIFFERENTIAL DIAGNOSIS
Usually related to MV diseases with diastolic murmur:
- Functional murmur: Carey Coomb's murmur due to acute rheumatic valvulitis
- Austin-Flint murmur of function MS in severe AR
- Left atrial myxoma
- Tricuspid stenosis
- Ball-valve thrombus
- Cor-triatriatum

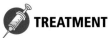 **TREATMENT**

MEDICATION
- In sinus rhythm: Diuretics if signs of pulmonary edema. β blockers to limit tachycardia with exertion. Digoxin for symptomatic relief.
- In atrial fibrillation: Rate control with digoxin, β blockers, or calcium channel blockers if blood pressure is imperative. Attempts to restore sinus rhythm are warranted, as these often improve symptoms.
- Medical management is used for patients with NYHA class I or II symptoms.
- Antibiotic prophylaxis against infective endocarditis

ADDITIONAL TREATMENT
General Measures
- May need antiarrhythmic therapy to maintain sinus rhythm in some settings
- Lifelong oral anticoagulation is indicated for rheumatic MS with a prior embolic event, or atrial fibrillation.
- Anticoagulation can be considered for patients with severe MS and LA dimension >55 mm, or LA enlargement and spontaneous echo contrast.
- Management of anemia if concurrently present

Issues for Referral
- Pregnancy
- Mechanical relief of obstruction: Balloon valvotomy or surgical relief of obstruction

Additional Therapies
Prophylaxis against recurrence of acute rheumatic fever with benzathine penicillin 1.2 MU deep I.M. q3wks
- For rheumatic fever without carditis: Prophylaxis for 5 years until age 20, whichever is greater
- With carditis: For 5 years or until age 30, whichever is greater. Life-long prophylaxis is favored by some.

SURGERY/OTHER PROCEDURES
- Balloon valvuloplasty is procedure of 1st choice if feasible:
  - Indications: Significant symptoms or complications of MS, MV orifice area <1 cm^2
  - Contraindications: Significant mitral regurgitation, LA thrombus
  - Worsened mitral regurgitation is the most common complication of balloon valvuloplasty.
- Open commissurotomy
- Mitral valve replacement (MVR) (3):
  - Indications: Significant MR, heavily calcified valve

IN-PATIENT CONSIDERATIONS
Initial Stabilization
- Management of pulmonary edema
- Management of A-fib with rapid ventricular rate

Admission Criteria
- Pulmonary edema/NYHA Class IV or worsening CHF
- A-fib with RVR

IV Fluids
None or restricted

Nursing
Propped-up positioning

Discharge Criteria
Resolution of acute problems

 ONGOING CARE

FOLLOW-UP RECOMMENDATIONS
- Every year after mitral valvuloplasty
- Closer follow-up required in pregnancy

Patient Monitoring
- Heart rate
- Anemia
- Potassium

DIET
Salt-restricted

PATIENT EDUCATION
Counseling of contraception, infectious endocarditis prophylaxis

PROGNOSIS
- The 10-year survival rate for asymptomatic persons is ~80%.
- The 10-year survival rate for patients with mild symptoms is ~60%.
- The 10-year survival rate among patients who develop congestive heart failure is 15%.

COMPLICATIONS
- Flash pulmonary edema
- Pulmonary hypertension
- Hemoptysis
- Dysphagia or hoarseness due to LA enlargement
- Recurrent bronchopulmonary infections
- Infective endocarditis
- Systemic emboli due to A-fib: Cerebral (most common), peripheral, visceral

REFERENCES
1. Movahed M. Increased prevalence of MS in women. *J Am Soc Echocardiography*. 2006;19(7): 911–3.
2. Feigenbaum H, et al. *Feigenbaum's Echocardiography*, 6th edition. Philadelphia: Lippincott Williams & Wilkins, 2005:312–24.
3. Kim JB. Comparison of long term outcome after mitral valve replacement and balloon mitral valvotomy. *Am J Cardiol*. 2007;99(11):1571–4.

ADDITIONAL READING
- Bonow RO, et al. Valvular heart. In: *Braunwald's Heart Disease: A Textbook of Cardiovascular Medicine*, 7th ed. Philadelphia: WB Saunders; 2005:1553–1602.
- Carabello BA. Modern management of mitral stenosis. *Circulation*. 2005;112(3):432–7.
- 2008 Focused update incorporated into the ACC/AHA 2006 Guidelines for the management of patients with Valvular Heart Disease. *J Am Coll Cardiol*. 2008;52:1–142.
- Valvular heart disease. *J Am Coll Cardiol*. 2009;53: A403–A418.

 CODES

ICD9
- 394.0 Mitral stenosis
- 424.0 Mitral valve disorders
- 746.5 Congenital mitral stenosis

CLINICAL PEARLS
- The longer the mid-diastolic murmur, the more severe the stenosis (most specific on physical exam).
- Atrial fibrillation causes disappearance of presystolic accentuation.
- Opening snap indicates that the valve cusps are pliable.
- Decreasing S_2-to-opening snap interval indicates more severe stenosis.
- Heart rate control is crucial in the management of MS.

M

MYASTHENIA GRAVIS

Daniela Levi

 BASICS

DESCRIPTION
- MG is an autoimmune disease characterized by antibody reaction to antigen epitopes of the acetylcholine receptor.
- Myasthenic crises are diagnosed when a patient with myasthenia develops respiratory muscle weakness and impending respiratory failure.
- It is the most common primary disorder of the neuromuscular junction.
- Myasthenia is a pure motor syndrome characterized by fluctuating skeletal muscle weakness.
- Common affected muscle groups are:
  - Extraocular
  - Pharyngeal
  - Facial
  - Respiratory musculature
- 2 clinical forms: Ocular and generalized:
  - Ocular MG (15%): Weakness limited to eyelids and extraocular muscles
  - Generalized MG (85%): Commonly affects ocular as well as a variable combination of bulbar, proximal limb, and respiratory muscles
- 50% of patients present with ptosis or diplopia:
  - 50% of patients who 1st present with ocular symptoms develop generalized MG within 2 years.
- Onset is typically mild and intermittent over many years:
  - May be sudden and severe
  - Usually triggered by an infection

EPIDEMIOLOGY
- This condition preferentially affects:
  - 20–40 years (female predominance)
  - 60–80 years (male predominance)
- Can occur at any age

Incidence
10–20 per million per year

Prevalence
10–20 per 100,000 in the U.S.

RISK FACTORS
- Familial MG
- Other autoimmune diseases
  - SLE, Sjögren syndrome, polymyositis
  - Autoimmune thyroid disease

Genetics
- Familial predisposition is seen in 5% of cases.
- Congenital MG syndrome describes a collection of rare hereditary disorders:
  - Is not immune-mediated
  - Results from the mutation of a component of the neuromuscular junction
  - Onset is usually at birth or in early childhood
  - Autosomal recessive

- Transient neonatal MG:
  - 10–20% of infants born to myasthenic mothers
  - Caused by transplacental passage of acetylcholine receptor antibodies
  - Resolves in weeks to months, and these infants do not have an increased risk for the long-term or future development of MG

GENERAL PREVENTION
- In most patients, the diagnosis of MG has been established when admitted with respiratory failure.
- Respiratory failure is usually triggered by an intercurrent infection.
- A large number of drugs have been reported to exacerbate myasthenia:
  - Aminoglycosides, macrolides, lidocaine, propranolol, quinidine, magnesium sulfate

PATHOPHYSIOLOGY
- This is a true autoimmune disease.
- Antibodies directed at myoid cells in the thymus (which express acetylcholine receptors) and attack the neuromuscular junction:
  - T cell-dependent antibodies mediate the attack on acetylcholine receptors (AChR)/receptor-associated proteins at the postsynaptic membrane of the neuromuscular junction.
- MuSK (muscle specific tyrosine kinase) antibodies:
  - Tyrosin related
  - In AChR-negative patients
  - Associated with more recurrences
- There is overrepresentation of human leukocyte antigen-1 (HLA-A1), HLA-B8, and HLA-DRw3:
  - HLA testing is not clinically useful.

ETIOLOGY
- Anti-AChR antibodies are present in most patients with generalized myasthenia.
- Ocular myasthenia is associated with Anti-AChR antibodies in ~60% of cases.

COMMONLY ASSOCIATED CONDITIONS
- Thymic hyperplasia (60–70% of MG patients)
- Thymoma (10–15% of MG patients)
- Autoimmune thyroid disease (3–8% of MG patients)
- Other autoimmune diseases (SLE, polymyositis, Sjögren)
- Cholinergic crisis (myosis, marked salivation, plugging, bronchospasm, fasciculation, cramps and diarrhea)

 DIAGNOSIS

HISTORY
- Gradual onset of diplopia, ptosis, difficulty with speech and secretions, proximal limb weakness, and ventilatory dysfunction
- Severity of weakness fluctuates during the day:
  - Least severe in the morning and worse as the day progresses
  - Increased fatigability with exercise
  - Improvement with rest
- Symptoms are transient, with asymptomatic periods lasting days or weeks.
- With progression of MG, asymptomatic periods shorten, and then are lost entirely (constant symptoms fluctuating from mild to severe).

PHYSICAL EXAM
- Common signs and symptoms are:
  - Ptosis:
    - Vertical gaze with "curtain phenomenon" (worsening ptosis)
  - Fluctuating diplopia
  - Marked weakness of oropharyngeal function:
    - Dysphagia
    - Dysarthria
  - Masseter muscle weakness:
    - Fatigable chewing
  - Nasopharyngeal weakness
    - Dysphonia
  - Neck weakness
  - Proximal limb weakness (arm >leg)
  - Respiratory weakness, impending failure:
    - Dyspnea and tachypnea with minimal effort
    - Use of sternocleidomastoid or scalene muscles by palpation
    - Staccato-like speech
    - Asynchronous, paradoxical breathing
  - Nonspecific signs: Tachycardia, restlessness, forehead sweating
- Tensilon (edrophonium) test:
  - Initial dose 2 mg IV can be followed by another 2 mg q60sec up to a maximum dose of 10 mg.
  - Improvement in ptosis is the only bedside objective parameter to follow.
  - A positive test shows improvement of strength within 30 seconds of administration.
  - Sensitivity 80–90%
  - Cardiac disease and bronchial asthma are relative contraindications.
  - Can trigger a cholinergic crisis.
  - Atropine 0.4–0.6 mg IV may be required as antidote.
- Ice pack test:
  - Can be used in patients with ptosis and contraindications to the Tensilon test
  - Ice pack applied to closed eyelid for 60 seconds; ice will decrease the ptosis
  - Sensitivity 80% in patients with prominent ptosis

DIAGNOSTIC TESTS & INTERPRETATION
- Edrophonium test (as described above)
- Measurement of anti-AChR antibodies
- Electromyography with repetitive stimulation
- Chest CT
- Vital capacity and negative inspiratory pressure

Lab
Initial lab tests
- Can include CBC, electrolytes, ABG, thyroid function tests, cultures, CXR and EKG
- AChR antibody:
  – 80–85% of all MG patients are seropositive:
  – Generalized myasthenia: 75–85%
  – Ocular myasthenia: Up to 60%
  – MG and thymoma: 98–100%
  – Poor correlation between antibody titer and disease severity
- MuSK antibody:
  – Used if MG suspected, patient seronegative
  – Present in 40–50% of seronegative patients with generalized MG
  – Absent in ocular MG

Follow-Up & Special Considerations
In a patient with known positive antibodies, the level correlates with disease activity.

Imaging
CT or MRI of anterior mediastinum to evaluate the thymus

Diagnostic Procedures/Other
- Electromyography:
  – Repetitive nerve stimulation (RNS):
    ○ Moderately sensitive for both generalized MG (75%) and ocular MG (50%).
    ○ Positive test shows a decremental response (>10%) at 3Hz.
  – Single-fiber EMG (SFEMG):
    ○ Assesses temporal variability between 2 muscle fibers within same motor unit.
    ○ Highly sensitive (90–95%), but less specific.
- Respiratory function tests:
  – Vital capacity FVC:
    ○ Critical value 15–20 mL/Kg (<12 mL/Kg need mechanical ventilation)
  – Negative inspiratory pressure (NIF) also called peak inspiratory pressure:
    ○ Critical values are −30 to −40 cm H_2O
  – Peak expiratory pressure:
    ○ Critical value 40 cm H_2O

Pathological Findings
- Muscle electron microscopy: Can show receptor infolding and synaptic cleft widening
- Immunofluorescence shows IgG antibodies on receptor membranes.

DIFFERENTIAL DIAGNOSIS
Other neuromuscular disorders that present as pure motor syndromes need to be ruled out.

 # TREATMENT

MEDICATION
First Line
Anticholinesterases:
- Neostigmine: Starting dose is 0.5 mg SC or IM q3h titrated to effect
- Pyridostigmine: Starting dose is 30 mg PO t.i.d.
  – Titrate dose to desired clinical effect and minimal side effect to a maximum dose of 120 mg q3–4h

Second Line
Immunosuppressives:
- Steroids are useful but may initially worsen weakness.
- Azathioprine, cyclophosphamide, cyclosporine

ADDITIONAL TREATMENT
- IVIG (IV γ-globulin): Total dose is 2 g/kg, usually over 2–5 days
- Plasma exchange: A typical course of treatment consists of 5 exchanges (3–5 L of plasma each) over 7–14 days:
  – Retrospective comparison of plasma exchange and IVIG:
    ○ Plasma exchange is associated with better ventilatory status at 2 weeks and functional outcome at 1 month.
    ○ Complication rate is lower with IVIG.
  – IVIG trial can follow plasmapheresis.
  – The effect of both treatments is seen typically in less than a week, and the benefit can last for 3–6 weeks.
- Ventilatory support:
  – Noninvasive ventilation in the form of BiPAP:
    ○ Before hypercapnia occurs
  – Mechanical ventilation:
    ○ May stop pyridostigmine briefly (restore receptor sensitivity to acetylcholine)

General Measures
- ICU during myasthenic or cholinergic crises:
  – May allow hypercapnia in the intensive care settings if the patient is alert and able to protect the airway.
- Inpatient for initiation of corticosteroids
- Outpatient follow-up every 3 months with stable patients

Issues for Referral
Referral is institution-specific and can include: Neurology, pulmonary, blood bank, CT surgery, ICU

SURGERY/OTHER PROCEDURES
Thymectomy is useful in patient <60 but should await recovery from myasthenic crisis:
- Perform multiple plasma exchanges prior to surgery.

IN-PATIENT CONSIDERATIONS
Admission Criteria
- Myasthenic or cholinergic crisis
- Management of pulmonary complications

 # ONGOING CARE

FOLLOW-UP RECOMMENDATIONS
Patient Monitoring
Typically, outpatient care involves monitoring of symptoms and respiratory function tests.

PROGNOSIS
Good overall; however, myasthenic crisis is associated with 4% mortality.

COMPLICATIONS
- Acute and chronic respiratory insufficiency due to atelectasis, aspiration, pneumonia
- Cholinergic crisis

ADDITIONAL READING
- McConville J, et al. Detection and characterization of MuSK antibodies in seronegative MG. *Ann Neurol.* 2004;55:580.
- Saperstein DS, et al. Management of MG. *Semin Neurol.* 2004;24:41.
- Seneviratne J. Noninvasive ventilation in myasthenic crisis. *Arch Neurol.* 2008;65:54.

 # CODES

ICD9
- 358.00 Myasthenia gravis without (acute) exacerbation
- 358.01 Myasthenia gravis with (acute) exacerbation
- 775.2 Neonatal myasthenia gravis

CLINICAL PEARLS
- Your patient is having a myasthenic crisis and not a cholinergic crisis.
- Can use BiPAP; however, a $PaCO_2$ of $\geq$50 torr at onset predicts BiPAP failure.
- Corticosteroids, aminoglycosides, macrolides, may precipitate ventilatory failure.

M

MYOCARDIAL INFARCTION, MECHANICAL COMPLICATIONS

Sajjad A. Sabir
Isaac Halickman

BASICS

DESCRIPTION
- In an era of early reperfusion therapy, mechanical complications of myocardial infarction (MI) have decreased, but remain a significant cause of mortality in patients with MI (1).
- Acute mechanical complications of MI include:
  - Left ventricular free wall rupture (LVFWR)
  - Ventricular septal rupture (VSR)
  - Mitral regurgitation (MR)
  - Right ventricular infarction (RVI)
  - Left ventricular (LV) failure with cardiogenic shock (discussed elsewhere)

LEFT VENTRICULAR FREE WALL RUPTURE
- 3.2–6.2% of all MI patients (2):
  - Marked reduction from 6.2% in pre-interventional era to 3.2% in early reperfusion era
  - Seen in 50% of patients within 5 days and in 90% of patients within 2 weeks of MI (6–9)
- Risk factors include (3–5):
  - First MI
  - Acute transmural MI
  - Age (>70)
  - Gender (Female > Male)
  - Single-vessel disease
  - Absence of LV hypertrophy
  - Anterior location
- 3 pathologic subsets of LVFWRs (10):
  - Type 1: Abrupt slit-like tear commonly associated with anterior infarcts and occurs within 24 hours; increased with thrombolytic use
  - Type II: Erosion of infarcted myocardium between normal and infarcted myocardium; occurs 1–3 days post-MI
  - Type III: Early aneurysm formation:
    ○ Occurs late
    ○ Decreased incidence with use of thrombolytics
- Acute rupture may present with:
  - Severe chest pain
  - Abrupt electromechanical dissociation or asystole
  - Hemodynamic collapse from hemopericardium
  - Death
- Subacute presentation may include:
  - Syncope
  - Persistent or recurrent chest pain
  - Shock
  - Arrhythmia
  - Agitation
  - Nausea and vomiting
- Physical exam findings may include:
  - Jugular venous distension
  - Pulsus paradoxus
  - Cardiogenic shock
  - Electromechanical dissociation
  - Arrhythmias

VENTRICULAR SEPTAL RUPTURE
- 0.2% of MI patients in the reperfusion era (11)

- Risk factors include (11):
  - Single-vessel disease, commonly left anterior descending artery (LAD)
  - Older age
  - Female gender
  - Hypertension
  - Absence of smoking history
  - Tachycardia
  - Killip class 3–4 CHF
- Rupture occurs at the border of necrotic and nonnecrotic myocardium.
- A simple VSR is characterized by a through-and-through communication across the septum.
- A complex rupture is characterized by a serpiginous rupture.
- Patients may present with:
  - Chest pain
  - Dyspnea
  - Biventricular failure
  - Hypotension
  - Shock
  - A new murmur
- Physical exam may demonstrate:
  - A harsh holosystolic murmur, often loudest at the lower left sternal border and associated parasternal systolic thrill
  - RV and LV S_3
  - Pulmonary edema
  - Cardiogenic shock

MITRAL REGURGITATION
- Incidence varies from 13–39% (12–13).
- Risk factors include:
  - Advanced age
  - Female sex
  - Large infarct
  - Previous MI
  - Recurrent ischemia
  - Multivessel disease
  - Congestive heart failure
- Causes of MR include:
  - Papillary muscle rupture
    ○ Life-threatening complication
    ○ Posteromedial papillary muscle rupture (supplied by posterior descending artery) much more common than anterolateral (dual supply by LAD and left circumflex arteries)
  - Incomplete closure of the valve
  - Dilated annulus from severe LV dysfunction
  - Chordae tendineae rupture
  - Worsening of chronic MR
- Presenting symptoms may include:
  - Sudden onset of dyspnea
  - Pulmonary edema or
  - Hypotension
- Physical exam may demonstrate:
  - A new pansystolic murmur loudest at apex with radiation to axilla in the case of posteromedial papillary muscle rupture
  - The murmur may be soft or absent in the setting of poor cardiac output

RIGHT VENTRICULAR INFARCTION
- Mild RV dysfunction is seen in ~35% of inferior MIs and clinically significant RV involvement is apparent in about 10% of inferoposterior MIs (14).
- Major risk factor is an inferoposterior MI.
- Severity of RV dysfunction depends on the location of the right coronary artery (RCA) occlusion, amount of collaterals from the LAD, and the degree of blood flow through the thebesian veins.
- Proximal RCA occlusions result in severe dysfunction.
- Patients may present with:
  - Hypotension
  - Elevated neck veins with clear lungs
  - Lack of dyspnea
  - Shock from severe RV failure
- Physical exam findings may include:
  - Jugular-venous distension with normal lung exam
  - RV S_3 gallop
  - Kussmaul's sign
  - Depending on degree of RV failure, tricuspid regurgitation may be present from RV dilation

GENERAL PREVENTION
- Risk factor modification and primary prevention against cardiovascular disease
- Early reperfusion therapy

COMMONLY ASSOCIATED CONDITIONS
- ST elevation myocardial or transmural infarction
- Hypertension
- Cardiac tamponade
- Electromechanical dissociation
- Cardiogenic shock

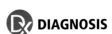

DIAGNOSIS

DIAGNOSTIC TESTS & INTERPRETATION
Lab
- Do not play an important role in initial diagnosis
- CBC, cardiac biomarkers, serum electrolytes, hsCRP, thyroid function tests
- Monitor hemoglobin and hematocrit
- Type and cross-match

Imaging
- Echocardiography is the diagnostic modality of choice (1)[C].
- If transthoracic echocardiogram (TTE) provides limited windows, consider transesophageal echocardiogram (TEE).
- TEE may determine the mechanism of MR (1)[C].
- ECG demonstrates inferior ST elevation with ST elevation in V4R lead in RVI (1)[B].

Diagnostic Procedures/Other
- LVFWR:
  - End-stage rupture may show bradycardia and EMD
  - If an uncertainty remains after an echocardiogram, perform emergent pericardiocentesis.
  - Hemodynamic signs of tamponade (equalization of diastolic pressures in all chambers) from a Swan-Ganz catheter

- VSR:
  - Pulmonary artery catheter to document left-to-right shunt ("step-up" in oxygen saturation from right atrium to right ventricle)
- MR/RVI:
  - Chest x-ray
  - Cardiac catheterization

DIFFERENTIAL DIAGNOSIS
- Cardiac tamponade
- Cardiogenic shock
- Septic shock
- Tension pneumothorax
- Pulmonary embolism
- Hypertrophic obstructive cardiomyopathy
- Nonischemic valvular heart disease
- Other mechanical complications of MI

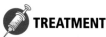 TREATMENT

- IV fluids in patients without evidence of volume overload (1)[C]
- Vasopressor support for hypotension that does not respond to volume loading (1)[C]
- Inotropic support (1)[B]
- IABC for hemodynamic stabilization (1)[B]
- Pulmonary artery catheter monitoring may be useful (1)[C]
- Oxygen supplementation to arterial saturation >90% for patients with pulmonary congestion (1)[C]
- Morphine sulfate for patients with pulmonary congestion (1)[C]
- Immediate revascularization with PCI or CABG for STEMI (1)[A]
- Immediate surgical correction of LVFWR (1)[B] and simultaneous CABG (1)[C]
- Immediate surgical correction of VSR (1)[B] and simultaneous CABG (1)[B]
- Patients with acute papillary muscle rupture should be considered for urgent cardiac surgical repair (1)[B].
- CABG surgery should be undertaken at the same time as mitral valve surgery (1)[B].
- In patients with RV infarction:
  - AV synchrony should be achieved and bradycardia should be corrected (1)[C].
  - RV preload should be optimized (1)[C].

ADDITIONAL TREATMENT
General Measures
- Standard supportive measures as indicated by the hemodynamic scenario
- ICU-level care if patient not already in ICU or CCU
- ACLS measures as indicated by clinical scenario

Issues for Referral
- All patients with MI should be evaluated by a cardiologist.
- Cardiothoracic surgery evaluation

IN-PATIENT CONSIDERATIONS
Initial Stabilization
- Hospitalization in a critical care facility
- Close telemetry and hemodynamic monitoring (1)[C]
- IV access for inotropic and vasopressor support
- ACLS measures as indicated by clinical scenario

 ONGOING CARE

FOLLOW-UP RECOMMENDATIONS
- Outpatient cardiology and cardiothoracic surgery referral
- Serial echocardiograms

PROGNOSIS
- Varies based on the type of complication
- Almost all are fatal without treatment

COMPLICATIONS
- Atrial and ventricular arrhythmias
- Heart failure
- Left ventricular thrombus
- Death

REFERENCES

1. Gueret P, et al. Echocardiographic assessment of the incidence of mechanical complications during the early phase of myocardial infarction in the reperfusion era: A French multicenter prospective registry. *Arch Cardiovasc Dis*. 2008;101(1):41–7.
2. Figueras J, et al. Changes in hospital mortality rates in 425 patients with acute ST-elevation myocardial infarction and cardiac rupture over a 30-year period. *Circulation*. 2008;118(25):2783–9.
3. Purcaro A, et al. Diagnostic criteria and management of subacute ventricular free wall rupture complicating acute myocardial infarction. *Am J Cardiol*. 1997; 80:397.
4. Batts KP, et al. Postinfarction rupture of the left ventricular free wall: Clinicopathologic correlates in 100 consecutive autopsy cases. *Hum Pathol*. 1990;21:530.
5. Oliva PB, et al. Cardiac rupture: A clinically predictable complication of acute myocardial infarction; report of 70 cases with clinicopathologic correlations. *J Am Coll Cardiol*. 1993;22:720.
6. Lopez-Sendon, et al. Diagnosis of subacute ventricular wall rupture after acute myocardial infarction: Sensitivity and specificity of clinical, hemodynamic, and echocardiographic criteria. *J Am Coll Cardiol*. 1992;19:1145.
7. Pohjola-Sintonen S, et al. Ventricular septal and free wall rupture complicating acute myocardial infarction: Experience in the Multicenter Investigation of Limitation of Infarct Size. *Am Heart J*. 1989;117:809.
8. Becker RC, et al., for the TIMI 9 Investigators. Fatal cardiac rupture among patients treated with thrombolytic agents and adjunctive thrombin antagonists. Observations from the Thrombolysis and Thrombin Inhibition in Myocardial Infarction 9 study. *J Am Coll Cardiol*. 1999;33:479.
9. Moreno R, et al. Primary angioplasty reduces the risk of left ventricular free wall rupture compared with thrombolysis in patients with acute myocardial infarction. *J Am Coll Cardiol*. 2002;39:598.
10. Becker AE, et al. Cardiac tamponade: A study of 50 hearts. *Eur J Cardiol*. 1975;3(4):349–58.
11. Crenshaw B, et al. Risk factors, angiographic patterns, and outcomes in patients with ventricular septal defect complicating acute myocardial infarction: GUSTO-I (Global Utilization of Streptokinase and TPA for Occluded Coronary Arteries) Trial Investigators. *Circulation*. 100. 27–32.2000; Abstract.
12. Lavie CJ, et al. Mechanical and electrical complications of acute myocardial infarction. *Mayo Clin Proc*. 1990;65:709.
13. Picard MH, et al. Echocardiographic predictors of survival and response to early revascularization in cardiogenic shock. *Circulation*. 2003;107:279.
14. Kinch J, et al. Right ventricular infarction. *N Engl J Med*. 1994;17:1211–7.

ADDITIONAL READING

- Antman EM, et al. ACC/AHA Guidelines for the management of patients with ST-elevation myocardial infarction. *Circulation*. 2004;110(5):588–636.

 CODES

ICD9
- 410.90 Acute myocardial infarction of unspecified site, episode of care unspecified
- 429.71 Certain sequelae of myocardial infarction, not elsewhere classified, acquired cardiac septal defect
- 429.79 Certain sequelae of myocardial infarction, not elsewhere classified, other

CLINICAL PEARLS
- A new cardiac murmur in patients with MI should always prompt further cardiac workup.
- IABC is contraindicated in aortic insufficiency.
- Intensity of the MR murmur does not always correlate with the severity of MR.
- In RV failure, increased RA pressure may lead to opening of PFO, causing right-to-left shunt, resulting in hypoxemia.

M

NECROSIS, RENAL CORTICAL

Brian Sherman
Roopa Kohli-Seth

BASICS

DESCRIPTION
- RCN is an extreme form of acute tubular necrosis and a rare cause of acute renal failure.
- Cortical necrosis is death of the tissue in the outer part of kidney (cortex). This is the result of severe ischemia of the small arteries that supply blood to the cortex. This causes acute kidney failure, typically bilateral, with cortical necrosis and is usually irreversible.
- Secondary to vascular spasm, microvascular injury, or intravascular coagulation
- RCN is usually extensive and bilateral, although focal and localized forms may occur.
- In most cases, the medulla, juxtamedullary cortex, and a thin rim of subcapsular cortex are spared.
- Usually, a number of etiologies that can cause severe hypotension can lead to this in the ICU.

EPIDEMIOLOGY
Incidence
- Incidence of RCN was found to be 0.2% in a study of 11,800 autopsies.
- In adults, sepsis causes 1/3 of all cases of renal cortical necrosis.
- Renal cortical necrosis can occur at any age. ~10% of the cases occur in children
- 20% of acute renal failure during the 3rd trimester of pregnancy is due to RCN.
  - RCN was observed by postmortem exam in 0.5% of infants aged ≤3 months at death.

Prevalence
- Frequency of RCN in all patients with acute renal failure is 1.9–2%.
- In adults, sepsis causes 1/3 of all cases of renal cortical necrosis. Other causes in adults include rejection of a transplanted kidney, burns, inflammation of the pancreas, injury, snakebite, use of certain drugs, and poisoning from certain chemicals.

RISK FACTORS
- Congenital heart disease
- Fetal–maternal transfusion
- Dehydration
- Perinatal asphyxia
- Anemia
- Placental hemorrhage
- Sepsis
- HUS
- Acute gastroenteritis with dehydration
- Placental abruption
- Infected abortion
- Prolonged intrauterine fetal death
- Severe eclampsia
- Shock
- Trauma
- Snakebite
- Hyperacute kidney transplant rejection
- Poisons
- Drugs (e.g., NSAIDs, calcineurin inhibitors)
- Contrast media

GENERAL PREVENTION
- Appropriate hydration, especially prior to and after contrast media
- Rapid resuscitation in case of sepsis or severe hypotension

PATHOPHYSIOLOGY
- Pathogenesis remains unclear; typically, the initiating factor is intense vasospasm of the small vessels. If this vasospasm is brief and vascular flow is reestablished, acute tubular necrosis results. Prolonged vasospasm can cause necrosis and thrombosis of the distal arterioles and glomeruli, and renal cortical necrosis ensues.
- RCN in placental abruption may be due to a combination of a hypercoagulable state, endothelial injury, and DIC.

ETIOLOGY
- Obstetric complications are the most common (50–70%) causes of RCN, and nonobstetric causes account for 20–30% of all cases of cortical necrosis.
- Septic abortions are a common cause, along with placental abruptions.
- Sepsis and septic shock
- Medications
- Venomous snake bites
- Hyperacute rejection of renal transplant graft

COMMONLY ASSOCIATED CONDITIONS
- Sepsis
- Endotoxemia
- Children with severe volume depletion

DIAGNOSIS

HISTORY
- Renal failure:
  - Oliguria
  - Hematuria
- Pregnancy:
  - Bleeding
  - Abortion
  - Symptoms of eclampsia
- Neonatal conditions:
  - Perinatal asphyxia
  - Bleeding
  - Cyanotic heart disease
- Childhood conditions:
  - Diarrhea
  - Vomiting
  - HUS
- Other:
  - Severe trauma
  - Snakebite
- Flank pain

PHYSICAL EXAM
- Blood pressure, including mildly high pressure or even low pressure
- Tachycardia
- Flank pain
- Abdominal tenderness
- Dark urine
- Kidney
- Pregnancy:
  - Lower abdominal tenderness
  - Contracted uterus
  - Vaginal bleeding
  - Abortion
  - Eclampsia

DIAGNOSTIC TESTS & INTERPRETATION
Lab
- Serum electrolyte measurements and urine electrolytes, creatinine, and microscopy:
  - Hypocalcemia
  - Hyperkalemia
  - Metabolic acidosis
  - Elevated creatinine
- CBC:
  - Thrombocytopenia.
- Coagulation studies
  - Fibrinogen levels
  - Increased fibrin-degradation products
- Urinalysis:
  - Hematuria
  - Proteinuria
  - RBC casts
  - Granular casts
- Bilirubin levels, LDH:
  - Signs of hemolytic anemia

Imaging
- X-ray: Thin cortical shells or tram lines caused by calcification are radiologic hallmark:
  - Develop 4–5 weeks later
- US:
  - Initially shows enlarged kidneys and reduced blood flow; may show hyper echoic structures in the cortex.
  - Cortical tissue becomes shrunken later in disease progression.
- CTA:
  - Confirmation radiological test, highest sensitivity
  - Absent opacification of the renal cortex
  - Enhancement of subcapsular and juxtamedullary areas and of the medulla without extravasation of contrast
- MRI:
  - Thin rim of low signal intensity along border of kidneys
  - Cortical patchy areas of low signal intensity

Diagnostic Procedures/Other
- Kidney biopsy:
  - Most accurate but severely invasive

Pathological Findings
- RCN is classified into 5 pathologic forms, depending on severity:
  - Focal pathologic form: Focally necrotic glomeruli without thrombosis and patchy necrosis of tubules
  - Minor pathologic form: Larger foci of necrosis with vascular and glomerular thrombi
  - Patchy pathologic form: Patches of necrosis occupying 2/3 of the cortex
  - Gross pathologic form: Almost the entire cortex is involved
  - Confluent pathologic form: Widespread glomerular and tubular necrosis with no arterial involvement

DIFFERENTIAL DIAGNOSIS
- Acute kidney injury (other):
  - Acute tubular necrosis
- Renal artery thromboembolism
- Renal infarction
- Renal vein thrombosis

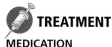

TREATMENT

MEDICATION
- Hydration with sodium chloride (1)[A]
- Renal replacement therapy (1)[A]:
  - Continuous vs. intermittent RRT (1)[C]
- Correction of electrolyte disturbances
- Stop offending drug; in the case of calcineurin inhibitors consider RH, erythropoietin (2)[C]

ADDITIONAL TREATMENT
General Measures
- Initiate dialysis early (3)[C].
- Treat the underlying cause.
- Restore hemodynamic stability.

Issues for Referral
- Nephrologist for hemodialysis or intensivist run CVVH:
  - Renal replacement therapy improves mortality and morbidity.
- Underlying condition may require ICU care.

SURGERY/OTHER PROCEDURES
May need access for dialysis

IN-PATIENT CONSIDERATIONS
Initial Stabilization
- Improve hemodynamics.
- Institute early goal-directed therapy if sepsis:
  - Fluids
  - Antibiotics
  - Correction of electrolytes
- Dialysis if immediate need secondary to electrolyte derangements
- Blood transfusions for severe anemia

Admission Criteria
Depends on the severity of the underlying condition

IV Fluids
Restoration of hemodynamic stability:
- Crystalloids
- Blood products
- Colloids

Nursing
Strict ins and outs

Discharge Criteria
Resolution of initial illness:
- A large percentage of patients will remain with kidney damage, some requiring dialysis; therefore, inability to correct kidney function should not preclude discharge.

ONGOING CARE

FOLLOW-UP RECOMMENDATIONS
- Patients remaining on dialysis will need care from nephrologist and consult with vascular surgery for evaluation for graft or AV fistula.
- Continue treating residual problems and follow-ups as necessary from primary condition.

Patient Monitoring
- Continued vigilance for worsening renal failure
- If on hemodialysis, treat as ESRD patient.

DIET
- Low-potassium
- Low-phosphorus

PROGNOSIS
- In untreated patients, the mortality rate exceeds 50%.
- 80% of patients live ≥1 year if treated:
  - Most people need permanent dialysis or kidney transplantation.

Pediatric Considerations
- 10% of the cases occur in infants and children.
- RCN in childhood is usually secondary to HUS or severe volume depletion.
- Newborns with deliveries complicated by premature detachment of the placenta

Pregnancy Considerations
- Occurrence peaks in women of childbearing age because of obstetric causes.
- 1/2 of cases in women follow complications of pregnancy, such as premature detachment or abnormal position of the placenta, bleeding from the uterus, infections immediately after childbirth, blockage of arteries by amniotic fluid, death of the fetus within the uterus, and preeclampsia.

COMPLICATIONS
- Acute renal failure is typical, with associated complications:
  - Electrolyte disturbances
- Chronic renal failure, occurring in 30–50% of patients, requires dialysis and transplantation.

REFERENCES
1. Kellum J, et al. BMJ Clinical Evidence, Acute renal failure Search date April 2007,
2. Pallet N, et al. Antiapoptotic properties of recombinant human erythropoietin protects against tubular cyclosporine toxicity. *Pharmacol Res.* 2010;61:71–75.
3. Schiffl H. Renal recovery from acute tubular necrosis requiring renal replacement therapy: A prospective study in critically ill patients. *Nephrol Dial Transplant.* 2006,21(5):1248–52.

ADDITIONAL READING
- Kamioka I, et al. Prognosis and pathological characteristics of five children with non-Shiga toxin-mediated hemolytic uremic syndrome. *Pediatr Int.* 2007;49(2):196–201.
- Mertens PRD, et al. Contrast-enhanced computed tomography for demonstration of bilateral renal cortical necrosis. *Clin Investig.* 1994;72(7): 499–501.
- Murry PT, et al., eds. *Intensive Care In Nephrology.* New York: Taylor/Informa Healthcare, 2006.

CODES

ICD9
- 583.6 Nephritis and nephropathy, not specified as acute or chronic, with lesion of renal cortical necrosis
- 584.5 Acute kidney failure with lesion of tubular necrosis

CLINICAL PEARLS
- DIC and endotoxemia become predictors of high risk.
- Consider the diagnosis in a pregnant woman with sudden onset of abdominal pain, a tender uterus, vaginal bleeding; high suspicion following illicit abortion.
- Consider the diagnosis in a newborn or young child with dehydration, oliguria, and hematuria.

N

NECROTIZING FASCIITIS

Raghu Seethala

BASICS

DESCRIPTION
- Necrotizing fasciitis is a virulent bacterial infection that results in progressive destruction of the subcutaneous tissue. Infection commonly progresses rapidly and extends beyond the superficial signs of infection.
- Recently the term necrotizing soft tissue infection (NSTI) has been proposed to include all forms of this disease, regardless of the anatomic depth of infection.

EPIDEMIOLOGY
Incidence
~1000 cases of NSTIs per year in the US (1)

RISK FACTORS
- Immunocompromised
- Diabetes
- Obesity
- Chronic renal failure
- HIV
- Alcohol abuse
- IV drug use
- Trauma
- Ruptured bowel

GENERAL PREVENTION
No definite recommendations regarding the use of chemoprophylaxis or prevention of necrotizing fasciitis

PATHOPHYSIOLOGY
Necrotizing fasciitis develops as bacteria gain entry to subcutaneous tissue through external trauma, perforated bowel, or the urogenital area. Bacterial pathogens then proliferate within subcutaneous tissue along superficial and deep fascial planes releasing bacterial toxins, which cause thrombosis of perforating vessels to the skin, leading to tissue ischemia, liquefactive necrosis, and systemic illness.

ETIOLOGY
- NSTI is classified into three categories based on the bacterial causative agent(s).
- Type I is the most common. It is a polymicrobial infection due to a mix of gram-positive cocci, gram-negative rods, and anaerobes. The following are common microbial causes: *Staphylococcus aureus, Bacteroides, Clostridium perfringens, Klebsiella, Escherichia coli, Acinetobacter, Pseudomonas.*
- Type II, which is less common, is typically monomicrobial caused by Group A *Streptococcus* with or without MRSA. Type II is unique because it could be associated with toxic shock syndrome.
- Type III is not universally agreed on as a separate classification. It is a monomicrobial infection by one of these organisms: *Vibrio vulnificus, Aeromonas, Clostridium perfringens.*

COMMONLY ASSOCIATED CONDITIONS
Cellulitis

DIAGNOSIS

HISTORY
- Presentation varies widely and initially can be subtle. Patients often complain of pain, anxiety, diaphoresis, malaise, anorexia, and pain out of proportion to physical exam.
- There may be an antecedent history of trauma, surgery, or IV drug use.
- Cellulitis that is rapidly progressing, not responding to antibiotics, or associated with systemic signs of sepsis should also raise index of suspicion.

PHYSICAL EXAM
- The physical exam is the most important factor in making the diagnosis of NSTI.
- Skin findings include:
  - Local erythema and swelling
  - Induration
  - Bullae
  - Crepitus
  - Pain out of proportion to skin findings
  - Pain beyond the margins of erythema
- Systemic findings include:
  - Fever
  - Tachycardia
  - Hypotension
  - Altered mental status

DIAGNOSTIC TESTS & INTERPRETATION
Lab
- CBC with differential: WBC >15,000 cells/mm^3 is a common finding.
- Electrolytes, BUN, creatinine:
  - Hyponatremia: Sodium <135 mmol/L is a common finding.
  - Renal insufficiency can occur from hypotension and sepsis.
  - Hypo- and hyperglycemia can be present.
- Blood cultures
- PT/PTT/INR: Coagulation factors may be abnormal due to DIC.
- Type and cross: Important to obtain initially because patients require prompt surgical intervention.
- ABG/lactate: A lactic acidosis may be present.
- Laboratory Risk Indicator for Necrotizing Fasciitis (LRINEC) score is a retrospectively devised scoring system to help make the diagnosis of NSTI. It consists of 6 parameters: C-reactive protein, WBC, hemoglobin, sodium, creatinine, and glucose. A score is assigned based on the value of each parameter. In the original study, a score of ≥6 is associated with a 92% positive predictive value and a 96% negative predictive value (2)[B]. This scoring system has not been validated in large, prospective studies.

Imaging
- No gold standard imaging study; imaging studies are not required because the diagnosis is mainly a clinical one, but certain radiographic findings can aid in making the diagnosis in equivocal cases.
- CT scan has an 80% sensitivity for making the diagnosis of NSTI. CT findings include fascial edema or thickening, abscess, and gas formation (1).
- On plain x-ray, the presence of subcutaneous gas is helpful but present in only 39% of patients with NSTI (2).
- Characteristic MRI finding is soft-tissue, fascial thickening. MRI has a 90–100% sensitivity and 50–85% specificity in detecting NSTI (1). MRI is not used often since patients can be unstable and critically ill and in need of rapid surgical intervention.

Diagnostic Procedures/Other
The gold standard for diagnosis and treatment is operative exploration. All patients require immediate surgical debridement. Findings present in the OR that confirm the diagnosis are presence of foul-smelling discharge "dishwater" fluid (brownish-tan color), necrosis or lack of bleeding, change in fascia from a tough and shiny white appearance to a dull gray, and a loss of normal resistance of the fascia to finger dissection (1).

Pathological Findings
- Superficial epidermal hyaline necrosis
- Dermal edema
- Polymorphonuclear infiltration into dermis
- Late stages: Inflammation and thrombosis of penetrating fascial vessels
- Sometimes microorganisms can be found within destroyed tissue.

DIFFERENTIAL DIAGNOSIS
- Cellulitis
- Myonecrosis
- Lymphedema
- Noninfectious fasciitis
- Phlegmasia cerulea dolens
- Myxedema

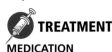

TREATMENT

MEDICATION
First Line
- The mainstay of treatment is surgical debridement, but antibiotics should be administered as soon as this diagnosis is entertained.
- Initial empiric IV antibiotic therapy should be broad spectrum to cover the various bacterial causative agents. Therapy can be tailored to specific pathogen when culture results are available (3)[C].

- Mixed infection:
  – Option 1:
    ○ Ampicillin-sulbactam 1.5–3.0 g q6–8h **or** piperacillin-tazobactam 3.375 g q6–8h **plus** clindamycin 600–900 mg q8h **plus** ciprofloxacin 400 mg q12h
  – Option 2:
    ○ Imipenem/cilastin 1 g q6–8h **or** meropenem 1 g q6–8h **or** ertapenem 1 g/d
  – Option 3:
    ○ Cefotaxime 2 g q6h **plus** metronidazole 500 mg q6h **or** clindamycin 600–900 mg q8h
- Streptococcus infection:
  – Penicillin 2–4 MU q4–6h **plus** clindamycin 600–900 mg q8h
- *S. aureus* infection:
  – Nafcillin 1–2 g q4h **or** oxacillin 1–2 g q4h **or** vancomycin (for MRSA) 30 mg/kg/d in 2 divided doses **or** clindamycin 600–900 mg q8h
- *Clostridium* infection:
  – Clindamycin 600–900 mg q8h **or** penicillin 2–4 MU q4–6h

Second Line
- Some retrospective studies and small prospective studies demonstrate potential benefit of intravenous immunoglobulin (IVIG) (2)[B].
- IVIG binds to bacterial exotoxins, thereby reducing toxin-induced tissue necrosis and decreasing cytokine production, thus suppressing the inflammatory response.

ADDITIONAL TREATMENT
General Measures
- Immediate surgical debridement is the mainstay of treatment.
- Hemodynamic stabilization with IV fluids and early antibiotics
- Electrolyte repletion

Issues for Referral
- Prompt surgical consultation
- Consider infectious disease consultation.

Additional Therapies
Hyperbaric oxygen therapy has been proposed as an adjunct therapy. Increased tissue oxygenation is purported to prevent the spread of bacteria and decrease exotoxin proliferation (2)[C]. Studies to date have revealed conflicting results.

SURGERY/OTHER PROCEDURES
- Surgical debridement is the cornerstone of treatment. Patients should go to the OR as soon as possible after diagnosis is made.
- All necrotic tissue should be excised. The margin of excision should extend until healthy bleeding tissue is encountered. This sometimes requires amputation.
- Patient should be taken back to OR daily or every other day to evaluate for spread of infection and determine if further debridement is needed. Rarely is surgical control achieved after one debridement.
- Once tissue has been fully debrided and infection is under control wound reconstruction via skin grafting can be undertaken.

IN-PATIENT CONSIDERATIONS
Initial Stabilization
- Consider intubation as needed for patients in shock with profound acid–base abnormalities or depressed mental status.
- Obtain large-bore IV access; consider central venous access and invasive arterial blood pressure monitoring as needed.
- Undertake aggressive IV fluid resuscitation to restore intravascular volume and maintain tissue perfusion and oxygenation.
- Administer vasopressors and inotropes as required to maintain tissue perfusion.

Admission Criteria
All patients require admission to an ICU.

IV Fluids
Volume expansion with crystalloid (NS or LR)

Nursing
- Patients usually require ICU-level care.
- Nursing staff should be familiar with surgical wound care.
- Emotional support to patients and families is essential as they often need to undergo amputations.

Discharge Criteria
Will vary on a case-by-case basis, usually after the active disease is resolved. Patients may need repeated readmissions for staged reconstructive surgeries.

 ONGOING CARE

FOLLOW-UP RECOMMENDATIONS
Patient Monitoring
- Usually require ICU level of care
- Careful monitoring of wound to assess for spread of necrosis and need for repeat surgical debridement

DIET
- Initially NPO for surgical debridement; early enteric nutrition is essential as there are large metabolic demands due to critical illness and the need for excessive tissue healing.
- Patient should be fed between surgical interventions either by mouth or NGT, OGT, if intubated.

PROGNOSIS
- Most important determinant of mortality is time to surgical debridement
- Mortality rate 24–34% (4)
- Independent predictors of mortality are (4)[B]:
  – WBC count >30,000 cells/mm^3
  – Creatinine >2.0 mg/dL at admission
  – Heart disease
  – Clostridial infection

COMPLICATIONS
- Septic shock
- Death
- Multiorgan failure
- Amputation
- Cosmetic and functional loss of tissue

REFERENCES
1. Sarani B, et al. Necrotizing fasciitis: Current concepts and review of the literature. *J Am Coll Surg.* 2009;208:279–88.
2. Phan HH, Cocanour CS. Necrotizing soft tissue infections in the intensive care unit. *Crit Care Med.* 2010;38:460–68.
3. Anaya DA, et al. Predictors of mortality and limb loss in necrotizing soft tissue infections. *Arch Surg.* 2005;140:151–7.
4. Stevens DL, et al. Practice guidelines for the diagnosis and management of skin and soft-tissue infections. *Clin Infect Dis.* 2005;41:1373–1406.

CODES

ICD9
728.86 Necrotizing fasciitis

CLINICAL PEARLS
- This is a rapidly progressing, severely ill state, in which pain is out of proportion to the findings of the physical exam and pain is present beyond the margins of erythema. These are important clinical clues to the diagnosis.
- Immediate surgical intervention is necessary to improve mortality.
- Broad-spectrum antibiotics must be administered early on.
- Consider IVIG for streptococcal or clostridial infection.

N

NEEDLESTICK INJURIES

Eliany Mejia Lopez
Jose R. Yunen

 BASICS

DESCRIPTION

A penetrating stab wound from a needle (or other sharp object) that may result in exposure to blood or other body fluids, commonly encountered by people handling needles in a medical facility, are an occupational hazard in the medical community.

- Risk of disease:
  - Fortunately, most needlestick injuries do not result in exposure to an infectious disease, and of those that do, the majority do not result in the transmission of infection.
  - The rate of occupational transmission from an:
    ○ HIV-positive source is 0.3% for a percutaneous exposure and 0.09% for a mucous membrane exposure.
    ○ HBV-positive source to a nonimmunized host is 6–24%
    ○ HCV-positive source is ~1–10%

EPIDEMIOLOGY

Incidence

- 600,000–800,000 such injuries occur annually, about 1/2 of which go unreported. A recent CDC study estimates that an average of 385,000 needlestick injuries occur annually in U.S. hospital settings.
- Most injuries involve nursing staff, but laboratory staff, physicians, and other health care workers are also injured.

RISK FACTORS

- The main group at risk is health care workers, but injuries also occur in other fields of work. Workers may acquire a blood-borne virus (BBV) infection if they are exposed to infected blood or body fluids: This could be either via the mucous membranes (eyes, mouth, and nose), through broken skin, or through an inoculation injury route.
- The specific risk of a single injury depends on:
  - Injuries with a hollow-bore needle
  - Deep penetration
  - Visible blood on the needle
  - A needle located in a deep artery or vein
  - Blood from terminally ill patients is known to increase the risk for HIV infection.

- Such injuries depend partly on the design and type of needle device used. In addition, these injuries have been associated with certain work practices: Recapping, transferring a body fluid between containers, and failing to properly dispose of used needles in puncture-resistant "sharps" containers.

GENERAL PREVENTION

- A comprehensive needlestick injury prevention program includes:
  - Employee training
  - Recommended guidelines
  - Safe recapping procedures
  - Effective disposal systems
  - Surveillance programs
  - Elimination of unnecessary use of needles
  - Implementation of devices with safety features
  - Safety promotion in the work environment
  - Outcome evaluation
- Some studies have shown that needleless or protected-needle IV systems decreased needlestick injuries related to IV connectors by 62–88%.
- In the U.S., the Needlestick Safety Act was signed in 2000 and Bloodborne Pathogens Standard in 2001, which mandate the use of safety devices and needle-removers with any sharps or needles.

PATHOPHYSIOLOGY

The main risk posed by needlestick injury is exposure to BBV. The major pathogens of concern in occupational body fluid exposures are HIV, HBV, and HCV. These pathogens require percutaneous or mucosal introduction for infectivity. The major target organs are the immune system (HIV) and the liver (hepatitis). Other microorganisms are involved to a lesser extent, such as fungi, tetanus, *S. aureus, S. pyogenes*, TB, and cutaneous gonorrhea. Many of these diseases were transmitted in rare, isolated events.

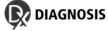 DIAGNOSIS

HISTORY

Should focus on the patient's medical history, immunizations, and risk factors for hepatitis and HIV.

PHYSICAL EXAM

- Evidence of the reported trauma.
- No abnormal physical findings are expected.

DIAGNOSTIC TESTS & INTERPRETATION

Lab

Initial lab tests

- HIV
- HAV IgM,
- Hepatitis B surface antibody
- HBsAg
- HB core IgM
- HCV
- Source patient (if available):
  - HIV
  - Hepatitis B antigen
  - Hepatitis C antibody
  - AST/ALT
  - Alkaline phosphatase

Follow-Up & Special Considerations

Hepatitis C antibody testing at 2, 4, and 8 weeks:

- Prior treatment with retrovirals:
  - CBC
  - HCG
  - Serum creatinine/BUN
  - UA
  - LFTs

TREATMENT

After a needlestick injury, prompt treatment must be initiated to minimize the risk of infection for the recipient.

MEDICATION
The need for tetanus and/or HBV prophylaxis is based on medical and immunization history. Unless the source is known to be negative for HBV, HCV, and HIV, postexposure prophylaxis (PEP) should be initiated, within 1 hour of the injury, at the emergency department.

First Line
Hepatitis B prophylaxis: Hepatitis B immune globulin (HBIG) and/or hepatitis B vaccine:
- 1 mL IM as early as possible (24 hours) following a needlestick
- 1-month booster: 1 mL
- 6-month booster: 1 mL

Pregnancy Considerations
- No contraindications during pregnancy and lactation
- HIV prophylaxis is based on an assessment of the risk by using the 3-step process developed by the CDC:
  - Step 1: Determine exposure code.
  - Step 2: Determine HIV status code of the source.
  - Step 3: Match exposure code with HIV status code to determine if any postexposure prophylaxis is indicated.
- Basic regimen:
  - HIV-PEP should be initiated as soon as possible, within hours and no later than 72 hours following the potential exposure.
  - 4 weeks of zidovudine (600 mg/d in 2–3 divided doses) and lamivudine (150 mg b.i.d.)
  - In January 2001, the CDC warned against using nevirapine for PEP because of the risk of liver damage.
- Expanded regimen:
  - 3-drug regimens, comprising 2 nucleoside-analogue reverse-transcriptase inhibitors (NRTIs) plus a boosted protease inhibitor, can be considered in situations where antiretroviral therapy resistance is known or suspected:
  - Basic regimen + either indinavir (800 mg q8h) or nelfinavir (750 mg 3 times/d).

Pregnancy Considerations
Category C: Fetal risk revealed in studies in animals but not established or not studied in humans; may use if benefits outweigh risk to fetus.

Second Line
- Tenofovir + lamivudine
- Stavudine + lamivudine
- Emtricitabine is an acceptable alternative to lamivudine.
- Hepatitis C prophylaxis:
  - There is no active HCV-PEP; early diagnosis and identification of chronic disease is required. If detected, referral for evaluation and treatment must be indicated.

ADDITIONAL TREATMENT
General Measures
- Tetanus prophylaxis is rarely required and is based on medical history.
- Health care providers should have been immunized against hepatitis B.
- Hepatitis A prophylaxis may need to be considered depending on the source–patient situation.

IN-PATIENT CONSIDERATIONS
Initial Stabilization
- Irrigate and clean wound.
- For a mucosal surface exposure or if the wound is large enough, irrigate with copious amounts of saline.

ONGOING CARE

FOLLOW-UP RECOMMENDATIONS
- Counseling and HIV testing by enzyme immunoassay to monitor for a possible seroconversion: At baseline, 6 and 12 weeks, and 6 months.
- Hepatitis C antibody testing at 2, 4, and 8 weeks.
- Follow-up with occupational health or infectious disease in 24–72 hours
- Patients who are prescribed PEP should be offered follow-up and clinical monitoring; the main purpose is to monitor adherence and to identify and manage side effects.

DIET
No special diet needed

PROGNOSIS
- Most needlestick injuries do not result in exposure to an infectious disease.
- Most health care workers with occupational exposure to body fluids do not develop disease.

COMPLICATIONS
Transmission of BBV (HIV, HCV, HBV) as explained above

ADDITIONAL READING

- Cardo DM, et al. A case-control study of HIV seroconversion in health care workers after percutaneous exposure. Centers for Disease Control and Prevention Needlestick Surveillance Group. *N Engl J Med*. 1997;337(21):1485–90.
- CDC. Public Health Service guidelines for the management of health-care worker exposures to HIV and recommendations for postexposure prophylaxis. Centers for Disease Control and Prevention. *MMWR Recomm Rep*. 1998;47(RR–7):1–33.
- CDC. Recommendations for follow-up of health-care workers after occupational exposure to hepatitis C virus. *MMWR Morb Mortal Wkly Rep*. 1997; 46(26):603–6.
- Post-exposure prophylaxis to prevent HIV infection. Joint WHO/ILO guidelines on post-exposure prophylaxis (PEP) to prevent IHV infection. Geneva, Switzerland; World Health Organization; 2007.
- Rosenstock L. Statement for the record on needlestick injuries. National Institute for Occupational Safety and Health Centers for Disease Control and Prevention. U.S. Department of Health and Human Services. Available at: http://www.hhs. gov/asl/testify/t000622a.html.
- Occupational exposure: http://www.cdc.gov/ mmwr/preview/mmwrhtmL/rr5409a1.htm

CODES

ICD9
- V01.79 Contact with or exposure to other viral diseases
- V15.85 Personal history of contact with and (suspected) exposure to potentially hazardous body fluids
- 879.8 Open wound(s) (multiple) of unspecified site(s), without mention of complication

N

NEPHRITIS, ACUTE INTERSTITIAL

Sindhura Gogineni
Roopa Kohli Seth

 BASICS

DESCRIPTION
- Pattern of acute kidney injury (AKI) is characterized histopathologically by inflammation and edema of the renal interstitium.
- Disease process also commonly involves adjacent renal tubules.

EPIDEMIOLOGY
Incidence
- 5–15% of hospitalized patients with AKI (1)
- 18.6% of elderly patients with AKI

RISK FACTORS
Factors leading to exposure of medications, infections, immune or neoplastic disorders

GENERAL PREVENTION
Avoiding exposure to nephrotoxic drugs

PATHOPHYSIOLOGY
- Diffuse or patchy infiltration of interstitium by inflammatory cells
- These inflammatory cells are triggered by drugs, infection, or immune processes.
- Inflammatory cells consist of T lymphocytes, monocytes, and occasionally plasma cells and neutrophils.

ETIOLOGY
- Drugs account for about 70% (2):
  - Antibiotics: Beta lactams, vancomycin cephalosporins, sulfonamides, ciprofloxacin, linezolid
  - Other: NSAIDs, proton pump inhibitors, diuretics, indinavir, allopurinol
- Immune reaction: Acute renal allograft rejection, SLE; Sjögren, Wegener syndromes
- Infection associated: *Legionella, Leptospirosis,* cytomegalovirus, streptococci, sarcoidosis
- Idiopathic
- TINU syndrome: Tubulointerstitial nephritis and uveitis

COMMONLY ASSOCIATED CONDITIONS
- Tubulointerstitial nephritis
- Drug reactions
- Sepsis

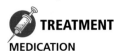 **DIAGNOSIS**

HISTORY
- Fever, skin rash, arthralgia: 10% of drug-induced
- Malaise, anorexia, nausea, vomiting
- Loin pain, dysuria, decreased or no urine output:
  - Onset in relation to medications, infection

PHYSICAL EXAM
- Maculopapular rash, joint tenderness
- Costovertebral angle tenderness (pyelonephritis)

DIAGNOSTIC TESTS & INTERPRETATION
Lab
Initial lab tests
- Chemistry:
  - Raise in BUN, serum creatinine
  - Hyperchloremic nonanion gap metabolic acidosis
  - May have hyponatremia, hyperkalemia
- CBC with differential:
  - Eosinophilia-associated with drug-induced AIK
  - Increased neutrophils associated with infections
- Urine analysis:
  - Isosthenuria is common.
  - Proteinuria: Usually <1 g/24 hr:
    ○ NSAID-associated; nephrotic range
  - Leukocytes or leukocyte casts:
    ○ Rare red blood cells
  - Eosinophiluria can be detected by Wright's stain or Hansel's stain.
  - Positive predictive value in diagnosis of AIN is 38%.
  - Urine sodium, osmolarity, FeNa- Rule out prerenal AIK. Urine Na is usually >40, urine osmolarity <400 m OsmL/kg, Fe Na >2%

Follow-Up & Special Considerations
Creatinine, urine output, electrolytes

Imaging
- No specific imaging study is useful for diagnosis.
- Gallinium-67 was proposed to differentiate from ATN. However, it has high false positivity, and is not routinely recommended.

Diagnostic Procedures/Other
- Renal biopsy: Gold standard for diagnosis
- Recommended especially in patients with no recovery of renal function even after withdrawal of suspected medication.

Pathological Findings
Infiltration of interstitium by inflammatory cells: T lymphocytes, monocytes, eosinophils, plasma cells, and neutrophils:
- Additional glomerular involvement: NSAIDs
- Granuloma: Granulomatous diseases

DIFFERENTIAL DIAGNOSIS
- Acute tubular necrosis
- Glomerulonephritis
- Vasculitis
- Renal artery or vein occlusion

TREATMENT

MEDICATION
First Line
Withdrawal of suspected medication

Second Line
Patients with no improvement of renal function within 2 weeks of discontinuation of offending drug should be started on steroid therapy:
- Methylprednisolone 250–500 mg/d for 3–4 consecutive days followed by oral prednisone 1 mg/kg/d tapering off over 8–12 weeks (3)[C]
- *OR* prednisone 1 mg/kg/d (to a maximum of 40–60 mg) for a minimum of 1–2 weeks, beginning a gradual taper after the serum creatinine has returned to or near baseline, for a total therapy duration of 2–3 months

ADDITIONAL TREATMENT
General Measures
Fluid and electrolyte management:
- Symptomatic treatment for fever and systemic symptoms

Issues for Referral
No improvement after withdrawal of suspected drug or treating the underlying etiology

Additional Therapies
- Steroid-resistant AIN: Mycophenolate 500–1000 mg b.i.d.
  - Monitor for side effects: Leukocyte counts and GI side effects.
- Dialysis (hemodynamically stable) or CVVH (hemodynamically unstable): AKI leading to hyperkalemia, acidosis, uremic symptoms, fluid overload, pericarditis

SURGERY/OTHER PROCEDURES
- Renal biopsy for diagnosis
- Dialysis access and dialysis for treatment of AKI

IN-PATIENT CONSIDERATIONS

Initial Stabilization
- Withdraw offending drug
- Treat underlying cause

Admission Criteria
RIFLE criteria: Patient at risk or above and greater severity of illness as per APACHE or sepsis-related organ failure assessment (SOFA).

RIFLE	Serum Creatinine (Cr) increase	Urine output
RISK (R)	Cr × 1.5	<0.5 mg/kg/hr × 6 hr
INJURY (I)	Cr × 2	<0.5 mg/kg/hr × 12 hr
FAILURE (F)	Cr × 3 or >4 mg/dL	<0.3 mg/kg/hr × 24 hr or anuria × 12 hr
Loss (L)	Persistent ARF = complete loss of renal function >4 wk	
End stage (E)	End stage renal disease	

IV Fluids
Isotonic fluids

Nursing
Strict quantification of input and output

Discharge Criteria
- Improvement of creatinine or urine output
- No electrolyte abnormalities.
- No uremic symptoms

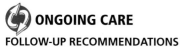

ONGOING CARE

FOLLOW-UP RECOMMENDATIONS

Patient Monitoring
- Creatinine, urine output, electrolytes every day at least until ICU discharge
- If BUN and creatinine are trending up, watch for signs and symptoms of uremia and fluid overload.

DIET
Prerenal diet: Low protein
- Low-potassium diet if hyperkalemia
- If patient is on tube feeding or TPN, protein should not be >1.5 g/kg body weight.

PATIENT EDUCATION
AKI, acute interstitial nephritis; its etiology and adverse effects:
- Avoid medications that might cause interstitial nephritis

PROGNOSIS
Serum creatinine remains elevated in 40% of patients:
- 10% of patients will need prolonged course of dialysis
- AIN associated with NSAIDs carries a poor prognosis.
- Comorbid conditions (sepsis, hypotension, diabetes) can lead to prolonged AKI and poor recovery.

COMPLICATIONS
Caused by direct and indirect effect of AKI

System	Mechanism	Complication
Cardiovascular	Fluid Overload	CHF Hypertension
Pulmonary	Fluid overload, cytokines	Pulmonary edema, acute lung injury
Gastrointestinal	Fluid overload, gut ischemia, reperfusion injury	Abdominal compartment syndrome, GI ulcer, and bleeding
Immune	WBC dysfunction	Infection
Hematological	Decreased RBC, Von Willebrand	Anemia, bleeding
Nervous system	Hyponatremia, acidosis, uremia	Seizures, altered mental status
Electrolyte	Hyponatremia, hyperkalemia	Arrhythmias
Acid–base	Impaired insulin resistance; downregulation of β-receptors	Hyperglycemia, decreased cardiac output, blood pressure.
Pharmacokinetic and dynamics	Increased volume of distribution; decreased availability, albumin binding, elimination	Underdosing or drug toxicity

REFERENCES
1. Michel DM, et al. Acute interstitial nephritis. *J AM Soc Nephrol*. 1998;9:506–15.
2. Baker RJ, et al. The changing profile of acute tubulointerstitial nephritis. *Nephrol Dial Transplant*. 2004;19:8.
3. Gonzalez E, et al. Early steroid treatment improves the recovery of renal function in patients with drug-induced acute interstitial nephritis. *Kidney Int*. 2008;73:940–6.

ADDITIONAL READING
Bellomo R, et al. Acute renal failure—Definition, outcome measures, animal models, fluid therapy and information technology needs: The Second International Consensus Conference of the Acute Dialysis Quality Initiative (ADQI) Group. *Crit Care*. 2004;8:R204–R212.

 ### See Also (Topic, Algorithm, Electronic Media Element)
- Acute renal failure
- CRRT

 ## CODES

ICD9
580.89 Acute glomerulonephritis with other specified pathological lesion in kidney

CLINICAL PEARLS
- AIN is an intrarenal cause of AKI characterized histopathologically by inflammation and edema of the renal interstitium.
- Improvement of renal function with the withdrawal of the offending drug or treating the underlying cause establishes a presumptive diagnosis.
- Identify and treat important complications of AIN/AKI: Acidosis, pericarditis, fluid overload, uremic symptoms, and hyperkalemia.

N

NEPHROTIC SYNDROME

Tzvi Y. Neuman
Roopa Kohli-Seth

 BASICS

DESCRIPTION
A rare syndrome of primary or secondary kidney disease leading to:
- Proteinuria
- Peripheral edema
- Hypoalbuminemia
- Hypercholesterolemia

EPIDEMIOLOGY
Incidence
- 3–4 new cases per 100,000 adults per year
- Males >Females
- Black males have a higher incidence of focal segmental glomerulonephritis

Prevalence
- Minimal change: 10% adults, 65% children
- Focal segmental glomerulosclerosis: 35% adults, 10% children
- Membranous glomerular disease: 30% adults, 5% children
- Membranoproliferative glomerular disease: 10% adults, 10% children
- Other proliferative kidney diseases: 15% adults, 10% children

RISK FACTORS
- Patients with chronic kidney disease who have heavy protein losses
- Black males with hypertension

Genetics
- NPHS2 gene variants are associated with nephrotic syndrome; the R229Q allele is under investigation for its role in the disease.
- Other genes under evaluation: Candidate gene, α-actinin-4, and those genes encoding for podocyte proteins (nephrin and podocin); transcription factor WT1; calcium channel TRPC6; enzyme phospholipase C-epsilon-1; and carnosinase

GENERAL PREVENTION
Good control and follow-up care of secondary causes

PATHOPHYSIOLOGY
- Increased glomerular permeability to large macromolecules, and loss of serum albumin and other proteins
- Interstitial edema due to decreased plasma oncotic pressure or urinary sodium retention at the renal tubules

ETIOLOGY
- Primary (idiopathic) glomerular disease:
  - Focal segmental glomerulosclerosis: Most common cause of idiopathic nephrotic syndrome in adults; strong association with hypertension and black race; may also be associated with HIV, reflux nephropathy, previous glomerular injury, NSAID use, or massive obesity
  - Membranous glomerular disease: Usually idiopathic; may be associated with HBV, autoimmune disease, thyroiditis, carcinoma, or certain drugs
  - Minimal change glomerular disease: An idiopathic condition; may also be associated with NSAID use or paraneoplastic effect of malignancy
  - Membranoproliferative glomerular disease due to damaged glomeruli
- Secondary causes:
  - Diabetes mellitus, SLE, amyloidosis, cancer (myeloma, lymphoma)
  - Drugs: Gold, antimicrobials, NSAIDs, penicillamine, captopril, tamoxifen, lithium
  - Infection: HIV, HBV, HCV, mycoplasma, Syphilis, malaria, schistosomiasis, filariasis, toxoplasmosis
  - Congenital diseases: Alport syndrome, congenital nephritic syndrome of Finnish type, Pierson syndrome, Nail-patella syndrome, Denys-Drash syndrome

COMMONLY ASSOCIATED CONDITIONS
- Diabetic nephropathy
- Light chain amyloid nephropathy

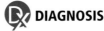 **DIAGNOSIS**

HISTORY
- Features of systemic disease process
- New-onset edema
- Drug history: Any new agents (prescription or OTC) introduced recently
- Infection, acute or chronic
- Diagnosis of cancer (particularly lung and colon)
- Family history (e.g., Alport syndrome)

PHYSICAL EXAM
- Edema (periorbital, lower extremity, genital, ascites, pleural effusions, pericardial effusion)
- Fatigue
- Leukonychia
- Breathlessness
- Elevated jugular venous pressure/distension
- Chest pain associated with thromboembolic event
- Evidence of acute renal failure
- Eruptive xanthomata
- Frothy urine

DIAGNOSTIC TESTS & INTERPRETATION
Lab
Initial lab tests
- Serum urea and creatinine, estimated GFR
- Urine analysis: Fat bodies, fatty casts with "Maltese cross" appearance noted under polarized light; evaluate hematuria or proteinuria; exclude urinary infection:
  - Proteinuria >3–3.5 g in 24 hours, or spot urine: Creatinine ratio >300–350 mg/mmol
- Serum albumin <25 g/L
- CBC, coagulation profile, liver function tests, serum calcium, CRP, ESR, glucose, lipids
- Serum electrophoresis, urine electrophoresis
- Autoimmune screen and hepatitis screen

Follow-Up & Special Considerations
Watch volume status and for evidence of thromboembolic event.

Imaging
Initial approach
- Renal US to asses renal size and morphology; Doppler technique to evaluate for thrombosis
- Abdominal US/renal vein Doppler/IVC venography/CT/MRI if suspicious for renal vein thrombosis

Follow-Up & Special Considerations
- Chest x-ray to evaluate for pleural effusion
- Consider Doppler US of lower extremities if suspicious for DVT.
- Consider V/Q scan or CT angiography to evaluate for pulmonary embolus.
- Echocardiogram to evaluate for pericardial effusion

Diagnostic Procedures/Other
Renal biopsy may be indicated to look for primary kidney disease:
- Light microscopy, histologic evaluation, immunofluorescence, immunoperoxidase, or electron microscopy evaluation

Pathological Findings
- Minimal change glomerular disease: Diffuse fusion of the epithelial foot processes on electron microscopy
- Focal segmental glomerulosclerosis: Some glomeruli with segmental areas of mesangial collapse and sclerosis seen on light microscopy
- Membranous glomerular disease: Thickening of the basement membrane without cellular infiltration or proliferation
- Membranoproliferative glomerular disease: "Tram-track" appearance under the microscope due to increased mesangial cellularity and immune complex deposition

DIFFERENTIAL DIAGNOSIS
Other edema states (cirrhosis, CHF), carcinoma, infection, malignant hypertension, polyarteritis nodosa, toxemia of pregnancy

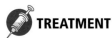

TREATMENT

MEDICATION

First Line

- Immunosuppression in certain patients:
  - Minimal change disease: Prednisone 1 mg/kg/d (1)[A]
    - Those with relapse who are steroid sensitive should receive a course of steroids until urine is protein free for 3 days followed by an alternate-day regimen of lower dose steroids for another month (1)[A]
    - Those who continue to be refractory should receive either cyclosporine or cyclophosphamide (1)[D], may also consider use of mycophenolate mofetil in such patients
  - Focal segmental glomerulonephritis: Prednisone 1 mg/kg/d (2)[D]; refractory cases may need cyclosporine (2)[D]
- Loop diuretics to reverse edema state (these are protein bound and can potentially be filtered across the glomerulus); use the IV route in refractory cases (3)[C]
- ACE inhibitors (ACE-I) or angiotensin II receptor blockers (ARBs) to treat proteinuria with or without hypertension (3)[A]

Second Line

- Thiazide diuretics
- Potassium-sparing diuretics
- IV albumin may improve diuresis by increasing the delivery of diuretic, as well as improve intravascular volume.

ADDITIONAL TREATMENT

General Measures

- Maintain negative sodium balance
- Reduce or eliminate proteinuria
- Treat underlying pathology

Issues for Referral

All new cases should be evaluated by a nephrologist to determine the need for renal biopsy.

COMPLEMENTARY & ALTERNATIVE THERAPIES

Chinese herbal preparation, Huangqi, may relieve symptoms of nephrotic syndrome.

SURGERY/OTHER PROCEDURES

- May require renal biopsy
- In severe uncontrollable proteinuria with complications of renal dysfunction or malnutrition, single or bilateral nephrectomy may be considered; renal embolization may be another option.

IN-PATIENT CONSIDERATIONS

Initial Stabilization

Treat inciting cause and associated complications

Admission Criteria

Usually a complication of nephrotic syndrome leading to other organ decompensation:

- Pleural effusion, congestive heart failure, hypertensive emergency, hemodynamic instability, significant thromboembolic disease, labile glucose, or acute coronary syndrome

IV Fluids

Not indicated unless the patient has intravascular volume depletion

Nursing

Ensure patient comfort, adherence to physician orders, and assist in patient education

Discharge Criteria

- Hemodynamic stability
- Control over inciting complications: Edema states, hyperglycemia, thromboembolic or coronary event, hypertension, or infectious process

ONGOING CARE

FOLLOW-UP RECOMMENDATIONS

- Prophylactic anticoagulation may be considered in patients with previous history of thrombosis and serum albumin <2 g/dL who have proteinuria >3–3.5 g/24-hour urine collection.
- Use of prophylactic antibiotics is not recommended.
- Use diuretics to maintain negative sodium balance.
- Use ACE-Is or ARBs to decrease proteinuria.
- Use statin therapy to treat dyslipidemia.
- Goal blood pressure is <130/80.

Patient Monitoring

Regular monitoring of plasma electrolytes and renal function

DIET

- Sodium intake <3 g/d
- Fluid restriction <1.5 L/d

PATIENT EDUCATION

Slow reversal of edema states:

- Target weight loss of 0.5–1 kg/d to prevent electrolyte disturbance and hemoconcentration

PROGNOSIS

- Minimal change disease has good outcome, with complete remission within 2 weeks to several months; does not progress to renal failure.
- Focal segmental glomerulosclerosis may progress to ESRD within 10 years.
- Membranous disease may spontaneously resolve; however, 50% may progress to renal failure within 10–20 years.

COMPLICATIONS

- Impaired thrombolytic activity, procoagulant diatheses:
  - Thromboembolism (venous DVT, pulmonary embolus or renal vein; arterial)
- Low serum IgG, reduced complement, and depressed T-cell function:
  - Bacterial infection (cellulitis, pneumonia, peritonitis)
  - Viral infection
- Hyperlipidemia may lead to increased cardiovascular abnormalities.
- Bone disease secondary to vitamin D loss
- Acute renal failure:
  - Spontaneous complication vs. overdiuresis; interstitial nephritis (secondary to diuretics, NSAIDs, sepsis, renal vein thrombosis)
- Muscle wasting

Pediatric Considerations

- Children with nephrotic syndrome usually present with minimal change disease; occurs predominantly in children aged 2–6 years (2 new cases per 100,000 persons per year).
- Children have an increased risk of pneumococcal peritonitis.

REFERENCES

1. Bargman JM. Management of minimal lesion glomerulonephritis: Evidence-based recommendations. *Kidney Int Suppl*. 1999;55(70):S3–S16.
2. Burgess E. Management of focal segmental glomerulosclerosis: Evidence-based recommendations. *Kidney Int Suppl*. 1999;55(70):S26–S32.
3. Philipneri M. Nephrotic syndrome: Drug therapy. Physicians' Information and Educational Resource. 2008. Accessed at http://pier.acponline.org/physicians/diseases/d651/d651.html

ADDITIONAL READING

- Hull RP, et al. Nephrotic syndrome in adults: Clinical review. *BMJ*. 2008;336:1185–9.
- Beck LH, et al. Glomerular and tubulointerstitial diseases. Primary Care: *Clin Office Pract*. 2008; 35:265–96.
- Yuan W, et al. Chinese herbal medicine: Huangqi type formulations for nephrotic syndrome. *Cochrane Database Syst Rev*. 2008;2.

CODES

ICD9

- 581.9 Nephrotic syndrome with unspecified pathological lesion in kidney
- 593.89 Other specified disorders of kidney and ureter
- 791.0 Proteinuria

CLINICAL PEARLS

- Expedient diagnosis with good clinical suspicion is vital.
- Use immunosuppression and control of volume state.
- Entertain early suspicion for thromboembolic event, infection, or volume overload.
- Treat with ACE-I or ARB; consistent follow-up with outpatient nephrology is important.

N

NEUROLEPTIC MALIGNANT SYDROME

Christopher R. Gilbert
Paul E. Marik

 BASICS

DESCRIPTION
- Idiosyncratic disorder characterized by mental status changes, dysautonomia, fevers, and rigidity
- Defined by the DSM-IV as (1)[C]:
  - Development of severe muscle rigidity and hyperthermia in association with neuroleptic medications.
  - Presence of ≥2 of the following:
    - Diaphoresis
    - Dysphagia
    - Elevated or labile blood pressure
    - Incontinence
    - Laboratory evidence of muscle injury
    - Leukocytosis
    - Mental status changes
    - Mutism
    - Tachycardia
    - Tremor
  - Above mentioned symptoms cannot be the result of underlying psychiatric, neurological, or medical diagnosis (including ingestions).
- Often presents acutely and, if unrecognized, can rapidly progress to multiorgan failure and death

EPIDEMIOLOGY
Incidence
- Rare disorder, occurring in 0.1–3% of the population receiving neuroleptic medications
- No predilection for specific age, sex, or type of psychiatric illness

RISK FACTORS
- Exposure to drugs known to cause NMS:
  - Large or escalating doses
  - Parental administration
- Volume depletion
- Preexisting agitated state
- Iron deficiency

Genetics
- Suggested familial predilection
- May be linked to *Taq*I A Dopamine D_2 receptor gene

GENERAL PREVENTION
Avoidance or close monitoring of patients on drugs known to cause NMS

PATHOPHYSIOLOGY
Unknown: Leading theory describes the blockade of dopamine receptors leading to hyperthermia and dysautonomia

ETIOLOGY
Related to medication usage, most commonly the typical antipsychotics, but other implicated:
- Haloperidol
- Chlorpromazine
- Olanzapine
- Risperidone
- Quetiapine
- Clozapine
- Metoclopramide
- Promethazine

COMMONLY ASSOCIATED CONDITIONS
- Occurs more commonly in patients with psychiatric disorders, as these patients are often on medications that predispose them to NMS.
- May also occur in patients with Parkinson disease, but this appears to be related to acute withdrawal of dopaminergic agents.

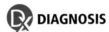 **DIAGNOSIS**

HISTORY
- Many patients describe increased agitation and feeling of doom.
- Others present with catatonia.
- Mental status changes, fevers, rigidity, and dysautonomia commonly present over a 24–72-hour period (1)[C].

PHYSICAL EXAM
- Most common presentation is a change in mental status, which can range from mild confusion to coma.
- Temperature of >38°C is often included in diagnostic criteria; however, temperatures of >40°C are not uncommon
- Muscle rigidity is often dramatic and described as "lead-pipe rigidity":
  - Often also accompanied by tremor
  - Less commonly accompanied by dyskinesia, chorea, trismus, or opisthotonus
- Dysautonomias commonly are tachycardia and blood pressure lability, but malignant arrhythmias and cardiac arrest may occur.

DIAGNOSTIC TESTS & INTERPRETATION
Lab
Initial lab tests
- If syndrome is suspected early, then initial labs may be within normal limits.
- Most striking and common abnormality is an elevated creatine kinase (some reports >100,000 IU/L).
- Other markers of liver damage, such as transaminases and lactate dehydrogenase, may be elevated.
- Common electrolyte abnormalities include hypo/hypernatremia, hyperkalemia, hypocalcemia, hypomagnesemia, and metabolic acidosis.
- Acute renal failure may also occur in the setting of volume depletion and rhabdomyolysis.

Follow-Up & Special Considerations
No diagnostic test is available for NMS; rather, the diagnosis is a clinical one.

Imaging
Radiological studies may be used to rule out other disorders.

Diagnostic Procedures/Other
- No specific diagnostic procedure is needed/available for diagnosis.
- Other procedures such as lumbar puncture, electroencephalogram, etc., may need to be performed to rule out other disorders.

DIFFERENTIAL DIAGNOSIS
- Serotonin syndrome
- Malignant catatonia
- Malignant hyperthermia
- Drug withdrawal (ETOH, opiate, baclofen)
- Drug intoxication (PCP, cocaine, ecstasy)
- Thyrotoxicosis
- Heat stroke
- Meningitis/encephalitis

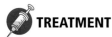

TREATMENT

MEDICATION

First Line
- Most important step is removal of suspected offending drug.
- No randomized trials to suggest any medications are beneficial for treatment:
  - Numerous case reports noting benefits of pharmacological treatments.
  - One recent review of 271 case reports noted increased mortality with dantrolene use and increased recovery time with use of dantrolene and other dopamine agonist (2)[C].

Second Line
- Suggested that treatment regimens should last for 10 days (1)[C]
- Dantrolene:
  - 2–3 mg/kg/d IV or 50–200 mg/d PO (1)[C]
- Bromocriptine:
  - 2.5–10 mg PO q6h (1)[C]

ADDITIONAL TREATMENT

Additional Therapies
- Mild doses of benzodiazepines (lorazepam 1–2 mg q4–6h) may improve symptoms and speed recovery (3)[C].
- Electroconvulsive therapy has been tried in small series with improved efficacy and decreased mortality (3,4)[C].
- In Parkinson patients with acute dopaminergic withdrawal, methylprednisolone (1000 mg for 3 days) decreased duration of illness and improved symptoms and laboratory values (5)[C].

IN-PATIENT CONSIDERATIONS

Initial Stabilization
- Should include basic ABC assessment
- Patients may present with respiratory failure or cardiac arrhythmias; treatment is supportive.
- Further stabilization includes correction of volume deficits and any major electrolyte abnormalities.
- Some experts suggest early intubation in patients who are unable to protect their airway or in those developing extreme rigidity.

Admission Criteria
- Most cases of suspected NMS should be monitored as an inpatient with a minimum of continuous cardiac monitoring.
- Many experts recommend critical care monitoring for any patient with progressive symptoms or lab abnormalities.

IV Fluids
- Aggressive volume resuscitation often is required secondary to volume deficit and continued ongoing losses (hyperthermia).
- May need to monitor for signs of volume overload in patients who develop renal failure, but volume overload on presentation is rare.

Nursing
- Frequent or continuous monitoring of heart rate, blood pressure, mental status, and respiratory status may be necessary.
- Frequent turning to prevent bedsores as patients are often too rigid to move or may be catatonic
- Aspiration precautions

Discharge Criteria
- Resolving electrolyte abnormalities and rhabdomyolysis that may be managed as an outpatient.
- Many patients are discharged to a psychiatric ward for further psychiatric evaluation/stabilization because medication changes are often necessary.

ONGOING CARE

FOLLOW-UP RECOMMENDATIONS
- Review of case reports of rechallenge with antipsychotics notes recurrence ranges ranging from 30–50%:
  - Increased with:
    - High-potency antipsychotics
    - High initial doses
    - Use of lithium
    - Decreased interval between NMS recovery and initiation of antipsychotic
- If reinitiation of antipsychotics is necessary, some suggest frequent follow-up to monitor symptoms, and creatine kinase levels should be monitored.

PATIENT EDUCATION
Patient and family members/caregivers should be warned of the possibility of recurrence of symptoms, along with the signs and symptoms of NMS.

PROGNOSIS
- If recognized early and offending drug removed, cases may be self-limited.
- Development of renal failure and further multiorgan failure are predictive of increased mortality.

COMPLICATIONS
- Renal failure
- Aspiration pneumonitis/pneumonia
- Venous thromboembolism
- Residual catatonia
- Persistent neurocognitive defects
- Multisystem organ failure; death

REFERENCES

1. Bhanushali MJ, et al. The evaluation and management of patients with neuroleptic malignant syndrome. *Neurol Clin N Am.* 2004;22:389–411.
2. Reulbach U, et al. Managing an effective treatment for neuroleptic malignant syndrome. *Critical Care.* 2007;11:1–6. http://ccforum.com/content/11/1/R4
3. Strawn JR, et al. Neuroleptic malignant syndrome. *Am J Psychiatry.* 2007;164:870–6.
4. Davis JM, et al. Electroconvulsive therapy in the treatment of the neuroleptic malignant syndrome. *Convulsive Ther.* 1991;7:111–20.
5. Sato Y, et al. Efficacy of methylprednisolone pulse therapy on neuroleptic malignant syndrome in Parkinson's disease. *J Neurol Neurosurg Psychiatry.* 2003;74:574–6.

ADDITIONAL READING

- http://www.ninds.nih.gov/disorders/neuroleptic_syndrome/neuroleptic_syndrome.htm

CODES

ICD9
333.92 Neuroleptic malignant syndrome

CLINICAL PEARLS

- Maintain a high clinical suspicion for NMS, as it can progress rapidly to death.
- The most common symptom is mental status change, with fever and rigidity also being common.
- More atypical presentations with lack of rigidity and/or normothermia have been reported, and therefore continued vigilance is required.
- Withdrawal of the offending drug and supportive care to prevent further complications are the most important aspect in these patients' care.

N

NONTHYROIDAL ILLNESS SYNDROME

Rodrigo Cavallazzi
Paul E. Marik

 BASICS

DESCRIPTION
- Nonthyroidal illness syndrome defines abnormalities in thyroid function tests that occur during starvation or in systemic nonthyroid illness.
- Nonthyroidal illness syndrome is also known as *euthyroid sick syndrome*.

EPIDEMIOLOGY
Incidence
Common disorder in critically ill patients
Prevalence
It has been reported in 44–75% of hospitalized patients.

RISK FACTORS
Severe illness and fasting
Genetics
It has been suggested that the paradoxically low or normal TSH observed in nonthyroidal illness syndrome may be caused by suppression of proTRH gene expression in the neurons of the hypothalamic paraventricular nucleus.

GENERAL PREVENTION
- Avoidance of drugs that impair thyroid function such as aspirin, phenytoin, carbamazepine, iodine, and dopamine.
- No specific measures are currently available to prevent nonthyroidal illness syndrome.

PATHOPHYSIOLOGY
Several factors contribute to the abnormalities seen in nonthyroidal illness syndrome:
- There is decreased conversion of T4 to T3 in extrathyroidal tissues due to diminished activity or concentration of iodothyronine 5'-monodeiodinase in tissues.
- Decreased serum albumin leads to alteration in serum binding of thyroid hormones.
- The decreased albumin level enhances the activity of compounds that are capable of displacing thyroid hormones from thyroid binding globulins.
- There is also evidence of cleavage of thyroxine-binding globulin by protease, which causes thyroxine-binding globulin to lose its T4 binding activity.
- There is reduced thyroid hormone output from the thyroid gland as a result of reduced hypothalamic mRNA for TRH.

ETIOLOGY
Etiology is multifactorial and changes according to specific diseases.

COMMONLY ASSOCIATED CONDITIONS
Fasting, critical illness in general, and specific disease states commonly associated with this disorder:
- Heart failure
- Renal disease
- Liver disease
- Psychiatric illness
- Burns
- Sepsis

DIAGNOSIS

HISTORY
- The diagnosis is suspected in a critically ill patient with abnormal thyroid function tests and no prior history of pituitary disease.
- In patients with abnormal thyroid function tests, history should focus on trying to identify a cause for the abnormality: Prior thyroid injury, goiter, drugs impairing thyroid function, and pituitary disorder.

PHYSICAL EXAM
- Inspection of the neck and thyroid palpation
- Common clinical exam findings of hypothyroidism are initially absent.
- Findings such as goiter or myxedema favor primary hypothyroidism rather than nonthyroidal illness syndrome.
- The hypermetabolic status of critical illness may mask hypothyroidism features such as bradycardia and weight gain.

DIAGNOSTIC TESTS & INTERPRETATION
Lab
Initial lab tests
- Initial lab tests include TSH, T4, free T4, T3, and cortisol level.
- Additional lab tests include reverse T3 (rT3) and cortisol levels.
- Low serum T3 is the most common abnormality.
- Serum rT3 is normal or elevated.
- An elevated serum rT3 level argues against the diagnosis of hypothyroidism.
- Serum T4 levels are reduced in proportion to the severity of the illness.

- TSH levels are usually normal or reduced but almost always inappropriately low for observed T3 and T4 levels (1)[C].
- Primary hypothyroidism is a strong possibility if TSH is above 25 μU/mL (2)[C].

Follow-Up & Special Considerations
- It is controversial whether patients with nonthyroidal illness syndrome become hypothyroid. However, if the illness is prolonged, there is evidence suggesting that they may become hypothyroid.
- It has been proposed that the changes in endocrine function seen during severe illness have a biphasic course.
- The 1st phase may represent an adaptive response of the organism, allowing reduced metabolic rate.
- The 2nd phase is likely to represent a maladaptive response since survival of critically ill patients is a relatively recent phenomenon.

Imaging
- There is no role for imaging in nonthyroidal illness syndrome.
- However, if there is suspicion of central hypopituitarism based on biochemistry, pituitary imaging should be performed.

Diagnostic Procedures/Other
- Serum cortisol level should be measured.
- Serum cortisol level tends to be elevated or high normal in nonthyroidal illness syndrome, whereas serum cortisol and gonadotropin levels are decreased in central hypothyroidism (2)[C].

DIFFERENTIAL DIAGNOSIS
- Primary hypothyroidism
- Secondary hypothyroidism
- Hyperthyroidism
- Thyroiditis
- Drug effects

TREATMENT

MEDICATION

First Line

- Thyroid hormone treatment in nonthyroidal illness syndrome is controversial.

- A few small randomized clinical trials have evaluated T3 repletion after CABG, and, while there was improvement in hemodynamic variables in some studies, there was no significant difference on perioperative morbidity and mortality (3)[B].
- A few clinical trials have evaluated either T3 or T4 repletion in critically ill patients. While most trials did not show a beneficial or harmful effect, 1 single trial showed increased mortality in a critically ill population with acute renal failure receiving T4 treatment (1,3)[B].
- Currently, treatment of nonthyroidal illness syndrome with thyroid hormone replacement or other medications cannot be routinely recommended (4)[B].

Second Line

- A clinical trial with a crossover design in 14 critically ill patients found that the GH-releasing peptide plus TRH combination reactivated the blunted GH and TSH secretion (5)[B].

- A placebo-controlled trial evaluated the effect of selenium supplementation on the thyroid hormone metabolism in critically ill trauma patients. Selenium was associated with earlier normalization with T4 and rT3.

ADDITIONAL TREATMENT

General Measures
- Treatment should be focused on the underlying critical illness.
- Avoid drugs that have important effects on thyroid function.

Additional Therapies
Special care should be given to the treatment of potentially associated adrenal insufficiency.

IN-PATIENT CONSIDERATIONS

Initial Stabilization
- Should include basic ABC assessment
- Avoid hypothermia
- Correct electrolyte disturbances

Admission Criteria
- Dictated by the underlying disease
- The presence of nonthyroidal illness syndrome per se does not indicate need for admission.
- However, it should be recognized that T4 levels below 4 mcg/d are associated with dismal prognosis.

Discharge Criteria
- In general, discharge criteria are not dictated by nonthyroidal illness syndrome. Rather, discharge depends on the resolution of the underlying critical illness.
- It is expected that, as the underlying disease improves, the thyroid function tests will normalize.

 ONGOING CARE

FOLLOW-UP RECOMMENDATIONS
It is recommended to monitor thyroid function tests during recovery.

Patient Monitoring
Patients should be monitored for clinical signs of hypothyroidism.

DIET
- Thyroid function is influenced by caloric content and dietary composition.
- Reduced carbohydrate intake causes decreased T3, increased rT3, and decreased thyroid globulin levels.

PATIENT EDUCATION
- Education for patient and family members should point out that nonthyroidal illness syndrome is a common condition in critically ill patients that does not typically require treatment because of absence of clinical hypothyroidism and lack of clinical benefit of studies evaluating thyroid hormone replacement.
- It should also be recognized that the presence of nonthyroidal illness syndrome may indicate that the underlying illness is severe.

PROGNOSIS
- It depends on the underlying critical illness.
- T4 levels $<4\ \mu g/dL$ and $<2\ \mu g/dL$ are associated with risk of death of 50% and 80%, respectively.

COMPLICATIONS
- Patients with prolonged nonthyroidal illness syndrome may become biochemically hypothyroid.
- Deleterious hemodynamic effects may develop as consequence of prolonged nonthyroidal illness syndrome.

REFERENCES
1. De Groot LJ. Non-thyroidal illness syndrome is a manifestation of hypothalamic-pituitary dysfunction, and in view of current evidence, should be treated with appropriate replacement therapies. *Crit Care Clin*. 2006;22(1):57–86, vi.
2. Chopra IJ. Clinical review 86: Euthyroid sick syndrome: Is it a misnomer? *J Clin Endocrinol Metab*. 1997;82(2):329–34.
3. AdLer SM, Wartofsky L. The nonthyroidal illness syndrome. *Endocrinol Metab Clin North Am*. 2007;36(3):657–72, vi.
4. Berger MM, et al. Influence of selenium supplements on the post-traumatic alterations of the thyroid axis: A placebo-controlled trial. *Intensive Care Med*. 2001;27(1):91–100.
5. Van den Berghe G, et al. Reactivation of pituitary hormone release and metabolic improvement by infusion of growth hormone-releasing peptide and thyrotropin-releasing hormone in patients with protracted critical illness. *J Clin Endocrinol Metab*. 1999;84(4):1311–23.

ADDITIONAL READING
- Lechan RM. The dilemma of the nonthyroidal illness syndrome. *Acta Biomed*. 2008;79(3):165–71.

 CODES

ICD9
790.94 Euthyroid sick syndrome

CLINICAL PEARLS

- Nonthyroidal illness syndrome is generally characterized by low serum T3, normal or low free T4 and TSH, and elevated rT3 levels.
- TSH levels are usually normal or reduced but almost always inappropriately low for observed T3 and T4 levels.
- TSH is undetectable in <7% of patients with nonthyroidal illness syndrome. If TSH is below 0.1 μU/mL, hyperthyroidism is likely to be present.
- If a patient is treated with thyroid hormone replacement, IV T3 administration is preferred over T4 because of diminished activity or concentration of iodothyronine 5'-monodeiodinase in tissues.

N

NUTRITION, ENTERAL

Pierre Singer
Haim Shapiro

 BASICS

DESCRIPTION
Nutrition through a nasogastric, nasojejunal, or percutaneous endoscopic gastrostomy (PEG)

EPIDEMIOLOGY
Incidence
Between 40% and 85% of critically ill patients

GENERAL PREVENTION
Early use of enteral feeding, prevention of intestinal atrophy, and putting the patient in a semisitting position (30–45 degrees) to prevent aspirations

ETIOLOGY
Protein energy malnutrition in critically ill patients not able to eat orally or take supplements

COMMONLY ASSOCIATED CONDITIONS
- Mechanical ventilation through an endotracheal tube or a tracheostomy
- Multiple trauma without GI lesions, burns, pneumonia

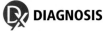 **DIAGNOSIS**

PHYSICAL EXAM
- Gastric residue <150 mL allows full enteral nutritional support. Gastric residue >500 mL or vomiting indicates that the patient should receive TPN after trying to feed through a nasojejunal tube.
- The position of the tube should be checked at every nurse shift and its permeability assessed as well.

DIAGNOSTIC TESTS & INTERPRETATION
Lab
Initial lab tests
CBC, SMA, INR, Ca^{++}, Phosphor, Mg, liver function tests

Follow-Up & Special Considerations
Daily SMA and Ca, P and Mg daily for the 1st 3 days, then twice a week for liver function tests, albumin, and total protein

Imaging
Initial approach
X-ray may be required according to various countries for nasogastric tubes but is mandatory in all the cases of jejunal tubes.

Follow-Up & Special Considerations
- Sinusitis should be suspected in case of fever.
- Caution for hypo/hypernatremia, kalemia, phosphatemia, magnesemia:
  – Hyperosmolar state
  – Elevated liver functions

Pathological Findings
Liver steatosis, hepatitis or cirrhosis

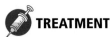 **TREATMENT**

MEDICATION
First Line
- Iso-osmotic polymeric formula
- For diabetic patients: Formulas low in carbohydrates and rich in fiber, monounsaturated fatty acids
- For patients suffering from ARDS and acute lung injury (ALI), a formula enriched in EPA and DHA

Second Line
Formula enriched in small peptides, MCT, and polychoses for patients with intestinal failure

ADDITIONAL TREATMENT

General Measures
- Prokinetics, such as metoproclamide or erythromycin to improve gastric emptying
- Nasojejunal tube if gastric residual volumes are too large.
- Glycemia control and insulin as required

COMPLEMENTARY & ALTERNATIVE THERAPIES
- TPN if energy requirements are not reached using enteral feeding.
- Calculate cumulative energy balance.

SURGERY/OTHER PROCEDURES
PEG if severe head trauma or CVA and chronically ill ventilated patient

IN-PATIENT CONSIDERATIONS

Initial Stabilization
- Required to meet calorie needs and administer essential amino acids, fatty acids, vitamins, and trace elements
- Dextrose required for the brain and the affected organs

Admission Criteria
All critically ill patients who do not eat and will not eat for the next 3 days and have a functional GI tract

IV Fluids
May be administered in addition:
- Water may be added in the enteral formula if required

Nursing
- Tube flushed every shift
- Gastric residue measured every shift

Discharge Criteria
- Stop enteral feeding if patient is able to eat orally.
- Stop if PN has to be administered.

 ## ONGOING CARE

FOLLOW-UP RECOMMENDATIONS
Assess enteral nutrition requirements every day.

Patient Monitoring
- Assess gastric residue
- Lab results

DIET
Assess ability to eat (intake)

PROGNOSIS
Able to provide the nutrients microelements and essential fatty acids

COMPLICATIONS
- Aspiration
- Intestinal ischemia
- Sinusitis
- Esophagitis
- Gastric erosion and perforation

ADDITIONAL READING

- ESPEN book: Basics in Clinical Nutrition
- Heyland, et al. Canadian guidelines. Retrieved from www.critcalcarenutrition.com
- Kreymann G, et al. ESPEN PN guidelines for EN. Clin Nutr. 2006 (in press).
- McClave SA, et al. Guidelines for the provision and administration of nutrition support therapy in the critically ill patient. *JPEN.* 2009;33:277–316.

 ### See Also (Topic, Algorithm, Electronic Media Element)

www.lll-nutrition.com

CODES

ICD9
- 260 Kwashiorkor
- 783.3 Feeding difficulties and mismanagement

CLINICAL PEARLS

- Avoid dextrose load and >350 g/d.
- The goal of PN is to provide energy and nutrients as required by the critically ill patient.
- Try to measure resting energy expenditure using indirect calorimetry. This will guide your prescription.
- Prevent refeeding syndrome by starting slowly and progressively parenteral nutrition in malnourished patients and by frequently measuring P, Mg, and Ca.

NUTRITION, PARENTERAL

Pierre Singer
Haim Shapiro

 BASICS

DESCRIPTION
Nutrition through a peripheral or a central venous catheter

EPIDEMIOLOGY
Incidence
Between 7% and 22% of critically ill patients

GENERAL PREVENTION
Early use of enteral feeding, preventing intestinal atrophy

ETIOLOGY
- Short-bowel syndrome
- Ileus
- Gastric emptying disorders and inadequate enteral calorie intake

COMMONLY ASSOCIATED CONDITIONS
- Severe sepsis requiring vasopressors
- Large administration of opiates
- GI surgery
- Pancreatitis:
  - Severe diarrhea

 DIAGNOSIS

DIAGNOSTIC TESTS & INTERPRETATION
Lab
Initial lab tests
CBC, SMA, INR, Ca^{++}, phosphorus (P), Mg, liver function tests
Follow-Up & Special Considerations
- Daily SMA and Ca, P, and Mg daily for the 1st 3 days, then twice a week for liver function tests
- Albumin and total protein

Imaging
Initial approach
Chest x-ray after central venous approach or PICC line
Follow-Up & Special Considerations
- Infectious to diagnose catheter-induced sepsis
- Caution for hypo/hyper natremia, kalemia, phosphatemia, magnesemia:
  - Hyperosmolar state
  - Elevated liver function

Pathological Findings
Liver steatosis, hepatitis, or cirrhosis

 TREATMENT

MEDICATION
- Dextrose 10% up to 70%
- IV fat emulsions including long-chain triglycerides or medium-chain triglycerides and fatty acids including saturated or mono/poly unsaturated fatty acids with double-chain starting at C3: Omega 3, or C6: omega 6, or C9: omega 9 fatty acids
- Amino acids, including the essential and nonessential amino acids, as well as (if required) alanyl-glutamyl dipeptide.

ADDITIONAL TREATMENT
General Measures
- Dedicated line
- Special dressing of the insertion site
- Glycemias repeated and insulin as required

IN-PATIENT CONSIDERATIONS

Initial Stabilization
- Meet caloric needs and administer essential amino acids, fatty acids, vitamins, and trace elements.
- Dextrose is required for the brain and the affected organs.

Admission Criteria
Not receiving enough via PO or enteral route for >48 hours, and will not eat normally within 10 days

IV Fluids
May be administered

Nursing
Dressing to be changed every 48 hours

Discharge Criteria
Stop PN if enteral or PO nutrition can meet the requirements:
- PN can be administered at home.

 ## ONGOING CARE

FOLLOW-UP RECOMMENDATIONS
Assess PN requirements every day.

Patient Monitoring
- Assess the dressing
- Lab results

DIET
Assess ability to eat (intake)

PATIENT EDUCATION
Home PN can be prescribed if the patient agrees and is competent.

PROGNOSIS
Can provide nutrients, microelements, and essential fatty acids

COMPLICATIONS
- Infections (MRSA, fungi, gram-negative)
- Liver function disturbances
- Hyperglycemia
- Hypertriglyceridemia

REFERENCES
1. Singer P, et al. ESPEN PN guidelines for PN. *Clin Nutr.* 2009 (in press)
2. Heyland, et al. Canadian guidelines. Accessed at www.critcalcarenutrition.com

ADDITIONAL READING
- *ESPEN Blue Book: Basics in Clinical Nutrition.* Geneva: ESPEN.

 ## See Also (Topic, Algorithm, Electronic Media Element)

www.lll-nutrition.com

 ## CODES

ICD9
- 560.9 Unspecified intestinal obstruction
- 579.3 Other and unspecified postsurgical nonabsorption
- 783.3 Feeding difficulties and mismanagement

CLINICAL PEARLS
- Avoid dextrose load and >350 g/d.
- The goal of PN is to provide energy and nutrients as required by critically ill patients.
- Try to measure resting energy expenditure using indirect calorimetry. This will guide your prescription.
- Prevent refeeding syndrome by starting PN slowly and progressively in malnourished patients and by frequently measuring P, Mg, and Ca.

N

NUTRITION, TOTAL PARENTERAL
Stephanie Whitener

 BASICS

DESCRIPTION
• When full nutritional support is not possible through enteral methods, intravenous delivery of nutrients can be used.
• The purpose of TPN is to provide the patient with nutritional requirements and appropriate amounts of protein, carbohydrates and fats to support metabolic needs.

EPIDEMIOLOGY
Prevalence
The prevalence of malnourishment is 30–50% for hospitalized patients; 40% of these patients arrive malnourished to the hospital.

RISK FACTORS
Dysfunction of the GI tract secondary to abdominal surgery, high-output enterocutaneous fistulas, malabsorptive states, and critical illness conditions. This can lead to poor nutritional status despite enteral intake.

GENERAL PREVENTION
Enteral feeding is always preferred over parenteral nutrition.

COMMONLY ASSOCIATED CONDITIONS
• Enterocutaneous fistulas
• Short bowel syndrome
• Patients with thermal injury who cannot tolerate enteral feeding
• Prolonged ileus
• Acute radiation and chemotherapy enteritis

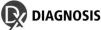 **DIAGNOSIS**

HISTORY
• Patients may describe a history of significant weight loss, inability to tolerate enteral feeding.
• Nature of the severity of the underlying disease should be assessed to determine if the patient is able to have enough nutritional intake to meet his/her metabolic needs.

PHYSICAL EXAM
• Weight loss of >10% usual body weight within 6 months or >5% within 1 month
• Cachexia as well as the presence of ascites or edema
• Skin changes and dry mucous membranes
• Poorly healing wounds
• Bruising or petechiae
• Wasting of musculoskeletal system, especially temporal muscles, deltoids, and suprascapular and infrascapular muscles.
• Physical signs of malnourishment do not manifest until an advanced state of deficiency has developed.

DIAGNOSTIC TESTS & INTERPRETATION
Lab
• Lower level of serum proteins such as serum albumin, prealbumin, and transferrin.
• C-reactive protein and alpha-1-acid glycoprotein

Diagnostic Procedures/Other
• Prognostic Nutritional Index (PNI) is a nutritional assessment tool that uses albumin and transferrin levels, triceps skinfold measurements and delayed hypersensitivity skin test reactivity to predict the risk of operative morbidity and mortality in relation to nutritional status.
• Prognostic Inflammatory and Nutritional Index uses markers of inflammation in combination with parametersof nutrition assessment to predict infectious complications and death

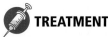 **TREATMENT**

ADDITIONAL TREATMENT
Issues for Referral
Nutritional support services can help to guide TPN ingredients for individual patient needs.

IN-PATIENT CONSIDERATIONS
Initial Stabilization
After assessment of nutritional status of the patient, and determination that TPN will be used as either a main source of nutrition or a supplement, the patient should have a central venous catheter placed to provide the route of administration for TPN.

Admission Criteria
Patients with critical illness and malnutrition can be admitted for optimization of nutrition.

IV Fluids
In order to avoid hypoglycemia, D5 or D10 infusions should be used for bridging whenever TPN dependent patients have their TPN stopped.

Nursing
• TPN ingredients are formulated daily.
• TPN is administered centrally via a central venous catheter, PICC line, or port-a-cath.

Discharge Criteria
TPN can be discontinued when the patient's nutritional status has improved or the underlying disease process has resolved or when the patient can receive nutrition through enteral feed.

ONGOING CARE

FOLLOW-UP RECOMMENDATIONS

Patient Monitoring

- Nutritional labs (albumin, prealbumin, electrolytes) should be monitored while patients are receiving TPN
- Continued assessment of the need for parenteral nutrition as well as the possibility of using enteral nutrition should be done while the patient is receiving TPN

DIET

- Standard TPN is made up of 500 mL of 10% amino acid and 500 mL of 50% dextrose with micronutrient repletion, electrolytes and trace elements.
  - 30–70% of total calories should come from glucose, 15–30% of total calories should come from fat and 5–10% of total calories should come from protein.
  - Electrolytes are added to TPN mixture.
  - Trace elements such as zinc, copper, chromium, manganese and selenium are also added.
  - Insulin can be added on a daily basis after assessment of the patients overall insulin requirement.

PROGNOSIS

There is a very strong association between malnutrition and postoperative morbidity and mortality in surgical patients.

COMPLICATIONS

- Most common complication is hyperglycemia
- Mechanical obstruction of the catheter delivering TPN
- Re-feeding syndrome (hypo-phosphatemia, hypokalemia and magnesemia with other clinical symptoms) may occur for patients who have not been consistently nourished for over 4-5 days prior to initiating TPN
- Infection—usually related to catheter used for carrier of TPN.
  - Catheter should be removed, infection should be treated and a new bag of TPN should be initiated.

REFERENCES

1. Martin K, et al. Assessing Appropriate Parenteral Nutrition Ordering Practices in Tertiary Care Medical Centers. *J Parenter Enteral Nutr*. 2011:35;122–30.
2. Kochever M, et al. ASPEN Statement of Parenteral Nutrition Standardization. *J Parenter Enteral Nutr*. 2007:31;441–48.
3. Heyland DK, et al. Total parenteral nutrition in the surgical patient: A meta-analysis. *Can J Surg*. 2001:44;102–11.

 CODES

ICD9

- 269.9 Unspecified nutritional deficiency
- 569.81 Fistula of intestine, excluding rectum and anus
- 579.9 Unspecified intestinal malabsorption

CLINICAL PEARLS

- Total parenteral nutrition is indicated for patients who have inadequate oral intake for >7–14 days because of nonfunctioning GI tract, intolerance to enteral feeding, inability to get enteral access or risk of enteral complications such as aspiration.
- TPN mixtures consist of amino acids, dextrose, fat solutions, micronutrients, and electrolytes in order to meet the patients' metabolic needs.
- Continual assessment of patient nutritional needs and adjustment of TPN composition is necessary in order to decrease the morbidity and mortality of malnourished patients.
- Hyperglycemia is the most common complication of TPN.

N

PACHYMENINIGITIS, HYPERTROPHIC CHRONIC

Patrick F. Walsh

BASICS

DESCRIPTION
- Localized or diffuse thickening of the dura matter, observed on T2 gadolinium-enhanced MRI images
- Headache and cranial nerve abnormalities are common:
  - Idiopathic, when no identifiable cause is found
  - Secondary dural thickening when identifiable causes co-exist; however, definite relationship is debatable

EPIDEMIOLOGY
Incidence
- Very low
- Age 36–80 years (most in 60s)
- Male = Female

Prevalence
- 65 cases reported in English literature during the past 8 years
- Literature consists of case reports only.

RISK FACTORS
- Idiopathic:
  - None
- Secondary:
  - Autoimmune disorders
  - Malignancy
  - Infection

Genetics
No genetic relationship suggested

GENERAL PREVENTION
- Can relapse when therapy discontinued. Seek medical attention if symptoms recur or worsen.
- May require additional immunosuppressants to prevent relapse or progression

PATHOPHYSIOLOGY
- Fibrous dural thickening at skull base may cause cranial nerve abnormality by:
  - Cranial nerve compression at foramen
  - Compromised blood flow to cranial nerve
  - Optic nerve compression in cavernous sinus may contribute to visual abnormalities.
- Intracranial involvement causes headache.
- Spine involvement may result in radiculomyelopathy.
- Involvement of cavernous sinus may result in thrombosis and its associated complications.

ETIOLOGY
- Idiopathic: Most likely results from an unknown autoimmune abnormality
- Secondary: Autoimmune, malignant, or infectious

COMMONLY ASSOCIATED CONDITIONS
Secondary coexisting conditions:
- Intracranial hypotension
- Malignancy:
  - Meningioma
  - Dural carcinomatosis
  - Lymphoma
  - Castleman disease
- Autoimmune/vasculitic disorders:
  - Wegener syndrome
  - RA
  - Sarcoid (neuro sarcoid)
  - Behçet disease
  - Polyarteritis
- Infection:
  - Syphilis
  - TB
  - Lyme disease
  - HTLV-1
  - Fungal
  - *Borrelia*
- Systemic fibrosing disorders:
  - Episcleritis
  - Sclerosing cholangitis
  - Mediastinal fibrosis
- Tolosa-Hunt syndrome

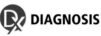

DIAGNOSIS

HISTORY
- Headache (HA) most common (95%):
  - HA worse at night and while recumbent
- Cranial nerve palsy (70%)
- Visual abnormality
- Blindness
- Gait ataxia
- Seizures
- Low grade fever

PHYSICAL EXAM
- Decreased visual acuity, blindness
- Weakness of facial muscles
- Decreased deep tendon reflexes
- Paresthesias
- Papilledema

DIAGNOSTIC TESTS & INTERPRETATION
Lab
- Diagnosis of exclusion
- ESR elevated in >50% of cases
- Important to eliminate other causes associated with secondary pachymeningitis
- MRI is study of choice.

Initial lab tests
Important to rule out other causes of dural thickening/enhancement on MRI:
- ANA, ANCA, RF, SS-A, SS-B, RNP
- Serum/immune electrophoresis
- ACE level
- Blood count, metabolic profile
- Studies for infectious etiology: CMV, HIV, HTLV-1, VDRL, TB, EBV, Borrelia, fungus, toxoplasmosis
- CSF for cell count, protein, glucose, cytology, PCR for viruses, Gram stain
- CSF culture for viral, bacterial, acid-fast, and fungal organisms

Imaging
Initial approach
- CT scan of head will show dural abnormality, but may miss tumors or lesions.
- MRI showing thick markedly hypointense pachymeninges on T2-weighted images with intense enhancement after administration of gadolinium is classic finding (1)[C]:
  - Pattern may be patchy or diffuse and commonly involves posterior fossa and skull base.
  - Spinal involvement is minimal, usually affects the cervical and high thoracic segments.
- Consider MRV for venous thrombosis.

Follow-Up & Special Considerations
Follow-up MRI imaging may correlate with clinical improvement in 1/2 of the cases.

Diagnostic Procedures/Other
- Dural biopsy:
  - Exclude neoplasia and infection
- Sample CSF
- EEG and nerve conduction studies depending on clinical context

Pathological Findings
- Thickened dense collagenous fibrosis with minimal cell infiltrate (1)[C]:
  - Some samples have lymphocytes or plasma cells.
- Granulomas, neoplasia, or infectious agents are consistent with secondary hypertrophic pachymeningitis.

DIFFERENTIAL DIAGNOSIS
- Intracranial hypotension
- Neoplasia
- Infection

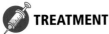 **TREATMENT**

MEDICATION

First Line
- Treat secondary underlying condition if present.
- No consensus in literature
- Steroids appear to be mainstay of treatment:
  - Dose equivalent to 1 mg/kg/d of prednisone
  - May consider pulse dose of methylprednisolone 1 g/d for 5 days prior to 1 mg/kg dose
- Duration:
  - Attempt to taper after 6–12 weeks.
  - If symptoms recur, stop taper and increase dose.
  - Some patients have completely stopped therapy with no relapse. Percentages vary according to small case reports

Second Line
- Methotrexate (2)[C]:
  - Used as steroid-sparing agents
  - Helpful in steroid refractory cases
- Azathioprine

ADDITIONAL TREATMENT

General Measures
- Mitigate side effects of steroids.
  - Calcium and vitamin D supplement
- Rule out TB before starting immunosuppressive therapy.
- Update immunizations.

Issues for Referral
- Neurology for seizure disorder
- Ophthalmology for visual disorders

Additional Therapies
- Physical therapy
- Rehabilitation facility

COMPLEMENTARY & ALTERNATIVE THERAPIES
None

SURGERY/OTHER PROCEDURES
Surgery on extremely rare occasion to relieve nerve root compression or elevated ICP

IN-PATIENT CONSIDERATIONS

Initial Stabilization
- Control seizure if present.
- Pain control for headache

Admission Criteria
- Inability for oral intake without aspiration
- Seizure disorder
- Intractable headache

IV Fluids
NS

Nursing
- Frequent neurochecks
- Pain control for headache

Discharge Criteria
- Acute problem resolving
- Will need specialized services for blindness and decreased visual acuity

 ONGOING CARE

FOLLOW-UP RECOMMENDATIONS
Care is provided on an outpatient basis.

Patient Monitoring
- Follow routine screening procedures appropriate for sex and age.
- Long-term side effects from steroids:
  - DEXA scans
  - Bisphosphonate therapy if needed
- End-organ damage from methotrexate:
  - Every 4–8 weeks, check CBC, UA, AST or ALT, creatinine
- End-organ damage from azathioprine:
  - CBC every 2 weeks with change in dose; every 1–3 months thereafter
  - Yearly ALT, creatinine, Pap smear
- Annual influenza vaccine if immunosuppressed

DIET
Low-fat, low-salt diet while on steroids:
- Monitor for weight gain

PATIENT EDUCATION
- Signs of myelosuppression:
  - Shortness of breath (SOB), nausea, vomiting, oral ulcers, fever
- Provide medication list to all physicians involved in your care.

PROGNOSIS
- From case studies ~30% recover with no need for further treatment (2)[C]:
  - Remainder have frequent relapses or remain on therapy indefinitely, some at lower doses.
- Visual acuity has improved in a few cases.

COMPLICATIONS
- Cerebral edema
- Worsening cranial nerve function
- Side effects of treatment

REFERENCES
1. Kupersmith MJ, et al. Idiopathic hypertrophic pachymeningitis. *Neurology.* 2004;62:686–94.
2. Bosman T, et al. Idiopathic hypertrophic cranial pachymeningitis treated with oral methotrexate: A case report and review of literature. *Rheumatol Int.* 2008;28:713–8.

ADDITIONAL READING
- Rudnik A, et al. Idiopathic hypertrophic pachymeningitis – case report and literature review. *Folia Neuropathol.* 2007;45:36–42.

 CODES

ICD9
322.9 Meningitis, unspecified

CLINICAL PEARLS
- Long history of headache and cranial nerves abnormalities with negative workup
- Thickened dura on imaging
- Think of chronic hypertrophic pachymeningitis.
- False-positive MRI enhancement of dura after lumbar puncture and CSF removal.

PANCREATITIS, ACUTE

Asaf Miller

 BASICS

DESCRIPTION
- Pancreatitis is an inflammatory disease of the pancreas that can be classified as acute or chronic.
- Acute pancreatitis is a rapidly developing process, usually associated with pain and alterations in exocrine function.
- It is a process that occurs in a gland that was morphologically and functionally normal before the attack, and it can resolve completely.
- It is usually a self-limiting disease from which the patient recovers without complication or intervention.
- However, it is potentially lethal, complicated by multisystem failure and sepsis that require intensive care and surgical debridement.

EPIDEMIOLOGY
Incidence
- The incidence of pancreatitis varies in different countries and depends on cause.
- Estimated incidence in the U.S. is 80/100000 per year.

ETIOLOGY
- Common causes:
  - Gallstones (30–60% of in most series)
  - Alcohol (15–30% in the U.S.)
  - Drugs: Azathioprine, thiazide diuretics, furosemide, methyldopa, isoniazid, valproic acid, estrogens, sulfonamides, tetracycline
  - Hypertriglyceridemia. Serum triglyceride levels are usually >1000 mg/dL
  - Endoscopic retrograde cholangiopancreatography (ERCP)
  - Trauma
  - Postoperative
- Uncommon causes:
  - Atheroembolic and hypoperfusion of pancreatic circulation.
  - Vasculitis and connective tissue disorders
  - Cancer of pancreas
  - Renal failure
  - Cystic fibrosis
  - Sphincter of Oddi dysfunction
  - Infections (cytomegalovirus, coxsackievirus, mumps, ascaris, Clonorchis)
  - Autoimmune pancreatitis
  - Hypercalcemia
  - Periampullary tumors
  - Perforated duodenal ulcer

DIAGNOSIS

HISTORY
- Abdominal pain typically is localized to the epigastrium and periumbilical region but can involve one or both upper quadrants. It can radiate to the chest, flanks, back, and lower abdomen. It is usually constant and worsens when the patient is supine.
- Relief can be obtained by sitting with flexed trunk and knees drawn upward. It may have a pleuritic component
- Nausea and vomiting
- Abdominal distention

PHYSICAL EXAM
- Diaphoresis
- Patients seem uncomfortable and anxious
- Low-grade fever
- Tachycardia and tachypnea
- Hypotension and shock due to hypovolemia and mediators that cause vasodilatation and increased permeability
- Abdominal tenderness with guarding; rebound can be present.
- Bowel sounds are diminished or absent.
- Abdominal distention
- Upper abdominal mass can be felt.
- Jaundice can be seen as a result of edema of the head of the pancreas, compressing the common bile duct.
- Green-brown discoloration of the flank (Turner's sign) and blue discoloration around the umbilicus (Cullen's sign) are seen in severe necrotizing pancreatitis.
- Unilateral (usually on the left side) or bilateral pleural effusion with pleuritic chest pain can be found.
- Atelectasis and rales at the lung base
- Erythematous subcutaneous fat nodules may occur

DIAGNOSTIC TESTS & INTERPRETATION
Lab
- General blood tests:
  - Leukocytosis
  - Metabolic acidosis
  - Hemoconcentration: elevated hemoglobin and hematocrit (>50%)
  - Elevated creatine and urea
  - Hypoalbuminemia (albumin <3 g/dL)
  - Hyperglycemia
  - Hypocalcemia
  - Hyperbilirubinemia
  - Elevated lactate dehydrogenase (>500 U/dL)
  - Hypertriglyceridemia
  - Hypoxemia may be an early sign for ARDS

- Specific blood tests:
  - Serum amylase:
    - Usually but not always elevated
    - There is no correlation between the degree of elevation to severity of pancreatitis.
    - After 72 hours, even in ongoing pancreatitis, amylase tends to return to normal.
    - There are other situations were amylase is elevated:
    - Pancreatic disease: Acute and chronic pancreatitis, pancreatic pseudocyst, abscess and necrosis, pancreatic trauma, and carcinoma
    - Nonpancreatic disorders: Renal failure, carcinoma of esophagus, ovary and lung, salivary gland disease (calculi, mumps etc.), macroamylasemia, pregnancy, DKA, intra-abdominal disease (peritonitis, perforation of peptic ulcer, aortic aneurism, intestinal obstruction), biliary disease.
- Other enzymes:
  - Lipase levels rise and tend to persist after serum amylase returns to normal.
  - Levels of other pancreatic enzymes (trypsinogen, chymotrypsinogen, elastase) can also be measured but have little role for clinical purpose.

Imaging
- Abdominal US is helpful in detecting gallbladder stones or bile duct dilatation. It can also detect pancreatic pseudocysts later in the course of the disease.
- CT is the modality of choice for diagnosis, severity and prognosis in acute pancreatitis. It should be used in patients with severe pancreatitis or suspected local complications.

DIFFERENTIAL DIAGNOSIS
Other diseases that cause abdominal pain, vomiting and tenderness. In some of these situations serum amylase is also elevated although to lesser extent than in pancreatitis, and CT shows normal appearing pancreas:
- Cholecystitis
- Cholangitis
- Perforated hollow viscus
- Mesenteric ischemia
- Bowel obstruction

TREATMENT

- In most patients, the disease is self-limited and subsides spontaneously within 1 week:
- Infected necrotizing pancreatitis:
  - Pancreatic necrosis is an area of nonviable pancreatic tissue that may be diffused or local.
  - Necrosis is present in 20–30% of patients, and has a mortality rate of up to 39%.
  - It is diagnosed by contrast-enhanced CT scan.
  - Infected pancreatitis is a diffused infection of an inflamed necrotic pancreas occurring in the first 2 weeks after the onset of pancreatitis.
  - Gram-negative intestinal bacteria and *Candida* are the most common pathogens.
  - Diagnosis of infected pancreas is done using CT-guided fine needle aspiration (FNA).
  - If the initial FNA is sterile, and fever and leukocytosis persist, reaspiration may be performed in a few days.
  - Antibiotic treatment is indicated but is inadequate as the sole treatment.
  - Unstable patients with infected necrotizing pancreatitis should be treated by surgical necrosectomy. Concomitant antibiotics should also be administered.
  - In stable patients, delaying surgery improves survival and decreases complication rate.
  - Recent trials suggest that percutaneous drainage with antibiotics is an acceptable option in the management of this population.
- Pancreatic pseudocyst and abscess:
  - Pseudocyst is a collection of pancreatic fluid, tissue, debris, and pancreatic enzyme that is enclosed by a wall of fibrous or granulation tissue without epithel. It is not usually present until after 4–6 weeks from the onset of pancreatitis. It can contain bacteria. When pus is present, the pseudocyst is called pancreatic abscess.
  - Pseudocysts can become symptomatic by causing abdominal pain or adjacent organ obstruction. They can also cause pancreatic duct obstruction.
  - A palpable mass may be found in the middle or left abdomen.
  - Amylase level is elevated in most cases.
  - US is useful in detecting pseudocyst.
  - Pseudocysts that do not cause symptoms can be watched, and many of them resolve spontaneously.
  - Stable patient with uncomplicated course (no hemorrhage, expansion, rupture, and infection) in whom serial US studies show pseudocyst shrinking are managed conservatively.
  - Otherwise, the pseudocyst should be drained by CT-guided aspiration or operation.

- Pancreatic ascites and pleural effusion:
  - Ascites is caused by disruption of the main pancreatic duct.
  - A clue to diagnosis is elevated serum amylase and an ascites fluid with high albumin levels (>30 g/L) and high levels of amylase (can be >20,000 U).
  - Treatment consists of NG suction, parenteral nutrition, and paracentesis.
  - Somatostatin inhibits pancreatic secretions.
  - If ascites accumulation continues after 3 weeks, surgical treatment consisting of main pancreatic duct stenting or operation should be considered.

ADDITIONAL TREATMENT
General Measures

- Analgesics: Meperidine rather than morphine is the narcotic drug of choice for gallstone pancreatitis because morphine contracts the sphincter of Oddi.
- IV fluids to maintain normal intravascular volume and electrolytes are essential in the early stages. They may halt disease progression.
- No oral alimentation for 3–5 days. Afterward, clear liquid diet and then normal feeding can be introduced. Nasojejunal feeding or parenteral nutrition may be used in severe protracted pancreatitis.
- NG suction is used by most clinicians to decrease of gastrin release as response to gastric contents from entering the duodenum. However, no proven advantage was shown.
- The use of prophylactic antibiotics is discouraged. Broad-spectrum antibiotics are recommended in infected necrotizing pancreatitis.
- Patient with severe pancreatitis should be admitted to ICU where careful monitoring is available.

ONGOING CARE

PROGNOSIS

- Most patients have a relatively mild, self-limited course that resolves with supportive treatment.
- 5–10% of patients have a severe attack associated with morbidity and mortality of approximately 40%.
- Clinical variables associated with worse prognosis are age >60 years, first attack of pancreatitis, obesity, postoperative pancreatitis, hypocalcemia.
- The Ranson and Imrie criteria are clinical and laboratory features available during the first 48 hours of diagnosis and useful in defining prognosis.
- Ranson criteria:
  - On admission: Age >55, WBC >16,000/mm^3, blood glucose >200 mg/dL, LDH >350 IU/L, AST >250 IU/L
  - During initial 48 hours: Hematocrit decrease >10%, BUN rise >5 mg/dL, serum Ca^{2+} <8 mg/dL, PO$_2$ <60 mm Hg, base deficit >4 mEq/L, fluid sequestration >6 L

- Imrie's criteria:
  - Age >55, WBC >15,000/mm^3, blood glucose >10 mmol/L, LDH >600 μg/L,
  - AST >100 μg/L, PO$_2$ <60 mm Hg, serum urea >16 mmol/L, Ca^{2+} <2 mmol/L, serum albumin <32 g/L
- The presence of <3 Ranson's or Imrie's criteria is associated with low morbidity and mortality, and the presence of ≥3 criteria is a sign of severe pancreatitis, with a high incidence of sepsis.
- APACHE 2 score is also useful as a prognostic marker in acute pancreatitis.

ADDITIONAL READING

- Bery AR, et al. Diagnostic tests and prognostic indicators in acute pancreatitis. *J R Coll Surg Edinb*. 1982;27:345.
- Buchler M, et al. Complications of acute pancreatitis and their management. *Curr Opin Gen Surg*. 1993; 1:282.
- Dervenis C, et al. Diagnosis, objective assessment of severity and management of acute pancreatitis. Santorini consensus conference. *Int J Pancreatol*. 1999;25:195.
- Freeny PC. Radiology of acute pancreatitis: Diagnosis, detection of complications, and interventional therapy. In Glazer G, Ranson JHC (eds.), *Acute Pancreatitis*. London: Bailliere Tindall, 1988; 275.
- Sarner M, et al. Classification of pancreatitis. *Gut*. 1984;25:756.
- Steer ML, et al. Where and how does pancreatitis begin? In Amman RW et al. (eds.), *Pancreatitis: Advances in Pathobiology Diagnosis and Treatment*. Falk Symposium 143. New York: Springer, 2005, 3–12.

 CODES

ICD9
- 577.0 Acute pancreatitis
- 577.1 Chronic pancreatitis

PARACENTESIS

Jose R. Yunen
Vicente San Martín

PROCEDURE

INDICATIONS

- Diagnostic: Determination of the etiology of ascites, diagnosis of infection in chronic ascites, diagnosis of intra-abdominal malignancy

- Therapeutic: Relief of respiratory distress due to ascites, decrease intra-abdominal pressure, and improve venous return

CONTRAINDICATIONS

- Coagulopathy
- Skin cellulitis over proposed incision site
- Pregnancy

- Acute abdominal process requiring surgical management
- Previous abdominal surgery with adhesions
- Distended bladder or bowel

TECHNIQUE

See algorithm.

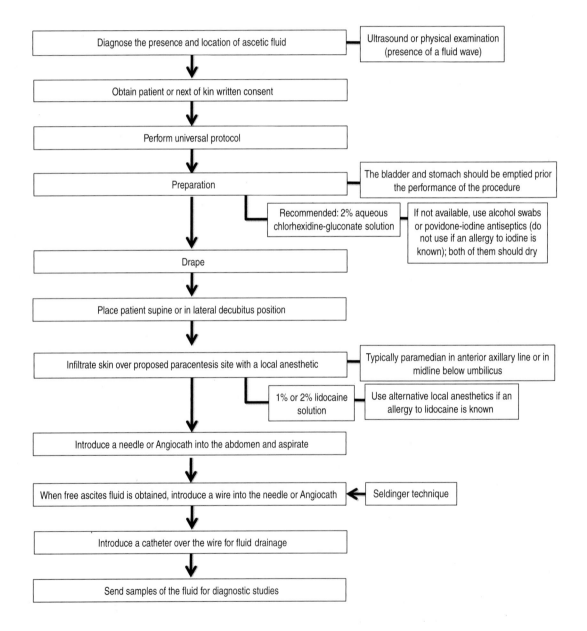

COMPLICATIONS
- Gastric or bowel perforation
- Peritonitis
- Intra-abdominal bleeding
- Postparacentesis hypotension

ADDITIONAL READING
- Thomsen T, et al. Paracentesis. *N Engl J Med*. 2006;355:e21.

P

PELVIC INFLAMMATORY DISEASE (PID) AND TUBO-OVARIAN ABSCESS (TOA)

Erika H. Banks

 BASICS

DESCRIPTION
- PID is an infection in the upper genital tract (uterus, fallopian tubes, and/or ovaries) originating from ascending spread of *Chlamydia trachomatis* (CT), *Neisseria gonorrhea* (GC), or other organisms colonizing cervix.
- Tubo-ovarian abscess (TOA) is an infection in the upper genital tract complicated by the collection of pus in an area created by adherence within the fallopian tubes and the ovaries.

Geriatric Considerations
PID should not occur in geriatric patients. If an abscess or infection occurs in a postmenopausal woman, suspect a gynecologic malignancy or a GI origin (diverticulitis).

Pregnancy Considerations
PID or TOA should not occur concomitant with a viable pregnancy after 12 weeks' gestation (unless after instrumentation or with IUD).

EPIDEMIOLOGY
Incidence
- 1 million cases of acute PID a year in the U.S.
- Annually, PID occurs in 1–2% of young, sexually active, reproductive age women a year in the U.S.

RISK FACTORS
- Younger menstruating women
- Multiple sexual partners (or partner with multiple partners)
- Correlated with low socioeconomic status
- Lack of barrier contraception
- History of PID
- Recent instrumentation (abortion, recent IUD placement, hysterosalpingogram)

Genetics
No genetic predisposition

GENERAL PREVENTION
- Abstinence, or monogamy with a tested monogamous partner
- Use of male latex condoms
- Screening for and early treatment of cervical colonization with CT and/or GC:
  - CDC recommends yearly chlamydia testing of all sexually active women ≤25.
  - Older women with risk factors for chlamydial infections (new sex partner or multiple sex partners)

PATHOPHYSIOLOGY
Ascending CT or GC cervical infection that causes a polymicrobial (aerobic and anaerobic) bacterial infection in the upper genital tract

ETIOLOGY
- 85% spontaneous in young sexually active females
- 15% following instrumentation

COMMONLY ASSOCIATED CONDITIONS
- TOA: A collection of pus in an area created by adherence of fallopian tubes, ovaries, and other pelvic organs
- Fitz-Hugh Curtis syndrome: Adhesions from liver edge to the anterior abdominal wall are evidence of perihepatic inflammation.

DIAGNOSIS (1)[C]

HISTORY
- Acute pelvic or lower abdominal pain
- Vaginal discharge
- Fever/chills

PHYSICAL EXAM
- Cervical motion tenderness
- Adnexal tenderness
- Fever
- Abdominal tenderness
- One of these 3 necessary for diagnosis:
  - Lower abdominal direct tenderness with or without rebound
  - Cervical motion tenderness
  - Adnexal tenderness
- Plus ≥1 of the following:
  - Oral temp >38.3°C
  - Gram stain of endocervix with gram-negative intracellular diplococci
  - Leukocytosis >10,000/mm^3
  - Purulent material from peritoneal cavity
  - Pelvic abscess on bimanual or sonography

DIAGNOSTIC TESTS & INTERPRETATION
Lab
Initial lab tests
- Cervical culture for GC and CT
- CBC shows leukocytosis (left shift)

Follow-Up & Special Considerations
- Baseline chemistries, liver function tests, coagulation profile, and serum lactate if evidence of sepsis
- Blood cultures prior to antibiotics for ill-appearing patient

Imaging
Initial approach
Pelvic (vaginal probe) US to rule out TOA
Follow-Up & Special Considerations
- If not responding to IV antibiotics, CT scan to evaluate for possible IR drainage
- Clinical improvement may take 72 hours, evidenced by resolution of abdominal pain, improved fevers, decreased WBC
- Patients who fail to demonstrate clinical improvement within 72 hours should undergo percutaneous drainage or surgical removal of TOA
- Clinical deterioration or development of an acute abdomen should prompt surgical intervention.

Diagnostic Procedures/Other
Diagnostic laparoscopy can be used to diagnose salpingitis if the presentation is atypical or the patient is unresponsive to initial treatment.

Pathological Findings
Purulent material in the peritoneal cavity

DIFFERENTIAL DIAGNOSIS
- Acute appendicitis
- Gastroenteritis
- Ectopic pregnancy
- Endometriosis
- Rupture or torsion of adnexal mass

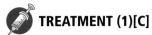 **TREATMENT (1)[C]**

MEDICATION
First Line
- Check CDC published recommendations as they are often updated as resistances develop.
- Oral therapy for outpatients or parenteral for inpatients
- Prompt initiation of 1st-line parenteral treatment (2010 CDC):
  - Cefotetan 2 g IV q12h *AND* doxycycline 100 mg PO or IV q12h
    OR
  - Cefoxitin 2 g IV q6h *AND* doxycycline 100 mg PO or IV q12h
    OR
  - Gentamicin 2 mg/kg load then 1.5 mg/kg q8h *AND* clindamycin 900 mg IV q8h:
    - This regimen is 1st-line for TOA but should *ADD* ampicillin for enterococcus coverage

Second Line
Ampicillin/Sulbactam 3 g IV q6h *AND* doxycycline 100 mg PO or IV q12h

ADDITIONAL TREATMENT

General Measures
- Initiate early goal-directed therapy for evidence of sepsis.
- Fluid resuscitation
- Hemodynamic, inotropic, and ventilatory support as indicated
- See Sepsis

Issues for Referral
- If unresponsive to IV antibiotics within 72 hours of treatment, consultation with:
  – Surgical team (gynecology)
  – Interventional radiology

Additional Therapies
Consider CT- or US-guided drainage if unresponsive and amenable

COMPLEMENTARY & ALTERNATIVE THERAPIES
None

SURGERY/OTHER PROCEDURES
- For sepsis unresponsive to IV antibiotics or rupture of TOA, proceed with laparotomy and extirpative surgery (generally TAH BSO).
- Surgery in the setting of PID/TOA can be difficult and morbid; therefore, it is used as a last resort.

IN-PATIENT CONSIDERATIONS

Initial Stabilization
Fluid resuscitation for febrile patients or those with nausea/vomiting

Admission Criteria
- Hospitalization to treat PID if woman is:
  – Severely ill (e.g., nausea, vomiting, or high fever)
  – Unresponsive to or unable to take PO antibiotics
  – Has an abscess in the adnexa (TOA)
  – Needs monitoring as PID not ruled in and to be sure that symptoms are not due to another condition that would require emergency surgery
  – HIV positive
- ICU admission for:
  – Hypotension not responsive to fluids
  – Vasoactive agents or inotropes required
  – Hypoxia, significant oxygen requirement
  – Mechanical ventilation
  – Invasive hemodynamic monitoring

IV Fluids
- Maintenance
- Replace losses if septic, febrile, vomiting

Nursing
- Vital signs and SaO$_2$
- Record I/Os
- Serial abdominal exams

Discharge Criteria
- Stable vital signs
- Adequate oxygenation
- Adequate urine output
- Normalization of laboratory parameters
- Improving pain

 ONGOING CARE

FOLLOW-UP RECOMMENDATIONS
Patient Monitoring
- Hospital discharge when afebrile with improvement of leukocytosis and resolution of pain
- Complete A 14-day course of antibiotics
- Short-term follow-up
- If TOA, follow-up US at 6 weeks

DIET
- NPO only if peritoneal signs, surgical abdomen or preoperative for surgical management
- Otherwise, regular diet

PATIENT EDUCATION
Condoms until both partners fully treated

PROGNOSIS
- If not recognized and treated in a timely fashion, PID can cause sepsis, septic shock, and death.
- Mortality rate for ruptured TOA is still 5–10%.
- 25% of patient with PID experience recurrence (younger women become reinfected twice as often as older women).

COMPLICATIONS
- Ectopic pregnancy (50% of ectopic pregnancies due to previous PID)
- Chronic pelvic pain (4-fold risk after a history of PID)
- Infertility (increases with recurrent infections)

REFERENCE
1. CDC. Updated recommended treatment regimes for gonococcal infections and associated conditions. U.S., April 2007.

ADDITIONAL READING
- Haggerty CL, et al. Newest approaches to treatment of pelvic inflammatory disease: A review of recent randomized clinical trials. *Clin Infect Dis*. 2007; 44:953–60.
- Lareau SM, et al. Pelvic inflammatory disease and tubo-ovarian abscess. *Infect Dis Clin N Am*. 2008; 22:693–708.

- McWilliams GDE, et al. Gynecologic emergencies. *Surg Clin N Am*. 2008;88:265–83.
- Trigg BG, et al. Sexually transmitted infections and pelvic inflammatory disease in women. *Med Clin N Am*. 2008;92:1083–111.
- Walter CK, et al. Antibiotic therapy for acute pelvic inflammatory disease: The 2006 Centers for Disease Control and Prevention Sexually Transmitted Diseases Treatment Guidelines. *Clin Infect Dis*. 2007;44(Supp 3):S111–S122.

 See Also (Topic, Algorithm, Electronic Media Element)

Sepsis

 CODES

ICD9
- 079.88 Other specified chlamydial infection
- 614.2 Salpingitis and oophoritis not specified as acute, subacute, or chronic
- 614.9 Unspecified inflammatory disease of female pelvic organs and tissues

CLINICAL PEARLS
- If not recognized and treated in a timely fashion, PID can cause sepsis, septic shock, and death.
- 1st-line treatment of PID and TOA is IV antibiotics and supportive care.
- Check current CDC recommendations for optimal antibiotic regimens as they are often updated due to resistance patterns.
- Patients who fail to demonstrate clinical improvement within 72 hours should undergo percutaneous drainage or surgical removal of TOA.
- Surgery in the setting of PID/TOA can be difficult; however, prompt surgical intervention should be initiated for:
  – Clinical deterioration
  – Development of an acute abdomen
  – Sepsis unresponsive to IV antibiotics
  – Rupture of TOA

P

PERICARDITIS
Hari Gnanasekeram

BASICS

DESCRIPTION
- Pericarditis is an inflammation of the layers of pericardium, with or without associated pericardial effusion.
- There is a broad spectrum of etiologies, but most common cases are viral or idiopathic.

EPIDEMIOLOGY
- ~ 1 per 1000 hospital admissions
- 1% of emergency room visits in patients with ST-segment elevation

RISK FACTORS
- Males > Females
- More common in adults than in children

Genetics
Unknown

PATHOPHYSIOLOGY
- Pericardium has an infiltration of polymorphonuclear (PMN) leukocytes and pericardial vascularization.
- Pericardium manifests a fibrinous reaction with exudates and adhesions.
- A serous or hemorrhagic effusion may develop.
- Granulomatous pericarditis occurs with tuberculosis, fungal infections, rheumatoid arthritis (RA), and sarcoidosis.

ETIOLOGY
- 26–86% of cases are idiopathic, mostly undiagnosed viral infections.
- Infection: Most common cause in 1–10% of cases.
- Viral etiologies include coxsackievirus B, echovirus, adenoviruses, influenza A and B, Enterovirus, mumps, Epstein-Barr, human immunodeficiency virus (HIV), herpes simplex type 1, Varicella-zoster, measles, parainfluenza type 2, and respiratory syncytial virus, cytomegalovirus, hepatitis A, B, and C.
- Bacteria account for 1–8% of cases and often cause purulent pericarditis.
- Organisms include gram-positive species such as *Streptococcus pneumoniae* and *Staphylococcus*.
- Gram-negative species include *Proteus, Escherichia coli, Pseudomonas, Klebsiella, Salmonella, Shigella, Neisseria meningitidis*, and *Haemophilus influenzae*.
- Tuberculosis

- Less commonly: *Legionella, Nocardia, Actinobacillus, Rickettsia, Borrelia burgdorferi* (Lyme borreliosis), *Listeria, Leptospira, Chlamydophila psittaci*, and *Treponema pallidum* (syphilis).
- Fungal etiologies include *Candida, histoplasmosis, Nocardia*, and *Aspergillus*
- Connective tissue disease: SLE, RA, scleroderma, acute rheumatic fever
- Drug-induced: Minoxidil, mesalamine hydralazine, bleomycin, phenytoin
- Malignancy: Most often hematologic, but may be metastasis to pericardium, or inflammation from contiguous tumor
- Uremia.
- Anticoagulant therapy
- Dissecting aortic aneurysm
- Diagnostic and surgical procedures causing postpericardiotomy syndrome
- Trauma
- Radiation
- Postmyocardial infarction (Dressler syndrome)
- Less commonly:
  - Gaucher disease
  - Pancreatitis
  - Myxedema
  - Parasites and protozoans

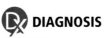

DIAGNOSIS

HISTORY
Preceding viral syndrome

PHYSICAL EXAM
- Pericardial friction rub is pathognomonic for acute pericarditis.
- Beck's triad (hypotension; elevated systemic venous pressure, jugular venous distention; muffled heart sounds) may occur in patients with cardiac tamponade.
- Pulsus paradoxus (defined as a >10 mm Hg decrease in arterial systolic pressure with inspiration)
- Tachypnea, tachycardia, and fever may be present.
- Arrhythmias occur in a minority of patients.

- S_3 may suggest myopericarditis.
- Signs and symptoms:
  - Generalized malaise and myalgias with fever
  - Chest pain is the cardinal symptom
  - Pain may be sharp, dull, aching, burning, or pressing. Usually precordial, and may have referral to the trapezius ridge.
  - Onset is usually sudden. Intensity varies, but may be severe. May be worse during inspiration, lying flat, during swallowing, and with body motion; may lessen when leaning forward.

DIAGNOSTIC TESTS & INTERPRETATION
Lab

- Elevated troponins (or creatine kinase) are commonly noted (1)[B].
- Increased ESR
- Elevated C-reactive protein with leukocytosis
- Tuberculosis and rheumatoid factor screen, ANA, and HIV serology may be helpful.
- Further viral serologies may be tested but are rarely helpful.

Imaging
- ECG:

  - Most common presentation is diffuse upward ST-segment elevation with PR-segment depression that may evolve through following 4 stages (1)[B]:

    o ST elevation with upright T waves in 90% cases
    o ST elevation normalizes over days.
    o Evolution to diffuse T wave inversions
    o Final normalization of ST-T wave changes
- Chest radiograph:
  - In initial stages, contributes little, but an enlarged cardiac silhouette suggests pericardial effusion.

- Echocardiogram:
  - Usually most helpful in the diagnosis of pericardial effusion and tamponade physiology (2)[B]
  - Pericardial thickening
  - Interventricular septal bounce
  - Abrupt cessation of diastolic expansion on M mode
  - Inspiratory rise and expiratory fall in tricuspid early diastolic, hepatic vein, and RV outflow velocities
- CT and MRI:
  - Inflamed pericardium with pericardial thickening >2 mm (>4 mm in 75% of cases).
  - Pericardial calcification up to 25% of cases (2)[B]

DIFFERENTIAL DIAGNOSIS
- Acute MI
- Aortic dissection with pericardial involvement
- Pulmonary embolism or pneumonia
- Pneumothorax
- Esophageal tear

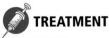

TREATMENT
MEDICATION
- Therapy is directed toward underlying disorder, with recovery expected within 14 days.
- NSAIDs are considered mainstay of therapy, with GI prophylaxis as appropriate (3)[B]:
  - Ibuprofen 300–800 mg q6–8h, as needed
  - Aspirin 500–1000 mg q6–8h can also be used (4)[B].
  - Colchicine (1–2 mg 1st day, with maintenance dose 0.5–1 mg/d) is effective for recurrences (3,5)[B].
  - Indomethacin 25–50 mg q6–8h can be used if others ineffective (3)[C]
  - Systemic prednisone treatment (1.5 mg/kg/d) can be used for recurrent symptoms, uremic or tuberculous pericarditis (3)[B]. Can be associated with increased rate of recurrence.

- Precautions:
  - Aspirin or NSAID allergy, history of gastritis or GI bleed.
  - ASA and NSAID can be used in 1st and 2nd trimester, not in 3rd (4).
  - Colchicine should be avoided in pregnancy (4).

ADDITIONAL TREATMENT
Issues for Referral
- Pericarditis with tamponade physiology requires referral for pericardiocentesis.
- Pericardiectomy for recurrent tamponade

IN-PATIENT CONSIDERATIONS
- Subacute onset with unstable hemodynamics and symptoms
- Recurrent severe pain
- Immunosuppressed state with fever >101°F.
- Failure to respond to NSAID therapy
- Cardiac tamponade with large pericardial effusion that does not resolve with medical therapy

ONGOING CARE
FOLLOW-UP RECOMMENDATIONS
Follow-up is rarely required unless symptoms recur or new symptoms develop.

Patient Monitoring
Can be followed on an outpatient basis symptomatically

DIET
Normal

PATIENT EDUCATION
Education for possible recurrent symptoms and to monitor alarm symptoms

PROGNOSIS
Complete resolution of symptoms usually within 2 weeks of therapy, especially after target treatment of underlying causative condition

COMPLICATIONS
- Recurrent pericarditis with underlying autoimmune process
- Cardiac tamponade
- Constrictive pericarditis; rare

REFERENCES
1. Newby L, et al. Troponins in pericarditis: Implications for diagnosis and management of chest pain patients.
2. Geoffrey C, et al. Management of constrictive pericarditis in the 21st century. *Curr T Options Cardiovasc Med*. 2007,9:436–42.
3. Brucato A, et al. Recurrent pericarditis: Infectious or autoimmune? *Autoimmun Rev*. 2008;8(1):44–7.
4. Brucato A, et al. Medical treatment of pericarditis during pregnancy. *Int J Cardiol*. 2009 Mar 25.
5. Imazio M, et al. Colchicine for pericarditis. *Eur Heart J*. 2009; 30(5):532–9.

CODES

ICD9
- 420.90 Acute pericarditis, unspecified
- 420.91 Acute idiopathic pericarditis
- 420.99 Other acute pericarditis

PERIPHERAL NEUROPATHY, CHEMOTHERAPY-INDUCED (CINP)

Zaid Said

BASICS

DESCRIPTION
- Peripheral neuropathy is a painful, common, and potentially dose-limiting side effect of treatment with several chemotherapeutic agents.
- CIPN is dose-related and cumulative and may be irreversible.

EPIDEMIOLOGY
Incidence
- Unknown
- Varies with the type of agent used, dose, duration of use, patient comorbidities, and other as-yet-unidentified risk factors.
- Incidence of peripheral neuropathy in some of the commonly used chemotherapeutic agents (1,2,3,4):
  - Paclitaxel: 56%
  - Docetaxel: 50%
  - Abraxane: 71%
  - Vinorelbine: 25%
  - Carboplatin: 4%

Prevalence
- Unknown
- Likely to rise dramatically as the number of neurotoxic agents increases and as patients live longer after diagnosis and treatment

RISK FACTORS
Comorbid conditions that appear to place patients at greater risk for CIPN include:
- Diabetes
- HIV
- Alcoholism
- Vitamin B deficiencies

Genetics
No known genetic pattern

PATHOPHYSIOLOGY
Neuropathy is caused by morphologic or functional abnormalities in peripheral nerves and is separated into:
- Axonopathy (axonal abnormalities)
- Myelinopathy (myelin sheath abnormalities) (5)

ETIOLOGY
Several chemotherapeutic agents can cause CIPN; the drugs most famously known to cause CIPN include:
- Taxanes: Paclitaxel (Taxol),
- docetaxel (Taxotere), and Abraxane
- Vinca alkaloids: Vincristine (Oncovin) and vinorelbine (Navelbine)
- Platinum-based chemotherapeutic agents: Cisplatin (Platinol), carboplatin (Paraplatin), oxaliplatin (Eloxatin)

COMMONLY ASSOCIATED CONDITIONS
- Different kinds of malignant tumors for which those medications are prescribed
- The risk increases in the presence of prior PN.

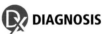

DIAGNOSIS

HISTORY
- Gradual onset
- Early symptoms are sensory
- Occurring in a stocking-glove distribution
- It starts distally then extending proximally with increasing cumulative dose
- Symptoms include:
  - Numbness, tingling and paraesthesias
  - Decrease touch perception
  - Burning/stabbing pain
  - Decrease proprioception
  - Difficulty ambulating with loss of deep tendon reflexes
- Motor component for the deficit including weakness of the distal muscles and usually a late presentation for the disease

PHYSICAL EXAM
- Decrease in the sensory functions (touch, vibration, and proprioception).
- Loss of deep tendon reflexes.
- In case of motor involvement, muscle weakness will be found.

DIAGNOSTIC TESTS & INTERPRETATION
Diagnostic Procedures/Other
- Electrophysiologic testing
- Nerve conduction study (NCS)
- Needle electromyography (EMG):
  - Axonal neuropathy is identified by NCS as a low compound muscle action potential and by needle EMG as fibrillation.
  - Pure demyelinating neuropathy is identified by NCS as slow conduction velocity and prolonged distal latencies and by needle EMG as no fibrillation or positive sharp wave activity (5).

Pathological Findings
Histologic exams of sural nerve or peroneal nerve from patients with taxane-induced neuropathy have identified:
- Axonal degeneration
- Reduced myelinated fiber density
- Loss of large fibers

DIFFERENTIAL DIAGNOSIS
Other causes of peripheral neuropathy

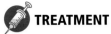

TREATMENT

MEDICATION

- Treatment is similar to that of non–cancer-related peripheral neuropathies.
- Relief of neuropathic pain using 10–50 mg of amitriptyline has been reported. Gabapentin 400 mg t.i.d. was also used to relieve severe myalgia (5).
- Neuroprotective agents:
  - Amifostine: May be particularly effective for prevention of peripheral neuropathy from platinum-based drugs. This drug was approved by the FDA for reducing renal toxicity during the administration of cisplatin and may also have neuroprotective properties (5).
  - Vitamin E: May reduce neurotoxicity, especially cisplatin-induced neurotoxicity. Utility had been proved in a randomized controlled study (6).
  - Glutamine may reduce the severity of peripheral neuropathy associated with high-dose paclitaxel. Studies are needed to validate its routine use for CIPN prevention (7,8).
  - Other agents can be helpful: Lamotrigine, BNP7787, AM424 (rhuLIF), but more data should be supplied (5).

COMPLEMENTARY & ALTERNATIVE THERAPIES

Physical and occupational therapy is very important to all patients with chronic peripheral neuropathies.

ONGOING CARE

PATIENT EDUCATION

- Education and counseling of the patient with chemotherapy-induced PN is very important since he or she could be experiencing a chronic long-term change of daily functioning.
- 2 areas that can directly impact this adjustment include physical and occupational therapy.

PROGNOSIS

- Most of the signs and symptoms will improve after treatment cessation or decreasing the dose.
- ~1/2 of the patients with PN by polyoxyethylated castor oil–based paclitaxel experienced the improvement of PN within 9 months after cessation of paclitaxel treatment (9).
- Patients on docetaxel who experienced neurotoxicity in clinical trials and for whom follow-up information on the complete resolution of the event was available had spontaneous reversal of symptoms with a median of 9 weeks from onset (range: 0–106 weeks) (2).

COMPLICATIONS

There is a great decrease in patients' function and daily activity.

REFERENCES

1. Abraxane Prescribing Information. Abraxis. Available at: http://www.fda.gov/cder/foi/label/2005/021660lbl.pdf. Accessed March 7, 2009.
2. Docetaxel Prescribing Information. Taxotere. Available at: http://www.fda.gov/cder/foi/label/2004/020449s028lbl.pdf. Accessed March 7, 2009.
3. Vinorelbine Drug Prescription. Navelbine. Available at: http://www.rxlist.com/navelbine-drug.htm.
4. Carboplatin Drug Prescription. Paraplatin. Available at: http://www.rxlist.com/paraplatin-drug.htm.
5. Lee JJ, Swain SM. Peripheral neuropathy induced by microtubule-stabilizing agents. *JCO*. 2006; 1633–42.
6. Argyriou AA, et al. Vitamin E for prophylaxis against chemotherapy-induced neuropathy: A randomized controlled trial. *Neurology*. 2005;64:26–31.
7. Vahdat L, et al. Reduction of paclitaxel-induced peripheral neuropathy with glutamine. *Clin Cancer Res*. 2001;7:1192–7.
8. Amara S. Oral glutamine for the prevention of chemotherapy-induced peripheral neuropathy. *Ann Pharmacother*. 2008;42(10):1481–5.
9. Postma TJ, et al. Paclitaxel-induced neuropathy. *Ann Oncol*. 1995;6:489–94.

ADDITIONAL READING

- Hensley ML, et al. American Society of Clinical Oncology clinical practice guidelines for the use of chemotherapy and radiotherapy protectants. *J Clin Oncol*. 1999;17:3333–55.

 # CODES

ICD9
357.6 Polyneuropathy due to drugs

PERITONITIS, SPONTANEOUS BACTERIAL

Amy Rezak
Rezak Askari

 BASICS

DESCRIPTION
Spontaneous bacterial peritonitis (SBP) is an acute infection of ascitic fluid without a clear source of contamination.

EPIDEMIOLOGY
Prevalence
In cirrhotic patients with ascites the prevalence has been reported to be approximately 10–30% (1).

RISK FACTORS
- Patients with cirrhotic or nephritic ascites
- Cirrhotic patients with gastrointestinal bleeding (up to 50% develop bacterial infections during hospitalization) (1).
- Previous SBP
- Recent instrumentation (endoscopy)

GENERAL PREVENTION
The administration of antibiotics has been shown to prevent recurrences in patients who have had SBP.

PATHOPHYSIOLOGY
- The pathophysiology remains unclear however, it is believed that bacteria (from bowel, urine, respiratory tract) may enter the circulation allowing hematogenous spread and this would ultimately colonize the ascites.
- Most typically a single organism is isolated.
- The most common organisms are: gram-negative bacilli such as Escherichia coli and gram positive organisms like streptococci and enterococci.

COMMONLY ASSOCIATED CONDITIONS
- Cirrhosis of the liver (most common)
- SBP also develops in patients with acute viral hepatitis, chronic active hepatitis, postnecrotic cirrhosis, metastatic malignant disease, congestive heart failure, systemic lupus erythematosus, lymphedema, but also in patients with no underlying disease.

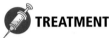 **DIAGNOSIS**

HISTORY
- Fever
- Abdominal pain, ileus
- Altered mental status
- Additional symptoms include diarrhea hypotension or hypothermia.

PHYSICAL EXAM
Peritoneal signs or diffuse abdominal pain may be present, however, their absence does not exclude the diagnosis of SBP.

DIAGNOSTIC TESTS & INTERPRETATION
Lab
- Elevated CBC,
- Check chemistry, LFTs, albumin, and blood cultures

Imaging
- CXR and Abdominal x-ray to rule out free intra-abdominal air.
- CT of abdomen with contrast to exclude intra-abdominal source.

Diagnostic Procedures/Other
- Paracentesis
- A polymorphonuclear (PMN) cell count of ascetic fluid >250 cells/mm^3 is diagnostic for SBP

DIFFERENTIAL DIAGNOSIS
- Secondary peritonitis (perforated viscus as a result of an ulcer, appendicitis, trauma or diverticulum)
- Portal hypertension
- Hepatitis

TREATMENT

MEDICATION
First Line
Third generation cephalosporins such as Cefotaxime for 5 days for patients (without Bacteremia)

Second Line
Ceftriaxone, Amoxicillin plus clavulanic acid, Ofloxacin.

COMPLEMENTARY & ALTERNATIVE THERAPIES
The use of intravenous albumin in cirrhotic patients with SPB has been shown to improve survival and decrease renal impairment (1).

IN-PATIENT CONSIDERATIONS
Initial Stabilization
- Obtain cultures, both blood and peritoneal
- Early empiric antibiotic coverage
- Repeat paracentesis may be performed after 2 days of initiating antibiotics and should demonstrate a reduction in PMN cell count.

Admission Criteria
Any patient with a history of cirrhosis and known ascites who develops fever, abdominal pain gastrointestinal bleeding. Intensive care maybe necessary if generalized sepsis ans septic shock develops.

IV Fluids
If the patient has an ileus or is unable to take PO, then maintenance IVF should be initiated

Discharge Criteria
Resolution of symptoms and completion of antibiotic therapy

 ## ONGOING CARE

FOLLOW-UP RECOMMENDATIONS
- Recurrence is common (up to 70% within one year); therefore antibiotic prophylaxis should be considered in patients who have had one or more episodes of SBP.
- Antibiotic prophylaxis is also recommended for cirrhotic patients with gastrointestinal bleeding. Recommended prophylaxis regimens include Norfloxacin, Ciprofloxacin or Bactrim.

Patient Monitoring
The patient should be monitored in an ICU setting if signs of peritonitis or sepsis are present

DIET
Salt restricted diet for patients with Cirrhosis and ascites.

PATIENT EDUCATION
Patients should be informed of their increased risk for developing a recurrence of SBP.

PROGNOSIS
The mortality of SBP is between 10–30%. The development of renal impairment is strongly associated with poor outcomes.

COMPLICATIONS
- Bacteremia
- Sepsis
- Hepatorenal Syndrome

REFERENCES

1. Parsi MA, Atreja A, Zein NN. 76. Spontaneous bacterial peritonitis: recent data on incidence and treatment. *Cleve Clin J Med*. 2004;71(7): 569–576.
2. Baron Miriam J, Kasper Dennis L, "Chapter 121. Intraabdominal Infections and Abscesses" (Chapter). Fauci AS, Braunwald E, Kasper DL, Hauser SL, Longo DL, Jameson JL, Loscalzo J: Harrison's Principles of Internal Medicine, 17e: http://www.accessmedicine.com.ezp-prod1. hul.harvard.edu/content.aspx?aID=2890287.
3. Warrell D, Cox T, Firth J, Benz E. (2003). *OXFORD TEXTBOOK OF MEDICINE* (4th). New York, NY; Oxford University Press. Retrieved May 31, 2011 from http://www.R2Library.com/marc_frame.aspx? ResourceID=107

 ## CODES

ICD9
- 567.23 Spontaneous bacterial peritonitis
- 571.6 Biliary cirrhosis
- 789.59 Other ascites

CLINICAL PEARLS

- More than 90% of SBP cases are monomicrobial
- Paracentesis should be performed to obtain a diagnosis
- Immediate antibiotic therapy should be initiated after cultures are obtained if SBP is suspected

PHEOCHROMOCYTOMA

Monvasi Pachinburavan
Paul E. Marik

 BASICS

DESCRIPTION
- Pheochromocytoma is a catecholamine-secreting neuroendocrine tumor that arises from the chromaffin cells of the adrenal medulla.
- Extraadrenal paragangliomas include extra-adrenal, catecholamine-producing, sympathetic paragangliomas, and parasympathetic paragangliomas that rarely produce catecholamines.
- Pheochromocytomas are termed malignant when there is evidence of invasion to adjacent organs or metastatic disease.

EPIDEMIOLOGY
Incidence
- 0.005–0.1% of the general population
- 0.1–0.2% of adult hypertensives

Prevalence
- 0.4% in patients with hypertension and symptoms suggestive of pheochromocytoma
- 4% in patients with incidentaloma

RISK FACTORS
- Patients with a history of familial pheochromocytoma
- Patients with a radiographically identified adrenal mass

Genetics
- 25% of pheochromocytomas are familial.
- Familial pheochromocytoma has been associated with germline mutation in 5 genes:
  - The VHL gene in von Hippel-Lindau disease
  - The NF1 gene in neurofibromatosis type 1
  - The RET gene in multiple endocrine neoplasia (MEN) type 2
  - Succinate dehydrogenase subunit B (SDHB) gene in familial paraganglioma syndrome
  - Succinate dehydrogenase subunit D (SDHD) gene in familial paraganglioma syndrome
- The SDHB gene is associated with an increased risk of malignant pheochromocytoma compared to SDHD.
- >90% of MEN type2 and VHL are benign. ~90% of NF1 are benign.

PATHOPHYSIOLOGY
The symptoms of pheochromocytoma are caused by excessive production and secretion of catecholamines by the chromaffin cells of the adrenal medulla.

ETIOLOGY
- Tumor of the chromaffin cells of the adrenal medulla
- 25% of cases may be associated with a germ line mutation.

COMMONLY ASSOCIATED CONDITIONS
- Von Hippel Lindau disease
- Neurofibromatosis type I
- MEN type 2
- Familial paraganglioma syndrome

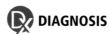 **DIAGNOSIS**

HISTORY
- Patients may have a family history of familial pheochromocytoma.
- Increased utilization of imaging studies has increased the incidence of adrenal incidentaloma found in asymptomatic patients.
- The presenting symptoms in pheochromocytoma are varied and can often be nonspecific:
  - Refractory or paroxysmal hypertension
  - Episodic headaches
  - Sweating
  - Tachycardia
  - Orthostatic hypotension
  - Blurred vision
  - Pallor
  - Flushing
  - Heat intolerance
  - Nausea
  - Abdominal pain
  - Glucose intolerance

PHYSICAL EXAM
- Tachycardia
- Paroxysmal hypertension
- Papilledema
- Abdominal mass

DIAGNOSTIC TESTS & INTERPRETATION
Lab
Initial lab tests
- Diagnosis of pheochromocytoma has 2 essential components: Demonstration of excessive catecholamine production and tumor localization.
- A 24-hour urinary measurement of fractionated metanephrine, catecholamines, and vanillylmandelic acid has been used as a gold standard for detecting excessive catecholamine production.
- Fractionated plasma free metanephrine is a less cumbersome alternative to 24-hour urine collection. This test also carries a high sensitivity and specificity; 99% and 89% respectively. It had been used more frequently as an initial screening tool for patients with high suspicion if pheochromocytoma.

Follow-Up & Special Considerations
Certain medications, such as tricyclic antidepressants, can interfere with measurement of urinary catecholamines.

Imaging
- Tumor localization determines the treatment of pheochromocytoma.
- A dedicated spiral CT scan with adrenal protocol using contrast can detect up to 0.5 cm masses with a sensitivity of ~95%.
- The MRI also has a sensitivity of ~90%. MRI has the advantage of no radiation exposure and better detection of vascular invasion.
- Both CT and MRI carry a relatively low specificity of 50–70%.
- I-MIBG scanning uses a SPECT scan. It can detect tumors in other parts of the body and metastasis. I-MIBG scanning carries a higher specificity of >95% but has lower sensitivity.
- PET scans have limited use in the evaluation of pheochromocytoma.

DIFFERENTIAL DIAGNOSIS
- For hypertension:
  - Essential hypertension
  - Renovascular hypertension
- For adrenal mass:
  - Adenoma
  - Metastatic disease

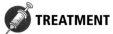

TREATMENT

MEDICATION
- α-Adrenergic blockade should be initiated prior to surgery.
- Phenoxybenzamine 10 mg b.i.d., titrated over 1–3 weeks to adequate blockade evidenced by orthostatic hypotension. Maximum dose 2 mg/kg/d.
- Selective α-1 blockers (prazosin, terazosin) can also be used.

ADDITIONAL TREATMENT
General Measures
- Patients with pheochromocytoma have long-term exposure to excessive catecholamines, leading to chronic vasoconstriction and volume contraction in addition to electrolyte abnormalities. Inadequate volume expansion may lead to BP lability in the intraoperative period.
- Patients should be aggressively resuscitated with fluids to ensure volume expansion prior to surgery. Electrolyte abnormalities should be corrected.

Issues for Referral
Surgery for pheochromocytoma should be performed by experienced surgeons and anesthesiologists.

Additional Therapies
- Surgical resection and debulking is the treatment of choice for pheochromocytoma.
- 2nd-line therapy for patients with unresectable and metastatic disease is I-MIBG therapy and combination chemotherapy with MIBG and CVD (cyclophosphamide, vincristine, and dacarbazine). Somatostatin analogs have also been used with limited success.

SURGERY/OTHER PROCEDURES
- Laparoscopy adrenalectomy remains the definitive treatment for pheochromocytoma. Surgical debulking is also used in advanced disease to lower catecholamine secretions. Surgery may cause release of catecholamines causing vasoconstriction leading to hypertensive crisis during surgery.
- Preoperative BP control with α-blockers and ensuring adequate intravascular volume are essential.

IN-PATIENT CONSIDERATIONS
Initial Stabilization
- BP control
- Judicious use of IV fluids to ensure volume expansion
- Correction of electrolyte imbalances
- Complete α-blockade prior to surgery

Admission Criteria
- Hypertensive urgencies and emergencies
- BP lability
- Electrolyte abnormalities requiring admission for correction

IV Fluids
Patients with pheochromocytoma have long-term exposure to excessive catecholamines leading to chronic vasoconstriction and volume contraction. Adequate volume expansion with aggressive fluid resuscitation is essential to preventing BP lability during the intraoperative and postoperative period.

Discharge Criteria
- Once BP is adequately controlled
- α-Blockade achieved
- After correction of electrolyte imbalances

ONGOING CARE

PATIENT EDUCATION
Patients should be given genetic counseling if familial pheochromocytoma is present.

PROGNOSIS
10-year survival for malignant pheochromocytoma is 40%.

ADDITIONAL READING

- Adler JT, et al. Pheochromocytoma: Current approaches and future directions. *Oncologist*. 2008;13:779–93.
- Mittendorf EA, et al. Pheochromocytoma: Advances in genetics, diagnosis, localization, and treatment. *Hematol Oncol Clin N Am*. 2007;21:509–25.
- Pacak K. Preoperative Management of the pheochromocytoma patient. *J Clin Endocrinol Metab*. 2007;92(11):4069–79.
- Scholz T, et al. Current treatment of malignant pheochromocytoma. *J Clin Endocrinol Metab*. 2007;92(4):1217–25.

CODES

ICD9
- 194.0 Malignant neoplasm of adrenal gland
- 227.0 Benign neoplasm of adrenal gland

CLINICAL PEARLS

Preoperative α-blockade and volume expansion are essential to prevent BP lability during surgery.

PLACENTA PREVIA

Pamela Tropper
Dena Goffman

 BASICS

DESCRIPTION
- Placental implantation over the internal os of the cervix
- Cervical dilatation, as with labor, causes the placenta to separate from the underlying tissue; massive bleeding may occur.

EPIDEMIOLOGY
Incidence
- 1 in 200
- Increasing incidence due to high cesarean delivery rates

RISK FACTORS
- Multiple gestation
- Previous uterine scar including prior cesarean deliveries
- Multiparity
- Advanced maternal age
- Smoking
- Fertility procedures including in vitro fertilization (IVF) and intracytoplasmic sperm injection (ICSI)

Genetics
No known genetic association

GENERAL PREVENTION
- Avoid unindicated cesarean delivery
- Smoking cessation prior to pregnancy

PATHOPHYSIOLOGY
- Complete previa: Placenta crosses the internal os. When the cervix dilates, hemorrhage ensues.
- Marginal previa: The placenta is adjacent to but does not cross the internal os.

ETIOLOGY
- Unknown
- Possible association with multiparity and multiple cesarean deliveries due to poor vascularity at sites of previous scarring

COMMONLY ASSOCIATED CONDITIONS
- Primary perinatal morbidity is secondary to prematurity (50% increase)
- Severe hemorrhage
- In the patient with a previous cesarean delivery, the presence of placenta previa greatly increases the risk of placenta accreta.

DIAGNOSIS (1,2)[B]

HISTORY
- Classic presentation is painless vaginal bleeding in the 3rd trimester.
- Prior bleeding in the pregnancy
- Postcoital bleeding

PHYSICAL EXAM

ALERT
- Do not do bimanual exam if placenta previa is suspected!
- Assess vital signs.
- Examine the patient for evidence of vaginal bleeding.
- Evaluate uterine tenderness and tone.
- Assess fetal presentation and heart rate.
- Determine gestational age.

DIAGNOSTIC TESTS & INTERPRETATION
Lab
Initial lab tests
- CBC
- Coagulation profile and fibrinogen
- Type and cross-match

Follow-Up & Special Considerations
- Coagulation profile in pregnancy differs from nonpregnant adults due to increases in multiple clotting factors: Fibrinogen is increased (680 mg/dL) and PTT decreased (24 seconds). Therefore, coagulopathy may be present at values different from nonpregnant adults.
- Transfusion should not be delayed in the presence of hemorrhage due to a normal hematocrit.
- RhoGAM should be given to nonsensitized Rh-negative mothers who are expectantly managed. Dosing should be determined by estimate of feto-maternal bleed by Kleihauer-Betke.

Imaging
Initial approach
- Diagnosis is made by vaginal US evaluating placental location in relation to the cervical os.
- Diagnosis of previa by abdominal US has a higher false-positive rate
- Sonographic confirmation of fetal gestational age and fetal lie

Follow-Up & Special Considerations
- In early pregnancy, placenta previa may be visualized by US.
- In the majority of these patients, the previa resolves spontaneously by the 3rd trimester.

Diagnostic Procedures/Other
- In the presence of placenta previa, especially in the presence of a scarred uterus, attention should be paid to the placental–uterine interface to rule out placenta accreta.
- MRI may be a useful adjunct to US in the evaluation of placenta accreta.

DIFFERENTIAL DIAGNOSIS
- Includes other sources of bleeding:
  - Placental abruption
  - Cervical or vaginal lesions/infection
  - Bloody show

TREATMENT (1,2)[B]

MEDICATION

- LR solution and/or Hespan until blood is available
- May need to use O-negative or type-specific uncross-matched blood if bleeding is profuse.

ADDITIONAL TREATMENT
General Measures
- Call for Help.
- 2 large-bore IVs
- Communication with anesthesia, nursing, operating room, interventional radiology
- Notify blood bank of potential need for blood and blood products.
- Blood loss may be significant.
- Maternal resuscitation should begin immediately while the diagnosis is being confirmed.
- Despite fetal status, the mother should be stabilized before any operative intervention.
- Depending on gestational age and condition of mother and fetus, there are 2 possible courses of management:
  – Expectant management if mother is stable, fetus is alive, and gestational age is early
  – Cesarean delivery if mother is unstable/hemorrhaging or there is fetal non reassuring status after the mother has been stabilized and the fetus is considered "viable" (i.e., with appropriate neonatal care the newborn is expected to survive)

Issues for Referral
- Maternal fetal medicine should be involved.
- Neonatology for resuscitation of the newborn
- Interventional radiology may be useful in cases where bleeding persists after delivery of the placenta but patient is stable and future fertility is desired.

SURGERY/OTHER PROCEDURES
- Due to its implantation in the lower uterine segment, bleeding may continue even after delivery of the placenta.
- The placenta may not separate easily due to invasion into the myometrium (placenta accreta).
- In either of these cases, techniques such as B-Lynch sutures, Bakri balloon tamponade, and other hemostatic mechanisms may be tried.
- Hysterectomy may be necessary and should be done in a timely fashion.

IN-PATIENT CONSIDERATIONS
Initial Stabilization
- Initial stabilization with fluid resuscitation
- Blood transfusion
- Correct coagulopathy

Admission Criteria
- Significant blood loss with change in vital signs
- Coagulation profile abnormalities
- Evidence of end-organ damage

IV Fluids
Appropriate maintenance and replacement of losses

Nursing
- q15min VS
- Monitor for evidence of vaginal bleeding.
- Monitor fundal height (should remain at level of umbilicus) a rising fundus may indicate bleeding into the uterine cavity.

Discharge Criteria
- Normal vital signs
- Stable hemoglobin/hematocrit x2
- Correction of coagulation abnormalities

 ONGOING CARE

FOLLOW-UP RECOMMENDATIONS
- Follow vital signs and urine output to be sure the patient is adequately hydrated and that blood transfusion has been adequate.
- 2-week follow-up in office to assess uterine size and bleeding

Patient Monitoring
Monitor vaginal bleeding; delayed PPH can occur.

DIET
Patients should be advised to eat iron-rich foods and supplements to maintain a normal hematocrit in anticipation of possible hemorrhage.

PATIENT EDUCATION
Recurrence risk of 4-8%

PROGNOSIS
The prognosis for placenta previa is generally good, although with a high incidence of prematurity, risk of blood transfusion, and possibility of hysterectomy.

COMPLICATIONS
- If the patient has been hypotensive, she may develop Sheehan syndrome:
  – Postpartum pituitary necrosis can result in pan-hypopituitarism and adrenal crisis.
  – An early sign may be failure to lactate.
- End-organ damage including renal failure, liver damage, ARDS, consumptive coagulopathy, cardiac ischemia, is possible with significant hemorrhage.

REFERENCES

1. Neilson JP. Interventions for suspected placenta previa. *Cochrane Database of Syst Rev*. 2003;2. (Level B)
2. Sinha P, Kuruba N. Ante-partum haemorrhage: An update. *J Obstet Gynaecol*. 2008;28:377–81. (Level B)

ADDITIONAL READING

- Bhide A, Thilaganathan B. Recent advances in the management of placenta previa. *Curr Opin Obstet Gynecol*. 2004;16(6):447–51.
- Oyelese Y, Smulian JC. Placenta previa, placenta accreta, and vasa previa. *Obstet Gynecol*. 2006; 107(4):927–41.

 See Also (Topic, Algorithm, Electronic Media Element)

Postpartum Hemorrhage

CODES

ICD9
- 641.00 Placenta previa without hemorrhage, unspecified as to episode of care
- 641.10 Hemorrhage from placenta previa, unspecified as to episode of care
- 762.0 Placenta previa affecting fetus or newborn

CLINICAL PEARLS
- Hemorrhage from placenta previa can be profuse.
- Early aggressive maternal resuscitation with hydration and blood transfusion is indicated.
- Definitive treatment of hemorrhage from placenta previa is surgical.

PLACENTAL ABRUPTION

Pamela Tropper
Dena Goffman

 BASICS

DESCRIPTION
Separation of the placenta from the uterus prior to delivery of the fetus

EPIDEMIOLOGY
Incidence
1 in 100 pregnancies

RISK FACTORS
- Chronic hypertension
- Preeclampsia/eclampsia
- Smoking
- Cocaine
- Multiple gestation
- Increasing maternal age and parity
- Polyhydramnios
- Prior history of abruption
- Thrombophilia
- Procedures:
  – Amniocentesis
  – Amnio reduction
- Trauma
  – Domestic violence
  – Motor vehicle accident

Genetics
Some cases associated with inherited thrombophilia

GENERAL PREVENTION
- Avoidance of smoking, cocaine
- Use of seatbelts

PATHOPHYSIOLOGY
- Placental separation occurs prior to delivery of the fetus.
- Presentations:
  – Concealed: Blood remains behind the placenta, little or no vaginal bleeding
  – Asymptomatic: Incidental finding after delivery
  – Classic: Vaginal bleeding with uterine tetany often associated with fetal distress or stillbirth
  – Chronic abruption: Small abruption occurs but delivery delayed, risk of intrauterine growth restriction (IUGR)

ETIOLOGY
Unknown

COMMONLY ASSOCIATED CONDITIONS
- Hypovolemic shock
- DIC
- Placenta previa
- Prematurity
- Intrauterine growth restriction
- Preeclampsia
- Eclampsia

DIAGNOSIS (1,2)[C]

HISTORY
- Sudden onset of uterine pain, constant or worsening with contractions
- Usually, vaginal bleeding but may be absent
- Recent trauma or cocaine use
- Smoker

PHYSICAL EXAM
- Tetanic uterus:
  – Contractions may be present but uterus does not relax between contractions.
- Vaginal bleeding
- Fetal status
- Hypovolemic shock may be present out of proportion to visible blood loss.
- Bleeding from IV sites

DIAGNOSTIC TESTS & INTERPRETATION
Lab
Initial lab tests
- CBC
- Type and cross
- Coagulation profile
- Kleihauer-Betke
- Clotting may be assessed rapidly at the bedside by collecting blood in test tube; if clotting takes >5 minutes, a coagulation defect is likely.

Follow-Up & Special Considerations
- DIC present in 30%
- Resolves after delivery; however, may worsen for 24 hours postpartum
- Requires plasma, factors, packed red blood cells, platelets depending on clinical condition
- If patient is RH-negative, requires RhoGAM; dose to be based on Kleihauer-Betke test.
- Preeclampsia may be present and should be appropriately and simultaneously managed.

Imaging
Initial approach
US can confirm the diagnosis of placental abruption, but only seen in 25% of cases.

ALERT
Failure to identify abruption by sonogram does not rule it out.

Follow-Up & Special Considerations
If patient remains undelivered, follow-up with serial US to rule out IUGR

DIFFERENTIAL DIAGNOSIS
- Other sources of 3rd trimester bleeding and/or pain:
  – Placenta previa
  – Uterine rupture
  – Preterm labor
  – Nongynecologic source of abdominal pain

TREATMENT (1,2)[C]

MEDICATION
- LR and/or Hespan until blood is available
- May require O-negative or type-specific, not cross-matched blood

ADDITIONAL TREATMENT
General Measures
- Stabilize mother.
- Mode of delivery depends on fetal status and gestational age.
- If fetus has died or status is reassuring, vaginal delivery is appropriate.
- If there is nonreassuring fetal status or the mother cannot be stabilized, cesarean section is indicated.
- Use of tocolytics is contraindicated.

SURGERY/OTHER PROCEDURES
- Postpartum bleeding may requires correction of clotting factors.
- Hemostatic techniques, such as B-lynch, may be indicated.
- Hysterectomy may be required.

ALERT
Follow patient with DIC with minimal surgical intervention, correct coagulopathy.

IN-PATIENT CONSIDERATIONS
Initial Stabilization
- Aggressive fluid resuscitation
- Blood transfusion
- Correct coagulopathy

Admission Criteria
- Patient requiring ICU admission for placental abruption will likely be delivered.
- Significant blood loss with change in vital signs
- Coagulation profile abnormalities
- Evidence of end-organ damage

IV Fluids
Appropriate maintenance and replacement of losses

Nursing
- q15min VS
- Monitor for evidence of vaginal bleeding.
- Monitor fundal height (should remain at level of umbilicus); a rising fundus may indicate bleeding into the uterine cavity.

Discharge Criteria
- Normal vital signs
- Stable hemoglobin/hematocrit x2
- Correction of coagulation abnormalities

ONGOING CARE

FOLLOW-UP RECOMMENDATIONS
- Follow vital signs and urine output to be sure the patient is adequately hydrated and that blood transfusion has been adequate.
- 2-week follow-up in office

Patient Monitoring
- Follow hematocrit and coagulation profile.
- Give support and assist with bereavement in cases of fetal demise.
- Follow for signs of Sheehan syndrome.

DIET
Antepartum folate may decrease risk of placental abruption.

PATIENT EDUCATION
- Recurrence risk is ~10% after 1 episode.
- 25% recurrence after 2 prior abruptions

PROGNOSIS
- Abruptions range from small and partial to complete and catastrophic.
- Large placental abruptions can result in maternal and fetal morbidity and mortality.

COMPLICATIONS
- Stillbirth
- Couvelaire uterus (extravasation of blood into uterine wall)
- Sheehan syndrome if patient was hypotensive:
  – Postpartum pituitary necrosis can result in pan-hypopituitarism and adrenal crisis.
  – An early sign may be failure to lactate.
- End-organ damage, including renal failure, liver damage, ARDS, consumptive coagulopathy, cardiac ischemia, is possible with significant hemorrhage.

REFERENCES
1. McDonald SD, et al. Risk of fetal death associated with maternal drug dependence and placental abruption: A population-based study. *J Obstet Gynaecol Can: JOGC*. 2007;29(7):556–9.
2. Sinha P, et al. Antepartum haemorrhage, an update. *J Obstet Gynaecol*. 2008;28(4):377–81.

ADDITIONAL READING
- Oyelese Y, et al. Placental abruption. *Obstet Gynecol*. 2006;108(4):1005–16.
- De Santis M, et al. Inherited and acquired thrombophilia: Pregnancy outcome and treatment. *Reprod Tox*. 2006;22(2):227–33.
- Sakornbut E, et al. Late pregnancy bleeding. *Am Fam Physician*. 2007;75(8):1199–206.

CODES

ICD9
- 641.20 Premature separation of placenta, unspecified as to episode of care
- 641.21 Premature separation of placenta, with delivery
- 641.23 Premature separation of placenta, antepartum

CLINICAL PEARLS
- Couvelaire uterus appears mottled and poorly perfused. Surgical intervention is *not* warranted.
- Mark the uterine fundus on the maternal abdomen with a marker. Increasing fundal size suggests concealed abruption.

PLEURAL EFFUSION

Balaram Anandamurthy
Robert E. Siegel

 BASICS

DESCRIPTION
- Pleural effusion is defined as an abnormal collection of fluid in the pleural space (bordered by the parietal and visceral pleura).
- ~1.3 million cases are seen in the U.S. each year. Heart failure is the leading cause of effusion, with 500,000 cases per year

PATHOPHYSIOLOGY
- The pleural space normally contains a very thin amount of low-protein fluid with a pH of ~7.6; it is formed by the capillaries of pleural membranes and absorbed by the lymphatics.
- Interstitial spaces of the lung and the peritoneal cavity also contribute to some fluid through the pores in the diaphragm.
- Excess production or decreased absorption results in an effusion.
- Pleural fluid is characterized as either transudate or exudate based on protein, lactate dehydrogenase (LDH), and cholesterol content.
- Transudates result from an imbalance of hydrostatic or oncotic pressure.
- Exudates result primarily from infection, inflammation, or invasion of pleura.

ETIOLOGY
- Transudative effusions may be seen in:
  - Congestive heart failure (CHF)
  - Cirrhosis
  - Atelectasis
  - Pulmonary embolism
  - Nephrotic syndrome
  - Hypoalbuminemia
  - Peritoneal dialysis
  - Myxedema
  - Constrictive pericarditis
- Exudative effusions may be seen in:
  - Parapneumonic effusions
  - Cancer, commonly of the lung, breast, GI tract and lymphoma
  - Tuberculosis
  - Pulmonary embolism
  - Esophageal perforation
  - Sarcoidosis
  - Thoracic duct injury resulting in chylous effusion
  - Autoimmune disorders such as rheumatoid arthritis

COMMONLY ASSOCIATED CONDITIONS
- CHF
- Pneumonia
- Empyema
- Cirrhosis
- Malignancy
- Trauma
- CABG

DIAGNOSIS

HISTORY
- Progressive dyspnea
- Cough, often nonproductive
- Pleuritic chest pain
  - Lower extremity edema, PND, orthopnea in CHF
  - Shortness of breath and weight loss in cancer
  - Pleuritic chest pain and cough in tuberculosis
  - Fever, chest pain, and cough in bacterial pneumonia

PHYSICAL EXAM
- Physical signs are usually absent in small effusions.
- With fluid of ~300 mL, decreased movement on the affected side, absent breath sounds, egophony above the level of effusion, and decreased vocal and tactile fremitus
- Large amounts of fluid in the pleural space may result in deviation of the trachea and mediastinum to the opposite side, with absent or diminished breath sounds on the side of effusion.
- S_3 gallop, jugular venous distension, anasarca may be seen in CHF.
- Pleural friction rub suggests inflammation of the pleura.

DIAGNOSTIC TESTS & INTERPRETATION
Lab
Initial lab tests
- All new pleural effusions in the outpatient setting mandate diagnostic thoracentesis.
- Critically ill patients often develop transudative or sympathetic pleural effusions. The decision to tap depends on the clinical suspicion for infection, esophageal leaks, etc., or the size.
- Sympathetic pleural effusions are exudative and caused by disease adjacent to the pleura (e.g., after subdiaphragmatic surgery, peritonitis, pancreatitis).
- Pleural fluid specimen should be sent for pH, protein, LDH, glucose, cholesterol, cell count with differential, Gram stain, culture, and cytology where appropriate.
- It may be reasonable to order LDH and protein initially, and the other tests later if the effusion turns out to be an exudate.
- To differentiate transudative from exudative effusions, Light's criteria may be used: Exudates meet one or more of the below criteria
  - Pleural fluid protein-to-serum protein ratio >0.5
  - Pleural fluid LDH-to-serum LDH ratio >0.6
  - Pleural fluid LDH >2/3 the upper limits of the laboratory's normal serum LDH.

- Light's criteria have higher sensitivity but lower specificity to diagnose exudates.
- Alternately, pleural fluid cholesterol >45 mg/dL, in addition to LDH >0.45 X serum value or protein >2.9 g/dL may be used to identify exudates.
- Triglyceride >100 mg/mL may be seen in chylous effusion.
- All available tests may misclassify effusion if the values are near cutoff point.
- Low glucose (<60 mg/dL) with low pH (<7.2) is typically seen in:
  - Rheumatoid arthritis
  - Empyema
  - Tuberculosis
  - Malignant effusion
  - Esophageal perforation
- Adenosine deaminase (ADA) and interferon-γ or culture for acid-fast bacilli may be sent to aid in the diagnosis of tuberculosis.
- Pleural fluid amylase more than serum amylase is seen in pancreatitis, esophageal rupture, or malignancy.

Imaging
Initial approach
- Chest x-ray: PA, AP, and lateral decubitus views. Effusion classically appears as a homogeneous opacity with a meniscus. The sensitivity is based on the amount of fluid in the hemithorax:
  - 50 mL results in blunting of posterior costophrenic angle on a lateral film.
  - ~200 mL results in obscuring the costophrenic angle and appearance of a meniscus on posteroanterior film.
  - 500 mL of fluid results in obscuring of hemidiaphragm.
  - 2000–2500 mL results in opacification of the entire hemithorax.
  - Free-flowing effusions thicker than 1 cm are ideal for thoracentesis.
- US:
  - Useful for detection of both free and loculated effusion
  - Can be helpful in differentiating complex effusions
  - Can be helpful in performing thoracentesis or chest tube insertion
- CT scan:
  - Very sensitive for small amounts of effusion
  - Helps in the management of loculated or recurrent effusion
  - Helps in distinguishing empyema from lung abscess
  - Evaluation of lung parenchyma, which is obscured by effusion on chest film
  - Helps in chest tube placement
- CTA to rule out pulmonary embolism should be considered if etiology of effusion is not clear.

Follow-Up & Special Considerations

Clinical re-evaluation in 24–48 hours for improvement of symptoms or if thoracentesis was delayed initially

Diagnostic Procedures/Other

- ~25% of effusion etiology remains undiagnosed even after performing all the available tests.
- Thoracoscopy and pleural biopsy may be considered in select cases.

Pathological Findings

- Gross appearance:
  – May be bloody in chest trauma, thoracic surgery, cancer, or ruptured aortic aneurysm
  – Purulent fluid, cloudy, or frank pus suggests empyema.
  – Milky fluid suggests chylothorax.
- Cytology with atypical appearing cells suggests malignancy. Immunocytochemistry may be used for identifying the type of cancer.

DIFFERENTIAL DIAGNOSIS

- Heart failure
- Pancreatitis
- Cirrhosis
- Esophageal rupture, microperforation, or postsurgical anastomotic leak
- Superior vena cava syndrome
- Collagen vascular disease like lupus, rheumatoid arthritis
- Pneumonia
- Empyema
- Lung abscess
- Hemothorax
- Thoracic duct injury; chylothorax

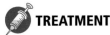 TREATMENT

MEDICATION

First Line

- Asymptomatic patients with uncomplicated heart failure or viral pleurisy can be observed with careful follow-up.
- Antibiotics: Empiric therapy is indicated in parapneumonic effusions, empyema, and esophageal microperforation or postsurgical leak.
- Diuretics in CHF and cirrhosis
- Anticoagulation for PE

Second Line

- Doxycycline, sterile talc, and bleomycin are useful sclerosing agents for pleurodesis.
- Intrapleural instillation of fibrinolytics for complicated parapneumonic effusions with poor chest tube drainage

ADDITIONAL TREATMENT

General Measures

- Should be individualized
- Based on the underlying etiology

Additional Therapies

- Thoracentesis is both diagnostic and therapeutic and also provides immediate relief of breathlessness:
  – The amount of fluid that needs to be drained is directed by the severity of symptoms and needs to be restricted to 1–1.5 L to prevent re-expansion pulmonary edema.
- Chest tube placement is indicated in empyema, hemothorax, or complicated effusions.
- Parapneumonic effusions are classified into 4 categories based on the amount and characteristics of the pleural fluid (3)[C]:
  – Category 1 (minimal, free-flowing effusion <10 mm on lateral decubitus) and category 2 (small-moderate effusion >10 mm and <1/2 hemithorax) may not need drainage procedures.
  – Category 3 (large, free-flowing effusions more than or equal to $1/2$ hemithorax, loculated effusions or effusions with thickened parietal pleura) and category 4 (pus) usually require drainage (chest tube/repeated therapeutic thoracentesis) or surgery.
- Malignant effusions (5)[B]:
  – Chest tube placement with sclerotherapy is successful in 60–90% of cases, but may need hospitalization for up to 1 week.
  – Long-term tunneled pleural drainage catheters can be performed on an outpatient basis and are effective in controlling symptoms in 80–100% of patients.
  – Both treatment options are of equal efficacy.

SURGERY/OTHER PROCEDURES

- Closed drainage and chest tube placement
- Video-assisted thoracoscopic surgery (VATS), open thoracotomy, and decortication may be considered as deemed necessary.

IN-PATIENT CONSIDERATIONS

Initial Stabilization

- Ensuring adequate oxygenation with supplemental oxygen
- Establishing good circulatory status and prevention of shock
- Sitting position to decrease the work of breathing.
- Therapeutic thoracentesis or chest tube insertion depending on suspected etiology or size
- Drainage of large pleural effusions may alleviate respiratory distress but response is variable.
- Large or massive simple (noninfected) pleural effusions are usually not the primary cause of respiratory failure or failure to wean.

IV Fluids

- Careful administration is warranted
- None in transudative effusions
- Goal-directed fluid resuscitation in hypotensive patients

 ONGOING CARE

PROGNOSIS

Depends on the underlying cause of the effusion; early diagnosis and prompt treatment improves clinical outcome, especially in empyema and hemothorax.

COMPLICATIONS

- Respiratory failure
- Trapped lung
- Empyema
- Pleural fibrosis
- Sepsis.

REFERENCES

1. Porcel JM, et al. Diagnostic approach to pleural effusion in adults. *Am Fam Physician*. 2006;73:7.
2. Blackwell C, et al. Pleural fluid volume estimation: A chest radiograph prediction rule. *Acad Radiol*. 1996;3:103–109.
3. Colice GL, et al. Medical and surgical treatment of parapneumonic effusions. *Chest*. 2000;118: 1158–71.
4. Light RW. Pleural effusion. *N Engl J Med*. 2002; 346(25):1971–7.
5. Spector S, et al. Management of malignant pleural effusion. *Semin Resp Crit Care Med*. 2008;29: 405–13.

ADDITIONAL READING

- Light R. Pleural disease. In Gibson PG, ed., *Evidence-based Respiratory Medicine* 2005. Hoboken NJ: Wiley-Blackwell, 2005:521–36.
- Medford A, et al. Pleural effusion. *Postgrad Med J*. 2005;81:702–10.

CODES

ICD9

- 428.0 Congestive heart failure, unspecified
- 511.81 Malignant pleural effusion
- 511.9 Unspecified pleural effusion

CLINICAL PEARLS

- Acute pulmonary embolism may result in either transudative or exudative effusion.
- Acute diuresis in CHF can raise pleural fluid protein to exudative grade.
- If pleural fluid analyses do not match the clinical picture, alternate diagnoses should be pursued.

PNEUMONIA, ACUTE EOSINOPHILIC

Jeff Marcus
Umesh Gidwani

 BASICS

DESCRIPTION
- Rare, idiopathic, acute-onset eosinophilic alveolitis that causes fever, dyspnea, and acute respiratory failure
- AEP occurs in the absence of infection, drugs, or other known causes of eosinophilic pneumonia
- Described very recently (1989) (1)
- Systems affected: Pulmonary

EPIDEMIOLOGY
Incidence
Incidence unknown:
- Highest incidence between 20 and 40 years (2)
- Male > Female (2:1) (3)

Prevalence
Extremely rare, probably <100 cases reported worldwide

RISK FACTORS
- Recent-onset smoking
- Environmental exposure: Dust, sand
- Drug inhalation: Cocaine, heroin
- Unusual outdoor activities (4):
  - Cave exploration
  - Plant repotting
  - Cleaning a smokehouse
  - Motor cross racing
  - Firework smoke inhalation

GENERAL PREVENTION
Avoidance of pathogenic inhaled antigens

PATHOPHYSIOLOGY
- A presumed inhalation of a toxic substance causes an extensive eosinophilic alveolitis due to a hypersensitivity reaction.
- Tissue pathology is related to the release of toxic eosinophilic products including:
  - Major basic protein, eosinophil cationic protein, and eosinophil-derived neurotoxin
- Tissue pathology may also be caused by the release of reactive oxygen species.

ETIOLOGY
- Unclear, but presumed hypersensitivity reaction to an inhaled agent as outlined above
- Temporal relation to onset of smoking

DIAGNOSIS

HISTORY
- Occurs in previously healthy individuals
- Inhalational exposure as listed above
- Febrile illness of <7 days
- Nonproductive cough
- Dyspnea
- Associated symptoms:
  - Malaise
  - Myalgias
  - Night sweats
  - Pleuritic chest pain

PHYSICAL EXAM
- Fever
- Tachypnea
- Bibasilar inspiratory crackles
- Hypoxemic respiratory failure
- Shock is very rare.

DIAGNOSTIC TESTS & INTERPRETATION
Lab
Initial lab tests
- CBC:
  - Initial neutrophilic leukocytosis
  - Eosinophil count rarely elevated

Follow-Up & Special Considerations
- Eosinophil count rises as disease progresses (5).
- IgE is elevated in the majority of patients
- Pulmonary function tests:
  - Rarely done; shows mild restrictive defect, reduced DLCO
  - Returns to normal after recovery (5)

Imaging
Initial approach
- Chest radiograph:
  - Bilateral alveolar and interstitial infiltrates (1,3,4)
  - Kerley B lines common
  - Pleural effusions in 50% of patients
- High-resolution chest CT:
  - Ground-glass and reticular opacities with air space consolidation, bilateral and patchy
  - Pleural effusions that are the last to resolve

Follow-Up & Special Considerations
Chest radiographs usually return to normal within 3 weeks (4,5).

Diagnostic Procedures/Other
- Bronchoscopy with BAL fluid (BALF) examination is the key to diagnosis:
  - BALF eosinophils >25% (4,5)
  - Elevated interleukin (IL-5); IL-1ra, vascular endothelial growth factor, and granulocyte macrophage colony stimulating factor are also elevated.

Pathological Findings
- Lung biopsy is only needed to exclude other diseases:
  - Acute and organizing diffuse alveolar damage (DAD)
  - Interstitial, alveolar, and bronchiolar infiltration with eosinophils
  - Severe extent of disease (>75% of tissue involved)
  - No granulomas or alveolar hemorrhage

DIFFERENTIAL DIAGNOSIS
Diagnosis of exclusion, so the following must be ruled out:
- Other causes of DAD (septic ARDS, hematopoietic stem-cell or solid organ transplantation, radiation damage, connective tissue disorders, etc.)
- Eosinophilic pneumonia caused by drugs (aspirin, ethambutol, penicillins, Bactrim, carbamazepine, etc.)
- Parasitic eosinophilic pneumonia (Löffler syndrome): *Ascaris, Strongyloides, Ancylostoma, Necator*
- Fungal eosinophilic pneumonia: Aspergillus, coccidioidomycosis
- Chronic eosinophilic pneumonia
- Other idiopathic interstitial pneumonias that cause acute respiratory failure (e.g., Hamman-Rich syndrome)

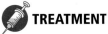

TREATMENT

MEDICATION

First Line

- IV corticosteroids: A common regimen is methylprednisolone 125 mg q6h until respiratory failure resolves
- Oral therapy may be initiated in the absence of respiratory failure
- Dramatic response, often within 12–48 hours

Second Line

Oral corticosteroids:

- Prednisone: 40–60 mg/d for 2–4 weeks beyond symptom resolution
- Taper prednisone course by 5 mg every week
- Relapse does not occur after stopping therapy

ADDITIONAL TREATMENT

General Measures

- There are no data on treatments other than corticosteroids.
- Many patients require full ventilator support.
- Some patients improve without corticosteroid therapy (5).

Issues for Referral

Patient with acute respiratory failure require intensive care (see chapter on ARDS).

IN-PATIENT CONSIDERATIONS

Initial Stabilization

- Airway management is essential in the setting of acute respiratory failure.
- Hemodynamic monitoring may be necessary, but shock is rare.

Admission Criteria

Patients without respiratory failure can be managed on a general medical floor.

IV Fluids

Standard fluid management in the setting of acute respiratory failure

Nursing

ICU-level nursing care in the setting of acute respiratory failure

Discharge Criteria

Recovery from respiratory failure after successful extubation

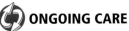

ONGOING CARE

FOLLOW-UP RECOMMENDATIONS

Avoidance of inciting airborne irritants listed above (including smoking)

Patient Monitoring

Outpatient tapering of corticosteroid therapy

DIET

No known necessary dietary restrictions or alterations

PATIENT EDUCATION

- Smoking cessation education if indicated
- Avoidance of dust, smoke, etc.

PROGNOSIS

- Recovery is rapid with appropriate therapy.
- There are no significant clinical sequelae after recovery.
- Death is exceptional.

COMPLICATIONS

Common complications from acute respiratory failure include:

- Ventilator-associated pneumonia
- Hospital-acquired pneumonia
- Delirium
- Complications from procedure (central line placement, intubation, etc.)

REFERENCES

1. Allen JN, et al. Acute eosinophilic pneumonia as a reversible cause of noninfectious respiratory failure. *N Engl J Med*. 1989;321:569.
2. Buchheit J, et al. Acute eosinophilic pneumonia and respiratory failure: A new syndrome? *Am Rev Respir Dis*. 1992;145:716.
3. Hayakawa H, et al. A clinical study of idiopathic eosinophilic pneumonia. *Chest*. 1994;105:1462.
4. Pope-Harman AL, et al. Acute eosinophilic pneumonia. A summary of 15 cases and review of the literature. *Medicine*. 1996;75:334.
5. Philit F, et al. Idiopathic acute eosinophilic pneumonia: A study of 22 patients. *Am J Respir Crit Care Med*. 2002;166:1235.

ADDITIONAL READING

- Allen J. Acute Eosinophilic pneumonia. *Semin Respir Crit Care Med*. 2006;27:142.

CODES

ICD9

518.3 Pulmonary eosinophilia

CLINICAL PEARLS

- AEP is a diagnosis of exclusion that requires an acute febrile illness, hypoxemic respiratory failure, diffuse pulmonary infiltrates, BAL eosinophilia >25%, lung biopsy with eosinophilic infiltrates, and absence of known causes of eosinophilic pneumonia.
- It is a rare and therefore poorly studied disease.
- The most recognized cause of AEP is new-onset smoking.
- Corticosteroids are the treatment of choice and should be tapered over 2–4 weeks.
- If patients fail to respond to corticosteroid therapy, an alternative diagnosis should be considered.
- Relapse does not occur after withdrawal of corticosteroids.

P

PNEUMONIA, ACUTE INTERSTITIAL

Umesh K. Gidwani

 BASICS

DESCRIPTION
- AIP is a rapidly progressive interstitial lung disease of unknown cause that has a high mortality.
- Also known as acute interstitial pneumonitis, Hamman-Rich syndrome, idiopathic ARDS

EPIDEMIOLOGY
Incidence
- The incidence of AIP is not known.
- Most patients are >40 years, and the mean age is ~50 years.
- Male = Female
- A syndrome similar to AIP was first described by Hamman and Rich.

Prevalence
The prevalence of AIP is unknown.

RISK FACTORS
- There are no established risk factors.
- Significantly, cigarette smoking is not a risk factor for AIP.

Genetics
No genetic links have been identified.

GENERAL PREVENTION
There are no proven risk factors and no known preventive strategies.

PATHOPHYSIOLOGY
- Widespread and diffuse damage to alveolar epithelium
- Diffuse distribution
- Rapidly progressive
- High mortality
- Differs from ARDS in that there is no identifiable cause

ETIOLOGY
The cause of AIP remains unknown.

DIAGNOSIS

HISTORY
The patient presents with severe exertional dyspnea that progresses rapidly within a few weeks. This may be preceded by a prodromal illness resembling a viral upper respiratory syndrome. Hypoxia and respiratory failure requiring mechanical ventilation ensue within a few weeks. Death can occur within 4–12 weeks.

PHYSICAL EXAM
- The patient is often tachypneic and hypoxic.
- Extensive bilateral crackles are heard on lung auscultation.
- Physical findings of lung consolidation may also be present.

DIAGNOSTIC TESTS & INTERPRETATION
Lab
Initial lab tests
ABGs:
- Moderate to severe hypoxia with a widened alveolar-arterial gradient

Follow-Up & Special Considerations
Pulmonary function tests:
- Restrictive pattern with low lung volumes
- Decreased diffusion capacity

Imaging
Initial approach
- Chest x-ray
- Progressive diffuse ground glass pattern +/- areas of consolidation

Follow-Up & Special Considerations
HRCT chest:
- Areas of "ground-glass" attenuation early in the exudative phase of the disease. Areas of consolidation are seen in the majority, but not all cases.
- Later in established cases, the areas of consolidation are replaced by ground-glass opacities. As the AIP organizes, there is distortion of the bronchovascular bundles and traction bronchiectasis.
- If the patient survives, the consolidation and ground-glass areas clear, and there are residual areas of hypoattenuation, lung cysts, and parenchymal distortion.

Diagnostic Procedures/Other
- BAL fluid shows RBCs and hemosiderin-laden macrophages reflecting alveolar hemorrhage.
- BAL fluid contains increased total cells, neutrophils, and occasionally lymphocytes
- Atypical pneumocytes and hyaline membrane fragments may be seen.
- Fiberoptic bronchoscopy with transbronchial biopsy OR open/video assisted lung biopsy to obtain tissue for histopathology

Pathological Findings
- Diffuse alveolar damage (DAD) is seen:
  - Temporally uniform changes that may reflect an episode of lung injury occurring at a single point of time
  - Diffuse alveolar septal thickening by fibroblast proliferation set in edematous stroma
  - Patchy airway organization and hyaline membrane formation
  - Presence of microthrombi within capillaries and small pulmonary arteries
- Differentiation from ARDS:
  - AIP is pathologically indistinguishable from ARDS.
  - DAD in the absence of an inciting cause is AIP (idiopathic ARDS).
- Differentiation from acute exacerbation of idiopathic pulmonary fibrosis (IPF):
  - In AIP, a temporally uniform DAD pattern is seen.
  - In acute exacerbation of IPF, there is DAD superimposed on the pathologic findings of usual interstitial pneumonitis (UIP), which include hyalinized collagenous fibrosis and honeycombing.

DIFFERENTIAL DIAGNOSIS
All causes of DAD:
- ARDS
- Accelerated worsening of UIP
- Collagen vascular disease
- Infections, especially *Pneumocystis carinii* and cytomegalovirus
- Acute eosinophilic pneumonia
- Drug-induced pneumonitis
- Hypersensitivity pneumonitis

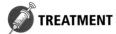

TREATMENT

MEDICATION

- The first line of the treatment of AIP is supportive care: Intubation, mechanical ventilation, and intensive care.
- There are no large-scale studies on drug treatment for AIP.
- Steroids: A trial of steroids, given in a high-dose, pulsed fashion over several months was shown to have some success in a retrospective chart review of 10 patients. These patients were admitted to the ICU, received lung biopsy early, and were started on 1 g/d IV methylprednisolone for 3 consecutive days followed by 1 mg/kg/d IV methylprednisolone or oral prednisolone for 4 weeks, with subsequent gradual tapering. The total duration of corticosteroid therapy in the survivors was 81 days (range, 28–126 days). 2 patients died within 32 days, 1 died at 75 months of pneumonia, and 7 survived past 78 months when the retrospective review period ended.

ADDITIONAL TREATMENT

General Measures

Supportive care including mechanical ventilatory support and attention to nutrition and prevention of complications

Additional Therapies

- Cyclophosphamide and cyclosporine have been used without much success.
- Inhaled nitric oxide and IV prostacyclin may be used to improve gas exchange in acute respiratory failure.

IN-PATIENT CONSIDERATIONS

Initial Stabilization

Intubation, mechanical ventilation, intensive care:

- Supportive care including attention to VTE, VAP, and stress ulcer prophylaxis; nutrition and blood glucose control
- A lung-protective strategy with low tidal volumes may be beneficial. In a randomized multicenter trial of 861 patients with ARDS on mechanical ventilation, 2 ventilatory strategies were compared. Traditional ventilation treatment, which involved an initial tidal volume of 12 mL/kg of predicted body weight and an airway pressure measured after a 0.5-second pause at the end of inspiration (plateau pressure) of $\leq$50 cm H_2O, was compared with ventilation with a lower tidal volume, which involved an initial tidal volume of 6 ml/kg of predicted body weight and a plateau pressure of $\leq$30 cm H_2O. A significant mortality benefit led to the trial being stopped early. Mortality was lower in the group treated with lower tidal volumes than in the group treated with traditional tidal volumes (31.0 vs. 39.8%, P = 0.007), and the number of days without ventilator use during the first 28 days after randomization was greater in this group (mean [$\pm$ SD], 12 $\pm$ 11 vs. 10 $\pm$ 11; P = 0.007).

Admission Criteria

Acute respiratory failure

IV Fluids

No particular strategy for fluid therapy in AIP has been studied, although lessons from the FACTT trial from the ARDSnet group may be applied here. In the FACTT trial, 1001 patients from 20 clinical centers who had acute lung injury (ALI) or ARDS were randomized to either conservative or liberal fluid management. No significant difference in 60-day mortality was observed between the 2 groups of patients. Patients who received conservative fluid management had improved lung function and shortened duration of mechanical ventilation and stay in the ICU, with no increase in nonpulmonary organ failure. Mortality at 60 days was 25% in the conservative group and 28% in the liberal group. Compared with patients in the liberal group, those in the conservative group showed improvements in oxygenation index and lung injury scores and had more ventilator-free days (14.6 vs. 12.1) and days out of the ICU (13.4 vs. 11.2) during the first 28 days. 10% of patients in the conservative group and 14% of patients in the liberal group experienced renal failure.

Nursing

ICU-level nursing care

Discharge Criteria

Recovery from respiratory failure

 ONGOING CARE

FOLLOW-UP RECOMMENDATIONS

Survivors may be left with residual lung parenchymal fibrosis.

Patient Monitoring

Periodic pulmonary function testing for survivors of AIP has not been studied.

PROGNOSIS

- Survival in AIP is worse than in ARDS, with a >50% mortality reported in the literature.
- Survivors may be left with residual lung parenchymal fibrosis.
- Recurrence of the disease in survivors has been reported.

COMPLICATIONS

- The common complications of acute respiratory failure are infections, stress ulcers, ventilator-associated pneumonia, and death.
- Survivors may have systemic complications, such as prolonged weakness and disability.
- There may be chronic respiratory insufficiency due to residual pulmonary fibrosis.

REFERENCES

1. Hamman L, et al. Fulminating diffuse interstitial fibrosis of the lungs. *Trans Am Clin Climatol Assoc.* 1935;51:154.
2. Hamman L , Rich AR. Acute diffuse interstitial fibrosis of the lungs. *Bull Johns Hopkins Hosp.* 1944;74:177.
3. Katzenstein AL, et al. Acute interstitial pneumonia. A clinicopathologic, ultrastructural, and cell kinetic study. *Am J Surg Pathol.* 1986;10:256–67.
4. Suh GY, et al. Early intervention can improve clinical outcome of acute interstitial pneumonia. *Chest.* 2006;129:753–61.
5. NIH/NHLBI ARDSnet. Ventilation with lower tidal volumes as compared with traditional tidal volumes for acute lung injury and the acute respiratory distress syndrome. *N Engl J Med.* 2000;342: 1301–8.
6. Weidemann HP, et al. Comparison of two fluid-management strategies in acute lung injury. *N Engl J Med.* 2006;354:2564–75.

ADDITIONAL READING

- American Thoracic Society/European Respiratory Society International Multidisciplinary Consensus Classification of the Idiopathic Interstitial Pneumonias. *Am J Respir Crit Care Med.* 2002; 165(2):277–304.

 CODES

ICD9
136.3 Pneumocystosis

CLINICAL PEARLS

- Rapidly progressive acute respiratory failure with a high mortality is common.
- API is caused by diffuse alveolar damage of unknown etiology.
- Mainstay of treatment is intubation, mechanical ventilation, and supportive care
- High-dose pulsed steroids may be helpful.
- Survivors may be left with residual lung parenchymal fibrosis.

PNEUMONIA, CRYPTOGENIC ORGANIZING

Sanjay Dhar
John Oropello

 BASICS

DESCRIPTION
- Characterized by endobronchial polypoid masses of fibroblastic tissue filling the lumens of terminal and respiratory bronchioles and extending in a continuous fashion into alveolar ducts and alveoli, representing an organizing pneumonia (1)[A]
- Clinico-radiological entity of unknown cause called cryptogenic organizing pneumonia (COP); also known as idiopathic bronchiolitis obliterans organizing pneumonia (BOOP)
- Flu-like illness, fever, bilateral crackles, increased ESR and patchy lung infiltrates are the usual presentation.
- A small percentage of patients may present with rapidly progressive BOOP with respiratory failure within 1–3 days of symptom onset.

PATHOPHYSIOLOGY
- Cryptogenic; cause is unknown.
- Organizing pneumonia is the pathological hallmark.
- Fibroinflammatory process in the lung
- Sequence: Alveolar injury, intra-alveolar clotting with deposition of fibrin, subsequent colonization with fibroblasts to produce a connective tissue matrix.

ETIOLOGY
When unknown, it is called cryptogenic organizing pneumonia.

COMMONLY ASSOCIATED CONDITIONS
- Most patients have idiopathic BOOP, but there are several known causes of BOOP, and several systemic disorders have BOOP as an associated primary pulmonary lesion.
- Immunosuppression-hematopoietic stem cell transplant, graft vs. host disease, liver transplant, renal transplant, non-Hodgkin lymphoma, malignancies in children, myelodysplastic syndrome, coronary artery bypass surgery, acquired immunodeficiency syndrome
- Radiation therapy (e.g., lung cancer, breast cancer)
- Infections: *Coxiella burnetii, Pseudomonas aeruginosa, Mycoplasma*, human herpesvirus 7, *Pneumocystis jiroveci*, influenza A virus, measles virus, parvovirus B19, human immunodeficiency virus (HIV), *Chlamydia* species, *Plasmodium vivax*,and *Plasmodium malariae*.
- Drugs: 5-aminosalicylic acid, acebutolol, amiodarone, amphotericin, bleomycin, busulphan, carbamazepine, cephalosporins, cocaine, doxorubicin, gold, interferon-α, interferon +: Cytosine, arabinoside, or ribavirin; interferon-β1a, L-tryptophan, methotrexate, minocycline, nitrofurantoin, paraquat, phenytoin, sotalol, sulfasalazine, tacrolimus, ticlopidine, vinbarbital-aprobarbital
- Connective tissue disorders: Rheumatoid arthritis, Sjögren syndrome, Behçet syndrome, SLE, antiphospholipid antibody syndrome, primary biliary cirrhosis, thyroiditis.
- Miscellaneous: Sarcoidosis, lung cancer, asthma, cystic fibrosis, idiopathic thrombocytopenic purpura, mixed cryoglobulinemia, sinusitis, menstruation, pregnancy

DIAGNOSIS

HISTORY
- Appears as subacute illness with duration of symptoms before diagnosis of about 2–6 months.
- Usual onset after viral illness
- Common symptoms: Cough (90%), dyspnea (80%), fever (60%), sputum expectoration, malaise, and weight loss (50%)
- Hemoptysis and chest pain are rare.
- No response to broad-spectrum antibiotics

PHYSICAL EXAM
- Fine crackles may be present at lung bases (75%).
- Clubbing is unusual.

DIAGNOSTIC TESTS & INTERPRETATION
Lab
Initial lab tests
- CBC: Leucocytosis with predominance of neutrophils
- ESR and CRP increased
- Resting alveolar arterial gradient widened
- Exercise-related hypoxemia

Follow-Up & Special Considerations
Bronchoalveolar lavage (BAL):
- Cytologic exam: Mixed cell pattern; increased lymphocytes 20–40%, neutrophils 10%, eosinophils 5%, foamy macrophages, occasionally mast cells and plasma cells.
- BAL may identify infections.
- CD4 to CD8 ratio in BAL is decreased.

Imaging
Initial approach
- Chest x-ray and CAT scan
- In immunocompetent patients, the CAT scan findings most commonly consist of multiple bilateral patchy air space opacities involving mainly subpleural and/or peribronchovascular regions.
  - In immunocompromised patients, findings are less characteristic, more commonly ground-glass attenuation or nodules.
  - Other findings described include diffuse interstitial opacities, mixed pattern of combined air space and interstitial opacities, bronchial wall thickening and dilatation, and focal lesions (2)[A].

Follow-Up & Special Considerations
Pulmonary function tests: Mild to moderate restrictive ventilatory defect.
- Smokers may exhibit an obstructive pattern.
- Carbon monoxide diffusing capacity is reduced.
- Resting or exercise-related hypoxemia

Diagnostic Procedures/Other
- Open lung biopsy
- Video-assisted thoracoscopic lung biopsy
- Transbronchial lung biopsy

Pathological Findings
- Lung biopsy specimens reveal intra-alveolar buds of granulation tissue consisting of fibroblasts and myoblasts.
- Organizing pneumonia is the most conspicuous feature of COP.

DIFFERENTIAL DIAGNOSIS
Primary pulmonary lymphomas, bronchoalveolar carcinomas, connective tissue disorders, radiation pneumonitis, idiopathic inflammatory myopathies, chronic interstitial pneumonias, usual interstitial pneumonias, hypogammaglobinemia:
- Every effort should be made to exclude an associated cause.

Geriatric Considerations
More commonly present with associated conditions

Pediatric Considerations
Associated with viral pneumonias (adenovirus) and hematological malignancies

Pregnancy Considerations
Has been reported to occur in pregnancy

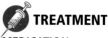 **TREATMENT**

MEDICATION
First Line
Corticosteroids are mainstay of treatment:

- Dosage generally is 1 mg/kg (60 mg/d) for 1–3 months, then 40 mg/d for 3 months, then 10–20 mg/d or every other day for a total of 1 year (3)[A].
- Duration of treatment varies usually between 6–12 months. A shorter course may be sufficient in certain situations.
- Clinical symptoms improve within 48 hours; radiological manifestations may take 4-6 weeks to resolve. Total and permanent recovery is seen in most patients somewhat dependent on the cause or associated condition (3)[A].

Second Line
- Cyclophosphamide, azathioprine, inhaled triamcinolone, macrolides have been used to treat BOOP (3,4)[B].
- Postinfection BOOP developing after bacterial agents (chlamydia, legionella, mycoplasma), viral agents (parainfluenza and adenovirus), parasitic agents (malaria), and fungal infections (*Cryptococcus neoformans* and *Pneumocystis jiroveci*) should be treated according to etiology of the causative agent.

ADDITIONAL TREATMENT
General Measures
- Symptoms should be controlled medically:
  - Hospitalization is warranted for unstable patients and invasive testing.
  - Severe hypoxemia, or need for ventilator support, or hemodynamically unstable patients must be managed in ICU.
  - Early pulmonary referral for BAL and definitive diagnosis by lung biopsy
- Standard bundle approach to prevent hospital-acquired infections
- Stress relaxation techniques may alleviate dyspnea/anxiety.

SURGERY/OTHER PROCEDURES
- Open lung biopsy:
  - BAL, transbronchial lung biopsy, percutaneous lung biopsy
- Clinical assessment at regular follow-up intervals, initially 2–4 weeks.
- Follow-up imaging to assess resolution of patchy alveolar infiltrates
- Patient monitoring may include:
  - Chest CT scan
  - BAL
  - Pulmonary function tests
  - Transbronchial lung biopsy
- Patient education on causative agents and associated conditions, avoidance of implicated drugs, paint aerosols, smoke inhalation, free-base cocaine:
  - Early recognition of complications
  - Compliance on treatment and follow-up visits

IN-PATIENT CONSIDERATIONS
Initial Stabilization
- Airway: Mechanical ventilation if clinically indicated may be the best initial step in stabilization.
- Breathing
- Circulation
- Monitoring-oxygenation, electrocardiogram

Admission Criteria
- Respiratory distress
- Hemodynamic instability
- Invasive diagnostic procedures

IV Fluids
- To maintain euvolemia/isotonic state
- Correct electrolyte abnormalities

 ONGOING CARE

DIET
- Aspiration precautions
- As tolerated

PROGNOSIS
- Good response to steroids in most patients
- Symptoms improve within 48 hours, although resolution of radiological pulmonary infiltrates takes several weeks.
- Symptoms may persist in 1/3.
- Frequent recurrence of symptoms after withdrawal of steroids, but usually respond to resumption of steroids with no adverse consequences
- May occasionally resolve spontaneously
- Factors associated with poor outcome include (5)[B]:
  - Interstitial pattern on imaging
  - Lack of lymphocytosis on BAL
  - Associated disorders
  - Scarring and remodeling of lung parenchyma in addition to organizing pneumonia.

COMPLICATIONS
- In presence of associated conditions, varies due to heterogeneity of disease:
- ARDS
- Ventilator-dependent respiratory failure
- In relation to procedures:
  - Pneumothorax
  - Bleeding
  - Infection
  - Lung collapse
  - Bronchopleural fistula

REFERENCES

1. Epler GR. Bronchiolitis obliterans organizing pneumonia. *Semin Respir Infect*. 1995;10(2): 65–77.
2. Lee KS. Cryptogenic organizing pneumonia: CT findings in 43 Patients. *Am J Roentgenol*. 1994; 162:543–6.
3. Epler GR. Bronchiolitis obliterans organizing pneumonia. *Arch Intern Med*. 2001;161:158–64.
4. Stover DE. A treatment alternative for bronchiolitis organizing pneumonia. *Chest*. 2008;128:3611–17.
5. Cordier JF. Organising pneumonia. *Thorax*. 2000;55:318–28.

ADDITIONAL READING

- Colby TV. Bronchiolitis pathologic considerations. *Am J Clin Pathol*. 1998;109(1):101–9.
- Epler GR, et al. Bronchiolitis obliterans organizing pneumonia. *N Engl J Med*. 1985;12(3):152–8.
- Epler GR. Bronchiolitis obliterans organizing pneumonia. *Arch Intern Med*. 2001;161(2):158–64.

 CODES

ICD9
516.8 Other specified alveolar and parietoalveolar pneumonopathies

CLINICAL PEARLS
- COP reflects inflammatory lung response to an initial injury of unknown cause.
- Organizing pneumonia is the hallmark of the disease.
- Identify determined cause or associated conditions.
- Rapid response to corticosteroids is noted.

PNEUMONIA, ICU

Devendra N. Amin

 BASICS

DESCRIPTION

- For the purpose of this chapter, pneumonia refers primarily to bacterial infection of the lower respiratory tract.
- Pneumonia requiring treatment in the ICU can have multiple etiologies.
- It is important to determine if it is a community-acquired pneumonia (CAP) or a health care-associated pneumonia (HCAP).
- Pneumonia developing in the ICU is a hospital-acquired pneumonia (HAP) and is defined as occurring ≥48 hours after admission.
- Ventilator-associated pneumonia (VAP) is defined as occurring >48–72 hours after intubation (1,2).

RISK FACTORS

- For multidrug-resistant (MDR) pathogens in HCAP patients:
  - Severe illness,
  - Prior broad-spectrum antibiotic (BSA) therapy
  - Poor functional status (2)
- Low risk for MDR pathogens: 1 risk factor
- High risk for MDR pathogens: 2 of 3 risk factors
- Modifiable risk factors:
  - Intubation and mechanical ventilation increases the risk of HAP/VAP 6–21-fold. Judicious use of noninvasive positive pressure ventilation (NIPPV) may reduce the need for intubation.
  - Orotracheal intubation is preferred to nasotracheal intubation to prevent sinusitis as a risk for VAP.
  - Once intubated, attempts must be instituted to prevent respiratory circuit condensate from draining back into the patient. Continuous aspiration of subglottic secretions can reduce the risk of VAP.
  - Minimizing sedation and using daily sedation vacation protocols with a daily weaning assessment help to accelerate weaning and extubation.
  - Daily oral care with chlorhexidine and maintaining the head of bed at 30 degrees of elevation or more unless contraindicated also reduces the incidence of VAP significantly.
  - Small bowel feeding is preferred to stomach feeding to reduce risk of gastric reflux and aspiration.
  - Although both H_2 blockers and proton pump inhibitors reduce the risk of upper GI bleeding in critically ill patients, both increase the risk of HAP/VAP.
  - Sucralfate has not been associated with a lower rate of VAP but a slightly higher rate of stress-related bleeding (2).

GENERAL PREVENTION

- Influenza vaccine
- Pneumococcal vaccine in appropriate groups

PATHOPHYSIOLOGY

- Bacterial pathogens in the lung produce a local inflammation, stimulating mucous hypersecretion; capillary leak can develop, producing alveolar and interstitial protein-rich edema. WBCs also enter the alveolar spaces and this combination results in consolidation. The loss of lung compliance and gas exchange worsens, producing hypoxia. Viral and mycoplasma pneumonias generally do not produce consolidation as infected alveolar walls do not exude into the alveolar spaces:
  - Worsening consolidation and bilateral involvement can result in hypoxic and hypercarbic respiratory failure that, in the presence of normal left-sided filling pressures and a PaO_2/FiO_2 ≤200 is defined as ARDS.
- HAP/VAP:
  - Early-onset HAP and VAP are defined as occurring within the 1st 4 days of hospitalization; these carry a better prognosis and are more likely to be caused by antibiotic-sensitive bacteria. Late-onset HAP and VAP (≥5 days) are more likely to be caused by MDR pathogens and are associated with increased patient mortality and morbidity. However, patients with early-onset HAP who have received prior antibiotics or who have had a prior hospitalization within the past 90 days are at greater risk for colonization and infection with MDR pathogens and should be treated similarly to patients with late-onset HAP or VAP (2).
- HAP, VAP, HCAP are caused by a wide spectrum of bacterial pathogens, may be polymicrobial, and are rarely due to viral or fungal pathogens in immunocompetent hosts. Common pathogens include aerobic gram-negative bacilli, such as *P. aeruginosa*, *Escherichia coli*, *Klebsiella pneumoniae*, and *Acinetobacter* spp. Infections due to gram-positive cocci, such as *Staphylococcus aureus*, particularly MRSA, have been rapidly emerging in the U.S. Pneumonia due to *S. aureus* is more common in patients with diabetes mellitus, head trauma, and those hospitalized in ICUs.
- The frequency of specific MDR pathogens causing HAP/VAP varies by ICU, hospital, patient population, exposure to antibiotics, type of ICU patient, and changes over time, thus emphasizing the need for timely, local surveillance data. HAP involving anaerobic organisms may follow aspiration in nonintubated patients, but is rare in patients with VAP (2).

- Factors in pathogenesis: Sources of pathogens for HAP/VAP include:
  - Health care devices, the environment (air, water, equipment, and fomites), and commonly the transfer of microorganisms between the patient and staff or other patients
  - Host and treatment-related colonization factors, severity of the patient's underlying disease, exposure to antibiotics, other medications, and exposure to invasive respiratory devices and equipment are important in the pathogenesis of HAP and VAP.
  - Aspiration of oropharyngeal pathogens, or leakage of secretions containing bacteria around the endotracheal tube cuff, are the primary routes of bacterial entry into the lower respiratory tract.
  - Inhalation or direct inoculation of pathogens into the lower airway, hematogenous spread from infected IV catheters, and bacterial translocation from the GI tract lumen are uncommon pathogenic mechanisms.
  - Infected biofilm in the endotracheal tube, with subsequent embolization to distal airways, may be important in the pathogenesis of VAP.
  - The stomach and sinuses are potential reservoirs of nosocomial pathogens that contribute to bacterial colonization of the oropharynx (2).

ETIOLOGY

- In hospitalized CAP patients, common organisms are: *Streptococcus pneumoniae*, *Haemophilus influenza*, *Mycoplasma pneumonia*, *Chlamydia pneumonia*, and *Legionella pneumonia*. Increasingly prevalent is *S. aureus*. Enteric gram-negative organisms and viruses have been seen in up to 10% of patients in some series. Aspiration pneumonia is also seen in up to 3–6% of patients. The etiologic organism is only identified in 20–70% of patients.
  - For CAP patients who require intensive care commonest organisms are: *S. pneumoniae*, *Legionella*, *H. influenzae*, *S. aureus*, and enteric gram-negative organisms. *Pseudomonas aeruginosa* and MSRA may be significant in patients with bronchiectasis.
  - 50–60% of patients with severe CAP have unknown etiology. Failure to identify the causative organism has not been associated with a different outcome than if a pathogen is identified. In severe CAP, outcome is similar for patients with and without an identified causative organism.
- Risk factors for CAP due to *P. aeruginosa* (1.5–5% of patients) are: ≥7 days of BSA, bronchiectasis, malnutrition, and diseases and therapies associated with neutrophil dysfunction (such as >10 mg of prednisone per day) (1).

PNEUMONIA, ICU

- Risk factors for CAP due to *S. aureus* (1–22% of patients) are recent influenza infection, diabetes mellitus, and renal failure.
- HCAP is defined as pneumonia occurring in any one of the following:
  – Acute care hospitalization within the last 90 calendar days
  – Residence in a nursing home or extended-care facility for any time in the last 90 days
  – Chronic dialysis within the last 30 days
  – Wound care, chemotherapy, tracheostomy care, or ventilator care provided by a health care professional in the last 30 days

COMMONLY ASSOCIATED CONDITIONS
- Diabetes
- Coronary artery disease
- COPD
- Renal failure

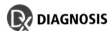 DIAGNOSIS

HISTORY
- Bacterial infection of the lungs produce, fever, chills, cough, often initially non productive, dyspnea, pleuritic chest pain, purulent sputum, sometimes bloody. Accompanied by tachycardia, tachypnea, and hypoxia.
- Patients may have myalgias and joint pains. Confusion can occur in the elderly. Additional history should include:
  – Vaccination status and smoking history
  – Travel, occupational exposure, and home environment (e.g., pets, especially birds); history can be diagnostic

PHYSICAL EXAM
- Fever with cold clammy skin, cyanosis
- Hypotension
- Tachycardia, tachypnea,
- Dullness to percussion over consolidated lung with Increased vocal resonance
- Bronchial breathing over consolidated lung
- Inspiratory crackles and possible pleural rub

DIAGNOSTIC TESTS & INTERPRETATION
Lab
Initial lab tests
- Pulse oximetry, ABG if a metabolic or respiratory acidosis are a possibility and if requiring ventilator support
- WBC, blood cultures (before antibiotics), procalcitonin
- Basic metabolic profile (look for hyponatremia and renal dysfunction)
- Urinary *Legionella* and pneumococcal antigens
- Sputum/respiratory secretion sample should be obtained as soon as possible but should not delay antibiotic administration.
- Testing for H5N1 (1,3,4,5)

Follow-Up & Special Considerations
VAP is the most widespread infection encountered in the ICU and is associated with significant morbidity, mortality, and cost. 10–20% of patients mechanically ventilated for >48 hours will develop VAP, increasing mortality 2-fold (6). Timely, appropriate antibiotic therapy improves patient survival in the presence of infection.

Imaging
Initial approach
- Chest radiograph: Preferably 2 views; diagnostic with areas of consolidation or air bronchogram.
- Parapneumonic effusions may be present.

Follow-Up & Special Considerations
- Repeat chest radiograph if clinically worsening
- Early CT chest for bilateral disease or in ARDS.

Diagnostic Procedures/Other
- Clinical: High sensitivity, low specificity:
  – New or progressive infiltrate and 2 of 3 clinical features: Fever >38°C, leukocytosis or leukopenia, purulent secretions. This can lead to an excessive use of antibiotics. Clinical Pulmonary Infection Score (CPIS) has been used to assist in the clinical diagnosis of VAP. However, while using CPIS to diagnose the presence of VAP results in fewer missed VAP episodes its use can result in patients being treated with antibiotics unnecessarily. A semiquantitative culture of tracheal aspirate if performed more than several hours after intubation may represent colonizing organisms rather than true infecting pathogen. However, a negative culture from tracheal aspirate in a patient without a recent change in antibiotics (72 hours) has a strong negative predictive value. This allows for quick initiation of ICU-specific BSA. De-escalation should be considered at 48–72 hours based on the culture results and clinical response (7,8).
- Microbiologic: High sensitivity and specificity.
- Bronchoalveolar lavage (BAL):
  – Once intubated for >6–12 hours, the endotracheal tube is colonized and pathogens from a routine irrigation of the endotracheal tube are unlikely to correspond to the causative pathogen; may result in overtreatment or wrong antibiotic choice. Recommended to obtain a blind protected bronchial lavage specimen (mini BAL), a bronchoscopically obtained BAL (should not be bloody), or a protected specimen brush (PSB) sample and send for quantitative culture. If positive for $\geq 10^4$ cfu/mL, it is indicative of the causative pathogen. $<10^4$ cfu/mL indicates colonization.
  – Conversely, a negative quantitative BAL specimen in a patient without a recent change in antibiotics in the previous 72 hours has a strong negative predictive value of 94% (2,7,8).

- Procalcitonin (PCT) measurement in CAP patients:
  – A normal (<0.05 ng/dL) to low (<0.25 ng/dL) procalcitonin also has a strong negative predictive value (88–95%) and is indicative of a nonbacterial process. Repeat procalcitonin at 6–12 hours. If still low, an alternative diagnosis should be considered. Not all infiltrates are caused by bacterial infection. If PCT levels are >0.25 ng/dL and/or rising, the likelihood of a bacterial infection is high (3,4,5).
- Diagnostic thoracentesis for moderate to large pleural effusion for suspected empyema

Pathological Findings
- As seen on chest radiograph, classically alveolar infiltrates with air bronchograms and sometimes with pleural effusion
- Positive sputum and blood cultures
- Hypoxia

DIFFERENTIAL DIAGNOSIS
- Viral pneumonia
- Aspiration pneumonia
- bronchiolitis obliterans organizing pneumonia (BOOP)
- Pulmonary embolism
- Lung neoplasm
- Pneumocystis pneumonia
- Hypersensitivity pneumonitis
- Sarcoidosis
- Tuberculosis

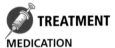 TREATMENT

MEDICATION
- Severe pneumonia (CAP) in ICU:
  – Goal is to give antibiotics as soon as possible within 6 hours of admission for CAP and HCAP, VAP, but within 1 hour for patients in septic shock (11,12,13)

First Line
- IV β-lactam: Ceftriaxone 1–2 g IV then daily 5–10 days AND
- IV fluoroquinolone: Levofloxacin 750 mg/d for 5–10 days OR
- IV macrolide: Azithromycin 500 mg/d for 5–7 days
- If MRSA is suspected:
  – Vancomycin 25 mg/kg IV, then q12h (renal adjustment needed) OR
  – Linezolid 600 mg IV q12h (tyramine-free diet)
- If at risk for *Pseudomonas*:
  – IV antipseudomonal β-lactam: Cefepime 1 g q12hr or Primaxin 50 0 mg q6hr or piperacillin/tazobactam 4.5 g q6hr, all for 10–12 days, AND
  – IV aminoglycoside: Gentamicin/tobramycin 5–7 mg/kg/d then daily renal evaluation OR
  – IV antipseudomonal fluoroquinolone: Ciprofloxacin 500 mg IV b.i.d. AND
  – Macrolide: Zithromax 500 mg/d IV OR
  – IV Fluoroquinolone: Levofloxacin 750 mg/d
  – For penicillin allergy use:
  – Aztreonam 1–2 g IV q6–12h (renal adjustment needed)
  – And a fluoroquinolone: Levofloxacin 750 mg/d IV (1).

- Severe pneumonia: HCAP, HAP, and VAP in ICU:
  - For patients with 0–1 risk factor for MDR organisms: Antibiotic choice is the same as for CAP
  - For patients with 2–3 risk factors for MDR organisms:
    ○ Cover for MRSA and gram-negative organisms. Choose one antibiotic from *A* and one combination from *B*:
    A: Vancomycin 25 mg/kg IV then q12h (renal adjustment and monitoring needed) *OR* linezolid 600 mg IV q12h; *If high risk for MDR organisms, double coverage for Pseudomonas/extended spectrum β-lactamase (ESBL)-producing pathogens and* Acinetobacter *spp.*
    B: Tobramycin 5–7 mg/kg/d IV (renal adjustment monitoring needed) *AND* piperacillin/tazobactam 4.5 g IV q6h *OR* cefepime 2g IV q12h
    For penicillin allergy, use: Tobramycin 5–7 mg/kg/d IV (renal adjustment monitoring needed) AND aztreonam 1–2 g IV q6–12h (renal adjustment needed)
    For suspected high-risk MDR pathogens: Tobramycin 5–7 mg/kg/d IV (renal adjustment monitoring needed) AND imipenem 1–2 g IV q6–12h (2).
- Monitor clinical response, cultures and drop in procalcitonin to help de-escalate antibiotic therapy at 48–72 hours optimal duration for antibiotics is 5–8 days, 10–14 days for ESBL pathogens and Pseudomonas sp.
- Duration of antibiotic treatment: Optimal duration in a clinically responding patient varies from 5–14 days. In addition to signs of clinical improvement, following drop in procalcitonin levels from peak level (usually seen in the 1st 24 hours) to a 90% reduction can more accurately define a day to discontinue antibiotics and reduce unnecessary antibiotic exposure without risk of recurrence of the pneumonia. If poor clinical response and PCT remains elevated at 48–72 hours, alternative antibiotic coverage should be aggressively reviewed (2,14,15,16).

COMPLEMENTARY & ALTERNATIVE THERAPIES FOR SEVERE CAP/HCAP/VAP

- Patients with severe CAP who received activated protein C had a survival benefit if they had an APACHE II score of >25 or pneumococcal infection, a PSI class of IV or V, or a CURB 65 of at least 3 (12).
- Systemic steroids in patients with CAP/HCAP/VAP complicated by septic shock requiring pressors also have been shown to be beneficial. The recommended dose is hydrocortisone 100 mg IV q8h. This should be weaned off over a few days once off inotropes and no longer in shock (11).

ADDITIONAL TREATMENT
General Measures
Pregnancy Considerations
- Maintaining good oxygenation is key to fetal survival.
- Ceftriaxone and azithromycin are category B; levofloxacin and moxifloxacin are category C; in pregnancy these should be used if the benefits outweigh the risks.

Additional Therapies
- Ventilator support for hypoxic respiratory failure, using low tidal volume, lung-protective strategies in developing ARDS (17)
- Maintain head of bed at 30 degrees; oral hygiene b.i.d. with chlorhexidine mouthwash
- For primarily bilateral dependent consolidation (ARDS), a patient with worsening hypoxia may benefit from prone ventilation if not responding to conventional ventilation (18).

SURGERY/OTHER PROCEDURES
- Diagnostic and/or therapeutic thoracentesis for moderate to large or increasing volume pleural effusion.
- To rule out empyema that would require chest tube thoracostomy for drainage

IN-PATIENT CONSIDERATIONS
Initial Stabilization
Oxygen to maintain adequate saturation 92–95% and to relieve dyspnea

Admission Criteria
- Assess severity for ICU admission.
- Admission to ICU is indicated for patients with severe CAP/HCAP. Using modified ATS criteria can guide appropriate admissions. Defined as the presence of either 1 of 2 major criteria or the presence of 3 minor criteria.
  - Major criteria include mechanical ventilation and septic shock with use of vasopressors.
  - Minor criteria include SBP) <90 mm Hg, DBP <60 mm Hg, multilobar disease, $PaO_2:FiO_2$ ratio <250, respiratory rate >30/min, BUN >19.1 mg/dL, confusion, and hypothermia with a temperature <36°C (1,9).
- Alternatively, use CURB 65 score for a quick but slightly less accurate prognosis and choice of location for a patient with CAP:
  - Determine severity of illness with CURB 65 score (CAP only) confusion, urea >19 mg/dL, respiratory rate >30/min, SBP <90 mm Hg,
  - Age >65, 1 point for each factor; 2 = mortality rate of 13%, 3 = mortality rate of 17%, 4–5 = mortality rate of 42–57%; admit to ICU if score is 4–5

- Clinical pulmonary infection score (CPIS) for VAP is diagnostic and management algorithm used when a microbiologic diagnosis is not available. Its accuracy is improved when microbiological data are available (see appendix for calculation) (10).

IV Fluids
NS/LR to maintain hydration, blood pressure, and urine output

 ## ONGOING CARE

DIET
If intubated with acute lung injury, preferably small bowel feeding tube, using a fish oil-rich formula (19)

PROGNOSIS
Variable, but worsens with delay in appropriate antibiotics

COMPLICATIONS
- Exudative pleural effusions
- Empyema thoracis
- Hypoxic respiratory failure
- Ventilator support
- ARDS
- SIADH

REFERENCES

1. Mandell LA, et al. Infectious Diseases Society of America/American Thoracic Society consensus guidelines on the management of community-acquired pneumonia in adults. *Clin Infect Dis.* 2007;44(Suppl 2):S27–72.
2. Guidelines for the Management of Adults with hospital-acquired, ventilator-associated, and healthcare-associated pneumonia. Official statement of the American Thoracic Society and the Infectious Diseases Society of America. *Am J Respir Crit Care Med.* 2005;171:388–416.
3. Niederman MS. Biological markers to determine eligibility in trials for community-acquired pneumonia: A focus on procalcitonin. *Clin Infect Dis.* 2008;47:S127–32.
4. Schuetz P, et al., for the ProHOSP Study Group. Effect of procalcitonin-based guidelines vs standard guidelines on antibiotic use in lower respiratory tract infections: The ProHOSP randomized controlled trial. *JAMA.* 2009;302(10):1059–66.
5. Bouadma L, et al. Use of procalcitonin to reduce patients' exposure to antibiotics in intensive care units (PRORATA trial): Multicentre randomised controlled trial. *Lancet.* 2010;375:463–74.

6. Chastre J, et al. Ventilator-associated pneumonia. *Am J Respir Crit Care Med*. 2002;165:867-903.

7. Baughman RP. Microbiologic diagnosis of ventilator associated pneumonia. *Clin Chest Med*. 2005 26:1.

8. Pugin J, et al. Diagnosis of ventilator-associated pneumonia by bacteriologic analysis of bronchoscopic and nonbronchoscopic "blind" bronchoalveolar lavage fluid. *Am Rev Respir Dis*. 1991;143:1121–22.

9. Singanayagam A, et al. Severity assessment in community acquired pneumonia: A review. *Q J Med*. 2009;102:379–88.

10. Fartoukh M, et al. Diagnosing pneumonia during mechanical ventilation: The clinical pulmonary infection score revisited. *Am J Respir Crit Care Med*. 2003;168:173–9.

11. Phillip Dellinger R, et al. Surviving Sepsis Campaign: International guidelines for management of severe sepsis and septic shock: 2008. *Crit Care Med*. 2008;36(1):296–327.

12. Laterre PF, et al. Severe community acquired-pneumonia as a cause of severe sepsis: Data from the PROWESS study. *Crit Care Med* 2005;33:952–61.

13. Kumar A, et al. Duration of hypotension before initiation of effective antimicrobial therapy is the critical determinant of survival in human septic shock. *Crit Care Med*. 2006;34:1589–96.

14. Chastre J, et al. Comparison of 8 vs 15 days of antibiotic therapy for ventilator-associated pneumonia in adults: A randomized trial. *JAMA*. 2003;290:2588–98.

15. Nobre V, et al. Use of procalcitonin to shorten antibiotic treatment duration in septic patients: A randomized trial. *Am J Respir Crit Care Med*. 2008;177:498–505.

16. Bouadma L, et al. Use of procalcitonin to reduce patients' exposure to antibiotics in intensive care units (PRORATA trial): A multicentre randomised controlled trial. *Lancet*. 2010;375:463–74.

17. Brower R, et al. Ventilation with lower tidal volumes as compared with traditional tidal volumes for acute lung injury and the acute respiratory distress syndrome. *N Engl J Med*. 2000;342:1301–08.

18. Mancebo J, et al. A multicenter trial of prolonged prone ventilation in severe acute respiratory distress syndrome. *Am J Respir Crit Care Med*. 2006;173(11):1233–9.

19. Singer P, et al. Benefit of an enteral diet enriched with eicosapentaenoic acid and gamma-linolenic acid in ventilated patients with acute lung injury. *Crit Care Med*. 2006; 34(4):1033–8.

ADDITIONAL READING

- Interim guidance for use of 23-valent pneumococcal polysaccharide vaccine during novel influenza A (H1N1) outbreak. Accessed at http://www.cdc.gov/h1n1flu/guidance/ppsv/h1n1.htm
- Severe Community-Acquired Pneumonia
- Infectious Disease Clinics of North America - Volume 23, Issue 3 (September 2009)
- Diaz E. Management of ventilator-associated pneumonia. *Infect Dis Clin N Am*. 2009;23(3):521–33.

 See Also (Topic, Algorithm, Electronic Media Element)

Appendix: Clinical Pulmonary Infection Score (CPIS)

Parameter	Score
Temperature (°C)	
≥ 36.5 and ≤ 38.4	0
≥ 38.5 and ≤ 38.9	1
≥ 39.0 or ≤ 36.5	2
WBC Count	
$\geq 4,000$ and $\leq 11,000$	0
$<4,000$ or $>11,000$	1
$<4,000$ or $>11,000$ & bands $\geq 50\%$	2
Tracheal Secretions	
None or scant	0
Nonpurulent	1
Purulent	2
PaO_2/FiO_2	
>240, ARDS* or pulmonary contusion	0
≤ 240 and no ARDS*	2
Chest Radiograph	
No infiltrate	0
Diffuse (or patchy) infiltrate	1
Localized infiltrate	2

*ARDS is defined as a $PaO_2:FiO_2 \leq 200$, PAOP ≤ 18 mm Hg, and acute bilateral infiltrates

Total CPIS	Action
≤ 6 and low suspicion for VAP	Evaluate for other potential sources of infection
≤ 6 and high suspicion For VAP	BAL or mini-BAL
>6	BAL or mini-BAL

For online calculation:
http://www.surgicalcriticalcare.net/Resources/CPIS.php

 CODES

ICD9
- 482.89 Pneumonia due to other specified bacteria
- 486 Pneumonia, organism unspecified
- 997.31 Ventilator associated pneumonia

CLINICAL PEARLS

- In patients with infiltrates and fever without leukocytosis and negative bacterial culture, a low or normal procalcitonin should emphasize the need to look for an alternative nonbacterial infection or inflammatory process. Viral or fungal infections and inflammatory processes such as BOOP should be considered.
- Bacteremia with rapidly progressive infiltrates has a worse prognosis.
- Late/delayed admission to ICU for severe pneumonia had a 47% vs. 23% mortality rate.
- Combination therapy is more effective in severe pneumococcal bacteremia CAP; mortality rate 23% vs. 55% for single-agent treatment.
- *S. pneumoniae* drug resistance is present to 2nd-generation cephalosporins, macrolides (low and high level), and now to fluoroquinolones. Know your local antibiogram and resistance patterns.
- Repeated courses of macrolides are major risk factor for resistance.
- Early mobilization reduces hospital length of stay in CAP.
- Pneumococcal vaccine reduces invasive pneumococcal disease in children and adults.
- Use of guidelines improves outcomes.
- Treatment failure is common.

PNEUMONIA, PNEUMOCYSTIS JIROVECI

Francisco Polanco
Jose R. Yunen

 BASICS

DESCRIPTION
- A form of pneumonia arising in immunosuppressed patients caused by *Pneumocystis jiroveci*. This is one of the most common opportunistic infections occurring in patients infected with HIV.
- Most common manifestation is pneumonia; in <3% of cases can cause organ involvement and disseminated disease.
- Synonym(s): *Pneumocystis carinii* pneumonia (PCP), Pneumocystis, Pulmonary pneumocystosis, Interstitial plasma cell pneumonia

EPIDEMIOLOGY
Incidence
- Pneumocystis pneumonia is the AIDS indicator disease in 43% of patients.
- Because of more effective prophylaxis and antiretroviral therapy, its incidence is decreasing.
- Predominant age and sex:
  - In HIV-infected children not taking prophylaxis, median age of onset is 5 months
  - In HIV-infected adults, may occur at any age
  - Male >Female

RISK FACTORS
- HIV patients with recurrent bacterial pneumonia, unintentional weight loss, oral thrush, and higher plasma HIV RNA
- Patients with a history of previous *Pneumocystis* pneumonia
- Non-HIV immunosuppressed patients:
  - Patients with hematologic or solid malignancies receiving chemotherapy or stem cell transplantation
  - Organ transplant recipients
  - Patients receiving immunosuppressive agents: High-dose corticosteroids most commonly implicated
  - Patients with congenital immunodeficiencies, neutropenia, malnutrition, premature birth

GENERAL PREVENTION
- All HIV patients with a history of *Pneumocystis* pneumonia, CD4 cells <200 cells/μL, or history of oropharyngeal candidiasis require prophylaxis.
- Prophylaxis may be discontinued in patients on antiretroviral therapy with CD4 cell counts >200 for a 3-month period.
- Prophylaxis:
  - TMP-SMX: 1 double-strength tablet daily is the preferred regimen; it also confers protection against toxoplasmosis.
  - If TMP-SMX cannot be administered, dapsone, aerosolized pentamidine, or atovaquone can be used.

ETIOLOGY
The ubiquitous *P. jiroveci* may cause infection in normal hosts (2/3 of young children have positive serology), but will rarely cause symptoms in immunocompetent people. Studies suggest person-to-person transmission is possible.

 DIAGNOSIS

- Usually insidious but occasionally abrupt in onset
- Progressive dyspnea, initially on exertion, that worsens within days to weeks
- Fever is apparent in the majority of cases.
- Weakness, fatigue, malaise
- Nonproductive cough or productive of scant whitish or clear sputum
- Tachypnea
- Diffuse dry rales

DIAGNOSTIC TESTS & INTERPRETATION
Lab
- ABGs reveal hypoxemia and increased alveolar–arterial gradient, which varies with severity of disease; this is the most characteristic laboratory abnormality
- Level of serum lactate dehydrogenase >500 mg/dL is common but nonspecific.

- CD4 cell count is generally <200.
- Sputum (induced) may reveal *Pneumocystis* on cytologic evaluation using various stains or direct immunofluorescent staining.
- Spontaneously expectorated sputum has very low sensitivity and should not be sent.

Imaging
- Chest radiograph shows bilateral diffuse interstitial or perihilar infiltrate in 75% of cases.
  - May also be normal or show unilateral disease, pleural effusions, abscesses or cavitations, pneumothorax, or lobar consolidations
- CT demonstrates patchy, ground-glass attenuation

Diagnostic Procedures/Other
- Fiberoptic bronchoscopy with bronchoalveolar lavage or transbronchial biopsy (90–100% sensitive) is the preferred method of diagnosis when sputum test results are negative.
- Open lung biopsy is rarely required.
- A test for *Pneumocystis* based on polymerase chain reaction may be useful in the future on sputum, bronchoalveolar fluid.

DIFFERENTIAL DIAGNOSIS
- Tuberculosis
- Mycobacterium avium intracellulare
- Viral pneumonia
- Fungal pneumonia
- Cytomegalovirus pneumonia

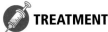 TREATMENT

MEDICATION
First Line
- TMP component: 15–20 mg/kg/d PO or IV divided into 3 or 4 doses
- SMX component 75–100 mg/kg/d PO or IV divided into 3 or 4 doses
- Alternative: TMP-SMX DS2 PO t.i.d.
- Dose of TMP-SMX should be reduced in patients with renal failure.
- Treatment duration: 14–21 days, usually 21 days in patients with AIDS
- Contraindications: Use with care in pregnant patient and infants <2 months.
- Precautions:
  - History of sulfa allergy
  - A high percentage of patients with AIDS will develop intolerance to TMP-SMX. Especially common are dermatologic reactions, hematologic toxicity, or fever.
  - Patients receiving this therapy must avoid direct sunlight.
- Significant possible interactions: Phenytoin, oral anticoagulants, oral sulfonylureas, digitalis

Second Line
- Pentamidine: 3–4 mg/kg/d IV over 60 minutes for 21 days
- Dapsone: 100 mg/d PO plus trimethoprim 15 mg/kg/d divided t.i.d. or q.i.d. Check glucose 6-phosphate dehydrogenase level before beginning dapsone because hemolysis may result.
- Clindamycin: 300–400 mg PO t.i.d.–q.i.d. plus primaquine 30 mg/d PO for 21 days
- Atovaquone suspension: 750 mg b.i.d. PO for 21 days
- Precautions: Pentamidine has greater toxicity than Bactrim: Hypotension, hyperglycemia, hypoglycemia, pancreatitis, rash, hepatic and renal dysfunction, thrombocytopenia

ADDITIONAL TREATMENT
Additional Therapies
Adjunctive corticosteroid (prednisone or methylprednisolone) therapy begun within 72 hours of diagnosis decreases mortality in AIDS patients (adults and children) with moderate to severe *Pneumocystis* pneumonia (those with room air PO_2 <70 mm Hg or A-a gradient >35 mm Hg). Prednisone dose: 40 mg b.i.d. days 1–5; 40 mg daily on days 6–10; 20 mg daily on days 11–21.

 ONGOING CARE

FOLLOW-UP RECOMMENDATIONS
All patients with PCP require secondary prophylaxis for life (after adequate treatment for PCP) unless CD4 cell count increases. (See General Prevention.)

DIET
No special diet needed

PATIENT EDUCATION
MedLine Plus. At: Http://www.nlm.nih.gov/medLineplus/pneumocystisinfections.htmL

PROGNOSIS
- Without treatment, fatal in immunocompromised hosts
- Mortality from 1st episode of *Pneumocystis* pneumonia is 10–15%. With prophylactic therapy, mean survival has increased.
- Patients requiring mechanical ventilation have 60–90% mortality rate.
- 40% of patients with *Pneumocystis* pneumonia will have a recurrence unless prophylaxis is given.

COMPLICATIONS
- Respiratory failure
- Pneumothorax (even after successful treatment)
- Extrapulmonary *Pneumocystis* pneumonia (especially in patients on inhaled pentamidine prophylaxis)

ADDITIONAL READING
- Briel M, et al. Adjunctive corticosteroids for Pneumocystis jiroveci pneumonia in patients with HIV-infection. *Cochrane Database Syst Rev.* 2009;1.
- CDC. Treating opportunistic infections among HIV-infected adults and adolescents: Recommendations from CDC, the National Institutes of Health, and the HIV Medicine Association/Infectious Disease Society of America. *MMWR.* 2009;58 (No. RR-4).
- Dohn MN, et al. Geographic clustering of *Pneumocystis carinii* pneumonia in patients with HIV infection. *Am J Respir Crit Care Med.* 2000;162: 1617–21.

 CODES

ICD9
- 042 Human immunodeficiency virus (hiv) disease
- 136.3 Pneumocystosis

CLINICAL PEARLS
- *P. jiroveci* infection is common and occurs at an early age; primary infection is largely asymptomatic. Symptomatic disease is rare and limited to immunocompromised individuals.
- *P. jiroveci* pneumonia is an AIDS-defining illness, most frequently when CD4 counts are <200 cells/μL.
- Initial lab evaluation shows hypoxemia on ABGs, increased A-a gradient, elevated LDH.

PNEUMONIA, VENTILATOR-ASSOCIATED

Oveys Mansuri

 BASICS

DESCRIPTION
VAP is a form of pneumonia that develops in patients who have been supported by mechanical ventilation for ≥48 hours. It is thought that mechanical ventilation plays a key role in its development.

EPIDEMIOLOGY
Incidence
- 9–27% of all intubated patients
- Cumulative risk:
  - 3%/day for 1st 5 days
  - 2%/day for days 6–10
  - 1%/day after day 10

Prevalence
- 38.1% of ICU patients
- 35.7 cases/1000 ventilator-days

RISK FACTORS
- Nonmodifiable:
  - Male sex, age >60, preexisting pulmonary disease, multiple organ system failure, coma, tracheostomy, reintubation, neurosurgery and head trauma
- Modifiable:
  - Supine position, gastric overdistension, contaminated ventilator circuit, frequent patient transfer, and low endotracheal tube cuff pressure

Geriatric Considerations
Increased risk secondary to prevalence of chronic diseases, especially COPD

Pediatric Considerations
Antibiotics being the mainstay of treatment, it is vitally important to use appropriate dosage adjustments by weight for pediatric patients.

Pregnancy Considerations
Important to consider pregnancy categorization of antibiotic agents before use; pharmacy consultation is recommended.

GENERAL PREVENTION
- Strict hand hygiene; universal precautions
- Strict contact precautions for patients with nosocomial infections
- Implementation of ventilator bundle
- Elevation of head of bed
- Oral care
- Sedation holidays
- Any steps that reduce the risks of aspiration associated with endotracheal tube
- Use of silver-coated endotracheal tube
- Stress ulcer prophylaxis
- Room and ventilator cleaning

PATHOPHYSIOLOGY
- Transmission of abnormal bacterial flora from the contaminated upper airway is thought to be the primary mechanism, combined with an impaired mucociliary clearance function of the lung in patients whose airway is instrumented with an endotracheal or tracheostomy tube.
- The immunosuppressive effects of critical illness may also play a role.

ETIOLOGY
- MRSA
- *Pseudomonas*
- *Klebsiella*
- *Serratia marcescens*
- *Enterobacter*
- *Stenotrophomonas*
- *Acinetobacter*
- VRE

COMMONLY ASSOCIATED CONDITIONS
- Prolonged intubation and dependence on mechanical ventilatory support
- Critical illness

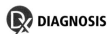 **DIAGNOSIS**

HISTORY
- Recent hospitalization or residence at a nursing home
- Intubation/tracheostomy
- Mechanical ventilation
- Recent antibiotic use
- Immunocompromised state
- Fever
- Sputum production consistent with infection

PHYSICAL EXAM
- Fevers
- Hypoxia/respiratory distress
- Change in quality/quantity of secretions

DIAGNOSTIC TESTS & INTERPRETATION
Lab
Initial lab tests
- Culture and Gram stain of deep sputum or endobronchial collection
- CBC to evaluate for elevated WBC and manual differential to look for bandemia
- Chemistry panel

Follow-Up & Special Considerations
- Biomarkers: Procalcitonin, soluble triggering receptor, and C-reactive protein
- No clear evidence in support of biomarkers to predict VAP. More research is needed.

Imaging
Initial approach
- Chest x-ray with rapid radiological read
- Chest CT (if there is uncertainty based on chest x-ray)

Follow-Up & Special Considerations
- Repeated sputum culture
- Repeat chest x-ray

Diagnostic Procedures/Other
Bronchoscopy to acquire BAL for culture and sensitivities or protected brush specimen (most sensitive if done before the start of antibiotics)

Pathological Findings
- Dense lung tissue inflammation
- Purulent airway secretions

DIFFERENTIAL DIAGNOSIS
- Aspiration pneumonia
- Bacterial pneumonia
- Community-acquired pneumonia
- Fungal pneumonia
- Viral pneumonia

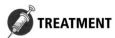

TREATMENT

MEDICATION

First Line
- Depends on culture and sensitivities
- Empiric therapy should be started early with any of the following options:
  - Ceftriaxone
  - Fluoroquinolones
  - Ampicillin-sulbactam
  - Ertapenem
- If the patients is critically ill and/or is unstable, the antibiotic regiment is a broad coverage of all possible nosocomial organisms.

Second Line
Combination therapy may be indicated for patients with suspicion of MDR in accordance with suspected infectious bacteria(s)

ADDITIONAL TREATMENT

General Measures
- Early empiric antibiotic therapy
- Follow-up of cultures and sensitivities and antibiotic modification in accordance with findings
- Implementation of *VAP bundles*: Minimize risk of aspiration, reduce colonization risks, minimize period of intubation with sedation holidays and weaning protocols.

Issues for Referral
- Infectious disease consultation as indicated
- Pulmonology and/or intensivist consultation with relation to ventilator weaning and complex ventilator management secondary to preexisting pulmonary disease
- May progress to ARDS

SURGERY/OTHER PROCEDURES
- Thoracentesis for removal of pleural (parapneumonic) effusions for infectious cause and/or clinical symptoms
- Thoracotomy for biopsy or surgical management of infection refractory to medical management

IN-PATIENT CONSIDERATIONS

Initial Stabilization
- Identification of primary infection
- Antibiotic therapy and source control
- Hemodynamic stabilization and resuscitation
- Mechanical ventilation modification as indicated

Admission Criteria
Patients with VAP will routinely be admitted to an ICU for management.

IV Fluids
- Adequate fluid resuscitation with use of crystalloid replacement (i.e., 0.9% NS or LR)
- Ensure appropriate access and consider central venous access if inadequate access or need for monitoring volume status (CVP).

Nursing
- Patient comfort
- Assure compliance with VAP bundle policies

Discharge Criteria
- Resolution of pneumonia or significant improvement allowing sub-ICU level of care
- Resolution of respiratory failure and no further dependence on mechanical ventilation and aggressive pulmonary toilet

 ONGOING CARE

FOLLOW-UP RECOMMENDATIONS
At discharge from ICU, generate detailed sign-out assuring safe and seamless transfer of care to floor or for discharge to home and follow-up with primary care physician.

Patient Monitoring
Continue close monitoring while in ICU.

DIET
- Maintain appropriate enteral feeding to optimize nutrition if no contraindications.
- Some studies demonstrate that early enteral feeding and nasoduodenal feeding lower VAP rates.

PROGNOSIS
VAP mortality: 27–76%

COMPLICATIONS
- Sepsis
- Shock
- ARDS
- Death

ADDITIONAL READING

- Albertos R, et al. Ventilator-associated pneumonia management in critical illness. *Curr Opin Gastroenterol*. 2011;27:160–66.
- Efrati S, et al. Ventilator-associated pneumonia: Current status and future recommendations. *J Clin Monitor Comput*. 2010;24:161–68.
- Lorente L, et al. New issues and controversies in the prevention of ventilator-associated pneumonia. *Am J Respir Crit Care Med*. 2010;182:870–6.
- Niel-Weise B, et al. An evidence-based recommendation on bed head elevation for mechanically ventilated patients. *Crit Care*. 2011;15:R111.
- Palazzo S, et al. Biomarkers for ventilator-associated pneumonia: Review of the literature. *Heart & Lung*. 2011;30:1–6.
- Safdar N, et al. Clinical and economic consequences of ventilator-associated pneumonia: A systematic review. *Crit Care Med*. 2005;33:2184–93.

 CODES

ICD9
- 486 Pneumonia, organism unspecified
- 997.31 Ventilator associated pneumonia

CLINICAL PEARLS
- Stabilize the patient's acute issues.
- Institute early empiric antibiotic therapy.
- Determine cultures and sensitivities and appropriate modification of antibiotic profile.
- Implement VAP bundle for prevention.

POISONING, ALCOHOL

Muhammad N. Athar
James A. Gasperino

 BASICS

DESCRIPTION
- Any alcohol can be toxic if ingested in large quantities.
- Toxic alcohol refers to ethanol, isopropanol, methanol, and ethylene glycol:
  - Ethanol is derived from the fermentation of sugars and cereals.It is available both as a beverage and as an ingredient in food extracts, cough and cold medications, and mouthwashes.
  - Isopropyl alcohol is commonly found in many mouthwashes, skin lotions, and rubbing alcohol.
  - Methyl alcohol is widely used as a solvent and paint remover. It is commonly used in photocopying and windshield washing fluids.Toxicity is primarily from ingestion but can also occur from prolonged inhalation or skin absorption.
  - Ethylene glycol is a colorless and odorless liquid commonly found in antifreeze.

EPIDEMIOLOGY
Incidence
- In 2005, 7394 cases of isopropanol, 807 cases of methanol, and 5469 cases of ethylene glycol ingestions were reported.
- Uncomplicated ethanol intoxication is responsible for 600,000 emergency department visits each year in the U.S.

Prevalence
>8 million Americans are believed to be dependent on alcohol.

RISK FACTORS
- Majority of isopropanol ingestions occur in children aged <6 years. Most methanol and ethylene glycol ingestions occur in adults >19 years.
- Chronic alcohol use

Genetics
Chronic alcoholics and those with severe liver disease have increased rates of metabolism.

GENERAL PREVENTION
- Mental status changes, hypothermia, and GI symptoms are clinical features of isopropyl alcohol poisoning.
- A normal serum anion gap and elevated serum osmolality are characteristic of isopropyl alcohol poisoning.
- The treatment of isopropyl alcohol poisoning is supportive, with hemodialysis reserved for severe cases that are associated with high isopropyl alcohol levels (i.e., >400 mg/dL), hypotension, prolonged coma, or hepatic or renal failure.

PATHOPHYSIOLOGY
- Ethanol is absorbed across the gastric mucosa and small intestines. Peak concentration is reached in 20–60 minutes. Once absorbed, it is converted to acetaldehyde, followed by conversion to acetate, which is then converted to acetyl coenzyme A and ultimately leads to production of carbon dioxide and water through a series of complex reactions.
- Isopropanol is rapidly absorbed across the gastric mucosa. Peak concentration is reached in 30–120 minutes. Isopropanol is primarily metabolized via alcohol dehydrogenase to acetone, the concentration of which peaks 4 hours after ingestion.
- Methanol is metabolized in the liver via alcohol dehydrogenase into formaldehyde, which is later converted to formic acid, which ultimately is metabolized to folic acid. Formic acid is responsible for the toxic effects of methanol.
- Ethylene glycol itself is nontoxic, but it is metabolized into toxic compounds. Ethylene glycol is oxidized via alcohol dehydrogenase into glycoaldehyde, which is later converted into glycolic acid; the last step is very rapid. The conversion of glycolic acid to glyoxylic acid is slower and is the rate-limiting step in the metabolism. Glyoxylic acid is later metabolized to oxalic acid.

 DIAGNOSIS

HISTORY
- Acute ethanol intoxication: Slurred speech, nystagmus, disinhibited behavior, incoordination, unsteady gait, memory impairment, stupor, or coma; hypotension may occur as well
- Methanol poisoning: Visual blurring, central scotomata, and blindness
- Ethylene glycol poisoning: Flank pain, hematuria, and oliguria
- Isopropyl alcohol poisoning: GI (nausea, vomiting, and abdominal pain) and CNS (depression of consciousness)
- Isopropyl alcohol is a 3× more potent CNS depressant than ethanol.

PHYSICAL EXAM
- Ethanol intoxication:
  - >25 mg/dL: Sense of warmth and well-being
  - 25–50 mg/dL: Euphoria and decreased judgment
  - 50–100 mg/dL: Incoordination, decreased reaction time, and ataxia
  - 100–250 mg/dL: Cerebellar dysfunction
  - >250 mg/dL: Coma
  - >400 mg/dL: Respiratory depression, loss of protective reflexes, and death

- Methanol or ethylene glycol poisoning:
  - CNS effects, such as inebriation, sedation, coma, seizures, hyperpnea (Kussmaul respirations), and hypotension.
  - Methanol hyperemia or disc pallor on funduscopic exam
- Isopropyl alcohol poisoning:
  - Mental status change and fruity breath odor suggesting acetone. Signs of shock, hematemesis, pulmonary edema, and hemorrhagic tracheobronchitis can be seen with massive ingestion.

DIAGNOSTIC TESTS & INTERPRETATION
Lab
- Basal metabolic profile
- Fingerstick glucose
- ABG
- Serum osmolality, osmolal gap
- Serum ethanol levels
- Serum methanol, ethylene glycol, and isopropyl alcohol concentrations
- Serum and urine ketones
- Special considerations:
  - Ethanol causes elevated anion gap, metabolic acidosis
  - Methanol and ethylene glycol cause elevated anion gap, metabolic acidosis, and osmolar gap.
  - Isopropyl alcohol causes an elevated osmolar gap, and when ingested alone, typically does not cause increased anion gap or metabolic acidosis

Imaging
Initial approach
- Chest radiograph
- CT of the head if decreased sensorium

Follow-Up & Special Considerations
- Blood ethanol levels
- EKG

DIFFERENTIAL DIAGNOSIS
- Other CNS depressants
- Metabolic acidosis with an increased anion gap and/or presence of an elevated osmolal gap is characteristic of methanol and ethylene glycol poisoning.
- Isopropyl alcohol presents with osmolar gap and absence of elevated anion gap, metabolic acidosis.

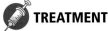 **TREATMENT**

MEDICATION
First Line
- Ethanol intoxication: Supportive, D5W for hypoglycemia
- Ethylene glycol and methanol poisoning:
  – The FDA has approved fomepizole for ethylene glycol and methanol poisoning.
  – The protocol consists of a 15 mg/kg IV loading dose followed by a 10 mg/kg IV bolus q12h for 4 doses (48 hours). The bolus dose should be increased to 15 mg/kg q12h to account for increased fomepizole metabolism.
  – Patients are treated until serum levels fall to <20 mg/dL.
  – ADH inhibition by ethanol loading (600 mg/kg IV) and maintenance infusion (e.g., 125–150 mg/kg/h) remains an alternative to fomepizole treatment for methanol and ethylene glycol poisoning.
  – Loading dose is adjusted if a measurable blood alcohol level is present.
  – Higher maintenance infusions are needed for alcoholics and patients receiving dialysis.
  – Maintain a target serum level of 100–200 mg/dL.
  – Oral ethanol dosing only if neither fomepizole nor IV ethanol is available.
- Isopropyl alcohol poisoning: Supportive with IV fluids

Second Line
- Methanol intoxication also requires cofactor therapy: Either folinic acid 50 mg IV or folic acid 50 mg IV q6h.
- Ethylene glycol poisoning patient should receive thiamine (100 mg IV) or pyridoxine (50 mg IV).
- Hemodialysis

ADDITIONAL TREATMENT
General Measures
- Stabilize ABCs.
- Indications for routine dialysis based on serum levels alone have been challenged.
- Administer IV fluids and atropine for initial treatment of hypotension and bradycardia.
- Methanol poisoning and ethylene glycol poisoning: Sodium bicarbonate to correct acidosis via IV bolus for pH <7.3

- GI decontamination with activated charcoal has role in alcohol intoxication due to rapid absorption of intoxicant from GI mucosa.
- Insert an arterial blood pressure catheter and central venous pressure line for close monitoring of hemodynamics.

Issues for Referral
- Toxicology consult
- Nephrology consult

IN-PATIENT CONSIDERATIONS
Initial Stabilization
As above

Admission Criteria
- Unable to protect airway
- Hypotension

IV Fluids
Isotonic saline

Nursing
Hemodynamic monitoring for hypotension and airway

Discharge Criteria
- Decreasing levels of alcohol and correction of acidosis
- Ability to protect airway

 ONGOING CARE

FOLLOW-UP RECOMMENDATIONS
Psychiatric follow-up for suicidal ingestion

Patient Monitoring
Ethanol co-ingestion may delay toxic manifestations of ethylene glycol and methanol ingestion.

PROGNOSIS
- Excellent if recognized early and treated aggressively
- In general, depends on the amount ingested

COMPLICATIONS
As above

ADDITIONAL READING
- Barceloux DG, et al. American Academy of Clinical Toxicology practice guidelines on the treatment of methanol poisoning. *J Toxicol Clin Toxicol*. 2002:40: 415.
- Barceloux DG, et al. American Academy of Clinical Toxicology practice guidelines on the treatment of ethylene glycol poisoning. *J Toxicol Clin Toxicol*. 1999;37:537.
- Brent J, et al. Fomepizole for the treatment of methanol poisoning. *N Engl J Med*. 2001;344: 424–9.
- Buchanan JA, Heard K. *Guide to Antidotes for Poisonings and Overdoses*. Nashville, TN: Cumberland Pharmaceuticals; 2008:28–29.
- Ethanol. In: Hoffman RS, Nelson LS, Howland MA, et al. (eds.). *Goldfrank's Manual of Toxicologic Emergencies*. New York: McGraw Hill, 2007:641–6.
- Fahlen M, et al. Gait disturbance, confusion, and coma in a 93-year-old blind woman. *Chest*. 120;295–7.
- Mokhlesi B, et al. Adult toxicology in critical care: part II: Specific poisonings. *Chest*. 2003;123: 897–922.
- *Nutrition and your health: Dietary guidelines for America. Home and Garden Bulletin*, 4th ed., no. 232. Washington, DC: US Department of Health and Human Services and the US Department of Agriculture (USDA); 1995.
- Pletcher MJ, et al. Uncomplicated alcohol intoxication in the emergency department: an analysis of the National Hospital Ambulatory Medical Care Survey. *Am J Med*. 2004;117:863.
- Stremski E, et al. Accidental isopropanol ingestion in children. *Pediatr Emerg Care*. 2000;16:238.

 CODES

ICD9
- 980.0 Toxic effect of ethyl alcohol
- 980.1 Toxic effect of methyl alcohol
- 980.2 Toxic effect of isopropyl alcohol

CLINICAL PEARLS
- Isopropyl alcohol causes elevated osmolar gap, without anion gap elevation or metabolic acidosis.
- Fomepizole is the treatment of choice for ethylene glycol and methanol poisoning.

POISONING, BENZODIAZEPINE

Muhammad N. Athar
James A. Gasperino

 BASICS

DESCRIPTION
- Benzodiazepines (BZDs) are sedative-hypnotic agents that have been in clinical use since the 1960s.
- BZDs are used for sedation and to treat anxiety, seizures, withdrawal states, insomnia, and drug-associated agitation.
- Widely prescribed

Geriatric Considerations
Action of long-acting BZDs can be prolonged due to reduced clearance by liver.

Pregnancy Considerations
Pregnancy risk: D

EPIDEMIOLOGY
- The Annual Reports of the American Association of Poison Control Centers National Data Collection System showed alprazolam was involved in 34 fatal deliberate self-poisonings over 10 years 1992–2001 compared with 30 fatal deliberate self-poisonings involving diazepam.
- Of the 72,978 single-substance BZD exposures that were reported to U.S. poison control centers in 2007, 269 resulted in major toxicity and 7 cases resulted in fatalities.

GENERAL PREVENTION
Keep medications out of reach of children.

PATHOPHYSIOLOGY
- BZDs exert their effect via modulation of the γ-aminobutyric acid A (GABA-A) receptor. GABA is the chief inhibitory neurotransmitter of the CNS.
- Short-acting BZDs (half-life <12 hours): Triazolam, oxazepam, and midazolam.
- Intermediate-acting BZDs (half-life 12–24 hours): Lorazepam and temazepam.
- Long-acting BZDs (half-life >24 hours): Diazepam and chlordiazepoxide.
- Absorption in the GI tract
- Highly lipophilic
- Highly protein bound
- Metabolism is primarily hepatic

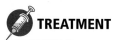 **DIAGNOSIS**

HISTORY
CNS depression with normal vital signs: Dizziness, confusion, drowsiness, blurred vision, unresponsiveness, anxiety, and agitation

PHYSICAL EXAM
Nystagmus, hallucinations, slurred speech, ataxia, coma, hypotonia, weakness, altered mental status, impairment of cognition, amnesia, respiratory depression, and hypotension

DIAGNOSTIC TESTS & INTERPRETATION
Lab
- Basal metabolic panel
- ABG
- Qualitative screening of urine or blood

Imaging
- Chest radiograph
- ECG

DIFFERENTIAL DIAGNOSIS
- Ethanol
- Barbiturates
- γ-Hydroxybutyrate
- Chloral hydrate

TREATMENT

MEDICATION
First Line
Supportive

Second Line
- Use of flumazenil is highly controversial.
- It is safe and effective when used to reverse the BZD given for procedural sedation.
- In adults, the recommended initial dose is 0.2 mg IV over 30 seconds.
- Repeated doses of 0.2 mg, to a maximum dose of 1 mg, can be given until the desired effect is achieved.
- Short half-life (0.7–1.3 hours) may need additional doses.

ADDITIONAL TREATMENT

General Measures
- Stabilize ABCs
- GI decontamination with activated charcoal is of no benefit in BZD overdose.
- Insert arterial blood pressure catheter and central venous pressure line for close monitoring of hemodynamics.

Issues for Referral
Toxicology consult if not responsive to initial medical therapy

IN-PATIENT CONSIDERATIONS

Initial Stabilization
As above

Admission Criteria
Unable to protect airway

IV Fluids
Isotonic saline

Nursing
Hemodynamic monitoring

Discharge Criteria
Clinical improvement, including signs, symptoms and neurological status

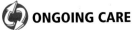 ONGOING CARE

FOLLOW-UP RECOMMENDATIONS
Psychiatric evaluation if suicidal ingestion

PATIENT EDUCATION
- Keep medications out of reach of children.
- Use with caution in patients with COPD, especially those with chronic hypercapnia.

PROGNOSIS
Good

COMPLICATIONS
Aspiration pneumonia

ADDITIONAL READING

- Bronstein AC, et al. 2007 Annual Report of the American Association of Poison Control Centers' National Poison Data System (NPDS): 25th Annual Report. *Clin Toxicol (Phila)*. 2008;46:927–1057.
- Isbister G, et al. Alprazolam is relatively more toxic than other benzodiazepines in overdose. *Br J Clin Pharmacol*. 2004;58:88–95.

- Seger DL. Flumazenil: Treatment or toxin. *J Toxicol Clin Toxicol*. 2004;42:209.
- Sedative-hypnotics. In: Hoffman RS et al., eds., *Goldfrank's Manual of Toxicologic Emergencies*. New York: McGraw Hill, 2007:615–22.
- Shalansky SJ, et al. Effect of flumazenil on benzodiazepine-induced respiratory depression. *Clin Pharm*. 1993;12:483.

 CODES

ICD9
969.4 Poisoning by benzodiazepine-based tranquilizers

CLINICAL PEARLS

The treatment is mainly supportive; treatment with flumazenil is controversial.

P

POISONING, BETA BLOCKER

Muhammad N. Athar
James A. Gasperino

 BASICS

DESCRIPTION
- βBlockers have been in clinical use for >40 years.
- Common indications include hypertension, ischemic heart disease, heart failure, arrhythmias, migraine headache, tremor, portal hypertension, and aortic dissection.

EPIDEMIOLOGY
Incidence
- The 2007 Annual Report of theAmerican Association of Poison Control Centers (AAPCC) National Poison Data System reported 9291 single exposures to β blockers leading to 413 minor outcomes, 631 moderate outcomes, 61 major outcomes, and 3 fatalities.
- According to the 2004 AAPCC toxic exposure review, 51% of all exposures and 47.6% of all overdose fatalities were in women.
- Of the fatalities reported to the 2004 AAPCC, 68% were in individuals <50 years of age and 43% were in children <6 years.
- The β blocker most implicated in fatalities is propranolol.

Prevalence
In 2007, the National Poison Data System reported 9291 single exposures to β blockers.

RISK FACTORS
- Cardiac patients
- Patient taking concomitant negative inotropic medications

Pregnancy Considerations
Pregnancy risk: C

GENERAL PREVENTION
Keep medications out of reach of children.

PATHOPHYSIOLOGY
- Competitive antagonism of the β receptor (β-1 found in cell membranes of heart muscle, eye, kidney; β-2 found in cell membranes of bronchial smooth muscle and liver and in peripheral vascular smooth muscle; β-3 found in adipose tissues) decreases cellular levels of cAMP.
- Membrane-stabilizing activity (e.g., propranolol, acebutolol) inhibits myocardial fast sodium channels, resulting in a wide QRS interval that may potentiate dysrhythmias.
- Lipophilic β blockers (e.g., propranolol) can rapidly cross the blood-brain barrier, leading to neurologic sequelae such as seizures and delirium.
- Agents with intrinsic sympathomimetic activity (acebutolol, pindolol) cause less bradycardia and hypotension.

ETIOLOGY
- In children, results from exposure to an adult's unattended medications
- In adults, is usually seen in suicide attempt or an accidental overdose of a routine medication

COMMONLY ASSOCIATED CONDITIONS
- Common co-ingestion with cardiac and analgesic medications
- Cardiac condition.

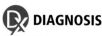 **DIAGNOSIS**

HISTORY
- Collect information regarding specific agent, amount ingested, time of ingestion, co-ingestion of other cardioactive agents
- Underlying cardiac disease (e.g., heart failure)
- Witnesses and EMS personnel may be helpful to recover pill bottles at the scene.
- Patient's pharmacy may provide valuable information regarding prescribed medications and the total number of pills dispensed.
- Ingestion of extended-release tablets, sotalol, or agents with membrane-stabilizing activity (e.g., propranolol or acebutolol) should be given special consideration.
- Symptoms occur within 2 hours following ingestion.
- Almost all develop symptoms within 6 hours of ingestion. Exceptions to this rule are ingestions of sustained-release medications and sotalol.
- Decreased level of consciousness, coma, and seizures (more common with lipid-soluble agents)

PHYSICAL EXAM
- Half-life is usually short (2–12 hours); however, it can be prolonged in overdose patients because of depressed cardiac output and reduced blood flow to the liver and kidneys.
- Bradycardia and hypotension secondary to negative inotropic effects
- Mental status changes including delirium, coma, and seizures
- Hypoglycemia
- Bronchospasm
- Ventricular dysrhythmias are seen more frequently with propranolol and acebutolol exposures because of their increased membrane-stabilizing activity.
- Agents like propranolol, because of increased lipophilicity and rapid diffusion into the CNS, are associated with neurologic effects in the absence of cerebral hypoperfusion.

DIAGNOSTIC TESTS & INTERPRETATION
Lab
Initial lab tests
- Serum β-blocker levels (assays not readily available)
- Fingerstick blood sugar
- Serum electrolytes including calcium, BUN, and creatinine
- Cardiac enzymes to rule out myocardial infarction in unstable patient
- Acetaminophen and salicylate levels because they are common co-ingestions
- Pregnancy test in women of childbearing age

Follow-Up & Special Considerations
- If calcium is administered repeatedly, levels should be measured q4–6h.
- If an insulin/glucose treatment regimen is used, glucose and potassium levels must be measured q30–60min.
- ECG monitoring for bradyarrhythmias and heart blocks.

Imaging
Initial approach
Plain chest radiography in patients with signs of pulmonary edema

Follow-Up & Special Considerations
Echocardiogram if cardiac failure with pulmonary edema

Diagnostic Procedures/Other
ECG

DIFFERENTIAL DIAGNOSIS
- Agents causing unexplained bradycardia and hypotension:
- Verapamil
- Diltiazem
- Digoxin
- Clonidine
- Cholinergic agents

TREATMENT

MEDICATION

First Line
- Glucagon bolus (2–5 mg IV over 1 min). If there is no clinical response (usually in 2–3 min), a second bolus dose of glucagon can be given. If there is a clinical response, glucagon infusion of 10 mg/h can be started.
- Calcium chloride (1 g of a 10% solution 10 mL is given as a slow push via a central venous catheter)
- Calcium gluconate should be used if no central IV access is available. 30 mL of 10% solution should be administered.
- Calcium should be avoided in cases of digoxin poisoning.

Second Line
- Epinephrine and dopamine for persistent hypotension
- High-dose insulin (e.g., 1 U/kg, 0.5–1 U/kg/h) and glucose (10% dextrose solution) should be considered for overdoses that are refractory to crystalloids, glucagon, and vasopressor infusions.
- Isoproterenol
- Milrinone
- Transcutaneous and transvenous pacemaker
- Intra-aortic balloon pump
- Hemodialysis may be useful in severe cases of atenolol, nadolol, and sotalol toxicity (low lipid solubility, low protein binding).
- Acebutolol is dialyzable.
- Propranolol, metoprolol, and timolol are not eliminated by hemodialysis.

ADDITIONAL TREATMENT

General Measures
- Stabilize ABCs
- IV fluids and atropine for initial treatment of hypotension and bradycardia
- GI decontamination with single-dose activated charcoal
- Consider whole-bowel irrigation if an extended-release preparation has been ingested
- Insertion of an arterial blood pressure catheter and central venous pressure line for close monitoring of hemodynamics

Issues for Referral
Toxicology consult if not responsive to initial medical therapy

Additional Therapies
- Sodium bicarbonate has been used successfully in patients with QRS prolongation.
- Magnesium infusion in ventricular arrhythmias, especially with sotalol overdose
- Benzodiazepines are the drugs of choice if seizures occur.
- Consider hemodialysis or hemoperfusion only when treatment with glucagon and other pharmacotherapy fails.

IN-PATIENT CONSIDERATIONS

Initial Stabilization
- IV fluids
- Use atropine in accordance with ACLS guidelines for symptomatic bradycardia.
- Atropine is given in a dose of 0.5–1 mg q3–5min up to a total of 0.03–0.04 mg/kg

Admission Criteria
- Hemodynamic instability
- Mental status change
- Asymptomatic patients with sotalol overdose

IV Fluids
NS

Nursing
Hemodynamic monitoring for hypotension, heart blocks, and seizures

Discharge Criteria
- Patients with sotalol overdose require at least 24 hours of in-house cardiac monitoring.
- Asymptomatic patients with overdose other than sotalol should be monitored for at least 6 hours in ED before discharge.
- In the symptomatic patient, continuous hemodynamic monitoring is required until the patient does not require pharmacologic assistance to maintain blood pressure.

ONGOING CARE

FOLLOW-UP RECOMMENDATIONS
Psychiatric follow-up for suicidal ingestion

PATIENT EDUCATION
- Keep medications out of reach of children.
- Elderly people may need assistance in medication intake if drug overdose was accidental.

PROGNOSIS
- Excellent if recognized early (within 6 hours) and treated
- Poor outcome related to underlying heart condition

COMPLICATIONS
- Cardiac failure
- Seizures

ADDITIONAL READING

- Bailey B. Glucagon in b-blocker and calcium channel blocker overdoses: A systematic review. *J Toxicol Clin Toxicol*. 2003;41:595.
- Bronstein AC, et al. 2007 Annual Report of the American Association of Poison Control Centers' National Poison Data System (NPDS): 25th Annual Report. *Clin Toxicol*. 2008;46:927–1057.
- DeWitt CR, et al. Pharmacology, pathophysiology and management of calcium channel blocker and β-blocker toxicity. *Toxicol Rev*. 2004;23:223–38.
- Holger JS, et al. Insulin versus vasopressin and epinephrine to treat beta-blocker toxicity. *Clin Toxicol (Phila)*. 2007;45:396.
- Love JN, et al. Acute beta blocker overdose: factors associated with the development of cardiovascular morbidity. *Clin Toxicol*. 2000;38:275–81.
- Wax PM, et al. Beta-blocker ingestion: an evidence-based consensus guideline for out-of-hospital management. *Clin Toxicol (Phila)*. 2005;43: 131.

See Also (Topic, Algorithm, Electronic Media Element)

- www.aapcc.org
- www.clintox.org
- http://circ.ahajournals.org/cgi/content/full/112/24_suppl/IV-67

CODES

ICD9
971.3 Poisoning by sympatholytics (antiadrenergics)

CLINICAL PEARLS

- The single most important factor associated with the development of cardiovascular morbidity in β-blocker ingestion is a history of a cardioactive co-ingestant, primarily calcium channel blockers, cyclic antidepressants, and neuroleptics.
- Toxicity from β-blocker exposure generally develops within 2 hours of ingestion.

POISONING, BIOCHEMICAL AGENT

Muhammad N. Athar
James A. Gasperino

 BASICS

DESCRIPTION
- Biochemical agents include biological agents and chemical agents that can be used in biochemical warfare.
- Increasing threat of the use of these agents by terrorists
- Biological agents are classified as category A, B, or C:
  - Category A: Smallpox, anthrax, plague, botulism, tularemia, Ebola, Marburg, Lassa, Junin, and related viruses
  - Category B: Q fever, brucellosis, glanders, melioidosis, psittacosis, typhus fever, eastern equine encephalitis, western equine encephalitis, Venezuelan equine encephalitis, ricin toxin, epsilon toxin of *Clostridium perfringens*, *Staphylococcus enterotoxin* B, *Salmonella* spp, *Shigella dysenteriae*, *Escherichia coli* O157:H7, *Vibrio cholerae*, *Cryptosporidium parvum*
  - Category C: Nipah virus, Hantaviruses, tickborne hemorrhagic fever viruses, tickborne encephalitis viruses, yellow fever, and MDR tuberculosis
- Chemical agents are classified as nerve agents (sarin, VX, and tabun), toxic asphyxiants (cyanide and arsine), pulmonary irritants (phosgene, chlorine, and ammonia), and blister agents (sulfur mustard).
- Simple asphyxiants act by displacing oxygen.
- Chemical asphyxiants interfere with utilization of oxygen.
- Biological weapons are more destructive and cheaper to produce than chemical weapons.

EPIDEMIOLOGY
Incidence
- Isolated reports and allegations of the use of biochemical agents in warfare in the 20th century
- 1993 report by the U.S. Congressional Office of Technology Assessment estimated that between 130,000 and 3,000,000 deaths could follow the aerosolized release of 100 kg of anthrax spores upwind of Washington, DC.
- Most likely agents in accidental release are CO, organic phosphorus pesticides, and chlorine.
- Most likely agents in act of terrorism are cyanide, sarin, and VX, phosgene, and sulfur mustard.

RISK FACTORS
Commonly sought agents by terrorists for their activities

PATHOPHYSIOLOGY
Varies depending on the agent exposed

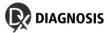 **DIAGNOSIS**

HISTORY & PHYSICAL EXAM
- The signature of a chemical agent release is the sudden onset of symptoms within minutes, with mass casualties; however, release of biological agents may take hours or days to become apparent.
- CDC has identified a number of high-priority organisms as category A agents such as smallpox, plague, botulism, tularemia, and anthrax.
- Smallpox is highly infectious and is characterized by high fever, headache, rigors, malaise, myalgias, vomiting, and GI symptoms complicated by delirium and erythematous exanthema, which can progress to pustular formation. Painful ulcerations of the tongue and oropharynx can also be seen.
- Anthrax, plague, and tularemia cause predominantly respiratory symptoms, fever, and painful lymphadenopathy. Widened mediastinum suggests inhalational anthrax.

- Botulism causes blurred vision, mydriasis, ptosis, dysphagia, dysarthria, dysphonia, and muscle weakness. Dry mouth, urinary retention, ileus, and constipation can be seen later.
- Category B biological agents of concern are ricin, staph enterotoxin B, *C. perfringens*, *Salmonella*, *Shigella*, *E. coli*, and *Vibrio*.
- Ricin: When ingested causes nausea, diarrhea, vomiting, fever, abdominal pain. Inhalational intake leads to chest tightness, coughing, weakness, nausea, and fever.
- Other category B agents produce mainly GI tract symptoms leading to dehydration, sepsis, septic shock, and MOF.
- Category C biological agents produce a variety of clinical conditions, most notably encephalitis.
- The main syndromes that suggest release of chemical agents are neurologic, pulmonary, skin, and eye symptoms.
- Nerve agents (sarin, etc.) produce diffuse muscle cramping, runny nose, difficulty breathing, eye pain, dimming of vision, sweating, muscle tremors followed by LOC, seizures, and flaccid paralysis.
- Toxic asphyxiants (cyanide, etc.) produce giddiness, palpitations, dizziness, nausea, vomiting, headache, eye irritation, hyperventilation, drowsiness followed by LOC, and death within 1–15 minutes. Metabolic acidosis with elevated venous blood O_2 level (arterialization of O_2) and "pink" skin are characteristic.
- Pulmonary irritants (phosgene, etc.) produce SOB, chest tightness, wheezing, laryngeal spasm, mucosal and dermal irritation and redness, followed by ARDS.
- Blister agents (sulfur mustard) produce mostly local symptoms of burning, itching, or red skin, mucosal irritation, swollen eyes, and sloughing of airway mucosa, with ARDS and neutropenia later in the course.

DIAGNOSTIC TESTS & INTERPRETATION
Lab
Initial lab tests
- CBC, basic metabolic panel, LFTs
- Urine and drug screen
- Blood cultures
- ABG
- CSF examination
- RBCs, serum cholinesterase levels, cyanide and thiocyanate levels when clinical condition demands

Follow-Up & Special Considerations
- In 1999, the CDC and the Association of Public Health Laboratories established the Laboratory Response Network (LRN) of about 120 laboratories.
- The LRNs are divided into levels A-D, based on capabilities. Level A laboratories are usually included in hospitals and clinics and are likely to be the 1st to the receive specimens in questions. Their role in detecting biological agents is to rule out and mostly refer to a laboratory within the network to confirm a diagnosis. Level B and C laboratories are those with increased capabilities to confirm diagnoses of a biological agent. They include state and county public health laboratories. Level D laboratories include national laboratories whose primary responsibility is to further characterize the agent.

Imaging
Chest radiograph

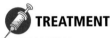

TREATMENT

MEDICATION
First Line
- First-line agent is the available antidote for that particular biochemical agent poisoning.
- Smallpox: VIG is available for use in case of accidental release.
- Anthrax: When susceptibilities are unknown, therapy with ciprofloxacin 400 mg IV b.i.d. or doxycycline 200 mg IVloading dose followed by 100 mg IV b.i.d. can be started.
- Botulism: A trivalent equine antitoxin (types A, B, and E) is available from the CDC.
- Tularemia and plague: Streptomycin (30 mg/kg/d IM divided b.i.d. for 10–14 days) is the drug of choice.
- Ricin: No antidote; mainly supportive management

- Nerve agents: Atropine and PAM. Atropine (2 mg) IV repeat q5min until effective:
  - Severe exposures to nerve agents may require 20–30 mg of atropine. Pralidoxime chloride (2–PAMCl) 600–1800 mg IM or 1.0 g IV over 20–30 minutes. Diazepam is used to control convulsive episodes.
- Simple asphyxiants: Remove from exposure, 100% oxygen by face mask, and intubation with 100% FiO_2if indicated.
- Pulmonary irritants: No specific antidote available. Treatment with 100% oxygen and management of ARDS.
- Blistering agents: No antidote available; supportive management.

Second Line
- Decontamination involves removing clothing and placing all items in plastic bags and showering using copious quantities of soap and water.
- Wash skin and shampoo with hypoallergenic liquid soap and copious tepid water in sequential steps of rinse, soap, rinse, wait 1 minute, then final additional rinse (20 minutes).
- Decontamination waste water may require special collection or treatment.

ADDITIONAL TREATMENT
General Measures
- Call the local health director; after-hours contact local health director via 911.
- If criminal activity is suspected, call your local law enforcement and the FBI.
- Alert local HAZMAT team via fire department at 911.

Issues for Referral
CDC Emergency Response Coordinating Group 770-488-7100

IN-PATIENT CONSIDERATIONS
Initial Stabilization
ABCs

Admission Criteria
- Unable to protect airways
- Unstable vital signs

IV Fluids
NSS

Nursing
Monitoring vital signs

Discharge Criteria
Stable blood pressure and able to maintain airway

 ## ONGOING CARE

FOLLOW-UP RECOMMENDATIONS
Psychiatric follow-up may be required for some affected individuals, for PTSD.

PROGNOSIS
- Depends on the biochemical agent
- Generally, biological exposures have better prognosis than chemical.

ADDITIONAL READING
- Greenfield RA, et al. Microbiological, biological, and chemical weapons of warfare and terrorism. *Am J Med Sci.* 2002;323;326–40.
- Kales SN, et al. Acute chemical emergencies. *N Engl J Med.* 2004;350:800.
- Karwa M, et al. Bioterrorism: Preparing for the impossible or the improbable. *Crit Care Med.* 2005;33:S75–95.
- North Carolina Statewide Program for Infection Control and Epidemiology (SPICE). http://www.unc.edu/depts/spice/
- www.bt.cdc.gov
- www.nfpa.org

CODES

ICD9
- 022.9 Anthrax, unspecified
- 050.9 Smallpox, unspecified
- 979.9 Poisoning by other and unspecified vaccines and biological substances

POISONING, CALCIUM CHANNEL BLOCKER

Muhammad N. Athar
James A. Gasperino

 BASICS

DESCRIPTION
Calcium channel blockers (CCBs) have been in clinical use for >25 years.

ALERT
CCB toxic syndromes are the most common cause of cardiac drug toxicity-related mortality.

Geriatric Considerations
Accidental overdose is very common.

Pediatric Considerations
In young children, calcium channel blockers have been reported to be fatal with single-tablet ingestions, especially with extended-release tablets causing delayed-onset hypotension.

EPIDEMIOLOGY
Incidence
- In 2006, the Annual Report of the American Association of Poison Control Centers (AAPCC) National Poison Data System reported 10,031 exposures to calcium channel blockers, resulting in 13 deaths and 316 major outcomes.
- In 2006, AAPCC reported 1363 exposures occurred in children <6 years (16% of reported cases).
- CCB toxicity has a high fatality rate.

Prevalence
In 2008, the AAPCC reported 10,398 exposures (4,840 single exposures) to CCBs, which resulted in 12 deaths.

RISK FACTORS
- Cardiac patients
- Patients on other negative inotropic drugs

Pregnancy Considerations
Pregnancy risk: C

GENERAL PREVENTION
Keep medications out of reach of children.

PATHOPHYSIOLOGY
- CCBs can be divided into 2 major categories: Dihydropyridines and nondihydropyridines, such as verapamil and diltiazem.
- CCBs have 4 cardiovascular effects: Peripheral vasodilatation, negative chronotropy, negative inotropy, and negative dromotropy.
- CCBs exert their effects by blocking the L-type calcium channels.

ETIOLOGY
- In children, results from exposure to an adult's unattended medications
- In adults, usually seen in suicide attempt or an accidental overdose of a routine medication

COMMONLY ASSOCIATED CONDITIONS
- Common co-ingestion with cardiac and analgesic medications
- Cardiac condition

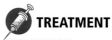 **DIAGNOSIS**

HISTORY
- Collect information regarding specific agent, amount ingested, time of ingestion, co-ingestion of other cardioactive agents.
- Underlying cardiac disease (e.g., heart failure)
- Witnesses and EMS personnel may be helpful to recover pill bottles at the scene.
- Patient's pharmacy may provide valuable information regarding prescribed medications and the total number of pills dispensed.
- Patients ingesting >5–10 × the usual dose can develop signs of severe intoxication.

PHYSICAL EXAM
- Dihydropyridine intoxication generally results in arterial vasodilation and reflex tachycardia.
- Nondihydropyridine (diltiazem and verapamil) toxicity causes peripheral vasodilation, decreased cardiac inotropy, and bradycardia.
- Classic triad of bradycardia, hypotension, and change in mental status is specific for diltiazem and verapamil.
- Jugular venous distension, rales on pulmonary examination, and signs of heart failure may be seen.
- CCB-toxic patients maintain a surprisingly clear mental status due to the neuroprotective effects of CCBs.
- Mental status changes include delirium, coma, and seizures once persistent hypotension leads to critically low cerebral perfusion occurs.
- Hyperglycemia secondary to inhibition of insulin release from pancreas

DIAGNOSTIC TESTS & INTERPRETATION
Lab
Initial lab tests
- Assays for CCBs are not routinely available.
- Fingerstick blood sugar
- Serum electrolytes including calcium, BUN, and creatinine
- Cardiac enzymes to rule out MI in unstable patient
- Acetaminophen and salicylate levels because they are common co-ingestions

Follow-Up & Special Considerations
- ECG monitoring for bradyarrhythmias and heart blocks
- Serum calcium and ECG for evidence of hypercalcemia in patients on calcium chloride infusion

Imaging
Initial approach
Plain chest radiograph in patients with signs of pulmonary edema

Follow-Up & Special Considerations
- Echocardiogram if cardiac failure with pulmonary edema
- If bowel obstruction is suspected, abdominal radiography is recommended.
- Color-flow vascular US of the intra-abdominal arterial supply may confirm bowel infarction.

Diagnostic Procedures/Other
ECG

DIFFERENTIAL DIAGNOSIS
Agents causing unexplained bradycardia and hypotension:
- β Blockers
- Digoxin
- Clonidine
- Cholinergic agents

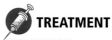 **TREATMENT**

MEDICATION
First Line
- Calcium chloride (via central venous access); the adult dose of calcium chloride is 10–20 mL of a 10% calcium chloride solution over 10 minutes. If no effect is noted, the dose can be repeated up to 4 times every 20 minutes.
- If calcium gluconate (via peripheral or central venous access) is used, the dose should be 30–60 mL of 10% calcium chloride because calcium gluconate has only 1/3 the calcium of calcium chloride.
- Calcium infusion: 0.4 mL/kg/h of calcium chloride or 1.2 mL/kg/h of calcium gluconate
- Glucagon: The dosing regimen is not well established; however, an initial 5 mg IV bolus is a reasonable start and may be repeated twice at 10-minute intervals.
- A glucagon infusion of 2–10 mg/h (50–100 μg/kg/h) has been suggested.

Second Line
- Epinephrine and dopamine for persistent hypotension
- High-dose insulin (e.g., 1 U/kg, 0.5–1 U/kg/h) and glucose (10% dextrose solution) should be considered for overdoses that are refractory to crystalloids, glucagon, and vasopressor infusions.
- Milrinone
- Transcutaneous and transvenous pacemaker
- Intra-aortic balloon pump for cardiogenic shock not responsive to medical therapy
- Hemodialysis has no role in CCB toxicity.

ADDITIONAL TREATMENT
General Measures
- Stabilize ABCs
- IV fluids and atropine for initial treatment of hypotension and bradycardia
- GI decontamination with activated charcoal
- Consider whole-bowel irrigation if an extended-release preparation has been ingested.
- Insertion of an arterial blood pressure catheter and central venous pressure line for close monitoring of hemodynamics

Issues for Referral
Toxicology consult if not responsive to initial medical therapy

IN-PATIENT CONSIDERATIONS
Initial Stabilization
- IV fluids
- Atropine should be given in accordance with ACLS guidelines for symptomatic bradycardia.
- Atropine may be ineffective in severe CCB overdose, although it may be effective if calcium is administered prior to atropine.
- Atropine is given in a dose of 0.5–1 mg every 3–5 minutes up to a total of 0.03–0.04 mg/kg.

Admission Criteria
- Hemodynamic instability
- Mental status change
- Observation in ICU for 6–12 hours in standard-release preparation overdose and for 24–36 hours in extended-release or once-a-day preparation overdose even if asymptomatic.

IV Fluids
NS

Nursing
Hemodynamic monitoring for hypotension, heart blocks, and seizures

Discharge Criteria
- Patients with immediate-release CCB ingestion who remain asymptomatic after 6–8 hours may be considered for discharge.
- If the CCB preparation was a sustained- or extended-release preparation, admission and cardiac monitoring for 24 hours are warranted.
- In the symptomatic patient, continuous hemodynamic monitoring is required until the patient does not require pharmacologic assistance to maintain blood pressure.

 ## ONGOING CARE

FOLLOW-UP RECOMMENDATIONS
Psychiatric follow-up for suicidal ingestion

Patient Monitoring
- Keep medications out of reach of children.
- Elderly people may need assistance in medication intake if drug overdose was accidental.

PATIENT EDUCATION
- Older patients should keep all medications away from children and use child-resistant caps if children live in or visit their home.
- Elderly people may need assistance in medication intake if drug overdose was accidental.

PROGNOSIS
- Excellent, if recognized early and treated aggressively
- Poor outcome is related to underlying heart condition.

COMPLICATIONS
- Cardiac failure
- Anoxic encephalopathy and seizures
- Bowel infarction with prolonged ischemia

ADDITIONAL READING

- Bailey B. Glucagon in b-blocker and calcium channel blocker overdoses: A systematic review. *J Toxicol Clin Toxicol*. 2003;41:595.
- Bronstein AC, et al. 2008 Annual Report of the American Association of Poison Control Centers' National Poison Data System (NPDS): 26th Annual *Report. Clin Toxicol (Phila)*. 2009;47:911–1084.
- DeWitt CR, et al. Pharmacology, pathophysiology and management of calcium channel blocker and β-blocker toxicity. *Toxicol Rev*. 2004; 23:223–38.
- Kerns W II, et al. Beta-blocker and calcium channel blocker toxicity. *Emerg Med Clin North Am*. 1994;12:365–90.

 ### See Also (Topic, Algorithm, Electronic Media Element)

- www.aapcc.org
- www.clintox.org
- http://circ.ahajournals.org/cgi/content/full/112/24_suppl/IV–67

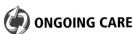 ## CODES

ICD9
972.9 Poisoning by other and unspecified agents primarily affecting the cardiovascular system

CLINICAL PEARLS
- CCB toxicity is more common in patients on other negative inotropic drugs.
- Calcium chloride is the best initial therapy.
- Initiate serum calcium and ECG monitoring for evidence of hypercalcemia in patients on calcium chloride infusion.

POISONING, CYANIDE

Aditya Kasarabada
James Gasperino

 BASICS

DESCRIPTION
- Occurs frequently with smoke inhalation, especially in enclosed spaces
- Sodium nitroprusside can cause cyanide poisoning during prolonged IV therapy (>5–10 μg/kg/min).
- Seen in foods such as cassava, papaya, peach, pear, apricot
- Solvents, plastics, electroplating, photography
- Cigarette smoking

EPIDEMIOLOGY
Incidence
- Underestimated, as death can be attributed to other causes such as ventricular tachycardia or ventricular fibrillation
- 5000–10,000 smoke inhalations
- 214 exposures in 2005

Prevalence
International industrial consumption of cyanide is estimated to be 1.5 million tons per year (mostly occupational exposures).

RISK FACTORS
- Chronic exposure: Smokers, dietary intake of cassava, nitroprusside therapy
- Acute exposure: Inhalation of smoke
- Household exposure: Acetonitrile-containing false-fingernail remover
- Occupational exposure: Jewelers exposed to metallic cyanide

Genetics
Predominant male preponderance for suicide with cyanide

GENERAL PREVENTION
- Install smoke alarms.
- Wear personal protective gear at work.
- Follow safe work practices.
- Monitor nitroprusside infusion closely.
- Prevent light decomposition of nitroprusside by using silver foil on IV tubing.

PATHOPHYSIOLOGY
- Inactivates metalloenzymes
- Inactivates cytochrome oxidases, which stops mitochondrial oxidative phosphorylation
- Shifts cellular metabolism from aerobic to anaerobic
- Results in accumulation of oxygen free radicals
- Inhibits GABA, reducing seizure threshold

ETIOLOGY
- Occurs frequently with smoke inhalation, especially in enclosed spaces
- Iatrogenic poisoning from prolonged IV therapy with sodium nitroprusside
- Intentional poisoning
- Industrial exposure
- Cigarette smoking

COMMONLY ASSOCIATED CONDITIONS
Associated with chronic cyanide exposure:
- Tobacco amblyopia
- Leber hereditary optic atrophy
- Tropical ataxic neuropathy

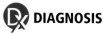 DIAGNOSIS

HISTORY
- Smoke inhalational injury
- Tachyphylaxis in an ICU patient on nitroprusside
- Generalized weakness, malaise, headache, dizziness, vertigo, abdominal pain, nausea, vomiting
- Generalized seizures, coma

PHYSICAL EXAM
- Nonspecific
- Falsely high pulse oximetry
- Cherry-red skin color, as oxygen cannot be extracted from hemoglobin
- Signs of inhalational injury such as soot in the nose, facial burns
- Bitter almond smell on breath
- Mydriasis
- Bright red retinal arteries, as oxygen cannot be extracted from hemoglobin

DIAGNOSTIC TESTS & INTERPRETATION
Lab
Initial lab tests
- Serum lactate levels >10 mmol/L in smoke inhalation or >6 mmol/L after suspected exposure suggest cyanide poisoning
- No cyanide poisoning if serum lactate is normal
- ABG with metabolic acidosis
- Difference between arterial and venous oxygen saturation <10% suggests cyanide poisoning, as oxygen is not being extracted
- Rule out other causes of metabolic acidosis.
- Carboxyhemoglobin levels in smoke inhalation
- Methemoglobin levels
- Blood cyanide levels may not be readily available or reliable.
- ECG

Follow-Up & Special Considerations
- Co-intoxication with carbon monoxide and cyanide.
- Formation of MetHb as part of treatment for cyanide toxicity
- Carboxy Hb and MetHb can be fatal

Imaging
Initial approach
Consider obtaining a CT of head for other causes of headache, dizziness, vertigo, seizures.

Follow-Up & Special Considerations
ICU monitoring

Diagnostic Procedures/Other
As above

DIFFERENTIAL DIAGNOSIS
- TCA overdose
- Carbon monoxide poisoning
- Organophosphates
- Salicylates

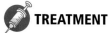

TREATMENT

MEDICATION

First Line
- Hydroxocobalamin directly binds cyanide to form cyanocobalamin, which is renally excreted (50 mg/kg or 5 g)
- Sodium thiosulfate is administered along with hydroxocobalamin (1.65 mL/kg IV of 25%), which acts as a sulfur donor for enzyme rhodanese, which converts cyanide to thiocyanate, which is renally excreted.
- May cause temporary reddish discoloration of skin, urine, and mucus membrane.

Second Line
- Cyanide antidote kit containing amyl nitrite pearls, sodium nitrite, and sodium thiosulfate
- Amyl nitrite and sodium nitrite induce methemoglobinemia
- Use nitrite with caution in burn patients as they can have concomitant carbon monoxide poisoning, further worsening hypoxia.
- Can cause vasodilatation and hypotension

ADDITIONAL TREATMENT

General Measures
- Avoid mouth-to-mouth resuscitation during CPR if cyanide poisoning suspected
- Supportive care
- Protect airway
- 100% oxygen
- Fluids and vasopressors as needed
- Control seizures
- Single dose of activated charcoal for oral ingestion (adults 50 mg, children 1 mg/kg up to a max of 50 g)

Issues for Referral
- Supportive management in ICU
- Time from exposure to clinical signs is often minutes.
- Clinical deterioration may occur rapidly.

Additional Therapies
- GI decontamination
- Supportive care

COMPLEMENTARY & ALTERNATIVE THERAPIES
Management of lactic acidosis

IN-PATIENT CONSIDERATIONS

Initial Stabilization
As above

Admission Criteria
Requires admission to ICU for close monitoring

IV Fluids
May be needed as part of supportive management to maintain hemodynamic stability

Discharge Criteria
When stable from a cardiopulmonary and neurological standpoint

ONGOING CARE

FOLLOW-UP RECOMMENDATIONS
Watch for acute and delayed neurological complications such as parkinsonism, ataxia

Patient Monitoring
- May need MRI or CT of head for neurological sequelae
- Imaging often shows injury to globus pallidus and putamen.

DIET
Dietary risk factors discussed above

PATIENT EDUCATION
- Install smoke alarms
- Personal protective gear at work
- Safe work practices

PROGNOSIS
Good, if therapy is instituted rapidly

COMPLICATIONS
As above

ADDITIONAL READING

- Annual Report of the American Association of Poison Control Centers Toxic Exposure Surveillance System. *Am J Emerg Med*. 2005;23:589–666.
- Borron SW, et al. Prospective study of hydroxocobalamin for acute cyanide poisoning in smoke inhalation. *Ann Emerg Med*. 2007;49:794.
- Cummings TF. The treatment of cyanide poisoning. *Occup Med*. 2004;54:82–85.
- Geller RJ, et al. Pediatric cyanide poisoning: causes, manifestations, management, and unmet needs. *Pediatrics*. 2006;118:2146–58.
- Mokhlesi B, et al. Adult toxicology in critical care: part II: specific poisonings. *Chest*. 2003;123:897–922.
- Morocco AP. Cyanides. *Crit Care Clin*. 2005;21:691–705, vi.

CODES

ICD9
989.0 Toxic effect of hydrocyanic acid and cyanides

CLINICAL PEARLS
- Occurs frequently with smoke inhalation
- Monitor patients with nitroprusside infusion closely.
- Normal serum lactate rules out cyanide poisoning.

POISONING, GAMMA HYDROXYBUTYRATE (GHB)

Muhammad N. Athar
James A. Gasperino

 BASICS

DESCRIPTION
- GHB is an analogue of γ-aminobutyric acid (GABA).
- It was initially used as anesthetic drug for sedation properties.
- GHB first gained popularity as a club drug used by young people at raves, parties, and bars.
- GHB was banned in the U.S. in 1992

EPIDEMIOLOGY
Incidence
National Institute of Drug Abuse (NIDA) 2006 survey indicated that 0.9% of 8th graders, 0.7% of 10th graders, and 1.1% of 12th graders reported GHB use.

Prevalence
- 79% of GHB users are male.
- 2/3 of patients presenting to the ED for GHB ingestion are aged 18–25 years.

RISK FACTORS
- Common date rape drug
- Use of co-intoxicants such as ethanol, MDMA (ecstasy), and methamphetamines is common.

Pediatric Considerations
Overdose with children common. Usually mistaken for water.

Pregnancy Considerations
GHB readily crosses placental barrier.

PATHOPHYSIOLOGY
- GHB is found naturally in the CNS, with the highest concentrations in basal ganglia.
- Repetitive movements may represent myoclonus.
- GHB also is found in the peripheral blood and readily crosses the blood–brain and placental barriers.
- GHB is rapidly absorbed after ingestion and takes 20–30 minutes to reach a maximal plasma concentration.
- The elimination half-life is 30 minutes.
- GHB is ultimately metabolized to CO_2 and eliminated through the lungs.
- GHB exerts neurological effects by binding to GABA-B receptors in the brain and inhibits norepinephrine release.

ETIOLOGY
- In children, exposure results from unattended medications.
- In adults, ingestion is either suicidal or accidental.

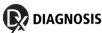 DIAGNOSIS

HISTORY
- Difficult to obtain because of patient's altered mental status
- Information should be obtained from paramedics, police, and the patient's employer, family, friends, primary care clinician, and pharmacist.
- History of date and rape goes together.
- History of GHB manufactured in a home lab is important since homemade GHB can be contaminated with sodium hydroxide (lye).
- CNS depression is the hallmark of GHB use.

PHYSICAL EXAM
- Neurologic findings: Euphoria followed by a period of depressed level of consciousness. Agitated delirium is also seen followed by stupor or coma. Seizure-like movements and myoclonus are common during the course of the intoxication.
- Aggressive, violent behavior
- Cardiovascular findings: Bradycardia is more common than hypotension.
- Pulmonary findings: Apnea and/or aspiration leading to respiratory compromise
- GI findings: Nausea and vomiting are common. Alkali burns to the lips, mouth, and GI tract can be seen when the GHB is contaminated by sodium hydroxide during the manufacturing process.
- Constitutional: Mild hypothermia

DIAGNOSTIC TESTS & INTERPRETATION
Lab
Initial lab tests
- No specific lab test
- CBC, serum electrolyte levels, liver function tests, toxicologic screens, ammonia level, ABG levels, osmolality, cultures, and pregnancy test may be obtained.

Follow-Up & Special Considerations
- Laboratory tests for GHB in serum or urine are not readily available.
- In rape victims targeted analysis of urine with gas chromatography/mass spectrometry (GC/MS) is needed for detection of GHB and must be specifically requested.

Imaging
- Brain CT to rule out trauma or stroke.
- CXR for aspiration

Diagnostic Procedures/Other
- ECG (U waves are frequently seen, even in the absence of hypokalemia).
- LP to rule out other causes of change in mental status

DIFFERENTIAL DIAGNOSIS
Other causes of altered mental status, stupor, and coma

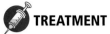 TREATMENT

MEDICATION
- No specific antidotes exist for GHB.
- Supportive management
- Airway patency and aspiration precautions are of paramount importance.
- Consider activated charcoal if co-ingestion is suspected.
- Gastric lavage is indicated only if ingestion of a lethal dose of another drug (acetaminophen, tricyclic antidepressant) occurred within 1 hour of presentation.
- Date rape victims should receive proper and prompt forensic and medical exam, sexually transmitted disease (STD) prophylaxis, pregnancy counseling, psychological or other supportive counseling and follow-up.

ADDITIONAL TREATMENT
General Measures
- As for all patients presenting with altered mental status 50 mL of D50W, thiamine 100 mg IV, and naloxone IV should be considered.
- Naloxone may be used cautiously as it can precipitate opioid withdrawal in chronic opioid users, resulting in vomiting, which may cause aspiration of gastric contents.

IN-PATIENT CONSIDERATIONS
Initial Stabilization
ABCs

Admission Criteria
- Severe symptoms
- Hemodynamic compromise

IV Fluids
NSS for hypotension

Nursing
Close monitoring for hypotension and respiratory failure

Discharge Criteria
When patient is able to protect the airway

 ONGOING CARE

FOLLOW-UP RECOMMENDATIONS
- United States Poison Control Network at 1-800-222-1222
- Psychiatric consultation for patients who are suicidal or depressed
- In suspicion of sexual assault, social services, police, and obstetrician/gynecologist should be consulted.

DIET
No specific dietary considerations

PATIENT EDUCATION
- Many patients mistakenly believe that GHB is a legal substance; thus educate on the legality of the drug.
- Patients who have used GHB in an attempt to increase growth hormone levels and enhance a bodybuilding need to be educated about the dangers of the drug.

PROGNOSIS
In isolated ingestion of GHB, prognosis is excellent.

COMPLICATIONS
- Respiratory depression
- Dose-related CNS depression
- Amnesia and hypotonia expected with exposures of 10 mg/kg
- Somnolence, drowsiness, dizziness, euphoria expected with exposures of 20–30 mg/kg
- Coma, bradycardia, Cheyne–Stokes respiration expected at exposures of 50–70 mg/kg
- Coma lasts <2 hours; full recovery usually in 8 hours
- Aspiration of gastric contents
- Withdrawal syndrome after chronic ingestion: Agitation, delirium, and visual and auditory hallucinations may last 5–15 days and require acute hospitalization.

ADDITIONAL READING
- Bravo DT et al. Reliable, sensitive, rapid and quantitative enzyme-based assay for gamma-hydroxybutyric acid (GHB). J Forensic Sci. 2004;49:379.
- Gamma hydroxybutyric acid. In Hoffman RS et al., eds., Goldfrank's manual of toxicologic emergencies. New York: McGraw-Hill, 2007:659–654.
- Gonzalez A, Nutt DJ. Gamma hydroxy butyrate abuse and dependency. J Psychopharmacol. 2005;19:195.
- Stillwell ME. Drug-facilitated sexual assault involving gamma-hydroxybutyric acid. J Forensic Sci. 2002;47(5):1133–4.

 CODES

ICD9
- 292.81 Drug-induced delirium
- 292.84 Drug-induced mood disorder
- 967.9 Poisoning by unspecified sedative or hypnotic

CLINICAL PEARLS
GHB is not detectable on routine hospital toxicology screens.

POISONING, LITHIUM

Muhammad N. Athar
James A. Gasperino

 BASICS

DESCRIPTION
- Widely used drug in the treatment of bipolar disease
- Narrow therapeutic index

ALERT
Low therapeutic index

Geriatric Considerations
Impaired renal function may increase toxicity.

EPIDEMIOLOGY
Incidence
- An estimated 10,000 toxic exposures occur per year.
- The mortality rate is ~25% with an acute overdose and 9% in patients intoxicated during maintenance therapy.

Prevalence
The American Association of Poison Control Centers Toxic Exposures Surveillance System reported 4954 cases of lithium exposure in 2002.

RISK FACTORS
- Acute renal failure
- Older age
- Volume depletion
- Concomitant use of NSAIDs or ACE inhibitors

Pregnancy Considerations
Pregnancy risk: D

GENERAL PREVENTION
- Frequent monitoring of blood levels because lithium has low therapeutic index
- Avoidance of volume depletion

PATHOPHYSIOLOGY
- The recommended therapeutic plasma lithium concentration is 0.6–1.2 mEq/L.
- Poor correlation with serum levels
- Toxicity develops when lithium distributes into cells.
- GI absorption is rapid.
- Peak plasma levels reached in 2–4 hours
- Lithium does not bind to protein and is freely distributed through the total body water.
- Plasma half-life is ~18 hours; may be prolonged in elderly persons and with delayed-release tablets.
- 100% excreted by the kidneys

ETIOLOGY
- Overdose
- Types of exposure are etiologically important.
- Acute vs. chronic exposure
- Acute on chronic exposure

DIAGNOSIS
- Mild toxicity (1.5–2.5 mEq/L)
- Moderate toxicity (2.5–3.5 mEq/L):
  - CNS effects include irregular coarse tremors, fascicular twitching, rigid motor agitation, muscle weakness, ataxia, sluggishness, and delirium.
  - GI effects include nausea, vomiting, and diarrhea.
  - Later cardiac effects include sinus bradycardia and hypotension.
- Severe intoxication (>3.5 mEq/L):
  - Seizures, stupor, and coma.
  - With severe intoxication, 10% risk of permanent neurologic sequelae (such as dementia and ataxia)
- Chronic: Usually precipitated with introduction of new medication that impairs renal function or causes a hypovolemic state

DIAGNOSTIC TESTS & INTERPRETATION
Lab
Initial lab tests
- Lithium levels in blood should be checked 12 hours postingestion.
- Basic metabolic panel
- Urinalysis, electrolyte levels, and renal function
- Thyroid function+

Follow-Up & Special Considerations
Lithium levels

Imaging
- Chest radiograph
- ECG
- CT scan of head

DIFFERENTIAL DIAGNOSIS
Acute lithium neurotoxicity may present with delirium, seizures, and EEG changes other than seizure activity (e.g., diffuse slowing).

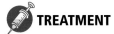 TREATMENT

MEDICATION
First Line
Hemodialysis: Lithium is readily dialyzed because of water solubility, low volume of distribution, and lack of protein binding.

Second Line
Continuous arteriovenous hemodiafiltration

ADDITIONAL TREATMENT
General Measures
- ABCs
- Gastric lavage may be attempted if the patient presents within 1 hour of ingestion
- Whole-bowel irrigation with polyethylene glycol lavage can be effective in preventing absorption from extended-release lithium.
- Restoration of sodium and water balance in hypovolemic subjects

Issues for Referral
- Toxicology consult for cases unresponsive to medical therapy
- Nephrology for hemodialysis

IN-PATIENT CONSIDERATIONS
Initial Stabilization
As above

Admission Criteria
Patients with severe intoxication or significant cardiac disease should be monitored in an ICU.

IV Fluids
Isotonic saline

Nursing
- Hemodynamic monitoring
- Monitoring for cardiac arrhythmias

Discharge Criteria
Resolution of clinical findings including seizures, mental status change, hemodynamic collapse

 ONGOING CARE

FOLLOW-UP RECOMMENDATIONS
Psychiatric evaluation for suicidal overdose

Patient Monitoring
- Lithium levels
- Predisposing factors for chronic toxicity: Dehydration, renal dysfunction, drug interactions, NSAIDs, diuretics, ACE inhibitors

PATIENT EDUCATION
Low therapeutic index of lithium

PROGNOSIS
10% develop chronic neurologic sequelae

COMPLICATIONS
- Truncal ataxia, nystagmus, short-term memory deficits
- SILENT (syndrome of irreversible lithium-effectuated neurotoxicity)

ADDITIONAL READING
- Goodman JW, et al. The role of continuous renal replacement therapy in the treatment of poisoning. *Semin Dial*. 2006;19:402.
- Hansen HE, et al. Lithium intoxication. Report of 23 cases and review of 100 cases from the literature. *Q J Med*. 1978;47:123.
- Lithium. In: Hoffman RS, Nelson LS, Howland MA, et al., eds., *Goldfrank's manual of toxicologic emergencies*. New York: McGraw Hill, 2007:591–4.
- Waring WS, et al. Pattern of lithium exposure predicts poisoning severity: Evaluation of referrals to a regional poisons unit. *Q J Med*. 2007;100:271–6.

 CODES

ICD9
- 969.8 Poisoning by other specified psychotropic agents
- 985.8 Toxic effect of other specified metals

CLINICAL PEARLS
- Acute toxicity may reveal higher levels, but fewer symptoms.
- Chronic exposure may reveal more symptoms, but lower levels.

POISONING, TCA

Muhammad N. Athar
James A. Gasperino

 BASICS

DESCRIPTION
Tricyclic antidepressants (TCAs) are used in the management of a wide range of psychiatric disorders.

EPIDEMIOLOGY
Incidence
The 2004 American Association of Poison Control Centers' (AAPCC) annual report on toxic exposures in the U.S. included 103,155 reported cases of antidepressant toxicity; 12,269 were due to TCAs, with a total of 86 deaths.

Prevalence
TCA toxicity accounts for ~12% of reported toxic exposures for antidepressants, but accounts for 29% of deaths due to antidepressant poisoning.

RISK FACTORS
- Suicidal intention
- Patients with underlying heart disease or cardiac arrhythmias or conduction disturbances could be especially sensitive to the toxic effects of TCAs.
- Individuals with underlying seizure disorders and taking TCAs may have a lowered seizure threshold.

Pregnancy Considerations
Pregnancy risk Category C

GENERAL PREVENTION
Keep medications out of reach of children.

PATHOPHYSIOLOGY
- Well absorbed orally
- Significant first-pass metabolism in the liver
- Large volume of distribution and long half-lives (>24 hours)
- Metabolized in the liver via glucuronic acid conjugation, later excreted through the kidneys
- 4 main pharmacologic properties:
  - Inhibition of norepinephrine and serotonin reuptake at nerve terminals
  - Blocks acetylcholine receptors (anticholinergic action)
  - Direct α-adrenergic blockade
  - Membrane-stabilizing effect on the myocardium by blocking the cardiac myocyte fast sodium channels (action similar to antiarrhythmic 1A)
- Readily penetrates into the CNS
- Therapeutic antidepressant activity is through increasing norepinephrine and serotonin at nerve terminals.

ETIOLOGY
Accidental/intentional overdose

 DIAGNOSIS

HISTORY
- Collect information regarding specific agent, amount ingested, time of ingestion, any co-ingestion.
- Underlying cardiac disease (e.g., heart failure)
- Witnesses and EMS personnel may be helpful to recover pill bottles at the scene.
- Patient's pharmacy may provide valuable information regarding prescribed medications and the total number of pills dispensed.

PHYSICAL EXAM
- Anticholinergic effect: Xerostomia, blurred vision, mydriasis, urinary retention, hypoactive or absent bowel sounds, pyrexia, myoclonic twitching
- Cardiovascular effects: Sinus tachycardia; prolonged PR, QRS, and QT intervals; heart block; peripheral vasodilatation; hypotension; cardiogenic shock; ventricular arrhythmias; asystole
- CNS effects: Drowsiness, extrapyramidal signs, rigidity, ophthalmoplegia, respiratory depression, delirium, seizure, coma

DIAGNOSTIC TESTS & INTERPRETATION
Lab
- Serum TCA levels correlate poorly with severity of toxicity
- Routine screening for other treatable toxins is recommended because multisubstance ingestion is common.
- Electrolyte, BUN, and creatinine levels
- Anion gap
- CBC count
- Alcohol level
- ABGs for evaluation of acidosis or hypoxia

Imaging
Initial approach
Chest radiograph

Follow-Up & Special Considerations
ECG
- Highly sensitive tool; can be used to rule out TCA toxicity
- QRS widening is a better predictor of toxicity than TCA levels.

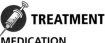 **TREATMENT**

MEDICATION
First Line
- Supportive
- IV hydration for hypotension
- Hypertonic sodium bicarbonate in patients with QRS widening >100 ms or a ventricular arrhythmia (1–2 mEq/kg rapid IV push)
- Vasopressors if unresponsive to fluid resuscitation (pressors of choice are norepinephrine and phenylephrine)
- Dopamine is not effective as a pressor because it depends on the release of endogenous norepinephrine for its action.

Second Line
- Lidocaine
- Magnesium sulfate

ADDITIONAL TREATMENT
General Measures
- ABCs
- Early intubation for patients with significant signs of toxicity
- IV fluids should be started for patients who are hypotensive.
- Orogastric lavage is beneficial only if patient presents early (<1 hour) after ingestion.
- Administer activated charcoal if patient presents within 2 hours of ingestion.

Issues for Referral
Toxicology consult if not responsive to initial medical therapy

Additional Therapies
- Seizures are treated with benzodiazepines.
- Risk of seizures and arrhythmias within the first 6–8 hours of ingestion
- Hemodialysis and hemoperfusion are ineffective.
- Tricyclic-specific fragment antigen binding fragments have been shown to reverse cardiotoxicity in animal model, but still in experimental stage

IN-PATIENT CONSIDERATIONS
Initial Stabilization
As above

Admission Criteria
- Altered mental status
- Hypotension
- Cardiac conduction abnormalities
- Seizures

IV Fluids
Isotonic saline

Nursing
Hemodynamic and cardiac monitoring

Discharge Criteria
- Able to protect airway
- No cardiac rhythm problem on ECG

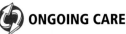 **ONGOING CARE**

FOLLOW-UP RECOMMENDATIONS
Psychiatric evaluation for attempted suicide

PATIENT EDUCATION
- Keep medications out of reach of children.
- Elderly people may need assistance in medication intake if drug overdose was accidental.

PROGNOSIS
- Excellent, if recognized early (70% of intentional TCA overdoses are fatal prior to arrival in the ED)
- In-hospital mortality is reported to be 2–3%.

COMPLICATIONS
- Seizures
- Heart blocks

ADDITIONAL READING
- Cyclic antidepressants. In: Hoffman RS, Nelson LS, Howland MA, et al., eds., *Goldfrank's Manual of Toxicologic Emergencies*. New York: McGraw Hill, 2007:608–14.
- Heard K, et al. A preliminary study of tricyclic antidepressant (TCA) ovine FAB for TCA toxicity. *Clin Toxicol (Phila)*. 2006;44:275–81.
- Kerr GW, et al. Tricyclic antidepressant overdose: A review. *Emerg Med J*. 2001;18:236–41.
- Watson WA, et al. 2004 Annual report of the American Association of Poison Control Centers Toxic Exposure Surveillance System. *Am J Emerg Med*. 2005;23:589–666.
- Woolf A, et al. Tricyclic antidepressant poisoning: An evidence-based consensus guideline for out-of-hospital management. *Clin Toxicol*. 2007;45:203–33.

 CODES

ICD9
969.05 Poisoning by tricyclic antidepressants

POLYNEUROPATHY, CRITICAL ILLNESS AND MYOPATHY

Alina Dulu

 BASICS

DESCRIPTION
Critical illness polyneuropathy (CIP) and myopathy (CIM; together CIPNM) are ICU-acquired neuromuscular disorders characterized by axonal degeneration disease and/or myopathy that is described in severely ill patients.

EPIDEMIOLOGY
Incidence
12–35% (1)

Prevalence
- 50% of patients who require >7 days of ICU care
- Electrophysiologic abnormalities consistent with CIPNM are seen in 80% of patients with systemic inflammatory response syndrome (SIRS) (2).
- Present in 60% of patients with ARDS.
- CIPNM can occur as early as 2–5 days in the presence of severe illness.
- Most often, it takes >1 week of mechanical ventilation to occur.

RISK FACTORS
- Severity and duration of the critical illness
- Multiple-organ system failure
- SIRS and severe sepsis
- Use of neuromuscular blocking agents, corticosteroids, cytotoxic drugs
- Status asthmaticus
- Bed rest and deep sedation (disuse atrophy)
- Severe malnourishment

GENERAL PREVENTION
- Avoid the use of amino glycoside antibiotics, neuromuscular-blocking agents, and high-dose corticosteroids alone and especially in combination.
- Tight glycemic control in ICU

PATHOPHYSIOLOGY
The mechanism of axonal injury in CIP is unknown, but there are assumptions:
- Perturbation in the microcirculation with resultant axonal injury and degeneration (3)
- Atrophy and loss of myosin cause weakness due to loss of force generation following muscle fiber action potentials.

ETIOLOGY
The causes are unknown, but suspected to be multiple and overlapping.

COMMONLY ASSOCIATED CONDITIONS
- Severe sepsis with multiorgan failure
- Septic encephalopathy
- Acute lung injury
- SIRS
- Uncontrolled hyperglycemia (4)

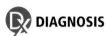 **DIAGNOSIS**

HISTORY
- Respiratory insufficiency
- Difficulty weaning from the ventilator when lung, chest wall, or cardiac causes are excluded
- Weakness
- Reduction in spontaneous movement of the limbs

PHYSICAL EXAM
- Symmetric flaccid weakness in all limbs
- Ranging from paresis to true quadriplegia
- Sparing of the facial muscles
- Depressed or absent reflexes bilaterally
- Muscle wasting of the limbs
- Fasciculations
- Mild sensory loss (difficult to assess in ICU patients)
- No autonomic abnormalities
- Respiratory insufficiency caused by weakness of diaphragm and intercostal muscles
- The Medical Research Council (MRC) score is used to document the extent of disease and follow changes over time
  - Exam of three muscle groups in each limb
  - Upper extremity: Wrist flexion, forearm flexion, shoulder abduction
  - Lower extremity: Ankle dorsiflexion, knee extension, hip flexion
  - On a 1–5 scale:
    - 0: No visible contraction
    - 1: Visible muscle contraction, but no limb movement
    - 2: Active movement, but not against gravity
    - 3: Active movement against gravity
    - 4: Active movement against gravity and resistance
    - 5: Active movement against full resistance

DIAGNOSTIC TESTS & INTERPRETATION
Lab
- No specific abnormal labs
- Serum creatine kinase is normal in most cases of CIM, but may be raised in necrotizing myopathy in the first week.
- Normal ESR
- Normal potassium, calcium, phosphorus, magnesium

Imaging
- MRI imaging of spine with gadolinium for differential diagnosis of tetraparesis
- Head CT to evaluate for acute CVA

Diagnostic Procedures/Other
- Electrophysiologic studies are the cornerstone of diagnosis:
  - Motor and sensory nerve conduction studies including phrenic nerve (NCS)
  - Electromyography including respiratory, diaphragmatic muscles (EMG)
  - Direct muscle stimulation
- Axonal degeneration of the motor neurons followed by the sensory neurons and sometimes myopathic altered motor unit potentials:
  - Preserved latencies with normal nerve conduction velocities
  - Decreased compound muscle action potential (CMAP)
  - Decreased sensory nerve action potential
  - Over time, fibrillation potentials will be evident on EMG needle exam.
  - Prolongation of the CMAP duration suggests an associated myopathy (CIM).
  - Repetitive nerve stimulation is normal.
- CIM:
  - Needle EMG exam contains fibrillation potentials and positive sharp waves in both the limb muscles and the diaphragms 2 to 3 weeks after the start of the process.
  - Loss of muscle responsiveness to direct stimulation
  - Short-duration, low-amplitude motor unit action potentials (MUPs) with early recruitment
- 50% of patients have electrophysiological abnormalities appearing before the clinical syndrome is evident.

Pathological Findings
- Nerve biopsies in CIP:
  - A primarily distal axonal degeneration of motor and sensory fibers
  - Neither demyelinating nor inflammatory features have been present
- Muscle biopsies in CIM:
  - Muscle fiber atrophy, preferentially type II fibers, occasional fiber necrosis and regeneration
  - Decreased reactivity in myofibrillar adenosine triphosphatase staining, corresponding to a selective pathognomonic loss of myosin filaments with preservation of thin (actin) myofilaments and Z discs

DIFFERENTIAL DIAGNOSIS
- Acute spinal cord pathology (transverse myelitis, epidural abscess)
- Mononeuropathies or plexopathies due to pressure palsies, compartment syndromes, porphyria
- Myopathy induced by long-term treatment with aminoglycoside antibiotics, neuromuscular-blocking agents, amiodarone alone or in combination with high-dose corticosteroids
- Neuromuscular junction disorders: Myasthenia gravis
- Inflammatory myopathies (polymyositis, dermatomyositis)
- Severe electrolyte abnormalities: Hypermagnesemia, hypokalemia, hypophosphatemia
- Guillain-Barré syndrome (GBS)
- Acute CVA
- Phrenic nerve injuries

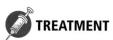 TREATMENT

MEDICATION
- No specific treatment has been demonstrated to hasten recovery.
- Supportive therapy
- Intensive insulin protocol to prevent or correct hyperglycemia reduced the incidence by neurophysiologic testing abnormalities from 52% to 29% (5).
- Treatment of the primary disease
- Early mobility, aggressive physical therapy

ADDITIONAL TREATMENT
General Measures
- Sedation protocols, daily interruption of sedative infusions for serial neuromuscular exam
- Routine implementation of the structured MRC exam

Issues for Referral
- Physical and rehabilitation therapy
- Surgery for early tracheotomy

SURGERY/OTHER PROCEDURES
Early tracheostomy

IN-PATIENT CONSIDERATIONS
Nursing
- Passive limb muscle stretching
- Active exercises with physical and occupational therapy
- Early mobilization out of bed

Discharge Criteria
Neurologically stable

 ONGOING CARE

PROGNOSIS
- Clinical recovery is nearly complete in CIP but gradual, over 2–3 months.
- The median hospital stay in patients with CIP is ~3 months.
- Increases mortality and length of hospital and ICU stay.
- Very few patients with severe disease remain quadriplegic with significant long-term functional disability.
- The outcome following CIM can be poor, particularly in the necrotizing variants.
- Electrodiagnostic testing may demonstrate residual nerve dysfunction several years after initial presentation.

COMPLICATIONS
- Patients with electrophysiologic evidence of CIP had a longer duration of mechanical ventilation.
- CIP and CIM is a frequent cause of neuromuscular weaning failure in critically ill patients, regardless of the type of primary illness.

REFERENCES
1. Lefaucheur JP, et al. Origin of ICU acquired paresis determined by direct muscle stimulation. *J Neurol Neurosurg Psychiatry*. 2006;77(4):500–6.
2. Deem S, et al. Acquired neuromuscular disorders in the intensive care unit. *Am J Respir Crit Care Med*. 2003;168:735–9.
3. Bolton CF, et al. Polyneuropathy in critically ill patients 1. *J Neurol Neurosurg Psychiatry*. 1984;47:1223–31.
4. Van den Berghe G, et al. Outcome benefit of intensive insulin therapy in the critically ill: Insulin dose versus glycemic control. *Crit Care Med*. 2003;31:359–66.
5. Van den Berghe G, et al. Intensive insulin therapy in the critically ill patient. *N Engl J Med*. 2001;345:1359–67.

ADDITIONAL READING
- Mason RJ, et al., eds. *Murray & Nadel's Textbook of Respiratory Medicine*, 4th ed. New York: Saunders, 2005.
- Samuels MA, et al., eds. *Office Practice of Neurology*, 2nd ed. New York: Churchill Livingstone, 2003.

 CODES

ICD9
- 357.82 Critical illness polyneuropathy
- 359.81 Critical illness myopathy

CLINICAL PEARLS
- Weakness acquired in the ICU due to CIPNM is three times more common than primary neuromuscular disorders such as GBS, myopathies, or motor neuron diseases
- CIPNM is diagnosed late because most of the time patients in the ICU are encephalopathic, confused, sedated, or intubated

POLYNEUROPHY, DEMYELINATING CHRONIC INFLAMMATORY

Alina Dulu

BASICS

DESCRIPTION
- A heterogeneous group of disorders of the peripheral nervous system whose common feature is multifocal demyelination of peripheral nerves
- Resembles AIDP; it has a more prolonged course, with slow progression, often relapsing and generally steroid-responsive:
  - The interval between onset of weakness and peak impairment is >4 weeks, averaging 3 months.

EPIDEMIOLOGY
- May affect individuals at any age
- The mean age has varied from 31.6–51.0 years.
- Slightly more common in men than in women

RISK FACTORS
Onset and relapses may be triggered by infections or immunizations.

PATHOPHYSIOLOGY
Both humoral and cell-mediated responses against a variety of myelin-derived antigens are detected in some CIDP patients.

ETIOLOGY
Autoimmune disorder

COMMONLY ASSOCIATED CONDITIONS
Frequent association with a systemic illness:
- Monoclonal gammopathy of undetermined significance (MGUS)
- Amyloidosis
- Multiple myeloma
- Lymphoma
- Systemic lupus erythematosus (SLE) and vasculitis
- Human immunodeficiency virus infections
- Malignancy

DIAGNOSIS

HISTORY
- Progressive or relapsing motor and sensory, rarely, only motor or sensory, dysfunction of more than one limb of a peripheral nerve nature, developing over at least 2 months
- Initial manifestation: Symmetrical motor or sensory symptoms
- Gait ataxia

PHYSICAL EXAM
- Diffuse weakness
- Abnormal tendon reflexes
- Sensory signs in more than 85% of patients:
  - Numbness and paresthesias of the feet and hands
- Facial weakness is common, particularly orbicularis oculi weakness
- Symptomatic dysautonomia is uncommon

DIAGNOSTIC TESTS & INTERPRETATION
Lab
Initial lab tests
CSF analysis:
- Elevated protein and cell count <10/mm^3
- Negative syphilis serology

Follow-Up & Special Considerations
- Serum protein electrophoresis for possible plasma cell dyscrasia
- ANA, ESR
- HIV antibody

Imaging
- MRI scan may demonstrate hypertrophy and gadolinium enhancement of cervical and lumbosacral nerve roots.
- Radiologic skeletal survey

Diagnostic Procedures/Other
- Electrophysiologic evidence of multifocal demyelination with superimposed axonal degeneration:
  - Slowing of motor conduction velocities
  - Prolonged or absent F waves,
  - Abnormal temporal dispersion
  - Partial conduction block.
- Sensory conduction study are abnormal.
- Needle EMG abnormalities:
  - Superimposed axonal degeneration and regeneration

Pathological Findings
- Nerve biopsy showing evidence of demyelination and remyelination
- Sural nerve biopsy for identifying vasculitis, amyloid deposits, cytoplasmic inclusions, neurofilamentous swollen axons, or evidence of other specific pathology
- Bone marrow biopsy

DIFFERENTIAL DIAGNOSIS
Investigation for SLE and other collagen vascular diseases, vasculitis, diabetes, HIV infection, or malignancy

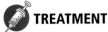 **TREATMENT**

MEDICATION

First Line
- Minor deficits at presentation may be observed without treatment.
- Patients who do not improve, continue to progress, or patients with moderate to severe deficits, should undergo treatment.
- The objective of the treatment is to prevent relapse.
- Immunosuppressive therapy is the mainstay of therapy.
- Corticosteroids (1)
- IVIg at 2 g/kg body weight over 2–3 consecutive days
- Plasma exchange: 1 plasma volume per exchange, 5 times over 2 weeks
- Cyclophosphamide (1–2 mg/kg/d or 1 g/m^2 body surface area
- Cyclosporin (3 to 5 mg/kg/d):
  - 40% of patients have a favorable response to oral corticosteroids

Second Line
Other immunosuppressants: Azathioprine, melphalan, mycophenolate mofetil, rituximab, and total lymphoid irradiation

ADDITIONAL TREATMENT

General Measures
Most treatment is in the outpatient setting.

Issues for Referral
- Physical and occupational therapy for rehabilitation, including supportive devices
- ENT/surgery for early tracheotomy and feeding gastrectomy for patients who require prolonged ventilatory support

IN-PATIENT CONSIDERATIONS

Initial Stabilization
Most or all treatment is in the outpatient setting.

Admission Criteria
- Admit to hospital for moderate to sever weakness attacks.
- Patients with rapidly worsening acute disease should be observed in ICU until the maximum extent of progression has been established.

Nursing
- Frequent repositioning of patient to minimize formation of pressure sores
- Pressure-induced ulnar or fibular nerve palsies are prevented by proper positioning and padding.
- Exposure keratitis in cases of facial plegia by using artificial tears and by taping the eyelids closed at night.

Discharge Criteria
Neurologically stable

 ONGOING CARE

FOLLOW-UP RECOMMENDATIONS

Patient Monitoring
- Patients receiving prednisone:
  - Interval weight, blood pressure, serum glucose, and potassium measurements
  - Should be placed on a high-protein, low-salt, low-fat diet
  - Supplemental calcium and vitamin D to reduce the risk of osteoporosis
- Patients treated with azathioprine:
  - Liver function studies and CBCs, repeated weekly for the 1st month and then at longer intervals
- Patients prescribed mycophenolate mofetil need monitoring for possible leukopenia.
- Patients on cyclosporin or cyclophosphamide need monitoring of renal and hematologic function.

PROGNOSIS
- >75% of patients develop at least moderate disability.
- Patients with mild impairment improve spontaneously.
- Mild or no disability in 87% of our patients (2)

COMPLICATIONS
- 5–12% of patients need respiratory support at some point in their course.
- Mortality during the first 5 years after diagnosis is <5%.

REFERENCES

1. Barohn RJ, et al. Chronic inflammatory demyelinating polyradiculoneuropathy: Clinical characteristics, course, and recommendations for diagnostic criteria. *Arch Neurol*. 1989;46:878–84.
2. Simmons Z, et al. Long-term follow-up of patients with chronic inflammatory demyelinating polyradiculoneuropathy, without and with monoclonal gammopathy. *Brain*. 1995;118:359–68.

ADDITIONAL READING
- Katirji B. *Neuromuscular Disorders in Clinical Practice*. Boston: Butterworth-Heinemann, 2002.
- Samuels MA. *Office Practice of Neurology*. Edinburgh: Churchill Livingston, 1996.

 CODES

ICD9
357.81 Chronic inflammatory demyelinating polyneuritis

CLINICAL PEARLS
CIDP is not simply a prolonged form of AIDP.

POST-CARDIAC SURGERY CARE

Luciano Lemos-Filho

 BASICS

DESCRIPTION

- Cardiac surgery in the modern era is made possible by cardiopulmonary bypass (CPB) intraoperatively and has become routine in the industrialized world.
- The cardiac surgery patient presents unique physiologic challenges in the postoperative period due to his primary pathology, exposure to CPB, and the surgical insult itself.

PATHOPHYSIOLOGY

- Preoperative pathology is critical to understanding postoperative physiology and expectations.
- Contact of blood with CPB can lead to platelet activation and dysfunction thus increasing bleeding risk; SIRS response, often with vasoplegic shock state; and pulmonary and renal injury.
- Blood loss and volume removal during surgery can predispose to hypovolemia.
- Cardioplegia can lead to cardiac dysfunction and need for inotropic support postoperatively.
- Surgery itself can lead to conduction abnormalities; pain and sympathetic surges can lead to postoperative atrial fibrillation.
- Bleeding/clotting into pericardium can lead to tamponade physiology.
- Therefore, the cardiac surgery patient can present with cardiogenic, vasodilatory, obstructive, and hypovolemic shock, or any combination thereof.

ETIOLOGY

Depends on particular complication

COMMONLY ASSOCIATED CONDITIONS

Often related to cardiac surgery; coronary bypass patients in particular often have coexisting:

- DM
- HTN
- PVD
- CRI
- Hyperlipidemia

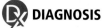 **DIAGNOSIS**

HISTORY

- It is paramount for the critical care practitioner to understand the procedure the patient underwent, including unexpected events, to anticipate complications postoperatively and interpret data in the correct context.
- Communication with anesthesiology is as important to understand airway issues, echocardiogram, and the physiology of the particular patient.
- Bedside face-to-face sign-out including surgery team, critical care, and anesthesia is thus encouraged.
- The sign-out should include the time on CPB and cross-clamp, the ejection fraction before and after, the current vasoactive meds, relevant labs and hemodynamics, and any residual pathology that was not corrected.

PHYSICAL EXAM

- Typically, cardiac surgery patients present to the ICU intubated (although in many centers they are extubated in the OR), and still under the effects of general anesthesia.
- The wound site will usually be covered but should be inspected externally for bleeding.
- Inspect monitoring catheters and their leveling.
- Chest tube output and quality is to be followed.
- Pulmonary artery catheter (PAC) is usually in place to allow serial measurement of cardiac output, mixed venous oxygen saturation, pulmonary artery and central venous pressures.

DIAGNOSTIC TESTS & INTERPRETATION

Lab

Initial lab tests

- CBC
- ABG with lactic acid
- Mixed venous gas
- Basic metabolic
- Liver panel
- Coagulation parameters

Follow-Up & Special Considerations

- Close follow-up of urine output, cardiac index, lactic acid as measures of perfusion
- Extubation should proceed as quickly as possible once patient is awake and tolerating spontaneous breathing test.

Imaging

Initial approach

Baseline CXR upon arrival to ICU to verify ETT, PAC, chest tube, and OG tube placement

Follow-Up & Special Considerations

- Close follow-up of labs, indices
- TEE in rare cases of decompensation immediately postop.

TREATMENT

MEDICATION

- Inotropes are divided into inopressors (epinephrine), inodilators (dobutamine, milrinone).
- Vasopressors: Vasopressin, norepinephrine
- Mixed: Dopamine
- Later in course, once off inotropes/pressors, β blockade for is used for blood pressure control and as prophylaxis for atrial fibrillation.

ADDITIONAL TREATMENT

General Measures
- Volume repletion
- Monitor chest tube output and transfuse as needed if bleeding or if Hgb <7.0.
- Over 200 mL/hr (or >50 cc/15 min), considered surgical bleeding; and usually requires return to OR.
- Early extubation is favored in the appropriate patient.

IN-PATIENT CONSIDERATIONS

Initial Stabilization
- Frequently, post-cardiac surgery patients require resuscitative efforts to correct the various possible shock states.

- IV fluids, especially in states of low CI with low CVP/filling pressures followed by:
  - Inotropic agents in cases of low CI when CVP is adequate (usually defined as 8–12 cm H_2O)
  - Pressor agents to maintain MAP >65 and goal urine output >0.5 mL/kg/hr
  - Typical goal CI >2.2
  - If no PAC is in place, assess with physical exam, urine output, lactate. If severe, TR PAC can be used to follow mixed venous saturation.
  - Rate stabilization with external pacing wires if necessary in cases of bradycardia or loss of atrial kick.

ONGOING CARE

COMPLICATIONS

- Atrial fibrillation
- Tamponade (typically clot rather than liquid tamponade in early postop period)
- Hemorrhage
- Acute respiratory failure
- Acute renal failure
- SIRS post CPB
- Arrhythmia requiring pacemaker

ADDITIONAL READING

Cohn L. Cardiac surgery in the adult. Accessed at http://cardiacsurgery.ctsnetbooks.org/current.shtmL#PART_II_PERIOPERATIVE_INTRAOPERATIVE_CARE

CODES

ICD9
- 785.51 Cardiogenic shock
- 997.1 Cardiac complications, not elsewhere classified
- 998.0 Postoperative shock, not elsewhere classified

CLINICAL PEARLS

- Distinction of right-heart failure from tamponade can be challenging in early postop period and often requires TEE.
- Tamponade is classically diagnosed with "equalization" of pressures (i.e., CVP, PA diastolic, PAOP within 5 mm H_2O of each other).

P

POSTOPERATIVE ANALGESIA

Seth Manoach

BASICS

DESCRIPTION
- IV opiates are the mainstay of postoperative pain management in the ICU.
- Secondary opiate anxiolytic effects are often desirable.
- Opiate respiratory depression and gut dysmotility must be carefully monitored and addressed.
- Inability to communicate pain does not mean absence of pain.

EPIDEMIOLOGY
Incidence
- ~50% of postoperative patients experience moderate pain, 20% experience severe pain, despite current analgesic practice.
- 40% of conscious patients experience severe pain "most of the time" during the 3 days before death.

ETIOLOGY
- Pain arises from direct trauma, distension, chemical or thermal event in periphery:
  - Local trauma and heat causes depolarization of rapid Aδ fibers.
  - Inflammatory cytokines, Δ pH/ion concentration cause depolarization of slow C-fibers.
- Peripheral nociceptive nerves synapse in dorsal horn of spinal cord.
- Axons of postsynaptic nerves ascend to contralateral thalamic nuclei.
- Thalamic nuclei project to parietal, frontal, and limbic cortex.
- Subcortical and cortical activation facilitates survival-adaptive perception, immediate and long-term aversive responses:
  - These are experienced in ICU patients as pain, anxiety, depressed mood.
- Pain increases the sympathomimetic, procoagulant, catabolic neuroendocrine response to surgery.

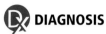

DIAGNOSIS

HISTORY
- Actively elicit complaints of pain.
- Patients may use gestures, communication boards, and visual analog scales.

PHYSICAL EXAM
Signs and symptoms depend on level of consciousness of patient:
- Mechanically ventilated, sedated, unconscious patients *may* manifest tachycardia or hypertension
- Unexplained agitation
- Restlessness
- Diaphoresis
- Increased minute ventilation

DIAGNOSTIC TESTS & INTERPRETATION

- IV opiates: Mainstay of postoperative pain treatment:
  - Critical respiratory depression can be reversed with naloxone.
  - Administer bowel regimen.
- Patient-controlled anesthesia (PCA) may be beneficial.
- Intrathecal and other neuraxial regimens may include local anesthetic and/or opioids.
- Frequently used narcotics:
  - Morphine: Most common agent:
    - If patient becomes hypotensive with use, may be volume depleted
  - Hydromorphone: 5 times more potent than morphine
  - Fentanyl is ideal for postop analgesia in ICU patients:
    - Context-sensitive half time: Functional half-life of fentanyl increases from 1 hour for 1st hour of infusion to >5 hour for prolonged (>8 hours) infusions.
    - Can transition to transdermal formulation or PO agent.
  - Meperidine:
    - Avoid use due to toxic metabolites.
    - Occasionally used for postoperative shivering

ADDITIONAL READING

- Berde C, et al. Opioid side effects—mechanism based therapy. *N Engl J Med*. 2008;358: 2400–2402.
- Lullman H, et al. *Color Atlas of Pharmacology*, 3rd ed. Stuttgart, New York: Thieme, 2005.
- Lynn J, et al. Perceptions of family members of the dying experience of older and seriously ill patients. *Ann Intern Med*. 1997;126:97–106.
- White PF, et al. Improving post-operative pain management: What are the unresolved issues? *Anesthesiology*. 2010;112:220–5.
- www.postoppain.org. Accessed May 10–12, 2010.

 CODES

ICD9

- 338.18 Other acute postoperative pain
- 338.28 Other chronic postoperative pain

CLINICAL PEARLS

- Pain is ubiquitous, underdetected, undertreated, and synergistic with anxiety in ICU.
- Opiates are mainstay of post-op ICU analgesia: Baseline infusion + episodic rescue dosing is the best approach.
- Respiratory depression and gut dysmotility are the principal adverse effects to be monitored and treated.

PREECLAMPSIA (PEC)

Juliana Gebb
Dena Goffman

 BASICS

DESCRIPTION

• New onset of hypertension and proteinuria after 20 weeks of gestation in a previously normotensive woman (may occur in pregnancy or up to 6–8 weeks postpartum)
• Systems affected: Cardiovascular, Renal, Pulmonary, Hepatic, Hematologic, Neurologic

EPIDEMIOLOGY
Incidence
5–8% of U.S. pregnancies (75% mild, 25% severe)

RISK FACTORS
• Nulliparity
• Chronic hypertension
• Pregestational diabetes
• Sickle cell disease
• Chronic renal disease
• Thrombophilia
• Antiphospholipid antibody syndrome
• Connective tissue disease
• Obesity
• Maternal age >40 or <18
• Personal history/1st-degree relative with PEC
• Multifetal gestation
• Hydrops fetalis
• Gestational trophoblastic disease

Genetics
Family history of PEC is a risk factor, but no clear genetic etiology has been described

GENERAL PREVENTION
• No preventative therapy has been shown to be effective in the overall pregnant population.
• Appropriate prenatal care can facilitate early recognition and appropriate treatment of PEC.

PATHOPHYSIOLOGY
• Hypothesized that abnormal placentation leads to an imbalance between antiangiogenic and angiogenic factors
• This imbalance results in vasoconstriction and leaky capillaries, leading to 3rd-spacing and possibly to:
  – Hemoconcentration
  – Renal insufficiency
  – Pulmonary edema
  – Subcapsular hematoma or liver rupture
  – Increased risk for thromboembolism
  – Oligohydramnios
  – Fetal growth restriction
  – Seizures
  – Intracranial hemorrhage
  – Hypertensive emergency
  – Hypertensive encephalopathy

COMMONLY ASSOCIATED CONDITIONS
• Chronic HTN, renal disease, diabetes, obesity
• Placental abruption seen in PEC

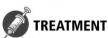 **DIAGNOSIS**

HISTORY
With severe PEC, patients may complain of headache, visual disturbances (scotomata and blurry vision), epigastric pain, nausea/vomiting, shortness of breath, decreased urine output, or may present with altered mental status.

PHYSICAL EXAM
• Mild PEC: Blood pressure (BP) >140/90 twice 6 hours apart
• Severe PEC: BP >160/110 twice 6 hours apart
• Hyperreflexia, epigastric tenderness, rales, peripheral edema, papilledema/retinal hemorrhages possible (more common with HTN encephalopathy, less common with eclampsia)

DIAGNOSTIC TESTS & INTERPRETATION
Lab
Initial lab tests
• CBC: May reveal hemoconcentration, thrombocytopenia, or hemolysis
• Comprehensive metabolic panel: May reveal elevated transaminases and/or BUN/creatinine
• LDH: Elevation suggests hemolysis
• Uric acid elevation
• Urine toxicology
• Urinalysis/24-hour urine collection for protein and creatinine:
  – Mild PEC: UA with 1+ protein or 24-hour urine protein ≥300 mg but <5 g
  – Severe PEC: UA with 3+ on 2 random samples 4 hours apart or 24-hour urine protein ≥5 g

Follow-Up & Special Considerations
• Check serial laboratory values for signs of HELLP (see HELLP chapter), renal insufficiency
• Criteria for severe PEC (one of the following):
  – BP >160/110
  – Oliguria (<500 cc/24 hours)
  – Cerebral or visual disturbances
  – Pulmonary edema
  – Epigastric pain
  – UA 3+ protein X 2 or 24-hour urine protein ≥5 g
  – Impaired liver function (transaminases 2x normal)
  – Thrombocytopenia (platelets <100 K)
  – Fetal growth restriction

Imaging
Initial approach
• Chest x-ray if shortness of breath or pulmonary findings
• Head CT if neurologic changes

Follow-Up & Special Considerations
• Posterior reversible encephalopathy syndrome (PRES):
  – Well-described entity in patients with PEC and eclampsia (see Eclampsia chapter)
  – Vasogenic edema due to acutely increased arterial BP that overwhelms autoregulatory capacity of cerebral vasculature

  – Typically presents with headache, visual changes (loss of acuity, visual neglect, homonymous hemianopia, cortical blindness), seizures, mental status changes
  – Prompt treatment of hypertension is critical in ensuring reversibility of deficits.
  – CT: Hypodensities of posterior white/gray matter; lesions are generally bilateral and parieto-occipital, but may involve temporal/frontal lobes, brainstem, cerebellum
  – T2-weighted MRI: Hyperintense signal

Diagnostic Procedures/Other
Hypertensive emergencies:
• Hypertensive encephalopathy
• Acute aortic dissection
• Pulmonary edema/respiratory failure
• Acute MI/unstable angina
• Eclampsia
• Acute renal failure
• Microangiopathic hemolytic anemia

DIFFERENTIAL DIAGNOSIS
• Chronic hypertension (onset prior to 20 weeks)
• Gestational hypertension (no proteinuria)
• TTP-HUS (generally no hepatic involvement)
• Acute fatty liver of pregnancy (low glucose)
• SLE exacerbation

TREATMENT

MEDICATION
First Line

• Magnesium sulfate: 4–6 g loading dose in 100 mL D5W over 20–30 minutes followed by 20 g in 500mL D5W at 50 cc/hr for seizure prophylaxis (2)[A]

• Delivery of the fetus depending on the gestational age and severity of disease (2)[C].

ALERT
Magnesium sulfate is contraindicated in patients with pulmonary edema. In patients with renal dysfunction or oliguria, magnesium levels must be followed and dose adjusted to avoid toxicity.

Second Line
Phenytoin: Use when magnesium sulfate is contraindicated (should not be used as 1st-line agent since proven inferior to magnesium for prevention of recurrent eclamptic seizures) (2)[B].

ADDITIONAL TREATMENT
General Measures
• Follow for signs/symptoms of HEELP, pulmonary edema, eclampsia, hypertensive crisis
• Follow for signs/symptoms of magnesium toxicity including hyporeflexia, somnolence, respiratory failure at toxic doses
• Antihypertensive medications given in PEC for sustained SBP >180 mm Hg or DBP >105–110 to prevent/terminate end-organ damage (2,4)[C]:
  – Hydralazine (5–10 mg IV q15–20min): Used commonly prior to ICU admission but meds listed below are preferred in ICU setting

– Labetalol: 20 mg IV initially followed by doubled dose 40 mg then 80 mg; 80 mg q10min until desired BP or max of 220 mg. Once BP has decreased to desired levels, can also be given as infusion or orally.

– Nifedipine: 10 mg capsules PO every 15–20 min to max of 30 mg): Has been shown to control BP more rapidly than IV labetalol (i.e., in 1 hour); also acts as a selective renal arteriolar vasodilator and natriuretic, thus improving urinary output

– Nicardipine: 5 mg/h initially, increasing infusion rate by 2.5 mg/h every 5 minutes to a maximum of 10 mg/h until desired BP reduction achieved

– Nitroprusside: 0.2 mcg/kg/min, increase to max of 5 mcg/kg/min): Alternative when nicardipine is not available or other meds have failed, but see alert.

ALERT
- Care should be taken not to decrease BP too drastically as this can impair uteroplacental, cerebral, myocardial, and renal blood flow. Goal should be diastolic BP >90 but <110.
- Sublingual nifedipine should be avoided as it may result in a precipitous and uncontrolled fall in BP.
- Fetal cyanide poisoning may occur with >4 hours of nitroprusside use.
- Nitroprusside increases intracranial pressure and should also be avoided in patients with recent MI, LV outflow obstruction, hypothyroidism.
- Nifedipine/nicardipine should be avoided while patient is on magnesium (combination may result in neuromuscular blockade, severe hypotension).

Issues for Referral
- Renal failure rarely requires hemodialysis.
- Anesthesia: Regional/neuraxial anesthesia is efficacious and safe in mild PEC or in severe PEC without coagulopathy (2)[A].

Additional Therapies
Furosemide is used in cases of pulmonary edema but with care as patients with PEC are intravascularly depleted and furosemide may lead to further renal impairment.

SURGERY/OTHER PROCEDURES
- Invasive hemodynamic monitoring (PA catheter) is rarely indicated in the setting of PEC; however, it can be considered for the management of especially difficult cases (2)[B].
- Patients with PEC often have laryngeal edema, making intubation and extubation challenging.

IN-PATIENT CONSIDERATIONS
Initial Stabilization
- Hypertensive crisis: Lower BP as directed above to terminate ongoing end-organ damage, but not to return BP to normal levels.
- Eclampsia: Magnesium sulfate should be started or rebolused; maternal stabilization is crucial prior to delivery of fetus.
- Fetal monitoring: FHR pattern used as a maternal "vital sign" but must stabilize mother prior to any fetal intervention; maternal stabilization generally improves fetal status.

Admission Criteria
- Hypertensive crisis
- Respiratory failure
- Status epilepticus (extremely rare with eclampsia so consider alternative diagnoses/ICH)
- Intracranial hemorrhage
- DIC

IV Fluids
Patients with PEC are intravascularly depleted and therefore require adequate hydration, but aggressive hydration must be avoided since PEC is associated with a hyperdynamic ventricular function with low pulmonary capillary wedge pressure. Aggressive hydration can cause the pulmonary capillary wedge pressure to increase significantly above normal levels.

Nursing
- Serial BP
- Detailed intake and output
- Foley catheter
- Familiarity with giving magnesium sulfate bolus/drip as improper dosing can be lethal
- Hourly reflex checks and urine output for patients on magnesium

Discharge Criteria
No further evidence of hypertensive crisis, stable BP, adequate urine output, improving laboratory values

 ONGOING CARE

FOLLOW-UP RECOMMENDATIONS
Close blood pressure monitoring

PATIENT EDUCATION
- Disease can rarely worsen in the postpartum period, so patients must know that signs and symptoms require immediate medical attention.
- Patients with PEC are at increased risk in a subsequent pregnancy.

PROGNOSIS
- PEC/eclampsia (particularly early onset): Increased future risk of HTN, ischemic heart disease, CVA, VTE; slight increased risk of ESRD
- PRES: Generally reversible, but cases of permanent deficit have been described.

COMPLICATIONS
- Hypertensive crisis
- Eclampsia
- Intracranial hemorrhage
- Renal, liver, or respiratory failure
- Liver rupture
- DIC
- Magnesium toxicity
- Intrauterine fetal demise
- Placental abruption
- Maternal death

REFERENCES

1. Bellamy L, et al. Pre-eclampsia and risk of cardiovascular disease and cancer in later life: Systematic review and meta-analysis. *Brit Med J.* 2007;335 (7627):974.
2. Diagnosis and management of preeclampsia and eclampsia. ACOG Practice Bulletin No. 33. American College of Obstetricians and Gynecologists. *Obstet Gynecol.* January 2002, Reaffirmed 2008.
3. Thackeray EM, et al. Posterior reversible encephalopathy syndrome in a patient with severe preeclampsia. *Anesth Analgesia.* 2007;105:184–6.
4. Vidaeff AC, et al. Acute hypertensive emergencies in pregnancy. *Crit Care Med.* 2005;33(10): S307–S312.

ADDITIONAL READING

- Fujitani S, et al. Hemodynamic assessment in a pregnant and peripartum patient. *Crit Care Med.* 2005;33(10):S354–S361.
- Sibai BM. Imitators of severe preeclampsia. *Obstet Gynecol.* 2007;109(4):956–66.
- Vidaeff AC, et al. Acute hypertensive emergencies in pregnancy. *Crit Care Med.* 2005;33(10):S307–S312.

 See Also (Topic, Algorithm, Electronic Media Element)

- HELLP
- Eclampsia
- Placental Abruption

 CODES

ICD9
- 642.40 Mild or unspecified pre-eclampsia, unspecified as to episode of care
- 642.41 Mild or unspecified pre-eclampsia, with delivery
- 642.42 Mild or unspecified pre-eclampsia, with delivery, with mention of postpartum complication

CLINICAL PEARLS

- PEC patients have hypertensive emergencies at lower BPs than do patients with chronic HTN.
- In PEC patients with hypertensive emergencies, BP should be lowered to prevent/halt end-organ damage but should not be lowered to normal levels.
- Antihypertensives are given for maternal benefit in cases of severe HTN but have not been shown to improve perinatal outcomes.
- Magnesium sulfate is the drug of choice for patients to prevent eclamptic seizures (except when pulmonary edema is present).
- Treatment of severe PEC involves delivery; whereas patients with TTP-HUS and SLE exacerbation are treated without delivery.

PROPOFOL INFUSION SYNDROME

Karim Djekidel
James Gasperino

 BASICS

DESCRIPTION
Rare but potentially deadly syndrome characterized by ≥2 of the following in a patient sedated with propofol:
- Arrhythmias (refractory bradycardia leading to asystole)
- Metabolic acidosis
- Rhabdomyolysis
- Hyperlipidemia
- Enlarged or fatty liver

EPIDEMIOLOGY
Incidence
Unknown

Prevalence
Unknown; see references for summary of case reports

RISK FACTORS
- Doses of >4 mg/kg/h (67 μg/kg/min) for >48 hours
- Concurrent use of glucocorticoids
- Concurrent use of catecholamines
- Poor nutritional status (low carbohydrate supply)
- Respiratory failure
- Severe head injury
- Impaired mitochondrial function

Genetics
- Medium-chain acyl coenzyme A dehydrogenase (MCAD) deficiency
- MCAD deficiency may be caused by a combination of 18 different MCAD gene variations.
- Genetic defects can lead to mitochondrial malfunction.

GENERAL PREVENTION
- Avoid doses >4 mg/kg/h regardless of duration.
- Switch to alternate agent if dosage limitations are reached without success.
- Early recognition: Labs, RBBB with coved ST elevation in V1–V3 (Brugada pattern) on ECG may be an early indicator of cardiac compromise.
- Adequate carbohydrate supplementation

PATHOPHYSIOLOGY
- The syndrome is usually associated with high doses of continuous propofol administration for prolonged periods (5 mg/kg/h for >48 hours)
- Unknown. Hypotheses considered: Mitochondrial enzyme inhibition, faulty fatty acid oxidation, existence of an unidentified metabolite

COMMONLY ASSOCIATED CONDITIONS
- Renal failure
- Metabolic acidosis
- Hyperkalemia
- Rhabdomyolysis
- Arrhythmias
- Myocardial failure
- Hepatomegaly
- Lipemia

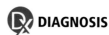 **DIAGNOSIS**

DIAGNOSTIC TESTS & INTERPRETATION
Lab
- Directed at detecting metabolic abnormalities and organ failure:
  - ABG for pH
  - Serum lactate
  - Creatine kinase
  - Liver function tests
  - Triglycerides
  - Electrolytes
  - Troponin I
  - Myoglobin

- Increased plasma malonyl carnitine and C5-acylcarnitine
- Downsloping ST-segment elevation in precordial leads V1 to V3:
  - Bradycardia
  - Atrial fibrillation
  - Ventricular and supraventricular tachycardia
  - Bundle branch block
  - Decreased mitochondrial complex IV activity
  - Decreased complex IV to cytochrome oxidase ratio of 0.004 (normal range, 0.014–0.034)

DIFFERENTIAL DIAGNOSIS
- Shock
- Sepsis
- Other causes of lactic acidosis
- Other causes of rhabdomyolysis

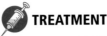 TREATMENT

ADDITIONAL TREATMENT
General Measures
Discontinuation of propofol

Additional Therapies
- Supportive care (IV crystalloids, colloids, vasopressors, inotropic agents, cardiac pacing)
- Hemodialysis/continuous renal replacement therapy
- Case reports of using ECMO successfully

Geriatric Considerations
Smaller volume of distribution and decreased clearance require dosage reductions.

Pediatric Considerations
Propofol should not be used for continuous sedation.

 ONGOING CARE

FOLLOW-UP RECOMMENDATIONS
Patient Monitoring
ABG, triglyceride levels, amylase, lipase

DIET
- Optimize nutritional status.
- Carbohydrate substitution at 6–8 mg/kg/min is also recommended, which might prevent propofol infusion syndrome

PATIENT EDUCATION
Inform of potential side effects of propofol.

PROGNOSIS
Poor

ADDITIONAL READING

- Corbett SM, et al. Propofol-related infusion syndrome in intensive care patients. *Pharmacotherapy*. 2008;28:250–8.
- Fudickar A, et al. Propofol infusion syndrome in anaesthesia and intensive care medicine. *Curr Opin Anesthesiol*. 2006;19:404–10.
- Kam PC, Cardone D. Propofol infusion syndrome. *Anaesthesia*. 2007;62:690–701.
- Rajda C, et al. Propofol infusion syndrome. *J Trauma Nurs*. 2008;15:118–22.
- Vincenzo F, La Manaca E. Propofol infusion syndrome: An overview of a perplexing disease. *Drug Saf*. 2008;31:292–303.
- Zaccheo MM, Bucher DH. Propofol infusion syndrome: A rare complication with potentially fatal results. *Crit Care Nurse*. 2008;28:18–25.

PSEUDOMONAS

Oveys Mansuri

 BASICS

DESCRIPTION
Gram-negative rod commonly associated with opportunistic nosocomial infections such as pneumonia, UTIs, and bacteremia

EPIDEMIOLOGY
Incidence
Bacteremia: Age-adjusted incidence per 100,000 person-years: 10.8 (males) and 3.7 (females)

Prevalence
- 4 per 1,000 discharges
- 4% of nosocomial bloodstream infections are caused by pseudomonas aeruginosa.

RISK FACTORS
- Immunocompromised patient
- Advanced age
- Severe burns
- Indwelling catheter
- Wounds contaminated with fresh water
- Cystic fibrosis
- IV drug abusers
- Exposure (recent or repeated) to broad spectrum antibiotics
- Recent hospitalization (or stay in long-term care facility)

Geriatric Considerations
- Consider malignancy, indwelling catheters for risk factors
- Adjust antibiotic dosing for renal impairment
- Recently, a trend is seen toward pneumonia in older patients.

Pediatric Considerations
- Cystic fibrosis patients have frequent, recurrent pseudomonas pneumonias.
- Adjust antibiotic dosing with relation to pediatric dosing guidelines.

Pregnancy Considerations
Consider antibiotic suitability in the pregnant patient.

GENERAL PREVENTION
- Contact precautions
- Hand-washing and hygiene, including glove use (universal precautions)
- Cleansing of environment and equipment to minimize intrahospital transfer from contaminated equipment (even faucet handles)

PATHOPHYSIOLOGY
- Virulence is dependent on multiple factors including exotoxins, endotoxin, external structure, and other secreted products.
- Initial infection is mediated by flagellum and motility.
- Thereafter, the mechanism of membrane-bound lipopolysaccharide and, in some part, expression of toxins determine pathogenicity of infection.

COMMONLY ASSOCIATED CONDITIONS
- Diabetes
- Malignancy
- Burns
- Cystic fibrosis
- Corneal ulcer
- Enteritis (Shanghai fever)
- Critical illness

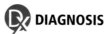 **DIAGNOSIS**

HISTORY
- Mental status changes, headache, confusion
- Valvular heart disease, history of prosthetic valves
- Productive cough, fever, ICU admission, mechanical ventilation, intubation, aspiration
- Exposure to fresh water (i.e., swimming)
- Medical devices, catheters
- Diarrhea (Shanghai fever)
- Frequency, urgency, and other UTI symptoms
- Burns, wounds, skin breakdown and subsequent exposure to contaminated water sources (hot tubs/swimming pools)

PHYSICAL EXAM
- Ophthalmic: Discharge with corneal ulceration
- Otoscopic: Erythema, swelling, inflammation, discharge consistent with malignant otitis externa
- Hypoxia secondary to pneumonia
- Pulmonary exam with rales, rhonchi, decreased breath sounds
- Cardiac exam with new murmur or change in baseline murmur
- Fever, tachycardia, hypotension with advanced infection, consistent with sepsis/shock
- Ecthyma gangrenosum lesions routinely found in skin folds (i.e., axilla, groin)

DIAGNOSTIC TESTS & INTERPRETATION
Lab
Initial lab tests
- CBC: Elevated WBC
- Blood cultures
- Urinalysis/urine culture
- Sputum/Respiratory secretions culture
- Wound and burn cultures:
  - Burn wound biopsies with quantitative cultures

Follow-Up & Special Considerations
Follow-up cultures maybe necessary

Imaging
Chest x-ray to evaluate for pneumonia

Diagnostic Procedures/Other
- Echo for evaluation of endocarditis if suspected
- Bronchoscopy for cultures if indicated

Pathological Findings
Necrotizing inflammation in advanced cases

DIFFERENTIAL DIAGNOSIS
- Acute respiratory distress syndrome
- Pneumonia (various etiologies)
- Sepsis

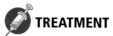 **TREATMENT**

MEDICATION
First Line
- Zosyn 3.375 g q6h or 4.5 g q8h
- Ceftazidime 2 g q8h
- Cefepime 2 g q12h
- Aztreonam 2 g q8h
- UTI: Ciprofloxacin 500 mg PO b.i.d.
- Pneumonia: Zosyn, cefepime, imipenem, meropenem, or aztreonam *AND* ciprofloxacin/levofloxacin or aminoglycoside+azithromycin per 2007 consensus guidelines:
  - Pseudomonas is highly likely to acquire resistance to antibiotics, hence patients with recurrent infections (like cystic fibrosis patients) will require detailed history of antibiotic use and pseudomonas resistance before deciding on the antibiotic of choice.

Second Line
- Gentamicin or tobramycin 3–5 mg/kg/d in 2–3 doses (if combination therapy indicated)
- Imipenem 500 mg q6h or meropenem 1 g q8h for multidrug-resistant infections
- Colistin inhaled: Multidrug resistant pseudomonas pneumonia failing IV treatment

ADDITIONAL TREATMENT

General Measures
- Early diagnosis and treatment/intervention
- Source control (remove foreign body, catheters, abscess)
- Combination therapy as indicated (combination antibiotics therapy; i.e., addition of aminoglycoside may be warranted in certain situations). Although there are no conclusive data in this regard, it is reasonable to administer dual-agent empiric therapy for critically ill patients.

Issues for Referral
- Ophthalmology consultation for eye infections and/or symptoms
- Infectious disease consultation for patients with extensive history of pseudomonas infections (cystis fibrosis patients)

SURGERY/OTHER PROCEDURES
- Removal of infected foreign body or medical device
- Surgical debridement of infected tissues/sites

IN-PATIENT CONSIDERATIONS

Initial Stabilization
- Identification of primary infection
- Early antibiotic therapy (combination) and source control
- Hemodynamic stabilization and resuscitation

Admission Criteria
- ICU admission for those with hemodynamic instability, need for frequent monitoring, respiratory failure, and other ICU needs
- Hospital admission is most likely warranted for most patients, due to the severity of disease.

IV Fluids
- Adequate fluid resuscitation with use of crystalloid replacement (i.e., 0.9% NS or LR)
- Ensure appropriate access and consider central venous access if inadequate access or need for monitoring volume status (CVP). Note the importance of expeditious removal of any infected lines or catheters.

Nursing
- Patient comfort
- Wound care of infected/debrided sites

Discharge Criteria
Resolution of systemic infection and improvement of local sites

ONGOING CARE

FOLLOW-UP RECOMMENDATIONS
- At discharge from ICU, generate detailed sign-out assuring safe and seamless transfer of care to floor or for discharge to home and follow-up with primary care physician.
- Many patients with recurrent pseudomonas infections require ongoing outpatient care (i.e. cystic fibrosis clinics).

Patient Monitoring
- Continue close monitoring while in ICU.
- Frequently exam of wounds suspected of infection

DIET
Maintain appropriate enteral feeding to optimize nutrition if no contraindications.

PATIENT EDUCATION
- Appropriate hygiene
- Hand-washing
- Contact precautions

PROGNOSIS
- Pseudomonas bacteremia: Prognosis is determined by overall patient condition and primary site of infection.
- Highly variable; 1 study found 30-day mortality at 39% for bacteremia.
- Studies demonstrated that early and appropriate antibiotic therapy can improve mortality.

COMPLICATIONS
- Brain abscess
- Endocarditis
- Bacteremia
- Septic shock/death
- Respiratory failure/mechanical ventilation
- Skin/soft tissue necrosis gangrene
- Typhlitis, bowel perforation, peritonitis

ADDITIONAL READING
- Agodi A. Pseudomonas aeruginosa carriage, colonization, and infection in ICU patients. *Intensive Care Med*. 2007;33:1155–61.
- Al-Hasan MN, et al. Incidence of Pseudomonas aeruginosa bacteremia: A population-based study. *AJM*. 121;8:702–8.
- Bertrand X. Endemicity, molecular diversity and colonization routes of Pseudomonas aeruginosa in intensive care units. *Int Care Med*. 2001;27:1263–68.
- Kwa ALH. Nebulized colistin in the treatment of pneumonia due to multidrug-resistant Acinetobacter baumannii and Pseudomonas aeruginosa. *Clin Infect Dis*. 2005;41:754–7.
- Reuter S, et al. Analysis of transmission pathways of Pseudomonas aeruginosa between patients and tap water outlets. *Crit Care Med*. 2002;30:2222–8.

CODES

ICD9
- 041.7 Pseudomonas infection in conditions classified elsewhere and of unspecified site
- 482.1 Pneumonia due to pseudomonas
- 599.0 Urinary tract infection, site not specified

CLINICAL PEARLS
- Early identification and acquisition of cultures
- Early (combination) empiric therapy and adjustment based on culture data
- Source elimination by way of catheter removal and/or surgical treatment of infected tissue/abscess
- Appropriate supportive care of all organ systems
- Multidisciplinary approach of care utilizing infectious disease, surgery, and intensivists as needed
- Patients with recurrent infections are likely to need long-term outpatient specialty care (cystic fibrosis clinics)

PULMONARY EMBOLISM AND DEEP VENOUS THROMBOSIS

Arif M. Shaik
Adel Bassily-Marcus

 BASICS

DESCRIPTION

- Venous thromboembolic disease (VTE) represents a spectrum of conditions that includes deep venous thrombosis (DVT) and pulmonary embolism (PE).
- PE remains the most common preventable cause of hospital death.
- Overall 3-month mortality with PE is 17% and if associated with hemodynamic instability is 31%.
- VTE is the 3rd most common acute cardiovascular disease after cardiac ischemic syndromes and stroke.
- Hospitalization increases VTE risk 260-fold.
- DVT has been estimated to develop in 30% of nonprophylaxed ICU patients within the 1st week.
- With prophylaxis, DVT occurs in 11% of ICU patients.
- ~10% of ICU patients have DVT on admission
- The most common DVT site is the calf vein. Veins of the pelvis are involved less commonly, and the inferior vena cava (IVC) is rarely involved.
- Up to 95% of PE originates from clots in proximal deep venous system of the lower limbs (popliteal, femoral, and iliac veins).
- Lower extremity DVT is found in 70% of patients with PE.
- 30% of patients with DVT have symptomatic PE, another 40% are asymptomatic.
- The estimated case fatality rate for PE (deaths/100 cases of PE) is 7–11%.
- Most deaths from PE occur within the 1st 2.5 hours after the diagnosis is made.
- 50% of PE cases have signs of right ventricular dysfunction, a poor prognostic sign.
- Upper extremity DVTs (UEDVT) represent 18% of all DVTs. PE develops in up to 36% of cases with mortality rate ranging from 15–50%, high because of major comorbidities. Central venous catheters are a potential major risk factor for thrombosis, with an incidence of 2–41%.
- 78–84% of large or fatal PE at autopsy were unsuspected antemortem.

PATHOPHYSIOLOGY

- Thrombosis in the veins is triggered by venostasis, hypercoagulability, and vascular endothelial injury. These 3 underlying causes are known as the Virchow triad.
- The most common gas exchange abnormalities are hypoxemia (decreased arterial PO_2) and an increased alveolar-arterial O_2 tension gradient.
- The greatest risk factor for VTE is recent major surgery.
- Hemodynamic consequences become apparent with >30–50% occlusion of the pulmonary arterial bed.
- The resultant increased right ventricular (RV) afterload with underfilling of the left ventricle decreases blood pressure and coronary flow contributing to RV ischemia. This worsens RV dysfunction and, in its most severe form, may result in with pulseless electrical activity and sudden death.
- Clinical risk factors: Major surgery, trauma, myocardial infarction, stroke, need for mechanical ventilation, neuromuscular blockers, presence of central venous catheter(s), exposure to platelet transfusion, and vasopressors
- Patient-related risk factors: Malignancy, prior VTE history, inherited coagulopathy, end-stage renal disease, heparin-induced thrombocytopenia

ETIOLOGY

- Hypercoagulable state:
  - Factor V Leiden (most common genetic risk factor for thrombophilia, autosomal dominant)
  - Prothrombin G20210A mutation
  - Antithrombin III deficiency
  - Protein C, S deficiency
  - Fibrinogen abnormality
  - Resistance to activated protein C
  - Primary Thrombocytosis

- Acquired factors:
  - Reduced mobility:
    - Fractures
    - Immobilization
    - Burns
    - Obesity
    - Old age
  - Malignancy (most common acquired risk factor):
    - Chemotherapy
  - Acute medical illness
  - Trauma/major surgery:
    - Spinal cord injury
    - Without prophylaxis, DVT incidence may be as high as 90%
    - Following elective hip surgery
    - Without prophylaxis, DVT incidence is 50%
    - Postoperative (major surgery): Without prophylaxis, event rate is 25%
  - Catheters (indwelling central venous catheters) are the most powerful risk factor for UEDVT
  - Pregnancy:
    - Postpartum period
    - Oral contraceptives
    - Estrogen replacements (high dose only)
  - Venous pacemakers
  - Venous stasis
  - Warfarin (first few days of therapy).

COMMONLY ASSOCIATED CONDITIONS

- Varicose veins (unclear if confer increased DVT risk)
- Hip, knee, and spine surgeries
- Malignancy: Pancreas, lung, and breast

DIAGNOSIS

It is now widely accepted that the clinical diagnosis of PE, although highly nonspecific, is the most important step in assessing the likelihood of PE.

HISTORY
- The classic triad of signs and symptoms of PE—hemoptysis, dyspnea, and chest pain—are neither sensitive nor specific.
- Pleuritic type of chest pain
- Orthopnea
- Nonproductive cough
- Circulatory collapse
- History of malignancy or oral contraceptive pills.
- Prior history of DVT and PE.
- Chest pain and dyspnea during pregnancy.
- Occasionally: Syncope, nausea, vomiting, dizziness, and seizures.
- Lower extremity swelling
- History of recent fractures, trauma, surgery

PHYSICAL EXAM
- Tachypnea
- Tachycardia
- Dyspnea at rest or with exertion
- Lower extremity edema, calf tenderness

DIAGNOSTIC TESTS & INTERPRETATION
Lab
Initial lab tests
- Hypoxemia, absent in 20% of patients with PE
- Normal alveolar–arterial oxygen gradient does not exclude PE.
- ABG shows slight alkalosis and raised alveolar–arterial oxygen gradient
- 12-lead ECG: Most common finding is sinus tachycardia
- The classic finding of right-heart strain demonstrated by an S_1-Q_3-T_3 pattern (present in only 26% of PE patients), T waves inversion in leads V1–V4, a QR pattern in lead V1, incomplete right bundle-branch block

- The D-dimer test misses 10% of patients with PE, while only 30% of patients with positive D-dimer findings have a confirmatory diagnosis of PE.
- There is no utility of using D-dimer tests in the assessment of thrombosis risk nor to diagnose thrombosis in medical-surgical critically ill patients.
- The utility of D-dimer test to rule out DVT is limited in hospitalized patients, in presence of malignancy or postoperatively.
- In critically ill patients, neither tests for hypercoagulability nor D-dimer levels predict patients at risk of DVT and therefore should not be used to guide diagnostic testing for DVT.

Follow-Up & Special Considerations
- Brain natriuretic peptides (BNP): An elevated BNP or N-terminal pro-BNP (NT-proBNP) predicts RV dysfunction and mortality.
- Serum troponins: Elevated serum troponin levels identify patients with PE who are at increased risk of death.
- Hypercoagulable state screening

Imaging
Initial approach
- Clinical assessment should be made before imaging.
- Chest x-ray: Normal in PE, occasional atelectasis, consolidation and elevated hemidiaphragm with lung infarcts seen
- Echocardiography is helpful in the diagnosis and management of acute RV dysfunction. Severe hypokinesis of the RV mid free wall, preserved apical contractility maybe specific for PE. Avoid volume loading in RV dilation with tricuspid regurgitation, paradoxical septal shift. A thrombus within the pulmonary artery or thrombus in transit through the right heart may be visualized. It provides rapid and accurate risk assessment at bedside, avoiding transporting unstable patients away from critical care areas. It has high specificity (82–100%), is relatively inexpensive, and can be followed serially over time.
- Compression US (CUS) has replaced venography to diagnose DVT. Intensivist-performed limited CUS can detect DVTs with good specificity and moderate sensitivity.

- CTA is the initial imaging modality of choice for stable patients with normal renal function, with a sensitivity of 96–100%, specificity 89–98%.
- V/Q scans fell into disfavor after PIOPED study. Only 13% were diagnosed by high probability for PE. Higher sensitivity has been reported in SPECT V/Q imaging.
- MRA should only be considered at centers that routinely perform it well and for patients who have contraindications to standard tests (difficult to obtain adequate quality images).

Follow-Up & Special Considerations
- Echocardiography may demonstrate right ventricular dysfunction in acute PE, predicting a higher mortality and possible benefit from thrombolytic therapy.
- MRI: Pulmonary emboli may be detected by using standard or gated spin-echo techniques
- CT venography was shown to increase the sensitivity of multidetector CTA for the detection of PE (where DVT was considered a surrogate for PE; not routinely considered because of very high radiation exposure).
- Prophylaxis:
  - VTE prophylaxis is the single most important safety measure in hospitalized patients.
  - Critically ill patients are at risk for VTE: ICU risk factors:
    ○ Mechanical ventilation
    ○ Use of paralytics
    ○ Central venous catheters
    ○ Severe sepsis
    ○ DIC
  - All ICU patients should receive thromboprophylaxis on admission (1)[A].
  - Unfractionated heparin (UH) 5,000 Units SC q8h (for high risk) or q12h (for moderate risk) has been the standard ICU prophylaxis.
  - For ICU patients at moderate risk for VTE (e.g., medically ill, postoperative patients), UH or low-molecular-weight heparin (LMWH) are recommended (2)[A].
  - For critically ill patients at high risk, LMWH thromboprophylaxis is recommended (2)[A].
  - SC heparin can prevent about 1/2 of all PEs and 2/3 of DVTs.

- Mechanical methods of prophylaxis alone are not as effective in ICU patients. Used when bleeding is a great concern.
- Extended prophylaxis for up to 28 days is recommended for high-risk patients undergoing general, gynecological, or orthopedic surgeries.
- New direct thrombin inhibitors and oral direct factor Xa inhibitors may soon be available for perioperative VTE prophylaxis.
- Coagulopathy does not protect against hospital-acquired VTE in chronic liver disease patients.
- Consider dose adjustment when using LMWH, fondaparinux, direct thrombin inhibitors, and other antithrombotic drugs in critically ill patients with renal impairment or in elderly patients. With reduced creatinine clearance, these drugs may accumulate and increase risk of bleeding. Each drug must be evaluated separately especially for various LMWHs.
- In selecting drugs for prophylaxis or treatment in critically ill patients, also consider the half-life of the drugs, as well as availability of reversal. UH half-life is 1.5 hours, the reversal is quick and complete using protamine sulfate (rarely used). LMWH half life is 4.5–7 hours; protamine does not reverse it completely (cannot reverse the small direct antithrombin effect).
- It is reasonable to consider anti-factor Xa activity testing when using LMWH in special groups (obesity, renal failure, older age).

Diagnostic Procedures/Other
- SPECT V/Q imaging may further improve the accuracy of pulmonary scintigraphy detected abnormalities particularly at the subsegmental level and in the lung bases.
- Conventional pulmonary angiography

Pathological Findings
- Bilateral pulmonary congestion and focal intra-alveolar hemorrhage
- A large saddle embolus can be seen at the bifurcation of the main pulmonary trunk with extension into and obstructing the right and left main pulmonary arteries
- Increase in the number of macrophages, mainly in the right ventricular wall; also some cases reported as having massive macrophage infiltration in the entire right ventricular wall, suggesting ischemia due to PE

DIFFERENTIAL DIAGNOSIS
- Acute hypoxia:
  - Pneumothorax
  - Pneumonia/aspiration pneumonitis
  - Pulmonary edema
  - ARDS/ALI
  - Sepsis/severe sepsis
  - Intrapulmonary shunt:
  - Hepatopulmonary syndrome
  - Pulmonary edema/CHF
  - Obstructive sleep apnea
  - Atelectasis
- Acute coronary syndrome, acute RV failure
- Aortic dissection
- Pneumonia
- Pericarditis
- Lower extremity pain:
  - Ruptured baker's cyst
  - Crystalline arthritis
  - Cellulitis
  - Postphlebitic syndrome

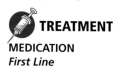

TREATMENT

MEDICATION

First Line

- IV heparin weight-based or SC, LMWH or SC unfractionated heparin (UFH), or SC factor Xa inhibitor (fondaparinux) are approved for initial therapy (2)[A]
- For treatment purposes, there is no discrimination between proximal and distal DVT, nor between symptomatic and asymptomatic; all these events receive the same treatment (2)[A].
- Benefits from heparin may be related to the reduction of late recurrences and not the prevention of early catastrophic result.
- The incidence of VTE recurrence was 3 times higher if APTT was not therapeutic within the 1st 24 hours (target aPTT 1.5–2 times normal).
- Heparin reduces the mortality rate of PE because it slows or prevents clot progression and reduces the risk of further embolism.

- Prompt effective anticoagulation (AC) has been shown to reduce the overall mortality rate from 30% to <10%
- Heparin is recommended for at least 5 days and until INR is ≥2 (with warfarin) for 24 hours (2)[A].
- The decision to use fibrinolytic therapy depends on severity of the PE, prognosis, and risk of bleeding.
- For the majority of patients with acute PE, fibrinolytic therapy is not recommended.
- Thrombolytic therapy is suggested for 2 groups of patients where it may be potentially beneficial: those who are hemodynamically unstable (2)[B], and those who have right-heart strain, (3)[B] unless contraindicated due to risk of bleeding.
- Symptomatic superficial vein thrombosis can be treated with fondaparinux 2.5 mg/d SC for 45 days (4)[A].

Second Line

- Early ambulation is recommended for patients with acute DVT and PE when feasible (5)[A].
- Warfarin interferes with hepatic synthesis of vitamin K–dependent coagulation factors; it can be started after 1 day on IV or SC full-dose AC.
- Heparin should be continued for the first 5–7 days of PO warfarin therapy, regardless of the PT time, to allow time for depletion of procoagulant vitamin K–dependent protein.
- Evidence suggests that 6 months of AC reduces rate of recurrence to 1/2 of the recurrence rate observed when only 6 weeks of AC is given. Long-term AC is indicated for patients with an irreversible underlying risk factor and recurrent DVT or recurrent PE.
- Duration of treatment differs with different situations:
  - Upper extremity DVT: AC for ≥3 months.
  - Lower extremity DVT and PE
    - Reversible cause: 3 months AC.
    - 1st unprovoked proximal DVT and PE
    - We recommend that after 3 months of AC therapy, all patients with unprovoked proximal DVT and PE should be evaluated for the risk–benefit ratio of long-term therapy.
    - 2nd unprovoked DVT and PE: Requires long-term treatment
    - Unprovoked deep DVT: 3 months AC
    - DVT and PE associated with cancer: LMWH recommended for 3 to 6 months and continuation of AC until cancer resolves.

Pregnancy Considerations

- In normal pregnancy, D-dimer levels increase with gestational age.
- In pregnant women and women of reproductive age, perfusion lung scanning may be the imaging test of choice rather than CT angiography due to concerns for radiation exposure.
- Once the diagnosis is confirmed, SC LMWH or IV heparin or SC UFH is started initially.
- Although SC LMWH is preferred (easier use), IV heparin is preferred in patients who have high bleeding risk, as it has short half-life and is reversible.
- SC LMWH and SC UFH should be stopped 24–36 hours prior to delivery. It should be restarted 12 hours and 6 hours after C-section and vaginal delivery, respectively, only if no significant bleeding occurred.

Geriatric Considerations

- Caution using SC LMWH as it is cleared by the kidneys; always adjust according to creatinine clearance.
- Risk of falls should be assessed when starting long-term AC.
- ##IVC filter is an option if contraindications for AC are present (e.g., fall risk).

ADDITIONAL TREATMENT
General Measures

- Oxygen; may need mechanical ventilation.
- IV fluids, caution in RV dysfunction. Absence of hemodynamic improvement after loading suggests ventricular independence physiology, cessation of fluid administration is advised.
- IVC filter (Greenfield filter) is indicated in the following settings:

  – Patients with acute venous thromboembolism who have an absolute contraindication to anticoagulant therapy (e.g., recent surgery, hemorrhagic stroke, or significant active or recent bleeding) (2)[A]

  – Patients with massive PE who survived but in whom recurrent embolism will be likely fatal
  – Patients with recurrent venous thromboembolism
- Management of secondary pulmonary HTN
- Elastic stockings and compression bandages should be used for symptomatic DVT to prevent postthrombotic syndrome.

SURGERY/OTHER PROCEDURES

- Pulmonary embolectomy is an option for massive PE with shock and presence of failure or contraindication of thrombolysis.
- Endovascular catheterization is not recommended for most patients.

 ## ONGOING CARE

DIET
Awareness of warfarin–food interaction

PROGNOSIS
- ~ 10% of patients who develop PE die within the 1st hour, and 30% die subsequently from recurrent embolism. Anticoagulant treatment decreases the mortality rate to <5%.
- PE resulting from UEDVT was not observed in patients who were treated with AC.

COMPLICATIONS
- DVT: Chronic venous ulcers, cellulitis
- PE: Cor pulmonale, right-side heart failure, secondary pulmonary hypertension.
- Recurrent thromboembolism

REFERENCES

1. Geerts WH, et al. Prevention of venous thromboembolism: The Seventh ACCP Conference on Antithrombotic and Thrombolytic Therapy. *Chest.* 2004;126(3 Suppl):338S–400S.
2. Kearon C, et al. Antithrombotic therapy for venous thromboembolic disease: American College of Chest Physicians Evidence-Based Clinical Practice Guidelines (8th Edition). *Chest.* 2008;133(6 Suppl): 454S–545S.
3. Goldhaber SZ. Thrombolytic therapy for patients with pulmonary embolism who are hemodynamically stable but have right ventricular dysfunction: Pro. *Arch Intern Med.* 2005;165(19): 2197–9.
4. Decousus H, et al. Fondaparinux for the treatment of superficial-vein thrombosis in the legs. *N Engl J Med.* 2010;363(13):1222–32.
5. Anderson CM, et al. Ambulation after deep vein thrombosis: A systematic review. *Physiother Can.* 2009;61(3):133–40.

ADDITIONAL READING

- Bourjeily G, et al. Pulmonary embolism in pregnancy. *Lancet.* 2010;375:500.
- Writing group for the christopher study Investigators. Effectiveness of managing suspected pulmonary embolism using an algorithm combining clinical probability, d-dimer testing, and computed tomography. *JAMA.* 2006;295:172–9.
- Paul DS, et al. Diagnostic pathways in acute pulmonary embolism: Recommendations of the PIOPED II investigators. *Am J Med.* 2006;119: 1048–55.

 ## CODES

ICD9
- 415.19 Other pulmonary embolism and infarction
- 453.40 Acute venous embolism and thrombosis of unspecified deep vessels of lower extremity
- 453.42 Acute venous embolism and thrombosis of deep vessels of distal lower extremity

CLINICAL PEARLS

- Aspirin alone is not recommended for DVT prophylaxis for any patient group.
- ECG changes are associated with more severe PE; their absence does not exclude PE.
- The use of thrombolysis in ICU patients remains controversial; mostly indicated in hemodynamically unstable patient with PE.
- Perfusion lung scanning and CT pulmonary angiography are the modalities most often used to diagnose PE.
- AC should be initiated immediately in any patient with a confirmed PE or high clinical suspicion and low bleeding risk.
- The clinical utility of D-dimer assays is limited by the nonspecificity of a positive result due to factors such as inflammation, trauma, and surgery.

PULMONARY FIBROSIS

Umesh Gidwani
Sasikanth Nallagatla

 BASICS

DESCRIPTION
Pulmonary fibrosis (PF) consists of a diverse group of disorders with overlapping clinical, radiographic, pathologic, and physiologic features of a variety of related clinical conditions characterized by cellular infiltration, scarring, and/or architectural disruption of the pulmonary parenchyma.

- Due to the overlap of these various conditions and a lack of standardized diagnostic criteria and terminology, confusion persisted in the classification and understanding of this condition. This problem was systematically addressed in 2001 by a consensus conference that sought to standardize definitions and terminology (1).
- Pulmonary fibrosis is the end-stage pathology of a group of disorders now classified as *diffuse parenchymal lung diseases* (DPLD).
- DPLD is further subclassified into idiopathic interstitial pneumonias (IIP), DPLD due to drugs or collagen vascular diseases, granulomatous DPLD (e.g., sarcoidosis), and DPLD due to diseases such as lymphangiomyomatosis, pulmonary Langerhans' cell histiocytosis, etc.
- The IIPs are sufficiently distinct to be further divided into two types: Idiopathic pulmonary fibrosis (IPF) and IIPs other than IPF
- For the purposes of clarity and brevity, further discussion is limited to IPF.
- IPF is a nonneoplastic pulmonary disease characterized by the formation of scar tissue within the lungs in the absence of any known provocation.
- IPF is also known as cryptogenic fibrosing alveolitis (CFA).

Geriatric Considerations
- Commonly seen in patients >50 years
- Both incidence and prevalence increase with age

Pediatric Considerations
Uncommon in pediatric population

Pregnancy Considerations
Women can have a successful pregnancy despite severe pulmonary dysfunction

EPIDEMIOLOGY
Incidence
Estimated incidence of 7–16 per 100,000

Prevalence
Estimated prevalence of 14–43 per 100,000 (2)

RISK FACTORS
- Cigarette smoking: Odds ratio of 2.3 (95% confidence interval, 1.3–3.8) (3)
- Exposure to viruses and environmental irritants have been implicated, but not conclusively linked.

Genetics
Up to 3% of cases of IPF cluster in families.

GENERAL PREVENTION
Avoid exposure to tobacco smoke and environmental irritants.

PATHOPHYSIOLOGY (4)
- IPF results from sequential acute lung injury.
- The resultant wound-healing response to this injury culminates in pulmonary fibrosis.
- Factors that modify the fibrotic response include the genetic background of the patient, the predominant inflammatory phenotype (Th1 or Th2), and environmental inflammatory triggers, such as cigarette smoking, viral infection, and respirable toxins.

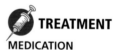 **DIAGNOSIS**

HISTORY
- Progressive dyspnea
- Nonproductive cough
- Abnormal CXR
- Occupational, social and family history may provide useful information

PHYSICAL EXAM
- Inspiratory crackles (common in IPF)
- Increased intensity P2, RV lift, TR murmur (in patients with pulmonary hypertension)
- Clubbing (up to 50% of IPF patients)

DIAGNOSTIC TESTS & INTERPRETATION
Lab
- Routine blood testing is rarely diagnostic.
- Elevated erythrocyte sedimentation rate and hypergammaglobulinemia may be found but are nondiagnostic.

Imaging
- Virtually all patients with IPF have an abnormal chest radiograph at the time of presentation.
- HRCT shows patchy peripheral reticular infiltrates with intralobular linear opacities, irregular septal thickening, subpleural honeycombing, and traction bronchiectasis (UIP pattern). Abnormalities are more prominent in the lower lobes. Ground-glass changes are absent.

Diagnostic Procedures/Other
- Transbronchial biopsy
- Surgical lung biopsy
- Pulmonary function tests:
  - PFTs reveal a restrictive pattern; decreased VC, RV and TLC), decreased DLCO, widened A-a gradient.
- Diagnosis without surgical lung biopsy (1):
  - Major criteria:
    - Exclusion of other known causes of ILD such as certain drug toxicities, environmental exposures, and connective tissue diseases
    - Abnormal pulmonary function studies that include evidence of restriction (reduced VC, often with an increased FEV1/FVC ratio) and impaired gas exchange [increased $P(A-a)O_2$, decreased PaO_2 with rest or exercise or decreased DLco]
    - Bibasilar reticular abnormalities with minimal ground-glass opacities on HRCT scans
    - Transbronchial lung biopsy or BAL showing no features to support an alternative diagnosis

- Minor criteria:
  - Age >50 years
  - Insidious onset of otherwise unexplained dyspnea or exertion
  - Duration of illness >3 months
  - Bibasilar, inspiratory crackles (dry or "Velcro"-type in quality)

Pathological Findings
- The pathological appearance of IPF is usual interstitial pneumonia (UIP). The cardinal feature of UIP is a bilateral, heterogeneous process, which predominates in the peripheral and subpleural regions of the lower lobes (5).
- Interstitial inflammation, fibrosis, and honeycomb change are seen at low magnification. Aggregates of proliferating fibroblasts and myofibroblasts within fibroblastic foci are noted. Alveolar walls are thickened by collagen, extracellular matrix, and mild-to-moderate infiltration by lymphocytes, plasma cells, and histocytes. Hyperplasia of type II pneumocytes is also noted. Honeycomb cysts are composed of cystic, fibrotic airspaces.

DIFFERENTIAL DIAGNOSIS
- Other DPLDs
- Other IIPs (DIP, AIP, NSIP, RB-ILD, COP, LIP)
- Connective tissue diseases
- Radiation pneumonitis
- Advanced sarcoidosis
- Infections
- Lymphangitic spread of cancer

TREATMENT

MEDICATION
- No large randomized trial has demonstrated benefit in primary outcomes. When possible, participation in a clinical trial is recommended.
- Combination therapy is preferred over monotherapy:
  - 1 recommended regimen is a combination of steroid, azathioprine, and N-acetylcysteine (NAC)
  - Prednisone 0.5 mg/kg/d until stability/improvement, then taper over 6 months
  - Azathioprine 2 mg/kg/d PO, starting at 50 mg/d, increasing by 25 mg increments every 1–2 weeks, to a maximum of 150 mg/d. Response to therapy may take 3–6 months
  - NAC 1800 mg/d PO
  - Therapy is discontinued for serious side effects or after 6 months with no response.
  - Therapy can be continued up to a year or more if there is good response.
- Antifibrotic agents like pirfenidone and bosentan have shown some benefit in IPF. Therapy can be continued up to a year or more if good response is obtained:
  - Pirfenidone treatment was associated with fewer exacerbations. Dose is 40 mg/kg/d (max 2403 mg/d). Approved in Japan (Oct. 2008), rejected by U.S. FDA (Mar. 2010).
  - Bosentan showed a trend toward delayed time to death or disease progression.

- Suppression of gastroesophageal reflux (present in 90% of cases) leads to decreased microaspiration and is associated with disease stabilization.
- Other immunomodulatory and anti-inflammatory agents such as colchicine, cyclophosphamide, D-penicillamine, methotrexate, interferon-γ, and etanercept have been tried but have not shown reproducible benefit.
- Several other novel therapeutic targets are being actively investigated.

ADDITIONAL TREATMENT
General Measures
Since no therapy has proved to be efficacious in this disease, the focus should be on supportive care and the prevention and management of complications.
- Supportive care:
  - Supplemental oxygen
  - Influenza and pneumococcal vaccination
  - Education about the condition and its expected management and course
  - Pulmonary rehabilitation
- Management of acute exacerbations:
  - An exacerbation is defined as a combination of *all* of the following (6):
    ○ Existing diagnosis of IPF, unexplained worsening of dyspnea within 30 days
    ○ HRCT with new bilateral ground-glass abnormality and/or consolidation superimposed on a UIP pattern
    ○ No evidence of pulmonary infection by endotracheal aspirate or BAL
    ○ Exclusion of alternative causes, including left-heart failure, pulmonary embolism, and other identifiable causes of acute lung injury
  - High-dose steroids: Prednisone 1 mg/kg/d
  - Broad-spectrum antibiotics
  - Assisted ventilation as needed
- Management of pulmonary hypertension:
  - Oxygen, anticoagulation, pulmonary vasodilators, lung transplantation

COMPLEMENTARY & ALTERNATIVE THERAPIES
- Pulmonary rehabilitation can be beneficial
- Advance care planning and palliative care referral given the generally poor prognosis is important

SURGERY/OTHER PROCEDURES
Lung transplantation is the only intervention with a known survival benefit.

IN-PATIENT CONSIDERATIONS
Initial Stabilization
- Supplemental oxygen to maintain PaO_2 >55 mm Hg or SaO_2 >90%
- Maintain cardiovascular stability
- Mechanical ventilation (MV) in severe cases
- Ventilator strategy
- MV:
  - The outcome of acute respiratory failure and MV in IPF patients is uniformly dismal, with reports of 100% mortality.
  - MV should only be initiated if lung transplantation is imminent, a reversible cause is definitely identified, or with the full knowledge of the patient that this intervention if futile.
  - Goal should be of maximizing oxygenation and minimizing barotrauma.
  - Noninvasive positive pressure ventilation (NIPPV) may be considered in mild cases to relieve dyspnea and improve oxygenation and may be used only in alert and cooperative patients.

Admission Criteria
- Acute respiratory failure
- Acute exacerbation of IPF
- Complications such as pulmonary embolism, pneumonia, cor pulmonale

IV Fluids
Per the protocol in your ICU

Nursing
Usual ICU nursing protocols for acute respiratory failure

Discharge Criteria
Resolution of the acute exacerbation

 ONGOING CARE
FOLLOW-UP RECOMMENDATIONS
- Monitor clinical, radiographic and physiologic parameters
- ABGs, PFTs, HRCT every 3–6 months in 1st few years
- Bone densitometry and PPD annually for patients on steroids
- Monitor blood counts for patients on immunosuppressive drugs
- 2D echo to monitor the development of pulmonary hypertension

DIET
- No specific dietary restrictions
- Some recommend antioxidant supplements (no evidence)

PATIENT EDUCATION
- Educate patients about the nature of the diagnosis and potential environmental irritants and toxins.
- Breathing exercises
- Taking medications

PROGNOSIS
- The median survival of patients with IPF is ~3 years after diagnosis or 5 years after the onset of symptoms.
- The 6-minute-walk test has emerged as an important addition to prognostic evaluation, with significant oxygen desaturation identifying a subgroup of patients with a much higher mortality (7).
- Exacerbation of IPF or acute respiratory failure in IPF have mortality of 57–91%.
- MV for acute respiratory failure in IPF has a mortality close to 100%.

COMPLICATIONS
- Progressive respiratory failure
- Pulmonary hypertension and right-heart failure
- Exacerbations and infections

REFERENCES
1. American Thoracic Society/European Respiratory Society. International multidisciplinary consensus classification of the idiopathic interstitial pneumonias. *Am J Respir Crit Care Med*. 2002;165:277.
2. Fernandez Perez ER, et al. Incidence, prevalence, and clinical course of idiopathic pulmonary fibrosis: A population-based study. *Chest*. 2010;137:129.
3. Baumgartner KB, et al. Cigarette smoking: A risk factor for idiopathic pulmonary fibrosis. *Am J Respir Crit Care Med*. 1997;155:242.
4. Gross TJ, et al. Idiopathic pulmonary fibrosis. *N Engl J Med*. 2001;345:517.
5. Katzenstein ALA, et al. Idiopathic pulmonary fibrosis: Clinical relevance of pathologic classification. *Am J Respir Crit Care Med*. 1998; 157,1301.
6. Collard HR, et al. for the Idiopathic Pulmonary Fibrosis Clinical Research Network Investigators. Acute exacerbations of idiopathic pulmonary fibrosis. *Am J Respir Crit Care Med*. 2007;176:636.
7. Hallstrand TS, et al. The timed walk test as a measure of severity and survival in idiopathic pulmonary fibrosis. *Eur Respir J*. 2005;25:96.

ADDITIONAL READING
- Meltzer EB, et al. Idiopathic pulmonary fibrosis. *Orphanet J Rare Dis*. 2008;3:8. Accessed at http://www.ojrd.com/content/3/1/8

CODES

ICD9
- 508.0 Acute pulmonary manifestations due to radiation
- 515 Postinflammatory pulmonary fibrosis
- 516.3 Idiopathic fibrosing alveolitis

CLINICAL PEARLS
- IPF is a rare nonneoplastic lung disease characterized by the formation of scar tissue within the lungs in the absence of any known provocation.
- Patients present with dyspnea, clubbing, hypoxia, and crackles on auscultation; reticular and subpleural abnormalities on HRCT; and a restrictive defect with reduced DLCO on PFT.
- Complications such a progressive respiratory failure, exacerbations, and pulmonary hypertension are common.
- Treatment options are limited and unsatisfactory, and patients should be evaluated for lung transplantation or prepared for end-of-life care as the prognosis is uniformly dismal.

PULMONARY VENTILATION, NONINVASIVE

Zinobia Khan
John Oropello

Noninvasive Pulmonary Ventilation is ventilation without the use of an artificial airway (oro-tracheal/naso-tracheal or tracheostomy tube). It is divided into two types.

(A) Noninvasive negative pressure ventilation works by lowering the pressure around the chest wall during inhalation and changing the pressure to atmospheric pressure during exhalation. These types of ventilators use negative extra-thoracic pressure to augment the tidal volume. The original, negative pressure ventilator, the iron lung, covered the entire body below the neck.

(B) Noninvasive positive pressure ventilation (NIPPV) utilizes noninvasive oro-nasal interfaces to ventilate and uses portable devices or ICU ventilators.

(B1) Conditions where NIPPV can be used (1)[A]:

• COPD exacerbations and post extubation
• Cardiogenic pulmonary edema (CPE)
• Immunocompromised patients

Other conditions where it can be considered (more randomized control trials are needed to determine the standard of care):

• Asthma
• Post operative respiratory failure
• Do not intubate (DNR) patients
• Extubation failure

(B2) Interfaces that are used:

• oronasal or full face masks (covers the nose and mouth and can be used initially in the acute setting in order to prevent air leakage from the mouth)
• nasal mask and nasal pillows (covers the nose only, most comfortable, can be use after the acute phase so that patients can expectorate and talk, it is the least claustrophobic interface). Nasal masks and nasal pillows can be used with chin-straps to have an effect similar to full face masks.
• total full face masks (seal around the perimeter of the face)
• oronasal masks can be used with a dental appliance

(B3) Modes of NIV
Continuous positive airway pressure (CPAP)

• high flow oxygen and positive end expiratory pressure (PEEP)
• may decrease or increase work ofbreathing (WOB), increases PaO_2, re-expand atelectasis
• use with CPE

Bi-level (inspiratory positive airway pressure [IPAP] and expiratory positive airway pressure [EPAP], EPAP = PEEP, IPAP-EPAP = pressure support [PS])

• decreases WOB, increases PaO_2, re-expand atelectasis, decrease $PaCO_2$.
• use in COPD

(B4) Types of respiratory failure that NIPPV can be used:

(B4a) Acute respiratory failure

• Types I, II and CPE
  Type I = hypoxemia, use CPAP ventilation
  Type II = hypoxemia and hypercarbia, use Bi-level ventilation
• Most studies in the acute cases have been done in patients with chronic obstructive pulmonary disease (COPD) exacerbations
• It is a safe and effective treatment if used in properly selected patients in acute respiratory failure

(B4a I) Patient inclusion in acute cases:

• Respiratory rate (RR)> 24
• Respiratory accessory muscles usage or abdominal paradox
• Arterial blood gas (ABG) abnormalities-pH< 7.35 but > 7.10, $PaCO_2$ > 45, PaO_2/FiO_2 < 200

(B4al1) Starting NIPPV in acute setting

• elevate head of the bed to prevent aspiration, preferably > 45 degrees
• use full face mask, make sure correct size is available

• ensure that the patient has adapted to the mask: explain the use of the mask, initially place the mask on the patients face without using the straps, to ease anxiety
• easier to start at lower pressure and titrate upwards to get a decrease in HR, decrease in RR, subjective improvement and comfort
• sufficient oxygen to keep O_2 > 90%, increase pressure by 2 cm. of water until O_2 < 0.6
• set a back up rate for apnea
• pulse oximetry can be used between ABG samples, it is not a replacement for ABG, adjust ventilator based on ABG findings.
• CPE patients usually need < 1/2 day while patients with COPD exacerbation may need > 2 days
• the patient can be tapered off the NIPPV as the underlying condition that caused the respiratory failure improves.

(B4al2) Follow-Up & Special Considerations

• Frequent examinations
• ABG q 1 hour × 2hours then q4 hrs

• Factors that predict sucess/failure (2)[B]:

  1. Acute phsiology and chronic health evaluation (APACHE) II score: < 29
  2. Glasgow coma scale (GCS) score: 15
  3. pH: > 7.30
  4. RR: < 30

• Better predictive value after 2 hours
• 97% success, after 2 hours, if all 4 factors are favorable; 99% failure after 2 hours if all 4 are unfavorable.

ALERT

• If the patient is deteriorating (increase WOB, worsening of ABG, subjective worsening, increasing HR and RR, changes in mental status) —intubate immediately.
• Outcomes are worse with delayed intubations. Delays result in emergent intubation and increases in morbidity and mortality (3)[B].

(B4al3) Clinical Pearls

- NIV is safe and effective in properly selected patients.
- Patients should be carefully monitored and intubations should not be delayed if needed.
- Ventilators and portable Bi-level devices can both be used

(B4a II) Contraindications to NIPPV:

- cardiac or respiratory arrest
- hemodynamic instability
- inability to protect airways
- no suitable interface secondary to facial abnormalities
- agitated/uncooperative patients
- altered mental status
- excessive secretions
- active vomiting
- consolidation on CXR
- pneumothorax
- recent facial, upper airway, or GI surgery

(B4b) Sub-acute respiratory failure

- weaning and COPD extubation

(B4c) Chronic respiratory failure

- Type II, sleep apnea, COPD, cystic fibrosis and neuromuscular diseases.
- In order to decrease high pressures, the mask can be used with a dental appliance.

(B5) Ventilator modes for NIPPV

1. Pressure-limited

- present in both critical care ventilators and portable devices
- more comfortable than volume-limited mode
- better than volume –limited mode to compensate for leaks.

- provides pressure support ventilation that delivers a set IPAP to assist spontaneous breathing.
- provides pressure control ventilation that delivers time-cycled preset IPAP with adjustable inspiratory (i): expiratory (e) ratio at a controlled rate.

2. Volume-limited

- present in both critical care ventilators and portable devices
- usually set in the assist control mode
- better than pressure-limited mode for patients with little or no spontaneous breathing
- tidal volume set at a higher level to compensate for leakage.
- results in a high inspiratory pressure which cases leaks and discomfort

(B6) Ventilator settings

- start at a low IPAP (8 cm. of H_2O) and titrate up to high IPAP (20 cm. of H_2O)and titrate down
- PEEP on Bi-level device, PEEP optional on volume-limited ventilator
- PEEP can be set at 5 cm. of H_2O in COPD patients

(B6a) Advantages of NIPPV versus conventional mechanical ventilation

- reduce the need for intubation, decrease complications related to intubation,
- patients can communicate, swallow, cough and expectorate
- reduces pneumonia and sinusitis

(B6b) Advantages of ventilators versus portable Bi-level devices

- delivers exact oxygen concentration
- separate inspiratory and expiratory tubing, which minimizes carbon dioxide rebreathing
- alarms are more advance and patients disconnection can be easily detected.

(B7) Complications of NIPPV

- Major
  - aspiration pneumonia
  - pneumothorax
  - hypotension secondary to reduced preload
- Air leak
- Mask-related
  - Discomfort
  - Claustrophobia
  - skin erythema and ulceration
- flow-related
  - nasal and oral dryness
  - eye irritation
  - nasal congestion
  - gastric insufflation

REFERENCES

1. Garpested E, Brennan J, Hill NS. Noninvasive ventilation for critical care. *Chest*. 2007;132: 711–720.
2. Confalonieri M, Garuti G, Cattaruzza MS, et al. A chart of failure risk for noninvasive ventilation in patients with COPD exacerbation. *Eur Respiratory J*. 2005;25:348–355.
3. Esteban A, Frutos-Vivar F, Ferguson ND, et al. *N Engl J Med*. 2004;350:2452–2460.

 CODES

ICD9

- 428.1 Left heart failure
- 493.90 Asthma, unspecified, unspecified
- 496 Chronic airway obstruction, not elsewhere classified

RENAL FAILURE, ACUTE

Arif M. Shaik
Roopa Kohli-Seth

 BASICS

DESCRIPTION
- Acute renal failure (ARF), also known as acute kidney injury, is an acute decline in glomerular filtration rate (GFR) from baseline, with or without oliguria/anuria.
- The resulting effects include impaired clearance and regulation of metabolic homeostasis, altered acid–base and electrolyte regulation, and impaired volume regulation.
- It is categorized into 3 types: Prerenal, renal, and postrenal.

EPIDEMIOLOGY
Incidence
- Community-acquired ARF is present in 1% of hospitalized admissions.
- Hospital-acquired ARF is estimated from 3–7%.
- Incidence in ICU is 25–30%

Prevalence
4% overall in medical-surgical ICU patients

RISK FACTORS
Advanced age, prior history of renal insufficiency, diabetes mellitus, uncontrolled hypertension (HTN), cirrhosis, congestive heart failure (CHF), dehydration, chronic infections, immune disorders (lupus, IG A nephropathy and scleroderma), and nephrotoxic drugs

Genetics
Genetic polymorphisms of proteins play a role in neonatal physiology and may contribute to individual susceptibility to both ARF and its risk factors.

GENERAL PREVENTION
- Ischemic causes can be prevented by maintaining adequate intravascular volume in high-risk patients, such as the elderly, those with pre-existing chronic kidney disease, and after major surgery and burns.
- The incidence of nephrotoxic ARF can be reduced by tailoring the administration (dose and frequency) of nephrotoxic drugs to body size and GFR.
- Diuretics, NSAIDs, ACE inhibitors, angiotensin receptor blockers (ARBs), and vasodilators should be used with caution in patients with hypovolemia or renovascular disease
- Hydration with isotonic sodium bicarbonate is effective in prevention of contrast media–induced nephropathy (1).

PATHOPHYSIOLOGY
ARF may occur in 3 clinical patterns:
- As an adaptive response to severe volume depletion and hypotension with structurally intact nephron
- In response to cytotoxic, ischemic, or inflammatory insults to the kidney with structural and functional damage
- Hydronephrosis with obstruction to the passage of urine

ETIOLOGY
- Prerenal: Conditions affecting the flow of blood before it reaches the kidneys:
  - Hypovolemia
  - Hemorrhage
  - Sepsis
  - Third spacing of fluids
  - Heart failure
  - Hepatorenal syndrome, which represents a form of prerenal azotemia not responsive to fluid administration; seen in cases of severe liver disease
- Renal: Conditions intrinsically affecting the kidney that prevent proper filtration of blood or production of urine:
  - Acute interstitial nephritis (AIN) is most common
  - Acute tubular necrosis (ATN)
  - Acute glomerulonephritis (GN)
  - Pigment induced nephropathy
  - Renovascular disease, especially bilateral renal artery stenosis
  - Other vascular diseases, including hemolytic uremic syndrome, thrombotic thrombocytopenic purpura (TTP), and scleroderma renal crisis
- Postrenal injury results from mechanical obstruction of the urinary outflow tract:
  - Bladder neck obstruction is the most common cause of postrenal ARF and is usually due to prostatic disease (e.g., hypertrophy, neoplasia, or infection)
  - Neurogenic bladder
  - Retroperitoneal fibrosis, lymphoma, tumor, strictures
  - Less common causes include blood clots and calculi

COMMONLY ASSOCIATED CONDITIONS
Infection, diabetes mellitus, and HTN

Geriatric Considerations
Elderly are 3.5 times more susceptible to ARF than their younger counterparts.

Pregnancy Considerations
ARF is seen in septic abortions, toxemia of pregnancy, antepartum and postpartum hemorrhages, and ischemic ATN of late pregnancy.

DIAGNOSIS

HISTORY
- Prerenal: Hypovolemia, increased thirst, decreased urine output, dizziness, vomiting, diarrhea, and hemorrhage
- Renal: Symptoms depend upon underlying pathology:
  - In acute interstitial disease, patient may present with rash, fevers, history of taking NSAIDs and antibiotics.

- In pigment-induced nephropathy, patient presents with muscular pain, excessive exercise, seizures, falls, and intoxications.
  - In glomerular disease, symptoms include edema, hematuria, and HTN.
  - In tubular disease, there is history of hypotension, recent surgery, hemorrhage, or sepsis (2,3)[B].
- Postrenal: Elderly men with prostate enlargements, flank pain with hematuria for renal calculi disease, and recent history of prior gynecological surgery and abdominopelvic malignancy

PHYSICAL EXAM
- Peripheral edema
- Oliguria (however, patients can have nonoliguric renal failure)
- Delirium, lethargy, seizures
- Tachypnea and tachycardia
- Anorexia, nausea, generalized fatigue
- Abdominal exam distension for bladder outlet obstruction, enlarged prostate and bruit for renovascular disease

DIAGNOSTIC TESTS & INTERPRETATION
Lab
Initial lab tests
- BUN and serum creatinine
  - The ratio of BUN to creatinine exceeds 20:1 in conditions that favor enhanced reabsorption of urea (e.g., volume contraction) and suggests prerenal ARF.
  - Ratio of <20:1 suggests renal and postrenal etiology.
- Urinalysis may reveal the presence of:
  - Hematuria (glomerular nephropathy)
  - Proteinuria (nephrotic syndrome),
  - Casts (e.g., granular casts in ATN, RBC casts in acute GN, WBC casts in AIN)
  - Eosinophiluria (AIN)
- Urinary sodium and urinary creatinine to calculate the fractional excretion of sodium (FE_{Na}) (FE_{Na} = Urine sodium/plasma sodium × Plasma creatinine/urine creatinine × 100):
  - The fractional excretion of sodium is
    - <1 in pre renal failure,
    - >1 in intrinsic renal failure in patients with urine output <400 mL/day
    - > 4 in postrenal

Follow-Up & Special Considerations
Serologic tests for antinuclear antibody (ANA), antineutrophilic cytoplasmic antibodies (ANCA), antiglomerular basement membrane (GBM) antibody, hepatitis, antistreptolysin (ASO), and complement levels may help exclude glomerular disease.

Imaging
Initial approach
- Renal US helps exclude existing renal disease (small kidneys) and obstruction, but the degree of hydronephrosis does not correlate with degree of obstruction.
- A plain film of the abdomen or unenhanced helical CT scan is a valuable initial screening technique in patients with suspected nephrolithiasis.

Follow-Up & Special Considerations
- A CT scan may be required to further evaluate cases of obstruction suggested on US (e.g., possible masses or stones).
- MRA is often used to assess patency of renal arteries and veins in patients with suspected vascular obstruction.

Diagnostic Procedures/Other
Biopsy is reserved for patients in whom prerenal and postrenal ARF have been excluded and the cause of intrinsic ARF is unclear:
- Renal biopsy is particularly useful when clinical assessment and laboratory investigations suggest diagnoses other than ischemic or nephrotoxic injury that may respond to disease-specific treatment.

DIFFERENTIAL DIAGNOSIS
- Chronic kidney disease: Elevation of creatinine and reduced renal function >3 months
- Increased muscle mass: Any elevation of creatinine is minor and typically nonacute.

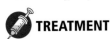 ## TREATMENT

MEDICATION
First Line
- Stop all nephrotoxic medications and contrast exposure (1,3)[A].
- Prerenal failure requires adequate IV hydration and correction of primary hypoperfusion:
  - Severe hypovolemia due to hemorrhage should be corrected with packed red cells, whereas isotonic saline is usually appropriate replacement for mild to moderate hemorrhage or plasma loss (e.g., burns, pancreatitis).
  - Renal hypoperfusion secondary to impaired left ventricular systolic function requires optimizing cardiac output and volume status by use of inotropes and diuretics.
- Intrinsic renal failure's management varies according to etiology:
  - Removal of offending drugs, when possible, is necessary in cases of AIN or drug-induced acute kidney injury (3)[A].
  - Acute GN and vasculitis management may also require corticosteroids, cytotoxic agents, or other immune-modifying drugs, depending on the specific diagnosis.
- Attempts should be made to relieve postrenal obstruction initially with Foley catheter before resorting to more definitive invasive procedures.

Second Line
- Metabolic acidosis is not usually treated unless serum bicarbonate concentration falls below 15 mmol/L or arterial pH falls below 7.2.
- Indications for renal replacement therapy include persistent hyperkalemia despite medical therapy, intractable metabolic acidosis, uremic encephalopathy, pericarditis, and intractable fluid overload. Intensity of renal replacement therapy does not alter morbidity in critical ill patients (4)[A].

ADDITIONAL TREATMENT
General Measures
Nutritional management during ARF is to provide sufficient calories and protein to minimize catabolism (3)[A].

Issues for Referral
- Renal replacement therapy
- Need for further workup and follow-up

COMPLEMENTARY & ALTERNATIVE THERAPIES
Different types of renal replacement therapies, such as CVVHD, CVVH, SLED, and SCUF

SURGERY/OTHER PROCEDURES
- Ureteric obstruction may be treated initially by percutaneous catheterization of the dilated renal pelvis or ureter.
- Obstructing lesions can often be removed percutaneously (e.g., calculus, sloughed papilla) or bypassed by insertion of a ureteric stent (e.g., carcinoma).

IN-PATIENT CONSIDERATIONS
Initial Stabilization
All severe electrolytes abnormality needs to be managed emergently.

Admission Criteria
ARF with intractable fluid overload and hyperkalemia not responding to medical treatment

IV Fluids
NS is used initially for volume expansion for correcting acute hypovolemia.

Nursing
Foley catheter placement and measurement of total input and output will help to maintain fluid management.

Discharge Criteria
Indices return to normal or reach steady-state stage

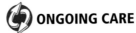 ## ONGOING CARE

FOLLOW-UP RECOMMENDATIONS
Follow-up with nephrologist and care according to the stage of renal failure

Patient Monitoring
- Monitor renal function and electrolytes.
- Modify dosage of renally excreted drugs

DIET
- Low-potassium and -sodium diet
- Fluid-restrictive diet

PATIENT EDUCATION
Avoiding NSAIDs and other common OTC medications, which are harmful.

PROGNOSIS
- Overall mortality rate in ARF is nearly 50%, varying from 60% in patients with ATN to 35% in patients with prerenal or postrenal ARF.
- Up to 7% of inpatient cases of ARF require renal replacement therapy (5)[B]. In-hospital mortality exceeds 50%, especially in those with multiorgan failure when ARF requires dialysis.

COMPLICATIONS
- Chronic renal failure
- Cardiopulmonary complications of ARF include arrhythmias, pericarditis, pericardial effusion, and pulmonary edema

REFERENCES
1. Pannu N, et al. Prophylaxis strategies for contrast-induced nephropathy. *JAMA*. 2006;295: 2765–79.
2. Lopes JA, et al. Acute renal failure in patients with sepsis. *Crit Care*. 2007;11:411.
3. Gill N, et al. Renal failure secondary to acute tubular necrosis: Epidemiology, diagnosis, and management. *Chest*. 2005;128:2847–63.
4. The VA/NIH Acute Renal Failure Trial Network. Intensity of renal support in critically ill patients with acute kidney injury. *N Engl J Med*. 2008;359:7–20.
5. Liangos O, et al. Epidemiology and outcomes of acute renal failure in hospitalized patients: A national survey. *Clin J Am Soc Nephrol*. 2006; 1(1):43–51.

ADDITIONAL READING
- National kidney foundations guidelines

 ## CODES

ICD9
- 584.5 Acute kidney failure with lesion of tubular necrosis
- 584.9 Acute kidney failure, unspecified

CLINICAL PEARLS
- Adequate IV hydration with isotonic saline is mandatory.
- Stop all nephrotoxic drugs at the onset of ARF.
- Adjust drug dosages according to creatinine clearance.

RENAL REPLACEMENT THERAPY

Arif Shaik
Roopa Kohli-Seth

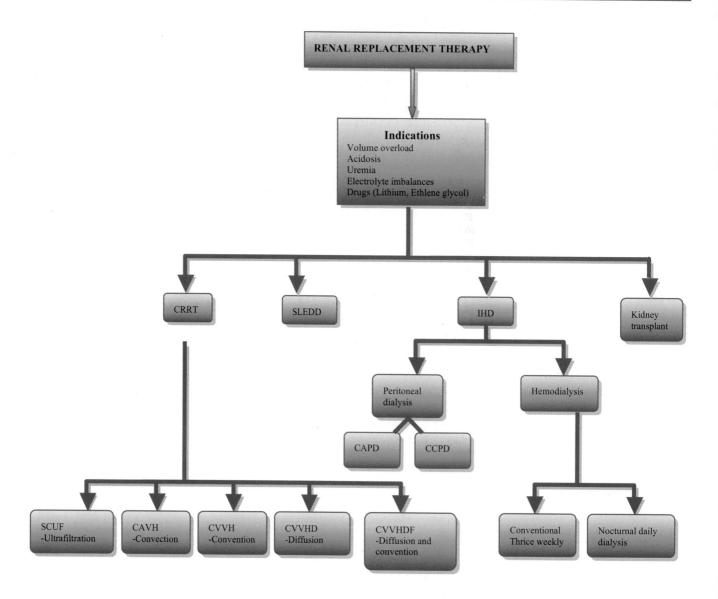

Renal Replacement Therapy (RRT):

- Renal replacement therapies are treatments for severe kidney failure, also called renal failure, stage 5 chronic kidney disease, and end-stage renal disease.
- As the kidneys lose their ability to function, fluid and waste products begin to build up in the blood. When these problems reach a critical stage, renal replacement therapy is required.
- Different types of RRT available and choosing appropriate therapy depends on patient factors like age, acute vs. chronic renal failure, inpatient vs. outpatient care, sepsis, and hemodynamic stability.
- Continuous renal replacement therapy (CRRT):
  - It permits fluid and solute removal with greater hemodynamic stability than intermittent hemodialysis. Continuous therapies closely mimic the native kidney in treating ARF and fluid overload

- The fluid infusion rate and composition of the replacement fluid can be adjusted based on the ultrafiltration rate, the volume of fluids and blood products administered through other IV lines to the patient, and the fluid balance goal (positive or negative).
- To normalize electrolytes and acid–base balance, an isotonic, buffered electrolyte solution is used as the replacement fluid
- Slow, gentle, and well tolerated by hypotensive patients
- Better control of uremia and clearance of solute from the extravascular compartment
- Remove large amounts of fluid and waste products over time.
- Although acute therapy of severe hyperkalemia, metabolic acidosis, or intoxications is more efficiently achieved with IHD, lesser abnormalities are corrected relatively quickly and controlled effectively with CRRT.

Different types of CRRT include:

- Slow continuous ultrafiltration (SCUF):
  - Safe management of fluid removal
  - Requires blood and effluent pump
  - UF rate ranges up to 2 L/hr
  - No dialysate and replacement fluids required.
  - Large fluid removal via ultra filtration
  - Blood flow rate for SCUF up to 200 ml/min
- Continuous arteriovenous hemofiltration (CAVH):
  - Solute clearance by convection
  - Replacement fluid required to prevent volume depletion
  - Similar to SCUF
- Continuous venovenous hemofiltration (CVVH):
  - Plasma water and solute are removed by convection and ultra filtration
  - Because it continues around the clock, CVVH is able to remove larger fluid volumes, which is a significant advantage with critical care patients on parenteral nutrition and multiple infusions

- It also may better preserve cerebral perfusion pressure
- Dialysate not required
- Replacement fluid necessary
- Ultrafiltrate produced is replaced by sterile solution (high ultrafiltrate rates).
- Enhanced clearance of autologous cytokines-thought to be involved in septic inflammatory response syndrome (SIRS)
- Continuous venovenous hemodialysis (CVVHD):.
  - Continuous diffusive dialysis
  - Dialysate required
  - Solute removal is directly proportional to dialysate flow rate
- Continuous venovenous hemodiafiltration (CVVHDF):
  - Solute removal by diffusion and convection
  - Safe fluid management
  - Combines CVVH and CVVHD therapies
  - UF rate ranges 12–20 L/24 hr
  - Uses dialysate and replacement solution.
- Sustained low-efficiency daily dialysis (SLEDD):
  - SLEDD has evolved as a conceptual and technical hybrid of continuous renal replacement therapy (CRRT) and intermittent haemodialysis (IHD).
  - A reduced rate of ultrafiltration for optimizing hemodynamic stability.
  - Low-efficiency solute removal to minimize solute disequilibrium.
  - Sustained treatment duration to maximize dialysis dose.
- Intermittent hemodialysis (IHD): Divided in 2 types—peritoneal and hemodialysis.

- Peritoneal dialysis:
  - Peritoneal lining acts as membrane to allow excess fluids and waste products to diffuse from the bloodstream into the dialysate.
  - Done by patients or family members at home. Catheter is necessary and inserted near umbilicus.
  - Manually performed 4–5 times daily.
  - Intra-abdominal sepsis is common with catheter infection.
  - Several different treatment schedules are possible:
    ○ Continuous ambulatory peritoneal dialysis (CAPD) involves multiple exchanges during the day (usually 4, but sometimes 3 or 5) with an overnight dwell. The dialysate is infused into the abdomen at bedtime and is drained upon awakening.
    ○ Continuous cycler peritoneal dialysis (CCPD) is an automated form of therapy in which a machine performs exchanges while the patient sleeps; there may be a long daytime dwell, and occasionally a manual daytime exchange is performed
- Hemodialysis:
  - Patient's blood is pumped through a dialysis machine to remove waste products and excess fluids. The machine works by putting the patient's blood in contact with a special solution, called *dialysate*. The blood is separated from the dialysate by a membrane that allows substances to move (diffuse) from the blood to the dialysate.

- Most efficient and large amount of fluids removed in 3–4 hours not suitable in unstable patients.
- Primarily used in end-stage renal disease patients.
- Need long-term access like temporal venous catheter, arteriovenous fistula, and arteriovenous graft
  ○ Conventional thrice weekly: Most common method as outpatient. Different baths used depending on patient's electrolytes.
  ○ Daily nocturnal dialysis: Occasionally used.
- Kidney transplantation:
  - It is considered the treatment of choice for many patients with severe chronic kidney disease because quality of life and survival are often improved, compared to patients who use dialysis.
  - There is a shortage of organs available for donation, so many patients who are candidates for transplantation are put on a transplant waiting list and require another form of renal replacement therapy until an organ is available.
  - Different options of transplant are living related, living unrelated, and cadaveric transplant.
  - Living organ donations function better and for a long time.

 CODES

ICD9
- 585.5 Chronic kidney disease, stage v
- 585.6 End stage renal disease
- 586 Renal failure, unspecified

RHABDOMYOLYSIS

Sudhanshu Jain
Roopa Kohli-Seth

 BASICS

DESCRIPTION
Muscle necrosis and release of intracellular muscle contents into the circulation

Pediatric Considerations
Inherited myopathies presents with recurrent episodes of rhabdomyolysis with minimal exertion during childhood.

EPIDEMIOLOGY
Incidence
- Annually, 26,000 cases reported in U.S.
- Accounts for 10–15% of all acute renal failure (ARF) causes
- Frequency of ARF in rhabdomyolysis is 30%.
- Young males more commonly affected

Prevalence
Exact prevalence is unknown.

RISK FACTORS
- Extreme physical exertion
- Hypothermia or hyperthermia
- Inhalational anesthetics
- Medications (neuroleptics, statins, etc.)
- Toxins (e.g., mushroom, carbon monoxide)
- Infections (especially viral infections)

Genetics
Inherited disorders associated with decreased energy production may cause rhabdomyolysis. These include disorders of carbohydrate metabolism, fatty acid oxidation, nucleoside metabolism, myopathies, and mitochondrial defects.

GENERAL PREVENTION
- Adequate volume resuscitation is initiated to prevent further muscle damage.
- Administration of free radical scavenger to prevent rhabdomyolysis may be useful in the future.

PATHOPHYSIOLOGY
- Direct cellular membrane damage or ATP depletion leads to intracellular calcium accumulation secondary to loss of ionic gradients created by sodium-potassium pumps and sodium-calcium channels.
- Raised intracellular calcium leads to greater activity of intracellular proteolytic enzymes, causing cell destruction and release of intracellular contents like myoglobin, aldolase, creatine kinase, aspartate transaminases, LDH, etc.

ETIOLOGY
- Traumatic:
  - Crush syndrome in multiple trauma syndrome
  - Tortured individuals/abused children
  - Immobilization
  - Prolonged surgical procedures
  - Compartment syndrome

- Nontraumatic:
  - Extreme physical exertion in untrained individual, in extremely hot, humid environment; in individuals with impaired sweating mechanism (heavy clothing or anticholinergic medications)
  - Sickle cell trait individuals, especially at high altitude
  - Hyperkinetic states like seizures (grand mal), delirium tremens, psychotic agitation, amphetamine overdose, status asthmaticus
  - Myopathies (recurrent rhabdomyolysis after exercise)
  - Disorders of glycogenolysis:
    - Myophosphorylase deficiency (McArdle disease, autosomal recessive), phosphorylase kinase deficiency
  - Disorders of glycolysis:
    - Phosphofructokinase deficiency, phosphoglycerate kinase deficiency, phosphoglycerate mutase deficiency, lactate dehydrogenase deficiency
  - Disorders of lipid metabolism:
  - Carnitine palmitoyltransferase deficiency (most common), carnitine deficiency, short- chain and long-chain acyl-CoA dehydrogenase deficiency
  - Disorders of purine metabolism:
  - Myoadenylate deaminase deficiency
  - Others:
    - Calcium adenosine triphosphate deficiency
    - Mitochondrial (defects in respiratory chain enzymes)
- Malignant hyperthermia:
  - Use of inhalational anesthetic agents in susceptible individuals
  - Autosomal dominant
  - Presents with fever, muscular rigidity, metabolic acidosis, and rhabdomyolysis)
- Neuroleptic malignant syndrome:
  - Exposure to neuroleptics and antiparkinsonian drugs
  - Presents with high fever, muscle contractions or tremors, and rhabdomyolysis
- Toxin-mediated:
  - Ethanol, methanol, ethylene glycol, isopropanol, heroin, methadone, barbiturates, cocaine, PCP, amphetamines, LSD, carbon monoxide, toluene, hemlock, herbs from quail bush, and snake, spider bites (especially black widow spider).
- Drug-mediated:
  - Statins, fibric acid derivative, quinine, colchicine, neuroleptics, antihistamines, amphotericin B, salicylates, caffeine, cyclic antidepressants, SSRIs, theophylline, aminocaproic acid, phenylpropanolamine, propofol
  - Drug–drug interaction: Protease inhibitors, erythromycin, gemfibrozil, and cyclosporine in combination with statins
- Infections:
  - Viral: Influenza A + B (most common), HIV, coxsackievirus, EBV, CMV, adenovirus, varicella zoster, West Nile virus, parainfluenza

- Bacterial: *Streptococcus pneumoniae, S. pyogenes, S. viridians*, Group B *Streptococcus; Staphylococcus aureus, Francisella tularensis, E. coli, Listeria* spp., *Salmonella* spp., *Clostridium perfringens, Clostridium tetani, Mycoplasma* spp., *Legionella* spp., *Bacillus* spp., *Brucella* spp., *Vibrio* spp., *Ehrlichiosis, Leptospira* spp.
  - Parasitic: *Plasmodium falciparum*
  - Fungal: *Candida, Aspergillus* spp.
- Electrolyte abnormalities:
  - Hypokalemia, hypophosphatemia,
  - Hypo-/hypernatremia
  - DKA and hyperosmolar diabetic coma
- Endocrine disorders:
  - Hypo-/hyperthyroidism
  - Pheochromocytoma
  - DKA
- Inflammatory myopathies: Polymyositis, dermatomyositis
- Capillary leak syndrome:
  - Recurrent increased capillary permeability causing interstitial fluid shift leading to edema and compartment syndrome
- Abrupt withdrawal of baclofen leading to severe muscle spasms

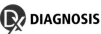 **DIAGNOSIS**

HISTORY
- Muscle weakness, swelling, and pain (localized or diffuse)
- Reddish-brown urine due to myoglobinuria, decreased urine output

PHYSICAL EXAM
- Motor weakness, tenderness, swelling, and erythema of overlying skin
- Compartment syndrome (worsening limb swelling and distal neurovascular compromise after fluid resuscitation, with intracompartmental pressures of 25–30 mm Hg within MAP)
- Signs of renal failure: Reddish-brown urine, edema, HTN, volume overload, decreased urine output

DIAGNOSTIC TESTS & INTERPRETATION
Lab
- Serum creatine kinase (100% sensitive)

  – 5–10x above normal in patients with risk factors or symptoms defines rhabdomyolysis. It peaks in 24 hours and decrease 30–40% per day after initial insult (1)[A]

- Myoglobin is an unreliable marker as its half-life is 1–3 hours and it is rapidly excreted in urine, leading to reddish-brown pigmenturia. Urine dipstick test positive in 50% of patients with rhabdomyolysis. It clears from circulation in 6 hours.
- Aldolase, LDH, SGOT are elevated (nonspecific markers).
- Cardiac troponin I is elevated in 33% of patients.
- Hyperkalemia, hyperphosphatemia
- Hypocalcemia (due to calcium deposits in damaged muscles and decreased bone responsiveness to parathyroid hormone)

- Hyperuricemia due to release of purines from damaged muscle cells; may also cause urate nephropathy
- Metabolic acidosis
- ARF in 30–40% patients (due to direct myoglobin toxicity, cast formation, and renal hypoperfusion)
- DIC (due to release of thromboplastin from damaged muscle cells)

Imaging
- Plays no role in diagnosis
- MRI useful in identifying etiologies like myositis, abscesses
- Renal US for workup of renal failure

Diagnostic Procedures/Other
- Intracompartmental pressure monitoring in patients with focal swelling
- Fasciotomy if intracompartmental pressures >25–30 mm Hg
- ECG

DIFFERENTIAL DIAGNOSIS
- Hemoglobinuria (hemolysis)
- Hematuria (renal cause, trauma)
- Acute intermittent porphyria
- Bilirubinemia
- Foods (e.g., beets)
- Drugs (e.g., vitamin B_{12}, rifampin, phenytoin, laxatives)

 TREATMENT

Fluid resuscitation with isotonic crystalloid is the mainstay of therapy for rhabdomyolysis, and studies suggest that the prognosis is better with early intervention.

MEDICATION
First Line
- Sodium bicarbonate:
  - Urinary alkalinization helps prevent heme protein precipitation.
  - Consider in patients with moderate to severe rhabdomyolysis and in patients with risk factors for developing ARF (preexisting renal disease, metabolic acidosis, dehydration) once adequate urine output is maintained (2)[C].
  - Use sodium bicarbonate drip (3 ampoules in 1 L of 5% dextrose or sterile water at initial infusion rate of 100 mL/hr) to achieve urinary pH $\geq$6.5.
  - Discontinue alkaline solution if symptomatic hypocalcemia or urinary pH<6.5 after 3–4 hours of infusion.
  - May cause alkalosis, decreased plasma potassium, hypocalcemia, and hypernatremia; caution in electrolyte imbalances, such as in patients with CHF, cirrhosis, edema, corticosteroid use, or renal failure; when administering, avoid extravasations because can cause tissue necrosis.
- Mannitol:
  - Use of diuretic in oliguric patients despite adequate volume repletion (3)[C]
  - Beneficial in severe CK elevations (>20,000 u/L) as it minimizes intratubular heme pigment deposition and acts as free radical scavenger

- Given 1 g/kg IV over 30 minutes, followed by 5 g/hr for a total of not more than 120 g/d.
- Monitor plasma osmolality, osmolal gap q4–6h.
- Discontinue mannitol if diuresis not achieved or osmolal gap >55 mosmol/kg (4)[B].
- Monitor cardiovascular status before and after rapid administration of mannitol for fulminating CHF due to sudden increase in extracellular fluid.

Second Line
Furosemide:
- Loop diuretic causes free water loss by inhibiting sodium and chloride reabsorption in the ascending loop of Henle and distal renal tubule
- Adult dose is 20–40 mg IV q2h p.r.n. to maintain urine output; can increase dose to desired urine output.

ADDITIONAL TREATMENT
- Once diuresis is established, continue aggressive fluid therapy until urine discoloration clears and serum CK <10000 u/L
- Serial CK measurements to asses for decreasing levels
- Monitor and treat hyperkalemia aggressively.
- Treat symptomatic hypocalcemia only (5)[B].
- Monitor for DIC (specially 3–5 days after initial insult) and treat with blood products for life-threatening hemorrhage.
- Consider hemodialysis for severe renal failure with uremic encephalopathy, pericardial effusion, refractory hyperkalemia, or metabolic acidosis and volume overload.
- Attempt to treat etiology and prevent further muscle damage.

SURGERY/OTHER PROCEDURES
Monitor for compartment syndrome and consider fasciotomy for intracompartmental pressures >35 mm Hg.

IN-PATIENT CONSIDERATIONS
Initial Stabilization
- Supportive care: ABC management; treat associated and causative conditions
- Establish diagnosis with history, physical, and laboratory markers.
- Mild to moderate cases with stable electrolytes can be admitted to medical floor.
- Severe cases with renal failure, hypotension, DIC, or refractory electrolyte abnormality should be admitted to ICU.

IV Fluids
Aggressive hydration to prevent heme-pigment induced ARF:
- NS infusion at 10–15 mL/kg/hr (some suggest 1–2 L/hr for initial period) to achieve urine output of 2–3 mL/kg/hr (some suggest 150–300 mL/hr) (1)[B]

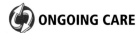 ONGOING CARE

PROGNOSIS
Depends on underlying etiology and comorbidities

COMPLICATIONS
- Death from hyperkalemia, renal failure
- Compartment syndrome
- DIC
- Hepatic insufficiency
- ARF

REFERENCES
1. Bagley WH, et al. Rhabdomyolysis. *Intern Emerg Med*. 2007;2(3):210–8.
2. Sauret JM, et al. Rhabdomyolysis. *Am Fam Physician*. 2002;65:907–12.
3. Heurta-Alardin AL, et al. Bench to bedside review: Rhabdomyolysis, an overview for clinicians. *Crit Care*. 2005;9:158–69.
4. Visweswaran P, et al. Rhabdomyolysis. *Crit Care Clin*. 1999;15:415–28.
5. Gabow PA, et al. The spectrum of Rhabdomyolysis. *Medicine* (Baltimore). 1982;61:141.

ADDITIONAL READING
- Vanholder R, et al. Rhabdomyolysis. *J Am Soc Nephrol*. 2000;11:1553–61.
- Zager RA. Rhabdomyolysis and myoglobinuric acute renal failure. *Kidney Int*. 1996;49:314–26.

 CODES

ICD9
- 728.88 Rhabdomyolysis
- 728.89 Other disorders of muscle, ligament, and fascia

CLINICAL PEARLS
- Rhabdomyolysis involves myocyte damage and release of intracellular contents into the circulation and toxic effects on distant organ systems.
- Diagnose is by clinical suspicion and elevated serum creatine kinase level.
- Renal failure occurs in 30–40% patients and can be prevented by aggressive hydration, urinary alkalinization, and mannitol therapy.
- Dialysis is indicated in refractory hyperkalemia, metabolic acidosis, and volume overload.
- Early diagnosis with aggressive treatment may decrease morbidity and mortality.

ROCKY MOUNTAIN SPOTTED FEVER

Sophia Koo

 BASICS

DESCRIPTION

Rocky Mountain Spotted Fever (RMSF) is a rickettsial illness transmitted by infected ticks. *Rickettsia rickettsii* infects endothelial cells and causes a diffuse small-vessel vasculitis with multiple end-organ manifestations. The diagnosis of RMSF can be challenging; the characteristic rash often appears after initial clinical presentation with fevers and other nonspecific symptoms and rapid diagnostic tests are not widely available. RMSF can be fulminant, with shock and multiorgan failure, particularly if appropriate antibiotic therapy is delayed.

EPIDEMIOLOGY
Incidence
- 8 cases per million people in 2008; has been rising over the past decade
- 92% of cases occur April–September (coinciding with peak adult and nymph tick activity), but sporadic cases reported are throughout the year.
- Highest rates in children, patients with exposure to dogs, grassy/wooded areas

Prevalence
- Transmitted by a variety of hard-bodied tick species, including the American dog tick (*Dermacentor variabilis*), the Rocky Mountain wood tick (*Dermacentor andersoni*), and the brown dog tick (*Rhipicephalus sanguineus*, reported as the vector for a cluster of cases in eastern Arizona).
- Cases are reported throughout the continental US, although 60% of cases are reported from Oklahoma, Missouri, Arkansas, Tennessee, North Carolina, and South Carolina.
- 6% spotted fever group seroprevalence in the military, particularly in men, ground combat specialists, recruits from endemic states

RISK FACTORS
Exposure to ticks and tick habitats

GENERAL PREVENTION
Tick precautions

PATHOPHYSIOLOGY
- The causative organism, *R. rickettsii*, invades endothelial cells, multiplies intracellularly, then spreads to adjacent cells and extracellular spaces.
- End result is a diffuse small-vessel vasculitis with multiple potential end-organ manifestations: Vasculitic rash, interstitial pneumonitis, myocarditis, renal failure, meningoencephalitis.
- Patients can develop fulminant shock and multiorgan failure.

ETIOLOGY
- Etiologic agent of RMSF is *R. rickettsii*, a fastidious, small (0.3 × 1.0 μm), pleomorphic gram-negative coccobacillus.
- All *Rickettsia* are obligate intracellular organisms, requiring eukaryotic host cells for growth.

COMMONLY ASSOCIATED CONDITIONS
RMSF is one member of the spotted fever group rickettsiae; several other members are known to cause RMSF-like illnesses in the US (*R. felis*, *R. parkeri*, *R. akari*, and *R. 364D*).

℞ DIAGNOSIS

HISTORY
- 99% of patients report fever.
- 80–90% have a diffuse maculopapular rash that appears 3–7 days after the onset of illness.
- 80–90% report headache.
- 70–90% report myalgias.
- General malaise
- Tick exposure history (not always apparent), occupation
- Travel history: Spotted fever group rickettsiae are geographically restricted; *R. rickettsiae*, *R. parkeri*, *R. felis*, *R. akari*, and *R. 364D* cause RMSF and milder RMSF-like illnesses in the continental US, but other spotted fever group rickettsial infections from other geographic locations (Mediterranean spotted fever, Israeli spotted fever, African tick bite fever, Astrakhan fever, etc.) can also present with fevers, rash, and systemic illness.

PHYSICAL EXAM
- Vital signs: Fevers, hemodynamics
- Careful dermatologic exam to assess for rash, especially the palms and soles (although only 50% of patients have a rash during the first 3 days of their illness); often blanching maculopapular eruption initially, then classic petechial rash
- Eschar at site of tick bite (rare in RMSF, more common with other clinically overlapping spotted fever group rickettsial illnesses such as the illness caused by *R. parkeri*, *R. akari*, and *R. 364D* in the US, African tick bite fever (*R. africae*), and Mediterranean spotted fever (*R. conorii*)
- Neurologic exam to assess for signs of meningoencephalitis
- Hepatosplenomegaly (nonspecific)

DIAGNOSTIC TESTS & INTERPRETATION
Lab
Initial lab tests
- CBC: Leukopenia, thrombocytopenia, anemia common, although nonspecific
- LFTs: Transaminase elevations common, but nonspecific
- Blood cultures (to assess for other etiologies of fever)
- *R. rickettsii* IgG and IgM by indirect immunofluorescence: Often not positive early in the acute phase of illness (50–60% of RMSF patients have +IgM by day 7–9, 75% by day 14), 4-fold change in IgG titers at 2–4 weeks required to confirm diagnosis (sensitivity of paired acute and convalescent serologies is 94–100%, specificity 100%), although there is a high level of serologic cross-reactivity between all members of the spotted fever group rickettsiae
- PCR of whole blood for *R. rickettsii*, ideally prior to initiation of antibiotic therapy

Follow-Up & Special Considerations
- Spotted fever group rickettsial illnesses are reportable illnesses.
- Convalescent serology 2–4 weeks after onset of illness to confirm RMSF diagnosis: Requires 4-fold rise in IgG titer

Imaging
As directed by history and exam findings: Chest x-ray to assess for pneumonitis; consider CNS imaging if the patient presents with meningoencephalitis.

Diagnostic Procedures/Other
Skin biopsy if rash is present

Pathological Findings
- Skin biopsy may show rickettsial forms in endothelial and vascular smooth muscle cells.
- Rickettsial PCR and immunohistochemistry can be performed in biopsy specimens, but these assays have low sensitivity, particularly with antibiotic therapy active against Rickettsiae, and are not widely available.

DIFFERENTIAL DIAGNOSIS
- Other spotted fever group rickettsioses
- Anaplasmosis/ehrlichiosis
- Meningococcemia
- Syphilis
- Leptospirosis

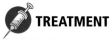 TREATMENT

MEDICATION
First Line
Doxycycline 100 mg b.i.d. for a minimum of 5–7 days (significantly lowers odds of mortality)

Second Line
Chloramphenicol 50–75 mg/kg/d for at least 7 days (should be considered a distant second choice)

ADDITIONAL TREATMENT
General Measures
Supportive care of shock, multiorgan failure

Issues for Referral
Dermatology and infectious diseases consultations are strongly recommended.

IN-PATIENT CONSIDERATIONS
Initial Stabilization
- If RMSF is a serious consideration on the differential, start empiric antibiotics: Delayed antibiotic therapy is associated with increased mortality and all diagnostic tests for RMSF take days to weeks to return.
- Supportive care if hemodynamic instability or multiorgan dysfunction are present

Admission Criteria
Recommend admission for diagnostic workup of fevers, rash, and systemic illness, which are nonspecific and can be manifestations of a wide array of infectious and noninfectious processes.

IV Fluids
As per protocol if patients not taking PO adequately

Nursing
No special considerations; consider ICU care in presence of any hemodynamic instability or severe end-organ dysfunction

Discharge Criteria
- Resolution of fevers
- Improving rash

 ONGOING CARE

FOLLOW-UP RECOMMENDATIONS
- Consider dermatology and infectious diseases follow-up.
- Convalescent *R. rickettsii* serologies 2–4 weeks after initial presentation of illness to confirm diagnosis of RMSF/spotted fever group rickettsiosis

DIET
No special restrictions

PROGNOSIS
- Historically associated with extremely high case fatality rates (25–30%); recent case fatality rates have declined to <0.5–5%, particularly with prompt recognition of RMSF-like syndromes and early initiation of effective antibiotic therapy.
- Higher odds ratios for mortality in patients >40, patients of African descent, patients with G6PD, and patients with fever >38°C on presentation, renal failure, or neurologic involvement

COMPLICATIONS
- Shock
- Multiorgan failure
- Death

ADDITIONAL READING
- Dantas-Torres F. Rocky Mountain spotted fever. *Lancet Infect Dis*. 2007;7:724–32.
- Walker DH. Rickettsiae and rickettsial infections: The current state of knowledge. *Clin Infect Dis*. 2007;45: S39–44.
- http://www.cdc.gov/rmsf/

 CODES

ICD9
- 082.0 Spotted fevers
- 083.8 Other specified rickettsioses

CLINICAL PEARLS

Classic triad of fever, rash, and headache is only present in about 50% of patients, and rash is often absent early in the course of illness. RMSF can be fulminant and fatal if appropriate antibiotic therapy is not administered in a timely fashion. If there is any clinical suspicion for RMSF, it is reasonable to treat empirically with doxycycline.

SEPSIS

Francisco Polanco
Jose R. Yunen

 BASICS

DESCRIPTION
- Sepsis is a clinical syndrome defined as the presence of systemic inflammatory response syndrome (SIRS) and source of infection.
- SIRS is an inflammatory response to multiple clinical insults, including infectious and noninfectious causes (e.g., pancreatitis, severe trauma or burn); it is defined as presence of the following criteria:
  - Temperature >38.3°C or <36°C
  - Heart rate >90/min
  - Respiratory rate >20/min
  - WBC count >12,000/mm^3 or <4,000/mm^3
- Severe sepsis occurs in the presence of organ dysfunction or hypotension, including:
  - Arterial hypoxemia (PaO$_2$/FiO$_2$ <300)
  - Urine output <0.5mL/kg/hr
  - INR >1.5 or PTT >60 sec
  - Thrombocytopenia <100,000/mm^3
- Septic shock: Systolic arterial pressure <90 mm Hg or a reduction in systolic blood pressure of >40 mm Hg unexplained by other causes, despite adequate fluid resuscitation.
- Synonym(s): Septicemia; Sepsis neonatorum

EPIDEMIOLOGY
Incidence
- 3 cases per 1,000 population
- 2 cases per 100 patients admitted to hospital

RISK FACTORS
- Positive blood cultures
- Age extremes
- Impaired host
- Critically ill patients
- Indwelling catheters
- Complicated labor and delivery
- Certain surgical procedures

Genetics
Single-nucleotide polymorphisms influence the risk for the development of sepsis and the risk of mortality from sepsis.

GENERAL PREVENTION
- Vaccination: Pneumococcal (population at risk), *Haemophilus influenzae* type B (infants, young children)
- Hand washing by health care workers
- Use of appropriate aseptic techniques and bundles during insertion of indwelling catheters

PATHOPHYSIOLOGY
In sepsis, the dysregulation of the inflammatory process is precipitated by an imbalance between pro- and anti-inflammatory mediators, resulting in widespread systemic tissue destruction and organ dysfunction.

ETIOLOGY
- Specific etiologic agents include:
  - Gram-positive organisms: Most commonly *Staphylococcus* spp., *Streptococcus* spp., *Enterococcus* spp.
  - Gram-negative organisms: Most commonly *Escherichia coli, Klebsiella* spp., *Proteus* spp., *Pseudomonas* spp.
  - Fungi: Most commonly *Candida* spp.
- Common sources of septicemia include:
  - Lungs
  - Urinary tract
  - Intra-abdominal
  - Intravascular catheters
  - Skin: Cellulitis, decubitus ulcer, gangrene
  - Heart valves

COMMONLY ASSOCIATED CONDITIONS
- Immunologic disorders: Neutropenia, HIV, hypo-/agammaglobulinemia, complement deficiency, splenectomy
- Diabetes mellitus
- Alcoholism
- Malignancy
- Cirrhosis
- Burns
- Multiple trauma
- IV drug abuse
- Malnutrition

 DIAGNOSIS

- Fever, chills, rigors
- Tachycardia
- Tachypnea
- Hypotension
- Confusion, agitation, restlessness
- Specific symptoms related to source of infection, including cough, SOB, dysuria, diarrhea

DIAGNOSTIC TESTS & INTERPRETATION
Lab
- Blood cultures before antibiotics administration
- ≥2 blood cultures should be obtained, and at least 1 from peripheral access
- Blood culture from any vascular access in place for more than 48 hours
- CBC with differential, C-reactive protein, coagulation profile (PT/INR/PTT)
- Electrolytes, BUN, creatinine, glucose, LFTs
- Lactic acid level, ABG
- Common findings: Leukocytosis, hyperglycemia, hypocalcemia, hypoxemia, respiratory alkalosis, metabolic acidosis
- Less common findings: Anemia, thrombocytopenia, prolonged PT, azotemia, hypoglycemia

Imaging
Relevant radiographs, US, CT, MRI should be performed to confirm and sample any source of infection

Diagnostic Procedures/Other
- Aspiration of potentially infected body fluids (pleural, peritoneal, CSF) when appropriate
- Drainage of potentially infected tissues (abscess, biliary tree, ulcers, others) when appropriate

DIFFERENTIAL DIAGNOSIS
- Shock from other etiologies (hypovolemic, cardiogenic)
- Localized infection
- Bacteremia without sepsis
- Viral infections (influenza, dengue, West Nile)
- Collagen vascular disease, vasculitis

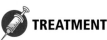 **TREATMENT**

MEDICATION
First Line
- Fluid resuscitation with crystalloid or colloid:
  - Fluids challenge of 1 L crystalloid or 300–500 mL colloid within 30 minutes)
  - Target CVP >8 mm Hg or >12 mm Hg for mechanically ventilated patients
- Vasopressors (target MAP >65 mm Hg):
  - Norepinephrine or dopamine are considered 1st choice; administer centrally if possible
  - Epinephrine, phenylephrine, and vasopressin should not be used as 1st choice.
  - Low-dose dopamine for renal protection is not recommended.
- Antibiotic therapy:
  - Should be broad-spectrum initially, focused on most likely pathogen
  - Reassess antibiotic choice using clinical data and microbiology to narrow coverage.
  - For severe sepsis and septic shock, antibiotics should be administered within 1 hour of admission.
  - *Pseudomonas* not suspected: Use 3rd-generation cephalosporin (ceftriaxone/cefotaxime), β-lactamase/β-lactamase inhibitor (piperacillin/tazobactam, ampicillin/sulbactam), or carbapenem (imipenem, meropenem); consider adding vancomycin if high prevalence of MRSA. In patients allergic to penicillin, ciprofloxacin or levofloxacin plus clindamycin can be used.
  - *Pseudomonas* suspected: Double pseudomonal coverage (ceftazidime, cefepime, or piperacillin-tazobactam plus either ciprofloxacin or aminoglycoside (amikacin/gentamicin)
  - Antifungals may be required if fungal infection is suspected (long-term antibiotic use, use of total parenteral nutrition, GI surgery or pathology)

- Source identification and control:
  - Specific site of infection should be identified as rapidly as possible, within 6 hours of presentation.
  - Surgical intervention is warranted for debridement of necrotic tissue or drainage of abscess.
  - Intravascular access devices should be removed if potentially infected.

Second Line
- Steroids:
  - Stress dose of steroids to be given only in septic shock patients with poor response to fluids and vasopressors
  - Hydrocortisone (150–300 mg/d) is preferred over dexamethasone
  - ACTH stimulation test is not recommended
- Glucose control:
  - Target glucose level <150 mg/dL
  - IV insulin therapy
  - Glucose levels q1–2h until glucose values and insulin infusion rates are stable
- Recombinant human activated protein C:
  - Consider in patients with sepsis-induced organ dysfunction (APACHE II score >25 or multiorgan dysfunction)
- Blood transfusion:
  - Red blood cells transfusion when hemoglobin decreases to <7 g/dL
  - Target hemoglobin: 7–9 g/dL

ADDITIONAL TREATMENT
Additional Therapies
- DVT prophylaxis:
  - Prophylaxis with either low-dose unfractionated heparin or low-molecular-weight heparin should be used, unless contraindicated.
  - Very high-risk patients should receive a combination of mechanical and pharmacological therapy.
- Stress ulcer prophylaxis:
  - H_2 blocker or proton pump inhibitors should be used.

ONGOING CARE
FOLLOW-UP RECOMMENDATIONS
Depending upon severity, transthoracic echocardiography is recommended for re-evaluation of asymptomatic patients:
- Every year for severe AS
- Every 1–2 years for moderate AS
- Every 3–5 years for mild AS.

DIET
- NPO initially
- Enteral feeds when possible

PATIENT EDUCATION
MedLine Plus. Accessed at http://www.nlm.nih.gov/medLineplus/sepsis.htmL

PROGNOSIS
- Mortality is 10–50%.
- Following factors have been associated with worse prognosis: Extreme ages, neutropenia, diabetes mellitus, alcoholism, renal failure

COMPLICATIONS
- Multiorgan failure
- ARDS
- DIC
- GI hemorrhage
- Death

ADDITIONAL READING
- Angus DC, et al. Epidemiology of severe sepsis in the United States: Analysis of incidence, outcome, and associated cost of care. *Crit Care Med*. 2001;29:1303.
- Dellinger RP, et al. Surviving Sepsis Campaign: International guidelines for management of severe sepsis and septic shock: 2008. *Crit Care Med*. 2008;36(1):296–327.

- Levy MM, et al. 2001 SCCM/ESICM/ACCP/ATS/SIS International Sepsis Definitions Conference. *Crit Care Med*. 2003;31:1250–6.
- Rivers E, et al. Early goal-directed therapy in the treatment of severe sepsis and septic shock. *N Engl J Med*. 2001;345:1368–77.
- Sprung CL, et al. Hydrocortisone therapy for patients with septic shock. *N Engl J Med*. 2008;358:111–24.

CODES

ICD9
- 038.9 Unspecified septicemia
- 995.90 Systemic inflammatory response syndrome, unspecified
- 995.91 Sepsis

CLINICAL PEARLS
- Sepsis is presence of SIRS associated with source of infection.
- Appropriate resuscitation during the 1st 6 hours is crucial.
- Delay in antimicrobial therapy increases mortality.
- Despite aggressive management and medicine advance, mortality rates for patients with severe sepsis and septic shock remains high.

S

SEPSIS IN THE OBSTETRIC PATIENT

Dena Goffman

BASICS

DESCRIPTION
- Systemic inflammatory response syndrome (SIRS): >2 of the following:
  - Temperature >38°C or <36°C
  - Heart rate >90 beats/min
  - Respiratory rate >20 breaths/min or $PaCO_2$ <32 mm Hg
  - WBC >12,000/mm^3, <4000/mm^3, or >10% immature forms
- Sepsis: Confirmed or suspected infection *PLUS* ≥2 SIRS criteria
- Severe sepsis: Sepsis with associated organ failure
- Septic shock: Sepsis with hypotension refractory to fluid resuscitation
- Multiple organ dysfunction syndrome (MODS)
- Important to note that no criteria for SIRS in pregnancy exist, and some of the physiologic changes of pregnancy will cause changes in the normal values for these parameters.
- The risk is attributing changes to pregnancy and missing sepsis in the obstetric patient.

EPIDEMIOLOGY
Incidence
- Bacteremia in 7.5/1000 obstetric admissions
- Sepsis only 8–10% of bacteremic OB patients
- Maternal sepsis is relatively infrequent
- Mortality rate ~3% (much lower than general medical patient)
- However, remains a leading cause of maternal mortality likely due to:
  - Delayed diagnosis
  - Failure of early aggressive treatment
  - End-organ dysfunction

RISK FACTORS
- Gram-negative organisms are most frequently isolated
- Infectious complications in pregnancy:
  - Asymptomatic bacteriuria, cystitis, pyelonephritis
  - Chorioamnionitis, septic abortion, endometritis, wound infection, necrotizing fasciitis
  - Pneumonia
  - Cholecystitis

Genetics
Patients with sickle cell disease and trait are more prone to GU infection in pregnancy

GENERAL PREVENTION
- Primary prevention:
  - Identify patients at risk for infection
  - Immunizations up to date
  - Screen urine in pregnancy (4–7% have asymptomatic bacteriuria and, if not treated, up to 40% of those will develop pyelonephritis.)
- Secondary prevention:
  - Early appropriate treatment of infection

PATHOPHYSIOLOGY
Physiological predisposition in pregnancy:
- Pyelonephritis: Reduction in renal concentrating ability, smooth muscle relaxation/ureteral dilatation, bladder flaccidity
- Chorioamnionitis/septic abortion: Decrease pH and increased glycogen in vagina epithelium
- Pneumonia: Elevation of diaphragm, delayed gastric emptying

ETIOLOGY
- Obstetric:
  - Chorioamnionitis
  - Septic abortion
  - Postpartum endometritis
  - Wound/episiotomy infection
  - Septic pelvic thrombophlebitis
- Nonobstetric:
  - UTI/pyelonephritis
  - Pneumonia
  - Appendicitis
  - Cholecystitis

COMMONLY ASSOCIATED CONDITIONS
- HIV infection
- Sickle cell disease
- Asplenia
- Chronic kidney disease
- Steroid use

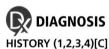

DIAGNOSIS

HISTORY (1,2,3,4)[C]
- Elicit localizing signs/symptoms to help identify infectious source and guide therapy:
  - Recent urinary tract or other infection
  - GU, GI, pulmonary complaints
  - Obstetric complaints (contractions, leaking fluid)

PHYSICAL EXAM (1,3)[c]
- Early findings include any of the following:
  - Fever, tachycardia, tachypnea, hypertension or hypotension, flushing, warm extremities, confusion
- As sepsis progresses:
  - Hypoperfusion, peripheral vasoconstriction, cyanosis, end-organ dysfunction
- Try to localize the source:
  - Fundal tenderness suggestive of chorioamnionitis in pregnancy or endometritis postpartum
  - Wounds should be evaluated for erythema, induration, drainage
  - CVA tenderness suggestive of pyelonephritis
  - Right-sided abdominal pain is likely to present in an atypical location in appendicitis, due to displacement by the gravid uterus.

DIAGNOSTIC TESTS & INTERPRETATION
Lab
Initial lab tests (1)[C]
- CBC, chemistries, LFTs, coagulation profile, serum lactate, ABG
- Blood and urine cultures before antibiotics
- Culture additional sites based on suspicion:
  - Wounds, respiratory secretions, cerebrospinal fluid
  - Amniocentesis can be performed for cell count, glucose, Gram stain, and culture for suspicion of chorioamnionitis.

Follow-Up & Special Considerations
- Labs should be followed serially.
- Important laboratory changes in normal pregnancy:
  - WBCs increase throughout pregnancy
  - Renal plasma flow/GFR increase; therefore BUN (4–7 mg/dL) and creatinine (0.4–0.7 mg/dL) are decreased in pregnancy.
  - Increased clotting factors and decreased fibrinolysis result in changes in coagulation profile and increased thrombotic risk.
  - Increased minute ventilation leads to decreased $PaCO_2$ (30 mm Hg) and compensatory decrease in serum bicarbonate (low 20s mEq/L) to maintain normal pH.

Imaging
Initial approach
- Chest x-ray (risk for ARDS)
- Appropriate additional imaging studies are based on suspected diagnosis.
- US, CT scan, and MRI can be used in pregnancy (5)[C].
- Use of iodinated contrast is safe in pregnancy and should be administered in the usual fashion (5)[C].

Follow-Up & Special Considerations
- Maternal stabilization and appropriate treatment are the priority.
- Fear of radiation of the pregnant patient can result in delay of diagnosis and treatment.
- Teratogenesis in the fetus is not a major concern after diagnostic pelvic CT studies (5)[C].
- Risk of carcinogenesis in the fetus is increased with radiation exposure but risk remains low (5)[C].

Diagnostic Procedures/Other
Consider amniocentesis (described above) for suspicion of chorioamnionitis.

DIFFERENTIAL DIAGNOSIS
- Sepsis/septic shock
- Hypovolemic shock
- Cardiogenic shock

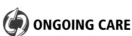

TREATMENT

ALERT
Maintenance of maternal blood pressure is a priority for uteroplacental perfusion.

MEDICATION
First Line
- Rapid IV fluid resuscitation with crystalloid (goal CVP 8–12 mm Hg) (1,2)[B]
- Vasopressor agents if fluid alone is unsuccessful (goal mean arterial pressure >65–70 mm Hg) (1,2)[B]
- Empiric broad-spectrum antibiotics (1,2)[C]:
  – Individualize based on likely source
  – Start within 1 hour

Second Line
- Blood products as needed (anemia, DIC) to HCT>30% (1,2)[C]:
  – Decision to transfuse is based on maternal/fetal status; threshold may be lower in the pregnant patient due to oxygen consumption and potential for blood loss with delivery.
- May require inotropic support with dobutamine (1,2)[C]
- Supplemental oxygen/ventilatory support (1,2)[C]
- Supportive care:
  – DVT prophylaxis is crucial in this hypercoagulable patient population (1,2)[A].
  – Stress ulcer prophylaxis (1,2)[A]
  – Glycemic control (1,2)[C]
- Prevent secondary infection
- Consider antenatal corticosteroids (betamethasone) for fetal benefit (1)[C]

ADDITIONAL TREATMENT
General Measures
Monitor effect of resuscitation:
- Improved maternal vital signs
- Urine output (>0.5 mL/kg/hr)
- Return of mental status to normal
- Return of fetal heart rate to normal

Issues for Referral
- Maternal fetal medicine specialist
- General surgery for nonobstetric surgical diagnosis
- Nutrition

Additional Therapies
Nutritional support is especially important in the pregnant patient if she is unable to eat for a prolonged period.

SURGERY/OTHER PROCEDURES
- Surgery is crucial for source control in surgical conditions.
- Prompt delivery is indicated if the source is believed to be intrauterine (chorioamnionitis).
- Intubation in gravid patient can be difficult due to edema/anatomical changes and has increased risk of aspiration. Experienced anesthesiologist is preferable for intubation.

IN-PATIENT CONSIDERATIONS
Initial Stabilization
Early goal-directed therapy for severe sepsis as in the nonpregnant patient with attention to:
- Optimizing maternal blood pressure for uteroplacental perfusion
- Maintaining maternal oxygenation SaO_2 >95% for fetal benefit

Admission Criteria
- Hypotension not responsive to fluids
- Vasoactive agents or inotropes required
- Hypoxia, significant oxygen requirement
- Mechanical ventilation
- Invasive hemodynamic monitoring

IV Fluids
- Crystalloids
- Follow intake and output

Nursing
- Follow blood pressure and SaO_2; goals are different than for the nonpregnant patient, for fetal benefit
- Left lateral positioning to optimize uteroplacental perfusion
- Observe for evidence of patient discomfort, palpable uterine contractions, vaginal bleeding, vaginal fluid discharge; systemic infection and critical illness can precipitate preterm labor

Discharge Criteria
- Stable vital signs
- Adequate oxygenation
- Adequate urine output
- Normalization of laboratory parameters

ONGOING CARE

FOLLOW-UP RECOMMENDATIONS
- Complete course of antibiotics as directed
- Close outpatient follow-up

DIET
As tolerated

PATIENT EDUCATION
Patient awareness of warning signs of recurrent infection, secondary infection

PROGNOSIS
- Favorable, as compared to nonpregnant patient with sepsis
- However, remains a leading cause of maternal mortality

COMPLICATIONS
- Maternal mortality
- ARDS/acute lung injury
- Renal failure
- Cholestasis, hyperbilirubinemia, jaundice
- DIC
- Nosocomial infections
- Preterm delivery and associated morbidities

REFERENCES

1. Guinn DA, et al. Early goal directed therapy for sepsis during pregnancy. *Obstet Gynecol Clin North Am*. 2007;34:459–79.
2. Fernandez-Perez ER, et al. Sepsis during pregnancy. *Criti Care Med*. 2005;33:S287–S293.
3. Paruk F. Infection in obstetric critical care. *Best Pract Res Clin Obstet Gynaecol*. 2008;22:865–83.
4. Sheffield JS. Sepsis and septic shock in pregnancy. *Crit Care Clin*. 2004;20:651–60.
5. Chen MM, et al. Guidelines for computed tomography and magnetic resonance imaging use during pregnancy and lactation. *Obstet Gynecol*. 2008;112:333–40.

ADDITIONAL READING
- American College of Obstetricians and Gynecologists. Critical care in pregnancy. ACOG Practice Bulletin No 100. *Obstet Gynecol*. 2009;113:443–50.

CODES

ICD9
- 647.80 Other specified infectious and parasitic diseases of mother, complicating pregnancy, childbirth, or the puerperium, unspecified as to episode of care
- 647.81 Other specified infectious and parasitic diseases of mother, with delivery
- 647.82 Other specified infectious and parasitic diseases of mother, with delivery, with mention of postpartum complication

CLINICAL PEARLS
- A high index of suspicion for sepsis in pregnant and postpartum patients is required since early identification and treatment improves outcome.
- Maintenance of maternal oxygenation and blood pressure are crucial for fetal benefit.
- Preterm labor and delivery may result from maternal sepsis.

SEROTONIN SYNDROME

Tajender S. Vasu
Paul Marik

 BASICS

DESCRIPTION

- Serotonin syndrome is characterized by a triad of neuromuscular hyperactivity, autonomic hyperactivity, and change in mental status.
- It is not an idiosyncratic drug reaction, but is a predictable response to serotonin excess in the CNS.
- It can occur from an overdose, drug interaction, or adverse drug effect involving serotonergic agents.
- Serotonin toxicity can be:
  - Mild: Serotonergic symptoms that may or may not concern the patient
  - Moderate: Toxicity causing significant distress but not life-threatening
  - Severe: Life-threatening toxicity causing severe hyperthermia, muscle rigidity, and multiorgan failure
- Most severe cases result from a drug combination, especially the combination of selective serotonin reuptake inhibitors (SSRI) and monoamine oxidase inhibitors (MAOI).

EPIDEMIOLOGY
Incidence
- The epidemiology is not completely known because >85% of physicians are unaware of this disorder.
- It occurs in ~15% of patients with SSRI overdose.

RISK FACTORS
Exposure to serotonergic drugs or drugs known to cause serotonin syndrome

Genetics
Unknown

GENERAL PREVENTION
Keep a high index of suspicion, and avoid the drugs known to cause serotonin syndrome.

PATHOPHYSIOLOGY
- Serotonin (5-hydroxytryptamine or 5-HT) is produced by decarboxylation and hydroxylation of L-tryptophan.
- Serotonin syndrome results from an excess of serotonin in the central nervous system that may result from:
  - Inhibition of serotonin metabolism (MAOI)
  - Inhibition of serotonin reuptake in nerve terminals (SSRI)
  - Increase in serotonin precursor (tryptophan), or serotonin release (serotonin-releasing agents)
- The excess serotonin in CNS stimulates the serotonin receptors found primarily in midline raphe nuclei, located in the brainstem.
- 7 subtypes of serotonin receptors (5-HT_1 to 5-HT_7), and 5-HT_{2A} receptors are mostly involved in the pathophysiology of serotonin toxicity.

ETIOLOGY
Serotonin syndrome may result from a large number of drugs and drug combinations:

- SSRIs: Fluoxetine, paroxetine, sertraline, citalopram, escitalopram
- Antidepressants: Venlafaxine, trazodone, nefazodone, clomipramine, St. John's wort
- Monoamine oxidase inhibitors: Phenelzine, moclobemide, tranylcypromine, clorgyline, isocarboxazid
- Antibiotics: Linezolid (a monoamine oxidase inhibitors), ritonavir (acts through inhibition of cytochrome P-450 $3A_4$)
- Serotonin-releasing agents: Fenfluramine, methylenedioxymethamphetamine (MDMA or ecstasy), amphetamine
- Other: Lithium, tryptophan, sumatriptan

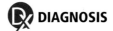 **DIAGNOSIS**

- 2 criteria may help in making the diagnosis of serotonin syndrome
- Sternbach's criteria:
  - Recent addition or increase in a known serotonergic agent
  - Absence of other possible etiologies (infection, substance abuse, or drug withdrawal)
  - No recent addition or increase of a neuroleptic agent
  - At least 3 of the following symptoms:
    ○ Mental status changes (confusion, hypomania)
    ○ Agitation
    ○ Myoclonus
    ○ Hyperreflexia
    ○ Diaphoresis
    ○ Shivering
    ○ Tremor
    ○ Diarrhea
    ○ Incoordination
    ○ Fever
- Hunter serotonin toxicity criteria: A history of exposure to serotonergic agents and the presence of any one of the following is diagnostic of serotonin toxicity:
  - Spontaneous clonus
  - Inducible clonus or ocular clonus with agitation or diaphoresis
  - Tremor and hyperreflexia
  - Hypertonia and hyperthermia (temperature >38°C) with inducible clonus or ocular clonus

HISTORY
- The history of exposure to drugs known to cause serotonin syndrome
- Clinical triad of neuromuscular hyperactivity, autonomic hyperactivity, and change in mental status:
  - Neuromuscular hyperactivity: Shivering, tremor, hypertonia, rigidity
  - Autonomic hyperactivity: Hyperthermia, flushing, diaphoresis, diarrhea
  - Mental status changes: Confusion, anxiety, agitation, hypomania
- Not all of these symptoms are present in every patient.

PHYSICAL EXAM
- Tachycardia, hypertension, mydriasis, hyperactive bowel sounds
- Hyperthermia develops in ~1/2 of cases and results from increased muscle activity due to agitation and tremor.
- Myoclonus, ocular clonus
- Hyperreflexia, clonus, hypertonicity:
  - These findings are greater in lower extremities than in upper extremities.
  - Sustained clonus is usually found at the ankles.

DIAGNOSTIC TESTS & INTERPRETATION
Lab
Most of the laboratory abnormalities are a consequence of poorly treated hyperthermia:
- Elevated serum creatinine and aminotransferase
- Metabolic acidosis
- Elevated serum creatine kinase

Imaging
Radiological studies may help to rule out other conditions.

Diagnostic Procedures/Other
- No laboratory test or procedure is diagnostic of serotonin syndrome.
- Diagnostic procedures like CT head, electroencephalogram, lumbar puncture etc., may help to rule out other disorders.

DIFFERENTIAL DIAGNOSIS
- Malignant hyperthermia
- Neuroleptic malignant syndrome
- Anticholinergic delirium
- Heat stroke
- CNS infection (meningitis/encephalitis)
- Sympathomimetic toxicity
- Acute baclofen withdrawal

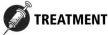 TREATMENT

MEDICATION

First Line
- Most important step is the removal of the offending drug.
- Mild cases (e.g., tremors and hyperreflexia) are managed with supportive care and treatment with benzodiazepines.
- Control of agitation with benzodiazepine is an essential step in the management (C).

Second Line
- 5-HT$_{2A}$ antagonists (cyproheptadine and chlorpromazine) have been used in moderate to severe cases (C).
- No randomized clinical trials demonstrate the effectiveness of 5-HT$_{2A}$ antagonists.
- Cyproheptadine is only available in oral form; the initial dose is 12 mg followed by 2 mg q2h until symptoms improve; patients may require up to 12–32 mg of the drug in a 24-hour period.
- Sublingual olanzapine (an atypical antipsychotic with 5-HT$_{2A}$ antagonist activity) has also been used.
- Chlorpromazine is the only 5-HT$_{2A}$ antagonist available in parenteral form; 50–100 mg of IM chlorpromazine may be administered.

IN-PATIENT CONSIDERATIONS

Initial Stabilization
- Focus on stabilization of ABCs.
- Supportive care including passive and active cooling of the patient, sedation, intubation, and muscle paralysis
- Physical restraints are discouraged because they can increase hyperthermia, rhabdomyolysis, and lactic acidosis [C].

Admission Criteria
- Most patients with mild serotonin toxicity should be observed in the hospital.
- Patients with severe toxicity, including hyperthermia, and rigidity, should be admitted to ICU for further management.

IV Fluids
Aggressive volume resuscitation is required because patients have volume loss due to hyperthermia.

Nursing
- Close monitoring of blood pressure, heart rate, and mental status
- Avoidance of physical restraints
- Frequent repositioning of the patients to prevent decubitus ulcers

Discharge Criteria
- Patients with moderate serotonin toxicity should be observed for 6 hours.
- Observation should be continued for 12 hours if a slow-release formulation such as venlafaxine has been ingested.
- After the control of hyperthermia, stabilization of electrolyte imbalance, and rhabdomyolysis, patients are discharged from ICU.

 ONGOING CARE

FOLLOW-UP RECOMMENDATIONS
Patients should have follow-up with a psychiatrist

PATIENT EDUCATION
Patients should be aware of the possibility of recurrence of the symptoms especially after re-exposure to serotonergic drugs.

PROGNOSIS
- Many mild cases resolve within 24 hours after the discontinuation of the precipitating drug.
- If unrecognized, severe serotonin toxicity is a potentially life-threatening disorder and may result in rhabdomyolysis, renal failure, and death.

COMPLICATIONS
- Rhabdomyolysis
- Renal failure
- Venous thromboembolism
- Decubitus ulcers
- Disseminated intravascular coagulation
- Seizures

ADDITIONAL READING
- Boyer EW, et al. The serotonin syndrome. *N Engl J Med*. 2005; 352:1112–20.
- Isbister GK, et al. Serotonin toxicity: A practical approach to diagnosis and treatment. *MJA*. 2007;187:361–5.
- Sternbach H. The serotonin syndrome. *Am J Psychiatry*. 1991;148:705–13.

 CODES

ICD9
333.99 Other extrapyramidal diseases and abnormal movement disorders

CLINICAL PEARLS
- Serotonin syndrome is characterized by a triad of neuromuscular hyperactivity, autonomic hyperactivity, and change in mental status.
- Early recognition is important because mild cases resolve after stopping the precipitating drug.
- Supportive care, including sedation, intubation, and muscle paralysis, is very important in the management of severe cases.
- If unrecognized, severe cases may progress to multiorgan failure and death.

S

SHOCK, ANAPHYLACTIC

Hiren Shingala

BASICS

DESCRIPTION
- Anaphylactic reaction: Acute, systemic type I allergic reaction with IgE-mediated basophil and mast cell degranulation
- Anaphylactoid reaction: Non-IgE mediated activation and degranulation of basophil and mast cells
- Both these reactions can result in shock: Cardiovascular collapse associated with respiratory and mucocutaneous manifestations

EPIDEMIOLOGY
Incidence
- Affects all ages
- Male = Female
- 21 cases per 100,000 person-years (1)
- Mortality: 0.65–2%

Prevalence
Lifetime prevalence: 1–2% of the population as a whole for anaphylaxis

RISK FACTORS
- Asthma
- Atopic allergies

PATHOPHYSIOLOGY
- Anaphylactic reaction:
  - Requires prior sensitization
  - Antigen binds to antigen-specific IgE attached to previously sensitized basophils and mast cells, resulting in release of mediators.
- Anaphylactoid reaction:
  - Does not require prior sensitization
  - Antigen directly releases mediators from basophils and mast cells.
- Common mediators: Histamine, leukotrienes, and prostaglandins
- Less common mediators: Neutral proteases, tryptase, chymase, cytokines, proteoglycans
- Physiologic effects of mediators:
  - Decreased vascular tone
  - Increased vascular permeability
  - Smooth muscle spasm in respiratory and GI tract
  - Increased mucus secretions
  - Stimulation of sensory nerve endings

ETIOLOGY
- IgE-mediated anaphylaxis:
  - Drugs: Penicillin, β-lactam antibiotics, sulfonamides, opioids, colloids, hypnotics, NSAIDs, aspirin, streptokinase, insulin
  - Food: Peanut (62% of anaphylaxis related to food), shellfish, tree nut, fish, egg, soy, milk
  - Insect stings (*Hymenoptera*)
  - Latex
- Anaphylactoid reactions:
  - Radiocontrast media (RCM)
  - Drugs: NSAIDs, aspirin, opioids, dextran, immunoglobulins, protamine, vancomycin, blood products

- Idiopathic: No etiology found despite meticulous efforts to search for it
- Special considerations:
  - Based on skin test, about 10% of patients allergic to a penicillin antibiotic are allergic to cephalosporins; but actual number might be lower (2).
  - Iodine is never a cause of anaphylaxis. It is an essential trace element found in human body. Patients who say they are "allergic" to Iodine typically have had reaction to RCM, shellfish, or contact reaction to povidone-iodine.
  - Shellfish or "iodine allergy" is not a contraindication to use of IV contrast and does not mandate a pretreatment regimen.
  - Use of low-instead of high-osmolarity contrast decreases incidence of reactions to ~0.5% from 1–3%.

DIAGNOSIS

HISTORY
- Symptoms typically occur within minutes of exposure, but can be delayed up to few hours, especially if allergen is ingested.
- Trigger is identified in majority of cases.
- Cardiovascular: Sense of impending doom, dizziness, syncope, chest pain, palpitation
- Respiratory: Throat tightness, shortness of breath, wheezing, hoarseness, sneezing, nasal congestion
- Mucocutaneous: Itching, flushing, urticaria
- GI: Nausea, vomiting, diarrhea, cramps
- Death can occur in less than 30 minutes.

PHYSICAL EXAM
- Patients are usually anxious unless in severe shock with obtundation.
- HEENT:
  - Nasal congestion, conjunctival injection
  - Angioedema
- Respiratory:
  - Wheezing (due to bronchospasm and airway edema)
  - Stridor (due to angioedema)
- Cardiovascular:
  - Hypotension (due to vasodilatation leading to capillary leak and fluid shifts to extravascular spaces)
  - Tachycardia (secondary to intravascular volume loss)
  - Shock can occur without any other manifestations.
- Skin:
  - Flushing
  - Urticaria: Anywhere in body, but commonly in palms, soles, and inner thighs

DIAGNOSTIC TESTS & INTERPRETATION
- Rapidly progressive and fatal; requires immediate treatment before any diagnostic studies are done
- Mainly clinical diagnosis: Allergen exposure, history, and physical exam
- Diagnostic tests may be beneficial in ruling out other diagnoses and if patient presents with typical anaphylaxis without any history of exposure to allergen.

Lab
Initial lab tests
- CBC: Nonspecific.
- Basic metabolic panel
- ECG and cardiac enzymes:
  - Useful in patients presenting with chest pain, shortness of breath, loss of consciousness, or in elderly patients with coexisting CHF or CAD.
- Serum and urine histamine levels:
  - Elevated in patients with anaphylactic shock, but are not readily available.
- Serum mast cell tryptase:
  - Levels are elevated transiently during reaction.
  - Might be helpful in diagnosis if it is uncertain.

Follow-Up & Special Considerations
Allergy panel testing/skin testing:
- Helps to identify particular allergen
- Generally reserved for outpatient subspecialist follow-up

Imaging
- Not required for diagnosis
- Chest x-ray:
  - Mainly to differentiate anaphylaxis from other respiratory causes

Diagnostic Procedures/Other
Pulmonary arterial catheterization:
- Not required for diagnosis
- Hemodynamic profile looks like distributive shock: Low blood pressure, low SVR, high cardiac output, low PAOP, low PASP and PADP

DIFFERENTIAL DIAGNOSIS
- Other types of shock: Hypovolemic, cardiogenic, obstructive, septic shock
- Status asthmaticus
- Epiglottitis
- Angioedema including hereditary angioedema
- Myocardial infarction
- Carcinoid syndrome
- Scombroid reaction

TREATMENT

MEDICATION
- Epinephrine:
  - Drug of choice for anaphylactic shock (3)[A], all other medications are adjunctive
  - Antagonizes most of the hemodynamic abnormalities in anaphylactic shock and causes bronchodilatation.
  - Dose:
    - 0.3–0.5 mL 1:1000 soln SC or IM q15min
    - 0.5–1 mL 1:10,000 soln IV; slow administration; repeat if needed
    - 0.3–0.5 mL 1:1000 soln SL q15min
  - Caution with IV injection: Extravasation can cause acute limb ischemia.
  - Commercial preparations are available that can be self-administered by patients upon onset of symptoms.
- H1 receptor blocker:
  - Mainly effective against cutaneous manifestations
  - Diphenhydramine is prototype
  - Dose (Diphenhydramine):
    - 25–50 mg q4–6h IV or PO as needed
    - Max 400 mg/d
  - Should be continued for 2–3 days
- H2 receptor blocker:
  - Additive effects with H1 receptor blockers
  - Ranitidine is prototype
  - Dose (Ranitidine):
    - 50 mg q4–6h IV/IM
    - 150 mg PO b.i.d.
    - Max 600 mg/d
- Corticosteroids:
  - Help in treating respiratory and cutaneous manifestations of anaphylaxis
  - Also helps to decrease incidence and severity of late phase reaction
  - Do not counteract cardiovascular effects acutely
  - Typical regimen is methylprednisolone 40–250 mg IV/IM q6h
  - Should be continued up to 4–5 days
- Bronchodilators:
  - To reverse bronchospasm
  - Dose is similar to those used to treat asthma
- Glucagon:
  - Used as an adjunct to epinephrine in patients with anaphylaxis who are taking β blockers
  - Dose: 1–5 mg initially; followed by infusion of 5–15 mcg/min until effect is achieved

ADDITIONAL TREATMENT
General Measures
- Avoidance of exposure to allergen
- Prehospital care:
  - Self-administration of epinephrine and diphenhydramine intramuscularly upon identification of first signs of anaphylaxis in a patient with known predisposition for anaphylaxis
  - Local treatment for insect stings
  - Basic life support

Issues for Referral
- All patients with anaphylactic shock should be referred to an intensivist.
- All patients with anaphylactic shock should be referred to allergist-immunologist.

SURGERY/OTHER PROCEDURES
Not required except to establish airway if endotracheal intubation fails

IN-PATIENT CONSIDERATIONS
Initial Stabilization
- On arrival to ED, assess ABCs.
- Assess airway patency; intubation or surgical airway might be necessary.
- Supplemental oxygen, supine or Trendelenburg position
- Large-bore IV lines with IV fluids
- Remove antigen source if possible (e.g., insect)
- Upon clinical diagnosis of anaphylactic shock, administer epinephrine, diphenhydramine, H2 antagonists, and IV steroids.

Admission Criteria
- All patients with anaphylactic shock need to be observed in hospital even if the episode resolves quickly with treatment.
- Patients with persistent hypotension will require admission to ICU.

special-considerations
- Increased severity with:
  - Congestive heart failure
  - Ischemic heart disease
  - β Blockers may limit the effectiveness of treatment with epinephrine, thus causing prolonged and severe hypotension.
  - Asthma
- Refractory hypotension will require large volume crystalloid resuscitation, multiple epinephrine injections, and continuous epinephrine infusion.
- If hypotension is refractory to above measures, consider starting continuous infusion of other vasopressors (e.g., dopamine, norepinephrine)
- Watch for cardiac arrhythmias with epinephrine in elderly patients and in patients with cardiac history. Use lowest possible dose.

IV Fluids
- Establish large-bore IV lines.
- Start crystalloids for hypotension.
- Individual fluid requirement varies by patient.
- Watch for signs of volume overload in patients with history of CHF.

 ## ONGOING CARE

FOLLOW-UP RECOMMENDATIONS
- Oral corticosteroids and oral antihistaminics should be continued for 3–5 days after discharge.
- Patient must be educated about signs and symptoms of anaphylaxis, given an epinephrine autoinjector, and instructed how to use it.
- Will need skin testing and/or IgE testing as outpatient with allergist/immunologist based on history.

DIET
If known, avoid food that patient is allergic to.

PROGNOSIS
- Excellent if patient receives immediate medical treatment
- Can reoccur on reexposure to inciting antigen

COMPLICATIONS
- Rare
- Respiratory failure from bronchospasm
- Cardiac arrhythmias

ADDITIONAL READING

- Anne S, et al. Risk of administering cephalosporin antibiotics to patients with histories of penicillin allergy. *Ann Allergy Asthma Immunol*. 1995;74(2): 167–70.
- Lieberman P, et al. The diagnosis and management of anaphylaxis. *J Allergy Clin Immunol*. 2005;115: S483–523.
- Yocum MW, et al. Epidemiology of anaphylaxis in Olmsted County: A population-based study. *J Allergy Clin Immunol*. 1999;104(2 Pt 1):452–6.

CODES

ICD9
- 995.0 Other anaphylactic shock, not elsewhere classified
- 995.60 Anaphylactic shock due to unspecified food

CLINICAL PEARLS
- Administer epinephrine and diphenhydramine immediately upon clinical suspicion of anaphylactic shock.
- Use glucagon as adjunct to epinephrine in patients with anaphylaxis who are taking β blockers.
- Observe patients in hospital even if anaphylactic shock reverses immediately with treatment.
- All patients with anaphylactic shock should be discharged with prescription of epinephrine autoinjector and proper education.

S

SHOCK, CARDIOGENIC

Themistoklis Nissirios

 BASICS

DESCRIPTION
Persistent hypotension and tissue hypoperfusion due to cardiac dysfunction in the presence of adequate intravascular volume and left ventricular (LV) filling pressure

EPIDEMIOLOGY
Incidence
7–8% of patients with acute myocardial infarction (MI)

RISK FACTORS
- Patients >75
- Hypertension
- Diabetes mellitus
- Dyslipidemia
- History of prior MI
- Prior coronary angioplasty
- History of congestive heart failure
- Anterior infarction
- Low ejection fraction
- High-grade coronary artery stenosis

GENERAL PREVENTION
- Education of the public, for early recognition of MI
- Hospital transport systems need to be developed to allow patients with STEMI to be transported directly to hospitals with PCI and coronary surgery capabilities.
- Recognition of failed thrombolysis for early transfer to tertiary centers with revascularization capabilities

PATHOPHYSIOLOGY
- Myocardial pathology:
  - MI or severe myocardial ischemia leading to impaired LV function, reduced systolic contractility, decreased cardiac output and arterial blood pressure
  - Coronary perfusion will decrease and further compromise coronary reserve.
  - Compensatory neurohormonal response with activation of the sympathetic and renin angiotensin systems, leading to systemic vasoconstriction, tachycardia, and fluid retention
- Cellular pathology:
  - Inadequate oxygen delivery to myocytes affects cellular ATP production.
  - Energy metabolism shifts from aerobic to anaerobic glycolysis, with resultant lactic acid production.
  - If hypoperfusion and ischemia are severe, myonecrosis ensues with mitochondrial swelling and subsequent plasma membrane disruption.

ETIOLOGY
- Acute MI:
  - Pump failure:
    ○ Large infarction
    ○ Smaller infarction with preexisting LV dysfunction
    ○ Infarction extension and expansion
    ○ Severe recurrent ischemia
  - Mechanical complications:
    ○ Acute mitral regurgitation caused by papillary muscle rupture
    ○ Ventricular septal defect
    ○ Free-wall rupture
    ○ Pericardial tamponade
  - Right ventricular infarction
- Other conditions:
  - End-stage cardiomyopathy
  - Myocarditis
  - Myocardial contusion
  - Prolonged cardiopulmonary bypass
  - Septic shock with severe myocardial depression
  - LV outflow tract obstruction
  - Aortic stenosis
  - Hypertrophic obstructive cardiomyopathy
  - Obstruction to LV filling
  - Mitral stenosis
  - Left atrial myxoma
  - Acute mitral regurgitation
  - Acute aortic insufficiency
  - Acute massive pulmonary embolism
  - Acute stress cardiomyopathy
  - Pheochromocytoma

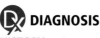 **DIAGNOSIS**

HISTORY
Focused history to exclude contributors for shock such as hypovolemia, hypoxia, sepsis, acidosis, pulmonary embolism, aortic dissection, abdominal aortic aneurysm rupture, and cardiac tamponade

PHYSICAL EXAM
- Ashen or cyanotic with cool skin and mottled extremities
- Rapid and faint peripheral pulses
- Jugular venous distention
- Rales
- Peripheral edema
- Tachycardia with narrow pulse pressure.
- Distant heart sounds, S3 and S4 present
- A systolic murmur is generally heard in patients with acute mitral regurgitation or ventricular septal rupture.

- Parasternal thrill indicates the presence of a ventricular septal defect, whereas the murmur of mitral regurgitation may be limited to early systole.
- A systolic murmur that becomes louder upon Valsalva and prompt standing, suggests hypertrophic obstructive cardiomyopathy (idiopathic hypertrophic subaortic stenosis).
- Altered mental status

DIAGNOSTIC TESTS & INTERPRETATION
Lab
- Biochemical profile: Electrolytes, renal function, and liver function tests
- CBC: Exclude anemia; high WBC may indicate an underlying infection; platelet count may be low because of coagulopathy related to sepsis.
- Cardiac enzymes
- ABGs
- Serum lactate level: Marker of hypoperfusion and indicator of prognosis

Imaging

- Rapid echocardiographic assessment is important (1)[B]:

  - Assessment of regional and global LV function, right ventricular size and function, the presence of mitral regurgitation and other valve abnormalities, pericardial effusion, and possible septal rupture
- A CXR can provide clues about the presence of LV failure (pulmonary vascular redistribution, interstitial pulmonary edema, Kerley B lines, cardiomegaly, bilateral pleural effusions), infection (pulmonary infiltrates), or aortic dissection (widened mediastinum).

Diagnostic Procedures/Other
- ECG may show ST-segment elevation, ST-segment depression, Q waves, or a new LBBB consistent with acute MI; T-wave inversion may also be seen in persons with myocardial ischemia.

- Invasive hemodynamic monitoring (2)[B]:

  - Assists in the precise measurement of volume status, left and right ventricular filling pressures, and cardiac output.
  - Sustained hypotension (SBP <90 mm Hg or a drop in mean blood pressure >30 mm Hg, both with a heart rate >60 bpm)
  - Decreased urine output (<0.5 mL/kg/h)
  - Increased PCWP (>15 mm Hg)
  - Increased right atrial pressure (>20 mm Hg)
  - Decreased cardiac output (cardiac index <2.1 L/min/m^2)
  - Increased systemic vascular resistance (>2100 dynes cm^2)

- High right-sided filling pressures in the absence of an elevated PCWP, when accompanied by electrocardiographic criteria, indicate RV infarction.
- Large V waves on the PCWP tracing suggest severe mitral regurgitation.
- A step-up in oxygen saturation between the right atrium and the right ventricle is diagnostic of ventricular septal rupture.
- Coronary artery angiography:
  - Assesses the anatomy of the coronary arteries and the need for urgent revascularization

Pathological Findings
Most pathological specimens are results of mechanical complications of STEMI, such as ventricular septal rupture, free wall rupture, and papillary muscle rupture.

DIFFERENTIAL DIAGNOSIS
- Myocardial infarction
- Myocardial ischemia
- Myocardial rupture
- Myocarditis
- Cardiogenic pulmonary edema
- Pulmonary embolism
- Septic shock
- Distributive shock
- Hemorrhagic shock
- Systemic inflammatory response syndrome

TREATMENT
MEDICATION
First Line
- Medication in acute coronary syndrome:
  - Aspirin
  - Heparin
  - Glycoproteins IIb/IIIa in non-STEMI
  - β-Blockers and nitrates should be avoided in the acute phase.
  - Patients who are unsuitable for invasive therapy should be treated with a thrombolytic agent in the absence of contraindications (Class I recommendation by ACC/AHA guidelines).
- Hemodynamic support:
  - Dopamine is the drug of choice:
    - Initiated at a rate of 5–10 mcg/kg/min IV
  - IV norepinephrine:
    - Initiated at a rate of 0.5 mcg/kg/min
    - Adjust dose to MAP of 60 mm Hg
  - Dobutamine:
    - Initiated at a rate of 0.5 mcg/kg/min, titrated to a maximum of 40 mcg/kg/min
  - Phosphodiesterase inhibitors:
    - Amrinone and milrinone

Second Line
- IV diuretics in patients with pulmonary edema and elevated PCWP
- IV amiodarone in patients with severe arrhythmias

ADDITIONAL TREATMENT
Additional Therapies
- Intra-aortic balloon counterpulsation (2)[B]:
  - Reduces systolic LV afterload and augments diastolic coronary perfusion pressure, increasing cardiac output and improving coronary artery blood flow; effective for the initial stabilization of patients with cardiogenic shock.
  - Complications:
    ○ Bleeding
    ○ Thrombocytopenia
    ○ Hemolysis
    ○ Leg ischemia
    ○ Aortic dissection
    ○ Femoral artery injury
    ○ Thromboembolism
    ○ Sepsis
  - Contraindications:
    ○ Severe aortic insufficiency
    ○ Severe peripheral vascular disease
    ○ Aortic aneurysm
- Ventricular assist devices (VADs) (3)[C]:
  - The use of VADs should be considered in patients with very low cardiac output (<1.2 L/min/m^2)
  - Effective as a bridge to cardiac transplant therapy

SURGERY/OTHER PROCEDURES
- Percutaneous coronary intervention has been shown to be safe and effective in treatment of acute MI complicated with cardiogenic shock, allowing for immediate definitive treatment (4)[A].
- Early surgical revascularization improves survival in patients with cardiogenic shock and failed angioplasty.

IN-PATIENT CONSIDERATIONS
Initial Stabilization
- Initial management with fluid resuscitation and supplemental oxygen; preload-reducing agents and diuretics must be avoided.
- Systolic blood pressure should be raised >90 mm Hg with vasopressors and/or inotropic drugs.

IV Fluids
Aggressive initial fluid resuscitation with normal saline unless frank pulmonary edema is present

Nursing
Experience with invasive hemodynamic monitoring

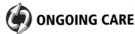

ONGOING CARE
FOLLOW-UP RECOMMENDATIONS
Patient Monitoring
ICU/CCU monitoring required

DIET
NPO until hemodynamic and neurologic stability

PROGNOSIS
Poor prognosis with 50–60% short-term mortality

COMPLICATIONS
- Right ventricular infarction
- Acute severe mitral regurgitation
- Postinfarction ventricular septal rupture
- LV free wall rupture
- Cardiac tamponade

REFERENCES
1. Berkowitz MJ, et al. Echocardiographic and angiographic correlations in patients with cardiogenic shock secondary to acute myocardial infarction. *Am J Cardiol*. 2006;98:1004–8.
2. Antman EM, et al. ACC/AHA guidelines for the management of patients with ST-elevation myocardial infarction: a report of the American College of Cardiology/American Heart Association Task Force on Practice Guidelines (Committee to Revise the 1999 Guidelines for the Management of patients with acute myocardial infarction). *J Am Coll Cardiol*. 2004;44:e1–211.
3. Duvernoy CS, et al. Management of cardiogenic shock attributable to acute myocardial infarction in the reperfusion era. *J Intens Care Med*. 2005; 4:188–98.
4. Hochman JS, et al., for the Should We Emergently Revascularize Occluded Coronaries for Cardiogenic Shock (SHOCK) Investigators. Early revascularization in acute myocardial infarction complicated by cardiogenic shock. *N Engl J Med*. 1999;341: 625–34.

 CODES

ICD9
785.51 Cardiogenic shock

CLINICAL PEARLS
- Early recognition and hemodynamic support is essential.
- Cardiogenic shock is the most common cause of death in patients with acute MI.
- Mortality is high, but IABP and early coronary interventions have improved the outcome.

S

SHOCK LIVER

Stephanie Whitener

 BASICS

DESCRIPTION
Shock liver, also called ischemic hepatitis, refers to diffuse hepatocyte injury leading to profound elevation of serum aminotransferases secondary to hypoperfusion.

EPIDEMIOLOGY
Incidence
- 26% in patients diagnosed with significant hypoperfusion
- 24% in patients not having shock but diagnosed with very low-flow states

Prevalence
0.6–1.5% in ICU setting

RISK FACTORS
- Patients who have preexisting liver disease and portal hypertension
- Patients who have preexisting congestion of the liver
- CHF resulting in either hypoperfusion or passive congestion of the liver
- Acute shock or episode of severe hypotension
- Resuscitation after cardiopulmonary arrest

GENERAL PREVENTION
Maintaining hemodynamic stability with adequate organ perfusion and cardiac output during acute episodes of shock

PATHOPHYSIOLOGY
- Hepatocytes are particularly vulnerable to hypoxemia from hypoperfusion because of the complex vascular system and high metabolic activity of the liver.
- Reperfusion injury also contributes to the pathology of shock liver and is mediated by the generation of reactive oxygen species that destroy the hepatocyte mitochondria and endoplasmic reticulum.

ETIOLOGY
- Acute shock and severe hypotension
- Venous congestion secondary to passive congestion due to CHF or sinusoidal obstruction syndrome
- Interruption of blood flow secondary to sickle cell crisis or hepatic artery thrombosis in patients after liver transplantation or portal vein thrombosis and rarely as part of generalized thrombosis secondary to heparin-induced thrombocytopenia

COMMONLY ASSOCIATED CONDITIONS
- All shock conditions
- Hypoperfusion states such as CHF, right heart failure with hepatic congestion
- Hepatic artery thrombosis

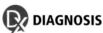 **DIAGNOSIS**

HISTORY
- Shock liver or ischemic hepatitis is seen after any cause of shock or hemodynamic instability:
  – However, some studies have shown that only 51% of cases of shock liver were preceded by severe hypotension or shock.

PHYSICAL EXAM
Usually not helpful; patients may demonstrate some right upper quadrant tenderness.

DIAGNOSTIC TESTS & INTERPRETATION
Lab
Initial lab tests
Liver function tests:
- Rapid rise in serum aminotransferase levels; peak levels are 25–250 times the upper limit of normal
- Early rise in lactate dehydrogenase levels

Follow-Up & Special Considerations
Shock liver can lead to liver failure or result in complete resolution of liver injury; liver function tests need to be followed.

Diagnostic Procedures/Other
- RUQ US with Doppler studies to evaluate the portal and hepatic veins as well as hepatic artery
- Echo to evaluate for suspected cardiac cause of hypoperfusion or shock state

Pathological Findings
The histologic finding in ischemic hepatitis/shock liver is necrosis of hepatocytes in zone 3 of the hepatic acinus.

DIFFERENTIAL DIAGNOSIS
- Acute viral hepatitis
- Acute drug or toxin-induced hepatic injury
- Acute exacerbation of autoimmune hepatitis
- Spontaneous reactivation of hepatitis B
- Budd-Chiari syndrome
- Hepatic sinusoidal obstruction syndrome
- Congestive hepatopathy

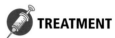 **TREATMENT**

MEDICATION
First Line
Supportive measures to restore adequate perfusion and cardiac output

Second Line
Treat underlying low-flow states such as CHF or hepatic artery thrombosis (1)[C].

ADDITIONAL TREATMENT
General Measures
Restore cardiac output and increase hepatic perfusion.

IN-PATIENT CONSIDERATIONS
Initial Stabilization
Restore cardiac output and organ perfusion.

Admission Criteria
Patients with shock liver most often require ICU level care due to underlying cause.

IV Fluids
Crystalloid or colloid infusions to restore cardiac output and organ perfusion

Discharge Criteria
Serum aminotransferase levels should normalize within 7–10 days once hemodynamic stability has been restored.

ONGOING CARE
FOLLOW-UP RECOMMENDATIONS
Patient Monitoring
- Follow liver function tests to establish a trend and monitor improvement.
- ICU-level hemodynamic monitoring is needed because of the shock state leading to shock liver and to assure its full resolution.

DIET
Patients are intolerant to enteric feeding due to their shock and severely impaired liver function.

PROGNOSIS
- The severity of the liver injury is associated with the duration of hypoperfusion or shock. The prognosis therefore is related to the overall prognosis of the patient's underlying condition.
- Most cases of ischemic hepatitis/shock liver are benign and self-limited. Aminotransferase elevations generally resolve within 7–10 days once hemodynamic stability has been restored.
- Severe cases can result in liver failure and death.

COMPLICATIONS
Patients with ischemic hepatitis superimposed on chronic CHF or with preexisting cirrhosis can develop fulminant hepatic failure:
- Mortality rates of 60–100% have been seen in patients with ischemic hepatitis complicating cirrhosis.

REFERENCES
1. Seeto RK, et al. Ischemic Hepatitis: Clinical presentation and pathogenesis. *AJM*. 2000;109: 109–13.
2. Henrion J, et al. Hypoxic hepatitis. Clinical and hemodynamic study in 142 consecutive cases. *Medicine*. 2003;82:392–406.
3. Birrer R, et al. Hypoxic hepatopathy: Pathophysiology and prognosis. *Intern Med*. 2007;1063–70.

CODES

ICD9
- 444.89 Embolism and thrombosis of other artery
- 573.3 Hepatitis, unspecified
- 785.50 Shock, unspecified

CLINICAL PEARLS
- Hypoperfusion to the liver leads to destruction of hepatocytes and profound elevations of aminotransferases.
- Severe hypotension/shock, as well as chronic hypoperfusion states such as CHF with hepatic congestion or right heart failure, can lead to the development of ischemic hepatitis.
- Hepatocytes are particularly vulnerable to damage secondary to hypoperfusion because of their complex vascular supply and high metabolic activity.
- Serum aminotransferase levels may peak at 25–250 times normal values but should normalize 7–10 days after reperfusion is established.
- Prevention and treatment are accomplished by supporting hemodynamics to restore perfusion to the liver.

S

SHOCK, SEPTIC
David J. Lundy

 BASICS

DESCRIPTION
- Septic shock is a complex disease in a spectrum ranging from the systemic inflammatory response syndrome to multiorgan failure and death.
- Septic shock is severe sepsis (infection with severe organ dysfunction) plus refractory hypotension.
- Circulatory derangements and increased metabolic demand cause an imbalance in oxygen demand/delivery leading to tissue hypoxia and organ dysfunction.

EPIDEMIOLOGY
Incidence
- ~ 751,000 cases of sepsis in the U.S. per year
- ~215,000 deaths per year (leading cause of death in the critically ill in the U.S.) (1)

RISK FACTORS
Risk factors for septic shock include preexisting comorbidities (diabetes, malignancy, etc.), extremes of age, and immune compromise

Genetics
Several genetic polymorphisms in cytokine and other receptors have been identified that modulate host response to infection. These may influence patient risk levels (2).

GENERAL PREVENTION
- Immunizations may help prevent infection in some patients, especially those immunocompromised or postsplenectomy.
- Early diagnosis and treatment of infections may prevent progression to septic shock.

PATHOPHYSIOLOGY
- Infection with any of a number of organisms (gram-negative, gram-positive, fungal) can lead to systemic infection:
  - Manifestations of septic shock are similar with different types of infecting organisms.
- Inflammation: Levels of many cytokines, including TNF-α IL-1, and IL-6 have been found to be elevated in patients with sepsis. However, inflammatory modulators are heterogeneously expressed (2).
- Immune function: As sepsis evolves, patients may shift from a proinflammatory to an antiinflammatory state, with a suppression of the immune system. Apoptosis of immune cells has been implicated in this process (2).
- Circulatory derangements:
  - Macrocirculation: Large vessels dilate, causing arterial hypotension
  - Microcirculation: Microvascular ($<100\ \mu$m) flow is heterogeneous, potentially leading to poor perfusion of capillary tissue beds and cellular hypoxia (3).

ETIOLOGY
Infection, coupled with an exaggerated host inflammatory response, leads to systemic hemodynamic derangements and cellular hypoxia:
- Common infection sites leading to septic shock (1):
  - Respiratory
  - Genitourinary
  - Intra-abdominal
  - Indwelling medical device
  - Wound/soft tissue
  - CNS
  - Endocarditis
- Common pathogens include gram-negative and gram-positive bacteria and fungi.

COMMONLY ASSOCIATED CONDITIONS
- Infection
- Systemic inflammatory response syndrome
- Severe sepsis
- Multiorgan failure

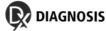 DIAGNOSIS

HISTORY
A history of symptoms of infection, fever, shortness of breath, indwelling medical devices, immune compromise, decreased mental status, decreased urine output are common in patients with septic shock.

PHYSICAL EXAM
- Signs of infection:
  - General: Fever, tachycardia
  - Site-specific: Rash, cellulitis, crackles suggestive of pneumonia, abdominal tenderness, CVA tenderness, meningeal signs
- Signs of hypoperfusion/shock:
  - Low urine output, change in mental status, cool/pale extremities, hypotension, tachycardia, hypoxia

DIAGNOSTIC TESTS & INTERPRETATION
Lab
Initial lab tests
- Obtain appropriate cultures prior to antibiotic administration:

  - $\geq$2 blood cultures (1 should be percutaneous and 1 from each vascular device in place) (4)[B].

  - Other cultures as clinically relevant (urine, sputum, wound, cerebrospinal fluid, etc.)
- CBC and differential suggesting infection.
- A metabolic panel and liver function tests may demonstrate organ dysfunction.
- ABG may demonstrate hypoxemia and acidosis.
- Urinalysis

- Serum lactate level (>4) (4)[B]

Follow-Up & Special Considerations
Follow culture results and sensitivities to tailor antibiotic regimen.

Imaging
Imaging studies should focus on identifying sources of infection (4)[B]:
- Chest radiography, bone scan, abdominal US, CT scan, MRI

Diagnostic Procedures/Other
- Lumbar puncture for suspected CNS infections
- Echocardiography for suspected endocarditis

DIFFERENTIAL DIAGNOSIS
Other shock etiologies such as cardiogenic, hypovolemic, obstructive, neurogenic, or other forms of distributive shock such as anaphylaxis

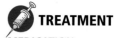 TREATMENT

MEDICATION
First Line
- Crystalloid or colloid IV fluids (4)[B]
- Antibiotic therapy: Begin IV broad-spectrum antibiotics within 1 hour of recognizing septic shock and deescalate based on culture and sensitivity results (4)[B].
- Vasopressors: Norepinephrine or dopamine to maintain mean arterial pressure >65 mm Hg if fluid resuscitation alone is inadequate (4)[B].
- Inotropes: Dobutamine for patients with myocardial dysfunction (high filling pressures and low cardiac output) (4)[B].
- Recombinant human activated protein C: Consider for patients with a high risk of death (APACHE II >25 or multiorgan failure) and no contraindications (4)[B].

Second Line
- Vasopressors: Epinephrine if pressure is not responsive to norepinephrine or dopamine (4)[B]:
  - Vasopressin (0.03 U/min) may be added to norepinephrine for refractory hypotension
- Steroids: Consider for patients with hypotension that responds poorly to fluid resuscitation and vasopressors (4)[B].

ADDITIONAL TREATMENT

General Measures

- Current recommendations focus on a protocol-driven resuscitation strategy focused on early targeting of specific parameters. During the 1st 6 hours of resuscitation, goals are:
  - central venous pressure: 8–12 mm Hg (4)[B].
  - Mean arterial pressure: ≥65 mm Hg (4)[B].
  - Urine output: ≥0.5 mL/kg/hr (4)[B].
  - Central venous oxygen saturation: ≥70% or mixed venous saturation ≥65% (4)[B]
- Identify and control source of infection as early as possible (4)[B].
- Remove any potentially infected intravascular devices (4)[B].

Issues for Referral

- Early critical care consultation
- Surgical consultation for source control when needed
- Nephrology consultation for renal failure and potential dialysis as warranted

Additional Therapies

- Supplemental oxygen
- Blood product transfusion for Hgb <7 or higher in select patients (4)[B]
- Mechanical ventilation if ARDS develops (4)[B]
- Glycemic control (4)[B]
- Hemodialysis or CVVH (4)[B]
- Deep vein thrombosis prophylaxis (4)[A]
- Stress ulcer prophylaxis (4)[A]

COMPLEMENTARY & ALTERNATIVE THERAPIES

The primary team should discuss individual prognosis of patients with septic shock with patients, family members, and caregivers to establish an appropriate level of care.

SURGERY/OTHER PROCEDURES

Surgery should be performed as early as possible for source control; based on source these may include:

- Wound debridement/abscess drainage
- Cholecystectomy/cholecystostomy for biliary sepsis
- Colectomy for toxic colitis
- Empyema drainage
- Pericardiocentesis
- Catheter or other device removal

IN-PATIENT CONSIDERATIONS

Initial Stabilization

Initial stabilization should include attention to ABCs:

- Advanced airway for severe respiratory compromise or decreased mental status
- Supplemental oxygen or mechanical ventilation as necessary
- Early IV access and circulatory support with fluid resuscitation and vasopressor/inotropic support if indicated

Admission Criteria

Any patient with suspected severe sepsis or shock should be admitted with a critical care consultation.

IV Fluids

IV fluids are given as boluses and continuous infusions to achieve/maintain central venous pressure and mean arterial pressure goals.

Nursing

Peripheral IV access, drawing labs (blood, urine etc.), administering fluids/medications, monitoring vital signs, monitoring intake and output, general nursing care

Discharge Criteria

Prior to discharge from an ICU, patients with septic shock should be hemodynamically stable without vasopressor support and on appropriate antibiotic therapy.

 ONGOING CARE

FOLLOW-UP RECOMMENDATIONS

Patients who have had septic shock may be at risk for additional episodes. Early signs of infection should be identified and aggressively treated. Appropriate immunizations and health maintenance should be followed

Patient Monitoring

Follow patients for evidence of clearance of infection.

DIET

Patients should be given a glucose source and IV insulin for control as necessary. Blood glucose levels should be checked q1–2h if needed to assure adequate control (4)[B].

PATIENT EDUCATION

Patients and families should be educated regarding the early recognition of the signs and symptoms of sepsis and septic shock. Furthermore, patients may take steps to prevent infection through appropriate immunizations, diligent wound care, and vigilant care of indwelling catheters/devices.

PROGNOSIS

- One randomized controlled trial demonstrated mortality rates improved from 46.5% to 30% with the application of an early endpoint-based resuscitation strategy.
- The prognosis may depend on the level of organ failure, the site of primary infection, comorbidities, success in source control, and speed of care (5).

COMPLICATIONS

Multiorgan failure, ARDS, death

Geriatric Considerations

Elderly patients may be at increased risk for both sepsis and septic shock. Due to diminished physiologic reserve, geriatric patients may have a more severe and sudden progression of disease than younger patients. Maintaining a high clinical index of suspicion is important in the elderly.

Pediatric Considerations

Despite being a major cause of mortality in children, overall mortality is lower than in adults. Diagnostic criteria require sepsis plus cardiovascular dysfunction or ARDS or dysfunction of 2 other organ systems (4).

REFERENCES

1. Angus DC, et al. Epidemiology of severe sepsis in the U.S.: Analysis of incidence, outcome, and associated costs of care. *Crit Care Med*. 2001; 29(7):1303–10.
2. Hotchkiss RS, et al. The pathophysiology and treatment of sepsis. *N Engl J Med*. 2003; 348(2):138–50.
3. Trzeciak S, et al. Early microcirculatory perfusion derangements in patients with severe sepsis and septic shock: Relationship to hemodynamics, oxygen transport, and survival. *Ann Emerg Med*. 2007;49(1):88–98, e81–82.
4. Dellinger RP, et al. Surviving Sepsis Campaign: International guidelines for management of severe sepsis and septic shock: 2008. *Crit Care Med*. 2008;36(1):296–327.
5. Rivers E,et al. Early goal-directed therapy in the treatment of severe sepsis and septic shock. *N Engl J Med*. 2001;345(19):1368–77.

 CODES

ICD9

- 038.9 Unspecified septicemia
- 785.52 Septic shock
- 995.90 Systemic inflammatory response syndrome, unspecified

CLINICAL PEARLS

- Septic shock is a common and deadly disease.
- Early, aggressive endpoint-based treatment algorithms targeting optimization of hemodynamic parameters and broad-spectrum antibiotic administration currently offers the best chance for a favorable outcome.

S

SHOCK, VASOACTIVE DRUGS IN CARDIOGENIC

Themiskolis Nissirios

 BASICS

DESCRIPTION
- Hemodynamic management of cardiogenic shock when fluids fail to restore tissue perfusion
- Vasoactive drug therapy in the treatment of cardiogenic shock aims to increase oxygen delivery above a critical threshold and increase mean arterial pressure (MAP) to a level that allows appropriate distribution of cardiac output for adequate organ perfusion.

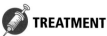 **TREATMENT**

MEDICATION
First Line
- Norepinephrine:
  - A potent α-adrenergic agonist with less marked β1-adrenergic agonistic properties and a short half-life
  - Initiated at 0.02–0.04 μg/kg/min to a dose that maintains adequate systemic blood pressure
  - Dose-related vasoconstriction
  - Used in patients with more severe hypotension
  - May be superior to dopamine in patients with cardiogenic shock (2)
  - Can be used in conjunction with dopamine and dobutamine; however, this may lead to worsening ischemia and serious arrhythmias (2)

- Dopamine:
  - Most commonly used positive inotrope(1)
  - Immediate precursor of both norepinephrine and epinephrine
  - Initiated at a dose of 3 mcg/kg/min while pulmonary capillary wedge and systemic arterial pressures, as well as cardiac output, are monitored.
  - Increase dose stepwise to 20 mcg/kg/min to reduce pulmonary capillary wedge pressure to ~20 mm Hg and elevate cardiac index to exceed 2 L/min/m
  - Low-dose (0.5–2 μg/kg/min):
    ○ Dopaminergic receptors are activated, leading to vasodilation of renal and mesenteric vascular beds
  - Intermediate-dose (5–10 μg/kg/min):
    ○ β-adrenergic receptors are activated, leading to positive inotropic and chronotropic effects on the myocardium
  - High-dose (10–20 μg/kg/min):
    ○ α-Adrenergic receptors are activated leading to systemic vasoconstriction
    ○ Significant risk of precipitating limb and end-organ ischemia and should be used cautiously
  - Gradually wean down to 3–5 μg/kg/min and then discontinue to avoid potential hypotensive effects of low-dose dopamine

- Dobutamine:
  - α- and β-Adrenergic agonistic activities
  - improves cardiac output through direct increases in inotropy and chronotropy and decreases in afterload
  - Initiated at 2 μg/kg/min and titrated upward according to the patient's response, usually to a maximum of 20 μg/kg/min
  - β-Adrenergic receptor stimulation increases myocardial contractility, with minimal peripheral vasodilation.
  - Tachyphylaxis may occur with infusions of >24–48 hours, because of receptor desensitization.

Second Line
- Milrinone:
  - 2nd-generation phosphodiesterase inhibitor
  - Prevents the breakdown of cyclic adenosine monophosphate (cAMP), raising intracellular calcium, thus increasing inotropy
  - Significant vasodilatory effect and relatively long plasma half-life make milrinone difficult to use as monotherapy.
  - Can be used with other inotropic agents to enhance myocardial contractility (2)
  - Loading dose of 0.5 mg/kg/min over 10 minutes, followed by a maintenance infusion of 0.375–0.75 mg/kg/min
  - Multiple side effects, including marked hypotension, atrial and ventricular arrhythmias (3)

- Epinephrine:
  – A potent α- and β-adrenergic agonist; may be used in patients with accompanied bradycardia
  – May cause atrial and ventricular tachyarrhythmias, severe hypertension, lactic acidosis, hypokalemia
  – Used in cases of extreme hemodynamic collapse, unresponsive to traditional agents

COMPLEMENTARY & ALTERNATIVE THERAPIES

- Levosimendan (4):
  – Calcium sensitizing agent, or inodilator
  – Bolus of 12–24 mg/kg over 10 minutes, or a continuous infusion at a rate of 0.05–0.10 mg/kg/min, titrated up to 0.2 mg/kg/min
  – Positive inotropy, by calcium sensitization of cardiac troponin C during systole
  – Also causes vasodilation due to the opening of adenosine triphosphate (ATP)-sensitive potassium channels in vascular smooth muscle and, in higher doses, to the inhibition of phosphodiesterase III
  – This leads to reduction of cardiac preload and afterload, enhancing coronary blood flow and increasing myocardial oxygen supply.
  – Not recommended for the sole treatment of cardiogenic shock because of its vasodilatory properties
  – Combined use of levosimendan with other vasoactive drugs may be considered.

REFERENCES

1. ADHERE Scientific Advisory Committee. Acute Decompensated Heart Failure National Registry (ADHERE(®)) Core Module Q1 2006 Final Cumulative National Benchmark Report: Scios, Inc.; July 2006.
2. De Backer D, et al. Comparison of dopamine and norepinephrine in the treatment of shock. *N Engl J Med* 2010;362:779–89.
3. Cuffe MS, et al. Short-term IV milrinone for acute exacerbation of chronic heart failure: A randomized controlled trial. *JAMA*. 2002;287:1541–7.
4. Moiseyev VS, et al. Safety and efficacy of a novel calcium sensitizer, levosimendan, in patients with left ventricular failure due to an acute myocardial infarction. A randomized, placebo-controlled, double-blind study (RUSSLAN). *Eur Heart J*. 2002;23(18):1422–32.

 CODES

ICD9
785.51 Cardiogenic shock

CLINICAL PEARLS

- Norepinephrine, dopamine and dobutamine are the agents of choice for cardiogenic shock.
- Doses should be adjusted to the lowest levels that improve tissue perfusion.
- Combination regimens can be used for an improved hemodynamic response.

S

SINUSITIS
B. Sharmila Mohanraj

 BASICS

DESCRIPTION
Sinusitis is defined as an inflammation of the paranasal sinuses. Acute viral sinusitis, a common cause of URIs, is complicated by bacterial superinfection in up to 2% of cases (1). This chapter focuses on nonviral causes of acute sinusitis as they pertain to the critically ill patient.

EPIDEMIOLOGY
Prevalence
- In 2009, acute sinusitis was estimated to affect >30 million people, (2) with up to 2% having bacterial involvement.
- In the ICU, up to 32% of intubated patients may develop clinical sinusitis. And as many as 75% may develop radiographic sinusitis (3).

RISK FACTORS
- Nasal intubation and use of nasoenteric tubes are significant risk factors. Also noted in 1 prospective cohort study are nasal colonization with gram-negative bacilli, sedation, or a GCS score ≤7 (3).
- Any other factors that lead to mucosal swelling (i.e., cystic fibrosis), local insult (i.e., facial trauma, dental procedures), or mechanical obstruction (i.e., tumor, nasal packing) may also be significant.
- Diabetes mellitus and immunosuppression are particular risk factors for fungal sinusitis.

GENERAL PREVENTION
Nasotracheal intubation should be avoided or used for a limited duration. Similarly, oral enteric feeding is preferable when possible.

PATHOPHYSIOLOGY
Sinus ostial obstruction (whether mechanical, from local insult, or from mucosal swelling), dysfunction of the ciliary apparatus, and viscous sinus secretions all contribute to the development of acute infection.

ETIOLOGY
- In community-acquired sinusitis, *Streptococcus pneumoniae* and *H. influenzae* account for the majority of isolates. Also seen are anaerobes, other *Strep.* spp., *M. catarrhalis,* and *S. aureus.*
- In nosocomial sinusitis, the predominant species are *Pseudomonas* spp. and *S. aureus*. Other common etiologies are other gram-negative bacilli and *Viridans streptococci*.
- Fungal sinusitis may be invasive or noninvasive (instead forms a mycelial mass). Typical pathogens include: *Mucor, Rhizopus, Fusarium, Pseudallescheria boydii*, and others. *Aspergillus* can cause an allergic fungal sinusitis.

DIAGNOSIS

HISTORY
There are no gold standard clinical signs or tests for sinusitis, making diagnosis a challenge, but several factors may be suggestive. Patients may complain of maxillary toothache, purulent rhinorrhea, hyposmia, or facial pain/fullness. Also correlated are poor response to decongestants and duration of symptoms >10 days.

PHYSICAL EXAM
- Most findings are nonspecific and similar to what may be seen with a simple viral URI; may observe nasal obstruction or abnormal transillumination of the sinuses.
- Necrotic eschars of the nasal mucosa or hard palate may be signs of invasive fungal disease.

DIAGNOSTIC TESTS & INTERPRETATION
Lab
No specific lab tests for acute sinusitis

Imaging
- Diagnosis is usually made clinically, but imaging may provide confirmation if symptoms are vague. Remember; however, that no imaging method is validated for the diagnosis of acute sinusitis, and findings may still be considered nonspecific.
- Imaging is often used with intubated patients, in whom history and exam are especially difficult. Also, it may be critical when evaluating for intracranial complications:
  - Plain radiographs may show the expected findings of pan-sinus opacification, air–fluid levels, and mucosal thickening.
  - Sinus CT is more often practical for the intubated patient and can demonstrate more detailed architecture. Bony erosion should raise suspicion for invasive fungal sinusitis.

Diagnostic Procedures/Other
- Sinus puncture and aspiration may help provide a microbiologic diagnosis; however, it is susceptible to contamination by nasal flora and, although a reference standard, is not considered a gold standard. Also, being invasive, it is typically reserved for patients who have failed 2 empiric courses of antibiotics.
- However, for suspected fungal sinusitis, early biopsy and culture of necrotic lesions is crucial.

Pathological Findings
- Mucosal hyphal invasion correlates with invasive fungal infection.
- Eosinophilic inflammatory infiltrates characterize allergic fungal sinusitis.

DIFFERENTIAL DIAGNOSIS
Signs and symptoms of acute bacterial sinusitis are difficult to differentiate from viral etiologies. Also the radiographic findings associated with sinusitis can often be seen in chronically intubated patients due to mechanical obstruction and supine position.

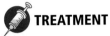

TREATMENT

MEDICATION

First Line

- Patients from the community with no recent antibiotics may be initiated on amoxicillin or amoxicillin/clavulanate. With a history of recent antibiotics, high-dose amoxicillin/clavulanate or a respiratory fluoroquinolone is suggested.
- In nosocomial settings, vancomycin and an antipseudomonal penicillin is a typical first-line choice. Carbapenems and aminoglycosides also achieve good sinus penetration if multidrug-resistant gram-negative bacilli are a concern.
- Duration is based on patient response; 10 days is typical with uncomplicated infection.
- Fungal therapy is pathogen-specific.

ADDITIONAL TREATMENT

General Measures

- Remove nasal tubes if feasible.
- Use semirecumbent positioning for intubated patients.

Issues for Referral

Otorhinolaryngology and infectious diseases consults are recommended for severe cases and critical for suspected fungal cases; ophthalmology and possibly neurosurgery if orbital or intracranial complications are present.

Additional Therapies

- Decongestants are often used although not well studied.
- Intranasal corticosteroids and antihistamines have shown inconsistent effectiveness.

SURGERY/OTHER PROCEDURES

- For acute bacterial sinusitis, surgical drainage may rarely be considered for severe cases refractory to courses of antibiotics (although there is a lack of evidence).
- Surgery is often necessary for management of intracranial complications.
- Aggressive debridement is the cornerstone of treatment for invasive fungal disease.

IN-PATIENT CONSIDERATIONS

Initial Stabilization

Patients presenting with intracranial complications, may require airway protection and possibly seizure management.

Admission Criteria

Based on evidence for severe infection or intracranial complications and signs of sepsis

IV Fluids

Associated sepsis may require aggressive resuscitation.

Discharge Criteria

Case-dependent

ONGOING CARE

FOLLOW-UP RECOMMENDATIONS

Clinical monitoring by subspecialists for severe cases

Patient Monitoring

With intracranial complications, may need follow-up imaging per subspecialists

DIET

Enteric diet once tolerating PO.

PATIENT EDUCATION

- http://www.ncbi.nlm.nih.gov/pubmedhealth/
- http://www.niaid.nih.gov
- http://www.cdc.gov
- http://www.entnet.org

PROGNOSIS

Intracranial complications and invasive fungal disease are associated with significant morbidity and mortality.

COMPLICATIONS

Include brain abscess, epidural abscess, meningitis, venous sinus thrombosis, orbital cellulitis, osteitis

REFERENCES

1. Sandy MA, et al. Acute community-acquired bacterial sinusitis: Continuing challenges and current management. *CID*. 2004;39:S151–8.
2. www.cdc.gov. DHHS: Summary health statistics for U.S. Adults. National Health Interview Survey, 2009.
3. Talmor M. Acute paranasal sinusitis in critically ill patients: Guidelines for prevention, diagnosis and treatment. *CID*. 1997;25:1441–6.

ADDITIONAL READING

- Infectious Diseases Society of America. Practice guidelines for acute and chronic rhinosinusitis. Projected publication, 2011.
- Mandell GL, et al. Principles and practice of infectious diseases. *Sinusitis*. New York: Churchill Linvingstone Elsevier, 2010;839–47.
- Rosenfeld RM, et al. Clinical practice guidelines: adult sinusitis. *Otolaryngol Head Neck Surg*. 2007; 137(3 Suppl):S1–31.
- Stein M, et al. Nosocomial sinusitis: A unique subset of sinusitis. *Curr Opin Infect Dis*. 2005;18:147–50.

 CODES

ICD9

- 461.8 Other acute sinusitis
- 461.9 Acute sinusitis, unspecified
- 477.8 Allergic rhinitis due to other allergen

CLINICAL PEARLS

- Avoidance of nasal tubes can help prevent nosocomial sinusitis.
- Invasive fungal sinusitis may be fulminant, requiring rapid diagnosis and early surgical intervention.

S

SMALL BOWEL OBSTRUCTION
Raghu Seethala

BASICS

DESCRIPTION
Small bowel obstruction (SBO) is a blockage of the small intestine due to various causes that results in an interruption in the normal flow of intestinal contents.

EPIDEMIOLOGY
Prevalence
The most common surgical disorder of the small intestine; in the US, it accounts for close to 20% of all acute surgical admissions.

RISK FACTORS
- Prior abdominal or pelvic surgery
- Intra-abdominal malignancy
- Hernia
- Inflammatory bowel disease
- Diverticulosis/diverticulitis
- Ingested foreign bodies

GENERAL PREVENTION
- Minimally invasive abdominal surgeries may reduce the formation of adhesions, thereby decreasing the subsequent risk of SBO.
- Seprafilm, a hyaluronic acid-carboxycellulose membrane, reduces the formation of severe adhesions, but has not been shown to prevent postsurgical small bowel obstruction (1)[B].

PATHOPHYSIOLOGY
- Obstruction results in dilation of the small bowel and stomach proximal to the blockage and collapse of the bowel distal to the blockage. As the proximal bowel dilates with intestinal secretions and swallowed air, intestinal contents do not pass through. This results in cessation of flatus and bowel movements. Patients will have repeated bouts of nausea and vomiting, leading to marked electrolyte and fluid abnormalities.
- Intestinal stasis then leads to the overgrowth of intestinal flora, which can lead to bacterial translocation.
- Bowel edema occurs, followed by the loss of the bowel's absorptive function, which leads to fluid sequestering in the bowel lumen.
- Progressive dilation of the bowel leads to increased luminal pressures. Increasing luminal pressures can then lead to reduced perfusion of the bowel, resulting in ischemia and necrosis.

ETIOLOGY
- Adhesions: Postoperative adhesions cause the majority of SBO.
- Neoplasm: 2nd most common cause of SBO.
- Hernias
- Strictures
- Trauma
- Foreign bodies
- Gallstone ileus
- Intussusception

Geriatric Considerations
- Patients commonly suffer from chronic constipation.
- Neoplasms of the bowel are more common.

Pediatric Considerations
- Intussusception
- Malrotation and midgut volvulus
- Duodenal atresia
- Incarcerated hernia

COMMONLY ASSOCIATED CONDITIONS
- Cancer
- Inflammatory bowel disease
- Diverticular disease
- Pica

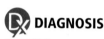

DIAGNOSIS

HISTORY
- Patients will often complain of nausea, vomiting, abdominal distension, abdominal pain, and obstipation.
- Abdominal pain is characterized as crampy and occurring in paroxysms every 5–15 minutes.

PHYSICAL EXAM
- Fever
- Tachycardia
- Abdomen:
  - Localized abdominal tenderness
  - Rebound tenderness or guarding
  - High-pitched bowel sounds
  - Abdominal distension
  - Rectal examination may reveal empty vault, or occult blood.

DIAGNOSTIC TESTS & INTERPRETATION
Lab
- CBC: Elevated WBC, elevated Hct from hemoconcentration
- Electrolytes, BUN/creatinine, glucose: Monitor for hypokalemia, prerenal azotemia
- ABG: Metabolic acidosis
- Lactate: Elevated lactate in cases of bowel ischemia
- Amylase: Can be elevated

Imaging
- X-ray: First-line study, nearly as sensitive as CT in differentiating obstruction from nonobstruction (1). In patients with high-grade obstruction, positive predictive value is 80% (2).
  - Plain films can appear normal in early obstruction and high jejunal or duodenal obstruction.
  - Upright chest: Evaluate for free air under the diaphragm.
  - Supine and upright abdominal films: Dilated loops of small bowel, multiple air fluid levels, paucity of air in the distal colon and rectum
- CT scan: Sensitive for detection of high-grade obstruction, sensitivity approaches 90% (2); in addition, CT can determine the cause, severity, and level of obstruction:
  - Transition point can be identified.
  - Absence of air or fluid in distal small bowel or large bowel signifies complete obstruction.
- Small bowel follow-through: Can be useful in diagnosing partial bowel obstruction. May also be useful in determining the need for surgery. Also has been shown to be therapeutic in partial SBO.
- MRI: Similar sensitivity to CT scan but logistical limitations preclude its use in routine diagnosis of SBO.

Pathological Findings
- Mucosal edema
- Ischemia/necrosis
- Hypersecretion

DIFFERENTIAL DIAGNOSIS
- Adynamic Ileus
- Mesenteric ischemia
- Perforated bowel
- Pancreatitis

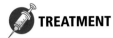 TREATMENT

Management is directed at correcting fluid and electrolyte abnormalities, decompressing the bowel, resting the bowel, and early surgical intervention when indicated.

MEDICATION

First Line
- Antibiotic therapy is indicated with gram-negative and anaerobic coverage if patient is septic or for prophylaxis prior to surgery.
- The role of routine antibiotics in SBO is controversial. Some think that antibiotics can protect against bacterial translocation and subsequent bacteremia (2)[C].

Second Line
Antiemetic therapy and pain medication should be administered as needed.

ADDITIONAL TREATMENT

General Measures
- Placement of nasogastric tube to decompress the stomach
- Foley catheter to strictly monitor urine output
- Resuscitation with IVF

- Initial nonoperative management can be attempted in partial SBO and SBO without peritonitis (2)[A].

Issues for Referral
Surgical consultation is required for each patient.

Additional Therapies
In patients being treated nonoperatively, the use of hypertonic water-soluble contrast agents, like Gastrografin, can lead to faster resolution of SBO and decreased length of stay (1)[B].

SURGERY/OTHER PROCEDURES
- Patients require surgical intervention when there are signs of peritonitis, hemodynamic instability, bowel ischemia, perforation, or severe metabolic acidosis.
- Patients treated nonoperatively who do not improve after 48 hours should be operated on.
- Operative procedure is dictated by etiology of obstruction. Operative treatment of most SBOs require laparotomy:
  – Lysis of adhesions
  – Reduction of hernia
  – Small bowel resection

- Laparoscopic treatment is effective in patients with mild abdominal distension, proximal obstruction, partial obstruction, and an anticipated single-band obstruction (1)[B].

IN-PATIENT CONSIDERATIONS

Initial Stabilization
- Obtain large-bore IV (18 g or larger) access for fluid resuscitation.
- Administer 0.9% NS or LR to correct volume deficit.
- Correct any electrolyte abnormalities.
- Place nasogastric tube to decompress the stomach.

Admission Criteria
All patients with SBO should be admitted.

IV Fluids
- Administer 0.9% NS or LR for initial resuscitation.
- While patient is NPO, give D5 1/2NS with 20–40 mEq K+/L at a maintenance rate.

Nursing
Strict measurement of inputs and outputs

Discharge Criteria
Resolution of SBO, tolerating PO with return of normal bowel function.

 ONGOING CARE

FOLLOW-UP RECOMMENDATIONS
Patients should follow-up with their surgeon 2–4 weeks after discharge from the hospital.

Patient Monitoring
Patients being treated nonoperatively need serial abdominal exams to evaluate for peritonitis, which would require surgery.

DIET
- NPO
- When patient has return of bowel function and is no longer nauseous or vomiting, advance diet slowly.

PROGNOSIS
- 3–6% of partial SBO will progress to strangulation.
- Nonstrangulated SBO has a mortality rate near 2%.
- Strangulated SBO has a mortality rate approximately 8% if surgery is performed within 36 hours; however, it is 25% if surgery occurs after 36 hours.

COMPLICATIONS
- Bowel ischemia
- Sepsis
- Risk of subsequent bowel obstruction

REFERENCES

1. Diaz JJ, et al. Guidelines for management of small bowel obstruction. *J Trauma*. 2008;64:1651–64.
2. Jackson PG, et al. Evaluation and management of intestinal obstruction. *Am Fam Physician*. 2011; 83:159–65.

 CODES

ICD9
- 560.9 Unspecified intestinal obstruction
- 568.0 Peritoneal adhesions (postoperative) (postinfection)
- 936 Foreign body in intestine and colon

CLINICAL PEARLS

- Periodic physical exam of the abdomen should be performed to monitor progression vs. improvement.
- Decompression of the proximal small bowel is required.
- Undertake early and aggressive fluid resuscitation and electrolyte repletion.
- Patients who are suspected to have bowel ischemia/strangulation need immediate surgical intervention.
- Patients not improving after 48 hours of conservative management need a surgical evaluation.

S

SPINAL CORD INJURY AND CAUDA EQUINA SYNDROME

Patrick F. Walsh

 BASICS

DESCRIPTION
- Penetrating or blunt force injury to spinal cord resulting in temporary or permanent neurologic deficit.
- May also be caused by ischemia, infection, or tumor invasion.
- Four types of forces are implicated in traumatic spinal cord injury (SCI):
  - Flexion/extension, vertical compression and longitudinal distraction, rotational, combined
- Injury to lumbar, sacral, coccygeal spinal nerves (roots) causes cauda equina syndrome.

EPIDEMIOLOGY
Incidence
- Males > Females (>3:1)
- 82% of males with SCI are 18–25 years
- 14,000 new cases per year
Prevalence
253,000 total cases in 2007

RISK FACTORS
- High-risk physical activity: Surfing/diving, football, winter sports, gymnastics, equestrian.
- Driving recklessly or while impaired
Genetics
No genetic cause identified

GENERAL PREVENTION
- Wear seat-belt and follow traffic laws.
- Utilize safety equipment in high-risk sports.

PATHOPHYSIOLOGY
- Mechanical disruption, transection, and distraction of neural elements usually occur with fracture or dislocation of spine. Compression by hematoma, abscess, and foreign body also occurs
- Spinal cord is organized into motor (descending) and sensory (ascending) tracts:
  - Corticospinal (descending) tracts decussate in medulla and descend through anterior spinal cord to synapse with motor neurons in anterior (ventral) horn.
  - Dorsal columns (ascending) carry light touch, proprioception, and vibration sense. These ascend and decussate in medulla before entering cortex.
  - Lateral spinothalamic (ascending) tracts carry pain and temperature sensation. They decussate ~3 segments above their entry into spinal cord.
  - Autonomic tracts located in anteromedial tract:
    ○ Sympathetic fibers exit C7–L1
    ○ Parasympathetic S2–S4
- Anterior spinal artery supplies anterior 2/3 of cord, and ischemia affects corticospinal, and lateral spinothalamic tracts. Posterior spinal arteries supply dorsal column:
  - Both arise from vertebral artery, with radicular arteries branching from aorta.
- Watershed area in midthoracic spine
- Shock may cause watershed-area ischemia.

- Arterial thrombi may cause infarct.
- Incomplete cord syndromes:
  - Central cord syndrome: Greater loss of upper extremity motor strength compared to lower, with some sensory loss. Forward fall with facial impact in elderly. History of cervical stenosis common. Some chance of recovery
  - Anterior cord syndrome usually caused by infarct with loss of motor function, and pain, and temperature sensation.
  - Brown-Séquard syndrome: Hemisection of cord with ipsilateral loss of motor function and position sense. Contralateral loss of pain and temperature sensation
- Cauda equina syndrome: Associated with injury to elongated lumbar and sacral spinal nerve roots. Unilateral lower motor neuron leg weakness, areflexic (lower motor neuron finding), with late bladder and bowel involvement. Perineal pain, no sexual dysfunction.
- Spinal cord concussion characterized by transient neurologic deficit.

ETIOLOGY
Trauma, ischemia, infection, malignancy

COMMONLY ASSOCIATED CONDITIONS
- Polytraumatic injuries with SCI:
  - Brain injury: 25%
  - Long-bone fracture: 15%
  - Fracture of another spinal segment: 10%
  - Pneumothorax, chest injury: 9%
  - Abdominal injury: 8%
  - Carotid and/or vertebral artery injury with:
    ○ C1–C3 fracture, C-spine subluxation
    ○ Fracture foramen transversarium
  - Neurogenic shock from impairment of descending sympathetic pathways causing relative bradycardia, vasodilation, hypotension, and hypothermia. Usually does not occur below T-6 (autonomic dysfunction)
  - Spinal shock is usually a transient physiologic depression of cord function resulting in complete loss of function, reflexes, and tone below lesion. Absence of bulbocavernosus reflex signifies continued spinal shock or injury at level of reflex arc. Presence of reflex signals termination of spinal shock, so any complete absence of distal motor or sensory loss is probably permanent.
- Nontraumatic:
  - Malignancy, ischemia, infection, emboli
  - RA: C-spine subluxation, C1 tenosynovitis
  - Down syndrome: Atlantoaxial subluxation

 DIAGNOSIS

ALERT
SCI patients can have significant other life-threatening injuries that are overlooked due to decreased pain sensation. Neurogenic shock is last consideration after all other causes are ruled out.

HISTORY
- Allergies
- Medication
- Past medical history, cancer, spinal stenosis, arthritis, infection
- Last meal, if airway may need to be secured
- Mechanism of injury, height of fall, how did patient land?

PHYSICAL EXAM
- Primary survey: Look for life-threatening injury
- Detailed secondary survey with careful neurological exam and documentation, label injury level according to lowest normal sensory and motor function. Reexamine hourly, record GCS
- Careful evaluation of respiratory status:
  - Above C6: Compromise of respiratory function
- Signs of infection, malignancy, RA, ischemia

DIAGNOSTIC TESTS & INTERPRETATION
Lab
Imaging is most important
Initial lab tests
- ABG, CBC, PT/INR, aPTT, BUN, creatinine
- Drug/ETOH screen, lactate or base deficit
Follow-Up & Special Considerations
FEV_1, vital capacity, liver function panel

Imaging
Initial approach

- Imaging is not required in awake and alert patients without distracting injury, neurological deficit, or neck pain or neck tenderness with full range of motion of C-spine (1)[A].

- X-ray: 3 views (anterior/posterior), lateral, odontoid) must include occiput to T1:
  – A/P and lateral x-ray for thoracic/lumbar spine
- CT scan has replaced routine radiology at most centers. Occiput to T1 with sagittal and coronal reconstruction images for CS (1)[A].
- Sensitivity for plain radiography was 52%, for CT scan C-spine it was 98% (2)[A].
- MRI is strongly suggested for ligamentous injury, soft tissue injury, neck pain with normal CT scan, a patient who is obtunded or comatose, who cannot participate in physical exam, or any abnormality on CT scan (1)[A].
- Abnormal segment noted on radiography with neurological deficit *must* have MRI (1)[A].
- MRI for spinal cord injury without radiologic abnormality (SCIWORA) from longitudinal distraction with/without flexion/extension

Follow-Up & Special Considerations
- Repeat imaging for worsening deficit
- Vascular imaging (vertebral, carotid artery)

Diagnostic Procedures/Other
Needle aspiration of abscess, tumor, or mass

Pathological Findings
- Fibrinoid necrosis in arteries
- Fusiform zone of spinal cord necrosis

DIFFERENTIAL DIAGNOSIS
Stroke in motor area, transverse myelitis

 TREATMENT

MEDICATION
- High-dose methylprednisolone based on Nation Acute Spinal Cord Injury Studies (NASCIS):
  – Dose 30 mg/kg bolus, then infuse 5.4 mg/kg/hr for 24 hours. Start within 8 hours of injury.
  – Recent reviews have cited concerns about design flaws and trial conduct
- American college of surgeons (ATLS) changed guideline to "a recommended treatment as opposed to "the recommended treatment."
- Congress of neurosurgeons: "Therapy should be undertaken with the knowledge that the evidence suggesting harmful side effects is more consistent than any suggestion of clinical benefit."

ADDITIONAL TREATMENT
General Measures
- Remove back board within 2 hours if possible.
- Rapid sequence intubation with in-line immobilization and laryngoscopy or fiberoptic intubation. Success depends on skill.
- Keep SBP >90 mm Hg and oxygen saturation >93% to prevent secondary injury.

Issues for Referral
Early transfer to trauma center or facility with neuron/ortho surgeons experienced in care of SCI

SURGERY/OTHER PROCEDURES
- Surgical stabilization for many C-spine injuries and other segments; timing is debatable (3)[A]
- Early tracheotomy, gastric feeding tube

IN-PATIENT CONSIDERATIONS
Initial Stabilization
- Volume resuscitation, euvolemia (4)[A]
- Vasopressors to keep SBP >90 mm Hg (4)[A]
- Atropine/cardiac pacing for bradycardia (4)[A]
- IPPB, bronchoscopy for secretions
- Prophylaxis for thromboembolism (4)[A]:
  – Use sequential compression devices
  – Once hemostasis is achieved, add LMWH
  – Bleeding risk >72 hours, consider IVC filter
- Stress ulcer prophylaxis
- VAP prevention
- Urinary tract catheterization
- Avoid succinylcholine after 1st 48 hours post SCI

Admission Criteria
Neurological deficit, respiratory compromise, shock, other life-threatening injuries

IV Fluids
NS

Nursing
- Pulmonary secretion management
- Log roll, assistance with patient transition
- Skin care, pressure reduction mattress
- Pain control

Discharge Criteria
Variable, from ventilator facility to directly home based on disability

 ONGOING CARE

FOLLOW-UP RECOMMENDATIONS
Patient will usually require in- or outpatient multidisciplinary care organized by social services and physicians caring for patient.

Patient Monitoring
ICU initially, then neuroscience unit

DIET
Early enteral feeding within 24–48 hours.

PATIENT EDUCATION
- Comprehensive training with patient and family on care of trach, catheters, and feeding tubes.
- Recognition of signs and symptoms skin breakdown, infection, and pneumonia

PROGNOSIS
- C–C3: 6.6 fold increased risk of death
- C4–C5: 2.5 fold increased risk of death
- C6–C8: 1.5 fold increased risk of death
- Deficits at 72 hours are usually irreversible

COMPLICATIONS
- Autonomic dysreflexia
- Coronary artery disease
- Bladder dysfunction
- UTI
- Vesicoureteral reflux
- Sexual dysfunction
- Osteoporosis
- Syringomyelia
- Thermoregulatory dysfunction

Pediatric Considerations
- SCIWORA is more common in children.
- Radiographic evaluation complicated by pseudosubluxation of C2 on C3 before age 7.
- Force is applied to neck with great angular momentum from relatively large head.

Geriatric Considerations
Spinal stenosis and fall forward with facial impact can cause central cord syndrome.

REFERENCES
1. Como JJ, et al. Practice management guidelines for identification of cervical spine injuries following trauma - update from the Eastern Association for the Surgery of Trauma Practice Management Guidelines Committee. East trauma practice guidelines. Accessed at www.east.org
2. Holmes JF, et al. Computed tomography versus plain radiography to screen for cervical spine injury: A meta-analysis. *J Trauma.* 2005;58:902–905.
3. LaRosa G, et al. Does early decompression improve neurological outcome of spinal cord injured patients? Appraisal of the literature using a meta-analytical approach. *Nature.* 2004;42(9): 503–12.
4. Wing PC, Dalsey WC, Alvarez E, Bombardier CH, Burns SP, Fitzpatrick MK, Green D, Huff JS, Kincaid MS, Lucke KT, Napolitano LM, Poelstra KA, Vaccaro A, Wilberger JE, Wuermser LA. *Early Acute Management in Adults with Spinal Cord Injury: A Clinical Practice Guideline for Health-Care Professionals.* Consortium for Spinal Cord Medicine, 2008.

ADDITIONAL READING
- http://www.spineuniverse.com/
- Stiell IG, et al. The Canadian C-Spine Rule versusthe NEXUS Low-Risk Criteria in Patients with Trauma. *N Engl J Med.* 2003;349:2510–8.

 CODES

ICD9
- 344.60 Cauda equina syndrome without mention of neurogenic bladder
- 952.9 Unspecified site of spinal cord injury without spinal bone injury
- 953.2 Injury to lumbar nerve root

CLINICAL PEARLS
- Injury to 1 segment mandates imaging of entire spine.
- Prevent secondary injury by avoiding hypotension/hypoxia.
- Early referral to trauma center is important.

SPIROMETRY

Ari Klapholz

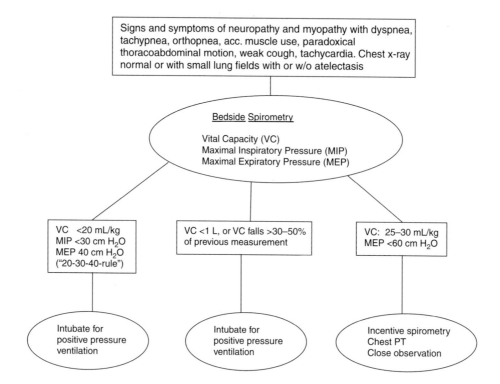

Signs and symptoms of neuropathy and myopathy with dyspnea, tachypnea, orthopnea, acc. muscle use, paradoxical thoracoabdominal motion, weak cough, tachycardia. Chest x-ray normal or with small lung fields with or w/o atelectasis

Bedside Spirometry

Vital Capacity (VC)
Maximal Inspiratory Pressure (MIP)
Maximal Expiratory Pressure (MEP)

VC   <20 mL/kg
MIP <30 cm H_2O
MEP 40 cm H_2O
("20-30-40-rule")

VC <1 L, or VC falls >30–50% of previous measurement

VC: 25–30 mL/kg
MEP <60 cm H_2O

Intubate for positive pressure ventilation

Intubate for positive pressure ventilation

Incentive spirometry
Chest PT
Close observation

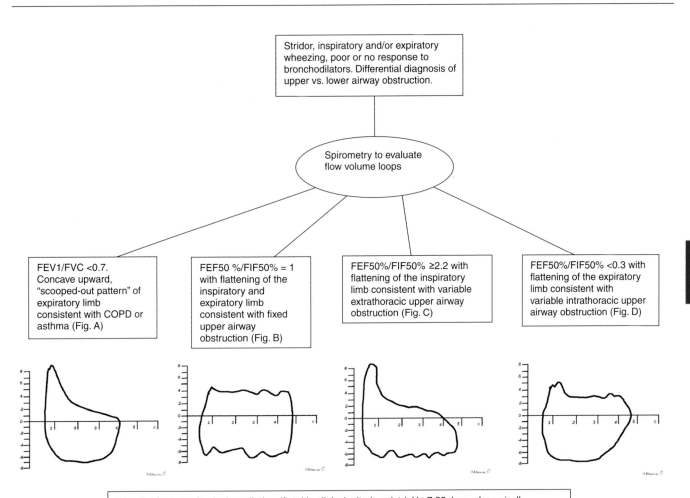

Stridor, inspiratory and/or expiratory wheezing, poor or no response to bronchodilators. Differential diagnosis of upper vs. lower airway obstruction.

Spirometry to evaluate flow volume loops

FEV1/FVC <0.7. Concave upward, "scooped-out pattern" of expiratory limb consistent with COPD or asthma (Fig. A)

FEF50 %/FIF50% = 1 with flattening of the inspiratory and expiratory limb consistent with fixed upper airway obstruction (Fig. B)

FEF50%/FIF50% ≥2.2 with flattening of the inspiratory limb consistent with variable extrathoracic upper airway obstruction (Fig. C)

FEF50%/FIF50% <0.3 with flattening of the expiratory limb consistent with variable intrathoracic upper airway obstruction (Fig. D)

Weaning from mechanical ventilation: If stable clinical criteria exist (pH ≥7.25, hemodynamically stable, oxygenation is adequate [PaO2/FIO2 ≥150]) and patient can initiate breath, proceed to spontaneous breathing trial (SBT). If risk of SBT failure is elevated, consider weaning indicators, such as the rapid shallow breathing index or the CROP index where tidal volume and maximal inspiratory pressure are utilized, respectively.

S

ST-SEGMENT ELEVATION MYOCARDIAL INFARCTION

Sweta Chandela

 BASICS

DESCRIPTION
STEMI results from sudden acute occlusion of at least 1 coronary artery and is distinguished from non-STEMI by the ECG:
- ECG shows ST-segment elevations in at least 2 contiguous leads, or new left bundle branch block
- Cardiac biomarkers will be elevated.
- Early reperfusion is usually the key to limiting infarct size.

EPIDEMIOLOGY
Incidence
~1,500,000 cases per year in U.S.

Prevalence
- >500 cases per 100,000 population
- Age 40–65 years, Males > Female
- Age >65 years, Males = Females

RISK FACTORS
- Age: Male >45 years; female >55 years
- Hypertension
- Diabetes, type 1 and 2; CAD equivalent
- Tobacco use
- Hyperlipidemia:
  - Elevated LDL
  - Low HDL
- Previous MI or stroke
- Family history of premature heart disease
- Framingham (and other) risk scores can be used to integrate multiple risk factors.
- Secondary factors:
  - Obesity; sedentary lifestyle
  - Elevated CRP
  - Increased level of stress

Genetics
- Maternal CAD is more strongly linked than paternal CAD as a risk factor/predisposition.
- Premature heart disease:
  - Male 1st-degree relative <55
  - Female 1st-degree relative <65

GENERAL PREVENTION
- Tobacco cessation
- Lipid control
- Aspirin 81 or 325 mg/d:
  - In patients with a Framingham risk score corresponding to a 10-year risk of coronary death or MI >10%.
  - Men 45–79 for reduction in MI
  - Women 55–79 years for reduction in MIs and ischemic strokes
- Prevention of diabetes, hypertension, stroke
- Diet
- Exercise:
  - At least 30 minutes of moderate physical activity on most days of the week

PATHOPHYSIOLOGY
- Atherosclerotic plaque rupture, atherothrombus formation, occlusion of coronary artery:
  - Plaque instability
  - Local endothelial and systemic inflammatory response
  - Increased thrombogenicity
  - Oxygen demand and supply mismatch

ETIOLOGY
- Atherosclerotic:
  - Plaque rupture and atherothrombi
  - Coronary stent thrombosis
  - Distal plaque embolization
- Nonatherosclerotic:
  - Coronary vasospasm
  - Cocaine/other drugs
  - Coronary artery dissection
  - Congenital coronary artery anomaly
  - Stress-induced (Takotsubo) cardiomyopathy
  - Proximal thoracic aortic aneurysm dissection
  - Vasculitis
  - Any condition that sufficiently increases myocardial oxygen demand or decreases myocardial oxygen supply

COMMONLY ASSOCIATED CONDITIONS
- Peripheral vascular disease
- Cerebrovascular accident
- Abdominal aortic aneurysm

DIAGNOSIS

HISTORY
- Angina pectoris of increased severity and duration, unresponsive to sublingual nitroglycerin:
  - Diaphoresis
  - Nausea/vomiting
  - Weakness
  - Palpitations
  - Presyncope
- Elderly, female, and diabetic patients may not have a classic presentation (i.e., silent MI)

PHYSICAL EXAM
- Hypertension/hypotension
- Tachycardia or bradycardia:
  - Inferior MI associated with Bezold-Jarisch reflex
  - Arrhythmias: Premature ventricular contractions, atrioventricular blocks (cannon a waves), atrial fibrillation, ventricular tachycardia, ventricular fibrillation
- Jugular venous distention
- Cardiac:
  - Displaced point of maximum intensity (PMI)
  - Soft S_1 and S_2
  - Mitral regurgitation murmur
  - Ventricular septal defect (VSD) murmur
  - S_3 and/or S_4 gallop
- Rales
- Decreased pulses
- Cold, clammy skin
- Peripheral edema

DIAGNOSTIC TESTS & INTERPRETATION
Lab
Initial lab tests
- Cardiac biomarkers
  - Troponin T or I: Positive in 3–6 hours after MI, peaks at 16 hours, trends down over 9–12 days
  - CK, creatine kinase: Positive in 4–8 hours after MI, peaks 18–24 hours, trends down over 3–4 days. CK MB band specific for myocardial tissue: >5% of total CK usually indicative of infarction
- CBC: Leukocytes elevated within hours of MI, peak 2–4 days, trend to normal over 1 week
- Electrolytes, BUN/creatinine
- INR
- Lipid profile
- Lactate

Follow-Up & Special Considerations
- Serial ECGs
- Serial cardiac biomarkers
- B-natriuretic peptide

Imaging
- ECG should be done within 10 minutes of presentation:
  - Peaked T waves, followed by ST-segment elevation, in at least 2 contiguous leads
  - New left bundle branch block is treated like a STEMI.
  - Evolution of MI shows T-wave inversion, followed by Q waves over 12–36 hours.
- Chest x-ray for cardiomegaly, pulmonary edema, right ventricular (RV) size

Diagnostic Procedures/Other
- Transthoracic echocardiogram:
  - Left ventricular (LV) function
  - RV function
  - Segmental wall motion abnormalities
  - Mitral regurgitation
  - Papillary muscle function
  - Cardiac tamponade
- Left ventriculography after coronary angiography for LV assessment

Pathological Findings
Myocardial necrosis

DIFFERENTIAL DIAGNOSIS
- Pericarditis
- Aortic stenosis
- Pleural pain
- Pulmonary embolism
- Aortic dissection
- Costochondritis
- Panic attack
- GI:
  - Cholecystitis
  - Peptic ulcer/gastroesophageal reflux
  - Gastritis
  - Esophagitis

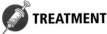 **TREATMENT**

MEDICATION
First Line
- Antianginal therapy:
  - Oxygen 2 L/min
  - Nitroglycerin sublingual 0.4 mg q5min for 3 doses, followed by IV drip
    - Avoid in RV infarction
    - Caution with phosphodiesterase inhibitors (treatment for erectile dysfunction)
    - Dose-dependent tolerance develops
    - Patients may complain of headache.
  - Morphine 2–4 mg q15min
- β-Blocker: Metoprolol 5 mg IV q5min for 3 doses, followed by PO dosing:
  - Mortality reduction with chronic PO use
  - Avoid in hypotension, bradycardia, evidence of AV node block on ECG, acute congestive heart failure, acute bronchospasm, cocaine
- Statins: Atorvastatin 80 mg PO q.d. or other statin:
  - Antiplatelet therapy:
    - Aspirin 325 mg PO chewed
    - Clopidogrel 300–600 mg loading dose
    - GP IIb/IIa inhibitor: Abciximab, eptifibatide
  - Antithrombins:
    - Unfractionated heparin by protocol
    - Low-molecular-weight heparin (enoxaparin) subcutaneous 1 mg/kg q12h
    - Direct thrombin inhibitors

- Reperfusion:
  - Percutaneous coronary intervention (PCI)
  - Fibrinolytics:
    - Tissue plasminogen activator given by 15 mg IV bolus, then 50 mg over 30 minutes, then 35 mg over 60 minutes
    - Retavase 10 units IV over 2 minutes followed by 2nd 10-unit infusion over 2 minutes 30 minutes later OR
    - Tenecteplase; dosing is weight based. See product package insert.
    - Contraindicated in recent head trauma, active internal bleeding, hemorrhagic CVA, pregnancy, persistent hypertension (>200/120 mm Hg); prolonged (>10 min) or traumatic CPR, trauma or major surgery within 2 weeks

Second Line
- Inotropic agents
- Diuretics
- Antiarrhythmics

ADDITIONAL TREATMENT
General Measures
- ER triage immediately based on symptoms and ECG
- Earliest reperfusion therapy with aim for total ischemic time <120 minutes, preferably <60 minutes
- Options for transportation of STEMI patients and initial reperfusion treatment goals:
  - EMS with fibrinolytic capability: Start prehospital fibrinolysis within 30 minutes of arrival on scene if patient qualifies
  - If no prehospital fibrinolysis and EMS transports to non-PCI-capable hospital, door-to-needle time for fibrinolysis should be <30 minutes
  - If no prehospital fibrinolysis and EMS transports to PCI-capable hospital, door-to-balloon time should be <90 minutes
  - If fibrinolysis is contraindicated or unsuccessful, interhospital transfer to PCI-capable facility; goal is 90 minutes to balloon

S

Issues for Referral
Non-PCI-capable facility

Additional Therapies
- Intra-aortic balloon pump:
  - Severe left main coronary artery stenosis
  - Severe LV dysfunction
  - Recurrent angina after revascularization
  - Recurrent ventricular tachycardia
- Temporary pacemaker

COMPLEMENTARY & ALTERNATIVE THERAPIES
Omega-3 fatty acids

SURGERY/OTHER PROCEDURES
- Cardiothoracic surgery in following cases:
  - Left main coronary artery stenosis >50%
  - Triple-vessel disease, especially in patients with diabetes and LV dysfunction
  - Papillary muscle rupture
  - Ventricular septal defect resulted from MI
  - Myocardial wall rupture
  - Coronary artery dissection
  - Cardiac tamponade not amenable to pericardiocentesis
  - Associated ascending aortic dissection
- Swan-Ganz catheter placement to monitor pulmonary artery pressure

IN-PATIENT CONSIDERATIONS
Initial Stabilization
- ABCs (ACLS)
- Achieve hemodynamic stability.
- Antianginal therapy
- Initial bed rest

Admission Criteria
All patients with STEMI are admitted to a CCU, then may be transferred to a telemetry monitor unit when clinically and hemodynamically stable with no further evidence of evolution of MI.

IV Fluids
- Avoid in severe LV dysfunction and CHF.
- Used to resuscitate in cases of RV infarction.
- May be used post coronary angiography/PTCI in cases of renal dysfunction

Discharge Criteria
- Complete resolution of chest pain, at rest and with exertion
- Hemodynamic stability
- Tolerance of all required medications

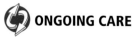 ONGOING CARE

Discharge regimen:
- Aspirin indefinitely (Class 1, Level A)
- β-Blocker (Class 1, Level A)
- Statin therapy when LDL >100 (Class 1, Level A)
- Clopidogrel 75 mg, for at least 1 month (Class 1, Level A) for medical therapy of CAD or bare metal stent, and ideally for 12 months (Class 1, Level B); at least 12 months for drug-eluting stent (Class 1, Level B)
- ACE inhibitor if LV ejection fraction is <40% or if concomitant diabetes mellitus or hypertension is present.
  - Blood pressure goal <140/90 mm Hg and <130/80 when chronic kidney disease or diabetes is present (Class 1, Level A).
  - Lipid management goals: LDL <100 (Class 1, Level A), <70 (Class 2a, Level A)
  - Diabetes management goal is hemoglobin A1c <7% (Class 1, Level A).
  - Tobacco cessation counseling
  - Lifestyle modification

FOLLOW-UP RECOMMENDATIONS
- Cardiology
- Electrophysiology if evidence of LV ejection fraction <35%, ICD

Patient Monitoring
- Transthoracic echocardiogram periodically to reassess LV function and segmental wall motion, LV thrombus.
- Post revascularization stress test for initiation of cardiac rehabilitation

DIET
- Low-fat/-cholesterol foods
  - Saturated fats: <7% of daily calories
  - Trans fats: <1% of daily calories
  - Total cholesterol: <200 mg/d
- Low carbohydrates:
  - Substitute in whole grains, multigrains, oats
  - High fiber
- Low sodium: <2300 mg/d
- High in fruit and vegetables
- Portion size control
- Eat fish containing omega-3 fatty acids.

PATIENT EDUCATION
Overall, therapeutic lifestyle modification and control of risk factors:
- Tobacco cessation
- Hypertension control
- Hyperlipidemia treatment goals
- Diabetes mellitus treatment goals
- Exercise and weight loss
- Stress reduction

PROGNOSIS

- Acute MI is the leading cause of death, in both men and women, worldwide.
- 30% of patients suffer death from acute MI; 1/2 of deaths occur within the 1st hour of symptom onset.
- 1-year mortality post MI can be as high as 21% especially with significant LV dysfunction (LVEF <30%).
- LV function is the most important prognostic indicator; others include:
  - Age
  - Ventricular arrhythmias post MI
  - Extent of myocardial revascularization
  - Recurrent ischemia post revascularization
  - Comorbid illnesses, specifically diabetes and hypertension
  - Compliance to therapy

COMPLICATIONS

- Cardiogenic shock
- Papillary muscle rupture
- Free wall aneurysm/rupture
- VSD
- Mitral valve incompetency
- Ventricular tachycardia/ventricular fibrillation
- Depression
- Dressler syndrome
- Death

ADDITIONAL READING

- Antman EM, et al. 2007 focused update of the ACC/AHA 2004 Guidelines for the Management of Patients with ST-Elevation Myocardial Infarction: a report of the American College of Cardiology/American Heart Association Task Force on Practice Guidelines. *J Am Col Cardiol*. 2008;51. Accessed www.acc.org/qualityandscience/clinical/statements.htm
- Faxon D, et al. Atherosclerotic vascular disease conference, writing group III: pathophysiology. *Circulation*. 2004;109:2617–25.
- Goodman SG, et al. Acute ST-segment myocardial infarction: American College of Chest Physicians Evidence-Based Clinical Practice Guidelines. *Chest*. 2008;133:708S.
- McCord J, et al. Management of cocaine-associated chest pain and myocardial infarction: A scientific statement from the American Heart Association Acute Cardiac Care Committee of the Council on Clinical Cardiology. *Circulation*. 2008; 117(14):1897–907.

 ## CODES

ICD9

- 410.90 Acute myocardial infarction of unspecified site, episode of care unspecified
- 410.91 Acute myocardial infarction of unspecified site, initial episode of care
- 410.92 Acute myocardial infarction of unspecified site, subsequent episode of care

CLINICAL PEARLS

Identify the MI territory from ECG leads:

- V1–V4 indicates anterior wall, which is supplied by left anterior descending artery and its branches.
- V5–V6, I, and avL indicates lateral wall, which is supplied by left circumflex artery and its branches.
- II,III, aVF indicates Inferior wall, which is supplied by right coronary artery and its branches.
- ST elevation in right-sided V3–V6 leads indicates RV infarction.

S

STATUS EPILEPTICUS
Claude Killu

BASICS

DESCRIPTION
Unremitting seizure with a duration >5–10 minutes or frequent clinical seizures without an interictal return to the baseline clinical state (1):

- Textbooks still define status as seizure activity lasting >30 minutes
- The Epilepsy Foundation Working Group on Status Epilepticus has recommended treating as status epilepticus any seizure activity that lasts >10 minutes.
- Refractory status epilepticus is ongoing seizures following 1st- and 2nd-line drug therapy.
- Nonconvulsive status epilepticus is mental status changes from baseline of at least 30–60 minutes, associated with ictal discharges.

EPIDEMIOLOGY
Incidence
100,000–200,000 episodes of status epilepticus in the U.S. annually.

- The annual incidence shows a bimodal distribution with peaks in neonates, children, and the elderly.

Prevalence
25% of status epilepticus cases occur in people diagnosed with epilepsy.

RISK FACTORS
- Status epilepticus will recur in ~1/3 of patients.
- Female gender and a failure to respond to the 1st drug administered for status epilepticus are risk factors for recurrence.

Genetics
Chronic epilepsy; status epilepticus may represent part of a patient's underlying epileptic syndrome (as with the Landau-Kleffner syndrome or Rasmussen's encephalitis), or may be associated with any of the generalized epilepsies.

GENERAL PREVENTION
Compliance with medications.

PATHOPHYSIOLOGY
Imbalance of excess excitation and reduced inhibition. Glutamate is the most common excitatory neurotransmitter and the NMDA receptor subtype is involved. γ-Aminobutyric acid (GABA) is the most common inhibitory neurotransmitter.

ETIOLOGY
- Antiepileptic drug noncompliance, withdrawal syndromes, structural brain injury, metabolic abnormalities, and overdose with drugs that lower the seizure threshold
- Medication like tacrolimus, cyclosporin, INH toxicity, cocaine and theophylline

COMMONLY ASSOCIATED CONDITIONS
Status epilepticus may represent part of a patient's underlying epileptic syndrome.

DIAGNOSIS

HISTORY
Noncompliance, overdose, metabolic disorder.

PHYSICAL EXAM
Assessment of the level of consciousness, observations for automatic movements or myoclonus, and any asymmetric features on exam that may indicate a focal structural lesion

DIAGNOSTIC TESTS & INTERPRETATION
Lab
Initial lab tests
- EEG that reveals continuous seizure activity is diagnostic of status epilepticus.
- Lumbar puncture in suspected infectious etiology.

Follow-Up & Special Considerations
- Clear ictal activity may not be seen during simple partial status epilepticus.
- EEG obtained over a short period of time and between seizures can miss intermittent ictal activity.

Imaging
Initial approach
MRI is the best tool to reveal the structural lesions that may trigger status epilepticus.

Follow-Up & Special Considerations
MRI may reveal areas of increased signal intensity on FLAIR, T2-, or diffusion-weighted images in the presence of status epilepticus.

Diagnostic Procedures/Other
Creatine kinase levels are typically markedly elevated after generalized convulsive epileptic seizures.

Pathological Findings
Neuronal death can occur after 30–60 minutes of continuous seizure activity. The pathologic hallmark of this phenomenon, cortical laminar necrosis, may also be seen on brain MRI.

DIFFERENTIAL DIAGNOSIS
3 most common forms of status epilepticus are: Simple partial, complex partial, and generalized tonic–clonic.

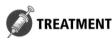

TREATMENT
MEDICATION
First Line

Benzodiazepines remain the 1st-line treatment for status epilepticus (2)[A]:

- Treatment with lorazepam alone was most effective in terminating seizures within 20 minutes and maintaining a seizure-free state in the 1st 60 minutes after treatment (3)[A].
- Dose of lorazepam, 2–4 mg IV over 2 minutes repeat every 5 minutes if still seizing to a total of 0.1 mg/kg

Second Line
- Given even if seizure is controlled with 1st-line therapy
- Need to monitor levels:
  - Phenytoin 20 mg/kg should be given slowly, not >50 mg/min because of risk of hypotension and cardiac arrhythmia (3)[B].
  - Fosphenytoin dose is 20 PE/kg, given at 150 mg/min IV drip or IM
- 3rd line:
  - Midazolam: Load 0.2 mg/kg, then start IV drip at 0.05–2 mg/kg/h
  - Propofol: Load 1 mg/kg; repeat to max 10 mg/kg, then continuous IV drip at 1–15 mg/kg/h
  - Barbiturates: Initial dose of phenobarbital is 20 mg/kg; infuse at a maximum of 100 mg/min(4)
- 4th line:
  - Pentobarbital 5 mg/kg bolus at 50 mg/min, then 1–3 mg/kg/h

- EEG monitoring for patients on 3rd and 4th line: Burst suppression pattern or seizure suppression are the electrophysiologic end points.
- Hemodynamic monitoring: Almost all patients on 3rd- and 4th-line medication will require vasopressor support (phenylephrine or dopamine) and mechanical ventilation.

ADDITIONAL TREATMENT
General Measures
Intubation and mechanical ventilatory support:
- Blood must be obtained for electrolyte, serum glucose, and toxicology studies, CBC, and a rapid "finger-stick" glucose.
- Vitamin B_6 for INH toxicity

Issues for Referral
Epileptologist

Additional Therapies
- Valproic acid, Topamax, Keppra, ketamine show promise
- Chloral hydrate, carbamazepine, or etomidate are less efficacious and should not be considered part of the routine management of status epilepticus.

COMPLEMENTARY & ALTERNATIVE THERAPIES
General anesthesia with isoflurane may be temporarily effective in stopping seizures.

SURGERY/OTHER PROCEDURES
Surgical removal of seizure-producing areas of the brain is an accepted form of treatment.

IN-PATIENT CONSIDERATIONS
Initial Stabilization
Hemodynamic and respiratory monitoring are also required to avoid side effects of therapy.

Admission Criteria
ICU

IV Fluids
Phenytoin must not be mixed with dextrose.

Nursing
Intensive care

Discharge Criteria
After clinical and electroencephalogram seizures stop:
- Patient with a flurry of seizures that are easily controlled might conceivably be discharged after several hours of observation.

 ONGOING CARE

FOLLOW-UP RECOMMENDATIONS
Serum drugs level monitoring

Patient Monitoring
Continuous EEG, cardiac, and respiratory

DIET
NPO during attack

PATIENT EDUCATION
Compliance with medication is most important.

PROGNOSIS
The mortality rate for adults who present with a 1st episode of status epilepticus is ~20%.

COMPLICATIONS
- Rhabdomyolysis, lactic acidosis, aspiration pneumonitis, neurogenic pulmonary edema, and respiratory failure may complicate convulsions.
- Mortality is high: ~20%.

REFERENCES

1. Lowenstein DH, et al. Status epilepticus. *N Engl J Med*. 1998;338:970.
2. Treiman DM. Pharmacokinetics and clinical use of benzodiazepines in the management of status epilepticus. *Epilepsia*. 1989;30(Suppl 2):s4.
3. Treiman DM, et al. A Comparison of four treatments for generalized convulsive status epilepticus. *N Engl J Med*. 1998;339:792.
4. Treatment of convulsive status epilepticus. Recommendations of the Epilepsy Foundation of America's Working Group on Status Epilepticus. *JAMA*. 1993;270:854.

ADDITIONAL READING

- Bleck TP. Management approaches to prolonged seizures and status epilepticus. *Epilepsia*. 1999;40(Suppl. 1):S59–S63.

 See Also (Topic, Algorithm, Electronic Media Element)

www.epilepsyfoundation.org

 CODES

ICD9
- 345.3 Grand mal status, epileptic
- 345.00 Generalized nonconvulsive epilepsy, without mention of intractable epilepsy
- 345.90 Epilepsy, unspecified, without mention of intractable epilepsy

CLINICAL PEARLS

- EEG is the best diagnostic tool.
- Note status of airway, respiration, blood pressure, and cardiac rhythm. Most patients require intubation.

STROKE, ISCHEMIC

H. Christian Schumacher
Raghad Said

 BASICS

DESCRIPTION
Ischemic stroke is defined as brain or retinal cell death due to prolonged ischemia (tissue-defined cerebral infarct).

EPIDEMIOLOGY
Incidence
88–191 per 100,000 (U.S.) for first ever stroke

Prevalence
3.3% in African Americans and 2.2% in whites (2)

RISK FACTORS
- >55
- Male > Female
- Hypertension, both systolic and diastolic
- Cigarette smoking
- Diabetes
- Nonvalvular atrial fibrillation
- Sickle cell anemia (1)

Genetics
- Genetic heritability of stroke risk factors
- Familial sharing of cultural/environmental and lifestyle factors

GENERAL PREVENTION
- Control of modifiable risk factors
- Aspirin is not recommended for the prevention of a 1st stroke in men.
- ASA is recommended for stroke prevention for women with higher risk.

PATHOPHYSIOLOGY
Reduced oxygen and nutritional supply due to a transient or permanent cerebral artery occlusion

ETIOLOGY
The etiologic classification is:
- Extracranial large artery atherosclerosis
- Intracranial large artery atherosclerosis
- Cardioaortic embolism
- Small artery occlusion (lacune)
- Other specific causes: Infectious vasculopathy, inflammatory vasculopathy, vasospasm, connective tissue disorders
- Cryptogenic or undetermined causes

COMMONLY ASSOCIATED CONDITIONS
- Hyperlipidemia
- Coronary artery disease
- Postmenopausal state
- Chronic kidney failure
- Obesity

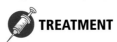 DIAGNOSIS

HISTORY
- Symptoms of cerebral infarct are typically associated with acute loss of function (negative symptoms).
- Positive symptoms (e.g., muscle twitching, progressive tingling, flashing lights in the visual field) should raise suspicion against CVA.
- Depending on the brain area involved, the following may occur in isolation or combined: Hemifacial weakness, amaurosis (curtain-like visual loss, loss of vision in ipsilateral eye after exposure to bright light, visual field deficit, double vision, hemiparesis, hemisensory loss, aphasia, dysarthria, ataxia
- Additional key components of history are:
  – Onset and duration of symptoms
  – Recent events: Previous TIA or stroke, MI, trauma, surgery, bleeding
  – Use of anticoagulants, antiplatelet agents

PHYSICAL EXAM
- Vital signs: Rhythm, BP and temperature
- Neurological exam to assess stroke severity and location: NIH Stroke Scale (NIHSS) helps to quantify neurological and facilitate communication between healthcare professionals.
- Cardiac exam may indicate arrhythmia or murmurs suggestive for a cardiac embolism.
- A carotid bruit may indicate carotid stenosis.

DIAGNOSTIC TESTS & INTERPRETATION
Lab
Initial lab tests
- All patients:
  – Chemistry profile, CBC, troponin- I, PT/INR, PTT, lipid panel
- Selected patients:
  – LFT, toxicology screen, blood alcohol level, pregnancy test, C-reactive protein, ESR, hypercoagulable workup, syphilis serology, homocysteine level, ABG

Follow-Up & Special Considerations
- EKG to rule out atrial fibrillation or acute MI
- Transthoracic and or transesophageal echocardiographyto rule out cardioembolic sources

Imaging
Initial approach

- Neuroimaging (3)[A]:
  – CT of the brain with no contrast: Rule out bleed
  – MRI: Preferred imaging modality

- Neurovascular imaging: To identify large intra- or extracranial stenosis or occlusion prior to intraarterial tPA or surgical interventions (3)[B]:
  – MRA of head and neck
  – CT angiography (CTA) of head and neck: Quality is comparable to conventional angiography
  – Conventional digital subtraction angiography

Follow-Up & Special Considerations
EEG: If seizures are suspected

Diagnostic Procedures/Other
- Carotid Doppler: Identify extracranial carotid and/or vertebral arteries stenosis
- Temporal artery biopsy may be considered if there is clinical suspicion for giant cell arteritis.

DIFFERENTIAL DIAGNOSIS
- Migraine with aura (visual, sensory or other)
- Hypoglycemia
- Seizures
- Subdural hematoma
- Epidural hematoma
- Syncope
- Transient global amnesia
- Conversion disorder
- Hypertensive encephalopathy

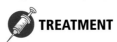 TREATMENT

ALERT
- The thrombolysis treatment window for some stroke patients may be extended to within 4.5 hours of symptom onset, according to a science advisory from the American Heart Association and American Stroke Association, published online in *Stroke*.
- The groups stressed, however, that therapy within 3 hours remains ideal "because the opportunity for improvement is greater with earlier treatment."
- According to the advisory, patients eligible for therapy with recombinant tissue plasminogen activator (rtPA) who are not treated within 3 hours can be treated up to 4.5 hours, unless they:
  – Are >80;
  – Are taking oral anticoagulants, regardless of the INR;
  – Have an NIH stroke scale score >25;
  – Have a history of both stroke and diabetes
  – For these groups, rtPA must be given within 3 hours.
- The relative utility of rtPA in this time window compared with other methods of thrombus dissolution or removal has not been established.
- No differences between the 3–4.5-hour cohort and the 3-hour cohort were apparent with respect to symptomatic intracerebral hemorrhage, mortality, or modified Rankin Scale score of 0–2 at 90 days.

MEDICATION

- rt-PA (3)[A]:
  – IV thrombolysis should only be performed by experienced physicians with this intervention.
  – Inclusion criteria are:
    ○ Diagnosis of ischemic stroke causing measurable neurological deficit that is not minor or clearing spontaneously
    ○ Caution should be exercised in treating patients with major deficits.
    ○ Onset of symptoms <3 hours before beginning treatment (see Alert)
    ○ Patient's or family's consent to therapy

– Contraindications are:
  ○ Symptoms suggestive of subarachnoid bleed
  ○ Head trauma or prior stroke or MI in the previous 3 months
  ○ GI or GU hemorrhage in previous 21 days
  ○ Major surgery in the previous 14 days
  ○ Arterial puncture at a noncompressible site in the previous 7 days
  ○ Previous intracranial hemorrhage
  ○ SBP <185 mm Hg and diastolic <110 mm Hg: If can lower BP within the window or treatment, patient becomes eligible (3)[B]
  ○ Active bleeding or acute trauma
  ○ Oral anticoagulant with INR >1.7
  ○ Heparin in last 48 hours with abnormal aPTT
  ○ Platelet count <100,000 mm³
  ○ Blood glucose concentration <50 mg/dL
  ○ Seizure with postictal impairment: If the residual impairment is not due to postictal states, patient might be eligible
  ○ CT showing a multilobar infarction (hypodensity >1/3 cerebral hemisphere)
– Dosing: 0.9 mg/kg (maximum dose 90 mg); give 10% of total dose as a IV bolus over 1 minute, followed by IV Infusion of the remaining 90% of the total dose over 60 minutes
– Hold treatment with antiplatelet agents or anticoagulants for 24–36 hours after rtPA
– IV rtPA significantly increased number of patient with favorable outcome at 3 months and 1 year.
– The frequency of symptomatic intracerebral hemorrhage at 24 hours after rtPA was 7.3% compared to 1.1%, with 30-day mortality of 60%.
– Side effects: Angioedema, systemic bleeding, and myocardial rupture in case of recent MI
• Anticoagulation:
  – Only indicated for secondary prevention of cardioembolic cerebral infarction
  – No anticoagulation should be given within 7–14 days after moderate to large ischemic stroke to avoid intracerebral bleed
  – Adjusted-dose warfarin (target INR 2.0–3.0)
  – Aspirin 325 mg q.d., if unable to take warfarin
  – If there is an ischemic stroke or systemic embolism despite adequate oral anticoagulation, aspirin 75–100 mg/d is reasonable while maintaining the INR at a target of 3.0.
• Antiplatelet agents:
  – Antiplatelet agents rather than oral anticoagulation are recommended for noncardioembolic ischemic strokes.
  – Aspirin (325 mg/d) given within 24–48 hours after stroke onset (3)[A]
  – The addition of clopidogrel to ASA increases the risk of hemorrhage and is not recommended (3)[C].
  – IV glycoprotein IIb/IIIa receptor is not recommended.

ADDITIONAL TREATMENT
General Measures
• Permissive hypertension: If the patient is not a candidate for IV t-PA or endovascular acute revascularization, and there is no other hypertensive emergency, BP up to 220/120 mm Hg is tolerated.
• If patient is a candidate for IV thrombolysis: Treat with IV labetalol (10–20 mg) or IV nicardipine (slow titration of 2.5–15 mg/hr) to achieve a SBP <185 mm Hg and DBP of <110 mm Hg

Issues for Referral
Referral to vascular surgeon in patients with significant hemodynamic extracranial carotid stenosis

Additional Therapies
Intra-arterial thrombolysis for patients who have major stroke of <6 hours' duration due to occlusions of the MCA and who are not otherwise candidates for IV rtPA [B]

COMPLEMENTARY & ALTERNATIVE THERAPIES
• Drug-induced hypertension is not recommended outside the setting of clinical trials.
• Insufficient evidence exists to recommend hypothermia for treatment of acute stroke.

SURGERY/OTHER PROCEDURES
• Patients with severe (>70%) extracranial carotid stenosis should be considered for carotid endarterectomy (CEA) or carotid artery stenting within 2 weeks rather than delaying therapy (4).
• Extracranial/intracranial bypass surgery is not routinely recommended (3)[C].
• Endovascular treatment of patients with symptomatic extracranial vertebral artery stenosis may be considered when symptoms reoccur despite maximal medical treatment.
• The usefulness of endovascular treatment in hemodynamically significant intracranial stenosis is uncertain and investigational.

IN-PATIENT CONSIDERATIONS
Initial Stabilization
• Manage ABCs.
• Rule out hypoglycemia.
• Obtain STAT head CT (3)[A].
• The goal is to complete an evaluation and to decide treatment within 60 minutes of the patient's arrival in an ED.

Admission Criteria
Patients undergoing IV thrombolysis need to be admitted to an ICU or a stroke unit.

IV Fluids
No hypotonic and dextrose containing fluids

Nursing
• DVT prophylaxis either with sequential compression devices and/or SC heparin
• Early mobilization in medically stable patients
• Incentive spirometry to prevent pneumonia
• Frequent positioning to avoid pressure ulcers
• Avoid prolong use of indwelling Foley catheter.
• Dysphagia screening before any PO intake

Discharge Criteria
Discharge is safe as soon as stroke workup is completed and individualized treatment for stroke prevention is initiated.

 ONGOING CARE

FOLLOW-UP RECOMMENDATIONS
Outpatient follow-up in 14 days after discharge

Patient Monitoring
Modifiable risk factors

DIET
NPO until medically stable

PATIENT EDUCATION
• Stroke warning signs and symptoms
• How to activate emergency medical system
• Need for follow-up after discharge
• Prescribed medications

PROGNOSIS
• In 2003, stroke accounted for 1 of every 15 deaths in the U.S.
• Stroke is the most common reason for persistent disability.
• 30-day mortality for ischemic stroke is 12%.

COMPLICATIONS
• Recurrent ischemic stroke
• Intracranial hypertension
• Symptomatic hemorrhagic infarct conversion
• Pneumonia
• Urinary tract infection
• Venous thromboembolism

REFERENCES
1. Thom T, et al. Heart disease and stroke statistics – 2006 update. Circulation. 2006;113:85–181.
2. Sacco RL, et al. Guidelines for the prevention of stroke in patients with ischemic stroke or transient ischemic attack: A statement for health care professionals from the American Heart Association/American Stroke Association Council on Stroke. Circulation. 2006;113:409–49.
3. Adams HP, et al. Guidelines for the early management of adults with ischemic stroke: Guideline from the American Heart Association/American Stroke Association Stroke Council. Stroke. 2007;38:1655–711.
4. Adams RJ, et al. Update to the AHA/ASA recommendations for the prevention of stroke in patients with stroke and transient ischemic attack. Stroke. 2008;39:1647–52.

ADDITIONAL READING
• Saver JL. Proposal for a universal definition of cerebral infarction. Stroke. 2008;39:3110–5.

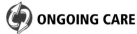 CODES

ICD9
434.91 Cerebral artery occlusion, unspecified with cerebral infarction

CLINICAL PEARLS
• An ischemic stroke is a medical emergency requiring a rapid work-up and management.
• IV thrombolysis is the standard of care in selected patients with an ischemic stroke when treatment can be initiated within 3 hours after onset; window is extended to 4.5 hours for specific patient population.
• Stroke etiology defines secondary stroke prevention treatment.

S

SUPERIOR VENA CAVA (SVC) SYNDROME

Rhonda D'Agostino
Nina D. Raoof

 BASICS

DESCRIPTION
- Obstruction of the superior vena cava either extrinsically (mass) or intrinsically (thrombus), resulting in a constellation of symptoms related to decreased venous return and airway obstruction
- May be acute or chronic depending on the underlying etiology

EPIDEMIOLOGY
Incidence
~ 15,000 cases annually in the U.S.

Prevalence
- Associated with underlying cause:
  - Age 40–60 (suspect malignant causes)
  - Age 30–40 (suspect nonmalignant causes)

RISK FACTORS
- Mediastinal tumor (lung, lymphoma, breast, germ cell, thymoma)
- Intravascular device (catheters, pacemakers)
- Aortic aneurysm
- Infectious or inflammatory mediastinitis
- Radiation to chest or mediastinum
- Vascular or cardiac surgery

Genetics
Associated with underlying cause

PATHOPHYSIOLOGY
- Malignancy-associated SVC syndrome: Obstruction of the SVC can be caused by invasion or extrinsic compression by tumors of the lung or mediastinum or by thrombosis of blood within the SVC.
- Intravascular devices may cause compromise of the SVC vessel wall leading to inflammation, fibrosis, and stenosis.
- The impaired venous return from the SVC results in increased collateral circulation to the IVC, azygous vein, and superficial venous vessels of the chest wall.
- The upper body venous pressure increases with edema of the head and neck and potentially may result in airway compromise.

ETIOLOGY
- ~60–85% due to malignancies (most frequently bronchogenic carcinoma)
- ~15–40% due to nonmalignant causes (intravascular device-related)
- Fibrosing mediastinitis from chest radiation, tuberculosis and histoplasmosis (rare)

COMMONLY ASSOCIATED CONDITIONS
- Upper airway obstruction
- Cerebral edema
- Pleural effusions
- Esophageal varices (rare)

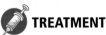 **DIAGNOSIS**

HISTORY
- Dyspnea (most common)
- Facial and neck swelling
- Cough
- Orthopnea
- Upper extremity swelling
- Syncope
- Head fullness, headache
- Stridor, hoarseness, or dysphagia
- Distorted vision
- Dizziness

PHYSICAL EXAM
- Facial, neck, or arm edema
- Distended neck veins
- Distended superficial chest veins
- Plethora
- Confusion
- Cyanosis

DIAGNOSTIC TESTS & INTERPRETATION
Imaging
Initial approach
- Chest x-ray: Mediastinal mass or widening, pleural effusion or lung mass
- Contrast-enhanced chest CT: Helps confirm diagnosis, define extent of venous blockage, and evaluate presence of collateral vessels
- MRI: For patients with contrast dye allergy
- Bilateral upper extremity venography

Follow-Up & Special Considerations
Fiberoptic laryngoscopy if airway patency is suspect

Diagnostic Procedures/Other
- Diagnostic thoracentesis with cytology
- Sputum cytology
- Biopsy of mediastinal mass
- Bronchoscopy or mediastinoscopy, if indicated
- Bone marrow biopsy: If lymphoma is suspected

Pathological Findings
As per underlying condition or malignancy

DIFFERENTIAL DIAGNOSIS
- Aortic aneurysm
- Paratracheal abscess
- Mediastinitis

TREATMENT

- Depends on specific etiology
- For malignancy-related SVC syndrome: Goals are to relieve symptoms and treat the underlying malignancy.
- For intravascular device-related SVC syndrome: Anticoagulation, percutaneous transluminal angioplasty, and/or metallic wall stents

MEDICATION
- Loop diuretics
- Glucocorticoids: For steroid-responsive lymphoma or thymoma, and for laryngeal edema if present after radiation therapy
- Chemotherapy: For underlying malignancy
- Thrombolytics: Catheter-directed or systemic
- Anticoagulation: Short-term after stent placement and after thrombolytic therapy
- Antiplatelet therapy (after stent placement)

ADDITIONAL TREATMENT
General Measures
- Elevation of the head of bed (HOB)
- Airway management with activation of difficult
- airway algorithm
- Diagnose underlying cause (tissue biopsy)
- 1st-line:
  - Remove catheters and/or wires
  - Urgent chemotherapy
  - Urgent radiotherapy
  - Endovascular stenting
  - Catheter-based thrombolytic therapy or mechanical thrombectomy
- 2nd-line:
  - Restenting
  - Synthetic graft
  - Spiral saphenous vein bypass graft
  - Vascular surgery

Issues for Referral
When surgical or interventional therapies are not available

Additional Therapies
- Large-bore peripheral IV access
- Central venous access (limited to the femoral vein)
- Avoid intramuscular injections in the arms

COMPLEMENTARY & ALTERNATIVE THERAPIES
Directed by malignancy

SURGERY/OTHER PROCEDURES
- Endovascular stenting
- Balloon angioplasty
- Mass resection
- Thrombectomy
- SVC reconstruction

IN-PATIENT CONSIDERATIONS
Initial Stabilization
- Airway management
- Intubation performed by an experienced operator
- Supplemental oxygen
- Contrast-enhanced CT scan
- Immediate US or venogram
- Remove indwelling upper extremity catheters.
- Vascular or thoracic surgery consult
- Diuretics
- Corticosteroids
- Thrombolysis
- Anticoagulation

Admission Criteria
- Stridor or dyspnea
- Hemodynamic compromise
- Sign/symptoms of cerebral edema (coma, headache, dizziness)

IV Fluids
None

Nursing
- Elevate head of bed.
- Supplemental oxygen
- Continuous cardiac monitoring
- Continuous oxygen saturation monitoring
- Low-salt diet

Discharge Criteria
Improvement or resolution of sign and symptoms

ONGOING CARE

FOLLOW-UP RECOMMENDATIONS
Patient Monitoring
- As determined by underlying condition.
- May include:
  - Long-term anticoagulation
  - Treatment for malignancy

PROGNOSIS
- Overall, as per underlying condition
- Presentation with SVC syndrome does not alter prognosis from malignancy:
  - SVC syndrome may recur if cancer progresses.
  - Relapse may occur both acutely after stent placement (in-stent thrombosis) or during long-term follow-up.

COMPLICATIONS
- Cerebral edema related to poor venous drainage
- Posttreatment complications:
  - Related to chemotherapy or radiation
  - Acute stent rethrombosis, malposition, or migration
  - Perforation during stent procedure
  - Cerebral hemorrhage following thrombolytic therapy
  - Complications related to surgical reconstruction (leak, infection, thrombosis)

ADDITIONAL READING

- Cheng S. Superior vena cava syndrome. A contemporary review of a historic disease. *Cardiol Rev.* 2009;17:16–23.
- Nguyen NP, et al. Safety and effectiveness of vascular endoprosthesis for malignant superior venal cava syndrome. *Thorax.* 2009; 64:174–8.
- Rice T. Pleural effusions in superior vena cava syndrome: Prevalence, characteristics and proposed pathophysiology. *Curr Opin Pulm Med.* 2007;13:324–7.
- Wilson LD, et al. Clinical practice. Superior vena cava syndrome with malignant causes. *N Engl J Med.* 2007;356:1862–9.
- Yu JB, et al. Superior vena cava syndrome—a proposed classification system and algorithm for management. *J Thorac Oncol.* 2008;3:811–4.

CODES

ICD9
459.2 Compression of vein

CLINICAL PEARLS

- SVC syndrome is most frequently caused by malignancy or thrombosis.
- Pathophysiology involves extrinsic compression or direct invasion of SVC by tumors or thrombosis from vessel wall injury or hypercoagulability in the presence of intravascular devices.
- Contrast-enhanced chest CT is the imaging modality of choice to confirm the diagnosis and define the extent of venous blockage and to assess collateral drainage.
- The severity of symptoms establishes the urgency of treatment.
- Treatment is directed at underlying pathologic process, including chemotherapy with or without radiotherapy.
- Emergent radiotherapy or endovascular wall stenting may be required for stridor or severe laryngeal edema, depressed mental status from cerebral edema, or cardiopulmonary collapse.

S

SYNDROME OF INAPPROPRIATE ANTIDIURETIC HORMONE (SIADH)

Nirav Mistry
Roopa Kohli-Seth

 BASICS

DESCRIPTION
Disease of impaired water excretion and an increase in total body water but no real change in body sodium levels, with resultant dilutional hyponatremia, hypo-osmolality, euvolemia, and inappropriately elevated urine osmolality. Caused by the inappropriate secretion of vasopressin

EPIDEMIOLOGY
Incidence
- Predominantly affects elderly females > males
- Usual hospital incidence, 30–35%

Prevalence
Hyponatremia (Na <130) reported between 2.4% and 16% in hospitalized patients

RISK FACTORS
- Head trauma
- Malignancy
- Medications (especially psych meds)
- Elderly age
- Postop status
- Hospitalization

GENERAL PREVENTION
Avoid medications that cause the syndrome.

PATHOPHYSIOLOGY
- Argininevasopressin (AVP), also known as antidiuretic hormone (ADH), is secreted from the posterior pituitary in response primarily to hyperosmolality and decreased volume (1)[A].
- AVP acts on the collecting ducts in the nephrons, causing water reabsorption.
- Inappropriate secretion of antidiuretic hormone (SIADH) is a state of pathological hormone excess resulting in dilutional hyponatremia and hypo-osmolality with euvolemia.

ETIOLOGY
- CNS disorders:
  - Head trauma/skull fractures
  - Subdural hematoma
  - Subarachnoid hemorrhage
  - Brain tumor: Primary or metastasis
  - Encephalitis/meningitis/cerebritis
  - Acute psychosis
  - Vasculitis
- Pulmonary lesions:
  - Viral/bacterial/fungal pneumonia
  - Abscess
  - Tuberculosis
  - Positive pressure ventilation
- Malignancy:
  - Bronchogenic carcinoma
  - Pancreatic carcinoma
  - Prostatic carcinoma
  - Renal cell carcinoma
  - Adenocarcinoma of colon
  - Thymoma
  - Osteosarcoma
  - Malignant lymphoma
  - Leukemia

- Drugs that increase ADH production:
  - Antidepressants:
    - Tricyclics
    - Monoamine oxidase inhibitors
    - SSRIs
  - Antineoplastics
  - Clofibrate neuroleptics
- Drugs that potentiate ADH action:
  - Carbamazepine
  - Chlorpropamide
  - Tolbutamide
  - Cyclophosphamide
  - NSAIDs
  - Somatostatin and analogues
- Miscellaneous:
  - Postoperative
  - Multiple sclerosis
  - Guillain-Barré syndrome
  - Acute intermittent porphyria
  - Stress
  - Pain
  - AIDS
  - Pregnancy (physiologic)

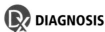 **DIAGNOSIS**

HISTORY
- Anorexia
- Abdominal pain/nausea/vomiting
- Agitation, confusion
- Hallucinations
- Incontinence
- Seizures
- Coma

PHYSICAL EXAM
- Coma
- Convulsions
- Low urine output
- Altered mental status/delirium
- Cranial nerve palsies
- Hypothermia
- Altered patterns of respiration (Cheyne-Stokes)

DIAGNOSTIC TESTS & INTERPRETATION
Lab
Initial lab tests

- Serum sodium level is low (1)[A].
- Serum osmolality (S_{osm}) is low <280 (2)[A].
- BUN/creatinine
- Urine osmolality (U_{osm}) is 100 + mOsm/kg
- Urinary Na >40 mEq/L (>40 mmol/L)
- Spot urine (1)[B] and spot Osm (1)[B]
- Serum glucose
- Thyroid function
- Morning cortisol
- Elevated serum ADH level
- Uric acid

Follow-Up & Special Considerations
- Water restriction trial:
  - Sodium will rise in response
  - Safe as long as patient does not have clinical signs of overt dehydration

Imaging
Imaging is usually not needed for diagnosis.

Diagnostic Procedures/Other
Chest x-rays, CT-scans, and MRI to rule out malignancies once SIADH is diagnosed

DIFFERENTIAL DIAGNOSIS
- Isotonic hyponatremia:
  - Hyperlipidemia
  - Hyperproteinemia
- Hypertonic hyponatremia (S_{osm} >295 mOsm/kg)
  - Hyperglycemia
  - Mannitol, sorbitol, glycerol, maltose
  - Radiocontrast agents
- Hypotonic hyponatremia (S_{osm} <280 mOsm/kg):
  - Hypovolemic:
    - Extrarenal salt loss (U_{Na+} <10 mEq/L): Dehydration, diarrhea, vomiting
    - Renal salt loss (U_{Na+} >20 mEq/L): Diuretics, ACE inhibitors, nephropathies, mineralocorticoid deficiency, cerebral sodium-wasting syndrome
  - Euvolemic:
    - SIADH
    - Postoperative hyponatremia
    - Hypothyroidism
    - Psychogenic polydipsia
    - Beer potomania
    - Idiosyncratic drug reaction (thiazides, ACE inhibitors)
    - Endurance exercise
  - Hypervolemic (edematous states):
    - Congestive heart failure
    - Liver disease
    - Nephrotic syndrome (rare)
    - Advanced renal failure

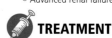 **TREATMENT**

MEDICATION
First Line
- Mainstay of treatment is fluid restriction.
- NS infusion trial in patients in which it is difficult to differentiate euvolemia from hypovolemia 3[A]
- Symptomatic hyponatremia:
  - Initial goal: Achieve serum sodium concentration of 125–130 mEq/L, guarding against overly rapid correction
  - Rate of sodium correction should be 0.5–1.0 mEq/L/h up to 12 mEq/L/h over 24 hours.
  - If CNS symptoms, hyponatremia should be immediately treated at any level of serum sodium concentration.
  - Hypertonic (e.g., 3%) saline (0.5–1.0 mL/kg IV) for severe hyponatremia with or without symptoms

- Asymptomatic hyponatremia:
  – Restrict water intake to 0.8–1.2 L/d
  – 0.9% saline may be used when serum sodium <120 mEq/L with unclear indication of patient's fluid status

Second Line
- Demeclocycline:
  – Inhibits effect of ADH on distal tubule
  – Useful for patients who cannot adhere to water restriction or need additional therapy
  – Onset of action may be 1 week; concentrating ability may be permanently impaired
- Lithium:
  – Blocks ADH at renal tubule
  – Use with caution to avoid lithium toxicity
- Vaptans:
  – Vasopressin-2 receptor competitive antagonists
  – Function by preventing water reabsorption in renal tubules
  – Drugs available in PO and IV forms

ADDITIONAL TREATMENT
General Measures
Stop the offending agent if cause is pharmacological.

Issues for Referral
- Surgical intervention may be needed.
- Neurosurgery to evaluate for CNS source
- Cardiothoracic or pulmonary for tumor etiology

SURGERY/OTHER PROCEDURES
Neurosurgery, general surgery, or CT surgery for various etiologies of SIADH

IN-PATIENT CONSIDERATIONS
Initial Stabilization
- Treat initial symptoms such as seizures, hypoxemia, etc. upon arrival to ED.
- Careful treatment with hypertonic saline
- Consultation with nephrology if indicated

Admission Criteria
- Symptomatic hyponatremia
- Moderate to severe hyponatremia

IV Fluids
- Mainstay of therapy is to limit fluid intake.
- If symptomatic hyponatremia, use hypertonic saline to minimal serum Na^+ 125.

Nursing
- Maintain strict fluid intake and output.
- Monitor respiratory status.
- Make frequent neurological assessments.
- Maintain fall precautions.

Discharge Criteria
Once serum sodium is stabilized and definitive treatment of serum sodium normalization is instituted

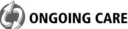 ONGOING CARE

FOLLOW-UP RECOMMENDATIONS
Patient Monitoring
- Frequent chemistries to follow treatment
- Therapy with demeclocycline in cirrhosis appears to increase risk of renal failure.
- Monitor lithium levels and toxicity.

DIET
Regular diet after discharge and definitive treatment is instituted.

PATIENT EDUCATION
- Patient to monitor for increase urine output or excess fluid intake
- Symptoms of lethargy should be reported
- Seizures

PROGNOSIS
- Higher mortality reported in patients admitted with hyponatremia
- Associated with underlying cause of SIADH

Pregnancy Considerations
Premenopausal women in whom hyponatremic encephalopathy develops from rapidly acquired hyponatremia (e.g., postoperative hyponatremia) are about 25 times more likely than postmenopausal women to die or to suffer permanent brain damage.

COMPLICATIONS
Central pontine myelinolysis may occur from osmotically induced demyelination as a result of overly rapid correction of serum sodium (an increase of >1 mEq/L/h, or 25 mEq/L within the first day of therapy).

REFERENCES
1. Decaux G, et al. Clinical laboratory evaluation of the syndrome of inappropriate secretion of antidiuretic hormone. *Clin J Am Soc Nephrol*. 2008;3(4):1175–84. Epub 2008 Apr 23.
2. Hannon M, et al. The syndrome of inappropriate antidiuretic hormone: Prevalence, causes and consequences. *Eur J Endocrinol*. 2010;162:S5–S12.
3. Sherlock M, et al. The syndrome of inappropriate antidiuretic hormone: Current and future management options. *Eur J Endocrinol*. 2010;162: S13–S18.

ADDITIONAL READING
- Frederick S, et al. Metabolic and endocrine emergencies (Chapter 41). In Stone CK, Humphries RL, eds., *Current Diagnosis & Treatment: Emergency Medicine*, 6th ed. Accessed at http://www.accessmedicine.com/content.aspx?aID=3112282
- Robinson AG. Posterior pituitary (neurohypophysis) (Chapter 6). In Gardner DG, Shoback D, eds., *Greenspan's Basic and Clinical Endocrinology*, 8th ed. Accessed at http://www.accessmedicine.com/content.aspx?aID = 2629091
- Syndrome of Inappropriate Antidiuretic Hormone (SIADH). Quick Answers to Medical Diagnosis and Therapy: Accessed at http://www.accessmedicine.com/quickam.aspx

 CODES

ICD9
- 253.6 Other disorders of neurohypophysis
- 276.1 Hyposmolality and/or hyponatremia

CLINICAL PEARLS
- SIADH is a common hyponatremic condition in hospital setting.
- It is the result of excess ADH secretion.
- Patients are normally euvolemic, hypo-osmolar, and hyponatremic.
- Primary treatment is fluid restriction.
- Hypertonic saline is used for severe symptoms.
- Rapid correction can lead to complications.

SYPHILIS
Timothy J. Henrich

BASICS

DESCRIPTION
- A systemic infectious disease caused by *Treponema pallidum*
- Transmitted sexually, maternal–fetal, and through contact with infected tissue
- Disease progresses through overlapping stages when untreated: Primary, secondary (both symptomatic), latent (asymptomatic), and tertiary (late):
  - Primary: Usually single painless chancre at point of entry; appears in days to weeks after exposure; heals without treatment in 3–6 weeks
  - Secondary: Rash (may be on palms or soles of feet), fever, adenopathy, headache. Weeks to months after initial exposure
  - Latent: Seroreactive without evidence of disease:
    - Early latent: Acquired within the last year (often difficult to diagnose unless documented prior syphilis testing)
    - Late latent or latent of unknown duration: Exposure >12 months prior to diagnosis
  - Tertiary (late): Years after initial exposure. May have negative serologies
    - Damage to multiple systems: Cardiovascular, CNS, and musculoskeletal
    - Causes gait disturbances (tabes dorsalis) and dementia (general paresis).
  - Neurosyphilis: CNS involvement of *T. pallidum*, can be symptomatic or asymptomatic. Timing can vary and can occur at any stage.

EPIDEMIOLOGY
Incidence
- Syphilis rate reached a nadir in 2000, but has subsequently been increasing (1).
- Increases in rates observed primarily among men (3.0 cases per 100,000 population in 2001 to 7.8 cases in 2009).
- In 2008: 63% of primary and secondary syphilis cases in men who have sex with men
- From 2004–2008, highest rate increase among individuals aged 15–24 years of age
- In 2009: 4.6 cases or primary and secondary per 100,000 population:
  - White, non-Hispanic: 2.1/100,000
  - African American: 19.2/100,000
  - Hispanic: 4.5/100,000
  - Asian/Pacific Islander: 1.6/100,000
  - American Indian/Alaska native: 2.4/100,000
  - Men: 7.8/100,000
  - Women: 1.4/100,000
  - Congenital: 10 cases/100,000 live births

Prevalence
- Predominant sex: Male > Female (6:1):
  - Male-to-female ratio relatively stable since 2003

RISK FACTORS
- Unprotected sex
- Men having sex with men
- Multiple sex partners
- HIV infection
- Exposure to infected body fluids
- IV drug use
- Transplacental transmission
- Inmates at adult correctional facilities

GENERAL PREVENTION
- Educate patient on the use of condoms and safer sex practices.
- Avoid contact with infected tissue.
- Screen and treat high-risk individuals and pregnant women or women planning on becoming pregnant.
- Provide educational materials to patients about sexually transmitted diseases (STDs).

PATHOPHYSIOLOGY
- Growth characteristics of *T. pallidum* largely unknown as unable to grow in culture
- No natural immunity to syphilis infection

ETIOLOGY
T. pallidum subspecies pallidum, spirochete

COMMONLY ASSOCIATED CONDITIONS
- HIV infection
- Viral hepatitis
- Other STDs

Pediatric Considerations
In noncongenital cases, consider child abuse.

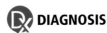

DIAGNOSIS

HISTORY
Previous sexual contact with partner with known infection or partner with high-risk sexual behavior

PHYSICAL EXAM
- Signs/symptoms depend on stage:
- Primary: After 2–3 week incubation, typically painless papule in groin or other inoculation site that ulcerates (usually single lesion, but sometimes >1). Associated with regional lymphadenopathy
- Secondary:
  - Rash: Skin or mucous membranes:
    - Diffuse red–brown macules or papules, including palms and soles
    - May appear with chancre or after it has healed
  - Nonspecific symptoms: Fever, adenopathy, malaise, anorexia, sore throat, headache
  - May have neurologic/ocular manifestations (e.g., meningitis, uveitis, meningovascular disease)
- Tertiary (late):
  - Gummatous syphilis (gummas may be external or visceral)
  - Cardiovascular (murmurs, heart failure)
  - Neurologic (late): General paresis, tabes dorsalis

DIAGNOSTIC TESTS & INTERPRETATION
Lab
- Dark-field microscopy demonstrating *T. pallidum* spirochetes in lesion exudate or tissue: Considered gold standard for diagnosis, although difficult to perform and not sensitive
- Initial screening tests can by either nontreponemal specific assays or by specific assays, such as enzyme or chemiluminescence antibody immunoassays
- Screening results should be followed by treponemal-specific testing; use of only one type of serologic test is insufficient (2).
- Nontreponemal tests (RPR or VDRL):
  - Nonspecific, false-positive results common; must confirm diagnosis with treponemal tests
  - Positive test should be quantified and titers followed at regular intervals after treatment (2).
  - Titers usually correlate with disease activity; 4-fold change demonstrates clinical significant difference (2).
  - Titer decreases with time or treatment; following adequate treatment for primary or secondary, a 4-fold decline should be noted after 6 months.
  - Absence of 4-fold decline indicates failure of treatment.
  - Titers eventually should be negative (see "Serofast reaction").
  - Titers of patients treated in latent stages decline gradually.
  - Prozone phenomenon: Negative results secondary to high titers of antibody; test diluted serum.
  - Serofast reaction: Persistently positive results years after successful treatment; new infection diagnosed by 4-fold rise in titer
  - Disorders that may alter lab results:
    - Pregnancy
    - Autoimmune disease
    - Systemic lupus erythematosus
    - Mononucleosis
    - Malaria
    - Leprosy
    - Viral pneumonia
    - Presence of cardiolipin antigens
    - Drug addiction
    - Acute febrile illness
    - HIV infection
- Enzyme or chemiluminescence antibody immunoassays:
  - Some laboratories now use as initial screening test as can be automated for high throughput
  - Often reflexed to RPR to obtain titer; useful in following treatment outcome or new infection
  - May stay positive for life after initial infection
- Confirmatory treponemal tests (confirmatory test after positive nontreponemal screening test); FTA-ABS, TP-PA, MHA-TP:
  - FTA-ABS (fluorescent treponemal antibody absorbed), TP-PA (*T. pallidum* particle agglutination), MHA-TP (microhemagglutination *T. pallidum* assay)
  - Confirmatory tests are not used for screening
  - Usually positive for life after treatment
  - Titers or levels of no benefit in 15–25% of patients treated during the primary stage; these patients revert to being serologically nonreactive after 2–3 years.
- Lumbar puncture:
  - Indicated for any patient who has clinical evidence of neurologic involvement or has syphilitic ocular or auditory manifestations
  - Some experts advise in all secondary and early latent cases without neurologic symptoms, but controversial.
  - Some experts advise in HIV-positive patients with late latent or latent of unknown duration.
  - In late latent or latent of unknown duration or when nonpenicillin therapy is planned
  - In treatment failures
  - If other evidence of active syphilis is present (e.g., aortitis, gumma, iritis)
  - In children with syphilis, after the newborn period, to rule out neurosyphilis
  - VDRL, not RPR, used on CSF; may be negative in neurosyphilis; highly specific but insensitive
  - Send fluid for protein, glucose, and cell count.
  - Monitor resolution by cell count at 6 months along with serologies as recommended (see "Patient Monitoring").
  - Negative FTA-ABS or MHA-TP on CSF excludes neurosyphilis (highly sensitive).
  - Positive FTA-ABS or MHA-TP on CSF not diagnostic because of high false-positive rate
  - Bloody tap, tuberculosis (TB), pyogenic or aseptic meningitis can result in false-positive VDRL.

Pregnancy Considerations
- All pregnant patients should be screened at 1st prenatal visit (3). If high exposure risk, repeat the tests at 28 weeks and at delivery.
- The same nontreponemal test for initial diagnosis also should be used for follow-up tests.

DIFFERENTIAL DIAGNOSIS
- Primary:
  - Chancroid
  - Lymphogranuloma venereum
  - Granuloma inguinale
  - Condyloma acuminata
  - Herpes simplex
  - Behçet syndrome
  - Carcinoma
  - Mycotic infection
  - Lichen planus
  - Psoriasis
  - Fungal infection
- Secondary:
  - Pityriasis rosea
  - Drug eruption
  - Psoriasis
  - Lichen planus
  - Viral exanthema
  - Stevens-Johnson syndrome
  - Pityriasis versicolor
  - Oral leukoplakia
- Other spirochetal disease (yaws, pinta)

 ## TREATMENT
MEDICATION
- Parenteral penicillin G is drug of choice for all stages (2)[A]. Choice of formulation is determined by the disease stage and clinical manifestations.
- Primary, secondary, early latent:
  - Benzathine penicillin G, 2.4 million units IM for 1 dose (2)[A]
  - Penicillin-allergic patients: Doxycycline, 100 mg PO b.i.d. × 2 weeks, or tetracycline, 500 mg PO q.i.d. × 2 weeks, or ceftriaxone, 1 g IM or IV daily × 10–14 days
  - Infants and children: Benzathine penicillin G 50,000 units/kg IM, up to the adult dose of 2.4 million units in a single dose (2)
- Late latent or latent of unknown duration and tertiary without evidence of neurosyphilis:
  - Benzathine penicillin G, 2.4 million units IM weekly × 3 doses (2)[A]
  - Penicillin-allergic patients: effectiveness of penicillin alternatives in the treatment of latent syphilis has not been well documented. Attempt desensitization and treatment with penicillin; doxycycline, 100 mg PO 2 b.i.d. × 28 days, or tetracycline, 500 mg PO × 28 days; adherence may be an issue.
  - Infants and children: Benzathine penicillin G 50,000 units/kg IM, up to the adult dose of 2.4 million units weekly × 3 doses (2).
- Neurosyphilis:
  - Aqueous crystalline penicillin G, 3–4 million units IV q4h or continuous infusion × 10–14 days
  - Procaine penicillin G, 2.4 million units IM daily in conjunction with probenecid, 500 mg PO q.i.d. × 10–14 days (if compliance can be ensured) (2)[A]
  - Penicillin-allergic patients: Attempt desensitization and treat with penicillin; ceftriaxone, 2 g/d IM or IV × 14 days

  - If late latent, latent of unknown duration, or tertiary in addition to neurosyphilis, consider also treating as recommended for late latent after completion of neurosyphilis treatment.
- Congenital:
  - Aqueous crystalline penicillin G, 50,000 units/kg/dose IV q12h × 1st 7 days of life and q8hs thereafter for a total of 10 days, or procaine penicillin G, 50,000 units/kg/dose IM daily × 10 days (2)
  - If negative CSF serologies, normal physical exam, serum titer the ≤4-fold the maternal titer: 50,000 units/kg benzathine penicillin G IM in single dose is also alternative depending on specific circumstances (2)[A]
- Older infants and children should be assessed whether they have congenital or acquired syphilis. Treatment is aqueous crystalline penicillin G 50,000 units/kg IV every 4–6 hours for 10 days (2).
- Pregnancy:
  - Treatment same as for nonpregnant patients
  - Serologies should be repeated at 28–32 weeks' gestation and at delivery
  - Some specialists recommend 2nd dose of 2.4 million units benzathine penicillin G 1 week after initial dose in 3rd trimester or with primary, secondary, or early latent syphilis.
  - Penicillin sensitivity: No proven alternatives to penicillin exist for treatment during pregnancy; consider desensitization and treatment with penicillin (2)[A].
- Contacts exposed to a patient in any disease stage should be evaluated and treated with a recommended regimen (2).
- Contraindications: Allergy to penicillin
- If >1 day of drug is missed, restart course.

ALERT
- HIV-infected and pregnant patients may show poor response to recommended IM doses.
- Do not give benzathine or procaine penicillins IV.

ADDITIONAL TREATMENT
General Measures
- Avoid intercourse until treatment is complete.
- Advise patients to inform sexual partners/contacts.

ALERT
- Syphilis in HIV-infected patient:
  - Treatment same as for HIV-negative patients
  - More often false-negative treponemal and nontreponemal tests or unusually high titers
  - Response to therapy is less predictable.
  - Early syphilis: Increased risk of neurosyphilis and higher rates of treatment failure
  - Neurosyphilis: Harder to treat; can occur up to 20 years after infection

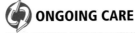 ## ONGOING CARE
FOLLOW-UP RECOMMENDATIONS
Repeat titers at 3, 6, 9, and 12 months after treatment; if >1 year's duration, check at 24 months also.

Patient Monitoring
- Use VDRL or RPR test to monitor therapy: 4-fold rise in titer indicates new infection, whereas failure to decrease 4-fold in 6 months is considered treatment failure (although definitive criteria for cure not established); titers not consistent between tests; always use same test, preferably the same lab, as initially used to perform the test.

- Retreat for persistent clinical signs or recurrence, 4-fold rise in titers, or failure of initially high titer to decrease 4-fold by 6 months.

DIET
Normal diet should continue as healing requires appropriate nutrition.

PATIENT EDUCATION
- Education of patient after treatment to avoid future STDs
- Consistent and correct use of latex condoms can reduce risk of acquiring further syphilis infections or other STDs.

PROGNOSIS
Excellent in all cases with appropriate treatment except patients with late syphilis complications and with HIV infection

COMPLICATIONS
- Jarisch-Herxheimer reaction: Common when starting treatment (of primary or secondary disease; less common with tertiary):
  - Lysis of treponemes and endotoxin release leading to fever, chills, headache, myalgias, new or worsening rash
  - Can be confused with drug reaction
  - Managed supportively
- Cardiovascular
- Cerebral vascular accidents
- Skin and connective tissue abnormalities
- Membranous glomerulonephritis
- Paroxysmal cold hemoglobinemia
- Meningitis and tabes dorsalis
- Irreversible organ damage
- Increased risk of HIV infection
- Congenital syphilis may lead to stillbirth, miscarriage, or infant death

REFERENCES
1. Centers for Disease Control and Prevention. *Sexually Transmitted Disease Surveillance 2009.* Atlanta: U.S. Department of Health and Human Services, 2010.
2. Sexually transmitted diseases treatment guidelines, 2010. *MMWR Recomm Rep.* 2010;59(RR-12): 26–40.
3. U.S. Preventive Services Task Force. Screening for syphilis infection in pregnancy: U.S. Preventive Services Task Force reaffirmation recommendation statement. *Ann Intern Med.* 2009;150:705–9.

 ## CODES

ICD9
- 091.2 Other primary syphilis
- 091.9 Unspecified secondary syphilis
- 647.00 Syphilis of mother, complicating pregnancy, childbirth, or the puerperium, unspecified as to episode of care

CLINICAL PEARLS
- Syphilis is the "great imitator" as it can affect nearly every organ/tissue in the body.
- Screen all pregnant women during 1st prenatal visit.
- Think about syphilis with rash of unclear origin or painless genital or anal ulcer.
- Test all patients with syphilis for HIV.

S

TEMPORAL ARTERITIS

Daniela Levi

BASICS

DESCRIPTION
- A systemic, granulomatous, predominantly large-vessel arteritis, most commonly affecting the branches of the cranial arteries (but may involve other aortic branches), seen primarily in the elderly
- Frequently associated with polymyalgia rheumatica (PMR)
- System(s) affected: Cardiovascular; Hemic/Lymphatic/Immunologic; Musculoskeletal; Nervous
- Synonym(s): Giant-cell arteritis; Horton headache

EPIDEMIOLOGY
- Predominant age: >60 (very rare <50 years).
- Incidence increases with age.
- Females > Males (2:1)

Pediatric Considerations
Does not occur in this age group

Geriatric Considerations
Incidence increases with age (twice as common in patients >80 years as it is in ages 50–59 years).

Incidence
More common in northern latitudes (15–30/100,000 person >50 years per year) vs. southern latitudes (<2/100,000 in some series)

RISK FACTORS
- Age >50 years
- Presence of polymyalgia rheumatica
- Heavy smoking and atherosclerosis in women but not in men

Genetics
May be important; several family clusters have been identified; Northern European descent

PATHOPHYSIOLOGY
- Panarteritis with mononuclear infiltrates penetrating all layers of the arterial wall:
  - A T-cell dependent disease (CD4+)
  - Dendritic cells activate the T cells in the arterial wall.
  - Activation of monocytes and macrophages lead to a systemic inflammatory syndrome.
  - The blood vessel determines the site-specificity of giant-cell arteritis.
  - Granuloma formation is a T cell-dependent process.

ETIOLOGY
- Cell-mediated immune response: CD4 cells
- Monocyte, macrophages, and dendritic cells
- Interferon γ, IL-1, 6, 12 production

COMMONLY ASSOCIATED CONDITIONS
Polymyalgia rheumatica

DIAGNOSIS

HISTORY
- Onset may be abrupt or insidious over months.
- Local:
  - Headache (usually unilateral temporal, may be generalized or occipital) seen in 2/3 of patients
  - Jaw/tongue "claudication" on mastication (fairly specific)
  - Visual disturbances: Early (amaurosis fugax, scotoma, diplopia) or late (ischemic optic neuritis, blindness)
  - Scalp tenderness
  - Swollen, red temporal artery (rare)
  - Decreased temporal artery pulse (may be increased early)
  - Sore throat, cough (10%)
  - Neurologic manifestations: Transient ischemic attack, stroke
- Systemic:
  - Polymyalgia rheumatica: Seen in 40–60%
  - Fever (low grade): 15% with fever of unknown origin
  - Fatigue/malaise
  - Weight loss/anorexia, arthralgias, myalgias, arthritis

PHYSICAL EXAM
- Tender temporal artery
- Proximal muscle tenderness with normal strength
- Loss of visual fields

DIAGNOSTIC TESTS & INTERPRETATION
Lab
- Erythrocyte sedimentation rate (ESR; Westergren) usually >50 mm/hr (may be >100 mm/hr):
  - Westergren ESR is preferable. If other ESR used (e.g., Wintrobe), then cannot use the listed guidelines for abnormalities.
  - ESR may be normal in <10% of patients.
  - Finding of a normal ESR is not compatible with the diagnosis of giant-cell arteritis
- C-reactive protein level has been found to be a sensitive indicator of disease.
- Interleukin-6 levels appear to be a sensitive indicator of active disease.
- Elevated alkaline phosphatase >1.5 times normal (unusual)
- Elevated aspartate aminotransferase >1.5 times normal (unusual)
- Anemia:
  - Mild to moderate
  - Normochromic/normocytic

- Mild leukocytosis
- Mild thrombocytosis
- Microscopic hematuria (30%)
- Drugs that may alter lab results: Prednisone, methotrexate, other immunosuppressives

Imaging
- Temporal arteriography (in selected cases)
- US is positive in 90%; may help to direct biopsy.
- Arteriography, CT, or MR angiography are required tests when suspected extracranial vasculitis:
  - On arteriography, typical finding is bilateral stenosis or occlusion of the subclavian, axillary, or brachial arteries.

Diagnostic Procedures/Other
- Temporal artery biopsy:
  - Minimum 2.5-cm segment of vessel with serial sections
  - Within 72 hours of starting steroids
  - If negative, must consider biopsy of contralateral artery (may increase yield up to 10–14%)

Pathological Findings
- Inflammatory infiltrate (either mononuclear cells or granulomas with giant multinucleated cells) seen in the intima and media of large vessels with resultant disruption of the internal elastic lamina
- Lesions may be isolated (e.g., skip lesions).
- Biopsy may not show evidence of active arteritis.
- Changes of healing arteritis or vasculitis support the diagnosis of giant-cell arteritis.

DIFFERENTIAL DIAGNOSIS

- Cerebral vasculitides
- Other causes of headache (tumor, other space-occupying lesions, sinusitis, cervical or temporomandibular joint arthritis)
- Cerebral vascular insufficiency
- Other connective tissue disease
- Retinal detachment or other causes of loss of vision
- Septic arteritis
- Embolic disease

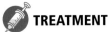 TREATMENT

MEDICATION
First Line
- Prednisone —early:
  - 60 mg/d; single morning dose (do not use every-other-day steroids)
  - Begin slow taper after 6–8 weeks if asymptomatic and ESR is decreased (occasionally patient may not normalize ESR).
- Prednisone —taper:
  - Taper initially by 5 mg every 2 weeks to dose of 25 mg. Then slow taper by 2.5-mg decrements every 2–4 weeks to a dose of 10–15 mg if guidelines described in preceding sections are met (must be individualized)
  - Continue 10–15 mg/d for several months to a year, with periodic attempts to taper (e.g., every 3–6 months) by 1–2 mg.
  - Use symptoms and ESR to help guide taper.
  - Average time to disease remission: 3–4 years, range 1–10 years
- Contraindications:
  - Systemic fungal infections, although physician must evaluate risks and benefits
  - Relative contraindications: Avoid, if possible, in patients with CHF, DM, systemic fungal or bacterial infection (must treat infection concurrently if steroids are necessary).
- Precautions:
  - Long-term steroid use:
    - Associated with several potentially severe adverse effects, including increased susceptibility to infection, glucose intolerance, adrenal suppression, muscle wasting, osteoporosis, peptic ulcer disease, sodium and water retention, cataracts, avascular necrosis, GI bleeding, psychosis, weight gain
    - Use lowest possible dose once there is successful taper and absence of symptoms.
    - On discontinuing, if the patient has received long-term therapy, taper slowly to avoid addisonian crisis. May need temporary stress-dose steroids for surgical procedures, accidents, or severe infections
- Significant possible interactions:
  - Refer to the manufacturer's literature.

Second Line
- Aspirin (low-dose 80–100 mg) decreases cranial ischemic events.
- Methotrexate, only if patient cannot use steroids (brittle DM, severe osteoporosis, CHF, etc.) or fails to respond to steroids. Recent studies vary in the efficacy of this treatment.

ADDITIONAL TREATMENT
General Measures
Institute surveillance for corticosteroid side effects, including monitoring serum glucose and osteoporosis screening.

SURGERY/OTHER PROCEDURES
Temporal artery biopsy

 ONGOING CARE

FOLLOW-UP RECOMMENDATIONS
Patient Monitoring
- ESR:
  - Repeat monthly initially and while tapering, then every 3 months.
- Follow visual/constitutional symptoms monthly initially, then as needed.

PROGNOSIS
- With early treatment, resolution of symptoms and preservation of vision
- Average duration of disease 3–4 years
- With no treatment, high risks of blindness and stroke
- Occasionally, ESR elevation is not related to giant-cell arteritis activity and cannot be used to monitor and/or adjust treatment.

COMPLICATIONS
- Complications related to steroids, particularly osteoporosis, infection, skin changes, salt retention, and glucose intolerance
- Exacerbation of disease during therapy or taper
- Blindness
- Stroke

ADDITIONAL READING
- Gonzales-Gay MA, et al. Giant cell arteritis: Disease patterns of clinical presentation in a series of 240 patients. *Medicine*. 2005;84:269.
- Hellman DB, Hunder GG. Giant cell arteritis and polymyalgia rheumatica. In: Harris ED et al., eds., *Textbook of Rheumatology*, 7th ed. Philadelphia: Saunders; 2005:1343–56.

- Hoffman GS, Stone JH. Disparate results in studies of methotrexate in the treatment of giant cell arteritis. *Arthritis Rheum*. 2002;46:1309.
- Hunder GG, et al. The American College of Rheumatology 1990 criteria for the classification of giant cell arteritis. *Arthritis Rheum*. 1990;33:1122–8.
- Lee MS, et al. Antiplatelet and anticoagulant therapy in giant cell arteritis. *Arthritis Rheum*. 2006;54:3306.
- Liozon E. Risk factors for visual loss in giant cell arteritis. *Am J Med*. 2001;111:211.
- Salvarani C. Polymyalgia and giant-cell arteritis. *N Engl J Med*. 2002;347:261.
- Weyland CM. Medium- and large-vessel vasculitis. *N Engl J Med*. 2003;439:160.

 CODES

ICD9
- 339.00 Cluster headache syndrome, unspecified
- 446.5 Giant cell arteritis

CLINICAL PEARLS
- If clinically active disease (headache, jaw claudication, elevated ESR), treat it as a giant-cell arteritis and use high-dose steroids.
- Normal ERS can virtually rule out temporal arteritis.
- Temporal arteritis has a strong association with polymyalgia rheumatica.

T

TETANUS

Amanda Kolb
David A. Chad

 BASICS

DESCRIPTION
- Severe toxic bacterial infection by *Clostridium tetani* characterized by intermittent tonic spasms of voluntary muscles
- 4 types:
  - Generalized
  - Localized
  - Cephalic (affects cranial nerves)
  - Neonatal (very high mortality)
- Usual course is acute, self-limited; 3–6 weeks duration; may be fatal
- System(s) affected: Nervous
- Synonym(s): Lockjaw (1)

Pediatric Considerations
- Mortality is high in young.
- Infection may enter through umbilical cord.

Pregnancy Considerations
- Must treat vigorously despite pregnancy
- Infection may enter uterus postpartum.
- Tetanus toxoid administered in 2nd and 3rd trimester of pregnancy if indicated or in higher risk patients will reduce neonatal tetanus deaths (2)[A].

EPIDEMIOLOGY
Incidence
- Rare in U.S.
- 700,000–1,000,000 cases annually worldwide

Prevalence
- Predominant age: >70% of cases in persons >50, less likely to have had vaccine booster
- Males > Females

RISK FACTORS
- Lack of vaccination/up-to-date booster
  - Age >40 makes adequate antibody coverage less likely
- Burns
- IV drug use
- Puncture wounds/crush injury/surgical wounds
- Early postpartum with an infected uterus
- Exposure of open wounds to soil/animal feces
- Frostbite
- Newborn (umbilicus stump entry)
- Skin ulcers
- Age >50
- Wound with low O_2 supply/chronic wounds

GENERAL PREVENTION
- Active immunization with tetanus toxoid:
  - DTaP (diphtheria and tetanus toxoid and acellular pertussis): For children 6 weeks–7 years of age. Primary series of 4 doses at 2, 4, 6, and 15–18 months. Follow with booster at 4 years of age.
  - Tdap (Tetanus, diphtheria, acellular pertussis): Give 1 dose at 11–12 years if 5 years since DTaP. Important for people in contact with infants <12 months and health care workers
  - Td boosters every 10 years (2)
- Wound debridement
- Passive immunization with tetanus immune globulin (TIG) postexposure
- Benzathine penicillin, penicillin G, erythromycin

PATHOPHYSIOLOGY
- Exotoxin tetanospasmin produced by germinating *C. tetani* spores enters body through wound, disseminates through blood and lymph.
- Incubation period is 4–14 days after injury.
- Tetanospasmin acts at motor neuron end-plates, enters CNS peripherally, travels centrally to brain and sympathetic nervous system, and alters neurotransmitter release.
- Blocks inhibitory neurons; results in unopposed muscle contraction/spasm/seizure (3)

ETIOLOGY
- Infection with *C. tetani* (anaerobic gram-positive bacilli) associated with foreign body that is contaminated by another bacteria in poorly vascularized tissue (*C. tetani* will not grow in healthy tissue on its own)
- Neurotoxin tetanospasmin causes symptoms.

COMMONLY ASSOCIATED CONDITIONS
See Risk Factors

 DIAGNOSIS

HISTORY
- Some penetrating injury (splinter, nail, IVDU) infected with *C. tetani* and co-infected with other bacteria in a region of relative hypoxia.
- History of contamination with soil/manure may increase risk as *C. tetani* spores are prevalent in the feces of domesticated animals.

PHYSICAL EXAM
- Arrhythmias
- Asphyxia
- Convulsions
- Cyanosis
- Dysphagia/drooling
- Fluctuating HTN/hypotension
- Hydrophobia
- Hyperhidrosis
- Hyperpyrexia
- Hyperreflexia
- Irritability
- Low-grade fever
- Muscular rigidity/spasticity
- Nuchal rigidity
- Opisthotonos
- Pain at wound site
- Painful tonic convulsions
- Risus sardonicus (fixed smile)
- Stiffness of the jaw (lockjaw)
- Sudden bradycardia/tachycardia
- Sudden cardiac arrest
- Tingling at wound site
- Trismus

DIAGNOSTIC TESTS & INTERPRETATION
Lab
- CBC: Polymorphonuclear leukocytosis
- Culture/Gram stain of *C. tetani* from wound will reveal anaerobic gram-positive large rods in only 30% of cultures; more often culture is negative.

Imaging
Diagnosis is clinically based; no definitive test.

Diagnostic Procedures/Other
- ECG: Supraventricular tachycardia, multifocal ventricular ectopia, bradycardia
- EEG sleeping pattern
- Spatula test: Touch oropharynx with tongue blade, if gag reflex elicited, test is negative; if patient bites down on blade, test is positive. 94% sensitive; 100% specific (4)
- Antitoxin assay (not readily available) levels >0.01 IU/mL are protective; tetanus less likely

DIFFERENTIAL DIAGNOSIS
- Acute dystonic reaction: Phenothiazines, metoclopramide, MAO inhibitors, SSRIs
- Subarachnoid hemorrhage
- Seizure disorder
- Meningoencephalitis
- Peritonsillar abscess
- Hypocalcemic tetany
- Strychnine poisoning
- Alcohol withdrawal
- Amyotrophic lateral sclerosis
- Conversion disorder

TREATMENT

MEDICATION
First Line
- Diazepam for muscle rigidity: 5–10 mg PO q4–6h p.r.n. if mild; mix 50–100 mg in 500 mL D5W and infuse at 40 mg/h if severe
- Tetanus toxoid in a previously immunized patient
- TIG: 3000–6000 U IM. May infiltrate the area around the wound with a portion of the dose
- Intrathecal immunoglobulin (1000 U lyophilized human immunoglobulin) reduces spasms, hospital stay, and respiratory assistance (NNT 4.2) (5)[A].
- Metronidazole may decrease mortality; some reviews consider it drug of choice. 1 g IV q12h not to exceed 4 g/d (6)[C].
- Penicillin G: 2 million U IV q6h. Traditionally considered drug of choice.
- Doxycycline 100 mg q12h, or clindamycin 150–300 mg IV q6h if penicillin-allergic
- Precautions: Do not use TIG IV. Administer IM in different location than toxoid to avoid reaction.

Second Line
- Equine tetanus antitoxin: 50,000 U IM, but only if TIG (human) is not available.
- Chlorpromazine/phenobarbitone for muscle rigidity; higher mortality and longer, more severe clinical course than diazepam(7)[A]

ADDITIONAL TREATMENT
General Measures
- Quiet observation
- Adequate caloric supply
- DVT and ulcer prophylaxis

Issues for Referral
- Primary physician should be ICU specialist.
- If respiratory symptoms are severe, consult pulmonologist.
- If considering intrathecal therapy, consult anesthesiologist.

Additional Therapies
Physical therapy once spasms resolve

SURGERY/OTHER PROCEDURES
- Wound debridement
- Tracheostomy if needed

IN-PATIENT CONSIDERATIONS
Initial Stabilization
- Intubation: Consider prophylactic intubation with moderate/severe symptoms:
  - Prepare for emergency surgical airway due to reflex laryngospasm.
- Anticonvulsants for muscle spasm/rigidity

Admission Criteria
Diagnosis of tetanus
IV Fluids
IV hydration necessary
Nursing
- Catheterize bladder.
- Maintain quiet, dark environment and minimize manipulation/procedures to avoid triggering spasm.

 # ONGOING CARE

FOLLOW-UP RECOMMENDATIONS
- Tetanus immunization series is necessary; infection does NOT confer immunity.
- Sequelae after infection are rare.

Patient Monitoring
Admit to ICU due to possible cardiac arrhythmias, autonomic dysfunction, and respiratory failure.

DIET
NPO until well, feed by NG/PEG tube

PATIENT EDUCATION
Importance of tetanus immunization

PROGNOSIS
- 25–50% mortality
- Poor prognostic factors:
  - Autonomic system involvement
  - Form of tetanus: Neonatal > generalized > cephalic > localized
  - Short incubation period
  - Patient's age
  - Severity of symptoms
  - Heart wound
- Recovery is complete if patient survives.

COMPLICATIONS
- Respiratory arrest
- Cardiac failure
- Pulmonary emboli
- Bacterial infection
- Dehydration
- Vertebral fractures
- Airway obstruction
- Anoxia
- Urinary retention
- Constipation
- Pneumonia
- Rhabdomyolysis

REFERENCES
1. CDC. Tetanus: US 1981–1984. Morb Mort Wkly Rep MMWR. 1985;34:602.
2. Demicheli V, et al. Vaccines for women to prevent neonatal tetanus. Cochrane Database Syst Rev. 2008;1:CD002959.
3. Tetanus. Epidemiology and prevention of vaccine-preventable diseases. Accessed at CDC Web site http://www.cdc.gov/vaccines/vpd-vac/tetanus 2008.
4. Apte NM, et al. Short report. The spatula test: A simple bedside test to diagnose tetanus. Am J Trop Med Hyg. 1995;53:386–7.
5. de Barros D, et al. Randomised controlled trial of tetanus treatment with antitetanus immunoglobulin by the intrathecal or intramuscular route. BMJ. 2004;328:615.
6. Ahmadsyah I, et al. Treatment of tetanus: An open study to compare the efficacy of procaine penicillin and metronidazole. Br Med J (Clin Res Ed). 1985;291:648.
7. Okoromah CAN, et al. Diazepam for treating tetanus. Cochrane Neonatal Group. Cochrane Database Syst Rev. 2008;1.

ADDITIONAL READING
- CDC. Summary of Recommendations for Childhood and Adolescent Immunizations. 2011. http://www.cdc.gov/vaccines/recs/schedules/child-schedule.htm

CODES

ICD9
037 Tetanus

CLINICAL PEARLS
- Tetanus is a self-limited infection caused by C. tetani; it can be severe and life-threatening.
- Infection is associated with contaminated wounds and unclear vaccination history.
- Immunization is essential to prevention.
- Diagnosis is clinical and must be considered in patients with muscle spasms despite lab results often being negative.
- Treatment involves neutralizing toxin, vaccinating, and providing antibiotics; however, supportive care is the mainstay of therapy to prevent complications.

THEOPHYLLINE OVERDOSE

Aditya Kasarabada
James Gasperino

 BASICS

DESCRIPTION
- Theophylline is a dimethylxanthine.
- Inhibits several members of the phosphodiesterase enzyme family
- Low therapeutic index
- Likelihood of toxic side effects increases at higher plasma concentrations but there is no predictable relationship.

EPIDEMIOLOGY
Incidence
- 757 reported overdose cases in 2004, of which 516 were unintentional
- 3 deaths in 2004

Prevalence
- ~30% of patients with theophylline concentrations >15 mg/L have signs of mild toxicity.
- 75–80% of patients with plasma levels ≥25 mg/L have side effects.

RISK FACTORS
- Plasma clearance decreases in drug interactions, smoking cessation, cirrhosis, acute hepatitis.
- Plasma clearance also decreases in CHF, hypothyroidism, acute pulmonary edema, sepsis, and shock.
- Predictors:
  - Peak serum concentration in acute intoxication
  - Age >60 years in chronic intoxication

Pregnancy Considerations
- Theophylline crosses the placenta.
- Adverse effects may be seen in the newborn.
- Use is generally safe at the recommended doses (serum concentrations 5–12 μg/mL).

GENERAL PREVENTION
Many medicines can interact with theophylline. Knowledge of all new prescription and over-the-counter medications is essential to avoid drug–drug interactions.

PATHOPHYSIOLOGY
- ~60% protein bound
- 85–90% eliminated by cytochrome P450 in the liver (CYP1A2)
- 10–15% urinary excretion
- CNS stimulation
- Cardiac stimulation
- Induces release of epinephrine
- Increases gastric acid secretion

ETIOLOGY
- Intoxication may result from either an acute ingestion or chronic use.
- Chronic intoxication may cause more severe clinical sequelae due to larger total body stores of drug.
- Patient and physician dosing errors decrease drug clearance and lead to the development of congestive heart failure or hepatic dysfunction.

COMMONLY ASSOCIATED CONDITIONS
Asthma

 DIAGNOSIS

HISTORY
- Mild toxicity includes nausea, vomiting, abdominal pain, tachycardia, and muscle tremor.
- Severe toxicity includes hypotension, cardiac arrhythmias, seizures, and death.
- Serum levels of 15 mg/L may cause anorexia, nausea, vomiting.
- Serum levels >40 mg/L may cause seizures and arrhythmias.

PHYSICAL EXAM
- Tremors, restlessness, agitation, seizures
- Sinus tachycardia, tachyarrhythmias
- Hypotension

DIAGNOSTIC TESTS & INTERPRETATION
Lab
Initial lab tests
- ECG to look for arrhythmias: Ventricular and supraventricular
- Basic chemistry for electrolyte imbalance
- Hypokalemia, hypercalcemia, hypomagnesemia, hypophosphatemia, hyperglycemia
- LFTs
- Serum theophylline level

Follow-Up & Special Considerations
- Serial BMP
- Theophylline levels

Imaging
CT of the head for other causes of seizures

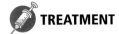 TREATMENT

Predominantly supportive care

MEDICATION

First Line
- Gastric decontamination
- Gastric lavage
- Multiple doses of activated charcoal
- Loading dose of 1 g/kg followed by 15 g every hour for 6–12 hours or 20 g q2h until plasma theophylline level is <20 mg/L
- Also useful in IV overdose

Second Line
- β-Blockers to control arrhythmias caused by excessive β-adrenergic stimulation
- Lidocaine for ventricular arrhythmias
- Diazepam and a barbiturate for refractory seizures
- Avoid phenytoin; can worsen theophylline-induced seizures

ADDITIONAL TREATMENT

General Measures
- Maintain airway.
- Support circulation.
- Correct electrolyte imbalance.
- Provide isotonic fluid boluses for hypotension.
- Resistant hypotension may require vasopressors with predominantly α-agonistic activity (e.g., dopamine, norepinephrine, phenylephrine).

Issues for Referral
Consult regional poison control.

Additional Therapies
- Hemodialysis
- Hemoperfusion (charcoal hemoperfusion is preferred)

- Indications for hemodialysis and/or hemoperfusion:
  – Patient is clinically unstable or has seizures, life-threatening hypotension, *AND/OR*
  – Plasma theophylline concentration >100 mg/L in acutely intoxicated patient
  – Plasma theophylline level >40 mg/dL in a chronically intoxicated patient >60 years
  – Plasma theophylline level >60 mg/dL in a chronically intoxicated patient <60 years

IN-PATIENT CONSIDERATIONS

Initial Stabilization
As above

Admission Criteria
- Admit all patients with signs and symptoms of toxicity.
- Admit patients with theophylline levels >30 mg/dL.

IV Fluids
Isotonic fluids

Nursing
Close monitoring for seizures and arrhythmias

 ONGOING CARE

FOLLOW-UP RECOMMENDATIONS
Serum theophylline levels in 24 hours

Patient Monitoring
- Heart rate
- Respiratory rate
- Monitor for CNS effect
- Serum theophylline levels

PATIENT EDUCATION
Advise patients on the wide range of symptoms caused by acute and chronic toxicity

PROGNOSIS
- Depends on severity of ingestion
- Refractory seizures may require neurologic evaluation and follow-up.

COMPLICATIONS
- Seizures
- Ventricular arrhythmias
- Supraventricular arrhythmias

ADDITIONAL READING

- Annual Report of the American Association of Poison Control Centers Toxic Exposure Surveillance System. *Am J Emerg Med*. 2005;23:589–666.
- Methylxanthines and selective β-adrenergic agonists. In: Hoffman RS, Nelson LS, Howland MA, et al., eds., *Goldfrank's Manual of Toxicologic Emergencies*. New York: McGraw Hill, 2007:553–9.
- Mokhlesi B, et al. Adult toxicology in critical care: Part II: Specific poisonings. *Chest*. 2003;123:897–922.
- Shannon M. Predictors of major toxicity after theophylline overdose. *Ann Intern Med*. 1993;119:1161–7.

 CODES

ICD9
974.1 Poisoning by purine derivative diuretics

CLINICAL PEARLS
- Theophylline has a low therapeutic index.
- In overdose, supportive care is primary treatment.
- Use activated charcoal.
- Observe for indications for hemodialysis and/or hemoperfusion.

T

THORACENTESIS

Jose R. Yunen
Vicente San Martín

PROCEDURE

INDICATIONS

- Diagnostic: Evaluation of pleural fluid to diagnose primary disease process
- Therapeutic: Drainage of fluid to improve respiratory status of the patient

CONTRAINDICATIONS

- Positive pressure ventilation (relative)
- Bleeding diathesis
- Bullous disease on the side of the effusion
- Small effusion with significant risk of injury to the lung during performance of the procedure

TECHNIQUE

See algorithm.

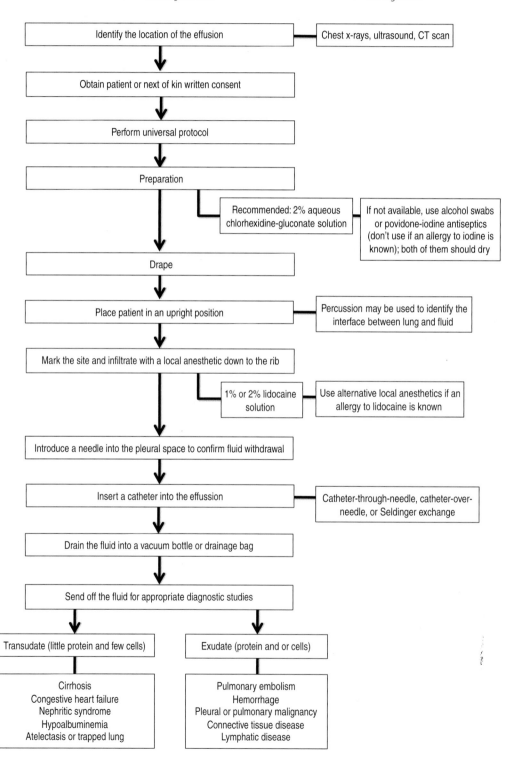

Identify the location of the effusion — Chest x-rays, ultrasound, CT scan

Obtain patient or next of kin written consent

Perform universal protocol

Preparation — Recommended: 2% aqueous chlorhexidine-gluconate solution — If not available, use alcohol swabs or povidone-iodine antiseptics (don't use if an allergy to iodine is known); both of them should dry

Drape

Place patient in an upright position — Percussion may be used to identify the interface between lung and fluid

Mark the site and infiltrate with a local anesthetic down to the rib — 1% or 2% lidocaine solution — Use alternative local anesthetics if an allergy to lidocaine is known

Introduce a needle into the pleural space to confirm fluid withdrawal

Insert a catheter into the effussion — Catheter-through-needle, catheter-over-needle, or Seldinger exchange

Drain the fluid into a vacuum bottle or drainage bag

Send off the fluid for appropriate diagnostic studies

Transudate (little protein and few cells):
Cirrhosis
Congestive heart failure
Nephritic syndrome
Hypoalbuminemia
Atelectasis or trapped lung

Exudate (protein and or cells):
Pulmonary embolism
Hemorrhage
Pleural or pulmonary malignancy
Connective tissue disease
Lymphatic disease

COMPLICATIONS
- Pneumothorax
- Re-expansion pulmonary edema

ADDITIONAL READING
- Thomsen T, et al. Thoracentesis. *N Engl J Med.* 2006;355:e16.

T

THROMBOCYTOPENIA, HEPARIN-INDUCED (HIT)

Stephen M. Pastores
Ann A. Jakubowski

BASICS

DESCRIPTION
- Two types:
  - HIT-1: Nonimmune, due to direct effect of heparin on platelet activation
  - HIT-II: Immune-mediated, due to formation of antibodies against a heparin-platelet 4 (PF4) complex
- HIT-1: Less thrombocytopenia; occurs within 2 days of starting heparin; platelets may recover without stopping heparin.
- HIT-II: Most serious type; more severe thrombocytopenia within 5–10 days of starting unfractionated heparin (UFH) or low-molecular-weight heparin (LMWH); UFH/LMWH must be discontinued; associated with venous and arterial thrombotic events
- System affected: Hematologic
- HIT generally refers to HIT-II

EPIDEMIOLOGY
Incidence
- Variable depending on the heparin formulation, duration of treatment and the clinical context in which heparin is administered (1)[A]
- 0.2–5% in patients exposed to UFH or LMWH for >4 days

Prevalence
Thrombosis within 30 days of HIT diagnosis, 53%

RISK FACTORS
- 10 × higher with UFH vs. LMWH
- Longer exposure to UFH/LMWH
- Prior exposure to UFH in patients receiving LMWH
- Surgical patients; orthopedic vs. cardiac
- Female patients

Genetics
- Polymorphisms of IgG Fc receptor, which deals with HIT antibody clearance
- Polymorphisms of platelet glycoproteins associated with risk of thrombosis in HIT

GENERAL PREVENTION
- Use LMWH rather than UFH for short-term anticoagulation.
- Limit UFH use to <5 days.
- Avoid use of UFH/LMWH in patients with documented history of HIT.
- Avoid heparin flushes in routine care of venous and arterial catheters (2)[B]; avoid heparin-coated catheters in documented HIT cases.

PATHOPHYSIOLOGY
- Premature removal of platelets from the circulation by the reticuloendothelial system and thrombosis
- IgG and IgM antibody response against PF4-heparin complex on the surface of platelets causes activation and aggregation of platelets.
- Theory related to thrombosis; platelet activation leads to production of prothrombotic platelet microparticles or release of procoagulants that promote thrombosis.
- PF4-heparin antibody complex activation of vascular endothelial surface induces release of von Willebrand factor, cytokines, adhesion molecules, and tissue factor.

ETIOLOGY
PF4-heparin complex on platelet surface induces antibody formation, which binds to the complex on platelets and results in platelet activation, aggregation, and clearance.

COMMONLY ASSOCIATED CONDITIONS
- Venous and arterial thrombosis, pulmonary emboli
- Postoperative state: Cardiac surgery, orthopedic surgery

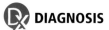

DIAGNOSIS

HISTORY
- Exposure to heparin (UFH > LMWH)
- Thrombocytopenia (<150,000/mm^3 or 50% decrease from baseline) typically occurs within 5–10 days after the initiation of UFH/LMWH.
- Earlier onset if heparin was administered in the previous 1–3 months and circulating antibodies are still present.
- 4Ts (thrombocytopenia, timing of platelet count fall, thrombosis or absence of other causes for thrombocytopenia) are useful for pretest probability assessment (2)[A].

PHYSICAL EXAM
- Excessive bruising at venipuncture site or sites of other trauma, petechiae
- Signs of venous and arterial thromboses, venous limb gangrene, cerebral sinus thrombosis
- Dyspnea +/− chest pain in association with pulmonary emboli
- Necrotic skin lesions at heparin injection sites
- Allergic reaction to heparin injection

DIAGNOSTIC TESTS & INTERPRETATION
Lab
Initial lab tests
- Platelet counts usually >20,000/μL with median platelet count nadir at 60,000/μL
- Serotonin release assay: Gold standard; functional test; >95% sensitivity and specificity; cumbersome, takes several days and fresh platelets are needed to perform test; used most often if ELISA results are questionable.
- ELISA immunoassay for anti-PF4/heparin antibodies: >90% sensitivity, 74–86% specificity; >95% negative predictive value, 50–93% positive predictive value; most commonly used in clinical practice
- Platelet aggregation test: Low sensitivity but >90% specificity.

Follow-Up & Special Considerations
- 10–20% ELISA results may be discordant with the serotonin release assay.
- In complex settings and/or when ELISA is marginally positive, functional assay helps to confirm or refute diagnosis of HIT.

Imaging
Appropriate venous and arterial imaging studies to evaluate for thrombosis (US, echocardiography, CT, MRI)

Pathological Findings
Related to venous and arterial thromboses

DIFFERENTIAL DIAGNOSIS
- Drug-induced thrombocytopenia other than heparin (e.g., glycoprotein IIb/IIIa antagonists, trimethoprim-sulfamethoxazole, valproic acid)
- Sepsis
- DIC
- Bone marrow disease
- Other immune causes of thrombocytopenia (e.g., thrombotic thrombocytopenic purpura/hemolytic uremic syndrome)
- HELLP syndrome (hemolysis with microangiopathic anemia, elevated liver enzymes, and low platelets in pregnancy)
- Catastrophic antiphospholipid antibody syndrome

TREATMENT

MEDICATION
First Line

- Direct thrombin inhibitors (DTIs): Lepirudin, argatroban, bivalirudin (3)[A]
- Lepirudin: Recombinant hirudin; 0.1 mg/kg/hr IV infusion with goal of aPTT 1.5–2.5 times baseline; in the setting of perceived life- or limb-threatening thrombosis, initiate 0.2 mg/kg IV bolus
- Caution with lepirudin in patients with renal insufficiency; recommend dose adjustment for creatinine >1.0 mg/dL as drug is renally cleared
- Antihirudin antibodies may develop (<0.2% risk of anaphylaxis)
- Argatroban: Small, synthetic molecule; cleared by hepatobiliary route; 2 μg/kg/min IV infusion with aPTT goal 1.5–3.0 times baseline
- Dose adjust argatroban (0.5 μg/kg/min IV infusion) with hepatic dysfunction (serum bilirubin >1.5 mg/dL) and in most critically ill patients
- Bivalirudin: Hirudin analog; approved only for HIT in patients undergoing percutaneous coronary intervention; 0.15 mg/kg/hr IV infusion with aPTT goal 1.5–2.5 times baseline

Second Line
Fondaparinux: Has been used but not FDA approved for HIT; long half-life and renal elimination may be important issues for ICU patients.

ADDITIONAL TREATMENT
General Measures
- Immediate cessation of all exposure to UFH/LMWH including heparin-bonded catheters and heparin flushes
- Platelet transfusions only for bleeding
- Postpone warfarin therapy in acute HIT until platelet count has risen to at least 150,000/mm³ (risk of venous limb gangrene with rapid fall in protein C levels)
- Careful overlap of DTI and warfarin should occur (over 5 days); maintain anticoagulation until the platelet count has reached a stable plateau within the normal range
- Use low initial doses of warfarin (<5 mg/d)
- Anticoagulation should be continued for at least 2–3 months in the absence of a thrombotic event and 3–6 months if thrombosis has occurred (3)[B].

Issues for Referral
- Questionable or complex cases of HIT should be referred to a hematology consultant.
- Limb-threatening thrombosis should prompt vascular surgery consultation.

IN-PATIENT CONSIDERATIONS
Initial Stabilization
- Initial diagnosis and management require hospitalization.
- Discontinue all forms of UFH/LMWH and initiate a non-heparin alternative anticoagulant (DTI).
- Evaluate for thrombosis/emboli as clinically indicated with lower extremity US, CT.

ONGOING CARE

FOLLOW-UP RECOMMENDATIONS
Outpatient clinic follow-up while on anticoagulation

Patient Monitoring
- Coagulation test monitoring (PT, INR, aPTT) at 2–3 weeks intervals while on anticoagulation
- Dose adjustments made depending on clinical signs and coagulation tests

DIET
Keep diet consistent, especially the amount of green vegetables while on warfarin.

PATIENT EDUCATION
- Inform patient of heparin allergy; avoid use of any form of heparin.
- Avoid NSAIDs (e.g., aspirin, ibuprofen), binge alcohol drinking, and certain herbal medicines while on warfarin.
- Inform primary physician of intake of any OTC medication or new medication.
- Pursue medical attention promptly for any significant trauma that can result in bleeding.

PROGNOSIS
HIT syndrome is self-limited but can be serious and life-threatening.

COMPLICATIONS
- Venous thromboses predominate in medical and orthopedic patients.
- Arterial and venous thromboses occur at a similar frequency in patients undergoing cardiac or vascular surgery.
- Limb ischemia may result in amputation.
- Thromboses in adrenal veins and central venous sinuses rare.

REFERENCES

1. Arepally GM, et al. Heparin-induced thrombocytopenia. *N Engl J Med*. 2006;355:809–17.
2. Napolitano LM, et al. Heparin-induced thrombocytopenia in the critical care setting: Diagnosis and management. *Crit Care Med*. 2006;34:2898–911.
3. Warkentin TE, et al. Treatment and prevention of heparin-induced thrombocytopenia. *Chest*. 2008; 133:340S–380S.

ADDITIONAL READING

- Hirsh J, et al. Parenteral anticoagulants: American College of Chest Physicians Evidence-Based Clinical Practice Guidelines (8th Edition). *Chest*. 2008;133: 141S–159S.

CODES

ICD9
- 289.84 Heparin-induced thrombocytopenia (HIT)
- 453.9 Embolism and thrombosis of unspecified site

CLINICAL PEARLS

- HIT is an immune-mediated thrombocytopenic disorder that occurs after exposure to heparin and can be associated with serious venous and arterial thromboses.
- Clinical 4Ts (thrombocytopenia, timing of platelet count fall, thrombosis and the absence of other causes for thrombocytopenia) are useful for pretest probability assessment (2)[A].
- All forms of heparin must be stopped in suspected or documented cases of HIT.
- Prompt recognition and treatment with direct thrombin inhibitors (mainly lepirudin, argatroban) can result in improved outcomes.

T

THROMBOCYTOPENIC PURPURA, IDIOPATHIC (ITP)

Louis P. Voigt
Stephen M. Pastores

BASICS

DESCRIPTION
- Acquired disorder manifested by thrombocytopenia (platelets <100,000/μL) in the absence of a clinically apparent condition or medication that may cause a low platelet count.
- May be acute or chronic (>6 months)
- System (s) affected: Heme/Lymphatic/Immunologic
- Synonym(s): Immune thrombocytopenic purpura, Werlhof disease, postinfectious thrombocytopenia

Pediatric Considerations
- May have a sudden onset in children and often occurs after an infectious illness
- Relatively benign in children and tends to resolve spontaneously after several months
- Children who develop severe thrombocytopenia (platelets <10,000/mm^3) or mucocutaneous hemorrhage require treatment.

Pregnancy Considerations
- ITP likely if thrombocytopenia occurs early during pregnancy or if platelet count is <50,000/μL
- Preeclampsia, HELLP syndrome, and gestational thrombocytopenia need to be excluded.
- Severe ITP (platelets <10,000/mm^3) places neonates at <1% increased risk of intracranial hemorrhage; C-section may be required.
- Observation, corticosteroids (prednisone), rituximab, and IV immunoglobulin are commonly used.
- Splenectomy should be deferred if possible, given the increased risk of fetal death and premature labor in early pregnancy.

EPIDEMIOLOGY
Incidence
- Children: 50 cases per 1,000,000 per year
- Adults: 60 cases per 1,000,000 per year

RISK FACTORS
- Age: Younger age (2–6 years), acute ITP; age >50 years, chronic ITP
- Female > Male (chronic ITP)
- Acute infection
- Hypersplenism
- Antiphospholipid antibody syndrome
- Preeclampsia
- HIV infection
- Cardiopulmonary bypass

Genetics
Familial cases and cases in monozygotic twins have been reported.

GENERAL PREVENTION
Avoid medications that inhibit platelet function or suppress the bone marrow.

PATHOPHYSIOLOGY
Related to the combination of increased platelet destruction by reticuloendothelial phagocytes and inhibition of megakaryocyte platelet production through the production of specific IgG autoantibodies by activated T cells in response to platelet membrane glycoproteins (1).

ETIOLOGY
Autoimmune: Involves IgG autoantibodies against glycoproteins in the platelet membrane that cause platelet uptake and destruction by the reticuloendothelial system

COMMONLY ASSOCIATED CONDITIONS
- Autoimmune hemolytic anemia (Evans syndrome)
- Sarcoidosis
- Graves disease
- Hashimoto thyroiditis
- SLE
- Infections due to:
  – Hepatitis C virus
  – HIV
  – *Helicobacter pylori*

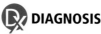
DIAGNOSIS

HISTORY
- Mucocutaneous bleeding: Epistaxis, gingival bleeding, menorrhagia, GI bleeding
- Easy bruisability
- Recent infection
- Exclude other causes of thrombocytopenia

PHYSICAL EXAM
- Petechiae
- Ecchymoses
- Purpura
- Conjunctival hemorrhage
- Signs of GI bleeding
- Absence of splenomegaly

DIAGNOSTIC TESTS & INTERPRETATION
Lab
Initial lab tests
CBC: Isolated thrombocytopenia (<100,000/μL):
- WBC and hemoglobin usually normal unless severe hemorrhage has occurred.
- PT, PTT normal

Follow-Up & Special Considerations
- Assay for antiplatelet autoantibodies is not used in clinical practice.
- Prolonged bleeding time (not useful if thrombocytopenia is present)

Imaging
CT of the head if intracranial bleeding is suspected.

Diagnostic Procedures/Other
- Bone marrow aspiration is not necessary in children and younger patients.
- Bone marrow exam advised in patients:
  – >60 years
  – With atypical presentation

Pathological Findings
- Peripheral blood smear shows decreased but large platelets; large immature platelets may be noted.
- Bone marrow shows normal or increased number of megakaryocytes.

DIFFERENTIAL DIAGNOSIS
- Pseudothrombocytopenia
- Drug-induced thrombocytopenia (including chemotherapeutic and immunosuppressive agents, heparin, quinidine)
- Infections
- Thrombotic thrombocytopenic purpura
- HIV/AIDS
- Lymphoma
- Leukemia
- Evans syndrome
- DIC

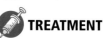
TREATMENT

- Treatment is dictated by severity of symptoms (bleeding):
  – Thrombocytopenia (<30,000/mm^3)
- Current treatment strategies focus on limiting platelet destruction.
- New treatment strategies center on increasing platelet production, but their long-term safety and efficacy are not well established.
- Asymptomatic patients can be observed.
- Patients require treatment in case of:
  – Severe thrombocytopenia (platelets <10,000/mm^3)
  – Frequent hemorrhage
  – Severe hemorrhage (e.g., GI bleeding, intracranial bleeding)
  – Certain surgical procedures, even if asymptomatic and/or with moderate platelet count

MEDICATION
First Line
- Prednisone 1–1.5 mg/kg/d PO for 2–4 weeks then taper (in adults): Acute ITP
- Methylprednisolone: 125–250 mg IV loading dose then 0.5–1.0 mg/kg IV q6h for 5 days in adults
- IV immunoglobulin (1 g/kg IV single dose or 400 mg/kg/d for 5 days)

Second Line
- Rituximab (anti-CD20 monoclonal antibody) for refractory ITP (2)[B]
- IV anti-Rho(D) immunoglobulin (75 mcg/kg) particularly in Rh+ patients
- Splenectomy for refractory cases

Third Line

- Thrombopoietin receptor agonists (3)[B]:
  - Romiplostim (AMG 531)
  - Eltrombopag

ADDITIONAL TREATMENT

General Measures

- Platelet transfusion as a temporizing/supportive measure for severe thrombocytopenia and major hemorrhage
- Remember to rule out IgA deficiency prior to administering IV immunoglobulin.
- Consider eradication of *H. pylori* for patients refractory to steroids or with relapsed ITP.

Issues for Referral

- Hematology consultation to assist in confirming diagnosis and decision-making regarding platelet transfusions
- Neurosurgery consultation in case of intracranial hemorrhage
- ICU admission warranted in cases of:
  - Neurologic symptoms
  - Internal hemorrhage
  - Emergent surgery
- ICU patients often treated with:
  - IV methylprednisolone at 1 g/d for 2–3 days
  - IV immunoglobulin at 1 g/kg/d for 2–3 days
  - Platelet transfusions

Additional Therapies

- Patients undergoing splenectomy should be vaccinated against *Streptococcus pneumoniae*, *Haemophilus influenzae*, and *Neisseria meningitides* at least 2 weeks prior to surgery.

COMPLEMENTARY & ALTERNATIVE THERAPIES

- Hematopoietic stem cell transplantation
- Plasmapheresis

SURGERY/OTHER PROCEDURES

- Splenectomy
- Surgical procedures warrant:
  - Platelet transfusion
  - IV methylprednisolone
  - IV immunoglobulin

IN-PATIENT CONSIDERATIONS

Initial Stabilization

- Depends on platelets count and clinical condition
- Platelets at <30,000 with active bleeding:
  - Methylprednisolone
  - IV immunoglobulin
  - Splenectomy
- Platelets at <30,000 without active bleeding:
  - Prednisone
  - Danazol
  - Dapsone

Admission Criteria

- Major hemorrhage
- Neurologic symptoms
- Severe thrombocytopenia (<10,000)
- Certain surgical procedures

Nursing

- Accidental fall prevention
- Skin care
- Monitor for:
  - Gum bleeding
  - Epistaxis
  - Hematuria

Discharge Criteria

- Variable
- Once platelet count is >20,000/mm^3
- When symptoms resolve

 ## ONGOING CARE

FOLLOW-UP RECOMMENDATIONS

- Close follow-up care by hematologist
- Intermittent CBC to monitor platelet count

Patient Monitoring

- Monitor for side effects of treatment
- Monitor for relapse or treatment failure:
  - Ecchymoses
  - Petechiae
  - Purpura

DIET

No special diet

PATIENT EDUCATION

Avoid medications that may worsen thrombocytopenia, trauma and contact sports

PROGNOSIS

- Mortality ranges from 0.1–5%.
- Mortality increases with age.
- Mortality higher in patients with refractory ITP.

COMPLICATIONS

- Related to ITP:
  - Frequent in cases of poor response to treatment and among the elderly
  - Recurrent bleeding
  - Intracranial hemorrhage (often fatal)
- Not related to ITP:
  - Corticosteroids and immunosuppressive agents increase the risks of infections.
  - Romiplostim and eltrombopag can cause thrombocytosis, bone marrow fibrosis, and rebound thrombocytopenia.
- Anti-D immunoglobulin can cause hemolysis.

REFERENCES

1. Cines DB, et al. Immune thrombocytopenic purpura. *N Engl J Med*. 2002;346(13):995–1008.
2. Cooper N, et al. The efficacy and safety of B-cell depletion with anti-CD20 monoclonal antibody in adults with chronic immune thrombocytopenic purpura. *Br J Haematol*. 2004;125(2):232–9.
3. Newland A. Emerging strategies to treat chronic immune thrombocytopenic purpura. *Eur J Haematol Suppl*. 2008;(69):27–33.

ADDITIONAL READING

- Bussel JB, et al. Eltrombopag for the treatment of chronic idiopathic thrombocytopenic purpura. *N Engl J Med*. 2007;357(22):2237–47.
- Guidelines for the investigation and management of idiopathic thrombocytopenic purpura in adults, children and in pregnancy. *Br J Haematol*. 2003; 120(4):574–96.
- Hino M, et al. Platelet recovery after eradication of Helicobacter pylori in patients with idiopathic thrombocytopenic purpura. *Ann Hematol*. 2003; 82(1):30–32.

 ### See Also (Topic, Algorithm, Electronic Media Element)

- http://www.itpfoundation.org/
- http://www.itpsupport.org.uk/

 ## CODES

ICD9

287.31 Immune thrombocytopenic purpura

CLINICAL PEARLS

- ITP is an autoimmune disease in which circulating antiplatelet antibodies accelerate peripheral destruction of platelets.
- The clinical presentation ranges from acute to insidious, and bleeding episodes may vary from minimal to severe.
- Oral or IV steroids are 1st-line therapy.
- Other treatment options include IV immunoglobulin, IV anti-Rho(D), rituximab, and splenectomy.
- Novel thrombopoietic agents include romiplostim and eltrombopag.

T.

THROMBOCYTOPENIC PURPURA, THROMBOTIC-HEMOLYTIC UREMIC SYNDROME (TTP-HUS)

Ashraf O. Rashid
Stephen M. Pastores

 BASICS

DESCRIPTION
- Multisystem syndromes characterized by thrombocytopenia, fevers, and microangiopathic hemolytic anemia
- TTP patients have predominantly neurological abnormalities
- HUS patients have predominantly acute renal failure
- System affected: Hematologic/Nervous/Renal

EPIDEMIOLOGY
Incidence
- Suspected TTP-HUS: 11 cases/million/year
- Idiopathic TTP-HUS: 4.5 cases/million/year

Prevalence
- More common in females in the fourth decade with a female-to-male ratio of 2:1 (ratio approaches 1:1 after the age of 60)
- More common in blacks than nonblacks (9:1 ratio)

RISK FACTORS
- Pregnancy
- Obesity
- Hematopoietic stem cell transplant
- Medications (e.g. quinine, clopidogrel, ticlopidine, cyclosporine, tacrolimus, valacyclovir, chemotherapeutic agents)
- Factor V Leiden mutation

Genetics
- Mutations of ADAMS-13 gene (A Disintegrin-like And Metalloprotease with Thrombospondin type 1 domains) on chromosome 9q34
- Autosomal recessive and autosomal dominant forms of familial HUS have been reported in children.

PATHOPHYSIOLOGY
- Involves deficiency of ADAMTS13 which is a metalloproteinase that cleaves the unusually large von Willebrand factor (ULVWf) multimers into the normal size range VWf multimers in plasma
- ADAMTS13 deficiency causes the accumulation of ULVWf multimers, platelet aggregation, and platelet clumping.

- An inhibitory autoantibody to ADAMTS13 may also be present in idiopathic TTP cases.
- Endothelial injury promotes platelet activation.
- Increased levels of plasminogen activator inhibitor type 1 (PAI-1) and decreased levels of a normal inhibitor of platelet aggregation may also play a role.

ETIOLOGY
- Hereditary: ADAMS-13 deficiency (rare) and known as Upshaw-Schulman syndrome (autosomal recessive).
- Idiopathic (acquired TTP): Circulating inhibitory antibodies (IgG) directed against ADAMS-13.
- Nonidiopathic: associated with other clinical conditions (malignancy, drugs, e.g., quinine)
- Shiga toxin-producing E. coli: most cases of childhood HUS and occasional adult cases

COMMONLY ASSOCIATED CONDITIONS
- HIV infection
- Autoimmune diseases
- Pregnancy and oral contraceptives
- Disseminated malignancy
- Complication of cancer therapy (mitomycin, cisplatin with or without bleomycin, gemcitabine) and following use of radiation and high-dose chemotherapy prior to hematopoietic stem cell transplantation

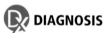 **DIAGNOSIS**

HISTORY
- Fever, malaise, weakness
- Abdominal pain, cardiac conduction abnormalities and hematuria
- Neurologic: headache, visual disturbances, sensory and motor deficits (including paresis), seizure, aphasia, and coma

PHYSICAL EXAM
- Sensory/motor deficits
- Abdominal tenderness
- Petechial hemorrhages mainly in lower extremities
- Signs of retinal ischemia

DIAGNOSTIC TESTS & INTERPRETATION
Lab
Initial lab tests
- Low platelet count, anemia
- Schistocytes and reticulocytes on peripheral blood smear
- ↓Hb, ↓Haptoglobin, hemoglobinuria, reticulocytosis
- ↑ LDH, ↑ unconjugated bilirubin
- Mild proteinuria, hematuria

Follow-Up & Special Considerations
- Negative direct Coombs' test
- Bleeding very rare despite low platelet counts
- Frank acute renal failure uncommon (<10%)
- PT, aPTT and INR usually normal

Imaging
Initial approach
Appropriate imaging studies to rule out other differential diagnoses (e.g., intracranial pathology in case of CNS deficit or malignancy).

Diagnostic Procedures/Other
- ADAMS-13 activity (<5% in 89% of cases)
- Presence of IgG antibodies (50% of cases)

Pathological Findings
Hyaline thrombi composed primarily of platelets in terminal arterioles and capillaries of affected organs

DIFFERENTIAL DIAGNOSIS
- Antiphospholipid syndrome
- Vasculitis
- Malignant hypertension
- Disseminated intravascular coagulation (DIC)
- Scleroderma
- Preeclampsia

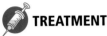 **TREATMENT**

MEDICATION

First Line
- Plasma exchange: treatment of choice
- Advantages: removal of ULVWf and circulating autoantibodies against ADAMS-13 and replacement of the patient's plasma with infusion of normal plasma supplies the missing ADAMTS13

Second Line
- Glucocorticoids (prednisone 1–2 mg/kg daily or methylprednisolone 125 mg IV twice daily): for cases of persistent thrombocytopenia. despite several days of plasma exchange
- Rituximab: anti-CD20 antibody; reserved for refractory or relapsing disease.
- Antiplatelet agents (aspirin, dipyridamole) may be of benefit when added to plasma exchange.

ADDITIONAL TREATMENT

General Measures
- Plasmapheresis is usually continued for 5–7 days until platelet counts recover; premature discontinuation may result in rapid relapse.
- Platelet transfusions should be avoided as these may cause worsening neurological symptoms and acute renal failure.

Issues for Referral
- A hematology consultant should be involved early in TTP-HUS cases.
- Acute renal failure may require referral to nephrologist for consideration of hemodialysis

Additional Therapies
- Vincristine
- Intravenous immune globulin (IVIG)

SURGERY/OTHER PROCEDURES
Splenectomy: for refractory cases

IN-PATIENT CONSIDERATIONS

Initial Stabilization
Untreated TTP has a 90% mortality rate and plasmapheresis should be considered early when there is a high index of suspicion.

Admission Criteria
Suspected cases of TTP should be managed in the ICU

IV Fluids
Appropriate IV hydration in patients with acute renal failure

 ONGOING CARE

FOLLOW-UP RECOMMENDATIONS
Outpatient follow-up to check for relapse

Patient Monitoring
Complete blood counts and LDH levels

DIET
Renal diet in case of acute renal failure.

PATIENT EDUCATION
- Avoid using offending drug(s)
- Seek prompt medical attention in the event of any systemic symptom suggestive of relapse
- Online support groups are available (e.g., http://www.ouhsc.edu/platelets/ and http://www.ttpnetwork.org.uk/)

PROGNOSIS
- Mortality rate has decreased from 90% to <20% after advent of plasmapheresis.
- Most of the patients have a single acute episode.
- Hereditary TTP is a chronic disease with frequent relapses every few weeks.
- Half of the patients with severe ADAMS-13 deficiency relapse, usually in the first year.
- Presence of severely reduced ADAMTS-13 activity as well as an inhibitor to ADAMTS-13 has been shown to be associated with a worse clinical outcome.

COMPLICATIONS
- Acute renal failure in <10% of cases; some progress to end stage renal disease
- Stroke
- Myocardial infarction

REFERENCES

1. Franchini M, et al. Advances in the pathogenesis, diagnosis and treatment of thrombotic thrombocytopenic purpura and hemolytic uremic syndrome. *Thromb Res.* 2006;118(2):177–84.
2. George JN. Thrombotic Thrombocytopenic Purpura. *N Engl J Med.* 2006;354:1927–35.
3. Michael M, et al. Interventions for hemolytic uremic syndrome and thrombotic thrombocytopenic purpura: a systematic review of randomized controlled trials. *Am J Kidney Dis.* 2009;53(2): 259–72.

ADDITIONAL READING

- Zheng XL, et al. Pathogenesis of thrombotic microangiopathies. *Annu Rev Pathol.* 2008; 3:249–227.

 CODES

ICD9
- 287.30 Primary thrombocytopenia, unspecified
- 287.33 Congenital and hereditary thrombocytopenic purpura
- 446.6 Thrombotic microangiopathy

CLINICAL PEARLS
- TTP-HUS are life-threatening multisystem disorders characterized by microangiopathic hemolytic anemia, thrombocytopenia, fever, renal dysfunction and neurological abnormalities.
- Pathophysiology is related to deficiency of ADAMST-13 and formation of platelet thrombi in affected organs.
- Treatment with plasma exchange has decreased mortality rate to 10–20%.
- Other treatment modalities include corticosteroids and rituximab for refractory cases.

T

THYROID STORM

Jacqueline B. Sutter
Paul E. Marik

 BASICS

DESCRIPTION
Thyroid storm represents a rare, extreme manifestation of thyrotoxicosis and is a life-threatening multisystemic disease.

EPIDEMIOLOGY
Incidence
- Overall incidence of hyperthyroidism is <1.5%, which represents mostly subclinical disease.
- Thyroid storm occurs in <10% of patients hospitalized for thyrotoxicosis.
- 20–30% of treated thyroid storm may progress to coma and death.
- Most common in 3rd–6th decades
- Previous association with hyperthyroid surgery is now uncommon.

Prevalence
- A rare disorder; 1–2% of patients with hyperthyroidism progress to thyroid storm.
- White and Hispanic populations have slightly higher prevalence than black populations.

RISK FACTORS
- Most common underlying cause of thyroid storm is Graves disease.
- Other precipitating factors associated with thyroid storm include: Infection, stress, DKA, labor, surgery, toxic ingestion of thyroid hormone, iodinated contrast studies and medications, cardiac and pulmonary disease

Genetics
- Thyrotoxic periodic paralysis (TPP):
  - Most commonly seen in Asian men
  - May be AD with incomplete penetrance
  - Presents with proximal symmetric muscle weakness, with possible progression to paralysis and hypokalemia

GENERAL PREVENTION
- Patient education in thyroid medication compliance
- Careful screening and treatment prior to thyroidectomy

PATHOPHYSIOLOGY
- Hypothalamus produces thyrotropin-releasing hormone (TRH), which stimulates the anterior pituitary gland to secrete thyroid-stimulating hormone (TSH), which subsequently activates the thyroid gland to release thyroid hormone.
- The thyroid gland produces thyroxine (T4), which is converted to the biologically active triiodothyronine (T3) primarily through deiodination by the liver and kidneys.
- A small amount of T3 is directly produced by the thyroid gland.
- Thyroid hormone is normally regulated by negative feedback of circulating free hormone:
  - Serum thyrotropin usually is undetectable with increases in T3/T4.

- Thyroid storm is believed to result from increase in free thyroid levels and possible increase in target-cell β-adrenergic receptor modifications in signaling pathways.

ETIOLOGY
- Autoimmune most common
- Other hyperthyroid conditions associated with thyrotoxicosis include:
  - Toxic multinodular goiter
  - Toxic adenoma
  - Molar pregnancy
  - Pituitary tumor
  - Pituitary resistance
- Drug-induced:
  - Supplemental iodine in deficient individuals
  - Contrast media in patients with underlying goiter
  - Amiodarone: Iodine-induced hyperthyroidism (type I) or inflammatory thyroiditis (type II)
  - Exogenous thyroid hormone consumption
- Infectious:
  - Bacterial or suppurative
  - Postviral

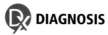 **DIAGNOSIS**

- Differential diagnosis includes: Sepsis, neurolept malignant syndrome, malignant hypertension, CHF, heat stroke, acute mania
- Must have a high index of suspicion

HISTORY
- History of thyroid disease or iodine ingestion (including amiodarone)
- Neuropsychiatric symptoms:
  - Ranges from anxiety or confusion to psychosis and even coma
  - Presence of alteration in mentation may be key feature in establishing diagnosis.
- GI symptoms:
  - Frequent bowel movements and diarrhea due to increased small bowel motor contraction
- Cardiovascular symptoms:
  - Palpitations
  - Chest pain
  - Dyspnea
- Constitutional symptoms:
  - Weight loss due to increased stimulation of lipolysis and lipogenesis
- Reproductive symptoms:
  - Oligomenorrhea
  - Decreased libido
- Ophthalmologic symptoms:
  - Diplopia
  - Eye irritation

PHYSICAL EXAM
- Cardinal features include mental status changes, fever, and tachycardia out of proportion to degree of fever.
- Presence of stigmata of Graves disease, including diffusely enlarged thyroid gland, ophthalmopathy, myopathy, apathy in elderly patients
- Warm, moist skin; widened pulse pressure; presence of shock
- Thyroid storm scoring system may be used to confirm diagnosis:
  - Temperature (99.0 ≥104.0°F): 5–30 pts
  - CNS effects (agitation-coma): 10–30 pts
  - GI dysfunction (diarrhea-jaundice): 10–20 pts
  - Tachycardia (99 ≥140): 5–25 pts
  - CHF (pedal edema; a-fib): 5–10 pts
  - History (negative-positive): 5–10 pts
  - Score >45, highly suggestive of diagnosis; 25–44, supportive ; score <25, unlikely

DIAGNOSTIC TESTS & INTERPRETATION
Lab
Initial lab tests
- Treatment must often be initiated before labs are available, so usually confirmatory.
- Little correlation exists between degree of elevation and manifestation of thyroid storm.
- Pattern of elevated free T4 and free T3 with depressed thyrotropin (<0.05 μU/mL) may be comparable to levels seen in thyrotoxicosis.
- Adrenocortical function is also affected due to acceleration of metabolism of endogenous cortisol and reserve may be diminished.
- Leukocytosis, elevated LFTS, hyperglycemia, and hypercalcemia may also be present.
- Hypokalemia in TPP

Follow-Up & Special Considerations
Avoid aspirin use, which can lead to decreased protein binding and subsequent increases in free T3 and T4 levels.

Imaging
- Chest radiography to identify pulmonary edema or precipitating pulmonary infection
- ECG:
  - Sinus tachycardia is most common
  - Atrial fibrillation
  - Rarely complete heart block
- Nuclear thyroid scan:
  - Diffuse uptake in Graves disease
  - Focal uptake in toxic nodular thyroiditis

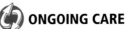

TREATMENT

MEDICATION

First Line

- Mainstay of therapy is aimed at reducing hormone synthesis, blockade of hormone release, and prevention of peripheral conversion of T4 to T3.

- Propylthiouracil (PTU) (1)[A]:
  - Thionamides prevent organification of iodine to tyrosine residues and the coupling of iodotyrosines, and should be administered 1st.
  - Also inhibits peripheral conversion of T4 to T3
  - Adults: 600–1200 mg loading dose followed by 200–250 mg PO q4–6h
  - Children: 6–10 years, 50–150 mg/d PO; >10 years, 150–300 mg/d PO; not established for use in <6 years
  - Has vitamin K activity; may affect levels of warfarin
  - Effects may be seen immediately but therapy usually is needed for 4–12 weeks

- Methimazole (1)[A]:
  - Also inhibits new hormone synthesis
  - Longer half-life permits less frequent dosing
  - Adults: 20–25 mg PO q6h initially

- Iodinated radiocontrast agents:
  - Inhibit thyroid hormone release and peripheral conversion of T4–T3 during first 1–3 weeks
  - Iopanoic acid (not available in U.S.) (1)[A]
  - Should be administered at least 1 hour after thionamide
  - 1 g PO q8 h for 24 hours, then 500 mg PO q12h

- Iodine (1)[A]:
  - Blocks thyroid release of T4 and T3
  - Lugol's solution: Adults/children: 10 gtt PO t.i.d. (can be added to IVF)
  - SSKI: Adults/children: 5 gtt PO q6h

- β-Adrenergic blocking agents for hyperadrenergic symptoms:
  - Propranolol is preferred due to ability to decrease peripheral conversion of T4–T3
  - Improves heart failure that is due to thyrotoxic tachycardia or myocardial depression
  - Adults: 60–80 mg PO q4h or 80–120 mg PO q6h

Second Line

- Glucocorticoids:
  - If hypotension is present or underlying adrenal insufficiency is suspected
  - Large doses of dexamethasone also inhibit hormone production and decrease peripheral conversion from T4–T3
  - Adults: 2 mg PO/IV q6h

Pregnancy Considerations

- PTU is drug of choice in women who are pregnant/breastfeeding (Pregnancy Category D).
- Iodide should not be avoided if possible in pregnancy as it may lead to goiter development in the fetus.

ADDITIONAL TREATMENT

General Measures

- Aggressively search for and treat any underlying infection or other precipitants.
- Provide supportive care and aggressive hydration.
- Use acetaminophen for treatment of hyperthermia.

COMPLEMENTARY & ALTERNATIVE THERAPIES

- Lithium carbonate:
  - Use in patients with thionamide or iodide therapy is contraindicated.
  - Also blocks release of hormone from thyroid gland and new hormone synthesis
  - Adults: 300 mg PO q8h
  - Levels should be monitored regularly to achieve levels 0.6–1.0 mEq/L

- Potassium perchlorate:
  - Use in combination with thionamide in type II amiodarone-induced thyrotoxicosis.
  - Inhibits iodide uptake by the thyroid gland
  - Adults 1 g PO q24h

- Cholestyramine:
  - Use in combination with thionamide.
  - Decreases reabsorption of thyroid hormone from enterohepatic circulation
  - Adults 4 g PO q6h

- Plasmapheresis, charcoal hemoperfusion, and plasma exchange may be used to rapidly reduce levels of thyroid hormone in refractory cases.

SURGERY/OTHER PROCEDURES

- Radioactive iodine ablation (1)[B]:
  - 80–90% will become euthyroid within 8 weeks after initial dose
  - Remainder will require one or more additional doses
  - Development or worsening of ophthalmopathy has been reported

- Thyroidectomy (1)[A]:
  - Curative in 90% of cases
  - Achievement of euthyroid state for weeks prior is optimal; if emergent, rapid lowering of thyroid hormone levels similar to treatment of thyroid storm

IN-PATIENT CONSIDERATIONS

Initial Stabilization

- Assess ABCs.
- Place on cardiac monitor and intubate if profoundly altered mental status is present.

Admission Criteria

Thyroid storm is a medical emergency that must be treated in the ICU.

IV Fluids

Aggressive hydration of up to 3–5 L/d crystalloid to compensate for insensible and GI losses

Nursing

- Aspiration and seizure precautions
- Frequent vital sign monitoring

Discharge Criteria

After initiation of antithyroid medication and maintenance of hemodynamic stability

ONGOING CARE

FOLLOW-UP RECOMMENDATIONS

Follow-up with endocrinology as definitive therapy with radioactive iodine may not be able to be performed until weeks to months after treatment for thyroid storm.

PROGNOSIS

- Usually fatal if untreated
- Early recognition greatly improves outcomes.
- Fatality in treated patients approaches 30% and usually is due to underlying illness.

COMPLICATIONS

- Surgery-related hypoparathyroidism, hypothyroidism, recurrent laryngeal nerve damage
- High-output cardiac failure
- Severe ophthalmopathy causing visual loss or diplopia
- Muscle wasting
- Pretibial myxedema

REFERENCES

1. Nayak B, et al. Thyrotoxicosis and thyroid storm. *Endocrinol Metab Clin N Am.* 2006;35:663–86.
2. Burch HB, et al. Life-threatening thyrotoxicosis. Thyroid storm. *Endocrinol Metab Clin North Am.* 1993;22(2):263–77.
3. Pimentel L, et al. Thyroid disease in the emergency department: A clinical and laboratory review. *J Emerg Med.* 2005(28);201–209.
4. Pearce EN. Diagnosis and management of thyrotoxicosis. *BMJ.* 2006(332):1369–73.

CODES

ICD9

- 242.00 Toxic diffuse goiter without mention of thyrotoxic crisis or storm
- 242.90 Thyrotoxicosis without mention of goiter or other cause, and without mention of thyrotoxic crisis or storm
- 242.91 Thyrotoxicosis without mention of goiter or other cause, with mention of thyrotoxic crisis or storm

CLINICAL PEARLS

- Autoimmune thyroiditis and toxic multinodular goiter are the most common underlying thyroid conditions in thyroid storm.
- Early recognition and initiation of antithyroid therapy is key to patient survival.
- Search for and treatment of precipitating factors are essential.

TICK DISEASES

Parul Kaushik

 BASICS

DESCRIPTION
- Ticks are the most common vectors of arthropod-borne diseases in the US.
- Ticks are divided into Ixodidae (hard ticks) and Argasidae (soft ticks).
- Common tick diseases in the US are Lyme disease, Rocky Mountain spotted fever (RMSF), human granulocytic anaplasmosis (HGA), human monocytic ehrlichiosis (HME), babesiosis, tick-borne relapsing fever (TBRF), tularemia, and Q fever.
- Tick paralysis is a toxin-mediated ascending paralysis that improves with removal of tick.

EPIDEMIOLOGY
Incidence
- Lyme disease is the most common tick disease in the US and the world.
- Although some diseases can occur year-round, peak season for most of the tick diseases is late spring and summer.
- The incidence of tick diseases is increasing due to:
  - Global warming
  - Increase in reservoirs, such as increase in deer population
  - Migration of people from urban to suburban areas
  - Patient/physician awareness

Prevalence
- Lyme disease, HGA, and babesiosis are endemic in northeast and upper midwestern states.
- HME is seen in south central, southwest, and midwestern areas.
- RMSF is found in most of the US states, and >60% of cases have been reported from North Carolina, Oklahoma, Arkansas, Tennessee, and Missouri.
- TBRF and Colorado tick fever (CTF) occur in wild and mountainous areas of western states.
- Tularemia has been reported from many US states but is most common in south central states.

RISK FACTORS
- Travel to endemic area
- Outdoor activities
- Dog owners are found at higher risk of contracting tick diseases.

GENERAL PREVENTION
Wearing light-colored clothes, using insect repellents such as DEET, performing regular tick checks, removing ticks attached to the body and scalp as soon as possible, and showering within 2 hours of coming indoors, especially between April and September, are considered effective preventive strategies.

PATHOPHYSIOLOGY
- Ticks can have 1-host or 3-host life cycle comprising stages of egg, larvae, nymph, and adult.
- Ticks at different stages can attach to the vertebrate host (such as humans) and transmit the organism that in turn attacks the target cells or organs (e.g., vascular endothelial cells in RMSF, leucocytes in ehrlichia diseases, erythrocytes in babesiosis, and bone marrow and lymph nodes in CTF).
- Incubation period varies for different diseases.

ETIOLOGY
- Lyme disease is caused by a spirochete, *Borrelia burgdorferi*; tick-borne relapsing fever is caused by *B. recurrentis,* and southern tick-associated rash illness (STARI) is caused by *B. lonestari*.
- Rickettsial illness such as RMSF is caused by *Rickettsia rickettsii*, small intracellular gram-negative bacteria, and Q fever is caused by *Coxiella burnetii*.
- HME and HGA are caused by *Ehrlichia chaffeensis* and *Anaplasma phagocytophilum,* respectively.
- Tularemia is caused by *Francisella tularensis*.
- CTF is caused by a retrovirus called Coltivirus and is transmitted by *Dermacentor andersoni*.
- Blacklegged tick (*Ixodes scapularis*) transmits Lyme disease, HGA, and babesiosis.
- Lone star tick (*Amblyomma americanum*) transmits HME.
- American dog tick (*Dermacentor variabilis*) transmits RMSF and tularemia.
- *Ornithodoros* tick transmits TBRF.

COMMONLY ASSOCIATED CONDITIONS
Ticks may transmit multiple infections simultaneously.

 DIAGNOSIS

HISTORY
- Often presents with a nonspecific febrile illness
- Fever, chills, headache, myalgia, malaise, and arthralgia.
- Nausea, vomiting, and abdominal pain may occur.
- Lethargy and confusion are seen in RMSF.

PHYSICAL EXAM
- Often unremarkable
- Rash can be present in some of these diseases:
  - 75% of patients with Lyme disease and STARI can present with red, expanding bull's eye lesion at the site of tick bite. Lyme disease can have several of these lesions, called erythema migrans (EM).
  - 90% of patients with RMSF have macular rash that starts from wrists, forearms, and ankles and spreads to the trunk. After 6 days of symptom onset, petechial rash can be seen.
  - In ulceroglandular disease, which is the most common manifestation of tularemia, patient presents with ulcerative lesion with central eschar associated with tender regional lymphadenopathy.
  - Up to 30% of patients with ehrlichiosis can have maculopapular or petechial rash.

- Cranial nerve palsies, joint pain, and effusion can occur in Lyme disease.

DIAGNOSTIC TESTS & INTERPRETATION
Lab
Initial lab tests
- CBC: Leukopenia and thrombocytopenia
- CMP: Elevated transaminases and creatinine
- Blood smear (in ehrlichia diseases, babesiosis and TBRF)
- Serologic studies, such as IgM and IgG, are often negative in the 1st 3–6 weeks.
- ELISA and Western blot tests are used to diagnose early and late disseminated Lyme disease.
- PCR testing

Follow-Up & Special Considerations
Serologies can be repeated a few weeks later to confirm the diagnosis, especially for RMSF, Lyme disease, and ehrlichia disease.

Imaging
Initial approach
- Chest x-ray
- CT head or MRI brain as needed
- Echocardiogram, if endocarditis due to Q fever is suspected

Follow-Up & Special Considerations
Based on the abnormality of initial Imaging

Diagnostic Procedures/Other
- Lumbar puncture in case of meningoencephalitis might show lymphocytic pleocytosis with elevated protein in CSF.
- Synovial fluid in Lyme arthritis has elevated WBC with a median of 25,000/mm with neutrophil predominance.

Pathological Findings
Synovial membrane biopsy in Lyme arthritis shows cellular hypertrophy, vascular proliferation, and mononuclear cell infiltrate.

DIFFERENTIAL DIAGNOSIS
- Viral syndrome and encephalitis
- Bacterial sepsis and meningitis
- Pneumonia
- Hepatitis
- Immune thrombocytopenic purpura
- Tick paralysis should be differentiated from other ascending paralysis such as Guillain-Barré syndrome.

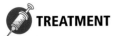

TREATMENT

MEDICATION

First Line
- Doxycycline 100 mg PO or IV b.i.d. or amoxicillin 500 mg PO t.i.d. for Lyme disease. Duration of treatment depends on the stage of disease.
- Doxycycline for RMSF, TBRF, Q fever, STARI, and ehrlichia diseases.
- Streptomycin for 10 days for tularemia
- Chronic Q fever or Coxiella endocarditis requires doxycycline and a quinolone for at least 4 years.
- Clindamycin and quinine for severe, and azithromycin and atovaquone are used for mild-moderate babesiosis.

Second Line
- Gentamicin can be used instead of streptomycin for tularemia.
- Tetracycline for 14 days might be used in mild-moderate cases of tularemia.
- Corticosteroids may be of benefit in encephalitis and vasculitis in RMSF.

ADDITIONAL TREATMENT

General Measures
- Supportive care, airway protection, and hemodynamic stability
- For CTF, the treatment is entirely supportive.

Issues for Referral
Infectious diseases consult is strongly recommended.

Pediatric Considerations
Doxycycline is the treatment of choice for RMSF and Q fever in children of all ages.

Pregnancy Considerations
- Lyme disease in pregnancy can cause fetal demise. It should be aggressively treated with 3 weeks of oral amoxicillin with cutaneous involvement or history of tick bite in endemic area.
- Doxycycline is contraindicated in pregnancy, so rifampin may be used for HME and HGA.

Additional Therapies
Exchange transfusion in babesiosis.

IN-PATIENT CONSIDERATIONS

Initial Stabilization
- Airway protection and circulatory support
- Institution of appropriate antibiotics as soon as possible

Admission Criteria
- Severe disease, presence of complications, and biochemical abnormalities
- Suspected cases of RMSF and tularemia should be admitted for monitoring and treatment.

IV Fluids
As per protocol if patient is unable to take PO

Nursing
May need ICU or neurologic monitoring in ICU, depending on clinical state and complications

Discharge Criteria
Resolution of symptoms

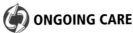

ONGOING CARE

FOLLOW-UP RECOMMENDATIONS
Patient may need to follow-up for repeat serological testing

PATIENT EDUCATION
- If tick is found attached to the skin, remove it as soon as possible using fine-tipped tweezers. Do not use bare hands to remove it.
- If there is fever or rash after a tick bite, see a doctor.
- Post Lyme syndrome, such as chronic fatigue syndrome and fibromyalgia, does not improve with prolonged courses of antibiotics.
- Lyme disease vaccine was removed from the market in 2002.
- Also see "General Prevention."

PROGNOSIS
- Variable, depending on the disease and complications
- Untreated RMSF has 30% mortality. Treatment with antibiotics decreases mortality to 3–5%. Elevated creatinine, immunosuppression, and patients with G6PD deficiency have worse outcome.

COMPLICATIONS
- Untreated Lyme disease may enter into early and late disseminated disease.
- Early disseminated disease is characterized by cranial nerve palsies, lymphocytic meningitis, conjunctivitis, and varying degrees of heart blocks.
- Late disseminated disease can manifest as monoarticular arthritis and cognitive impairment.
- DIC, stupor, coma, acute kidney injury, and multiorgan failure can occur in RMSF.
- Neurologic complication and severe depression can be seen in TBRF.
- Endocarditis with Coxiella
- ARDS, hepatic and renal failure, meningoencephalitis are seen with ehrlichia diseases.

ADDITIONAL READING
- Centers for Disease Control and Prevention. 2011. Ticks. Retrieved from http://www.cdc.gov/ticks/index.html
- Traub SJ, et al. Tick-borne diseases. In: Auerbach PS, ed. *Wilderness Medicine*, 5th Ed. Philadelphia. Elsevier, 2007.
- http://www.cdc.gov/ncidod/dvbid/lyme
- http://www.emedicinehealth.com/ticks/article_em.htm

 See Also (Topic, Algorithm, Electronic Media Element)

See "Ehrlichia" and "Babesia."

 CODES

ICD9
- 082.0 Spotted fevers
- 082.9 Tick-borne rickettsiosis, unspecified
- 088.81 Lyme disease

CLINICAL PEARLS
- Tularemia is a bioterrorism category A disease. *Francisella tularensis* is highly infectious. If made airborne, it can rapidly cause severe respiratory illness and hemodynamic collapse.
- Some of the tick diseases, such as tularemia, Q fever, and RMSF, are reportable diseases.

TOXIC SHOCK SYNDROME

Oveys Mansuri

 BASICS

DESCRIPTION

Toxin-mediated acute illness secondary to infection from *Staphylococcus aureus* or group A *Streptococcus* (GAS) characterized by fever, rash, hypotension/shock, multiorgan system failure, and eventual desquamation of the skin

EPIDEMIOLOGY

Incidence

1–2/100,000 women 15–44 years of age

RISK FACTORS

- Menstruating females (higher risk for those using high-absorbancy tampons)
- Females using barrier contraception
- Nasal surgery with packing
- Postoperative wound infections
- Postpartum state

Geriatric Considerations

Consider surgical site infections and any nonhealing wounds

Pediatric Considerations

May occur after varicella

Pregnancy Considerations

Postpartum and post–cesarian section

GENERAL PREVENTION

- Awareness of early symptoms of severe infection
- Knowledge of immunosuppressed state
- Recognition of foreign body sources (i.e., tampons, intrauterine devices)

PATHOPHYSIOLOGY

- Infection with *S. aureus* or GAS results in production of exotoxins that are absorbed systemically.
- *S. aureus* exotoxins TSST-1 and SEB are most common.
- These toxins function as superantigens, acting directly on T-cell receptors, activating a large portion of the T-cell population. This will lead to high levels of cytokine (interferon-γ, IL2, TNF) production in an uncontrolled fashion and will result in a shock state.

ETIOLOGY

Exotoxins of:

- S. aureus
- Group A Streptococcus (GAS) (M protein important as determinant of virulence)

COMMONLY ASSOCIATED CONDITIONS

- HIV
- Diabetes
- Recent history of chicken pox
- NSAID use

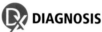 **DIAGNOSIS**

HISTORY

- 20% of patient have generalized flu-like symptoms (fevers, chills, nausea/vomiting, diarrhea).
- Sudden onset of fever, rash, hypotension/shock, end-organ failure
- Tampon use
- Underlying infection and/or abscess
- Postsurgical or postprocedure wounds
- Soft tissue infections, including cellulitis

PHYSICAL EXAM

- Fever
- Shock present within a 4–8 hour period of illness
- Thorough examination of all wounds, surgical or nonsurgical
- Vaginal exam
- Altered mental status (confusion is present in >50% of patients)
- Skin symptoms: Erythema, rash, bullae, desquamation

DIAGNOSTIC TESTS & INTERPRETATION

Lab

- CBC with elevated WBC
- Chemistry panel: Elevated BUN and serum Cr, electrolyte abnormalities
- LFTs: Elevated liver function tests
- Coagulation: Elevated studies
- Urinalysis: Myoglobinuria, hemoglobinuria
- Microbiology: Blood cultures (GAS+, Staph rarely positive), wound cultures and Gram stain

Imaging

Chest x-ray to evaluate for ARDS if indicated

Pathological Findings

Skin: Necrolysis of keratinocytes at different levels of epidermis, perivascular lymphocytic infiltrate, thrombi in superficial capillaries

DIFFERENTIAL DIAGNOSIS

- Cellulitis
- Gas gangrene
- Stevens-Johnson syndrome
- Kawasaki disease
- Drug reactions
- Septic shock
- Meningococcal infections
- Infectious mononucleosis

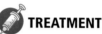 **TREATMENT**

MEDICATION

First Line

- GAS: Clindamycin 600–900 mg IV q8h; some recommend adding penicillin G 4 million U IV q4h [10–14 days of total treatment]
- STTS: Nafcillin or oxacillin 2 g IV q4h (vancomycin for patients with penicillin allergy); 10–14 days of total treatment; may also add clindamycin during initial illness to reduce synthesis of TSST-1

Second Line

IVIG (2 g/kg initially, then 0.4 g/kg over 6 hours for up to 5 days)

ADDITIONAL TREATMENT

General Measures

- Toxic shock is clinically identical to septic shock, hence the "Sepsis management bundle" should be implemented for its management (see Surviving Sepsis Campaign Guidelines)
- Manage septic shock-associated end-organ system dysfunction with supportive care and intervention as needed.

Issues for Referral

- Surgical consultation
- Infectious disease consultation
- ICU consultation

SURGERY/OTHER PROCEDURES
Prompt surgical evaluation and debridement as necessary; may require repeat exams and debridement

IN-PATIENT CONSIDERATIONS
Initial Stabilization
- Antibiotic therapy and source control
- Hemodynamic stabilization and resuscitation
- Tight blood glucose control
- Support of organ systems (i.e., mechanical ventilation, dialysis)
- Follow the guidelines of the "Sepsis management bundle" (see Surviving Sepsis Campaign Guidelines)

Admission Criteria
Most, if not all, patients with a working diagnosis of TSS should be admitted to and cared for in an ICU in consultation with a surgeon, infectious disease specialist, and intensivists.

IV Fluids
- Adequate fluid resuscitation with use of crystalloid replacement (i.e., 0.9% NS or LR)
- Ensure appropriate access and consider central venous access if inadequate access or need for monitoring volume status (CVP)
- Patients refractory to volume support may require vasopressor/vasoconstrictor support.
- Stress dose steroid therapy may also be considered in patients refractory to above measures.

Nursing
- Patient comfort
- Meticulous wound care in consultation with surgeons (if indicated)

Discharge Criteria
Resolution or shock and significant improvement of impaired end-organ functions

 ## ONGOING CARE

FOLLOW-UP RECOMMENDATIONS
At discharge from ICU, generate detailed sign-out assuring safe and seamless transfer of care to floor or for discharge to home and follow-up with primary care physician.

Patient Monitoring
- Continue close monitoring while in ICU
- Arterial line, central venous access with CVP monitoring
- Close and frequent monitoring of urine output
- Frequent examination of wounds and for extension/progression of infection

DIET
Maintain appropriate enteral feeding to optimize nutrition if no contraindications.

PATIENT EDUCATION
- Early recognition of signs/symptoms
- Education for the use of tampons

PROGNOSIS
- 5% of all cases are fatal
- Staphylococcal: 3% mortality, streptococcal: 30% mortality

COMPLICATIONS
- Risk of recurrent episodes of STSS
- End-organ dysfunction/failure may persist
- Shock, ARDS, ARF, DIC
- Death

ADDITIONAL READING
- Conway EE, et al. Toxic shock syndrome following influenza A in a child. *Crit Care Med*. 1991;19(1): 123–5.
- Darenberg J, et al. Intravenous immunoglobulin G therapy in streptococcal toxic shock syndrome: A European randomized, double-blind, placebo-controlled trial. *CID*. 2003;37:333–40.
- Tilanus AMR, et al. Severe group A streptococcal toxic shock syndrome presenting as primary peritonitis: A case report and brief review of the literature. *Int J Infect Dis*. 2010;14S:e208–e12.

 ## CODES

ICD9
- 040.82 Toxic shock syndrome
- 041.00 Streptococcus infection in conditions classified elsewhere and of unspecified site, streptococcus, unspecified
- 041.11 Methicillin susceptible Staphylococcus aureus

CLINICAL PEARLS
- Toxin-mediated illness secondary to infection from *S. aureus* or group A *Streptococcus* (GAS)
- Characterized by sudden onset of shock symptoms (starting with fevers/chills, vomiting/diarrhea, rash)
- Rapid deterioration to hypotension/shock, multiorgan system failure, and eventual desquamation
- Physical exam is focused on soft-tissue infection, postsurgical wounds, and retained foreign body (i.e., tampons).
- Fundamentals of therapy: ICU admission, resuscitation, source control/surgical debridement, antibiotic therapy
- Multidisciplinary approach involving intensivist, surgeon, infectious disease specialist, and other specialists as needed:
  - May have to minimize or eliminate use of tampons
  - Use of antibiotics may be advised during menstrual periods for defined period after recovery

TOXICITY, ACETAMINOPHEN

Muhammad N. Athar
James A. Gasperino

 BASICS

DESCRIPTION
- Acetaminophen is the most widely used analgesic in the US.
- Leading cause for calls to poison control centers (>100,000/year)

EPIDEMIOLOGY
Incidence
In 2003, >1200 cases of severe hepatic injury and 21 deaths were attributed to acetaminophen intoxication, accounting for 23% of all pharmaceutical-related deaths.

Prevalence
- Data from the US Acute Liver Failure Study Group Registry implicate acetaminophen poisoning in ~50% of all acute liver failure cases in this country.
- Accounts for >56,000 emergency room visits, 2600 hospitalizations, and an estimated 458 deaths due to acute liver failure each year.

RISK FACTORS
- Old age
- Tobacco use
- Drugs delaying gastric emptying (e.g., opiates, anticholinergic agents)
- Cytochrome P450 enzyme–inducing drugs (e.g., isoniazid, rifampin, phenytoin, carbamazepine)
- Drugs competing with sulfation and glucuronidation pathway (TMP-SMX, zidovudine)
- Malnutrition

Pregnancy Considerations
Pregnancy risk: B

Genetics
- Gilbert's syndrome (impaired glucuronidation)
- Polymorphisms in the cytochrome isoenzymes

GENERAL PREVENTION
Keep medications out of reach of children.

PATHOPHYSIOLOGY
- Therapeutic maximum recommended daily doses are 80 mg/kg in children and 4 g in adults.
- Toxicity is likely to occur in adults with ingestion of >12 g in 24 hours.
- Completely absorbed from the GI tract.
- Peak levels in blood in 30 minutes–2 hours after an oral therapeutic dose.
- Therapeutic serum levels range from 10–20 μg/mL.
- Levels in toxic ingestions reached at 4 hours of ingestion.
- Half-lives range from 2–4 hours but may be delayed in extended-release preparations.

- At therapeutic doses, 90% is metabolized in the liver to sulfate and glucuronide conjugates and excreted in the urine.
- 2% is excreted in the urine unchanged.
- The remaining 8% is metabolized via hepatic cytochrome P450 (CYP2E1, CYP1A2, CYP3A4) subfamilies into a toxic N-acetyl-p-benzoquinoneimine (NAPQI).
- At therapeutic doses, NAPQI is conjugated with hepatic glutathione to nontoxic cysteine and mercaptate that are excreted in the urine.
- In toxic doses, the sulfation and glucuronidation pathways are saturated, and metabolization to NAPQI via the cytochrome P450 enzymes is increased.
- Depletion of hepatic glutathione stores to 70–80% leads to reaction of NAPQI to hepatocytes, causing injury.

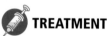 **DIAGNOSIS**

- Collect information regarding amount ingested and time of ingestion.
- Stage I (0.5–24 hours): Nausea, vomiting, diaphoresis, pallor, lethargy, and malaise. Laboratory results are normal.
- Stage II (24–72 hours): RUQ pain
- Stage III (72–96 hours): Encephalopathy, bleeding, jaundice
- Stage IV (4 days–2 weeks): Recovery

DIAGNOSTIC TESTS & INTERPRETATION
Lab
Initial lab tests
- Serum acetaminophen concentration 4 hours after the time of ingestion
- The level should be plotted on modified Rumack-Matthew nomogram.
- Liver enzymes
- PT, PTT, INR
- Renal functions

Follow-Up & Special Considerations
- Serum acetaminophen concentration at 8 hours or 4 hours after first level if extended-release tablet was ingested
- AST, ALT, and bilirubin
- PT, PTT, INR
- Test of renal function

Imaging
CT scan of head for altered mental status

Diagnostic Procedures/Other
ICP monitor

DIFFERENTIAL DIAGNOSIS
- Causes of acute liver failure
- Causes of acute renal failure

TREATMENT

MEDICATION
First Line
- N-acetylcysteine (NAC) is the treatment of choice.
- In acute ingestion, acetaminophen levels are plotted on modified Rumack-Matthew nomogram, and if levels are in "possible risk" for hepatotoxicity area on nomogram, treatment with NAC is standard of care.
- Rumack-Matthew nomogram is not used for extended-release preparation or for chronic ingestions.
- Serum acetaminophen levels obtained prior to 4 hours postingestion are not reliable due to ongoing drug absorption and distribution.
- NAC is also given in single ingestion of >150 mg/kg, for serum acetaminophen levels >10 μg/mL, and evidence of hepatotoxicity:
  - NAC increases glutathione stores, thus conjugating NAPQI to nontoxic substances that are excreted by kidneys.
  - NAC has powerful anti-inflammatory and antioxidant effects.
  - Death is extremely rare if NAC is administered within 8–10 hours of overdose. Efficacy is reduced if administered after 8 hours of ingestion.
  - In oral dose, NAC is available as a 10% or 20% (10- or 20-g/100 mL) solution.
  - 72-hour oral course given as a 140-mg/kg loading dose followed by 17 doses of 70 mg/kg q4h (total dose 1330 mg/kg)
  - In IV dose, NAC is supplied in 30-mL vials containing 20% (200 mg/mL) of NAC (Acetadote).

– IV dose is loading dose of 150 mg/kg in 200 mL of D5W over 60 minutes followed by 50 mg/kg in 500 mL of D5W over 4 hours, followed by 100 mg/kg in 1 L of D5W over the next 16 hours.
– IV dose preferred when patient has intractable vomiting, GI bleeding, bowel obstruction, and acute liver failure.
– NAC should be administered until death or recovery and an INR <2.0.

Second Line
• Cimetidine, an inhibitor of CYP isoenzymes: 300 mg q6h
• Cysteamine and methionine
• Hemodialysis and hemoperfusion

ADDITIONAL TREATMENT
General Measures
• Stabilize airway, breathing, and circulation
• IV fluids
• GI decontamination with activated charcoal (AC)
• AC adsorbs 50–90% of acetaminophen dose if administered within 4 hours.
• Consideration should be given to whole-bowel irrigation if an extended-release preparation has been ingested
• Insert arterial blood pressure catheter and central venous pressure line for close monitoring of hemodynamics.
• FFP for management of bleeding

Issues for Referral
• Early referral to liver transplant institute if unresponsive to medical therapy.
• King's College criteria generally accepted for liver transplant referral (arterial pH <7.3 or grade III/IV encephalopathy plus PTT >100 seconds plus serum creatinine >3.4 mg/dL)

COMPLEMENTARY & ALTERNATIVE THERAPIES
Bioartificial livers

SURGERY/OTHER PROCEDURES
• ICP monitoring may be necessary.
• Liver transplant

IN-PATIENT CONSIDERATIONS
Initial Stabilization
As above

Admission Criteria
• Signs of acetaminophen-induced acute liver failure
• Mechanical ventilation and cardiovascular support
• IV NAC use
• Although definitive treatment guidelines are not well established for patients who present with chronic or repeated ingestions of acetaminophen, transaminase elevation (>50 IU/L) and an acetaminophen level >10 mg/L on presentation have been suggested as indications for treating with NAC.

IV Fluids
• Isotonic
• D5W with NAC

Nursing
Close monitoring for hypotension and liver failure

Discharge Criteria
Decreasing levels of acetaminophen and clinical improvement, including signs, symptoms, and laboratories abnormalities

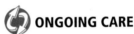 ONGOING CARE

FOLLOW-UP RECOMMENDATIONS
Serum acetaminophen in 24 hours
Patient Monitoring
• Heart rate
• Respiratory rate
• Monitor for ICP
• Serum acetaminophen levels

DIET
Not applicable

PATIENT EDUCATION
Chronic excessive alcohol use may predispose individuals to the hepatic toxic effects of acetaminophen at doses within the high therapeutic range.

PROGNOSIS
Generally good if the antidote NAC is administered within 10 hours of ingestion

COMPLICATIONS
• Hepatic encephalopathy
• Cerebral edema
• Acute renal failure (ATN)

ADDITIONAL READING

• Acetaminophen. In: Hoffman RS, Nelson LS, Howland MA, et al. (eds). *Goldfrank's Manual of Toxicologic Emergencies*. New York: McGraw Hill, 2007:291–300.
• Detry O, et al. Clinical use of a bioartificial liver in the treatment of acetaminophen-induced fulminant hepatic failure. *Am Surg*. 1999;65:934.
• Lee WM. Acetaminophen and the U.S. Acute Liver Failure Study Group: Lowering the risks of hepatic failure. *Hepatology*. 2004;40:6–9.
• Mokhlesi B, et al. Adult toxicology in critical care: part II: specific poisonings. *Chest*. 2003;123: 897–922.
• Prescott LF, et al. Intravenous N-acetylcysteine: The treatment of choice for paracetamol poisoning. *BMJ*. 1979;2:1097–1100.

 CODES

ICD9
• 572.8 Other sequelae of chronic liver disease
• 965.4 Poisoning by aromatic analgesics, not elsewhere classified

CLINICAL PEARLS
• In acute ingestion, acetaminophen levels are plotted on modified Rumack-Matthew nomogram; serum acetaminophen levels obtained prior to 4 hours postingestion are not reliable.
• N-acetylcysteine (NAC) is the treatment of choice.
• Rumack-Matthew nomogram is not used for extended-release preparation or for chronic ingestions.

T

TOXICITY, ANTI-NEOPLASTIC DRUG-INDUCED PULMONARY

Shenaz Georgilis
Saraswathi Devi V. Muppana

BASICS

DESCRIPTION
- Antineoplastic agent-induced pulmonary toxicity is an important cause of respiratory failure (RF) and usually a diagnosis of exclusion.
- Involves parenchyma, pleura, airways, pulmonary vascular system, and mediastinum.
- System affected: Pulmonary

EPIDEMIOLOGY
Incidence
- Variable depending on previous history of radiation, chemotherapy, and/or pulmonary disease
- 10% of patients develop pulmonary toxicity.
- Underdiagnosed worldwide

Prevalence
- Common in patients with underlying pulmonary disease, elderly, and pediatric population
- Highly drug and dose dependent

RISK FACTORS
- Age (for bleomycin, age >70)
- Chemotherapy
- Cumulative dose (BCNU; >1500 mg/m^2)
- Oxygen therapy (bleomycin)
- Combination therapy:
  - Cisplatin/cyclophosphamide + bleomycin
  - Melphalan/epirubicin + radiation
- Prior or concurrent radiation therapy
- Occupational factors (asbestos exposure)
- Previous lung damage (pulmonary fibrosis [PF], COPD, infection, smoking)
- Pulmonary metastatic disease
- Poor functional status

Genetics
- No direct identifiable genetic links
- Underlying disease process (sarcoid in African Americans) may cause increase incidence of pulmonary toxicity.

GENERAL PREVENTION
- Awareness of chemotherapeutic agents, their adverse and synergistic effects
- Careful selection of patients, treatment and stabilization of underlying lung disease

PATHOPHYSIOLOGY
- Hypersensitivity reaction: Methotrexate, etoposide, temozolomide
- Oxidant injury: Mitomycin-C
- Pulmonary vascular damage: Bevazucimab, thalidomide
- Neurogenic pulmonary edema: All-trans-retinoic acid (ATRA), cytarabine, intrathecal methotrexate
- Direct toxic effects: Chromosomal injury due to bleomycin

ETIOLOGY
History of receiving antineoplastic agents

COMMONLY ASSOCIATED CONDITIONS
- Alkylating agents:
  - Busulfan: Alveolar proteinosis
  - Cyclophosphamide: Diffuse alveolar
  - damage (DAD), PF
  - Ifosfamide: Acute pneumonitis (AP)
  - Methemoglobinemia
  - Oxaliplatin: AP, PF, eosinophilic pneumonia (EP), severe anaphylactic reactions
  - Temozolomide: AP
- Antibiotics:
  - Bleomycin: AP (increased with high oxygen exposure)
  - Mitomycin-C, mitoxantrone: AP
  - Doxorubicin: Organizing pneumonia (OP)
- Antimetabolites:
  - Methotrexate (MTX): AP
  - Cytosine arabinoside (Ara-C): AP, DAD, diffuse alveolar hemorrhage (DAH), pulmonary edema/ARDS
- Monoclonal antibodies:
  - Bevazucimab: Pulmonary hemorrhage (PH), Hemoptysis, DVT, Pulmonary embolism (PE)
  - Trastuzumab: Acute lung injury (ALI), AP, OP, bronchospasm
- Nitrosamines:
  - BCNU/carmustine: PF, pneumothorax
- Nucleoside analogs:
  - Gemcitabine: Capillary leak and pulmonary edema, DAD, DAH
- Podophyllotoxin:
  - Etoposide: AP, DAD, bronchospasm
- Rapamycin analogs:
  - Temsirolimus and everolimus: AP
- Taxanes:
  - Paclitaxel and docetaxel: AP, PF
- Topoisomerase I inhibitors:
  - Irinotecan: Pneumonitis (moderate to severe) and RF
  - Topotecan: Bronchiolitis and OP
- Thalidomide: DVT, PE, AP, OP
- Tyrosine kinase inhibitors (2):
  - Gefitinib: AP, DAD, DAH, PF
  - Erlotinib: AP, ARDS
  - Imatinib: AP, fluid retention, PE
- Radiation recall pneumonitis (1):
  - Previous radiation therapy to chest
  - Initiation of chemotherapy
  - Chest imaging: Pulmonary infiltrates in the exact location as radiation field
  - Agents associated: Adriamycin, carmustine, etoposide, doxorubicin, gefitinib, gemcitabine, paclitaxel, and trastuzumab (3)

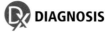

DIAGNOSIS

HISTORY
- History of cancer
- Initiation or continuing treatment with chemotherapy
- Lack of an alternative explanation for respiratory failure

PHYSICAL EXAM
- Nonspecific symptoms
- Fever, nonproductive cough, dyspnea, crackles, decreased breath sounds, hypoxemia
- DVT: Bevazucimab, thalidomide
- Hemoptysis: Bevazucimab
- Bronchospasm: Gemcitabine, trastuzumab
- Pleural effusion: Gemcitabine, imatinib, taxanes, thalidomide
- Noncardiogenic pulmonary edema: Ara-C
- RF and ARDS: Irinotecan, everolimus

DIAGNOSTIC TESTS & INTERPRETATION
Lab
Initial lab tests
- ABG: Hypoxemia at rest
- CBC: Leucocytosis, eosinophilia (MTX)
- Elevated ESR and C-reactive protein
- Elevated serum Krebs von den Lunge-6 (KL-6): Nonspecific, seen in chemotherapy and radiation-induced lung toxicity

Follow-Up & Special Considerations
Pulmonary function tests (PFT): Baseline for diffusing capacity for carbon monoxide (DLCO) and lung volumes

Imaging
Initial approach
Chest x-ray and CT: Diffuse or patchy, unilateral or bilateral, ground-glass opacities or consolidations, or pleural effusions

Follow-Up & Special Considerations
Surveillance of lung function with diffusing capacity, lung volumes, and CT scans

Diagnostic Procedures/Other
- PFT: Initial decrease in DLCO followed by reduced lung volume
- Bronchoscopy, bronchoalveolar lavage (BAL)
- BAL cell counts: Neutrophilia (bleomycin) lymphocytosis (methotrexate), eosinophilia (oxaliplatin), blast cells (ATRA-induced pulmonary syndrome)
  - Positive lymphocyte stimulation test
  - Low CD4+/CD8+ lymphocyte ratio.

- BAL to exclude:
  - Infections (positive cultures, serology)
  - Alveolar hemorrhage (hemorrhagic BAL return and hemosiderin-laden macrophages)
  - Lymphangitic spread of cancer (presence of malignant cells)
- Echocardiogram to exclude:
  - Cardiogenic pulmonary edema
- Transbronchial or open lung biopsy:
  - May show nonspecific pneumonitis, OP, EP, PF, DAD
  - To exclude pneumonia, vasculitis, lymphangitic carcinomatosis

Pathological Findings
- Interstitial inflammatory reaction
- Septal wall fibrin and collagen deposition
- Lung remodeling leading to severe fibrosis

DIFFERENTIAL DIAGNOSIS
- Infectious:
  - Typical and atypical pulmonary infections
- Noninfectious:
- Inflammatory
  - Alveolar hemorrhage
  - Cardiogenic pulmonary edema
  - ARDS
  - Alveolar proteinosis
- Autoimmune:
  - Collagen-vascular disease associated with interstitial lung disease
- Vascular:
  - Pulmonary vasculitis syndrome
  - Pulmonary embolism
  - Pulmonary hypertension
- Malignant:
  - Lymphangitic spread of cancer to lungs

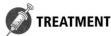 TREATMENT

MEDICATION
First Line
- Discontinue offending agent.
- Oral or systemic steroids (0.5–1 mg/kg/d), depending on the severity. Contraindicated in documented hypersensitivity, fungal, viral infections, GI bleeding.
  - Precaution: Abrupt discontinuation may cause adrenal crisis

Second Line
- Treat concomitant respiratory infections.
- Supportive care with mechanical ventilation
- Avoid high inspired oxygen concentrations in patients receiving bleomycin and mitomycin-c.
- Diuretics
- Bronchodilators

ADDITIONAL TREATMENT
General Measures
- Prescribing the lowest possible dose
- Regular monitoring to aid in early lung toxicity

Issues for Referral
- Complex cases of pulmonary toxicity should be referred to a pulmonologist.
- ICU consultation/admission for patients with severe respiratory distress or failure

Additional Therapies
- Smoking cessation
- Control of underlying lung disease

SURGERY/OTHER PROCEDURES
Video-assisted thoracoscopic surgery (VATS) or open lung biopsy

IN-PATIENT CONSIDERATIONS
Initial Stabilization
- Discontinuation of the offending agent
- Steroid therapy
- Intubation/mechanical ventilation
- Broad-spectrum antibiotics (if indicated)
- Bronchodilators

Admission Criteria
- Hypoxemia
- Severe hemoptysis
- Pulmonary thromboembolic disease,
- RF, ARDS

IV Fluids
Restriction of IVF fluids

Nursing
- Chest physiotherapy
- Monitor fluid status

Discharge Criteria
- Control of hemoptysis, minimum oxygen requirement, able to tolerate feeds
- Instructions to return immediately with worsening dyspnea, cough, fever

 ONGOING CARE

FOLLOW-UP RECOMMENDATIONS
PFT and CT scans

Patient Monitoring
Initially monthly outpatient visits: PFT (DLCO and LV), 6-minute walk test, chest radiographs

DIET
Low carbohydrate diet in COPD patients

PATIENT EDUCATION
- Influenza and pneumococcal vaccine
- Antismoking counseling
- Early recognition of chemotherapy-induced lung toxicity
- Patients with documented drug toxicity should avoid the specific drug in future.

PROGNOSIS
Patients with severe lung toxicity and irreversible fibrosis may be considered for lung transplantation.

COMPLICATIONS
- Pulmonary fibrosis
- RF requiring mechanical ventilation
- Pulmonary embolism, pulmonary hypertension
- Pneumothorax
- Pneumonia

REFERENCES
1. Bobbak V, et al. Pulmonary complications of novel antineoplastic agents for solid tumors. *Chest.* 2008;133(2):528–38.
2. Dimopoulou I, et al. Pulmonary toxicity from novel antineoplastic agents. *Ann Oncol.* 2006;17(3): 372–9.
3. Meadors M, et al. Pulmonary toxicity of chemotherapy. *Semin Oncol.* 2006;33(1):98–105.

ADDITIONAL READING

www.pneumotox.com

 CODES

ICD9
- 478.8 Upper respiratory tract hypersensitivity reaction, site unspecified
- 518.81 Acute respiratory failure
- 963.1 Poisoning by antineoplastic and immunosuppressive drugs

CLINICAL PEARLS
- Comprehensive understanding of drug-specific pulmonary toxicities and high index of suspicion are needed to make appropriate diagnosis.
- Pneumonia, cardiogenic pulmonary edema, and diffuse alveolar hemorrhage must be excluded.
- Open lung biopsy may be necessary in select cases to exclude alternate diagnoses.
- Antineoplastic agent-induced pneumonitis and respiratory failure should be considered in patients receiving chemotherapeutic agents.
- Cessation of the implicated causative agent and treatment with systemic steroids may result in rapid improvement.

T

TOXICITY, ASPIRIN

Muhammad N. Athar
James A. Gasperino

 BASICS

DESCRIPTION
- Aspirin is a widely prescribed antiplatelet therapy.
- Methyl salicylate (oil of wintergreen) is a common ingredient in liniments and ointments used for musculoskeletal pain.
- One teaspoon (5 mL) of oil of wintergreen contains 7 g of salicylate, which is the equivalent of 21.7 adult aspirin tablets.

Pediatric Considerations
- Aspirin causes Reye's syndrome in children.
- 3 g of aspirin intake can be fatal in children.

Pregnancy Considerations
Pregnancy risk: C

EPIDEMIOLOGY
Incidence
- In 2004, poison control centers in the US reported 40,405 human exposures to salicylates.
- Of these exposures, 25,239 were unintentional; 44% involved children <6 years.
- Aspirin as a single agent was involved in 18,181 cases (45%). Aspirin in combination with other drugs contributed 9267 cases (23%).
- Methyl salicylate was involved in 12,005 cases (30%), and other nonaspirin salicylates accounted for 952 cases (2%).
- 1% mortality rate

Prevalence
In 2004, 3804 cases of salicylate exposure resulting in moderate toxicity were reported and 1% with severe toxicity. There were 64 deaths (0.2%).

RISK FACTORS
Patients with poor pulmonary reserve have a high risk of respiratory failure.

GENERAL PREVENTION
Keep medications out of reach of children.

PATHOPHYSIOLOGY
- Aspirin is rapidly absorbed in the stomach, and peak blood levels occur within 1 hour.
- 90% of salicylate is protein bound and therefore limited to the vascular space.
- Aspirin is partially glycinated in the liver to salicyluric acid, which is excreted by the kidneys.
- Only a small amount of drug is excreted unchanged in the urine.
- Stimulates chemoreceptor trigger zone in the medulla.
- Respiratory centers are directly stimulated.
- Inhibition of cyclo oxygenase results in decreased synthesis of prostaglandins, prostacyclin, and thromboxanes.
- Interferes with cellular metabolism, causing metabolic acidosis
- Usual therapeutic levels are 10–30 mg/dL.
- Salicylate ingestion is considered toxic if patient is symptomatic, if >150 mg/kg has been ingested, or if levels are >35 mg/dL at 6 hours after ingestion.

ETIOLOGY
- In adults ingestion is typically suicidal or accidental.
- 150–300 mg/kg is considered mild to moderate toxicity.
- 301–500 mg/kg is considered serious toxicity.
- >500 mg/kg is potentially lethal toxicity.

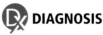 **DIAGNOSIS**

HISTORY
- Early symptoms: Tinnitus, fever, vertigo, nausea, vomiting, and diarrhea
- Altered mental status, coma, and seizures
- Hypoglycemic and coagulopathic symptoms secondary to hepatotoxicity

PHYSICAL EXAM
- Hyperventilation initially followed by respiratory arrest
- Hyperthermia
- Tachycardia and hypotension
- Dysrhythmias

DIAGNOSTIC TESTS & INTERPRETATION
Lab
Initial lab tests
- Serum salicylate levels
- Basic metabolic profile
- ABG (increased anion gap, metabolic acidosis, and respiratory alkalosis)
- PTT, PT, and INR

Follow-Up & Special Considerations
- Repeat salicylate levels every 2 hours until normal.
- Monitor potassium levels frequently after bicarbonate therapy.

Imaging
- Chest radiograph
- CT of head
- US of abdomen

DIFFERENTIAL DIAGNOSIS
- Caffeine intoxication
- Other causes of respiratory failure, pulmonary edema, and cerebral edema

TREATMENT

MEDICATION

First Line
- Sodium bicarbonate to alkalinize the urine
  - Bolus therapy 2–3 mEq/kg of NaHCO$_3$ IV push followed by infusion of 132 mEq NaHCO$_3$ in 1 L of D5W at 250 mL/h
- Hypokalemia may be a severe iatrogenic complication in patients treated with urinary alkalinization.

Second Line
- Hemodialysis if levels are >100 mg/dL
- Other indications are pulmonary or cerebral edema, renal insufficiency that interferes with salicylate excretion, and any clinical deterioration despite aggressive and appropriate supportive care.

ADDITIONAL TREATMENT

General Measures
- Stabilize ABCs.
- Intubation should be avoided if possible because aspirin stimulates respiratory center in medulla, causing massive increase in minute ventilation.
- GI decontamination with activated charcoal in dose of 1 g/kg body weight. Multiple doses may be required.
- Supplemental glucose with D5W infusion

Issues for Referral
- Toxicology consults if not responsive to medical therapy
- Nephrology consults if hemodialysis is indicated

IN-PATIENT CONSIDERATIONS

Initial Stabilization
ABCs

Admission Criteria
- Infants and elderly persons
- Individuals with chronic salicylism
- Those with ingestions of sustained-release products
- Respiratory failure
- Patients requiring hemodialysis

IV Fluids
- NaHCO$_3$ in D5W
- Isotonic saline may be cautiously used as there is potential to cause pulmonary edema.

Nursing
Close monitoring for hypotension, hypoglycemia, and respiratory failure

Discharge Criteria
Based on resolution of clinical manifestations of poisoning, including clinical signs, symptoms, and acid–base status

ONGOING CARE

FOLLOW-UP RECOMMENDATIONS
Consult psychiatric service for patients with intentional overdose.

Patient Monitoring
- Vital signs
- Salicylate levels in blood

PATIENT EDUCATION
- Numerous OTC medications contain aspirin or related compounds; accidental overdose remains a problem in adult populations.
- Patients with chronic health problems who take multiple medications should carefully record the use of all OTC medications and discuss possible drug–drug interactions with their poison control specialist/primary care physicians.

PROGNOSIS
Good, if treated early before development of complications

COMPLICATIONS
- Cerebral edema
- Noncardiogenic pulmonary edema
- GI hemorrhage and perforation
- DIC

ADDITIONAL READING

- Botma M, et al. Laryngeal oedema caused by accidental ingestion of Oil of Wintergreen. *Int J Pediatr Otorhinolaryngol*. 2001;58:229.
- Chyka PA, et al. Salicylate poisoning: An evidence-based consensus guideline for out-of-hospital management. *Clin Toxicol (Phil)*. 2007;45:95–131.
- Greenberg MI, et al. Deleterious effects of endotracheal intubation in salicylate poisoning. *Ann Emerg Med*. 2003;41:583.
- Proudfoot AT, et al. Position paper on urine alkalinization. *J Toxicol Clin Toxicol*. 2004;42:1.
- Salicylates. In: Hoffman RS, Nelson LS, Howland MA, et al. (eds.). *Goldfrank's Manual of Toxicologic Emergencies*. New York: McGraw Hill, 2007: 305–309

CODES

ICD9
- 331.81 Reye's syndrome
- 965.1 Poisoning by salicylates

CLINICAL PEARLS

Frequently misdiagnosed as dementia, acute psychosis, encephalopathy, alcoholic ketoacidosis, and sepsis

T

TOXICITY, NITROPRUSSIDE

Maher Dahdel

 BASICS

DESCRIPTION

- Sodium nitroprusside (SNP) is a potent arterial and venous vasodilator that is given IV, and has an onset of action <90 seconds and a serum half-life of 2 minutes.
- Nitroprusside is cyanogenic, containing 44% cyanide (CN^-) by weight. Some of the administered SNP releases CN^- into the circulation right away. Additional CN^- is produced when SNP is metabolized in the vascular tissue. The CN^- is metabolized in the liver to thiocyanate, which is slowly cleared by the kidneys.
- Both thiocyanate and cyanide can cause toxicity.

RISK FACTORS

- Infusion rate >2 mcg/kg/min
- Liver dysfunction
- Renal dysfunction
- Hyponatremia
- Inadequate bioavailability of thiosulfate:
  - Malnutrition
  - Surgery
  - Diuretics use

Genetics

- The risk is increased in individuals with abnormal cyanide-thiocyanate pathways, or decreased availability of hepatic rhodanese enzyme:
  - Congenital Leber's optic atrophy
  - Tobacco amblyopia

GENERAL PREVENTION

- Careful monitoring of dosage, particularly in patients susceptible to toxicity
- Substitution of alternative vasodilators as soon as feasible
- Concomitant infusion of sodium thiosulfate to provide a continuous source of sulfur donors
- Use of hydroxocobalamin (vitamin B_{12a}).

PATHOPHYSIOLOGY

- Once SNP is infused, it interacts with oxyhemoglobin, a molecule of cyanmethemoglobin, and four free CN^- ions. The free CN binds avidly to ferric ion (Fe^{+++}) in methemoglobin (MetHgb) to form additional cyanmethemoglobin. When CN is infused or generated within the bloodstream, essentially all of it is bound to MetHgb in RBCs until RBC MetHgb has been saturated.
- Thiosulfate reacts with cyanide to produce thiocyanate; thiocyanate is eliminated in the urine.
- Cyanide not otherwise removed binds to Fe^{+++} in cytochromes, inhibiting mitochondrial oxygen utilization, causing hypoxic damage, and leading to metabolic (lactic) acidosis and a narrow arteriovenous O_2 difference. Cyanide also inhibits a number of nonelectronic-chain enzymes.
- The major mechanism for the removal of cyanide involves the enzyme rhodanese, which is widely distributed, especially in hepatic cells.
- The amount of cyanide generated depends on the dose and rate of administration of SNP.
- Thiocyanate toxicity may occur in patients with renal insufficiency, especially with the use of thiosulfate.
- Methemoglobinemia may also occur.

ETIOLOGY

SNP toxicity happens when the production rate of cyanide and/or thiocyanate exceeds their elimination rate.

COMMONLY ASSOCIATED CONDITIONS

- Hypertensive emergencies:
  - Hypertensive encephalopathy
  - Pheochromocytoma
  - Intracranial hemorrhage
  - Aortic dissection
  - Postoperative status
  - Preeclampsia/eclampsia

- Acute and chronic heart failure
- Induced intraoperative hypotension:
  - Orthopedic surgeries
  - Neurosurgeries especially spinal
  - Aortic surgeries
  - Pheochromocytoma resection
  - CABG
  - Ophthalmic surgeries to control intraocular pressure

ALERT

- Contraindications to SNP:
  - Hepatic failure
  - Renal failure
  - Severe aortic stenosis
  - Untreated coarctation of aorta
  - Increased intracranial pressure
  - Poor cerebral perfusion
  - Symptomatic carotid artery stenosis

Pregnancy Considerations

SNP should be used with caution in pregnant women secondary to fetal cyanide toxicity:

- This risk can be decreased by the use of a small dose for short period.

Geriatric Considerations

- Geriatric patients need close monitoring for the development of cyanide toxicity due to age-related renal and hepatic insufficiency.
- Older patients are more sensitive to hypotensive effects of SNP.

DIAGNOSIS

- Signs of cyanide toxicity:
- Onset of toxicity takes minutes to hours.
- Hypoxemia
- Severe metabolic lactic acidosis
- CNS dysfunction:
  – Mental status changes
  – Seizure
  – Coma
  – Subarachnoid hemorrhage
- Cardiovascular instability:
  – Tachycardia
  – Ventricular arrhythmias
  – Hypotension
  – Nonspecific ST-T changes on ECG
  – Unexplained death
- Unexplained diffuse bowel necrosis
- Methemoglobinemia
- Thiocyanate toxicity:
  – Fatigue
  – Tinnitus
  – Nausea/vomiting
  – Neurotoxicity
  – Clinical hypothyroidism
- Other adverse effects of SNP:
  – Rebound hypertension
  – Coronary steal
  – Increased intracranial pressure
  – Increased intrapulmonary shunt with ablation of hypoxic pulmonary vasoconstriction
  – Platelet dysfunction
  – Reflux sympathetic activation

DIAGNOSTIC TESTS & INTERPRETATION
Lab
ABG:

- The arterial base deficit usually correlates well with increased blood lactate concentration.
- Elevated venous O_2 saturation secondary to the inability of tissues to extract oxygen from erythrocytes

Diagnostic Procedures/Other
Measurement of cyanide in blood is of limited clinical utility due to the time delay before the results can be known.

TREATMENT
MEDICATION
First Line
- Discontinue the infusion of SNP.
- Oxygen 100% despite normal O_2 saturation
- Correction of the metabolic acidosis with sodium bicarbonate as needed
- 3% sodium nitrate 4–6 mg/kg slow IV infusion
  – Produces MetHgb to bind CN
- Sodium thiosulfate 150–200 mg/kg IV infusion over 15 minutes:
  – Consider hydroxocobalamin (vitamin B12a) 25 reacts with cyanide to produce cyanocobalamin (vitamin B_{12})

Second Line
Consider hemodialysis or peritoneal dialysis if thiocyanate toxicity is suspected.

ADDITIONAL READING

- Elkayam U, et al. Vasodilators in the management of acute heart failure. *Crit Care Med*. 2008;36.
- Friederich JA, et al. Sodium nitroprusside: Twenty years and counting. *Anesth Analg*. 1995;81(1): 152–62.
- Robin ED, et al. Nitroprusside-related cyanide poisoning. *Chest*. 1992;102;1842–5
- Testa LD, et al. Pharmacologic drugs for controlled hypotension. *J Clin Anesth*. 1995;7:326–37.

CODES

ICD9
972.6 Poisoning by other antihypertensive agents

CLINICAL PEARLS

- It is difficult to predict the development of cyanide toxicity.
- If suspected, start thiosulfate immediately; do not wait for the laboratory confirmation of cyanide toxicity.
- Methemoglobinemia should be suspected in patients who have received >10 mg/kg sodium nitroprusside and who exhibit signs of hypoxemia despite adequate cardiac output and arterial PaO_2.

T

TOXICOLOGY & TOXIDROMES, GENERAL

Muhammad N. Athar
James A. Gasperino

 BASICS

DESCRIPTION
- Poisoning results from intentional or unintentional ingestion, inhalation, or contact.
- Toxic complications can also result from therapeutic use of medications.
- Mortality is low.
- ICU resources are used increasingly because of need for monitoring.
- Owing to lack of RCTs, limited evidence-based data are available on management of poisoning.
- Current recommendations are based on extrapolation of data from animal models, human volunteer studies, case reports, pharmacokinetics of the drug, pathophysiology of toxidrome, and consensus opinions.

EPIDEMIOLOGY
Incidence
- 2–5 million poisonings and drug overdoses occur annually in the U.S.
- Overall mortality rate is >0.05%.
- Mortality rate for hospitalized patients is ~1–2%.
- Fatalities most commonly result from carbon monoxide poisoning, ingestion of analgesics, sedative-hypnotics, antipsychotics, antidepressants, street drugs, cardiovascular drugs, and alcohols.

Prevalence
- Analysis of 2007 data from US poisoning center revealed:
- 95% of episodes caused minor or no effects.
- 90.9% were acute ingestions.
- 90.6% involved a single substance.
- 83.2% were unintentional.
- 8.4% were suspected cases of suicidal ideation.
- 73.3% of fatalities were in ages 20–59 years.
- 51.2% of exposures were in children <6 years.
- 12.5% of all exposure were analgesics.
- Most common exposures in children <6 years were cosmetics/personal care products.

RISK FACTORS
- Population at risk is elderly and children.
- Major depression

GENERAL PREVENTION
Keep medications out of reach of children.

ETIOLOGY
- 2007 AAPCC report implicated poisons:
- Analgesics (12%)
- Cosmetics (9.2%)
- Household cleaning substances (8.7%)
- Sedative-hypnotics and antipsychotics (6.2%)
- Foreign bodies (5.1%)
- Plants (4.7%)
- Cough and cold preparations (4.5%)

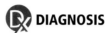 DIAGNOSIS

HISTORY
- Often unreliable when provided by a patient following intentional ingestion
- Information should be obtained from paramedics, police, and the patient's employer, family, friends, primary care clinician, and pharmacist.
- Focus on events surrounding the exposure and course of symptom development.
- Search the exposure environment for pill bottles.
- Suicide note may provide clues to etiologic agent.
- Regional poison control center can help in diagnosis of unknown agent.

PHYSICAL EXAM
- Focused exam: Detect life-threatening conditions and identify toxidrome.
- Mental status, vital signs, and papillary exam are useful to classify state of physiologic excitation or depression.
- Physiologic excitation is manifested by CNS stimulation and increased pulse, blood pressure, respiratory rate and depth, and temperature. Most commonly caused by anticholinergic, sympathomimetic, or central hallucinogenic agents or by drug withdrawal states.
- Physiologic depression is manifested by a depressed mental status, blood pressure, pulse, respiratory rate and depth, and temperature. Most commonly caused by cholinergic, sympatholytic, opiate, or sedative-hypnotic agents, or alcohols.
- Mixed physiologic effects occur in polydrug overdoses or following exposure to certain metabolic poisons (e.g., hypoglycemic agents, salicylates, cyanide), membrane-active agents (e.g., volatile inhalants, antiarrhythmic drugs, local anesthetic agents), heavy metals (e.g., iron, arsenic, mercury, lead), or agents with multiple mechanisms of action (e.g., tricyclic antidepressants).

- To enable rapid diagnosis of poisoning, the clinical features can also be grouped into 5 "toxidromes":
  - Cholinergic toxidrome: Salivation, lacrimation, urination, defecation, GI upsets, bradycardia, fasciculations, confusion, and miosis
  - Anticholinergic toxidrome: Dry skin, hyperthermia, mydriasis, tachycardia, delirium, thirst, and urinary retention.
  - Sympathomimetic toxidrome: Hypertension, tachycardia, seizures, CNS excitation, mydriasis, and diaphoresis.
  - Narcotic toxidrome: Miosis, respiratory depression, decreased level of consciousness, hypotension, and hyporeflexia.
  - Sedative-hypnotic toxidrome: Depressed level of consciousness, respiratory depression, hypotension, and hyporeflexia.

DIAGNOSTIC TESTS & INTERPRETATION
Lab
- Basic metabolic panel
- Routine urine toxicology screen
- Comprehensive toxicologic screening on blood and urine in patients with unexplained toxicity
- Urine pregnancy testing in all women of childbearing age
- Serum osmolality, ketones, creatine kinase, liver function tests, amylase, calcium, and magnesium
- ABG, co-oximetry, and serum lactate

Imaging
- Chest radiograph (radiopaque toxins, drug body packets, noncardiogenic pulmonary edema, or ARDS)
- Abdominal US can identify some enteric-coated and sustained-release formulations.

Diagnostic Procedures/Other
ECG

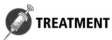 TREATMENT

General Measures
- Gastric decontamination:
  - After initial patient stabilization, decontamination is a priority.
  - Copious water or saline irrigation for topical exposures
  - Activated charcoal for ingestions should be given within 1 hour of ingestion in a dose of 1 mg/kg body weight.
  - Substances not adsorbed by activated charcoal are iron, lithium, cyanide, strong acid or base, alcohols, and hydrocarbons.
  - Syrup of ipecac is not recommended because of potential side effects.

– Gastric lavage, however, is contraindicated in ingestions of acid, alkali, or hydrocarbons.

– Whole-bowel irrigation may be performed for sustained-release or enteric-coated drugs, iron tablets, and illicit drug packets.

– Cathartics can be used; however, no clinical study has demonstrated beneficial effect.

– Endoscopy and surgery may be required.

• Antidotes:

– Antidote administration is appropriate if an antidote is available for the ingested poison.

– Antidotes dramatically reduce morbidity and mortality in certain intoxications.

– They are used in only about 1% of cases.

– Antidotes reduce or reverse poison effects by preventing absorption, bind and neutralize poisons directly, antagonize end-organ effects, or inhibit conversion to more toxic metabolites.

• Enhanced elimination:

– Multiple-dose activated charcoal

– Forced diuresis

– Urine ion trapping

– Hemodialysis, hemoperfusion, and hemofiltration

– Exchange transfusion

• Supportive care:

– Airway protection performed early in patient with depressed mental status because of the high risk for aspiration

– Hypotension is managed initially with IV fluids and followed by vasopressors.

– Hypertension in agitated patients is best treated with nonspecific sedatives such as a benzodiazepine.

– Ventricular tachycardias are treated with standard doses of lidocaine.

– Bradyarrhythmias associated with hypotension are generally treated with atropine or temporary pacing.

– Seizures generally are best treated with benzodiazepines followed by barbiturates if necessary.

– Drug-associated agitated behavior is generally best treated with benzodiazepine administration and/or haloperidol as needed.

Issues for Referral
Unknown pills or chemicals can be identified by consultation with a regional poison control center through a toll-free line (1-800-222-1222).

IN-PATIENT CONSIDERATIONS
Initial Stabilization
• ICU admission criteria must consider characteristics of the offending agent, patient factors, and the need for specialized monitoring

• ABCs

• In poisoned obtunded patient, hypertonic dextrose, thiamine, and naloxone may be considered.

Admission Criteria
• CNS depression (Glasgow Coma Scale $\leq$6)

• Agitation requiring chemical or physical restraint

• Respiratory depression (PCO$_2$ >45 mm Hg), hypoxia or respiratory failure (ARDS), and/or endotracheal intubation

• Hypotension (SBP $\leq$80 mm Hg)

• Seizures

• 2nd- or 3rd-degree AV block on ECG

• Nonsinus cardiac rhythm on ECG

• Significant acid–base disturbances (e.g., metabolic acidosis with pH $\leq$7.2)

• Significant metabolic abnormalities requiring close monitoring or aggressive correction

• Extremes of temperature (e.g., hyperthermia with temperature >104°F)

• Poisoning with ingested drug packets and sustained-release preparations

• Quantitative level of drug that predicts unfavorable outcome

• Need for invasive hemodynamic monitoring (e.g., pulmonary artery catheter or arterial line) or cardiac pacing

• Need for whole-bowel irrigation to enhance GI elimination of poison

• Need for emergency hemodialysis, hemoperfusion, hemofiltration

• Need for emergency antidote that requires close monitoring (e.g., crotalid antivenin, Digibind, physostigmine, naloxone drip)

• Ischemic chest pain from toxin (e.g., cocaine, carbon monoxide)

• TCA or other drug exposure with QRS >120 ms or QTc >500 ms

Nursing
• Vital signs

• Cardiac rhythm monitoring

• Strict I/O

Discharge Criteria
• Stable vital signs

• Able to maintain airway

• No metabolic abnormality

• Normal ECG

• For TCA overdose, cardiac monitoring is suggested for an additional 24 hours after normalization of the ECG and other signs of toxicity.

 ## ONGOING CARE

FOLLOW-UP RECOMMENDATIONS
Psychiatry evaluation for suicidal ingestion

ADDITIONAL READING

• Brett AS, et al. Predicting the clinical course in intentional drug overdose: Implications for use of the intensive care unit. *Arch Intern Med*. 1987;147:133.

• Bronstein AC, et al. 2007 Annual Report of the American Association of Poison Control Centers' National Poison Data System (NPDS): 25th Annual Report. *Clin Toxicol (Phila)*. 2008;46:927–1057.

• Initial evaluation of the patient: Vital signs and toxic syndromes. In: Hoffman RS et al., eds., *Goldfrank's manual of toxicologic emergencies*. New York: McGraw Hill, 2007:19–23.

 ## CODES

ICD9
• 967.9 Poisoning by unspecified sedative or hypnotic

• 977.9 Poisoning by unspecified drug or medicinal substance

• 986 Toxic effect of carbon monoxide

TRACHEOSTOMY

Claude Killu

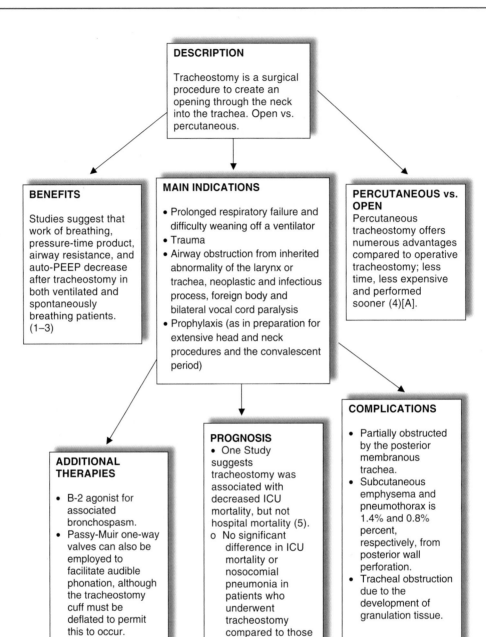

DESCRIPTION

Tracheostomy is a surgical procedure to create an opening through the neck into the trachea. Open vs. percutaneous.

BENEFITS

Studies suggest that work of breathing, pressure-time product, airway resistance, and auto-PEEP decrease after tracheostomy in both ventilated and spontaneously breathing patients. (1–3)

MAIN INDICATIONS

- Prolonged respiratory failure and difficulty weaning off a ventilator
- Trauma
- Airway obstruction from inherited abnormality of the larynx or trachea, neoplastic and infectious process, foreign body and bilateral vocal cord paralysis
- Prophylaxis (as in preparation for extensive head and neck procedures and the convalescent period)

PERCUTANEOUS vs. OPEN

Percutaneous tracheostomy offers numerous advantages compared to operative tracheostomy; less time, less expensive and performed sooner (4)[A].

ADDITIONAL THERAPIES

- B-2 agonist for associated bronchospasm.
- Passy-Muir one-way valves can also be employed to facilitate audible phonation, although the tracheostomy cuff must be deflated to permit this to occur.

PROGNOSIS
- One Study suggests tracheostomy was associated with decreased ICU mortality, but not hospital mortality (5).
  o No significant difference in ICU mortality or nosocomial pneumonia in patients who underwent tracheostomy compared to those who did not (6).

COMPLICATIONS

- Partially obstructed by the posterior membranous trachea.
- Subcutaneous emphysema and pneumothorax is 1.4% and 0.8% percent, respectively, from posterior wall perforation.
- Tracheal obstruction due to the development of granulation tissue.

ALERT
- Massive hemorrhage due to a tracheoarterial fistula is the most devastating complication.

Pediatric Considerations
The great vessels (i.e., carotid arteries, internal jugular veins) could be damaged with deep dissection.

REFERENCES

1. Elpem EH, et al. Pulmonary aspiration in mechanically ventilated patients with tracheostomies. *Chest*. 1994;105:563.
2. Leder SB. Incidence and type of aspiration in acute care patients requiring mechanical ventilation via a new tracheotomy. *Chest*. 2002;122:1721.
3. DeVita MA, et al. Swallowing disorders in patients with prolonged orotracheal intubation or tracheostomy tubes. *Crit Care Med*. 1990;18:1328.
4. Freeman BD, et al. A meta-analysis of prospective trials comparing percutaneous and surgical tracheostomy in critically ill patients. *Chest*. 2000;118:1412.
5. Frutos-Vivar F, et al. Outcome of mechanically ventilated patients who require a tracheostomy. *Crit Care Med*. 2005;33:290.
6. Terragni PP, et al. Early vs late tracheotomy for prevention of pneumonia in mechanically ventilated adult ICU patients: a randomized controlled trial. *JAMA* 2010;303:1483–9.

ADDITIONAL READING

- De Leyn P, et al. Tracheostomy: Clinical review and guidelines. *Eur J Cardiothorac Surg*. 2007;32(3): 412–21.

 See Also (Topic, Algorithm, Electronic Media Element)

www.hopkinsmedicine.org/tracheostomy

 CODES

ICD9
447.2 Rupture of artery

CLINICAL PEARLS

- Tracheostomy improves comfort and decreases work of breathing but does not decrease aspiration risk.
- Percutaneous tracheostomy is faster, yields a better cosmetic result.
- Early tracheostomy—at 7 days—is reasonable if the mechanical ventilation is expected to be >14 days. It may be associated with more rapid weaning and a decreased duration of ICU stay.

T

TRANSFUSION THERAPY AND REACTIONS

Mladen Sokolovic
Stephen M. Pastores

 BASICS

DESCRIPTION
Anemia, thrombocytopenia, and coagulopathy are frequently encountered problems in the ICU, and often necessitate transfusion of blood products.

Red Blood Cells
- Reasons for anemia in critical illness:
  - Diminished erythropoietin production and sensitivity
  - Functional iron deficiency
  - Bone marrow suppression
  - Nutritional deficiency
  - Increased RBC destruction
  - Occult or overt blood losses, including loss related to diagnostic phlebotomy
- Compensatory mechanisms for anemia include increasing cardiac output, peripheral vascular changes, and increasing oxygen extraction.
- Indications for RBC transfusion in the critically ill include active bleeding; hemoglobin <7 mg/dL in hemodynamically stable ICU, trauma, and surgical patients; and hemoglobin <10 mg/dL with coronary ischemia, limited cardiopulmonary reserve, or advanced age (1)[B].
- Fresh whole blood is difficult to obtain and should be used only to support massively bleeding patients; packed RBCs are commonly used; PRBC 1U = 250–350 mL.
- Must be ABO compatible. O Rh-negative is universal donor in emergencies. O Rh-positive can be used, except in women of childbearing age.
- Issues with RBC transfusion: Immunosuppression related to WBC exposure and sensitization and RBC storage lesion
- Restrictive RBC transfusion strategy (hemoglobin <7 g/dL to keep level of 7–9 g/dL) was at least as effective and likely superior to liberal transfusion strategy (hemoglobin <10 g/dL to keep level of 10–12 g/dL) (1)[B].

Platelets
- Risk of hemorrhage increases as functional platelet concentrations decline.
- ABO matched platelets preferable, but unmatched platelets can be used in emergencies. HLA matched platelets are needed in alloimmunized patients exhibiting refractoriness to platelet transfusion.
- 1 unit = 200–250 mL per 5–6 unit pool
- Indications for platelet transfusion depending on platelet count (2)[B]:
  - <5000 to prevent spontaneous bleeding
  - <20,000 with concomitant infection or increased risk of bleeding
  - <50,000 with bleeding or before a surgical procedure
  - <100,000 with intracranial bleed
  - Massive RBC transfusion to avoid dilutional thrombocytopenia

- Transfuse at higher thresholds if concomitant conditions that affect platelet function are present (NSAIDs, GP IIb/IIIa inhibitors, uremia, coagulopathy, infection, extracorporal circuits).
- Consumptive coagulopathies (TTP/HUS, HIT, HELLP) are relative contraindications for platelet transfusion.

Fresh Frozen Plasma (FFP)
- FFP contains all coagulation factors in different concentrations; usually used to correct hemostasis in bleeding that arises from malfunction, underproduction, consumptions, and inhibition of coagulation factors.
- Must be ABO but not Rh compatible. AB is universal donor type in emergencies.
- 1 unit = 200–250 mL
- Indications for FFP:
  - Multiple clotting factor deficiencies in liver disease, DIC, TTP/HUS (with plasmapheresis)
  - Warfarin reversal with bleeding
  - Prophylactic correction of coagulopathy prior to invasive procedure
  - Massive blood transfusions and INR >2 (3)[B]
- Not indicated for volume resuscitation or merely to correct INR in absence of bleeding

Cryoprecipitate
- Rich in von Willebrand factor (vWF), factors VIII, XIII, and fibrinogen (200 mg of fibrinogen and 100 U of factor VIII per 15 mL bag)
- Indications:
  - Bleeding in von Willebrand disease
  - Factor XIII deficiency
  - Hemophilia A only if factor VIII concentrate unavailable
- Concentrates of miscellaneous plasma clotting factors are also available and used in specific deficiencies.

Transfusion Reactions
- Clinically detectable transfusion reactions occur in ~20% of patients; severe reactions occur in 1–2%.
- In the ICU, acute transfusion reactions are more challenging due to atypical presentation, frequent inability of patients to report symptoms, and difficulty distinguishing adverse transfusion reaction from underlying illness.

Geriatric Considerations
Elderly are at higher risk for transfusion reaction and have poorer prognosis.

EPIDEMIOLOGY
Incidence
- Acute transfusion reactions:
  - Acute hemolytic reaction: 1/250,000–1 million units
  - Anaphylaxis: 1/150,000 units
  - Febrile reaction: 1/100–200 units
  - Allergic/urticarial reaction: 1/200 units
  - Transfusion related acute lung injury: (TRALI) 1/5000–8000 units
  - Bacterial infection, PRBCs: 1/500,000 units
  - Bacterial infection, platelets: 1/5000 units
  - Exact incidence of volume overload, thrombocytopenia, coagulopathy, hypocalcemia, and hyperkalemia is unclear.

- Other infectious and delayed reactions:
  - HIV: 1/1.2–2.4 million units
  - Hepatitis B: 1/220,000 units
  - Hepatitis C: 1/1–1.6million units
  - HTLV I and II: 1/600,000
  - CMV incidence varies; significant in immunosuppressed recipients.
  - Delayed hemolytic reaction: 1/1000 units
  - Transfusion-associated graft-versus-host disease (TA-GVHD) is probably underrecognized.
  - West Nile, malaria, babesiosis, Chagas disease, parvo B19; case reports

RISK FACTORS
- Multiple blood product transfusions
- IgA deficiency
- Multiparous women
- Old blood
- At risk for TA-GVHD: Neonates, leukemia/lymphoma patients, bone marrow and solid organ transplant recipients

GENERAL PREVENTION
- Adhere to evidence-based transfusion guidelines.
- Strictly follow protocol for patient identification, blood sample, and blood product bag labeling.
- Inquire about history of previous reactions.
- Transfuse autologous blood when possible.
- Leukoreduction decreases likelihood of febrile reactions, CMV, and immunosuppression.

ETIOLOGY
- Acute hemolytic reaction: Most often due to ABO incompatibility. Recipients preformed complement activating antibodies attach to antigens on donor's RBCs, causing intravascular hemolysis. Most common cause is human error; more likely to occur in ED, ICU, and OR.
- Delayed hemolysis: Antibody formed by prior transfusion reactivates 2–10 days post transfusion, causing hemolysis.
- Anaphylaxis: Recipient produces IgE antibody to an antigen that recipient's plasma does not contain (IgA deficiency).
- Urticaria: Hypersensitivity reaction probably caused by similar mechanism to anaphylaxis
- Febrile reaction: Caused either by released cytokines from donor's blood or by recipient produced antibody to donor leukocyte antigens
- TRALI: Caused by antibodies to recipient or donor's leukocyte HLA antigens, causing them to aggregate in pulmonary vasculature
- Bacterial infections: *Staphylococcus*, *Streptococcus*, gram-negatives, and *Yersinia enterocolitica* have been reported with PRBC and platelet transfusions (3)[B].
- TA-GVHD: Donor's viable T lymphocytes engraft and cause rejection of host tissue.

COMMONLY ASSOCIATED CONDITIONS
- DIC
- Renal failure
- Bone marrow failure

DIAGNOSIS

HISTORY
- Acute hemolytic reaction symptoms: Fever, chills, flank pain, anxiety, nausea, dyspnea.
- Anaphylaxis symptoms: Malaise, flushing, dyspnea, nausea, vomiting, diarrhea
- Allergic/urticarial reaction: Hives, pruritus shortly after transfusion.
- Febrile reaction: Fever 1–6 hours after the transfusion but no signs of hemolysis/anaphylaxis
- TRALI: Cough, dyspnea, fever, increased oxygen requirements
- Bacterial contamination: Fever, hypotension
- TA-GVHD: Fever, rash, diarrhea 8–30 days posttransfusion

PHYSICAL EXAM
In comatose or sedated patients, the transfusion reaction symptoms may not be obvious and clues may be provided by signs such as:
- Rash
- Fever
- Jaundice
- Hypotension
- Increase in oxygen demand
- Worsening pulmonary infiltrates
- Red urine
- Oozing from puncture sites

DIAGNOSTIC TESTS & INTERPRETATION
Lab
- Worsening anemia
- Thrombocytopenia (DIC)
- Hyperbilirubinemia
- High LDH
- Low haptoglobin
- Positive Coombs
- Hemoglobinuria
- Elevated urea and creatinine
- Detection of specific antibodies
- Elevated transaminases
- Gram stain to detect bacterial contamination

Imaging
TRALI: New bilateral lung infiltrates on chest x-ray

DIFFERENTIAL DIAGNOSIS
- Allergic reactions to other therapies
- Hemolysis due to medications
- Thrombocytopenia due to medications, sepsis, hypersplenism
- Fluid overload due to crystalloids/colloids
- Elevated bilirubin/transaminases due to acalculous cholecystitis

TREATMENT

ALERT
Whenever a transfusion reaction is suspected, STOP the transfusion!

MEDICATION
- Acute hemolytic reaction: Oxygen, IV fluids
- Anaphylaxis: Epinephrine, hydrocortisone, H_1 antihistamine
- Urticaria: Antihistamine
- Febrile reaction: Antipyretic, meperidine (rigors)
- TRALI: Oxygen; might require intubation and mechanical ventilation, IV fluids
- Bacterial contamination: Start empiric antibiotics to cover common gram-positive/-negative offenders.

ADDITIONAL TREATMENT
General Measures
- After stopping the transfusion, follow the hospital transfusion reaction protocol.
- Rule out human error.
- Monitor vital signs and urine output.
- IV fluid and vasopressors if needed to support blood pressure and urine output.
- Treat DIC with supportive therapy and blood products when indicated.

ONGOING CARE

PATIENT EDUCATION
- Patient must be educated to report any unusual symptoms with transfusion.
- Patient should report blood product reaction to health care providers in the future.

PROGNOSIS
- Mortality and morbidity are directly related to the amount of incompatible blood transfused in case of acute hemolysis.
- TRALI is usually self-limited but mortality of up to 10% has been reported.
- Most of the reactions are self-limited, and prognosis is good unless complications such as renal failure develop.

COMPLICATIONS
- DIC
- Renal failure
- Immunosuppression
- Iron overload

REFERENCES
1. Hebert PC, et al. A multicenter, randomized, controlled clinical trial of transfusion requirements in critical care. *N Engl J Med*. 1999;340:409–17.
2. Schiffer CA, et al. Platelet transfusion for patients with cancer: Clinical practice guidelines of the American Society of Clinical Oncology. *J Clin Oncol*. 2001;19:1519–38.
3. MacLennan S, et al. Risks of fresh frozen plasma and platelets. *J Trauma*. 2006;60:S46–S50.

ADDITIONAL READING
- Critical Issues in Hematology: Anemia, thrombocytopenia, coagulopathy and blood product transfusions in critically ill patients. *Clin Chest Med*. 2003;24:607–22.
- Marik PE, et al. Efficacy of red blood cell transfusion in the critically ill: A systematic review of the literature. *Crit Care Med*. 2008;36(9):2667–74.

CODES

ICD9
- 999.49 Anaphalylactic reaction due to other serum
- 999.80 Transfusion reaction, unspecified
- 999.83 Hemolytic transfusion reaction, incompatibility unspecified

CLINICAL PEARLS
- Adhere to evidence-based transfusion guidelines.
- Whenever a transfusion reaction is suspected, STOP the transfusion!
- In comatose or sedated patients, the transfusion reaction symptoms may not be obvious and clues may be provided by signs (rash, fever, jaundice, hypotension, increase in oxygen demand, worsening pulmonary infiltrates, red urine, or oozing from puncture sites).

T

TRANSFUSION-RELATED ACUTE LUNG INJURY

Sanjay Chawla

 BASICS

DESCRIPTION
- Acute onset of noncardiogenic pulmonary edema during or within 6 hours of transfusion of blood products.
- System(s) affected: Lung
- Synonym(s): TRALI

EPIDEMIOLOGY
Incidence
- Exact incidence is unknown because of underrecognition and underreporting.
- Overall estimate: 1 in 5,000 or between 0.02–0.05% per blood product transfused or between 0.04–0.16% per patient transfused (1,2)[A]
  - 1 in 432 units of whole blood platelets
  - 1 in 2,000 plasma containing components
  - 1 in 7,900 units of fresh frozen plasma (FFP)
  - 1 in 557,000 units of packed red blood cells (RBC)

Prevalence
- TRALI is the leading cause of transfusion- related death as reported to the US FDA since 2003.
- Accounts for more deaths than all other causes of transfusion associated deaths combined

RISK FACTORS
- Receiving transfusion of blood or blood components containing >50 mL of plasma, including whole blood, RBC, FFP, random or single donor platelets, granulocytes, stem cells, cryoprecipitate, and IV immunoglobulin (3)[A]
- Recent surgery, sepsis, trauma, massive transfusions, hematologic malignancies, and cardiac disease
- Multiparity of the blood donor and age of the blood products

GENERAL PREVENTION
- Deferral of high-risk donors or those implicated in a TRALI case although this may severely reduce the number of potential donors.
  - High-risk donors may include multiparous women or individuals who have antibodies to leukocyte antigens, such as human neutrophil antigens (HNA) or human leukocyte antigens (HLA) class I or II:
    - Limit transfusions according to evidence-based guidelines.
    - Consider washing cellular components to remove antibodies, lipids, and other biologic response modifiers from the plasma fraction of a blood product.
    - Use fresher blood products.

PATHOPHYSIOLOGY
- Exact mechanism of TRALI is not known.
- Antibody-mediated (1-event model):
  - Passive transfer of leukoagglutinating antibodies that bind to recipient neutrophils contained in the plasma portion of transfused products
  - Neutrophils are activated and sequestered in the pulmonary capillaries, where mediators are produced that lead to vascular injury and permeability from oxidases and proteases.
  - In 60–90% of cases, leukocyte antibodies have been found in the implicated donor, with the corresponding antigen in the recipient. However, in 5–10% of cases, TRALI may occur from recipient antibodies reacting to donor leukocytes (2)[B].
- Nonantibody mediated (2-event model): Based on cases in which donor antibodies or cognate antigen are not detected:
  - Initial event includes recent surgery, hypoxia, sepsis, trauma, massive transfusions, cardiopulmonary disease, or cardiopulmonary bypass.
  - In these conditions, the vascular endothelium is activated, resulting in cytokine release and adhesion molecule expression, which then leads to neutrophil sequestration in the lung.
  - The 2nd event occurs with the transfusion of stored blood products, which contain various biologic response modifiers that lead to neutrophil activation and release of oxidases and proteases.
- TRALI can occur in neutropenic patients either due to vascular endothelial growth factor (VEGF) or anti-HLA II antibodies that react with HLA II antigens on pulmonary endothelial cells (2)[B].

ETIOLOGY
- Two different, but not mutually exclusive, hypotheses have been postulated:
  - Anti-HLA antibodies present in the transfused products react with the recipient's own blood cells, inducing release of inflammatory mediators.
  - Bioactive lipids present during storage of blood products cause neutrophil activation in patients with pulmonary endothelial activation.

COMMONLY ASSOCIATED CONDITIONS
- Respiratory failure
- Concomitant fluid overload
- Cardiovascular instability that may require vasopressor and inotropic support

 DIAGNOSIS

HISTORY
- Acute onset of dyspnea either during or within 6 hours of transfusion without a preexisting risk for ALI
- If there is a preexisting risk factor for ALI, then a diagnosis of possible TRALI can be made.

PHYSICAL EXAM
- Tachypnea
- Frothy pulmonary secretions
- Diffuse rales
- Hypoxemia
- Cyanosis
- Hypotension
- Tachycardia
- Fever

DIAGNOSTIC TESTS & INTERPRETATION
Lab
Initial lab tests
No initial specific lab tests to confirm a diagnosis of TRALI:
- Suggestive findings include transient acute leukopenia, neutropenia, hypoalbuminemia, and hypocomplementemia.
- ABG or pulse oximetry: Hypoxemia with PaO_2:FiO_2 ratio <300 or oxygen saturation of <90% on room air.

Follow-Up & Special Considerations
- Detection of HLA I or II antibodies or neutrophil-specific antibodies in the donor plasma and the presence of the corresponding antigen on recipient neutrophils (not required for immediate diagnosis since results will not be readily available)
- Further testing by blood bank/transfusion service may identify antibody/antigen cognates.

Imaging
Chest x-ray shows bilateral alveolar opacities in the mid and upper lung fields with a normal cardiac silhouette and no evidence of pulmonary vessel engorgement.

Diagnostic Procedures/Other
Exclude volume overload or hydrostatic pulmonary edema:
- Echocardiogram may reveal normal systolic function; however, hydrostatic pulmonary edema may still exist due to diastolic dysfunction.
- Serum B-type natriuretic peptide (BNP) levels >100 pg/dL may be helpful to distinguish circulatory overload:
  - Invasive measurements, if available, are normal, including central venous pressure (CVP) and pulmonary artery occlusion pressure (PAOP).
  - Undiluted sample of pulmonary edema fluid will have a ratio of edema fluid protein to plasma protein of >0.75 in TRALI, whereas hydrostatic pulmonary edema will have a ratio of <0.65 (2,4)[A].

Pathological Findings
- Gross inspection: Heavy, edematous lungs with evidence of hemorrhage.
- Microscopic: Interstitial and intra-alveolar edema with leukocyte infiltration dilated pulmonary capillaries and extravasated RBCs and neutrophils.

DIFFERENTIAL DIAGNOSIS
- Transfusion-associated circulatory overload (TACO)
- Allergy/anaphylactic reaction
- Transfusion of contaminated blood products
- Hemolytic transfusion reaction

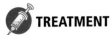 TREATMENT

MEDICATION
Supplemental oxygen to maintain oxygenation.

ADDITIONAL TREATMENT
General Measures
- Treatment is primarily supportive.
- Stop current transfusion and return the blood product to the blood bank/transfusion service.
- Avoid diuretics unless there is good evidence that the patient has cardiogenic pulmonary edema or concomitant circulatory overload.
- Use of diuretics in TRALI may lead to hypovolemia (2)[C].

Issues for Referral
Immediate notification of blood bank/transfusion service so that the implicated product can be evaluated for the presence of antibodies or contamination.

Additional Therapies
- Ventilatory support with either noninvasive ventilation or intubation and mechanical ventilation in severe cases
- In patients who require mechanical ventilation, a low tidal volume strategy of 6 mL/kg of predicted body weight with a targeted plateau pressure of <30 cm H_2O should be employed (4)[A].
- Glucocorticoids have been used in case reports; however, there are no randomized controlled studies to support or refute their use in TRALI (2,4)[B].

IN-PATIENT CONSIDERATIONS
Initial Stabilization
- Oxygen supplementation to correct hypoxemia
- Assisted ventilation by noninvasive ventilation or intubation and mechanical ventilation

Admission Criteria
High oxygen requirements, need for assisted ventilation, or hemodynamic instability

IV Fluids
- Isotonic fluids to maintain blood pressure and urine output
- Limit further fluid administration if there is evidence of circulatory overload.

Nursing
Frequent monitoring of oxygenation and cardiovascular status

Discharge Criteria
Resolution of respiratory and cardiovascular issues and reduction in oxygen requirements

 ONGOING CARE

FOLLOW-UP RECOMMENDATIONS
No special requirements once the episode has resolved

Patient Monitoring
- Continuous pulse oximetry or serial ABGs
- Serial blood pressure measurements
- Urine output

DIET
- No specific restrictions unless pulmonary function is compromised and risk for intubation is high.
- Patients requiring noninvasive support should remain NPO.

PROGNOSIS
- Most patients will have complete resolution within 96 hours and long-term lung function is not impaired.
- Generally good outcomes, with reported mortality rates of 5–10%, which are lower when compared to other forms of ALI/ARDS (2,4)[A].

COMPLICATIONS
Respiratory insufficiency or failure requiring intubation in the acute setting

REFERENCES
1. Toy P, et al. The National Heart Lung and Blood Institute Working Group on TRALI. Transfusion-related acute lung injury: Definition and review. *Crit Care Med*. 2005;33:721–6.
2. Jawa RS, et al. Transfusion-related acute lung injury. *J Intensive Care Med*. 2008;23:109–21.
3. Boshkov LK. Transfusion-related acute lung injury and the ICU. *Crit Care Clin*. 2005;21:479–95.
4. Looney MR, et al. Transfusion-related acute lung injury: A review. *Chest*. 2004;126:249–58.

ADDITIONAL READING
- Farmer JC, et al. Transfusion-related acute lung injury and other pulmonary complications of blood transfusion in the critically ill patient. *Crit Care Med*. 2006;34:S95–173.
- Triulzi DJ. Transfusion-related acute lung injury: Current concepts for the clinician. *Anesth Analg*. 2009;108:770–6.
- Wallis JP. Transfusion-related acute lung injury (TRALI): Presentation, epidemiology and treatment. *Intensive Care Med*. 2007;33(Suppl 1):S12–S16.

 CODES

ICD9
- 514 Pulmonary congestion and hypostasis
- 518.7 Transfusion related acute lung injury (TRALI)

CLINICAL PEARLS
- TRALI is a serious, potentially life-threatening form of noncardiogenic pulmonary edema temporally related to blood transfusion.
- Pathogenesis predominantly involves leukocyte antibodies in donor plasma directed at HLA class I or II, or neutrophil-specific antigens and activation of pulmonary endothelium.
- Management is primarily supportive, with oxygen supplementation and institution of mechanical ventilation in severe cases.
- Most patients have complete resolution within several days without long-term sequelae.

T

TRANSPLANTATION, HEMATOPOIETIC CELL

Rajesh Rethnam
Saraswathi V. Muppana
Stephen M. Pastores

 BASICS

DESCRIPTION
- Infusion of previously harvested patient bone marrow or peripheral blood stem cells (autologous HCT) or a donor's bone marrow, peripheral blood, and umbilical cord blood (allogeneic HCT) following myeloablative chemoradiation therapy (1)
- Potentially curative treatment for malignant, nonmalignant disorders and congenital immune deficiencies
- System(s) affected: Hematologic

EPIDEMIOLOGY
Incidence
30,000 autologous HCT (auto-HCT) and 15,000 allogeneic HCT (allo-HCT) are performed annually worldwide.

Prevalence
- Peripheral blood stem cells are the main source of stem cells for auto-HCT (PBSCT).
- Other sources of stem cells include bone marrow and umbilical cord blood.

RISK FACTORS
- General:
  - Patient age
  - Intensity of preparative regimens
  - Type and stage of underlying disease
  - Presence of comorbidities
- Infection:
  - Myeloablation
  - Neutropenia
  - Immunosuppressive therapy for GVHD
  - Prior infection with herpes group of viruses
  - Colonization with opportunistic fungi
  - Prior tuberculosis exposure
  - Presence of a central venous catheter
- Acute GVHD:
  - HLA mismatched graft, matched unrelated donor (MUD), older patients
- Chronic GVHD:
  - Acute GVHD (greatest risk), older patients, PBSCT, MUD
- Hepatic veno-occlusive disease (VOD):
  - Hepatitis B and C, pretransplant single-dose radiation therapy, busulphan, cytarabine, female gender (secondary to progesterone), presence of C282Y allele

Genetics
- Allo HCT: Major histocompatibility antigens (HLA) encoded by the HLA-complex genes on chromosome 6 accounts for GVHD.
- Variations in donor or recipient genes that encode the protein NOD2/CARD15 are associated with severe GVHD.

GENERAL PREVENTION
- Use of lower doses of chemotherapy and radiation in nonmyeloablative or "mini" allo- HCT may prevent GVHD.
- Antibacterial and antifungal prophylaxis during pre-engraftment period
- Routine screening for cytomegalovirus (CMV) viremia and antiviral prophylaxis in seropositive patients or in negative patients receiving graft from a positive donor:
  - Use of filtered blood products for CMV-negative patients receiving HCT from a negative donor.
  - Donor vaccination before HSCT is of proven value for prophylaxis of infections with viral hepatitis B, *Haemophilus influenzae*, *Streptococcus pneumoniae*; with conjugated vaccine and tetanus.

PATHOPHYSIOLOGY
- Infection: Shift in equilibrium between host defenses and pathogenicity of microorganism
- Acute GVHD: Release of tumor necrosis factor (TNF) and interleukin-1 (IL-1), provoking an increase in major histocompatibility complex (MHC) expression causing tissue damage.
- Involves skin, intestine, liver
- Chronic GVHD: Fibrosis, lichenoid skin, or mucous membrane changes
- VOD: Cellular injury and obstruction of the hepatic vein sinuses, also called sinusoidal obstruction syndrome (SOS).

ETIOLOGY
- Indications for auto-HCT:
  - Cancers:
    - Multiple myeloma (MM)
    - Non-Hodgkin's lymphoma (NHL)
    - Hodgkin's lymphoma (HL)
    - Acute myeloid leukemia (AML)
    - Neuroblastoma
    - Ovarian cancer
    - Germ cell tumors
  - Other diseases:
    - Autoimmune diseases
    - Amyloidosis
- Indications for allo-HCT:
  - Cancers
    - Acute leukemia: myeloid, lymphoblastic
    - Chronic leukemia: myeloid, lymphocytic
    - Myelodysplastic syndromes
    - Myeloproliferative disorders
    - Multiple myeloma, Hodgkin's and non-Hodgkin's lymphoma
    - Juvenile chronic myeloid leukemia

  - Other Diseases:
    - Aplastic anemia
    - Paroxysmal nocturnal hemoglobinuria
    - Sickle cell and Fanconi's anemia
    - Blackfan-Diamond syndrome
    - Thalassemia major
    - Severe combined immunodeficiency
    - Wiskott-Aldrich syndrome
    - Inborn errors of metabolism

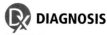 DIAGNOSIS

HISTORY
- History of HCT
- Neutropenic enterocolitis (typhlitis): Fever, abdominal pain, nausea, vomiting
- Fever, oral ulcers, skin rash, diarrhea (1st 3 months post HCT: Infections, acute GVHD)
- Right upper quadrant pain, jaundice (hepatic VOD)

PHYSICAL EXAM
- Infection: Inspection of central venous catheter sites, signs suggestive of pneumonia, hepatitis, or colitis
- GVHD: Skin lesions, oropharyngeal ulcers (mucositis)
- Hepatic VOD: Hepatomegaly, right upper quadrant tenderness, jaundice, ascites, fluid retention

DIAGNOSTIC TESTS & INTERPRETATION
Lab
Initial lab tests
- Pretransplantation period: Screening for baseline host status (neutropenia) and for heterogenous infections, mainly aerobic gram-negative bacilli.
- Pre-engraftment period ($\sim$0–30 days post HCT):
  - Bacterial cultures: Blood, urine, sputum (gram-positive organisms, mainly *Staphylococcus*)
  - Serology for opportunistic (*Aspergillus*, *Cryptococcus*)and invasive fungal infections (*Aspergillus*, *Candida*)
  - Mycobacterial infections: Positive purified test
  - Serology for herpes simplex virus (HSV)
- Postengraftment period: 30–100 days post HCT:
  - Serology, PCR for CMV, adenovirus, HHV-6
  - Nasopharyngeal swab for community-acquired viruses such as respiratory syncytial virus (RSV), influenza, parainfluenza
  - Serum LDH, ABG (hypoxemia) for *Pneumocystis jiroveci* (PCP)
- Late posttransplant period ($\geq$100 days post HCT):
  - Cultures for viral, bacterial, fungal infections
- VOD: Hyperbilirubinemia

Follow-Up & Special Considerations
Engraftment: Period in which absolute granulocyte count (AGC) is >500/mm^3 and platelet count >20,000x10^6, both sustained with no transfusion requirement for 3 days

Imaging
Initial approach
- Chest x-ray, CT: Idiopathic pulmonary syndrome (diffuse infiltrates), pneumonia (consolidation), viral pneumonitis (diffuse ground-glass opacities)
- Abdominal US: Hepatomegaly and ascites in hepatic VOD

- Doppler US: Abnormal portal vein waveform, marked thickening of the gallbladder wall, and hepatic artery resistance index >0.75 in VOD
- CT: Cecal masses and pneumatosis of intestinal wall in typhlitis

Follow-Up & Special Considerations
VOD: Increased serum procollagen type III, low antithrombin (AT) levels

Diagnostic Procedures/Other
- Bronchoscopy, BAL: To exclude bacterial, fungal, viral infections, diffuse alveolar hemorrhage (DAH)
- Skin, rectal, liver biopsy for GVHD
- Liver biopsy for VOD

Pathological Findings
- Skin, rectal biopsy for GVHD: Crypt cell necrosis and death (apoptosis)
- Liver biopsy for VOD: Zonal liver disruption and centrilobular hemorrhagic necrosis

DIFFERENTIAL DIAGNOSIS
- Acute GVHD: Drug rash, Steven-Johnson syndrome
- Chronic GVHA: Scleroderma, Sjögren syndrome
- Hepatic VOD: Budd-Chiari (hepatic vein and IVC obstruction)

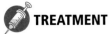 TREATMENT

MEDICATION
First Line
- Infection: Prophylactic/empiric broad-spectrum antimicrobials, antifungals, antivirals
- Recombinant hematopoietic growth factor (granulocyte colony stimulating factor; GCSF)
- Acute GVHD: High-dose steroids, antithymocyte globulin, gut decontamination with metronidazole, IV immunoglobulin
- Chronic GVHD: Long-term steroids and immunosuppressive therapy
- VOD: Anticoagulants or defibrotide (may increase bleeding complications), ursodiol
- Transplantation-related lung injury: Corticosteroids with etanercept (TNF inhibitor)

Second Line
- Oral mucositis: Topical and systemic pain medications, palifermin (recombinant human keratinocyte growth factor)
- Intestinal mucositis: TPN

ADDITIONAL TREATMENT
General Measures
- Social and psychological support improves survival and quality of life.
- Advanced care planning while patient is competent to ensure the care is consistent with patient's wishes.

Issues for Referral
- Dermatologist (acute GVHD)
- Gastroenterologist (intestinal mucositis)
- Pulmonologist (respiratory issues)
- Critical care consultation/admission for life-threatening complications

Additional Therapies
Growth hormone replacement therapy should be considered in children.

SURGERY/OTHER PROCEDURES
- Mediport or Hickman catheter for venous access
- Video-assisted thoracoscopic surgery (VATS), lung biopsy for post-HCT pulmonary complications

IN-PATIENT CONSIDERATIONS
Initial Stabilization
- Intubation and mechanical ventilation in case of respiratory failure
- Broad-spectrum antibiotics, antifungals, antivirals for suspected sepsis

Admission Criteria
- ICU admission warranted for:
- Respiratory failure/pneumonia
- Sepsis
- Mucositis
- Intra cranial hemorrhage
- Acute GVHD
- Cardiac dysfunction
- Veno-occlusive disease of liver
- Adverse reactions to drugs

IV Fluids
- VOD: Fluid restriction
- Mucositis: IV fluids to prevent dehydration

Nursing
- Frequent hand washing
- Care for mucositis
- Care of catheters (venous, arterial, Foley catheter)

Discharge Criteria
- Hemodynamic stabilization
- Able to tolerate feeds
- Balanced fluid status

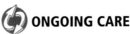 ONGOING CARE

FOLLOW-UP RECOMMENDATIONS
- Pulmonary function tests: Restrictive defect
- Revaccination with childhood vaccines: (measles and polio) once they are off immunosuppressive therapy

Patient Monitoring
- Hypothyroidism, sexual problems, depression
- Clinic visit 1–3 times a week for the first 4 weeks, then once a month for 6 months with blood tests to check blood counts, renal function, liver function, cyclosporine level. (2)

DIET
Neutropenic diet during pre-engraftment period

PATIENT EDUCATION
- Neutropenic precautions
- Adverse effects of chemotherapy, radiation
- Discussion on how to avoid infectious exposures from environment, safe sex practices, pet safety, food and water safety, and travel safety.
- Need for vaccination posttransplantation
- Early symptoms of HCT complications
- Must avoid carcinogens, particularly tobacco.

PROGNOSIS
- Variable; depends upon disease type, stage, stem cell source, HLA-matched status (for allogeneic HCST), and conditioning regimen
- Higher severity of illness score on ICU admission; need for mechanical ventilation or vasoactive agents portends poor outcome (3)

COMPLICATIONS
- Relapse
- Rejection
- Infections (bacterial, fungal, viral)
- Sepsis syndromes
- GVHD: Acute, chronic
- Hepatic veno-occlusive disease
- Mucositis
- Noninfectious: DAH, IPS, ARDS, drug toxicity, bronchiolitis obliterans
- Posttransplant lymphoproliferative disorder

REFERENCES
1. Copeland EA. Hematopoietic stem-cell transplantation. N Engl J Med. 2006;354:1813–26.
2. Rizzo JD et al. Recommended screening and preventive practices for long-term survivors after hematopoietic cell transplantation. Biol Blood Marrow Transplant. 2006;12(2):138–51.
3. McArdle JR. Critical care outcomes in the hematologic transplant recipient. Clin Chest Med. 2009;30(1):155–67.

ADDITIONAL READING
See Also (Topic, Algorithm, Electronic Media Element)
- http://stemcells.nih.gov
- http://www.cancer.gov/cancertopics/factsheet/therapy/bone-marrow-transplant

 CODES

ICD9
- 201.90 Hodgkin's disease, unspecified type, unspecified site
- 202.80 Other malignant lymphomas, unspecified site
- 203.00 Multiple myeloma, without mention of having achieved remission

CLINICAL PEARLS
- HCT is a potentially curative treatment for malignant and nonmalignant disorders and congenital immune deficiencies.
- Infections, GVHD (acute and chronic), hepatic VOD, and pulmonary complications are important complications and have temporal relationship to HCT.
- HCT patients who develop respiratory failure requiring mechanical ventilation, shock requiring vasoactive agents, and renal failure necessitating dialysis have poor outcomes in the ICU.

T

TRANSVENOUS TEMPORARY PACING

Victor Matos

PROCEDURE

INDICATIONS

- Asystole
- Symptomatic bradycardia (BP <80 mm Hg) (<50 BPM)
- Bifascicular or trifascicular block
- 2nd-degree AV block (Mobitz II)

- 2nd–3rd-degree AV block
- Probably helpful in: RBBB + LABBB or LPBBB (new or unknown); RBBB + 1st-degree AV block; LBBB (new or unknown); incessant ventricular tachycardia; recurrent sinus pause (>3 sec)

CONTRAINDICATIONS

- Coagulopathy
- Infection in the skin or subcutaneous tissues around cannulation site

- Contralateral carotid disease (internal jugular cannulation contraindicated)
- Diseased or absent contralateral lung (subclavian cannulation contraindicated)
- Ipsilateral pneumothorax (subclavian cannulation contraindicated)

TECHNIQUE

See algorithm.

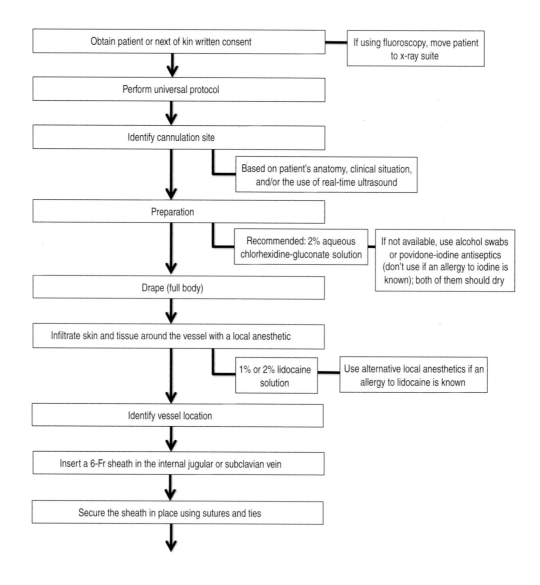

476

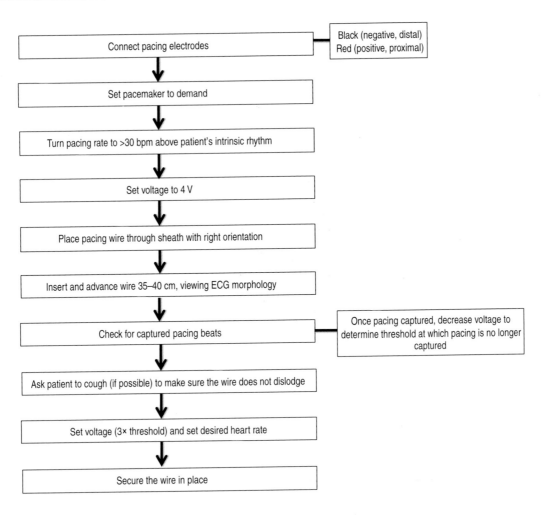

Connect pacing electrodes — Black (negative, distal) / Red (positive, proximal)

Set pacemaker to demand

Turn pacing rate to >30 bpm above patient's intrinsic rhythm

Set voltage to 4 V

Place pacing wire through sheath with right orientation

Insert and advance wire 35–40 cm, viewing ECG morphology

Check for captured pacing beats — Once pacing captured, decrease voltage to determine threshold at which pacing is no longer captured

Ask patient to cough (if possible) to make sure the wire does not dislodge

Set voltage (3× threshold) and set desired heart rate

Secure the wire in place

COMPLICATIONS
- Air embolism
- Pneumothorax
- Arterial puncture (if arterial cannulation do not remove the catheter; vascular surgery advice)
- Infection and thrombosis (delayed complications)
- Arrhythmias
- Myocardial perforation
- Dislodgement of wire
- Failure to pace

T

TRAUMA

Ronen Dudaie
Ariel L. Shiloh

BASICS

DESCRIPTION
- Trauma is defined as a body wound produced by sudden physical injury.
- Mechanism of injury:
  - Kinetic:
    - Blunt
    - Crush
    - Acceleration/deceleration
    - Penetrating
  - Thermal
  - Electrical
  - Chemical
  - Radiant
  - Asphyxiation

EPIDEMIOLOGY
- Leading cause of death in those aged <44.
- Accounts for 1 of 6 hospital admissions.
- 20% are admitted to ICU.

DIAGNOSIS

- Primary Assessment "ABCDE" and physical exam
- A: Airway evaluation and maintenance with cervical spine protection:
  - Patency
  - Voice
  - Stridor
  - Foreign body
- B: Breathing and ventilation:
  - Visual inspection
  - Palpation
  - Percussion
  - Auscultation
  - Subcutaneous emphysema and tracheal deviation must be identified if present.
- C: Circulation with hemorrhage control:
  - 2 large-bore peripheral IVs
  - Control external bleeding.
  - Assess for shock.
- D: Disability (neurologic evaluation):
  - Assess "AVPU": Alert, verbal stimuli response, painful stimuli response, or unresponsive
  - Glasgow Coma Scale

- E: Exposure/environmental control:
  - Remove clothing to assess for additional injuries and after exposure, address hypothermia or hyperthermia.
- Secondary assessment:
  - Head-to-toe evaluation
  - Focused and brief medical history:
    - "AMPLE": Allergy, medications/drugs, PMH, last meal, and related event
  - Imaging:
    - FAST exam: Focused Assessment with Sonography in Trauma
    - Diagnostic x-rays
    - CT as indicated
  - If at any time during the secondary survey the patient deteriorates, another primary survey is carried out as a potential life threat may be present.

DIAGNOSTIC TESTS & INTERPRETATION
Lab
- CBC
- ABO type and screen
- ABG
- Basic metabolic
- Coagulation panel
- CPK

TREATMENT

- ICU management: Tertiary evaluation
- Full reassessment on arrival to the ICU
- Obtain further medical history if possible.
  - Evaluate alcohol and drug dependence: Present in >30% of trauma patients
- Patient can be pre- or postsurgical:
  - Damage-control surgery for immediate life-threatening injuries requires continued postoperative resuscitation in the ICU.
  - Definitive surgery can be completed once acidosis, hypothermia, and coagulopathy are corrected.
- Exclude any undiagnosed injuries:
  - Head injury:
    - CT head scan
    - ICP monitoring
  - Spinal cord injury: CT/MRI spine
  - Aortic rupture: CT thorax, transesophageal echo, angiography, MRI thorax (imaging studies are based on patient stability)
  - Intra-abdominal injury
    - Ultrasound, CT abdomen/pelvis
    - Bladder pressure
  - Pulmonary contusion: Radiographic findings may be delayed after injury.
  - Rhabdomyolysis: Serial CPK measurements

ONGOING CARE

COMPLICATIONS

- Transfusion-associated complications:
  - Transfusion-related acute lung injury
  - Coagulopathy
- Contrast-induced nephropathy:
  - Serial creatinine and urine output measurement
- Abdominal compartment syndrome:
  - Bladder pressure monitoring
- Venous-thromboembolic disease:
  - Evaluation of potential contraindications to standard prophylaxis and appropriate therapeutic interventions:
    - Antiembolism stocking and sequential compression devices
    - Lower extremity US
    - Low-molecular-weight and unfractionated heparin
    - Removable IVC filter
- Stress-related mucosal disease:
  - H_2 blockers
- Ventilator-associated pneumonia (VAP):
  - Standard patient safety VAP precautions

ADDITIONAL READING

- American College of Surgeons. *ATLS, Advanced Trauma Life Support for Doctors*, 8th edition. Washington D.C.: American College of Surgeons, 2002.
- Parr MJ, et al. Damage control surgery and intensive care. *Injury.* 2004;35(7):7–22.
- Richards CF, et al. Initial management of the trauma patient. *Crit Care Clin.* 2004;201(1)1–11.

CODES

ICD9

- 879.8 Open wound(s) (multiple) of unspecified site(s), without mention of complication
- 929.9 Crushing injury of unspecified site
- 949.0 Burn of unspecified site, unspecified degree

T

TUBERCULOSIS

Lhissa Santana

 BASICS

DESCRIPTION
- TB is a potentially fatal contagious disease that can affect almost any part of the body, mainly the lungs. It is caused by a bacterial microorganism, the tubercle bacillus or *Mycobacterium tuberculosis*, through airborne inhalation from a person with active tuberculosis.
- 1/3 of the world's population is thought to be infected with *M. tuberculosis,* and new infections occur at a rate of about 1 per second.
- Latent infection:
  - Positive PPD but no symptoms
  - Negative chest radiograph
  - Noninfectious
- Active disease:
  - Occurs in 10% of infected individuals without preventive therapy
  - Risk increases with immunosuppression and is highest within 2 years of infection
  - 85% of cases are pulmonary
- Primary: Disease resulting from initial infection.
- Recrudescent: Active disease occurring after period of latent, asymptomatic infection
- Miliary: Disseminated disease
- Synonym(s): Phthisis pulmonale, Scrofula, Consumption

EPIDEMIOLOGY
Incidence
- Annual incidence rate:
  - 363 per 100,000 in Africa
  - 32 per 100,000 in the Americas
  - 3.8 per 100,000 in the U.S. in 2009, lowest rate ever recorded in the states
- The incidence of multidrug-resistant (MDR) TB cases has decreased in the U.S. from 2.5% (407 cases) in 1993 to 1.0% (86 cases) in 2008.

Prevalence
- Worldwide, 9.4 million cases occur every year and almost 2 million deaths are related to TB.
- ~30–40% of AIDS patients worldwide also have TB.
- TB is a leading cause of death among people with HIV/AIDS.

RISK FACTORS
- For infection:
  - Demographics: Homelessness, minority
  - Institutionalization (prison, nursing home)
  - Immigrant within 5 years (Asia, Latin America, Africa)
  - Health care workers
- For development of disease:
  - Patients with silicosis have ~30x greater risk for developing pulmonary TB.
  - Patients with end-stage renal disease on hemodialysis have an increased risk of 10–25x over the general population
  - Immunocompromised patients, HIV/AIDS; hematologic and reticuloendothelial diseases, such as leukemia and Hodgkin disease; prolonged corticosteroid use; intestinal bypass; chronic malabsorption syndromes; vitamin D deficiency, and low body weight
  - Other conditions: IV drug abuse; recent TB infection or a history of inadequately treated TB; chest x-ray suggestive of previous infection

GENERAL PREVENTION
- Identify and treat people with TB and their contacts.
- Vaccinate children to protect them from TB: Use BCG vaccine (live attenuated *Mycobacterium bovis*); 50% efficacy preventing pulmonary disease, prevents 80% of TB meningitis and miliary disease in children.
- In the U.S., consider BCG for children with negative PPD and HIV tests with unavoidable high risk, and for health care workers at high risk for drug-resistant infection.
- Several new vaccines are being developed: The first recombinant tuberculosis vaccine, rBCG30, entered clinical trials in the U.S. in 2004.
- A 2005 study showed that a DNA TB vaccine given with conventional chemotherapy can accelerate the disappearance of bacteria as well as protect against reinfection in mice.
- A very promising TB vaccine, MVA85A, is currently in phase II trials in South Africa and is based on a genetically modified *vaccinia* virus.

ETIOLOGY
- *M. tuberculosis*
- *M. bovis*
- *M. africanum*

DIAGNOSIS

HISTORY
- Cough
- Hemoptysis
- Fever and night sweats
- Weight loss
- Malaise
- Painless adenopathy
- Pleuritic chest pain
- Hepatosplenomegaly
- Late findings: Renal, bone, or CNS disease

PHYSICAL EXAM
- Usually unremarkable
- Rales on lung exam
- Specific findings based on organ involved

DIAGNOSTIC TESTS & INTERPRETATION
Lab
- Interferon-γ release assays (IGRAs) measure how the immune system reacts to the bacteria: QuantiFERON-TB Gold test (QFT-G) and T-SPOT. TB (not affected by BCG vaccine)
- Microbiological smears and cultures
- Nucleic acid amplification (Enhanced Amplified Mycobacterium Tuberculosis Direct Test and Amplicor Mycobacterium Tuberculosis Test)
- Persons with TB should be tested for HIV; if positive, get CD4 count.
- Baseline liver enzymes, bilirubin, creatinine, CBC with platelet count
- If using ethambutol: Baseline visual acuity and color discrimination

- If high risk: Test for hepatitis B and C
- If extrapulmonary suspected: Urine, CSF, bone marrow, and liver biopsy for culture
- Nonspecific laboratory findings include:
  - Anemia
  - Monocytosis
  - Thrombocytosis
  - Hypergammaglobulinemia
  - SIADH
  - Sterile pyuria
  - Steroids: False-negative skin test
- Factors that may yield false-negative skin test:
  - Recent viral infections
  - New (<10 weeks) infection
  - Severe malnutrition
  - HIV
  - Anergy
  - Age <6 months
  - Overwhelming TB

Imaging
- Chest radiograph in active pulmonary TB: Infiltrates or consolidations and/or cavities are often seen in the upper lungs with or without mediastinal or hilar lymphadenopathy.
- Lesions may appear anywhere in the lungs.
- In HIV patients and other immunosuppressed persons, any abnormality may indicate TB or the chest x-ray may appear normal.

Diagnostic Procedures/Other
- PPD: 5 units (0.1 cc) intermediate-strength intradermal injection into volar forearm. Measure induration at 48–72 hours
- PPD positive if induration:
  - >5 mm and HIV infection (or suspected), immunosuppressed recent TB contact, clinical evidence of disease on chest film
  - >10 mm, and age <4 years or other risk factors
  - >15 mm and age >4 years and no risk factors
  - 2-step test if patient has no recent PPD, age >55, nursing home resident, prison inmate, or health care worker. Administer 2nd test 1–3 weeks after initial one; interpret as usual.
- Drugs that may alter PPD results:
  - BCG: False-positive skin test, but unreliable and should not influence decision to treat latent tuberculosis infection
- 3 different morning sputum samples for acid-fast bacilli (AFB) stain and culture; use aerosol induction, gastric aspirate (children), or bronchoalveolar lavage if needed

- If positive AFB, begin treatment immediately.
- Culture and sensitivity guide treatment.
- AFB stains positive.
- Biopsy may show granulomas with central caseating necrosis.

DIFFERENTIAL DIAGNOSIS
- Other pneumonias
- Lymphomas
- Fungal infections, especially other atypical *Mycobacteria* or *Nocardia*

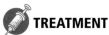 **TREATMENT**

MEDICATION
First Line
- Regimen 1 (preferred):
  - Initial phase: Isoniazid (INH), rifampin (RIF), pyrazinamide (PZA), and ethambutol (EMB) once daily for 8 weeks
  - Continuation phase: INH/RIF daily for 18 weeks. Or INH/RIF twice weekly for 18 weeks (only use for HIV+ if CD4 >100), OR INH/rifapentine once weekly for 18 weeks (acceptable alternative for HIV− patients only)
- Regimen 2:
  - Initial phase: INH/RIF/PZA/EMB daily for 2 weeks, then twice weekly for 6 weeks
  - Continuation phase: INH/RIF twice weekly for 18 wks (HIV+ patients only if CD4 >100), OR INH/rifapentine once weekly for 18 weeks (acceptable alternative for HIV− patients only)
- Regimen 3 (acceptable alternative):
  - Initial phase: INH/RIF/PZA/EMB daily for 8 weeks
  - Continuation phase: INH/RIF 3 times weekly for 18 weeks
- Regimen 4 (only when unable to give preferred regimen):
  - Initial phase: INH/RIF/EMB daily for 8 weeks
  - Continuation phase: INH/RIF daily or twice weekly for 31 weeks (1)[B]
  - No studies proving efficacy of 5-times weekly regimen, but clinical evidence suggests it [C]. Directly observed therapy (DOT) required for nondaily regimens.
- Latent tuberculosis should be treated with isoniazid 300 mg/d for adults, and 10–15 mg/kg (not to exceed 300 mg/d) in children for 6–12 months with DOT.
- Contraindications:
  - RIF: Avoid if patient taking antiretrovirals
  - EMB: May cause optic neuritis. Avoid unless patient is old enough to cooperate in visual acuity and color testing.
- Precautions:
  - INH, RIF, PZA: May cause hepatitis. Caution if liver disease.
  - RIF: Colors urine, tears, and secretions orange; can stain contact lenses.
  - INH: Peripheral neuritis and hypersensitivity possible. Treat with pyridoxine.
  - PZA: May increase uric acid; unclear safety during pregnancy [C]

- Significant possible interactions: Rifamycin alters level of phenytoin, antivirals, and other drugs metabolized by liver and may inactivate birth control pills (recommend a barrier method).

Second Line
- Steroids: Use only with concurrent anti-TB therapy; recommended for TB meningitis or pericarditis (3)[B]
- Streptomycin: Caution—ototoxic and nephrotoxic; do not use in pregnancy.
- HAART: Presence of active TB in HIV patients is an indication to start HIV medications.

ADDITIONAL TREATMENT
General Measures
- If clinical suspicion is present, treat immediately.
- Prescribing physician is responsible for treatment completion.
- Inpatient: Use personal sealed respirators, negative-pressure ventilation, ultraviolet.
- Ambulatory patients: Use mask and tissues.
- Not infectious if favorable clinical response after 2–3 weeks of therapy and 3 negative AFB smears

 ONGOING CARE

FOLLOW-UP RECOMMENDATIONS
Patient Monitoring
- Assess monthly for treatment adherence and adverse effects.
- Check liver enzymes if symptomatic, HIV+, chronic liver disease, alcohol use, pregnant, or postpartum. Temporarily discontinue medications if enzymes are >5× upper limit.
- If culture is positive after 2 months of therapy, reassess drug sensitivity and initiate DOT.
- Chest radiograph at 3 months

PATIENT EDUCATION
MedLine Plus. At: http://www.nlm.nih.gov/medLineplus/tuberculosis.htmL

PROGNOSIS
- Generally few complications and full resolution of infection if drugs are taken appropriately.
- If untreated, can lead to multiple complications, including death.
- The risk of reactivation increases with immunosuppression, such as that caused by infection with HIV. In patients co-infected with *M. tuberculosis* and HIV, the risk of reactivation increases to 10% per year.

COMPLICATIONS
- Cavitary lesions can be secondarily infected.
- Drug resistance is declining in U.S. At risk if HIV+, treatment taken improperly, or if from an area with high incidence of resistance.

REFERENCES
1. American Thoracic Society, CDC, and the Infectious Diseases Society. Treatment of tuberculosis. *Morb Mort Wkly Rep MMWR.* 2003;52(RR11):1–77.
2. CDC. Decrease in reported tuberculosis cases. *Morb Mort Wkly Rep MMWR.* 2010;59(10):289–94.
3. Guidelines for preventing the transmission of Mycobacterium tuberculosis in health-care settings. *Morb Mort Wkly Rep MMWR.* 2005;54(RR-17):1–141.
4. Mazurek GH, et al. Guidelines for using the QuantiFERON-TB Gold test for detecting Mycobacterium tuberculosis infection, U.S. *Morb Mort Wkly Rep MMWR.* 2005;54:49–55.

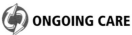 **CODES**

ICD9
- 011.90 Unspecified pulmonary tuberculosis, confirmation unspecified
- 017.20 Tuberculosis of peripheral lymph nodes, unspecified examination
- 795.5 Nonspecific reaction to tuberculin skin test without active tuberculosis

CLINICAL PEARLS
- Have high suspicion for TB in patients displaying a chronic cough and having 1 of the following risk factors: Homelessness, ethnic minority, immigrant from a country with high TB incidence, prisoner, HIV positive, or immunosuppressed.
- Preferred treatment regimen is INH, RIF, PZA, and EMB once daily for 8 weeks; then INH/RIF once daily for 18 weeks.
- DOT is required for all children, those who have difficulty understanding the therapy regimen, and institutionalized patients; it is highly recommended for any patient who may have trouble with compliance.

T

TUBULAR NECROSIS, ACUTE

Joseph Ng
Roopa Kohli-Seth

 BASICS

DESCRIPTION
- ATN usually occurs after an acute ischemic or toxic event, and it has a well-defined sequence of events.
- The initiation phase is characterized by an acute decrease in GFR to very low levels, with a sudden increase in serum creatinine and blood urea nitrogen.
- The maintenance phase: sustained severe reduction in GFR:
  - Continues for a variable length of time, most commonly 1–2 weeks.
  - Because the filtration rate is so low during the maintenance phase, the creatinine and BUN continue to rise.
- The recovery phase: Tubular function is restored, increase in urine volume (if oliguria was present during the maintenance phase), and a gradual decrease in BUN and serum creatinine to preinjury levels.
- ATN is characterized by epithelial cell injury leading to impaired reabsorption of sodium, with urine sodium concentration greater >40 mEq/L and a fractional excretion of sodium >2%
- Most cases of ATN can be linked to renal ischemia, use of nephrotoxic agents, or sepsis.

EPIDEMIOLOGY
Incidence
- 2–5% of patients in a tertiary care hospital
- Incidence in the surgical or medical ICU may exceed 20–30%.
- 10% of hospital-acquired ARF is due to radiocontrast administration.
- 10–15% of patients have aminoglycosides antibiotic-associated nephrotoxicity leading to ARF.

RISK FACTORS
- Renal hypoperfusion
- Sepsis/septic shock
- Myoglobinuria
- Hemoglobinuria
- Tumor lysis syndrome
- Radiographic contrast material
- Antibiotics
- Chemotherapeutic agents
- NSAIDs
- ACE inhibitors
- Chronic kidney disease
- Diabetes mellitus
- Congestive heart failure
- Volume depletion
- Use of statins
- Cocaine use

GENERAL PREVENTION
- Maintenance of renal tubular perfusion is important in preventing ischemic ATN (1)[A].
- Radiocontrast nephropathy is one of the forms of ARF most amenable to preventative measures:
  - Intravascular volume expansion with IV fluids 1 mg/kg/hr, for 12 hours before and 12 hours after administration of radiocontrast
  - Some studies suggest that isotonic sodium bicarbonate may be superior to sodium chloride, but this has not been definitively established.
  - N-acetylcysteine may offer protection from radiocontrast nephropathy. Clinical trials, however, have failed to conclusively demonstrate beneficial effect
- Discontinue diuretics and NSAIDs prior to radiocontrast administration.
- Use once-daily dosing of aminoglycosides instead of multiple daily dosing.
- Rhabdomyolysis/myoglobinuria-induced ATN can be avoided by aggressively administering large volumes of isotonic electrolyte solution to maintain intravascular volume.

PATHOPHYSIOLOGY
- Ischemic ATN:
  - Reduced filtration due to hypoperfusion
  - Casts and debris obstruction of the tubule lumen, causing back leak of filtrate through the damaged epithelium
- Radiocontrast-induced ATN:
  - Renal medullar vasoconstriction
  - Direct epithelial cell toxicity
- Aminoglycoside-induced ATN:
  - Accumulation of aminoglycosides in proximal tubular cells causing toxicity as concentrations rise
- Myoglobinuric ATN:
  - Myoglobin-induced tubular damage when filtered large quantities

ETIOLOGY
- ATN caused by aminoglycosides usually develops 7–10 days after initiation of therapy:
  - Typically nonoliguric
- Radiocontrast nephropathy is an abrupt decline in kidney function 24–72 hours after radiocontrast administration.
- Myoglobinuric ATN is caused when myoglobin is filtered in large quantities by the kidney and causes tubular damage.

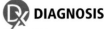 **DIAGNOSIS**

HISTORY
- Hypotensive event
- Recent surgery
- Radiocontrast infusion
- Rhabdomyolytic event
- Use of nephrotoxic medications

DIAGNOSTIC TESTS & INTERPRETATION
Lab
Initial lab tests
- Microscopic urine sediment analysis:
  - Shows pigmented granular casts
- Urine sodium
- Urine creatinine
- Urine osmolality
- Fractional excretion of sodium (low)
- Specific gravity of urine
- Levels of CPK

Follow-Up & Special Considerations
- Fractional excretion of sodium (FENA) >2%
- Urine sodium concentration >40 mEq/L
- Specific gravity of approximately 1.010
- BUN/Creat ratio 10:1

Imaging
- Renal US
- Duplex US of the renal artery to rule out stenosis or thrombosis
- Radiocontrast studies (IV pyelography, CT scan, angiography):
  - These may worsen renal insufficiency.

Pathological Findings
- Biopsy is rarely done.
- Earliest finding could be loss of the cellular brush border.
- Loss of tubular cells or denuded tubules on biopsy
- Tubular cells reveal swelling, formation of blebs over the cellular surface, and exfoliation of the tubular cells into the lumina.

DIFFERENTIAL DIAGNOSIS
- ARF
- Azotemia
- Chronic renal failure
- Acute glomerulonephritis
- Interstitial nephritis
- Prerenal azotemia
- Acute interstitial nephritis
- Renal vasculitis
- Obstructive uropathy

TREATMENT

MEDICATION

- Clinical data in use of "renal-dose" dopamine does not support widespread use in established ATN (2)[C]:
  - If dopamine is considered, limit to 24–48 hour infusion.
- Early dialysis before uremic symptoms arise (2)[B]
- Diuretics to convert the patient from an oliguric to a nonoliguric state is controversial (2)[C]:
  - Increasing urinary volume can make it easier to address problems of volume overload, hyperkalemia, and metabolic acidosis.
  - It may also provide room for TPN (2)[A].

ADDITIONAL TREATMENT

General Measures

- Fluid balance:
  - Trial of Isotonic fluid
  - Carefully monitor intake/output and weights (2)[A].
- Electrolytes and acid–base balance (2)[A]:
  - Hyperkalemia and hyponatremia
  - Keep serum bicarbonate >15 mEq/L.
  - Only treat hypocalcemia if symptomatic or IV bicarbonate is required.
- Uremia and nutrition:
  - 1–1.8 g/kg/d of protein
  - Initiate early and maintain caloric intake (2)[A].
  - Carbohydrates at least 100 g/d
- Drugs:
  - Stop magnesium-containing medications.
  - Adjust all medications for renal failure and readjust as it improves (2)[A].
- Hemodialysis and continuous hemofiltration have no role in preventing radiocontrast nephropathy.

Issues for Referral

Primarily renal dysfunction:

- Need for hemodialysis should be evaluated.

IN-PATIENT CONSIDERATIONS

Initial Stabilization

- Other reasons for ARF should be evaluated.
- Serum chemistry should be done immediately, then any electrolyte abnormalities corrected.

Admission Criteria

- Severity of ATN is dependent on the underlying primary disease.
- If no obvious reasons for ATN are suspected, a thorough workup should be performed:
  - Electrolyte abnormalities, as well as their complications, need to be addressed.

IV Fluids

- Isotonic crystalloid or isotonic sodium bicarbonate solution to hydrate
- If rhabdomyolysis is suspected, isotonic fluid should be administered to titrate for at least 150 mL of urine output per hour unless the patient is already anuric.
- Small fluid trial initially if oliguric
- If patient continues to be oliguric, fluid restrict to avoid overload.

ONGOING CARE

FOLLOW-UP RECOMMENDATIONS

Adjust dosage of medications according to renal function.

Patient Monitoring

- Fluid in/out as well as weights need to be carefully monitored.
- Symptoms related to electrolyte disturbances

PROGNOSIS

- Clinical studies have shown that ARF directly contributes to mortality:
  - 50% of patients die.
  - 25% have complete recovery.
  - 5% have no recovery.
  - 20% incomplete recovery (15% stable function, 5% function regresses)
- Patients with aminoglycosides-associated ATN:
  - Critically ill patients with normal renal function prior to the renal insults who survive the illness causing the ATN will most likely regain sufficient renal function (1)[A].
- Patients with radiocontrast-induced ATN:
  - Serum creatinine typically peaks within 3–5 days and returns to baseline by 7–10 days

COMPLICATIONS

- Fluid overload
- Electrolyte disturbances
- Permanent renal dysfunction requiring dialysis

REFERENCES

1. CSR. Prevention of radiocontrast-induced nephropathy *Catheter Cardiovasc Interv.* 2003;58(4):532–8.
2. Lameire N, et al. Acute renal failure. *Lancet.* 2005;365:417–30.
3. Schiffl H. Renal recovery from acute tubular necrosis requiring renal replacement therapy: A prospective study in critically ill patients. *Nephrol Dialysis Transplant.* 2006;21(5):1248–52.

ADDITIONAL READING

- Kellum JA. Acute kidney injury. *Crit Care Med.* 2008;36(4 Suppl):S141–5.

CODES

ICD9

- 584.5 Acute kidney failure with lesion of tubular necrosis
- 958.5 Traumatic anuria
- 997.5 Urinary complications, not elsewhere classified

CLINICAL PEARLS

- Conservative management predominates for ATN. This includes dialysis support as needed, with prevention of complications.
- Data support a trial of isotonic fluid repletion for ATN.
- Use of loop diuretics and "renal dose" dopamines have not been proved to be of any benefit.
- Azotemic patients who need radiocontrast procedures should receive a protocol of IV hydration, as well as the use of nonionic contrast material and the lowest dose possible.
- N-acetylcysteine for 48 hours before the procedure, as well as special hydration with sodium bicarbonate, still warrants further study (3)[C].
- FENA may be low in radiocontrast-induced nephropathy.

T

TULAREMIA

Francisco Bautista
Jose R. Yunen

 BASICS

DESCRIPTION
A rare but potentially life-threatening zoonosis caused by the bacterium *Francisella tularensis*, usually transmitted by hard ticks (*Dermacentor*). Characterized by ulcerative lesion in the points of inoculation accompanied by local and regional lymphadenopathy, as well as by nonspecific signs and symptoms like fever, lethargy, anorexia, and septicemia. Diagnosing tularemia is a challenge.

EPIDEMIOLOGY
Incidence
- A few hundred cases of tularemia are reported annually in the U.S.; up to 50% of the cases occur in Arkansas, Missouri, and Oklahoma.
- Most patients acquire the disease by cutaneous inoculation.

RISK FACTORS
- Laboratory workers, landscapers, farmers, veterinarians, hunters, trappers, cooks, and meat handlers.
- In 2000, tularemia was reinstated as a reportable disease by the CDC due to its biological weapon potential.

GENERAL PREVENTION
- People at high risk, particularly laboratory personnel, can be immunized with a live attenuated strain of *F. Tularensis* available from the U.S. Army Medical Research Institute of Infectious Diseases; this produces partial immunity.
- Avoid direct contact with blood and flesh of infected animals, rabbits, muskrats, and other wild animals.

PATHOPHYSIOLOGY
- *F. tularemia* is a highly infectious bacterium that penetrates the skin and mucosa yet also is transmitted by inhalation of 10–50 organisms.
- According to the form of transmission tularemia is divided in 6 forms: Ulceroglandular, oculoglandular, typhoidal, glandular, oropharyngeal, pneumonic
- Ulceroglandular form: Representing 75–85% of cases in which the organism spreads via the proximal lymphatic system; causes regional lymph nodes hypertrophy and necrosis
- Typhoidal (or septicemic) form: >5% of cases. This form is more severe, and often includes pneumonia. Ingestion may be the mode of transmission; requires enormous amounts of organism to cause infection.
- Oculoglandular: >1% of the cases. Usually cause by direct contact to the eye, due to rubbing in infectious materials.

ETIOLOGY
- *F. tularensis* is a facultative intracellular, gram-negative bacterium.
- It can persist for weeks to months in mud, water, and decomposing cadavers.
- In U.S., there are 2 types of *F. tularensis*, type A and type B. The type A produces a more severe disease.

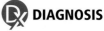 **DIAGNOSIS**

HISTORY
- Clinical manifestations are related entirely to the form of the disease.
- Ulceroglandular: Starts as a papule that turns into an indurated erythematous exudative ulcer that does not heal and takes the aspect of punch-out lesion between the 1st and 3rd week. The base of the ulcer becomes black, and the lymph nodes around it tend to swell but may drain spontaneously. Is possible to have all the symptoms of tularemia without the typical skin lesions, this is call *glandular tularemia*.
- Typhoidal: Sustained fever, headache, weight loss, and malaise are usually the most frequent manifestations. There are no cutaneous or lymphoid lesions.
- Oculoglandular: Granulomatous lesions in the eyelids, accompanied by adenopathy; preauricular corneal perforation is possible.

PHYSICAL EXAM
- Findings in tularemia vary according to different clinical presentation. Adenopathy, fever, ulcers, papules, myalgia, tend to appear in most forms.
- Pharyngitis and diarrhea are usually only seen in children.

DIAGNOSTIC TESTS & INTERPRETATION
Diagnostic Procedures/Other
- Definitive diagnosis usually is established by serologic testing, which ranges from ELISA to very sensitive PCR testing.
- Samples should be taken in pairs, with 2-week intervals, looking for increase in agglutination titers.
- A 4-fold increase in the titers or a single titer of 1:160 accompanied by suggestive clinical history and physical findings make the diagnosis.

DIFFERENTIAL DIAGNOSIS
- Impetigo
- Carbuncle
- Plague
- Syphilis
- Tick-borne diseases: Rocky Mountains Spotted Fever, Lyme, Q fever
- Cat scratch fever

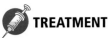 TREATMENT

MEDICATION
First Line
- Aminoglycosides are the drugs of choice. Both have shown to be effective.
  - Streptomycin: 1–2 g IM divided b.i.d. for 7–14 days or until patient is afebrile for 5–7 days
  - Gentamicin 5 mg/kg/d IV/IM q8h
- Fluoroquinolones may be an alternative in patients who cannot tolerate aminoglycosides.

Second Line
- Tetracycline and doxycycline have been used, but they have a higher recurrence rate than conventional therapy.
- Both levofloxacin and ciprofloxacin have been used clinically with success. In fact, in a large outbreak in Spain (142 cases), ciprofloxacin had the lowest treatment failure rate with the fewest side effects.

 ONGOING CARE

PATIENT EDUCATION
- Hands should be washed thoroughly after contact with possible sources.
- Because the primary vectors are ticks and deer flies, wearing protection outdoors is recommended.

PROGNOSIS
Worldwide mortality rate in those without treatment is around 8%, in those who receive treatment, mortality is <1%. The prognosis tends to be worse when there is a delay in the diagnosis and treatment.

COMPLICATIONS
- Pericarditis
- Meningitis
- Osteomyelitis
- Pneumonia

ADDITIONAL READING
- Braunwald E, et al., eds. *Harrison's Principles of Internal Medicine*, 15th ed. New York: McGraw-Hill, 2001.
- CDC. Tularemia associated with a hamster bite–Colorado, 2004. *MMWR Morb Mortal Wkly Rep*. 2005;53(51):1202–3.
- Morse SA, et al., eds. *Jawetz, Melnick & Adelberg's Medical Microbiology*, 22nd ed. New York: McGraw-Hill, 2001.
- Perez-Castrillon JL, et al. Tularemia epidemic in northwestern Spain: Clinical description and therapeutic response. *Clin Infect Dis*. 2001;33(4): 573–6.
- Ryan KJ, et al., eds. *Sherris Medical Microbiology*, 4th ed. New York: McGraw Hill, 2004:488–90.

 CODES

ICD9
- 021.0 Ulceroglandular tularemia
- 021.3 Oculoglandular tularemia
- 021.9 Unspecified tularemia

CLINICAL PEARLS
- Elevated titer in the absence of clinical tularemia does not establish a diagnosis.

T

TUMOR LYSIS SYNDROME

Raghukumar D. Thirumala
Stephen M. Pastores

 BASICS

DESCRIPTION
- Oncologic emergency caused by massive tumor cell lysis and release of potassium, phosphate, and nucleic acids into the blood
- Occurs most often after initiation of chemotherapy in patients with high-grade lymphomas and acute lymphoblastic leukemia but can occur spontaneously.
- Prevention is key to management with aggressive IV hydration and use of hypouricemic agents (allopurinol or rasburicase).
- System(s) affected: Hematologic, Renal

EPIDEMIOLOGY
Incidence
- Variable, depending on whether laboratory or clinical criteria are used
- Laboratory evidence of tumor lysis is more common than clinical syndrome (1).
- Laboratory evidence may be as high as 30% in Burkitt's lymphoma, 42% in non-Hodgkin's lymphoma.
- Reported in 50% of cases with acute leukemia

Prevalence
- Varies among different malignancies
- Higher frequency in bulky, aggressive, and chemosensitive tumors

RISK FACTORS
- Intrinsic tumor-related factors associated with high risk include:
  - High tumor cell proliferation rate
  - Tumor chemosensitivity
  - Large tumor burden (bulky disease >10 cm in diameter and/or WBC count >50,000 per μL)
  - Increased LDH levels
- Clinical characteristics predisposing to the development of tumor lysis syndrome:
  - Pre-existing decrease in renal function
  - Oliguria and/or acidic urine
  - Volume depletion
  - Pretreatment hyperuricemia or hyperphosphatemia (2)

Risk Stratification of Patients
- Based on type of malignancy and WBC counts
- Low-risk patients: Indolent NHL and slowly proliferative malignancies
- Intermediate-risk patients: Diffuse large-cell B-cell lymphoma and rapidly proliferative malignancies
- High-risk: Burkitt's lymphoma, lymphoblastic lymphoma, B-ALL

GENERAL PREVENTION
- Identification of high risk patients
- Aggressive hydration and diuresis
- Allopurinol (xanthine oxidase inhibitor): Blocks conversion of xanthine and hypoxanthine to uric acid
  - Rasburicase (recombinant urate oxidase)
  - Urinary alkalinization with either acetazolamide and/or sodium bicarbonate is controversial.

PATHOPHYSIOLOGY
Rapid lysis of tumor cells releases massive quantities of intracellular contents (potassium, phosphorus and nucleic acids) into the bloodstream resulting in hyperkalemia, hyperphosphatemia, secondary hypocalcemia, hyperuricemia, and acute renal failure.

ETIOLOGY
Occurs as a result of tumor hypoxia or with the use of chemotherapy, radiation, or embolization of the tumor.

COMMONLY ASSOCIATED CONDITIONS
- Acute lymphoblastic leukemia (ALL)
- Non-Hodgkin's lymphomas, particularly Burkitt's lymphoma
- Acute myeloid leukemia (AML)
- Chronic lymphocytic leukemia (CLL)
- Plasma cell disorders
- Solid tumors (rarely)

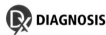 **DIAGNOSIS**

HISTORY
- Clinical manifestations may include nausea, vomiting, diarrhea, abdominal pain, anorexia, lethargy, edema, fluid overload, dysuria, flank pain, or hematuria
- Muscle cramps, tetany
- Seizures, syncope
- Cardiac dysrhythmias, sudden death

PHYSICAL EXAM
- Cardiac exam: Look for arrhythmias
- Watch for signs of fluid overload
- Neuro exam: Mental status and neuromuscular and sensory exam
- Signs of uremia

DIAGNOSTIC TESTS & INTERPRETATION
Lab
Initial lab tests
- Serum electrolytes, BUN, creatinine
- Serum uric acid
- Urinalysis
- ECG

Follow-Up & Special Considerations
- Serum creatinine, BUN, potassium, LDH, uric acid, calcium and phosphorus should be determined before therapy and q4–6h for the 1st 48–72 hours after initiation of tumor therapy.
- Urine pH

Imaging
Initial approach
- Chest x-ray
- US of kidneys for renal failure
- CT abdomen and pelvis for mass lesions

Follow-Up & Special Considerations
- Monitor urine output to assess adequacy of hydration.
- Continuous cardiac monitoring to identify arrhythmia

Pathological Findings
Uric acid crystals in the distal tubular lumen, tubular epithelial cells, and renal pelvis/ureters.

DIFFERENTIAL DIAGNOSIS
- Prerenal cause of acute renal failure
- Postrenal urinary tract obstruction from tumor
- Renal failure due to tumor infiltration, chemotherapy, or radiocontrast administration

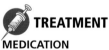 **TREATMENT**

MEDICATION
First Line
- Allopurinol:
  - Blocks conversion of xanthine and hypoxanthine to uric acid
  - Dose: 10 mg/kg/d divided q8h PO.
  - In intermediate-risk patients: Start within 12–24 hours prior to induction chemotherapy and continue for 3–7 days
  - Dose reduction (50%) recommended in renal failure.
- Rasburicase:
  - Recombinant urate oxidase used in high-risk patients and pediatric patients with hyperuricemia associated with TLS (2)[A]
  - Recommended dose: 0.15–0.2 mg/kg once daily as IV infusion over 30 minutes for 5 days

– Potential serious adverse reactions are rare and include anaphylaxis, rash, methemoglobinemia, hemolysis, sepsis.
– Avoid in G6PD-deficient patients, pregnant and lactating patients, asthma or atopic allergy.
– FDA approved in 2002 for pediatric patients with lymphoma, leukemia; not yet FDA approved for use in adult patients; insufficient data in geriatric patients to determine response to treatment.

Second Line
- Aggressive IV fluid hydration (2–3 L/m^2/d) with NS or D5/25% NS
- Maintain urine output within a range of 80–100 mL/m^2/hr.
- If necessary, use diuretics to maintain urine output.
- Urinary alkalinization with either acetazolamide and/or sodium bicarbonate is not currently recommended, except in metabolic acidosis.

ADDITIONAL TREATMENT
General Measures
- Low-risk patients require observation.
- Intermediate-risk patients: Aggressive hydration and allopurinol, with addition of rasburicase if hyperuricemia develops
- High-risk patients: Treat with hydration and rasburicase (3).

Issues for Referral
- High-risk patients should preferably be treated in oncology unit or ICU with monitoring and dialysis facilities.
- Renal consult should be obtained for refractory hyperphosphatemia and/or dialysis.

Additional Therapies
- Hyperphosphatemia should be treated with phosphate binders and/or hemodialysis.
- Hyperkalemic patients are treated with sodium polystyrene sulfonate if asymptomatic, and sodium bicarbonate and/or calcium gluconate if ECG changes.
- Symptomatic hypocalcemia patients are treated with calcium gluconate, administered with ECG monitoring.
- Hemodialysis might be needed for worsening uremia/electrolyte abnormalities.
- Dialysis use has reduced since introduction of rasburicase, although 3% of patients still require this procedure.

SURGERY/OTHER PROCEDURES
Central venous catheter or dialysis catheter placement for hyperkalemia or renal failure

IN-PATIENT CONSIDERATIONS
Initial Stabilization
- Initial diagnosis and management require hospitalization.
- Risk stratification guides optimal use of prophylactic measures and implementation of proper treatment.

Admission Criteria
- High-risk patients or laboratory/clinical evidence of TLS
- Intermediate-risk patients

IV Fluids
- Choice of fluid depends on the clinical circumstances.
- Use 0.9 NS as replacement fluid to maintain intravascular volume.
- Avoid potassium and calcium in the IV fluids due to risk of hyperkalemia and hyperphosphatemia with calcium phosphate precipitation when tumor lysis starts.

Nursing
- Frequent monitoring of fluid intake and output
- Frequent blood draws for monitoring serum electrolytes

Discharge Criteria
Patients can be discharged to a general medical floor or home once electrolyte abnormalities and/or symptoms resolve and renal function is stable.

 ONGOING CARE

FOLLOW-UP RECOMMENDATIONS
Patient Monitoring
Patient should be admitted to an ICU or monitored nursing area of the hospital.

DIET
Restrict foods high in potassium, phosphorus, and uric acid.

PATIENT EDUCATION
Need for adequate hydration, monitoring of intake and output, use of allopurinol, and need for follow-up

PROGNOSIS
Early recognition of high-risk patients and aggressive treatment results in better outcomes.

COMPLICATIONS
- Uremia and oliguric renal failure
- Severe electrolyte disturbances
- Iatrogenic complications

REFERENCES
1. Hochberg J, et al. Tumor lysis syndrome: Current perspective. *Haematologica.* 2008;93(1):9–13.
2. Coiffier B, et al. Guidelines for the management of pediatric and adult tumor lysis syndrome: An evidence-based review. *J Clin Oncol.* 2008;26(16): 2767–78.
3. Coiffier B, et al. Management of tumor lysis syndrome in adults. *Expert Rev Anticancer Ther.* 2007;7(2):233–9.

ADDITIONAL READING
- Cairo MS, et al. Tumor lysis syndrome: New therapeutic strategies and classification. *Br J Haematol.* 2004;127:3–11.

 ## CODES

ICD9
277.89 Other specified disorders of metabolism

CLINICAL PEARLS
- Tumor lysis syndrome is a potentially life-threatening complication that may occur after initiation of chemotherapy for high-grade lymphomas and acute leukemias.
- Metabolic abnormalities include hyperkalemia, hyperphosphatemia, hypocalcemia, and hyperuricemia.
- Key to management is prevention with identification of high-risk patients and initiation of prophylactic measures, including IV hydration and use of allopurinol or rasburicase.
- Rasburicase is FDA approved for the prevention and treatment of hyperuricemia and tumor lysis syndrome in patients with leukemia, lymphoma, or solid tumor receiving chemotherapy.

T

UNSTABLE ANGINA & NON-ST ELEVATION MYOCARDIAL INFARCTION

Sweta Chandela

 BASICS

DESCRIPTION
- Unstable angina (UA) and non–ST-segment elevation myocardial infarction (NSTEMI) patients have symptoms characteristic of acute myocardial ischemia, with positive cardiac biomarkers and/or ECG changes.
- ECG changes may consist of ST-segment depression, and new or worsening T wave inversions.
- NSTEMI is distinguished from UA by positive cardiac biomarkers.
- May represent subendocardial ischemia from reduced, but not completely occluded, coronary blood flow.
- Previously referred to as a non-Q wave MI.

EPIDEMIOLOGY
Incidence
1,260,000 new and recurrent coronary attacks per year:
- An estimated 500,000 new cases of stable angina occur each year.

Prevalence
16,800,000 patients with angina, heart attacks, and CAD

RISK FACTORS
- Age: Male >45 years; female >55 years
- Hypertension
- Diabetes, type 1 and 2; CAD equivalent
- Tobacco use
- Hyperlipidemia:
  - Elevated LDL
  - Low HDL
- Previous MI or stroke
- Family history of premature heart disease
- Secondary factors:
  - Obesity; sedentary lifestyle
  - Elevated CRP
  - Increased level of stress

Genetics
- Maternal history of CAD is more strongly linked than paternal CAD.
- Premature heart disease:
  - Male 1st-degree relative <55
  - Female 1st-degree relative <65

GENERAL PREVENTION
- Lipid control (LDL<130)
- Aspirin 81 or 325 mg daily:
  - Framingham risk score assessment
  - Men age 45–79 years for reduction in myocardial infarction
  - Women age 55–79 years for reduction in myocardial infarctions and ischemic strokes
- Prevention of diabetes, hypertension, stroke

PATHOPHYSIOLOGY
- Myocardial oxygen demand exceeds supply.
- Atherosclerotic plaque disruption, activation of local endothelial and systemic inflammatory responses, formation of atherothrombi, and transient occlusion of coronary artery resulting in decreased myocardial perfusion

ETIOLOGY
- Atherosclerosis
- Coronary vasospasm
- Cocaine/other drugs
- Anemia
- Postsurgical complication
- Shock: Septic, hypovolemia
- Systemic diseases that increase risk of atherosclerosis (i.e., SLE and rheumatoid arthritis)

COMMONLY ASSOCIATED CONDITIONS
- Peripheral vascular disease
- Cerebrovascular disease
- Abdominal aortic aneurysm

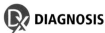 **DIAGNOSIS**

HISTORY
- Angina pectoris is retrosternal pain typically described as crushing, squeezing, or pressure-like and often demonstrated with a clenched fist over the chest (Levine's sign).
- Angina is unstable when accompanied by at least 1 of the following features:
  - Occurrence at rest
  - Occurrence with minimal exertion and no relief with rest
  - >20 minutes duration
  - Angina incompletely relieved by sublingual nitroglycerin (3 doses taken 5 minutes apart)
  - Severe in intensity or new onset
  - Crescendo pattern
- Additional features include:
  - Radiation of pain to neck or jaw, and ulnar distribution of left arm
  - Associated symptoms: Diaphoresis, nausea, vomiting, dyspnea, sometimes palpitations and rarely syncope
- Females, elderly, and diabetic patients may not present with typical chest pain.

PHYSICAL EXAM
- Vital signs:
  - Tachycardia
  - Normotensive, hypo- or hypertensive
- Neck: jugular venous distention
- Cardiac:
  - May be normal
  - Mitral regurgitation, new or worsening grade
  - S_3 gallop
  - Displaced PMI
- Lung: Rales
- Extremities: Peripheral edema
- Skin: Cold, clammy
- Vascular: Diminished pulses

DIAGNOSTIC TESTS & INTERPRETATION
Lab
Initial lab tests
- Cardiac biomarkers q6–8h:
  - Troponin T or I: Positive in 3–6 hours after MI, peaks at 16 hours, trends down over 9–12 days
  - CK, creatine kinase: Positive in 4–8 hours after MI, peaks 18–24 hours, trends down over 3–4 days.
  - CK-MB, band-specific for myocyte necrosis
- Electrolytes
- CBC

Follow-Up & Special Considerations
- Serial ECG if initial ECG showed ischemic changes, and for persistent or recurrent angina
- Serial cardiac enzymes
- Left bundle branch block on baseline ECG; refer to specific criteria to diagnose ischemia

Imaging
Initial approach
- ECG within 10 minutes of presentation
- Chest x-ray
  - Cardiomegaly
  - Pulmonary edema
  - Right ventricular enlargement on lateral film
  - Wide mediastinum

Follow-Up & Special Considerations
TIMI risk score assessment for management decision with early invasive vs. conservative strategy:
- TIMI score of 6–7 was associated with 40.9% risk of a primary endpoint (ischemic events, acute myocardial infarction, death, etc.).

Diagnostic Procedures/Other
- Transthoracic echocardiogram
- Cardiac catheterization
  - Coronary angiography
  - Left ventriculography for function and wall motion assessment

Pathological Findings
Myocardial cell necrosis

DIFFERENTIAL DIAGNOSIS
- Pericarditis
- Aortic stenosis
- Pleural pain
- Pulmonary embolism
- Aortic dissection
- Costochondritis
- Panic attack
- GI:
  - Cholecystitis
  - Peptic ulcer/gastroesophageal reflux
  - Gastritis
  - Esophagitis

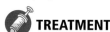 **TREATMENT**

MEDICATION
First Line
- Oxygen 2 L/min:
- Aspirin 325 mg, PO or chewable
- Nitroglycerin sublingual 0.4 mg q5min for 3 doses, followed by IV drip:
  - Avoid in right ventricular infarction
  - Caution with phosphodiesterase inhibitors (treatment for erectile dysfunction and pulmonary hypertension)
  - Dose-dependent tolerance develops.
  - Patients may complain of headache.
- Morphine 2–4 mg q15min
- β-Blocker: Metoprolol 5 mg IV q5min for 3 doses (Class 2a, Level B), followed by 50 mg PO q6h (Class 1, Level B) 15 minutes after last IV dose:
  - Mortality reduction
  - Avoid in hypotension, bradycardia, evidence of AV node block on ECG, acute congestive heart failure, acute bronchospasm, cocaine-induced MI
- Statins: Atorvastatin 80 mg PO q.d. or other statin

Second Line
High-risk USA/NSTEMI patients:
- Clopidogrel 300 mg, loading dose
- GP IIb/IIa inhibitor: abciximab (ReoPro), eptifibatide (Integrilin)
- Anticoagulation:
  – Unfractionated heparin (UFH) by protocol
  – Low-molecular-weight heparin (LMWH), enoxaparin subcutaneous 1 mg/kg q12h
  – Direct thrombin inhibitors

ADDITIONAL TREATMENT
General Measures
- Initial conservative strategy:
  – Aspirin (Class 1, Level A), clopidogrel if aspirin-intolerant (Class 1, Level A)
  – Anticoagulation with UFH or LMWH (Class 1, Level A), or fondaparinux (Class 1, Level B), but enoxaparin and fondaparinux are preferred (Class 2a, Level B)
  – Clopidogrel (Class 1, Level A)
  – Consider adding eptifibatide or tirofiban (Class 2b, Level B).
  – Assess need for coronary angiography.
- Initial invasive strategy:
  – Aspirin (Class 1, Level A), clopidogrel if aspirin-intolerant (Class 1, Level A)
  – Anticoagulation with UFH or LMWH (Class 1, Level A), bivalirudin or fondaparinux (Class 1, Level B)
  – Prior to angiography, initiate at least 1 (Class 1, Level A) or both (Class 2a, Level b) of the following:
    ○ Clopidogrel, an additional 300 mg for a total of 600mg loading dose
    ○ GP IIb/IIIa inhibitor
    ○ Delay to angiography, high-risk features, and early recurrent ischemic discomfort favor administering both.
- Arrhythmia management as needed

Issues for Referral
- Transfer to PCI-capable facility if coronary angiography shows coronary stenosis amenable to PTCI.
- Patients with risk factors who present with chest pain and have no ECG findings consistent with ischemia and negative cardiac biomarkers should have provocative testing: Exercise or pharmacologic stress test and nuclear imaging
- Cardiothoracic surgery:
  – Left main coronary artery stenosis >50%
  – Triple vessel disease, especially in patients with diabetes and LV dysfunction

COMPLEMENTARY & ALTERNATIVE THERAPIES
Omega 3 fatty acid supplements

SURGERY/OTHER PROCEDURES
- Cardiothoracic surgery with following anatomy:
  – Left main coronary artery stenosis >50%
  – Triple vessel disease, especially in patients with diabetes and LV dysfunction

IN-PATIENT CONSIDERATIONS
Initial Stabilization
- ABCs
- Antianginal therapy

Admission Criteria
All patients with ACS should be admitted to a cardiac care unit.

IV Fluids
- Avoid in cases of severe LV dysfunction and CHF
- Used to resuscitate in cases of RV infarction
- May be used before coronary angiography/PTCI in cases of renal dysfunction

Discharge Criteria
- All ACS patients should remain in hospital until cardiac biomarkers are trending down, and ECG should have stabilized.
- Complete resolution of chest pain, at rest and with exertion
- Hemodynamic stability

 ONGOING CARE

Discharge regimen:
- NSTEMI patients should be prescribed:
  – Aspirin indefinitely (Class 1, Level A)
  – β-Blocker (Class 1, Level A)
  – Statin therapy when LDL >100, (Class 1, Level A)
  – Clopidogrel 75 mg, for at least 1 month (Class 1, Level A) for medical therapy of CAD or bare-metal stent, and ideally for 12 months (Class 1, Level B); 12 months for drug-eluting stent (Class 1, Level B)
  – ACE inhibitor if LV ejection fraction is <40% or if concomitant diabetes mellitus or hypertension is present.
- Blood pressure goal <140/90 mm Hg and <130/80 mm Hg when chronic kidney disease or diabetes is present (Class 1, Level A)
- Lipid management goals LDL <100 (Class 1, Level A), <70 (Class 1, 2a, Level A)
- Diabetes management goal is hemoglobin A1C <7% (Class 1, Level A)
- Tobacco cessation counseling
- Lifestyle modification:
  – Prudent diet
  – Exercise

FOLLOW-UP RECOMMENDATIONS
Cardiologist

Patient Monitoring
Telemetry

DIET
- Low-fat/-cholesterol foods:
  – Saturated fats <7% of daily calories
  – Trans fats <1% of daily calories
  – Total cholesterol <200 mg/d
- Low carbohydrates:
  – Substitute in whole grains, multigrains, oats
  – High fiber
- Low sodium: <2300 mg/d
- High in fruit and vegetables
- Portion size control

PATIENT EDUCATION
- Overall therapeutic lifestyle modification and control of risk factors:
  – Tobacco cessation
  – Hypertension control
  – Hyperlipidemia treatment goals of LDL <70
  – Diabetes mellitus treatment goals
  – Exercise and weight loss
- Stress reduction

PROGNOSIS
TIMI risk score can identify high-risk patients.

COMPLICATIONS
- CHF
- Pericarditis
- Increased risk for STEMI in 4–6 week period

ADDITIONAL READING
- Braunwald E, et al. ACC/AHA 2002 guideline update for the management of patients with unstable angina and non-ST-segment elevation myocardial infarction—summary article: A report of the American College of Cardiology/American Heart Association task force on practice guidelines (Committee on the Management of Patients With Unstable Angina). *J Am Coll Cardiol*. 2002;40: 1366–74.
- Peterson ED, et al. Association between hospital performance and outcomes among patients with acute coronary syndromes. *JAMA*. 2006;295: 1912–20.
- Mehta RH, et al. Recent trends in the care of patients with non-ST-segment elevation acute coronary syndromes: Insights from the CRUSADE Initiative. *Arch Intern Med*. 2006;166:2027–34.
- Armstrong PW, et al. Acute coronary syndromes in the GUSTO-IIb trial: Prognostic insights and impact of recurrent ischemia. *Circulation*. 1998;98:1860–8.
- Kwong RY, et al. Detecting acute coronary syndrome in the emergency department with cardiac magnetic resonance imaging. *Circulation*. 2003;107:531–7.
- Antman EM, et al. The TIMI risk score for unstable angina/non-ST elevation MI: A method for prognostication and therapeutic decision making. *JAMA*. 2000;284(7):835–42.

 CODES

ICD9
- 410.90 Acute myocardial infarction of unspecified site, episode of care unspecified
- 410.91 Acute myocardial infarction of unspecified site, initial episode of care
- 411.1 Intermediate coronary syndrome

CLINICAL PEARLS
- Variant angina (Prinzmetal angina):
  – Occurs primarily at rest
  – Triggered by smoking
  – Due to coronary vasospasm
- 7 TIMI risk score predictor variables:
  – Age ≥65
  – At least 3 risk factors for coronary artery disease
  – Prior coronary stenosis ≥50%
  – ST-segment deviation on ECG at presentation
  – At least 2 anginal events in prior 24 hours
  – Use of aspirin in prior 7 days
  – Elevated serum cardiac markers

U

BASICS

DESCRIPTION

Vancomycin-resistant enterococcus (VRE) is a resistant form of enterococcus, commonly found in hospitals and long-term facilities. It leads to health care–associated (nosocomial) infections often resulting in urinary tract infections, bacteremias, and other clinically significant processes.

EPIDEMIOLOGY

Incidence

Increasing in ICU patients: ~15%

Prevalence

>28% of the enterococcal infections in ICU patients are now vancomycin-resistant.

RISK FACTORS

- Prior, recent antibiotic therapy
- Prolonged hospitalization
- End-stage renal disease
- Cancer
- Immunosuppression
- Indwelling catheters and prosthetic devices
- Residence at long-term care facilities

Geriatric Considerations

Exposed prosthetics or catheter infections

Pediatric Considerations

Antibiotics being the mainstay of treatment, it is vitally important to use appropriate dosage adjustments by weight for pediatric patients.

Pregnancy Considerations

Important to consider pregnancy categorization of antibiotic agents before use; pharmacy consultation is recommended.

Genetics

- Vancomycin inhibits bacterial cell-wall synthesis via binding to D-alanyl-D-alanine units.
- Vancomycin resistance gene clusters (vanA [most common], vanB, and vanD) modify binding site to D-alanyl-D-lactate, thereby reducing vancomycin binding.
- This resistance increases vancomycin MIC by 1,000 times.

GENERAL PREVENTION

- Hand hygiene: Strict universal precautions
- Contact precautions
- Surveillance via rectal swab/stool sample
- Daily chlorhexidine bathing
- Limited use of vancomycin

PATHOPHYSIOLOGY

Resistance caused by genetic alteration of enterococcal cell wall proteins resulting in modification of a peptide, practically preventing vancomycin binding to the bacteria, thus allowing cell-wall synthesis to continue.

ETIOLOGY

VRE originates from intestinal flora and spreads to other areas (i.e., urinary tract infection, wounds, intra-abdominal process).

COMMONLY ASSOCIATED CONDITIONS

- Prior antibiotic exposure
- Critical illness

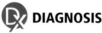 **DIAGNOSIS**

HISTORY

- General signs of infections and malaise
- Report of fever
- Abdominal pain
- Diarrhea
- Flank pain
- Prosthetics and/or catheters
- Recent hospitalizations
- Recent antibiotic therapy

PHYSICAL EXAM

- May present with altered mental status
- Examination of surgical incisions/wounds for signs of infection
- Fever/hypotension
- Abdominal tenderness/peritonitis
- Close exam of sites of prosthesis for swelling, tenderness, erythema, or fluid collection over area
- Inspection of catheter sites, central access for signs of infection
- Auscultation of heart sounds for new murmurs

DIAGNOSTIC TESTS & INTERPRETATION

Lab

Initial lab tests

- Culture and Gram stain from wound, drainage, and blood/urine/sputum, or from prosthetic sites as indicated
- CBC to evaluate for elevated WBC and manual differential to determine left shift (bandemia)
- Blood culture to rule out VRE bacteremia (high risk of endocarditis)
- Chemistry panel

Follow-Up & Special Considerations

Repeated blood cultures are necessary to rule out ongoing bacteremia and to demonstrate its resolution.

Imaging

- CT abdomen/pelvis: If history/physical exam suggestive of intra-abdominal process or source, also if no other clear identifiable source
- Ultrasound: Evaluation of abdomen for abscess; may be used in lieu of CT scan to minimize radiation exposure and/or IV contrast nephrotoxicity

Diagnostic Procedures/Other

Echocardiogram for patients with bacteremia or concern for endocarditis; echo is only indicated if the patient is acutely ill or of the physical exam is nondiagnostic but heart valve damage is very likely or if the degree of heart valve damage has to be established.

Pathological Findings

Abscesses at the site of infections and vegetation on heart valves if endocarditis occurs

DIFFERENTIAL DIAGNOSIS

- Other bacterial infections leading to similar clinical manifestation (MRSA, *E. coli*, *Pseudomonas*, etc.)
- Endocarditis
- Peritonitis
- Sepsis
- Abscess
- Urinary tract infection
- Wound infection

TREATMENT

MEDICATION
- Linezolid 600 mg PO/IV b.i.d.
- Daptomycin 4–8 mg/kg/d IV
- Tigecycline 100 mg IV once, then 50 mg IV b.i.d.

ADDITIONAL TREATMENT
General Measures
- Opening of abscesses as part of source control
- Removal of foreign body, prosthetic, catheter as part of source control

Issues for Referral
- Cardiology or cardiac surgical consults for severe endocarditis
- Interventional radiology consult for drainage of certain abscesses

SURGERY/OTHER PROCEDURES
- Surgical source control
- Incision and drainage of skin and soft tissue infection/abscess
- IR guided drainage of intra-abdominal abscess
- Removal of prosthesis and/or catheters (i.e., tunneled central line):
  – Obtain deep tissue cultures.
  – Frequently change dressing of open/incised areas.
  – Maintain drainage of abscesses.

IN-PATIENT CONSIDERATIONS
Initial Stabilization
- Identification of primary infection
- Antibiotic therapy and source control
- Hemodynamic stabilization and resuscitation

Admission Criteria
ICU admission for those with hemodynamic instability, need for frequent monitoring, respiratory failure, and other intensive care needs

IV Fluids
- Adequate fluid resuscitation with use of crystalloid replacement (i.e., 0.9% NS or LR)
- Ensure appropriate access and consider central venous access if inadequate access or need for monitoring volume status (CVP). Note the benefits of prior removal of any infected lines or catheters.

Nursing
Patient comfort, pain management

Discharge Criteria
Resolution or significant improvement in reason for admission to the ICU

 ONGOING CARE

FOLLOW-UP RECOMMENDATIONS
- At discharge from ICU, generate detailed sign-out assuring safe and seamless transfer of care to floor or for discharge to home and follow-up with primary care physician.
- Long-term antibiotic therapy may be necessary (and may require the placement of a PICC line).

Patient Monitoring
- Continue close monitoring while in ICU
- Frequent examination of wounds suspected of infection

DIET
Maintain appropriate enteral feeding to optimize nutrition if no contraindications.

PATIENT EDUCATION
- Appropriate hygiene
- Hand-washing
- Contact precautions

PROGNOSIS
Variable. Some patients can be cured, others may succumb to the infection and be refractory to medical and/or surgical management. The prognosis is determined by the site of VRE infection (endocarditis vs. superficial wound infection) and by the patient's overall medical condition and underlying diseases.

COMPLICATIONS
- Bacteremia
- Endocarditis
- Sepsis/Shock
- Death

REFERENCES
1. Climo MW, et al. The effect of daily bathing with chlorhexidine on the acquisition of methicillin-resistant Staphylococcus aureus, vancomycin-resistant Enterococcus, and healthcare-associated bloodstream infections: Results of a quasi-experimental multicenter trial. *Crit Care Med*. 2009;37:1858–65.
2. Huskins WC, et al. Intervention to reduce transmission of resistant bacteria in intensive care. *N Engl J Med*. 2011;364:1407–18.
3. Lin MY, Hayden MK. Methicillin-resistant Staphylococcus aureus and vancomycin-resistant enterococcus: Recognition and prevention in intensive care units. *Crit Care Med*. 2010;38(Suppl):S335–44.

ADDITIONAL READING
- Steinmetz MP, et al. Successful treatment of vancomycin-resistant enterococcus meningitis with linezolid: Case report and review of the literature. *Crit Care Med*. 2001;29:2383–5.

CODES

ICD9
041.04 Streptococcus infection in conditions classified elsewhere and of unspecified site, streptococcus, group d {enterococcus}

CLINICAL PEARLS
- Stabilize patient for any acute issues.
- Identify source and site of infection.
- Fundamentals of therapy are source control/surgical intervention as indicated, antibiotic therapy.

VENOUS AIR EMBOLISM

Irina Petrenko
John Oropello

BASICS

DESCRIPTION
- Venous air embolism (VAE) occurs when air enters the venous system via venous access devices, a surgical procedure, or CO_2 insufflation (e.g., laparoscopic surgery, trauma, or barotrauma).
- ~50 mL of air can cause hypotension and dysrhythmias, and >300 mL of air can be lethal.

PATHOPHYSIOLOGY
- The morbidity and mortality of VAE are directly related to the volume and rate of air entrainment:
  - Upon entry into the venous system, air is transported to the right atrium and ventricle. A large bolus of air entering the venous system can cause an air lock in the right atrium and ventricle, leading to outflow tract obstruction, decreased pulmonary venous return, and decreased left ventricular preload and cardiac output. Air entering the pulmonary arteries causes interference with gas exchange and pulmonary hypertension. These factors can lead to hypoxemia, cardiac arrhythmias, and cardiac failure and arrest.
  - Arterial gas embolism can occur via a patent foramen ovale (PFO) (present in ~27% of the general population) or via pulmonary arterial circulation (barotrauma, anatomic shunts). Arterial air may travel via the coronary arteries (typically RCA), leading to acute inferior wall MI, or systemically leading to seizure, stroke, or mesenteric infarction.

ETIOLOGY
- A direct communication between a source of air and the vasculature must exist.
- A pressure gradient favoring the passage of air into the circulation (rather than bleeding from the vessel) must be present.

COMMONLY ASSOCIATED CONDITIONS
- History of venous access procedure (insertion or removal), recent surgery, or trauma
- Medical conditions:
  - History of PFO (in arterial embolism)
  - Severe barotrauma/high airway pressures (pneumomediastinum, subcutaneous emphysema, pneumopericardium, pneumothorax, and pneumoperitoneum)

DIAGNOSIS

HISTORY
Sudden onset of following symptoms intraoperatively, postoperatively, during any endoscopic procedure; after central venous catheter insertion, access, or removal; IV contrast injection; home infusion therapy; or during mechanical ventilation:
- Dyspnea (100% incidence)
- Sense of doom, dizziness
- Substernal chest pain
- "Sucking" sound. A gasp or cough is sometimes reported when a bolus of air enters the pulmonary circulation.

PHYSICAL EXAM
- Neurologic:
  - Changes in mental status, focal neurological deficits: Hemiparesis or hemianopia due to cerebral infarction, and seizure activity
- Pulmonary:
  - Tachypnea, wheeze, rales, respiratory failure
- Cardiovascular system:
  - Hypotension, tachycardia, mill wheel murmur (churning sound heard throughout the entire cardiac cycle; caused by the movement of air bubbles in the right ventricle), signs of right-heart failure (JVD), shock
- Skin:
  - Crepitus over superficial vessels, livedo reticularis (arterial air embolism to the mammary arteries)
- Ocular:
  - Air bubbles within the retinal arteries

DIAGNOSTIC TESTS & INTERPRETATION
Lab
Initial lab tests
- ECG changes:
  - Sinus tachycardia
  - Right-heart strain (peaked P-wave)
  - Nonspecific ST-segment and T-wave changes; Q-wave ST elevations suggest coronary artery air embolism.
- CBC: Decreased platelet count
- ABGs:
  - Hypoxemia, hypercapnia, and metabolic acidosis

Follow-Up & Special Considerations
Similar findings can be present with many other medical conditions; compatible clinical scenarios with additional investigations for confirmation of air embolism are necessary for diagnosis.

Imaging
Initial approach
- Radiographic finding:
  - Normal (most common finding)
  - Pulmonary (alveolar) edema
- Other rarely reported findings include:
  - Air in the main pulmonary artery, focal oligemia (especially upper lobes Westermark sign), atelectasis, intracardiac air, air in the hepatic circulation, pulmonary artery enlargement
- End-tidal CO_2 monitoring:
  - Used as a monitoring technique during procedures with high incidence of VAE
  - A decrease in 2 mm Hg $ETCO_2$ can be an indicator of VAE but it is nonspecific.
- Transthoracic echocardiography:
  - Detects air in right atrium or ventricle, acute right ventricular dilation and pulmonary artery hypertension; detects PFO
- Transesophageal echocardiography:
  - The most sensitive monitoring modality for VAE; can detect as little as 0.02 mL/kg of air
- CT:
  - May detect air emboli in the central venous system (especially the axillary and subclavian veins), right ventricle, or pulmonary artery. The specificity of these findings is greatest when large defects are detected because small (<1 mL), asymptomatic air emboli occur during the performance of 10–25% of contrast-enhanced CT scans.

Follow-Up & Special Considerations
- False-negative studies with HCRT can lead to inappropriate management.
- Nonspecific presentations require high index of suspicion if clinical scenario is consistent with higher risk of VAE.

Diagnostic Procedures/Other
- Precordial Doppler US:
  - Used as a monitoring technique; can detect as little as 0.25 mL of air with high sensitivity and specificity (>90%)
- Esophageal stethoscope:
  - The sensitivity of the esophageal stethoscope has been shown to be very low in detecting a mill wheel murmur.
- Pulmonary artery catheter (if PA catheter is in place). A rise in pulmonary artery pressure is a nonspecific finding; sensitivity 45%

- V/Q scan:
  – Mimics those seen in pulmonary thromboembolism but the perfusion defects due to air embolism resolve more rapidly, frequently within 24 hours
- End-tidal nitrogen:
  – increases with VAE
  – Not widely available but is the most sensitive VAE detection method

DIFFERENTIAL DIAGNOSIS
- Acute respiratory failure/respiratory arrest
- Cardiogenic pulmonary edema
- Noncardiogenic pulmonary edema (ARDS)
- Acute core pulmonale
- Acute coronary syndrome
- Cardiac arrest
- Cerebrovascular accident
- Seizures

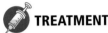 TREATMENT

MEDICATION
First Line
In vasodilatory shock:
- IV infusion norepinephrine 0.5–1 mcg/min; refractory shock may require up to 30 mcg/min
- Adverse reactions: HTN, arrhythmias, asthma exacerbation, anaphylaxis

Second Line
- IV infusion dopamine 20–50 mcg/kg/min:
  – Adverse reaction: Anaphylaxis, asthma exacerbation, extravasations, necrosis, gangrene
- IV phenylephrine 0.1–0.5 mg or, in refractory shock, 100–180 mcg/min:
  – Adverse reactions: Anaphylaxis, asthma exacerbation, tachycardia, arrhythmias, MI
- IV vasopressin 0.01–0.04 units/min:
  – Adverse reactions: Anaphylaxis, asthma exacerbation, tachycardia, arrhythmias, bradycardia, MI
- Adjunctive therapy:
  – Glucocorticoids, heparin, or lidocaine are not effective.

ADDITIONAL TREATMENT
General Measures
- Consider transfer to a hyperbaric chamber if immediately available and patient is stable. Potential benefits include:
  – Compression of existing air bubbles
  – Establishment of a high diffusion gradient to speed dissolution of existing bubbles
  – Improved oxygenation of ischemic tissues and lowered intracranial pressure
- CPR, if required

SURGERY/OTHER PROCEDURES
Central venous catheter or PA catheter placement to attempt evacuation of air if one is not already in place:
- Multilumen catheters or Swan-Ganz catheters have been shown be ineffective in aspirating air, with success rates between 6% and 16%.
- The highest reported success rates in aspirating air (30–60%) are with the Bunegin-Albin multiorifice catheter (Cook Critical Care, Bloomington, IN)

IN-PATIENT CONSIDERATIONS
Initial Stabilization
- If opening in venous catheter is detected, immediately clamp or close catheter.
- If a catheter has just been removed, place immediate occlusive pressure dressing over the site.
- Protect airway and administer oxygen:
  – Administer 100% oxygen and intubate for significant respiratory distress or refractory hypoxemia
- Promptly place patient in Trendelenburg (head down) position and rotate toward the left lateral decubitus position (Durant's maneuver).
- Establish IV accesses for IVF administration:
  – Maintain systemic arterial pressure with fluid resuscitation and vasopressors/β-adrenergic agents and CPR if necessary.
- May attempt to aspirate air via a preexisting central line but this is usually unsuccessful

IV Fluids
- IV fluid to increase intravascular volume and maintain MAP >65 mm Hg: 0.9% sodium chloride at 20 mL/kg as a initial bolus
- Other IV isotonic crystalloids can also be administered:
  – LR
  – Plasmalyte

 ONGOING CARE

DIET
Nothing to be consumed until after treatment

PROGNOSIS
- High mortality rate within first 48 hours
- Survivors may have a complete to partial resolution of symptoms with adequate treatment.

COMPLICATIONS
- Respiratory failure
- MI
- Long-term neurological impairment
- Death

ADDITIONAL READING
- Kapoor T, et al. Air embolism as a cause of the systemic inflammatory response syndrome: A case report. *Crit Care.* 2003;7:R98–R100.
- Leslie K, et al. Venous air embolism and the sitting position: A case series. *J Clin Neurosci.* 2006;13: 419–22.
- Mirski MA, et al. Diagnosis and treatment of vascular air embolism. *Anesthesiology.* 2007;106: 164–77.

 See Also (Topic, Algorithm, Electronic Media Element)

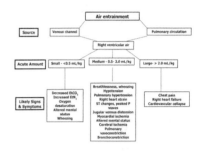

CODES
ICD9
958.0 Air embolism as an early complication of trauma

CLINICAL PEARLS
- Patients with any condition that disrupts veins, allowing a blood–air interface above the level of the right atrium or under higher pressures are at risk for air emboli.
- Sudden unexplained cardiopulmonary dysfunction with focal neurological findings during or soon after surgical procedures should suggest air embolism.

V

VENTILATION, DISCONTINUING (WEANING FROM) MECHANICAL

Neena Kumar
John Oropello

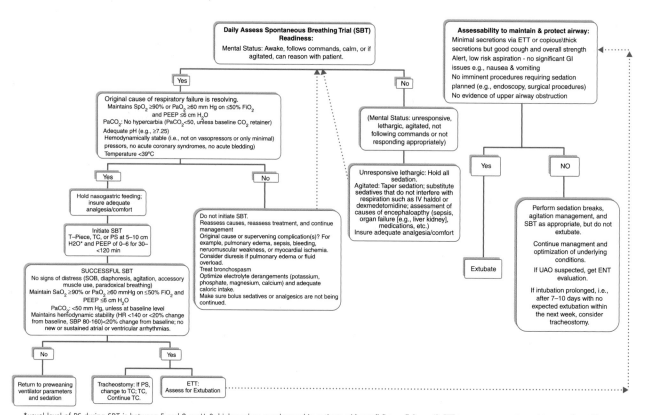

*usual level of PS during SBT is between 5 and 8 cm H_2O; higher values may be used in patients with small (i.e., <7.0-mm ID ETT to overcome greater resistance to flow. ** T-piece = endotracheal tube connected to humidified oxygen wall outlet, not through the ventilator system. (ETT, endotracheal tube; TC, tracheostomy collar; PEEP, positive end expiratory pressure; PS, pressure support; SpO_2, pulse oximeter hemoglobin-oxygen saturation.)

REFERENCES

1. MacIntyre NR, et al. Evidence-based guidelines for weaning and discontinuing ventilatory support: a collective task force facilitated by the American College of Chest Physicians; the American Association for Respiratory Care; and the American College of Critical Care Medicine. *Chest.* 2001;120:375S–95S.

2. Hooper MH, et al. Sedation and weaning from mechanical ventilation: linking spontaneous awakening trials and spontaneous breathing trials to improve patient outcomes. *Crit Care Clin.* 2009;25:515–25, viii.

ADDITIONAL READING

• Blackwood B, et al. Protocolized versus non-protocolized weaning for reducing the duration of mechanical ventilation in critically ill adult patients. *Cochrane Database Syst Rev.* 2010:CD006904.

CLINICAL PEARLS

• Assessment for sedation break and SBT should be performed in the early morning because most patients are more awake during the day.

• The SBT is a more reliable predictor of weaning success than conventional weaning parameters (e.g., tidal volume, respiratory rate, respiratory minute volume, maximal inspiratory pressure, etc.).

• Synchronized intermittent mandatory ventilation (SIMV) may prolong the time spent on ventilator. A SBT via either PS or T-piece (TC if tracheostomy) is currently the preferred method for weaning.

• T-piece or TC SBT has the advantage of avoiding the ventilator circuit and PS which some patients do not tolerate.

• PS has the advantage of alarms by monitoring respiratory parameters via the ventilator circuit.

• Continuous positive airway pressure (CPAP) alone as a weaning mode may increase the work of breathing in some patients; PS is preferred.

• Individualized approaches are needed in terms of the length of the SBT, the level of PS (cm H_2O), and determining the success of the SBT.

• A 70–85% rate of successful extubation is commonly reported using current SBT weaning techniques.

V

VENTILATION, MECHANICAL

Omar Rahman

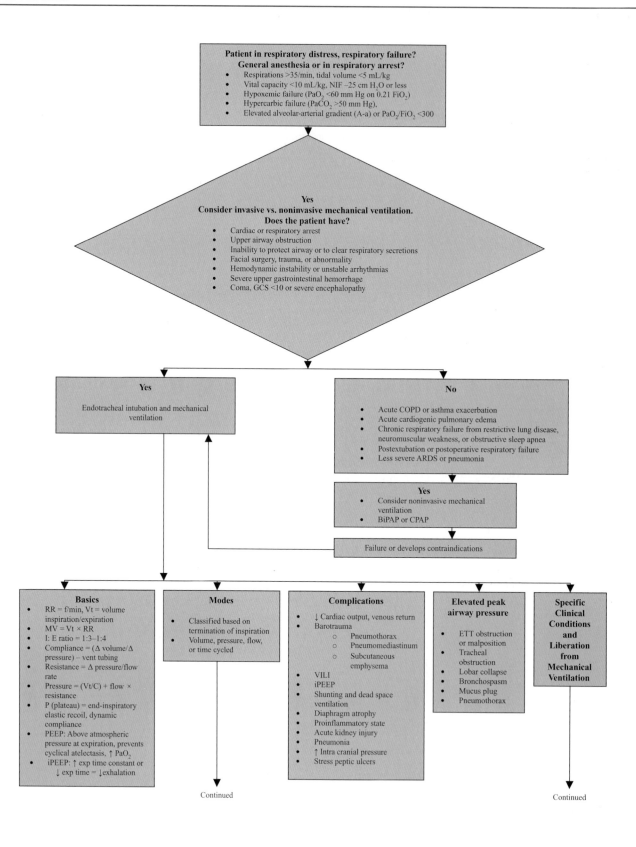

Patient in respiratory distress, respiratory failure?
General anesthesia or in respiratory arrest?
- Respirations >35/min, tidal volume <5 mL/kg
- Vital capacity <10 mL/kg, NIF –25 cm H_2O or less
- Hypoxemic failure (PaO_2 <60 mm Hg on 0.21 FiO_2)
- Hypercarbic failure ($PaCO_2$ >50 mm Hg),
- Elevated alveolar-arterial gradient (A-a) or PaO_2/FiO_2 <300

Yes
Consider invasive vs. noninvasive mechanical ventilation.
Does the patient have?
- Cardiac or respiratory arrest
- Upper airway obstruction
- Inability to protect airway or to clear respiratory secretions
- Facial surgery, trauma, or abnormality
- Hemodynamic instability or unstable arrhythmias
- Severe upper gastrointestinal hemorrhage
- Coma, GCS <10 or severe encephalopathy

Yes
Endotracheal intubation and mechanical ventilation

No
- Acute COPD or asthma exacerbation
- Acute cardiogenic pulmonary edema
- Chronic respiratory failure from restrictive lung disease, neuromuscular weakness, or obstructive sleep apnea
- Postextubation or postoperative respiratory failure
- Less severe ARDS or pneumonia

Yes
- Consider noninvasive mechanical ventilation
- BiPAP or CPAP

Failure or develops contraindications

Basics
- RR = f/min, Vt = volume inspiration/expiration
- MV = Vt × RR
- I: E ratio = 1:3–1:4
- Compliance = (Δ volume/Δ pressure) – vent tubing
- Resistance = Δ pressure/flow rate
- Pressure = (Vt/C) + flow × resistance
- P (plateau) = end-inspiratory elastic recoil, dynamic compliance
- PEEP: Above atmospheric pressure at expiration, prevents cyclical atelectasis, ↑ PaO_2
- iPEEP: ↑ exp time constant or ↓ exp time = ↓ exhalation

Modes
- Classified based on termination of inspiration
- Volume, pressure, flow, or time cycled

Continued

Complications
- ↓ Cardiac output, venous return
- Barotrauma
  - Pneumothorax
  - Pneumomediastinum
  - Subcutaneous emphysema
- VILI
- iPEEP
- Shunting and dead space ventilation
- Diaphragm atrophy
- Proinflammatory state
- Acute kidney injury
- Pneumonia
- ↑ Intra cranial pressure
- Stress peptic ulcers

Elevated peak airway pressure
- ETT obstruction or malposition
- Tracheal obstruction
- Lobar collapse
- Bronchospasm
- Mucus plug
- Pneumothorax

Specific Clinical Conditions and Liberation from Mechanical Ventilation

Continued

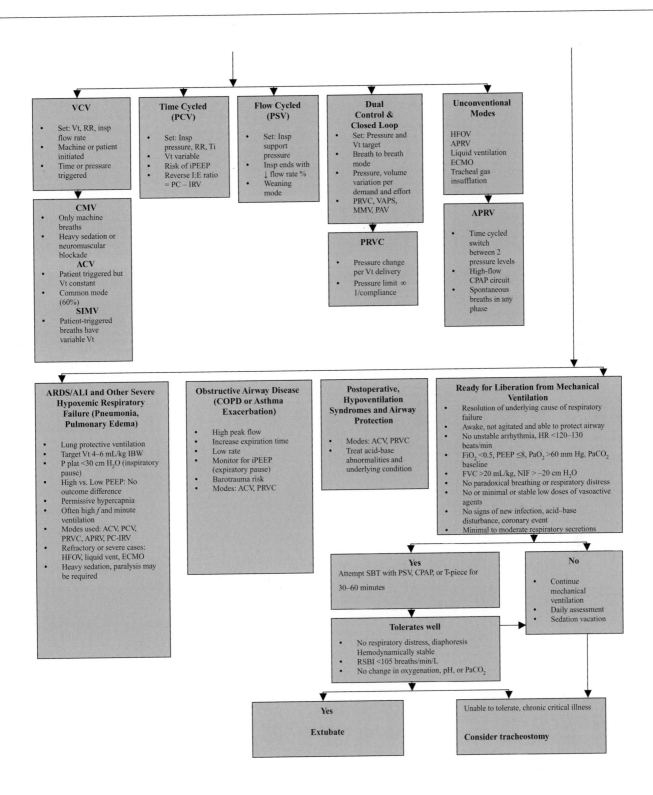

VCV
- Set: Vt, RR, insp flow rate
- Machine or patient initiated
- Time or pressure triggered

CMV
- Only machine breaths
- Heavy sedation or neuromuscular blockade

ACV
- Patient triggered but Vt constant
- Common mode (60%)

SIMV
- Patient-triggered breaths have variable Vt

Time Cycled (PCV)
- Set: Insp pressure, RR, Ti
- Vt variable
- Risk of iPEEP
- Reverse I:E ratio = PC – IRV

Flow Cycled (PSV)
- Set: Insp support pressure
- Insp ends with ↓ flow rate %
- Weaning mode

Dual Control & Closed Loop
- Set: Pressure and Vt target
- Breath to breath mode
- Pressure, volume variation per demand and effort
- PRVC, VAPS, MMV, PAV

PRVC
- Pressure change per Vt delivery
- Pressure limit ∞ 1/compliance

Unconventional Modes
- HFOV
- APRV
- Liquid ventilation
- ECMO
- Tracheal gas insufflation

APRV
- Time cycled switch between 2 pressure levels
- High-flow CPAP circuit
- Spontaneous breaths in any phase

ARDS/ALI and Other Severe Hypoxemic Respiratory Failure (Pneumonia, Pulmonary Edema)
- Lung protective ventilation
- Target Vt 4–6 mL/kg IBW
- P plat <30 cm H_2O (inspiratory pause)
- High vs. Low PEEP: No outcome difference
- Permissive hypercapnia
- Often high f and minute ventilation
- Modes used: ACV, PCV, PRVC, APRV, PC-IRV
- Refractory or severe cases: HFOV, liquid vent, ECMO
- Heavy sedation, paralysis may be required

Obstructive Airway Disease (COPD or Asthma Exacerbation)
- High peak flow
- Increase expiration time
- Low rate
- Monitor for iPEEP (expiratory pause)
- Barotrauma risk
- Modes: ACV, PRVC

Postoperative, Hypoventilation Syndromes and Airway Protection
- Modes: ACV, PRVC
- Treat acid-base abnormalities and underlying condition

Ready for Liberation from Mechanical Ventilation
- Resolution of underlying cause of respiratory failure
- Awake, not agitated and able to protect airway
- No unstable arrhythmia, HR <120–130 beats/min
- FiO_2 <0.5, PEEP ≤8, PaO_2 >60 mm Hg, $PaCO_2$ baseline
- FVC >20 mL/kg, NIF > −20 cm H_2O
- No paradoxical breathing or respiratory distress
- No or minimal or stable low doses of vasoactive agents
- No signs of new infection, acid–base disturbance, coronary event
- Minimal to moderate respiratory secretions

Yes
Attempt SBT with PSV, CPAP, or T-piece for 30–60 minutes

No
- Continue mechanical ventilation
- Daily assessment
- Sedation vacation

Tolerates well
- No respiratory distress, diaphoresis Hemodynamically stable
- RSBI <105 breaths/min/L
- No change in oxygenation, pH, or $PaCO_2$

Yes

Extubate

Unable to tolerate, chronic critical illness

Consider tracheostomy

V

VENTILATOR EMERGENCIES, MANAGEMENT OF

Steven Chao
Umesh K. Gidwani

Sudden respiratory distress in ventilated patients

A. Yes:
Disconnect patient from the ventilator.
Begin manual ventilation with 100% O_2 resuscitation bag mask (use PEEP valve if patient on PEEP >10 cm H_2O) & evaluate compliance/resistance through bag ventilation.
Check airway patency by passing suction catheter.
Perform a rapid physical examination and assess monitored alarms and indexes.

1. Patient respiratory distress relieved by manual ventilation.

No: Patient-related causes

a. Artificial airway problem:
(1) ETT migration, kinking, biting by patient, mucous plugging
Reposition ETT, bite-block, change ETT

b. Bronchospasm (high PIP with normal plateau):
(1) Asthma/COPD → bronchodilator; steroid
(2) Cardiac asthma → bronchodilator, diuretic

c. Secretions:
Suction, humidification, bronchoscopy if atelectasis by mucous plugging

d. Pneumothorax:
(1) Tension pneumothorax → immediate needle decompression 2nd ICS at midclavicular line

e. Pulmonary edema:
Diuretic, morphine, nitroglycerine

f. Abnormal respiratory drive:
Metabolic acidosis, CNS disorder, pain, anxiety → treat underlying etiology

g. Dynamic hyperinflation/auto PEEP (Exp. Flow not reaching zero):
Lowering inspiratory time (Ti), minute ventilation (Ve), Raw

Yes: Ventilator-related causes

a. System leaks:
Check circuit connection, closed suction catheter, HMEs nebulizer chamber

b. Inadequate FiO_2:
Check O_2 source and O_2 sensor calibration.
If needed, change ventilator.
nebulizer chamber

c. Inadequate flow setting (suggested by concave inspiratory pressure curve):
Raise the flow and change flow pattern to descending ramp.
Or, change pressure-regulated volume control (PRVC) mode.

d. Inappropriate trigger sensitivity
Correct accordingly by increasing or decreasing sensitivity.
Auto PEEP or water in inspiratory line make ventilator not sensing patient effort

B. No:
Common ventilator alarms

1. Low pressure, low PEEP, low Vt, low Ve:
a. Is the patient disconnected?
(1) Yes → Reconnect
b. Is there a leak in the patient circuit?
(1) Yes → Eliminate the leak
(2) No → Check for cuffleak, pilot balloon valve
Inflate cuff and check pressure, change ETT.
c. Is the flow sensor malfunctioning?
(1) Yes → Clear sensor and recalibrate. Replace if Needed.
d. Is the alarm set inappropriately?
(1) Yes → Reset the alarm.

2. High-pressure alarms:
a. Check endotracheal tube patency
If secretion → suction
If obstructed → change ETT
b. Check patient circuit.
Drain condensate if present and inspect for kink in circuit.
c. Increase Raw (airway resistance).
Assess and correct for bronchospasm, secretion, and pulmonary edema.
d. Decrease compliance.
Assess and correct for pneumonia, ARDS, and pleural effusion.
e. Patient-ventilator asynchrony
f. Exhalation valve malfunction:
Fix or replace the valve/change ventilator
g. Alarm set too low:
Increase the alarm setting.

3. Apnea alarm:
a. If weaning on CPAP → stop sedative and retry when patient more awake.
b. Patient disconnection or leak in circuit → reconnect patient or fix the leak.
c. Ventilator insensitive to patient effort → reset sensitivity.
d. Flow or pressure sensor malfunction → recalibrate or replace sensor (or ventilator).

4. Inverse I:E ratio indicator alarm:
a. Volume control ventilation:
Decrease inspiratory time Ti.
Increase flow or decrease tidal volume or rate
b. Pressure control ventilation:
If IRV is desired → activate inverse ratio Function.

5. Low gas source pressure or power input alarm:
a. Check 50-psi gas source or hose connection.
b. Check electrical power supply and reconnect if needed.
c. Try reset button → if alarm continue → replace ventilator

V

VENTRICULAR ASSIST DEVICES

M. Kamran Athar

 BASICS

DESCRIPTION
- Ventricular assist devices are mechanical pumps that take over the function of the damaged ventricle and restore normal hemodynamics and end-organ blood flow (1).
- These devices are useful in 2 groups of patients:
  - Patients with cardiogenic shock who require ventricular assistance to allow the heart to *rest* and *recover* its function.
  - Patients with myocardial infarction (M), acute myocarditis, and end-stage heart disease, who require mechanical support as a *bridge* to transplantation.
  - Some centers are placing assist devices in selected patients not eligible for transplantation as *destination* therapy.

EPIDEMIOLOGY
- Types:
  - Extracorporeal nonpulsatile:
    - Use centrifugal or axial flow pumps
    - Can provide univentricular or biventricular support
  - Extracorporeal pulsatile:
    - Use pneumatic pumps and can provide right and/or left heart support
    - Implantable
    - Total artificial heart
- Wearable left ventricular assist devices:
  - ThermoCardio systems HeartMate 1205 VE device
  - Novacor N100 left ventricular assist system[1]
  - Both devices are implanted through a median sternotomy.
  - Inflow cannula is inserted into the LV apex.
  - Outflow cannula is anastomosed to ascending aorta.
  - Pumping chamber is placed within abdominal wall.
  - Operate either in a fixed-rate mode or an automatic mode.
- Percutaneous LVADs:
  - Attractive alternatives to surgically implanted devices
  - Can be placed quickly
  - Can be used as a bridge to transplantation
- TandemHeart:
  - Left atrial to femoral arterial bypass system
  - Inflow cannula is inserted trans-septally via femoral vein into left atrium.
  - Output is delivered by a centrifugal pump via a cannula to the femoral artery.
  - Can provide up to 5 L/min of blood flow
  - Preliminary results show improved hemodynamics and reduction in serum lactate levels in patients with cardiogenic shock (2).

- Impella Recover Device:
  - Uses an axial flow pump
  - Can be used for either left or right ventricular assist
  - The inflow cannula with its axial pump is inserted across the aortic valve.
  - Blood is drawn through a distal port of the device from within the LV and then pumped into the aorta through the proximal port of the device.
  - Only small studies so far (3)
- Continuous aortic flow augmentation (CAFA):
  - Does not provide direct augmentation of cardiac output
  - Consists of a centrifugal pump that draws blood from a cannula placed in the left femoral artery.
  - Blood is then returned to the descending aorta via an outflow cannula in the right femoral artery.
  - Rates of blood flow are between 1.1–1.5 L/min
  - Suggested *mechanisms of action* include:
    - Direct ventricular afterload reduction
    - Stimulation of NO production due to increased aortic shear stress leading to vasodilatation and increased renal perfusion
  - MOMENTUM trial showed that CAFA improved CI and PCWP, but no difference in the primary efficacy endpoint (composite of technical, hemodynamic, and clinical success) (4).
- Extracorporeal membrane oxygenation:
  - Uses conventional cardiopulmonary bypass technology for circulatory support and extracorporeal oxygenation
  - Can be provided via a venous–arterial cannulation setup that provides both respiratory and circulatory support, OR
  - Veno-venous cannulation setup that provides only respiratory support
  - Right atrium and aorta are used in the OR, while femoral vein and femoral artery are used for percutaneous insertion.
  - Most often used mechanical circulatory support in pediatric units (5)
  - Limited data on ECMO use in adult patients outside of the OR
  - In a retrospective study of post cardiac surgery patients, 5-year survival was 74% (6).
  - Optimal use of ECMO in nonoperative setting appears to be short-term circulatory support for refractory shock.

PATHOPHYSIOLOGY
- Unloading of the left ventricle by LVAD:
  - This attenuates myocardial histologic abnormalities caused by HF, with normalization of fiber orientation, regression of myocyte hypertrophy, and reduction in myocyte wavy fibers and contraction-band necrosis.
- Prolonged LV unloading:
  - Reverses LV dilatation, shown by an improvement in end-diastolic P-V relationship
  - Improves efficiency of mitochondria
  - Reduces neuroendocrine abnormalities
  - In some cases, improved myocardial function can allow removal of the device, a scenario termed "bridge to myocardial recovery."

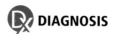 **DIAGNOSIS**

HISTORY
- Patients needing VADs may have diverse clinical presentation.
- Patients can present acutely with chest pain and SOB with signs/symptoms of cardiogenic shock.
- Patients with chronic heart failure can present with acute decompensation.
- Patients may have undergone cardiac bypass or may require mechanical support following percutaneous revascularization.

PHYSICAL EXAM
Will be consistent with signs of CHF and/or cardiogenic shock

DIAGNOSTIC TESTS & INTERPRETATION
Lab
- CBC, BMP, cardiac enzymes, BNP
- A 12-lead ECG should be performed.

Imaging
A 2-D echocardiogram should be performed.

Diagnostic Procedures/Other
Cardiac catheterization, depending upon the clinical setting

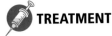 **TREATMENT**

- LVADs as a bridge to transplantation:
  - Patient selection:
    - Crucial in determining outcome of patients who receive LVAD; 1/3 of the patients do not survive to transplantation.
    - The main hemodynamic criteria include SBP <80, PCWP >20, CI <2 L/min/m^2 despite maximal inotropic and/or IABP support.
    - Patients with MS or AI may require correction of the valvular lesion before implantation.
    - Bypass of RCA lesion may be needed to optimize perioperative right-sided heart function.
    - Intracardiac septal defects should be repaired at the time of implantation to avoid right-to-left shunt.
  - Patient factors associated with adverse outcomes:
    - Renal dysfunction: Serum Cr >3 mg/dL. Some data show that BUN was more predictive of an adverse outcome.(7)
    - RAP >23 ± 6, RVEDV >200 mL, or RVESV >177 mL (8)
    - Mechanical ventilation and/or FiO$_2$ >70%
    - Reoperation/sternotomy
    - Peak O$_2$ consumption <10 mL/kg/min on cardiopulmonary stress testing
  - Contraindications to LVAD implantation and cardiac transplantation:
    - Irreversible major neurologic deficits
    - Severe obstructive or restrictive pulmonary disease
    - Dialysis dependence and
    - Hepatic insufficiency with PT >16 sec
- LVAD for treatment of cardiogenic shock:
  - Small studies have shown improved hemodynamics with percutaneous LVAD insertion (TandemHeart) (9,10)
  - Postcardiotomy patients showed improved survival with Impella device, when residual cardiac function was able to provide a CO of at least 1 L/min (3).
- VADs as long-term treatment for end-stage heart failure:
  - A RCT comparing LVAD with optimum medical therapy in patients ineligible for cardiac transplantation showed survival benefit and an improved quality of life, although 2-year survival was low with and without LVAD (23% and 6%) (11).
  - These findings suggest possible use of LVAD as long-term myocardial replacement therapy.
- LVADs and systemic anticoagulation:
  - Extracorporeal nonpulsatile and pulsatile devices require systemic anticoagulation.
  - Implantable pulsatile devices, like the HeartMate system, use textured biologic surfaces and may not require systemic anticoagulation.
  - For the total artificial heart, systemic anticoagulation is required.

 ONGOING CARE

COMPLICATIONS
- Early:
  - Bleeding:
    - Most common complication
    - Risk of major hemorrhage has decreased with the use of aprotinin (serine protease inhibitor)
  - Right-sided heart failure:
    - Usually associated with perioperative hemorrhage and the need for blood transfusion
    - Cytokine-mediated, especially TNF-α, which can induce pulmonary hypertension
    - Use of inhaled nitric oxide (INO) has reduced the need for placement of RVAD.
  - Air embolism
  - Progressive multiorgan failure
- Late:
  - Thromboembolism:
    - Historically the incidence was 20%.
    - The incidence has declined significantly due to the use of textured blood-contacting surfaces.
    - Most patients require aspirin alone and do not need long-term anticoagulation.
  - Infection (both nosocomial and device-related)
  - Device-related include those related to drive line require local wound care and antibiotics; those related to the abdominal-wall pocket holding the device may require open drainage, debridement, and rerouting of drive line through a fresh exit site.
  - Device malfunction:
    - Anecdotal reports
    - None compromised cardiac output.
    - All were easily repairable.

REFERENCES

1. Goldstein DJ, et al. Implantable left ventricular assist devices. *N Engl J Med*. 1998;339:1522–33.
2. Thiele H, et al. Reversal of cardiogenic shock by percutaneous left atrial-to-femoral arterial bypass assistance. *Circulation*. 2001;104:2917–22.
3. Cheng JM, den Uil CA, Hoeks SE, et al. Percutaneous left ventricular assist devices vs. intra-aortic balloon pump counterpulsation for treatment of cardiogenic shock: a meta-analysis of controlled trials. *Eur Heart J*. 2009;30:2102–8.
4. Greenberg B, et al. Effect of continuous aortic flow augmentation in patients with exacerbation of heart failure inadequately responsive to medical therapy. Results of the Multicenter trial of the Orqis Medical Cancion system for the Enhanced treatment of heart failure unresponsive to Medical Therapy (MOMENTUM). *Circulation*. 2008;118:1241–9.
5. Baldwin JT, et al. The National Heart, Lung and Blood Institute Pediatric Circulatory Support Program. *Circulation*. 2006;113:147–55.
6. Doll N, et al: Five-year results of 219 consecutive patients treated with extracorporeal membrane oxygenation for refractory postoperative cardiogenic shock. *Ann Thorac Surg*. 2004;77:151–7.
7. Farrar DJ. Preoperative predictors of survival in patients with Thoratec ventricular assist devices as a bridge heart transplantation: Thoratec Ventricular assist DevicePrincipal investigators. *J Heart Lung Transplant*. 1994;13:93–100.
8. Fukamachi K, et al. Preoperative risk factors for right ventricular failure after implantable left ventricular assist device insertion. *Ann Thorac Surg*. 1999;68:2181–4.
9. Burkhoff D, et al. A randomized multicenter clinical study to evaluate the safety and efficacy of the TandemHeart percutaneous ventricular assist device versus conventional therapy with intraaortic balloon pumping for treatment of cardiogenic shock. *Am Heart J*. 2006;152:469 e1–469 e8.
10. Thiele H, et al. Randomized comparison of intraaortic balloon support with a percutaneous left ventricular assist device in patients with revascularized acute myocardial infarction complicated by cardiogenic shock. *Eur Heart J*. 2005;26:1276–83.
11. Rose EA, et al. Long-term use of a left ventricular assist device for end-stage heart failure. *N Engl J Med*. 2001;345:1435–43.

 CODES

ICD9
- 410.90 Acute myocardial infarction of unspecified site, episode of care unspecified
- 428.9 Heart failure, unspecified
- 785.51 Cardiogenic shock

CLINICAL PEARLS
- Patient selection is a critical determinant of outcome in patients receiving LVAD.
- Most deaths are due to renal failure, RV failure, multiorgan failure, and infection in the period between device insertion and transplantation.

V

WITHDRAWAL, MODERATE AND SEVERE ALCOHOL

Fred DiBlasio Jr.
Raghad Said

BASICS

DESCRIPTION
Alcohol withdrawal (AW) syndrome is a cluster of symptoms that occurs in alcohol-dependent people after cessation or reduction in alcohol use.

EPIDEMIOLOGY
Incidence
~ 500,000 episodes of AW severe enough to require pharmacologic treatment occur each year.

Prevalence
* 8 million are alcohol dependent in the U.S.
* 5 % develop delirium tremens (DT) during withdrawal.
* Although men have a higher prevalence of alcohol dependence than women, gender differences regarding development of DT are unclear.

RISK FACTORS
* History of sustained drinking
* History of previous DT
* Presence of concurrent illness
* Withdrawal with elevated alcohol level
* >2 days since the last drink

Genetics
Genetic predisposition may play a role

GENERAL PREVENTION
* All inpatients should be screened for alcohol dependence.
* Asymptomatic patients with a history of prolonged, heavy alcohol consumption, DT, or seizures, who are admitted to the hospital for other reasons, can be prophylactically treated with PO chlordiazepoxide (50–100 mg q6h for 1 day, followed by 25–50 mg q6h for 2 more days. Additional doses of 25–50 mg can be given every hour as needed.

PATHOPHYSIOLOGY
* EtOH binds GABA receptors, the major inhibitory neurotransmitter in the brain, with resultant influx of chloride ions.
* Glutamate is a major excitatory amino acid:
  - EtOH inhibits NMDA-type of glutamate receptor, which mediates glutamate-induced excitation, with upregulation of this receptor.
* During EtOH withdrawal, the loss of GABA stimulation causes a reduction in chloride flux and is associated with tremors, diaphoresis, tachycardia, anxiety, and seizures. In addition, the lack of inhibition of the NMDA receptors may lead to seizures and delirium

ETIOLOGY
Abrupt cessation unmasks the adaptive responses to chronic EtOH use, resulting in overactivity of the central nervous system.

COMMONLY ASSOCIATED CONDITIONS
* Pancreatitis
* Cirrhosis
* Head trauma (SDH, epidural hematoma)
* GI bleed
* Alcoholic ketoacidosis

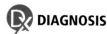

DIAGNOSIS

HISTORY
* A strong history of consistent intake and abrupt cessation of alcohol use
* No alternate etiology to account for symptoms
* Clinical Institute Withdrawal Assessment for Alcohol, Revised (CIWA-Ar) (1)[A]: Survey of 10 items can be administered rapidly at the bedside to assess the severity of alcohol withdrawal:
  - Items include nausea and vomiting, anxiety, tremor, sweating, auditory disturbances, visual disturbances, tactile disturbances, headache, agitation, and clouding of sensorium.
  - 0–7 points for each item except the last, which is assigned 0–4 points, with a total possible score of 67.
  - High reliability, reproducibility, and validity; has been shown to be usable in detox units, psych units, and med-surg wards

PHYSICAL EXAM
* Spectrum of signs and symptoms ranges from anxiety, decreased cognition, and tremulousness through increasing irritability and hyperactivity to full-blown DT:
  - Major withdrawal occurs 10–72 hours after the last drink
  - DT is an acute organic psychosis that is usually manifest within 24–72 hours after last drink but may occur up to 7–10 days later.
  - DT manifests as agitation, confusion, hallucinations, fever, and autonomic hyperactivity (tachycardia and hypertension).

DIAGNOSTIC TESTS & INTERPRETATION
Lab
Initial lab tests
Serum ethanol level, CBC, serum electrolytes, bicarbonate, BUN and creatinine, hepatic function tests, ABG, urine toxicology

Follow-Up & Special Considerations
* Most patients in AW are hypovolemic due to diaphoresis, hyperthermia, vomiting, and tachypnea.
* Hypokalemia is common because of renal and extrarenal losses, altered aldosterone levels, and changes in potassium distribution across the cell membrane.
* Hypomagnesemia is common and may predispose to arrhythmias and seizures.
* Hypophosphatemia may occur due to malnutrition, may be symptomatic, and if severe, may lead to cardiopulmonary failure and rhabdomyolysis.

Imaging
* Chest x-ray to rule out aspiration
* CT head to rule out other causes for change in mental status

Diagnostic Procedures/Other
Lumbar puncture to rule out CNS infection

DIFFERENTIAL DIAGNOSIS
* Alcoholic hallucinosis describes visual hallucinations developing within 12–24 hours of abstinence and resolving within 24–48 hours; mental status and vital signs are usually normal.
* Withdrawal seizures are brief generalized tonic–clonic convulsions that usually occur within 2–48 hours after last drink. If left untreated (with benzodiazepine), will lead to DT in some patients
* Infection (e.g., meningitis)
* Trauma (e.g., intracranial hemorrhage)
* Drug overdose
* Metabolic derangements (e.g., hypoglycemia)
* Hepatic failure can mimic or coexist with AW

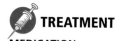

TREATMENT

MEDICATION
First Line
* Long-acting benzodiazepines (diazepam, lorazepam, chlordiazepoxide) are backbone of treatment (2)[A].
* Benzodiazepines act on the GABA receptor and produce cross-tolerance to EtOH.
* Symptom-guided dosing (Librium 50–100 mg PO q1–2h until symptoms are controlled, then p.r.n. based on symptoms) appears to reduce total usage over fixed-dose schedules (50 mg PO q6h for 4 doses, then 25 mg q6h for 8 doses; additional 25–50 mg doses p.r.n.)
* All patients with seizures or DT require IV therapy with benzodiazepines.
* IV midazolam can be used in critically ill.

Second Line
* Phenobarbital: Increases the affinity of GABA binding to its receptor; this increases the inhibitory effect needed to counteract the excitatory surge during DT (3)[C]:
  - Used for DT refractory to aggressive treatment with high-dose benzodiazepines
  - Incidence of respiratory depression and coma during treatment is much higher with the use of phenobarbital versus BZD.
  - Long half-life (80–120 hours) may result in difficulties in titrating an effective dose for sedating and waking a patient.
  - Half-life increases in cirrhosis and old age.
* Propofol can open chloride channels in the absence of GABA and antagonize the excitatory amino acids that are upregulated during alcohol withdrawal; used in refractory DT (4)[C].
* There are limited data on anticonvulsants like carbamazepine vs. placebo for alcohol withdrawal syndrome, but comparisons with other drugs show no clear differences (5)[C].

- Haloperidol is used to control psychiatric symptoms associated with DT, such as anxiousness, hallucinations and combativeness:
  - Used only as adjunctive therapy with BZD because its mechanism of action does not target the GABAA or NMDA receptors (3)[C]
  - The usual dose is 2–20 mg IV q1h p.r.n.
  - Side effects: QT prolongation, lowering seizure threshold, and interference with heat dissipation
- IV ethanol is not superior to benzodiazepines in EtOH withdrawal prophylaxis and is difficult to titrate (6).
- Dexmedetomidine has been demonstrated in case reports to be useful in treatment of alcohol and other withdrawal syndromes (7)[C].

ADDITIONAL TREATMENT
General Measures
- β blockers (atenolol 50–100 mg PO q.d.)
- Clonidine (0.2 mg PO b.i.d.) or in patch formulation suppresses CV signs of withdrawal and has some anxiolytic effect.

Issues for Referral
- Obtain assistance from a medical toxicologist or poison control center in cases of refractory DT.
- Consider DT refractory if >50 mg diazepam or 10 mg lorazepam is required to control the symptoms of severe withdrawal during the 1st hour of treatment, or doses of diazepam >200 mg or lorazepam 40 mg fail to control symptoms during initial 3–4 hours of treatment.
- Etiology is low endogenous GABA levels or acquired conformational changes in the GABA receptor

Additional Therapies
Physical restraints only as a last resort as they frequently increase agitation and create loss of mobility, increase pressure ulcers, aspiration, and prolonged delirium

COMPLEMENTARY & ALTERNATIVE THERAPIES
- Thiamine 100 mg PO/IV/IM q.d. PRIOR to glucose administration to prevent Wernicke's encephalopathy
- Folate 1 mg PO/IV q.d.
- IV magnesium to replace total body deficit and prevent liver damage even if blood level is normal

IN-PATIENT CONSIDERATIONS
Initial Stabilization
- Maintain ABCs
- Endotracheal intubation and mechanical ventilation are frequently necessary if phenobarbital or propofol are used.

Admission Criteria
- ICU admission:
  - Need for close neurologic monitoring in severe acute delirium and potential for seizure
  - Need for high-dose sedatives that may precipitate respiratory failure

- Cardiac disease
- Hemodynamic instability
- Marked acid–base disturbances
- Severe electrolyte abnormalities
- Respiratory insufficiency
- Severe sepsis
- Suspicion of GI pathology (pancreatitis, bleeding, hepatic insufficiency)
- Hyperthermia (T >39°C [103°F])
- Evidence of rhabdomyolysis
- Renal insufficiency
- Withdrawal despite elevated blood ethanol level
- Prior withdrawal complications (e.g. DT's)
- CIWA scale can be used to stratify patients into mild, moderate, and severe withdrawal and to quantify response to treatment.

IV Fluids
- Aggressive IV hydration is warranted.
- Requirements range from 4–10 L in 1st 24 hours.
- 5% dextrose (in 0.90% or 0.45% saline) should be used to prevent hypoglycemia.

Nursing
- Appropriate sedative dosing
- Evaluation as frequently as q10–15min is appropriate for severe symptoms
- Interval of 4–6 hours reasonable for stable patients with mild symptoms

Discharge Criteria
Medical stability

 ## ONGOING CARE

FOLLOW-UP RECOMMENDATIONS
Long-term alcohol cessation counseling

DIET
General diet, provided mental status will tolerate without significant risk of aspiration

PATIENT EDUCATION
Risk for recurrent episodes of withdrawal should be emphasized.

PROGNOSIS
- Despite appropriate treatment, the current mortality for patients with DT ranges from 5–15%.
- Older age, preexisting pulmonary disease, core body temperature >40°C (104°F), and coexisting liver disease are associated with a greater risk of mortality.

COMPLICATIONS
- Alcoholic hypoglycemia
- Arrhythmias
- Aspiration pneumonia
- Failure to identify an underlying illness that led to the cessation of alcohol use, such as pancreatitis, hepatitis, or CNS injury or infection
- Thiamine deficiency can lead to:
  - Wernicke's encephalopathy: Ataxia, confusion, ophthalmoplegia, impairment of short-term memory
  - Korsakoff's syndrome: Anterograde and retrograde amnesia, severe memory loss confabulation, lack of insight, apathy

REFERENCES
1. Sullivan JT, et al. Assessment of alcohol withdrawal: The revised clinical institute withdrawal assessment for alcohol scale (CIWA-Ar).r J Addict. 1989;84(11):1353–7.
2. Ntais C, et al. Benzodiazepines for alcohol withdrawal. Cochrane Database Sys Rev. 2005;3:CD005063
3. DeBellis R, et al. Management of delirium tremens. J Intensive Care Med. 2005;20(3):164–73.
4. McCowan C, et al. Refractory delirium tremens treated with propofol: A case series. Crit Care Med. 2000;28(6):1781.
5. Polycarpou A, et al. Anticonvulsants for alcohol withdrawal. Cochrane Database Syst Rev. 2005;CD005064.
6. Weinberg JA, et al. Comparison of IV ethanol versus diazepam for alcohol withdrawal prophylaxis in the trauma ICU: Results of a randomized trial. J Trauma. 2008;64(1):99–104.
7. Darrouj J, et al. Dexmedetomidine infusion as adjunctive therapy to benzodiazepines for acute alcohol withdrawal. Ann Pharmacother. 2008; 42(11):1703–5.

ADDITIONAL READING
Moss M, et al. Alcohol abuse in the critically ill patient. Lancet. 2006;368(9554):2231–42.

 ### See Also (Topic, Algorithm, Electronic Media Element)

National Institute on Alcohol Abuse and Alcoholism: http://pubs.niaaa.nih.gov/publications/Practitioner/CliniciansGuide2005/PrescribingMeds.pdf.

 ## CODES

ICD9
- 291.0 Alcohol withdrawal delirium
- 291.3 Alcohol-induced psychotic disorder with hallucinations
- 291.81 Alcohol withdrawal

CLINICAL PEARLS
- Long-acting benzodiazepines are backbone of treatment.
- Certain vitamins (thiamine and folate) are also an important part of the management of AW syndrome.
- Thiamine should be administrated prior to glucose to prevent Wernicke's encephalopathy.

W

INDEX